Refractive Keratotomy

for myopia and astigmatism

TEXT TITLE AND COVER PHOTOGRAPHS

This book concerns refractive keratotomy, a subject that includes radial keratotomy to correct myopia, transverse keratotomy to correct astigmatism, combined radial and transverse keratotomy procedures, and hexagonal keratotomy to correct hyperopia or presbyopia. We have selected the term *refractive keratotomy* because it subsumes all these different procedures and is technically accurate. Commonly the term *radial keratotomy* is used to designate all types of incisional procedures to correct myopia and astigmatism, but this is technically inaccurate. Radial keratotomy refers only to radial or semiradial incisions. Astigmatic keratotomy refers to incision patterns specifically designed to correct astigmatism. Fortunately the abbreviation *RK* stands for both refractive keratotomy and radial keratotomy, and therefore the useful shorthand does not have to be changed. Throughout the text we attempt to use the term *refractive keratotomy* when we are talking generically about incisions to correct myopia and astigmatism, the term *radial keratotomy* when we are talking only about radial incisions, the term *astigmatic keratotomy* when we are designating any of the patterns of keratotomy designed to correct astigmatism, and *transverse keratotomy* when we are talking about straight or arcuate incisions made perpendicular to the steep corneal meridian.

The photographs on the cover and spine are finite element computational models of radial and transverse keratotomy. The computer-generated graphics demonstrate the external view of one quarter of the cornea. The finite element mesh is visualized by the intersecting lines, with the mesh more tightly concentrated in the more important central part of the cornea. The color-coding represents the relative amount of stress on the tissue; yellow, red, and white represent areas of greater stress, and shades of blue represent areas of less stress.

Front cover: Graphic model of radial keratotomy showing the concentration of sheer stress as varying on either side of the peripheral portion of the incision.

Spine: Model of transverse arcuate keratotomy for the correction of astigmatism shows the changes in meridional stress, with high stress concentrations central to the end of the incision and lower stress concentration peripheral to the end of the incision. (Courtesy of Khalil Hanna and Francois Jouve.)

Refractive Keratotomy
for myopia and astigmatism

George O. Waring III, M.D., F.A.C.S.

Professor of Ophthalmology
Director, Refractive Surgery
Department of Ophthalmology
The Robert W. Woodruff Health Sciences Center
Emory University School of Medicine
Atlanta, Georgia

with 1650 illustrations and 56 four-color plates

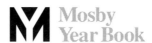
Mosby
Year Book

St. Louis   Baltimore   Boston   Chicago   London   Philadelphia   Sydney   Toronto

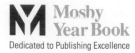
Mosby
Year Book
Dedicated to Publishing Excellence

Editor: Kimberly Kist
Developmental Editor: Maureen Slaten
Project Manager: Patricia Tannian
Production Editor: John Casey
Book Design: Liz Fett

Printed in the United States of America.
Mosby–Year Book, Inc.
11830 Westline Industrial Drive, St. Louis, Missouri 63146

Library of Congress Cataloging in Publication Data

Waring, George O., 1941-
    Refractive keratotomy for myopia and astigmatism / George Oral
Waring III.
    Includes bibliographical references and index.
    ISBN 0-8016-5349-5
    1. Keratotomy, Radial.   2. Myopia—Surgery.   3. Astigmatism—
Surgery.   I. Title.
    [DNLM: 1. Astigmatism—surgery.   2. Keratotomy, Radial
3. Myopia—surgery.   WW 320 W276r]
RE336.W35
617.77′55—dc20
DNLM/DLC
for Library of Congress   91-27325
                                                                                CIP

CL/MY 9 8 7 6 5 4 3 2 1

Dedication

(In this dedication, I rejoice
At the chance to be George Waring's voice
And mirror George's attitude
In expressing his deep gratitude
To those whose love and inspiration
He is proud to recognize on this occasion.

One would have to be a wizard
To write this book from A to Izzard
Without those whom he's recognizing
In these simple words of my devising.

If George had penned these words instead
This is what he would have said:)

To my dear wife, Susanne, I now raise high my glass
Without her this volume would not come to pass.
When it sought to engulf me, and I cried "authorcide,"
She was there to restore me—the consummate bride.
While from me, who was first among all of her suitors,
She got nights at the office, red eyes from computers.
Sussi pressed the right buttons to ease my distress
With sustenance, et al.—the "et al." you can guess.

And to this panegyric, I hasten to add
A tribute in love to my mother and dad:

To my mother:
Who coached and cajoled me to help make me literate . . .
Those hours were precious, now that I considerate it.

To my father:
Whose labors to school me he never regretted.
They were labors of love, and I never forget it.

Also for **Peter Laibson,** a standing ovation.
He tutored me into this lifetime vocation.
For, during my tenure in training at Wills,
He fostered my writing and clinical skills
And led me by hand through the ophthalmic catechism
With carrot and stick—and some well-deserved criticism.

It affords me great pleasure to give recognition
To staff, fellows, colleagues—in fact, each physician,
Each faculty member, my allies at Emory,
Whose steadfast support will be etched in my memory
For the times when I sought funds I thought were acquisible,
For when I was tardy or, worse yet, invisible.
Their patience, forbearance, and collegiality
Have helped raise this book from a dream to reality.

And, lastly I dedicate this book **to my peers,**
That small, hardy band of RK pioneers,
Those numerous colleagues whose dogged persistence
Has brought this new surgery into existence
Who sought for the truth in an orderly way
And shared what they learned in the I.S.R.K.*
And I even include all the gadflies cantankerous
And, likewise, those !?#@*! whose voices were rancorous.

To all of those whom I've included above,
I dedicate this book with respect and with love.

George O. Waring III

(I think that includes all to whom George gave credit.
At any rate, that is how George would have said it.
As for your humble scrivener, he is moved to confess
He's still "from Missouri" as this goes to press.

Ben Milder)

*International Society of Refractive Keratoplasty

About the Author

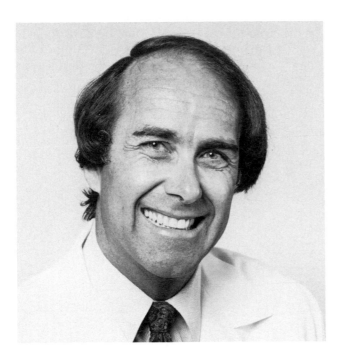

George Oral Waring III was born in Buffalo, New York, received his B.S. degree with honors from Wheaton College, and attained his M.D. degree from Baylor Medical College. His residency at Wills Eye Hospital was followed by a Heed fellowship in corneal disease under the direction of Peter Laibson, M.D.

Dr. Waring began his academic career at the University of California at Davis in 1974 and joined Emory University in 1979, where he is presently professor of ophthalmology and director of refractive surgery and tends a busy consulting practice. He is an active member of numerous professional societies including Diplomat of the American Board of Ophthalmology, American Ophthalmological Society, Fellow of the American Academy of Ophthalmology, Fellow of the American College of Surgeons, Trustee of the International Society of Refractive Keratoplasty, Royal Society of Medicine, and Société Française d'Ophtalmologie.

His broad-ranging research in corneal disease and surgery has included National Institute of Health grants to study radial keratomy (as director of the PERK study), excimer laser corneal surgery, intracorneal lenses (with Dr. Bernard McCarey), lipid corneal dystrophy in dogs, the biochemistry of Descemet's membrane (with Dr. Cristina Kenney), and high-risk corneal transplantation (Collaborative Corneal Transplantation study).

Dr. Waring has a special interest in ophthalmic publishing and editorial activities. He is editor-in-chief of *Refractive and Corneal Surgery* and serves on approximately a dozen editorial boards. He has published over 200 peer-reviewed articles and book chapters.

He has received numerous awards including the Society of Heed Fellows Outstanding Ophthalmology Honor Award, 1978-1979, the American Academy of Opthalmology Honor Award in 1981 and Senior Honor Award in 1991, a Gold Medal for Outstanding Contribution in Ophthalmology in Florence, Italy, in 1989, and an Honorary Medal from Ain Shams University in Egypt in 1989. Dr. Waring's love of teaching and travel has taken him to over 350 ophthalmic meetings in over 35 countries. He has helped train over 50 corneal fellows at Emory.

Dr. Waring is married to Susanne Gardner, a Doctor of Pharmacy and clinical assistant professor of ophthalmology at Emory. She publishes and edits *Ocular Therapeutics and Management*. Dr. Waring pursues his recreational activities with his three teenage children, George, Tim, and Joy. He plays squash regularly, helicopter skis in the Canadian Rockies, and has kayaked in the American Sierras and Rockies (Grand Canyon), the Swiss Alps, and the Nepali Himalayas.

Contributors

Koichiro Akiyama, M.D.[†]
Akiyama Ophthalmic Clinic
Yokohama, Japan

Shuichi Akiyama, M.D.
Akiyama Ophthalmic Clinic
Yokohama, Japan

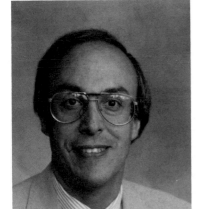

Perry S. Binder, M.D., F.A.C.S.
Associate Clinical Professor, Department of Ophthalmology
University of California, San Diego;
Director, Ophthalmic Surgery and Research
Sharp Cabrillo Hospital, San Diego, California

Dr. Binder received his B.S. degree in microbiology in 1964, and his M.S. degree in microbiology in 1968 from the University of Illinois. He received his M.D. degree from Northwestern University Medical School in 1969. Following his internship at UCLA and his ophthalmology residency at the University of Southern California, Dr. Binder completed a 1-year fellowship in corneal diseases at the University of Florida in Gainesville. He was a full-time faculty member in the Division of Ophthalmology at the University of California in San Diego from 1974 to 1981. Since that time he has been in full-time private practive at Eye Care of La Jolla in San Diego and is an associate clinical professor in the Department of Ophthalmology at the University of California in San Diego.

Dr. Binder is president of the National Vision Research Institute at the Sharp Cabrillo Hospital in San Diego. He served on the board of the Contact Lens Association of Ophthalmologists from 1976 to 1987, including a term as president in 1986. He has been a member of the Board of the International Society of Refractive Keratoplasty since its inception in 1979 and is currently finishing his second year as president. He served as the director of the Cornea Section for the Association for Research in Vision and Ophthalmology in 1986. He has been a member of the editorial board of over 10 journals and has published over 200 scientific articles in the field of contact lenses, corneal surgery, ocular infections, and refractive corneal surgery.

†Deceased (see p. 179).

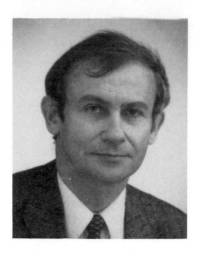

Philippe G. Ciarlet, Ph.D.
Professor and Director, Laboratoire d'Analyse Numérique
Université Pierre et Marie Curie
Paris, France

Dr. Ciarlet was named a professor in 1973 and director of the Laboratoire d'Analyse Numérique in 1981. He received the Prix Jaffé, one of the great prizes of the French Academy of Sciences, in 1989.

Dr. Ciarlet is a corresponding member of the French Academy of Sciences and has published 10 books.

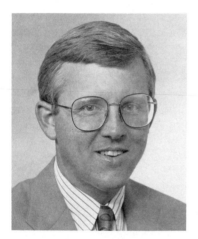

William S. Duffey, Jr., J.D.
Partner, King & Spalding
Atlanta, Georgia

Mr. Duffey received his B.A. degree, with honors, from Drake University in 1973 and his J.D. degree, cum laude, from the University of South Carolina School of Law in 1977. He served as a member of the United States Air Force Judge Advocate General Corps from 1978 through 1981, after which he joined King & Spalding in Atlanta. Mr. Duffey's practice focuses on complex civil and criminal litigation, including complex antitrust cases. He was a member of the defense team in the *Vest v. Waring* case, which is discussed in Chapter 9.

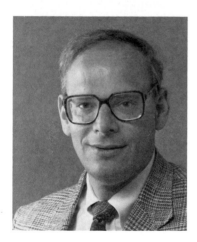

Richard A. Eiferman, M.D., F.A.C.S.
Professor of Ophthalmology
Department of Ophthalmology and Visual Sciences
School of Medicine, University of Louisville
Louisville, Kentucky

Dr. Eiferman graduated from the Medical College of Wisconsin in 1972 and completed his residency in Milwaukee in 1976. He completed a 1-year corneal external fellowship at Wills Eye Hospital under the direction of Peter Laibson. He joined the faculty at the University of Louisville, Department of Ophthalmology and Visual Sciences, in 1977. In addition to his professorship Dr. Eiferman is currently medical director of the Kentucky Lions Eye Bank and chief of ophthalmology at the Veterans Administration Medical Center. His research interest is in the area of wound healing.

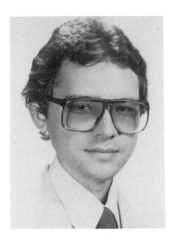

Francisco E. Fantes, M.D.
Chief of Ophthalmology, Department of Ophthalmology
Centro Medico Docenta La Trinidad
Caracas, Venezuela

Dr. Fantes completed a residency in ophthalmology at Bascom Palmer Eye Institute in Miami in 1987 and a 2-year corneal fellowship at Emory University in Atlanta in 1989. During his years at Emory he worked in excimer laser research with George O. Waring III, M.D. His main interest is excimer laser–cornea interactions and large area ablations. Dr. Fantes is currently chief of ophthalmology at the Centro Medico Docente La Trinidad in Caracas.

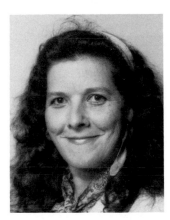

Mary C. Gemmill, C.O.M.T.
Chief Technologist, Supervisor of Paramedical Personnel
PERK Clinical Coordinator
Department of Ophthalmology, Emory University
Atlanta, Georgia

Ms. Gemmill has held her current positions for the Section of Ophthalmology since 1987. After obtaining a B.S. degree in biology from Western Maryland College in 1975, she studied at the Emory Orthoptic/Ophthalmic Technology Program and received certification as an orthoptist and an ophthalmic technician in 1979. She updated her certification to ophthalmic technologist in 1980.

Ms. Gemmill has been employed by the Emory Clinic since completion of the program in 1979, working in the subspecialties of cornea, pediatrics, glaucoma, and neurophthalmology. She was the clinical coordinator for the Prism Adaptation Trial from 1983 to 1984 and has been the PERK clinical coordinator and cornea clinical research coordinator since 1986. Ms. Gemmill is currently coordinating the Photorefractive Keratectomy Study.

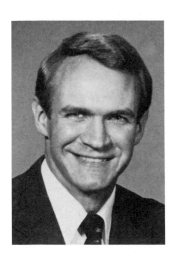

David L. Guyton, M.D.
Professor of Ophthalmology, The Wilmer Ophthalmological Institute
The Johns Hopkins University
Baltimore, Maryland

Dr. Guyton received his M.D. degree from Harvard Medical School in 1969, pursued bioengineering studies at the National Institutes of Health, and began ophthalmology residency at the Wilmer Institute of The Johns Hopkins University in 1973. Following a fellowship in strabismus and chief residency at the Wilmer Institute, he joined the full-time faculty in Wilmer and is currently professor of ophthalmology, serving as director of the Strabismus Service and of the Laboratory of Ophthalmic Optics.

Dr. Guyton is best known for his applied research in ophthalmic optics, developing the American Optical SR-IV Programmed Subjective Refractor and the Mentor Guyton/Minkowski Potential Acuity Meter. He is the most active teacher of ophthalmic optics in the United States today, teaching widely in basic science cources and review courses.

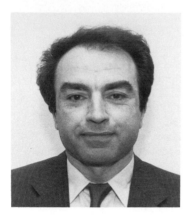

Khalil D. Hanna, M.D.
Associate Professor, Department of Ophthalmology
Emory University, Atlanta, Georgia;
Associate Professor, Ophtalmologie Service, Hotel-Dieu Hospital
Paris, France

Dr. Hanna is a part-time associate professor at Emory University in Atlanta and a research consultant with the IBM Scientific Center in Paris. Since 1987 he has been involved in a joint research project between Emory University and Hotel-Dieu Hospital on computer modeling of corneal surgery and excimer laser surgery.

Since 1985 Dr. Hanna has directed a research program and laboratory at Hotel-Dieu on applications of the excimer laser to the cornea, focusing primarily on excimer laser photorefractive keratectomy. He designed a flexible computer-controlled excimer laser delivery system for this purpose. He has also developed a suction mechanical trephine for corneal transplantation. Since 1984 Dr. Hanna's research has also included computer simulation of eye surgery.

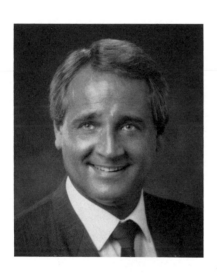

Jack T. Holladay, M.D.
Professor, Department of Ophthalmology
Hermann Eye Center, The Medical School
The University of Texas Health Science Center at Houston
Houston, Texas

Dr. Holladay is a clinical professor of ophthalmology at the University of Texas Medical School at Houston, Hermann Eye Center. His expertise in ophthalmic optics has resulted in his participation in the FDA ophthalmic device panel, the ANSI committee, which sets standards for intraocular lenses. He is also Editor of the Basic and Clinical Science Course book from the Academy of Ophthalmology. Dr. Holladay has authored many articles on the optics of intraocular lenses, cornea, multifocal lenses, and optical changes following radial keratotomy, as well as on devising an accurate formula for intraocular lens power calculations. His ability to clearly explain complex optical principles, making them useful for clinical application, is reflected in his writings and presentations.

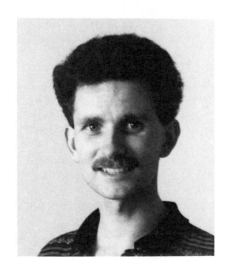

Francois E. Jouve
Research Engineer, Centre de Mathématiques Appliquées
Ecole Polytechnique
Palaiseau Cedex, France

Francois Jouve was born in Paris in 1963. He majored in applied mathematics at Ecole Normale Supézienze from 1983 to 1987. Since 1985 he has been working on the mathematical model of the eye with Drs. Khalil Hanna, Philippe Ciarlet, and George O. Waring III. His doctoral thesis on this subject will be completed in 1991.

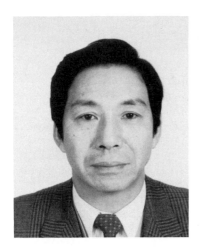

Atsushi Kanai, M.D.
Professor and Chairman, Department of Ophthalmology, Juntendo University
Tokyo, Japan

Dr. Kanai graduated from the School of Medicine at Juntendo University in 1963. He worked in the Department of Ophthalmology at Florida State University from 1968 to 1971. After returning to Japan he worked as an assistant professor in the Department of Ophthalmology at Juntendo University from 1971 to 1979, when he was appointed associate professor. Also in 1979 Dr. Kanai returned to the United States for 1 year to work with Professor H.E. Kaufman in the Department of Ophthalmology at Louisiana State University. In 1980 Dr. Kanai returned to Japan and worked with Professor Akira Nakajima at Juntendo University until Dr. Nakajima retired in March 1989. Dr. Kanai was appointed professor and chairman in October 1989.

Michael P. Kennedy, J.D.
Charter Medical Company
Macon, Georgia

Pamela Edwards Klein, M.Ed.
Whitefish Bay, Wisconsin;
Formerly, Research Associate, The Wilmer Ophthalmological Institute
The Johns Hopkins University
Baltimore, Maryland

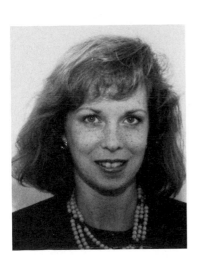

Ms. Klein received her B.A. degree in psychology from James Madison University and her M.Ed. in counseling from the University of Virginia. During graduate work her area of primary interest was health care services counseling.

For 10 years Ms. Klein has worked in clinical research in the fields of genetics, neurology, and ophthalmology. She has developed and written numerous patient information booklets and brochures. Most recently she was the project coordinator of a multicenter clinical trial at the Wilmer Institute concerning the immunology of corneal transplant rejection.

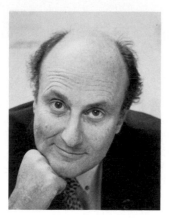

Michael H. Kutner, Ph.D.
Professor and Director, Division of Biostatistics
Department of Epidemiology and Biostatistics, Emory University
Atlanta, Georgia

Dr. Kutner received his doctoral degree in 1971 from Texas A & M University. His research interests have been primarily in linear statistical models. He has been a member of the Emory University Arts and Sciences graduate faculty since 1971 and has served as the chief biostatistician at the Clinical Research Center of Emory University Hospital since 1974.

Dr. Kutner has co-authored over 100 papers and two popular textbooks, *Applied Linear Statistical Models* and *Applied Linear Regression Models* with John Neter and William Wasserman. Dr. Kutner was elected a fellow of the American Statistical Association in 1984 and was the recipient of the H.O. Hartley Award. He has been actively involved in the American Statistical Association and the Biometric Society. He has served on the board of directors of ASA and has been an associate editor of *The American Statistician.*

He currently serves as co-principal investigator for the Statistical Coordinating Center for the Prospective Evaluation of Radial Keratotomy (PERK) study.

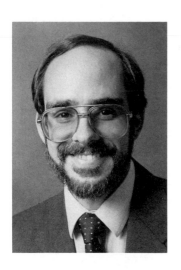

Michael J. Lynn, M.S.
Department of Epidemiology and Biostatistics, Emory University
Atlanta, Georgia

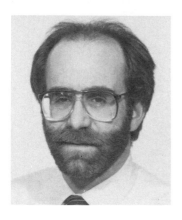

Jan A. Markowitz, Ph.D.
Instructor, The Wilmer Ophthalmological Institute
The Johns Hopkins University
Baltimore, Maryland

Dr. Markowitz is a graduate of the University of Rhode Island and received his Sc.M. and Ph.D. from the Department of Epidemiology, School of Hygiene and Public Health, at The Johns Hopkins University.

Since 1984 Dr. Markowitz has been a member of the faculty at The Wilmer Ophthalmological Institute at The Johns Hopkins University. His interests have been in the design and operation of clinical trials in ophthalmology and in the epidemiology of eye diseases. He has been involved in the Macular Photocoagulation Study, the Collaborative Ocular Melanoma Study, and the Studies of the Ocular Complications of AIDS.

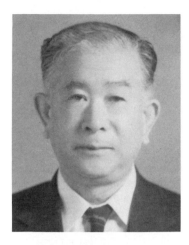

Akira Nakajima, M.D.
Professor Emeritus, Department of Ophthalmology
Juntendo University
Tokyo, Japan

Dr. Nakajima was a graduate in medicine from the University of Tokyo, where he also completed his postgraduate training and obtained a doctorate in science. He was professor and chairman of the Department of Ophthalmology at Juntendo University from 1960 to 1989 and was appointed professor emeritus in March 1989.

Dr. Nakajima was awarded the Gonin Medal at the XXI ICO Congress in Rome in 1986 and the Jose Rizal Medal at the XI APAO Congress in Kuala Lumpur in 1987. He is currently president of the International Council of Ophthalmology, senior vice president of the International Agency for the Prevention of Blindness, and president of the select body, Academia Ophthalmologica Internationalis.

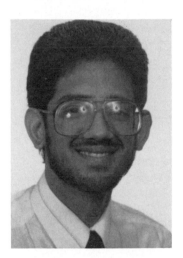

Azhar Nizam, M.S.
Senior Associate, Department of Epidemiology and Biostatistics
Emory University
Atlanta, Georgia

Mr. Nizam provides statistical and computing support for the Prospective Evaluation of Radial Keratotomy (PERK) study at Emory University and teaches introductory statistics and personal and statistical computing to graduate students. He earned his B.A. degree in mathematics and economics from Grinnell College in Iowa in 1985 and his M.S. degree in statistics from the University of South Carolina in 1987.

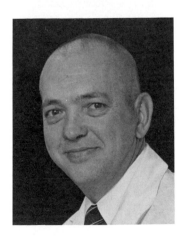

Robert E. Nordquist, Ph.D.
Professor of Ophthalmology, Department of Ophthalmology;
Director of Research, Dean A. McGee Eye Institute
University of Oklahoma Health Sciences Center
Oklahoma City, Oklahoma

Dr. Nordquist is an experimental pathologist who concentrates on ultrastructural morphology and wound healing. He is the recipient of the Cora Snetcher Professorship in Research Ophthalmology.

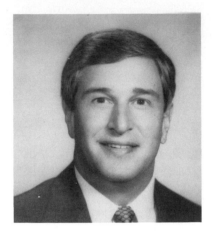

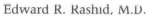

Associate Clinical Professor, Department of Ophthalmology
The University of Texas Health Science Center at San Antonio
San Antonio, Texas

Dr. Rashid attended Northwestern University Medical School in Chicago and graduated with his medical degree in 1976. After a year of internship in internal medicine he began his residency training at Wilford Hall USAF Medical Center in San Antonio. Upon completion of his ophthalmology residency, Dr. Rashid entered fellowship training in 1980 at Emory University in cornea and external diseases of the eye. Upon completion of his fellowship training he became chief of the cornea and external disease section at Wilford Hall USAF Medical Center, the only residency training program in the U.S. Air Force. During this time he was also the residency training director for the Ophthalmology program. In 1987 Dr. Rashid completed another fellowship in corneal refractive surgery, both at Emory University in Atlanta and several other university locations. He returned to Wilford Hall as the vice chairman of the Department of Ophthalmology and special consultant to the USAF surgeon general in cornea and external diseases of the eye. He is currently in private practice in San Antonio, where he also holds an associate professorship at The University of Texas.

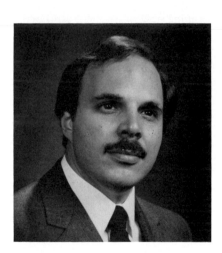

Donald R. Sanders, M.D., Ph.D.
Associate Professor, Department of Ophthalmology
University of Illinois at Chicago
Chicago, Illinois

Dr. Sanders received his B.S. degree in biological sciences from the University of Illinois at Chicago in 1971 and his M.D. degree from the same university in 1973. While at the University of Illinois School of Medicine, Dr. Sanders was enrolled in the Edmond J. James Scholar Program for Independent Study. He completed his internship at Northwestern University Hospital in 1974 and his residency in ophthalmology at the University of Illinois Eye and Ear Infirmary in 1977. He received certification from the American Board of Ophthalmology in 1978. In 1984 Dr. Sanders earned a doctoral degree in pharmacology from the University of Illinois at Chicago Health Sciences Center.

Dr. Sanders served as an assistant professor at the University of Illinois at Chicago Department of Ophthalmology from 1977 to 1981 and has served as an associate professor since 1981. He also served as chief of ophthalmology at the VA Westside Hospital from 1977 to 1987.

Dr. Sanders is the author of over 100 journal articles and books. Many relate to refractive surgery and the use of computers in ophthalmology. He is also the chief medical editor of *Ocular Surgery News*.

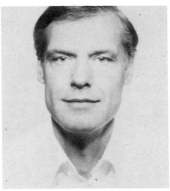

Bernd H. Schimmelpfennig, M.D.
Private Practice;
Lecturer, Eye Department, University of Zurich
Zurich, Switzerland

Dr. Schimmelpfennig was born in Germany. In 1961 he escaped from East Germany and studied medicine in West Berlin and Kiel. He worked at the university eye department in Zurich from 1971 to 1977. He was a post-doctoral fellow at Stanford University from 1977 to 1979. Since 1988 Dr. Schimmelpfennig has been in private practice as an eye surgeon with teaching responsibilities at the University of Zurich.

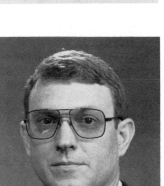

Gregory S. Schultz, Ph.D.
Professor of Obstetrics/Gynecology and Ophthalmology
Department of Obstetrics/Gynecology and Ophthalmology
University of Florida
Gainesville, Florida

Dr. Schultz received his doctoral degree in biochemistry from Oklahoma State University. After completing postdoctoral research in cell biology at Yale University, Dr. Schultz was appointed assistant professor of biochemistry at the University of Louisville.

Dr. Schultz's research interests center on the role of peptide growth factors and their receptors in the regulation of cell growth in wound healing.

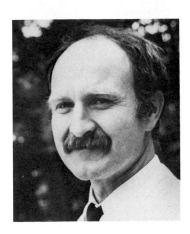

Theo Wolfgang Seiler, M.D., Ph.D.
Professor of Ophthalmology, Universitäts-Augenklinik Charlottenburg
Freie Universität Berlin
Berlin, Germany

Dr. Seiler received his Ph.D. degree in experimental physics in 1975 and his M.D. degree in ophthalmology in 1981 from Freie University in Berlin. Since 1981 he has run a laboratory in ophthalmic applications of lasers and bioengineering. His interest in excimer lasers began in 1983, and he has developed a technique for making linear excisions with the laser and for doing large area ablation (photorefractive keratectomy). Dr. Seiler was the first ophthalmic surgeon to perform excimer laser ablations in humans and has extensive experience in the treatment of myopia and corneal astigmatism with the excimer laser.

Dr. Seiler received the Theodor Axenfeld Award in 1989.

Hirohiko Shibata, M.D.
Akiyama Ophthalmic Clinic
Yokohama, Japan

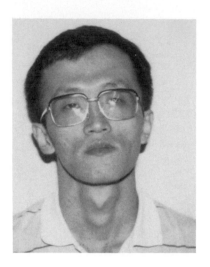

Jung-Woog Shin, M.S.
Graduate Student, School of Mechanical Engineering
Georgia Institute of Technology
Atlanta, Georgia

Mr. Shin was born in Busan, South Korea. He received his BSME degree in 1983 from Seoul National University in Seoul, Korea. From 1983 to 1985 he worked as an engineer in the CAD/CAM division at Seoul Electron Ltd. In 1987 Mr. Shin received his MSME degree from the Georgia Institute of Technology in Atlanta.

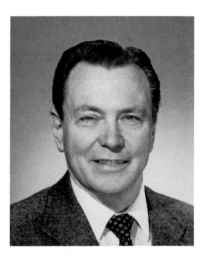

Spencer P. Thornton, M.D., F.A.C.S.
Director, Cataract and Corneal Surgery Service
Department of Ophthalmology, Baptist Hospital
Nashville, Tennessee

Dr. Thornton received his medical training at Bowman Gray School of Medicine of Wake Forest University and his residency in ophthalmology at Vanderbilt University Hospital in Nashville. He took additional training in anterior segment surgery, lens implantation, and refractive surgery.

Dr. Thornton is associate editor of the *Journal of Cataract and Refractive Surgery* in addition to serving on the editorial boards of *Refractive and Corneal Surgery* and *Ocular Surgery News.* He has published extensively in journals, authored numerous book chapters, and lectured in major universities worldwide. He has also served on the board of the American Society of Cataract and Refractive Surgery and the International Society of Refractive Keratoplasty. His major interests are accommodation, intraocular lenses, and refractive surgery.

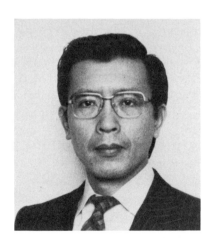

Hiroshi Uozato, Ph.D.
Associate Professor and Research Director
Department of Ophthalmology, Nara Medical University
Kashihara, Nara, Japan

Dr. Uozato received his B.S. degree, magna cum laude, in 1972 and his M.S. degree, summa cum laude, in 1974 from the Osaka Institute of Technology. He was awarded his doctoral degree, summa cum laude, in 1978 from the University of Osaka Prefecture.

In 1974 Dr. Uozato worked as a research assistant in the Department of Mechanical Engineering at the Osaka Institute of Technology. In 1978 he was named assistant professor in the Department of Ophthalmology at Nara Medical University and was appointed associate professor and research director in 1986. In 1988 he was named co-director for the Computerized Hospital Information Service at Nara Medical University Hospital.

Dr. Uozato is the author of numerous books and journal articles and has given over 200 presentations. He is the holder of seven patents.

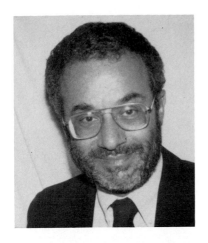

Raymond P. Vito, Ph.D.
Associate Professor, Department of Mechanical Engineering
Georgia Institute of Technology
Atlanta, Georgia

Dr. Vito was born in Buffalo, New York, and received his B.S. and M.S. degrees in engineering science from the State University of New York at Buffalo. He continued his studies at Cornell University and received his doctoral degree in theoretical and applied mechanics in 1972. After a year as a postdoctoral fellow at McMaster University, Dr. Vito joined the faculty of the Georgia Institute of Technology. His research interests are in biomechanics, especially measurement of the mechanical properties of living tissues.

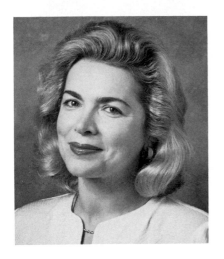

Susanne K. Gardner, D.Pharm.
Assistant Clinical Professor of Ophthalmology
Department of Ophthalmology, Emory University
Atlanta, Georgia

Dr. Gardner is the editor of *Ocular Therapeutics and Management,* a subscription newsletter that addresses the drug therapy of ocular diseases. She was born in Germany and has lived in the United States since childhood. Dr. Gardner received her graduate degree from the University of Michigan at Ann Arbor.

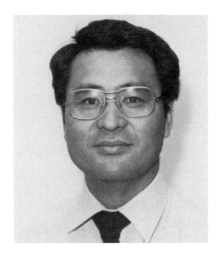

Tatsuo Yamaguchi, M.D., Ph.D.
Assistant Professor, Department of Ophthalmology
Juntendo University
Tokyo, Japan

Dr. Yamaguchi received his M.D. degree in 1971 from Juntendo University, and received his doctoral degree in 1985. From 1980 to 1985 he worked as an assistant professor in the Department of Ophthalmology at Louisiana State University and was appointed a clinical assistant professor in 1985. In that same year he was also appointed an assistant professor in the Department of Ophthalmology at Juntendo University. Since 1988 Dr. Yamaguchi has also worked in the Department of Ophthalmology at St. Luke's International Hospital in Tokyo.

Preface

Of Mountain Climbing
and Book Writing

Mountain climbers are my heroes. They strive to the summit with enormous individual dedication, will power, skill, and persistence. They plan, they climb, they endure, they descend—all in the midst of everyday obligations to family, profession, friends, and finances. The breadth of skills required of successful alpinists is extraordinary: fund-raising, interpersonal relations, technical knowledge of equipment, understanding of weather and terrain, persistent training and prolonged endurance, and exquisite intuition and judgment. Above all, each climber exercises that essential quality for success: putting one foot in front of the other all the way to the top. Writing books has much in common with climbing mountains.

I have never climbed high, but I have spent hours reading and vicariously summiting solo with Messner on Everest[1] and Nanga Parbat,[2] with Bass on the seven summits,[3] and with many others.[4-7] Their sufferings, privations, and achievements provided inspiration for me as I wrote this book.

In the beginning both climbers and authors let romantic ideas block out the reality ahead. These simplistic fantasies are fostered by previous climbers who have strutted past 8,000 meters and by myriad published authors. They did it. It can't be that hard. Of course, the first few days on the mountain and the first chapter or two of the book snuff out these idealistic illusions.

Modern alpine climbing often shuns the siege tactic of employing myriad Sherpas who carry loads to fixed camps in support of a team of climbers. Instead an intrepid group of individuals use "modern fair means" of carrying everything themselves, ascending quickly without oxygen, and bivouacking along the way. I used this approach to complete this book, carefully selecting reliable colleagues, who have expended enormous personal effort to create the best possible book on refractive keratotomy. My writing compatriots have been uniformly superior, each investing precious time, thought, and knowledge and tolerating my harassment, rewrites, and updates.

Fully aware that numerous books have been published on radial and astigmatic keratotomy, my goal has been to creatively assemble information on the subject with a breadth and depth that would be distinctive, authoritative, and comprehensive. In a sense, I avoided the classic direct route of ascent and sought to climb the mountain the hard way, along a new line, where most extreme conditions challenge finely tuned skills.

Plans that seem practical early in an ascent must be changed as the realities of the terrain, weather, and resources shape the climb. What is charted as the goal of 1 day's effort may become a week's work because of storm or avalanche. Messner experienced this halfway up Everest:

About 100 meters above the campsite I decide that climbing up the ridge is becoming too dangerous. Also too strenuous, for there the snow lies partially knee-deep. All the hollows are filled in. And above me a single giant-sized trough. Not only the avalanche danger, but the exertion above deters me. A feeling of hopelessness grips me as I poke the right ski stick into the floury mess. Snow slap danger! The topmost layer is firm but gives way with a crack when I step on it. Underneath the snow is grainy. On my own, under these conditions, I would quickly tire myself out.

Then I see that on the North Face the snow slabs have gone. What luck! There the foundation is hard. Yes, that's the way! Without thinking much I begin to cross the North Face.[1]

Conditions and information changed during the writing of this book. New data, technical advances, and alterations in understanding all required revisions and additions that could not wait for a second edition. So, in creating this book, we also undertook mid-climb changes of direction that carved out a new, creative route of ascent: the sections on astigmatism, laser corneal surgery, and biomechanics and computer modeling were conceived and added after formatting the initial outline. That this decision added a year to the production and publication of the book is unfortunate; that it adds contemporary breadth and depth yields a substantial benefit for you, the reader.

The economics of climbing and writing are complex. Few climbers can afford to support the equipment, supplies, travel, and ongoing expenses of a long ascent with their own financial resources and without external sponsorship. The conflict that emerges in writing a book such as this, whose sales number only a few thousand, is obvious. The publisher must restrain costs to keep the price of the book at an acceptable level for the ophthalmic public, yet he must ensure a profit. Most universities do not support the writing of books because books do not represent original scholarly activity. Few agencies provide grants for writing medical books; the Commonwealth Fund is an exception, and I appreciate their support. In essence, writing scientific books is one of those scholarly activities for which no one wants to pay.

The analogy between mountain climbing and book writing becomes more pertinent and obvious when we consider the daily activities of each. The boring repetitive tasks of putting one foot in front of the other and one thought after another call on sheer persistence to overcome aching body, wandering mind, and homesick heart. Messner:

I progress so slowly! How long my pauses to breathe are each time I don't know. With the ski sticks I succeed in going 15 paces, then I must rest for several minutes . . . step by step, fatigue.[1]

During the preparation of this book, calls for retreat dogged my colleagues and me from those who believed the text was "good enough." But the inclusion of insufficient and inadequate information in the book would have been tantamount to failing to reach the summit. Even so, I remained intensely aware that useful information was being omitted, that new articles were not integrated with the old, that inadequate expression of some concepts persisted in the text, and that better illustrations were available but time to include them was not. Nevertheless, I often forced myself to add one more reference, one more section, or one more chapter to craft the best possible text, sharing the climber's exasperating experience of climbing past "one more ridge," only to find another rise or two on the way to the summit.

Climbers bivouac, spending miserable, fearful, and fatiguing nights in frigid temperatures tethered on narrow ledges overlooking precipitous drops with minimal warmth and protection. Writers bivouac too. I wrote straight through the night or slept on the floor of my (warm) office more often than I care to admit, sometimes with my intrepid wife, Susanne—an option not available to the climber!

And there's the waiting. Friends, family, and employers wait for mountaineers. Family, patients, staff, colleagues, editors, and publishers wait for the writer. To all those who have waited for me and my colleagues during the preparation of this book, I am grateful.

Paradoxically, the climber who ascends above 8,000 meters spends less than an hour at the top—a painful and momentary revelry. The sense of accomplishment fades quickly as the "victor" realizes that he must now descend safely. The author "summits" after completion of the last chapter, but his joy is short-lived when he realizes he must proofread and update the edited manuscripts, pick his way through the galleys, rearrange the dummy layouts, and scrutinize details of the page proofs. I am sure that there are authors whose books have been completed but never published. Fortunately that fate did not meet *Refractive Keratotomy for Myopia and Astigmatism*, thanks to the diligent and persistent work of Katherine Lindstrom and her staff at Emory University and of John Casey, Maureen Slaten, Kim Kist, and others at Mosby—Year Book, Inc.

Just as no climber conquers a mountain, no author exhausts a subject. But both processes satisfy personal aspirations and longings. Friends, family, and colleagues have challenged me, "Why did you spend 5 years completing a book on one operation? Think of all you could have done with that time!" Both the climber and the writer think of the lost possibilities, but neither can resist stretching to the fullest their faculties and aptitudes; neither can resist the call to forge a new route or to assemble information in a new way. Messner expressed it articulately:

I must go, and yet each smallest chore is an effort. Up here life is brutally balanced between exhaustion and will-power; self-conquest becomes a compulsion. Why don't I go down? There is no occasion to. I cannot simply give up without a reason. I wanted to make the climb. I still want to. Curiosity, the game, ambition—all these superficial incentives have vanished, gone. Whatever it is that drives me is planted much deeper than I or the magnifying glass of the psychologists can detect. Day by day, hour by hour, minute by minute, step by step, I force myself to do something against which my body rebels.[1]

In the end, there is a difference. For the mountaineer, the final judgment about his activity resides mainly in his own heart and mind. For the author it resides in the opinion of the readers and scholars who use his work. I hope you will conclude that the time and work involved in completing *Refractive Keratotomy for Myopia and Astigmatism* was worth it.

George O. Waring III

REFERENCES

1. Messner R: The crystal horizon, Seattle, 1989, The Mountaineers.
2. Messner R: Solo Nanga Parbat, London, 1980, Kay and Ward.
3. Bass D: The seven summits, New York, 1986, Warner.
4. Craig RW: Storm and sorrow in the high pamirs, Seattle, 1977, The Mountaineers.
5. Gillett N and Reynolds J: Everest grand circle, Seattle, 1985, The Mountaineers.
6. Boardman P: The shining mountain: two men on Changbang's west wall, New York, 1985, Vintage Books.
7. Curran J: K 2, triumph and tragedy, Seattle, 1987, The Mountaineers.

Acknowledgments

Throughout this book I acknowledge the contributions and sources of information at the beginning of each chapter.

Here, I'm glad to acknowledge the many individuals who have contributed to the overall preparation of the text. Katherine Lindstrom edited the book in the Department of Ophthalmology at Emory University, corralling myriad details and multiple contributors and herding enormous volumes of information into a meaningful and understandable whole. Brenda Summer shouldered the yeoman's task of typing and repeatedly retyping the manuscript with a diligence rare in today's workplace.

Stephen Gordon prepared the majority of the illustrations, contributing creatively to the content and layout of many and doggedly executing multiple revisions of most. I especially appreciate his long-term dedication, without which this book would be less valuable for the reader.

The staff at Mosby–Year Book have helped guide the growth of the text from its initial plan as a 500-page textbook to its present comprehensive format. Publisher George Stamathis, Managing Editors Eugenia Klein and Kim Kist, as well as Maureen Slaten, John Casey, and Tim Sainz expertly carried the book through the multiple phases of publication. I appreciate their flexibility and forbearance.

My colleagues in the PERK study provided the initial impetus and sustained effort and support for a decade that allowed the PERK study to compile the most thorough existing data base about radial keratotomy. The Emory coordinating centers' staff included Ceretha Cartwright, John Carter, Mike Lynn, Michael Kutner, Steve Moffitt, Portia Griffin, Agar Nizam, Brooke Fielding, Vickie Rice-Santos, and Phyllis Newman. The investigators and coordinators at the clinical centers, the Data and Safety Monitoring Board and the Clinical Monitors, are acknowledged in Chapter 8, Development of Refractive Keratotomy in the United States, 1978-1990. Without the funding of the National Eye Institute of the United States National Institutes of Health and the active collaboration of Drs. Carl Kupfer, Robert Sperduto, Ralph Helmsen, Robert Mowery, and their staffs, the PERK study would not have come to fruition.

Nancy Hayes, Darla Loga, Susie Frease, Phyllis Lee, Rochelle Kraehe, Pamela O'Hagan, Lynn Ohl, Edith Barron, and Wendy Wiley added the burden of this book to their daily secretarial and administrative duties, ensuring its successful completion. Patricia Bennett, Sandy Ericson, Mary Gemmill, and numerous technical staff and postdoctoral corneal fellows expertly helped manage my clinical practice, allowing me time to prepare this text. I appreciate especially the support of the three other faculty members on the Corneal and Refractive Service at the Emory Clinic—Drs. Louis Wilson, Doyle Stulting, and Dwight Cavanagh—whose unflagging collegial support in both clinical practice and ophthalmic research have fostered my interest in keratotomy and have freed up time for the completion of this book.

The staff in the Medical Illustration Department of Emory University—Grover Hogan, Nancy Mathews, Patsy Bryan, Chuck Bogle, Charles Boyter, Joey Schroth, and Alan Foust—provided expert, artistic, and technical assistance, often under the pressure of crash deadlines. The Ophthalmic Photography Department—Jim Gilman, Ray Swords, Steve Carlton, Kevin Ott, Dan Boyles, Stephanie Mize, Angela Varvel, Glenn Holley, and Mark Maio—assisted with much of the clinical photography and preparation of figures in the text.

In an era of stringent cutbacks in academic and publishing budgets, I could not have completed this book without grants from enlightened colleagues in industry, including Alcon, Inc., Pharmacia, Inc., and Cooper Vision. Both the American Academy of Ophthalmology and the Commonwealth Fund provided additional support.

Contents in Brief

Contents

**SECTION III   Patient Selection and Planning
for Refractive Keratotomy**

**10   Patient Educational Materials for
Refractive Keratotomy, 281**
Pamela Edwards Klein
Jan A. Markowitz

**11   Refractive Keratotomy, the Law of
Informed Consent, and Medical
Malpractice, 299**
William S. Duffey, Jr.
Michael P. Kennedy

**12   Examination and Selection of Patients for
Refractive Keratotomy, 309**
George O. Waring III

16 Centering Corneal Surgical Procedures, 491

Hiroshi Uozato
David L. Guyton
George O. Waring III

17 Atlas of Surgical Techniques of Radial Keratotomy, 507

George O. Waring III

18 Repeated Surgery for Residual Myopia and Hyperopia after Refractive Corneal Surgery, 641

George O. Waring III

24   Stability of Refraction after Refractive Keratotomy, 937

George O. Waring III
Michael J. Lynn
Michael H. Kutner

APPENDICES

Refractive Keratotomy

for myopia and astigmatism

Myopia

Myopia: A Brief Overview

George O. Waring III

TERMINOLOGY

The term "myopia" comes from the Greek *myopia*, which means to squint. This derivation presumably alludes to squinting of the eyelids, which produces horizontal stenopaic slits that improve the visual acuity of uncorrected myopic individuals. Myopia is colloquially known as nearsightedness because myopic persons have good uncorrected visual acuity at a near distance—within an arm's length.

The history of myopia and the ideas concerning its pathogenesis and function have been thoroughly summarized by van Alpen[59] and Duke-Elder.[16] Since the days of the Greeks, myopia has been described and written about. Galen attributed ocular refraction and its abnormalities to the composition and quantity of the fluids in the eye. In the early seventeenth century Kepler made major contributions to defining refraction of the eye and observed that in myopic eyes parallel rays of light were focused in front of the retina. By the eighteenth century it was well established that myopic globes were longer than normal. As instruments capable of measuring the refractive elements of the eye were developed in the nineteenth and twentieth centuries, it became apparent that eyes with less than 4.00 to 5.00 diopters (D) of myopia had normal measurements for the refractive power of the cornea and lens and the length of the globe but that these measurements were improperly correlated to produce myopia. On the other hand, eyes with greater amounts of myopia had severe axial elongation of the globe, as discussed in Chapter 3, Optics and Corneal Topography of Radial Keratotomy.

BACKGROUND AND ACKNOWLEDGMENTS
To write a book on keratotomy for myopia and astigmatism without surveying these refractive disorders would indeed be "shortsighted." Therefore I include a brief summary of myopia here. In 1985 Brian J. Curtin published his superbly integrated book that summarized the world's literature on the myopias.[13] Much of the material presented here that concerns aspects of myopia distinctly relevant to radial keratotomy is drawn selectively from Curtin's book. (Background on astigmatism is presented in Chapter 31, Keratotomy for Astigmatism.) Marshall Parks and Burton Kushner provided information on the accommodative convergence/accommodation (AC/A) ratio and myopia.

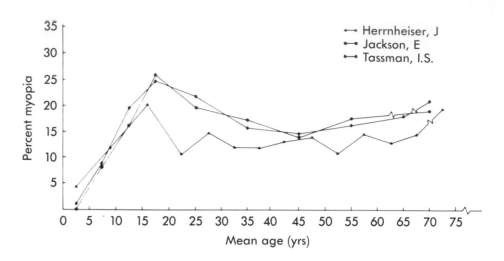

Figure 1-1
Prevalence of myopia increases until the late teens and then levels off. Three large studies. (From Herrnheiser J: Z Heilk 1892;13:342; Jackson E: JAMA 1932;98:132; Tassman IS: Am J Ophthalmol 1932;15:1044.)

SOCIOLOGIC ASPECTS OF MYOPIA
Prevalence of myopia

Studies of the prevalence of myopia have reported highly variable results, depending on the study methods, the age of the population, the definition of myopia, the examination conditions, and the racial composition and socioeconomic status of the study group.

Effect of age

In general, myopia is common in the premature infant, not so common in the newborn infant, and rare by age 6 months. Myopia demonstrates a sharp rise in incidence from ages 5 to 20 years and then a gradual decline in incidence throughout middle and advancing age. Approximately 20% to 40% of newborn infants are nearsighted.[12,20] The full-term infant may be expected to have about 2.00 D of hyperopia on the average, with an incidence of myopia ranging from 4% to 6%, then falling during the first 6 months of life.

The prevalence of myopia is greatest in adolescence, reaching approximately 25% and reflecting the tendency for hyperopia to decrease and myopia to increase during this time of development. Sorsby[52] followed 130 myopic children for 3 to 5 years observing that 65% showed an increase in myopia from −0.75 D to more than −4.00 D.[2,25] This trend of a gradual increase in the prevalence of myopia in the population peaks at about 20 years of age for an estimated overall adult prevalence of 20% (Fig. 1-1).

There are substantial differences in the prevalence of myopia among racial and ethnic groups. The highest prevalence of myopia is among Oriental races, reaching 50% to 70% of Chinese[17,44] and 30% of Japanese.[56] Eskimos, Native Americans, and black Africans generally have a low prevalence of myopia, although recent studies have identified an increase in myopia among Eskimos.[40]

Many studies of Europeans have identified an overall prevalence rate of 10% to 20%.[3] In the United States, prevalence figures are similar to those in Europe. Tassman[57] examined 10,153 patients in Philadelphia, finding a 17% prevalence of myopia. Jackson[32,33] examined his private patients in Denver, finding a 19.6% prevalence. Newcome[41] found a prevalence of 23.7% in a study of 1000 consecutive patients from the U.S. Army Ophthalmology Department.

The most recently published data on the prevalence of myopia in the United States are from the study by Sperduto and colleagues,[54] which uses data collected by the National Center of Health Statistics during the National Health and Nutrition Examination Survey

Table 1-1

Estimated Prevalence (%) of Specific Levels of Myopia by Age in the United States From 1971 to 1972

Myopia (diopters)	All ages	Age (yr)				
		12 to 17	18 to 24	25 to 34	35 to 44	45 to 54
<2.00						
OD*	13.4	11.1	11.7	13.1	15.9	15.8
OS†	13.2	11.0	11.6	13.4	14.9	15.4
2.00-7.90						
OD	11.4	12.5	15.8	10.7	8.4	8.9
OS	10.7	12.4	15.0	9.7	7.8	8.3
≥7.90						
OD	0.2	0.4	0.3	0.3	0.2	0
OS	0.4	0.4	0.7	0.2	0.7	0

From Sperduto RD et al: Arch Ophthalmol 1983;101:405.
*Oculus dexter, or right eye.
†Oculus sinister, or left eye.

from 1971 to 1972 (Table 1-1). The survey involved a national probability sample of 14,147 persons aged 1 to 74 years who were selected to represent the 192.7 million persons in the civilian, noninstitutionalized population at that time. Adequate data on refraction were available on approximately 56% of this population. The prevalence of any degree of myopia in persons between ages 12 and 54 years was 25%, with approximately twice as many whites being myopic as blacks (26% versus 12%). Those with higher annual incomes had more myopia than those with lower annual incomes (>$10,000 = 28%, <$5,000 = 17%), and 10 times as many people with high educational levels had myopia as those with low educational levels had (ninth grade education or more = 30%, eighth grade education or less = 3%).

Applying these figures to the population eligible for radial keratotomy reveals a prevalence of myopia between 2.00 and 8.00 D in approximately 10% of individuals aged 25 to 54 years. The population of people between 21 and 50 years of age in the United States (the ages during which radial keratotomy is most frequently performed) is approximately 111,670,000.[58] Of these individuals, 10% form a population of 11,167,000 eligible for radial keratotomy in the United States. These rough estimates can be computed on a worldwide basis. There are approximately 1,929,228,000 individuals in the world between ages 20 and 50 years.[15] Assuming a 10% prevalence of my-

Table 1-2

Estimates of Prevalence of Impairment from Visual Disorders: Impaired Vision

Type of eye affection	Impaired vision (in thousands)
Glaucoma	1,070
Cataract (prenatal, other)	1,711
Retinal disorder (prenatal, diabetic, other)	815
Retrolental fibroplasia	19
Myopia	715
Cornea or sclera	294
Uveitis	285
Optic nerve disease	121
Multiple affections	90
Refractive errors with lesser disability	1,662
Other affections	3,656
Unknown	221
Total (all affections)	10,659

From Support for Vision Research: Washington, DC, Department of Health, Education and Welfare, Publication No NIM 76-1098, 1976, U.S. Government Printing Office.

Table 1-3

Myopia as a Cause of World Blindness

Country or territory	Ranking as cause of blindness	Percentage of population affected
United States	7th	3
Hong Kong	5th	8
Japan	5th	8.4
Sri Lanka	5th	Not reported
Denmark	3rd	Not reported
Germany, Democratic Republic	1st or 2nd	14.7 or 13.9
Germany, Federal Republic	7th	6.6
Malta	1st	19.4
Poland	3rd	11
Union of Soviet Socialist Republics	2nd	Not reported

From Lim AS and Jones BR: Vision 1981;1:101.

opia between −2.00 and −8.00 D (a probable underestimate given the higher prevalence of myopia in Oriental populations), approximately 192,922,800 individuals might be eligible for radial keratotomy worldwide. This might form a partial explanation for the establishment of assembly-line techniques for performing radial keratotomy in major cities in the Soviet Union, where a single clinic performs 30 to 50 operations daily.[17a]

Visual disability and blindness from myopia

Refractive errors are the most common cause of impaired vision in the United States, and myopia is the fifth most common cause[13] (Table 1-2). Approximately 75% of teenagers who wear corrective lenses are myopic.

Although the vast majority of myopes have refractive disorders that can potentially be managed by radial keratotomy, a small group with high myopia, particularly those with pathologic myopia, have a truly vision-threatening disorder. Pathologic myopia is the eighth most frequent cause of severe visual impairment and the seventh most frequent cause of legal blindness in the United States. One problem in determining the role of myopia in blindness is classifying the cause of the blindness. For example, retinal detachment or optic nerve disease associated with myopia may not be grouped under the category of myopia itself, and thus results in underestimation of the effect of this pathologic process. In general, myopia is certainly among the five leading causes of blindness in the world (Table 1-3).

Blindness caused by myopia occurs at an earlier age than blindness caused by most other primary ocular disorders. It generally occurs a decade earlier than blindness caused by diabetic retinopathy, glaucoma, cataract, and age-related maculopathy. Thus the socioeconomic impact of myopic blindness is greater, since it tends to strike individuals during their most productive years.

Economic aspects of myopia

In his text Curtin emphasizes the impact of myopia as a socioeconomic problem: "Throughout life the myope has a financial burden of purchasing, and the inconvenience of servicing, a variety of visual aids. These may take the form of spectacles or corneal lenses. The myopes account for a large share of the optical aid market in the United States, which in recent years has exceeded four billion dollars in annual sales."[13]

In individual terms, assuming a male myope acquires the first spectacle correction at 9 years of age and wears them for 60 years, he can expect to replace the glasses 20 times (every 3 years) at a cost of approximately $150 per replacement. This is an approximate lifetime expense of $3000. Of course if contact lenses are worn, the cost rises to include the approximate $100 for examinations and $175 for rigid, gas-permeable contact lenses, which themselves are replaced approximately every 2 years. Assuming a myope might wear contact lenses for approximately 30 years (age 15 years to age 45 years), the expense for contact lenses could amount to $4200 plus expenses for backup glasses.

Looking at the surgical side and conservatively estimating one in 10 individuals in the United States to be myopic, approximately 11,167,000 individuals are potential candidates for radial keratotomy surgery, which, at approximately $1200 per eye, represents a potential surgical market of about $13.4 billion, or more than $1.1 million for each of the 12,000 ophthalmic surgeons in the United States. Of course given current techniques, only a small fraction of the myopic population will elect keratotomy, and furthermore, only approximately 10% of ophthalmic surgeons perform the operation regularly. Nevertheless, this potentially lucrative market has caught the fancy of some ophthalmic surgeons and medical marketers who have centered practices and surgical clinics on radial keratotomy.

These figures are relevant only in the United States, but when one considers the figures for Europe and especially Asia, it is clear that the management of refractive errors, whether optically or surgically, is truly a multibillion-dollar market.

CAUSE OF MYOPIA

Several factors account for the multiplicity and conflicting nature of theories of the cause of myopia, including the relative absence of laboratory experimentation, absence of controlled studies, failure to include the various components of refraction in assessment, and lack of distinction between the different types of clinical myopia. Thus there is a bewildering array of pathogenic theories that can only be summarized here.

Germinal dysgenesis theories

It has been proposed that primary abnormal development of the mesectomally derived sclera accounts for the thinning and ectasia of the sclera that contribute to increased axial length in high myopia. However, it has also been proposed that abnormal scleral development induced by disorders of neuroectoderm accounts for this thinning and ectasia.

Heredity

No doubt heredity plays an important role in determining the ocular refraction, but there is no clear-cut mode of inheritance for myopia. The role of heredity is documented most substantively in studies of monozygotic and dizygotic twins that show that monozygotic twins are much more likely to have similar refractive errors than dizygotic twins.[18,53] As the amount of myopia increases, however, the similarity of refractive errors between monozygotic twin pairs decreases but still remains higher than one finds in dizygotic twins.[36,37] For example, both Waardenburg[60] and von Rotth[47] found 1.00 D or less difference in the refraction of more than 90% of monozygotic twins.

Genealogic studies

Several studies of the inheritance of refractive errors in families have demonstrated a significant familial prevalence of myopia, although they have not identified a single mendelian mode of inheritance. The most frequent conclusion from these investigations is that autosomal-dominant transmission of low myopia with incomplete penetrance occurs. In fact, wide variation in the degree of myopia exists within families, as reviewed by Clausen.[10] Goldschmidt[18] has concluded that it is extremely unlikely that a common genetic background for low and high myopia exists and that it is not likely that myopia is a product of a single gene. Curtin concluded, "It is clear that the etiology of myopia is based principally upon heredity. This has been amply demonstrated in twin studies. At the same time, it would appear that in the higher orders of myopia, environment has a substantial impact upon the magnitude of the refractive error."[13]

Myopia associated with systemic and ophthalmic disorders

Approximately 30 systemic disorders (such as different types of albinism, Down syndrome, the Ehlers-Danlos syndrome, and Wagner-like vitreoretinal degenerations) and 20 ocular disorders (such as tapetoretinal degenerations and keratoconus) are associated with myopia. In most of these disorders keratotomy would be inappropriate.

Myopia as a disorder of growth

Little evidence supports myopia as a manifestation of abnormal systemic growth, and its relationship to the growth of specific ocular tissues is speculative at best.

Effect of environment on myopia

Curtin observed, "The number and disarray of [environmental] theories defy the talents of the most organized minds."[13] The most common environmental theory is probably that of increased scleral stress produced by both the convergence of the extraocular muscles and the increased tone of the ciliary muscle; each occurs during the accommodative convergence associated with near work. This helps explain the classic association of the onset of myopia with schooling. However, no conclusive evidence implicates near work as a clear-cut cause for myopia. Whether environmental factors produce weakness of the posterior sclera leading to increased axial length myopia is unknown.

The vast majority of other environmental theories rest on the premise that increased intraocular pressure produces expansion of the globe.

Ocular response to visual input

Myopia can be induced by ocular occlusion during the early months of postnatal development and particularly by lid suturing in a variety of laboratory animals including monkeys. This observation illustrates the importance of the retina as an active tissue capable of influencing ocular growth. Criswell and Goss have reviewed the literature on this subject.[11] In all animals myopia is produced by an increased axial diameter of the eye, which results from an expansion of the posterior segment. These observations are somewhat supported by human clinical studies, in which eyes with visual deprivation from ptosis or corneal scarring have been found to be more myopic than normal.[29,45]

Effect of near work on myopia

The role of near work in the pathogenesis of myopia is a subject of continual debate. Researchers generally agree that near work does not play a role in the cause or progression of pathologic myopia. But numerous clinical ophthalmologists share a pervasive conviction that near work can cause myopia in certain persons. An increased prevalence of myopia is associated with an increased amount of schooling, but whether this is a cause and effect relationship is a matter of debate. A similar debate, fueled by longitudinal studies that document the progression of myopia in individuals with occupations involving intensive close work, surrounds the effect of occupation on myopia. For example, Joffe[34] compared two groups of Russian workers and found that 49% of those whose occupations involved close work were myopic, compared with only 11% of those whose occupations did not. Among the strongest evidence supporting the effect of ocular use on refraction is the comparison of the refractive state of fixing and nonfixing eyes in the same individual. For example, Lepard[38] studied 55 patients with monocular amblyopia, checking their refractions every 2 years until age 25 years. The fixing eyes of these individuals showed a 2.00 to 3.00 D shift toward myopia, whereas the fellow nonfixing eye maintained a relatively stable refraction.

Application to radial keratotomy

There is little doubt that both genetic factors and environmental factors influence the appearance and progression of myopia, but the exact mechanisms by which these forces operate are not fully understood.

The importance of the pathogenesis of myopia for keratotomy surgery lies primarily in consideration of the progression of myopia. The well-documented progression of myopia during childhood and adolescence makes consideration of surgery during this time impractical, particularly because the amount of progression for an individual cannot be predicted in advance and because there are no clear-cut environmental factors that can be manipulated to stop the progression of myopia. Since radial keratotomy is not an adjustable procedure, it is best to wait until the myopia is stable before performing the surgery. Nevertheless, a few surgeons perform radial keratotomy in teenagers.[41a]

CLASSIFICATION OF MYOPIA

Classically myopia has been divided into two groups on the basis of the refractive error—low myopia (physiologic, simple, or school myopia) and high myopia (pathologic or degenerative myopia). However, Curtin convincingly defines a third group—intermediate myopia.[13] The characteristics of these three groups are laid out in Table 1-4. Although the three groups form a continuum, there are features that allow most eyes to be placed in one of the three groups.

Simple myopia is also called physiologic myopia

Table 1-4

Curtin Classification of Myopia

	Simple	Intermediate	Pathologic
Synonyms	Physiologic School Low	Low	Degenerative Malignant High
Refractive range (D)	−0.25 to −5.00	−3.00 to −10.00	−8.00 to −30.00
Components of refraction			
Cornea	Normal	Normal	Normal to steep
Anterior chamber depth	Normal	Normal	Normal to deep
Lens	Normal	Normal	Normal to steep
Axial length (mm)	Normal (22 to 25)	Elongated (24 to 32)	Very elongated (>30)
Posterior fundus appearance	Normal	Scleral crescent Tesselated	Scleral crescent Tesselated Posterior staphyloma
Associated ocular disease	Few	Few	Chronic open-angle glaucoma Peripheral retinal degeneration Retinal detachment Macular degeneration Breaks in Bruch's membrane Chorioretinal atrophy

because all the refractive components and structural aspects of the eye are normal; there is simply an improper correlation of the refractive power of the cornea and lens, the depth of the anterior chamber, and the length of the globe, which produces myopia. Intermediate myopia is so called because it lies between the physiologic and pathologic varieties, being distinguished by the presence of a scleral crescent adjacent to the optic nerve and a tesselated (tigroid) fundus, both resulting from some elongation of the globe. Intermediate myopia was first described only in 1967,[42] and little is known about the distinctive characteristics of this group because almost no studies of myopia or myopia surgery have divided the lower myopia patients into physiologic and intermediate groups. Pathologic high myopia is characterized by a posterior staphyloma with the secondary consequences of chorioretinal degeneration. The age at onset of most physiologic and intermediate myopia is between 5 and 12 years. In general the earlier the onset is, the longer the progression continues. The vast majority of myopic eyes amenable to treatment by radial keratotomy are in the physiologic and intermediate groups, simply because radial keratotomy is capable only of correcting myopia of up to 10.00 D, with the optimal range being less

than 6.00 D. No studies have indicated a differential response of the three types of myopia to keratotomy surgery.

The pathophysiology of these three groups is probably distinctive. The eye with simple myopia is structurally normal. Intermediate myopia demonstrates definite structural changes that probably result from a prolongation of the natural growth of the sclera in the oral-equatorial region, making the axial length too long for compensation by the refractive elements of the eye. These eyes probably have an increased incidence of glaucoma and retinal detachment. Pathologic myopia results from posterior ectasia of the sclera, the cause of which is uncertain, producing not only a high refractive error, but also a much higher rate of chronic open-angle glaucoma, retinal detachment, and chorioretinal degeneration than one sees in the normal population.

There are two other small groups of myopia: (1) congenital myopia, which is present in about 6% of newborns and disappears in the early months of life, presumedly from an initial lack of correlation between the ocular refraction and the axial length, and (2) the rare adult-onset physiologic myopia that is often associated with occupations requiring near work.

CLINICAL CHARACTERISTICS OF SIMPLE AND INTERMEDIATE MYOPIA
Visual acuity

There is good correlation between the amount of myopia, as modified by the amount of astigmatism, and the uncorrected visual acuity (Fig. 1-2). For example, Hirsch[24] found a correlation coefficient of +0.95 for the log of the amount of myopia versus uncorrected visual acuity.

Spectacle correction of myopia minifies the retinal image and at higher corrections may therefore decrease visual acuity somewhat—a problem overcome by the use of contact lenses.

Motility and the accommodative convergence/accommodation ratio

Because myopes have a far point close to infinity, they develop less need for accommodative effort. For near vision there is less stimulus for accommodation despite the demand for convergence; the accommodative convergence/accommodation (AC/A) ratio decreases with an increase in uncorrected myopia.

The reduced accommodation needed in myopia results in a decreased accommodative convergence that may lead to an exophoria when accommodative effort is abandoned. On the other hand, an uncorrected myopic person with a high AC/A ratio may be affected when a spectacle correction is used; the glasses will create a demand for more accommodation, resulting in an increase in accommodative convergence with resultant esophoria or esotropia at near distances. For example, a child with −2.00 D of myopia who develops an esophoria after glasses are prescribed may be prescribed bifocals by an optometrist who is concerned about a high AC/A ratio. However, the AC/A ratio is pliable, and having the patient read with the myopic glasses worn constantly for a few days will result in the disappearance of the esophoria because the AC/A relationship returns to normal. There is little information about the pliability of the AC/A ratio in adults. Some writers think this becomes important in the presbyopic age-group where the increased accommodative demand may stimulate even more accommodative convergence and produce a frank esotropia requiring the early institution of a reading aid.[22,23] However, many older individuals develop exophoria.

These factors may become important in radial keratotomy where overcorrection will stimulate the need for more accommodation and possibly more accommodative convergence. There are no published studies of the AC/A ratio or of motility before and after radial keratotomy. Symptomatic esophoria has not been reported in patients with residual myopia or emmetropia after radial keratotomy. Maybe the AC/A ratio is pliable in the third to fifth decades of life.

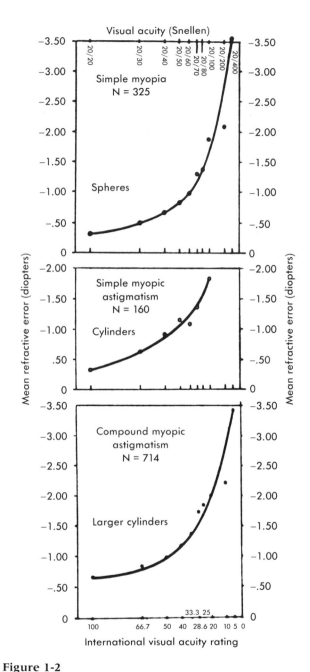

Figure 1-2
Mean visual acuities for specified refractions of three types of myopia. *N,* Number of cases. (From Crawford JS, Shagass C, and Pashby TJ: Am J Ophthalmol 1945; 28:1220.)

Intraocular pressure

Intraocular pressure is more likely to be elevated in eyes with myopia, and such eyes have an increased risk of developing chronic open-angle glaucoma, particularly after 30 years of age.[1,35] For example, Perkins and Phelps[44] found that among myopes, ocular hypertension led to visual field defects in one of three eyes, which is much more prevalent than in people with emmetropia (visual field defects in one of 20 eyes) and in people with hyperopia (visual field defects in one in 40 eyes).

Pigmentary glaucoma characteristically occurs in young male myopes.[39] Eyes with low-tension glaucoma are more likely to have myopia.

In general the ocular rigidity decreases as the amount of myopia increases, presumedly because the scleral wall is thinner and more distensible. Thus greater care must be taken in measuring the intraocular pressure in higher myopes, and applanation tonometry should be used to avoid underestimating the true intraocular pressure.

Changes in the vitreous body

Liquefaction of the vitreous with the formation of syneretic cavities, collapse of the vitreous gel, posterior detachment of the vitreous face, and increase of vitreous filaments and nodules occurs more commonly in myopic eyes.[50] This gives rise to the common complaint of vitreous floaters, which result from seeing the shadows cast on the retina by the condensed vitreous elements as they move back and forth during ocular saccades, particularly when the patient is looking at a

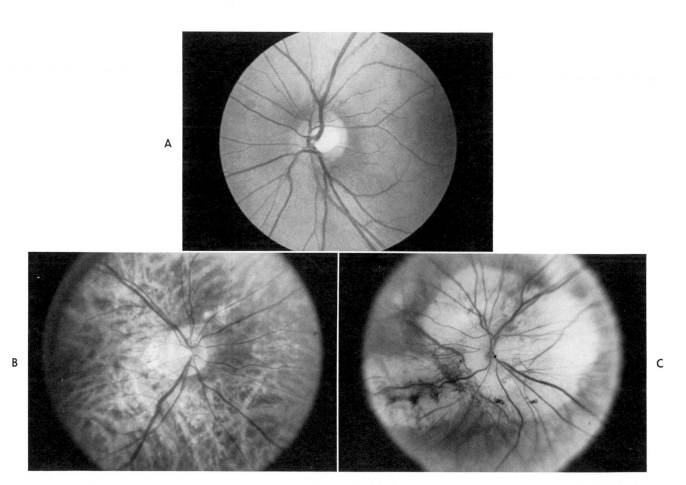

Figure 1-3
Appearance of the optic disc and posterior pole of the fundus in three types of myopia. **A,** Simple physiologic myopia shows a normal optic disc and cup/disc ratio with no peripapillary changes. **B,** Intermediate myopia shows scleral and pigment epithelial crescents adjacent to the optic disc along with a tessellated fundus. **C,** Pathologic degenerative myopia shows degeneration of the retina, retina pigment epithelium, and choloid producing the geographic atrophic areas throughout the posterior pole. (Photographs courtesy of James Gilman, CRA.)

bright background. The surgeon who performs keratotomies will be asked frequently about these phenomena and should take the time to explain them to the inquisitive patient rather than simply dismissing them as a normal phenomenon to be ignored. Patients should be warned that a marked increase in vitreous floaters associated with flashing lights should trigger an immediate ophthalmic consultation to search for a retinal detachment.

Myopic crescent

The slight retraction of the retina and the pigment epithelium from the temporal side of the optic disc forms a quarter moon–shaped crescent of choroidea, sclera, or both (Fig. 1-3). Simple myopia is not manifest as this crescent to any notable degree, but eyes with intermediate myopia have a crescent that is rarely wider than one-third the diameter of the disc. In some cases the crescent can extend nasally or form an annulus around the optic nerve.[14] In general the extent of the myopic crescent is proportionate to the amount of myopia and the elongation of the globe, but there is considerable variability in individual cases.

On the nasal side of the disc there is often an arcuate elevation or mound, sometimes with the choroidal and retinal tissues overriding the margin of the disc—a configuration called supertraction.

The myopic crescent and supertraction may result from an abnormal asymmetric growth of the temporal part of the sclera. The configuration gives rise to the illusion that the optic disc is tilted nasally, but such tilting is usually found only in eyes with the true posterior staphyloma of pathologic myopia.

Lattice retinal degeneration and retinal detachment

Myopic eyes have an increased predisposition for retinal detachment; lattice degeneration occurs in approximately one-fourth of myopic eyes,[8] retinal breaks

Table 1-5
Probability of Retinal Detachment in Eyes of Various Refractions

Refraction (D)	Probability of retinal detachment
≥ +5.00	1/63,636
0 to +4.75	1/48,913
0 to −4.75	1/6,662
−5.00 to −9.75	1/1,335
≥ −10.00	1/148

From Perkins ES: Sight Sav Rev 1979;49:11.

occur in approximately 10% of myopic eyes,[30] and retinal detachment occurs more frequently in myopic eyes than in emmetropic eyes. Half of myopic detachments occur in eyes with refraction of −4.00 D or less.[9] Perkins has observed that the probability of retinal detachment increases with the amount of myopia[43] (Table 1-5).

Thus the surgeon who performs radial keratotomy also undertakes the total eye care of the patient with myopia and is responsible for doing a complete fundus examination to detect and appropriately manage these vision-threatening disorders.

Axial length

Stenstrom has observed[55] that eyes with an axial length less than 25.5 mm displayed physiologic myopia, that in eyes with an axial length between 20.5 and 32.5 mm intermediate myopia is predominant, and that eyes with an axial length greater than 32.5 mm are more likely to have pathologic myopia. The general cutoff to distinguish eyes that are more likely to develop chorioretinal degeneration is 26 to 27 mm.

Onset and progression of physiologic and intermediate myopia

Childhood myopia usually has its insidious onset between 5 and 13 years of age, generally remaining undetected until the child complains of blurred vision in school, at which time the refraction is often −1.00 D or more. Thereafter the myopia tends to progress up to the age of 20 to 25 years, at which time it generally stabilizes. Once childhood myopia is established and becomes slightly progressive, it does not reverse direction to produce decreasing myopia.

The greatest increase in myopia occurs at the end of the first decade up to approximately 14 years of age. For example, Brown and Kronfeld[6] found that 63% of myopes between 7 and 12 years of age showed progression of myopia with the rate being greatest by 13 years of age. Other studies* support these findings (Fig. 1-4).

There is great variability of progression for individual eyes in this course. The variability depends on how much initial hyperopia was present to act as a buffer, the rate of growth of the axial length of the eye, and the rate at which a decrease in the refractive power of the cornea and the lens can compensate for increasing axial length. In general, myopia that has an earlier onset and a greater early rate of progression tends to show a greater total increase in axial length and to develop a myopic crescent characteristic of intermediate myopia. On the other hand, myopia that

*References 4, 7, 21, 25-28, 31, 42, 49, 51, 52.

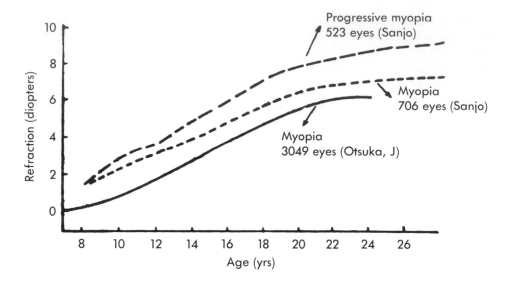

Figure 1-4
Course of myopic refraction observed in three large Japanese studies. Each plot reveals that maximal progression occurred between 14 and 18 years of age. (From Otsuka J: Acta Soc Ophthalmol Jpn 1967;71:1.)

has a later onset and a slower progression will develop less total axial elongation and probably remain in the simple, or physiologic, myopia group. Currently no clear data enable an ophthalmologist to identify eyes that have low myopia and a normal fundus in early childhood but will progress later to intermediate or pathologic types.

Brown[5,6] has calculated the rate of change of refraction in atropinized eyes from birth to age 50 years (Table 1-6) as greater than −0.10 D a year up to age 20 years—indicating a clinically meaningful amount of progression during that time, and as less than −0.05 D a year from age 21 to 51 years, indicating relative stability of refraction during this period.

Buckler's[7] study of longitudinal changes in refraction in 120 eyes demonstrated that hyperopic eyes tend to remain stable throughout life, whereas eyes that are emmetropic or myopic in childhood tend to show increasing myopia until they stabilize at about 20 years of age. However, the individual lines in Buckler's graph show some eyes that continue to become more myopic into the third and fourth decades, with the amount of myopic progression being roughly proportionate to the amount of myopia in the first and second decades of life.

Sako[48] studied the prevalence of myopia in approximately 10,000 Japanese students, observing a prevalence of 7.85% in primary schools, 24.7% in junior high schools, and 33.45% in senior high schools, with girls having 2% to 5% higher incidence of myopia than boys. This emphasizes the relationship of the progression of myopia to increasing age and educational status.

Table 1-6

Average Yearly Changes in Refraction: Atropinized Eyes

Age (yr)	Refraction change (D)
Birth to 7	+0.18*
8 to 13	−0.23
14 to 20	−0.14
21 to 33	−0.04
34 to 42	+0.03
43 to 51	−0.03

From Brown EVL: Arch Ophthalmol 1938; 19:719.
*Two thirds of those less than 8 years of age had strabismus.

No conclusive evidence associates the progression of myopia with general growth or somatic characteristics.[48]

Information on the progression and stabilization of physiologic and intermediate myopia is important to refractive surgeons because they need to identify the time of stable myopia so that radial keratotomy can be done for a known refractive error. To perform radial keratotomy on an eye with progressing myopia is ill advised because a perfect result based on the calculations will be ruined by future progression of myopia. Of course if such patients are overcorrected, future progression could work in their favors. This subject is discussed further in Chapter 12, Examination and Selection of Patients for Refractive Keratotomy.

In addition, information on the progression of and time for stabilization of physiologic and intermediate

Selected Methods Used to Correct or Reduce the Progression of Physiologic and Intermediate Myopia*[1,19]

Optical correction

Spectacle lenses
  Minus lenses to correct myopia
  Plus lenses or bifocals to reduce accommodation
  Base-in prisms to reduce convergence
Contact lenses
  Standard rigid, gas-permeable and soft minus lenses
  Orthokeratology to flatten the cornea
Undercorrection to decrease accommodation and correction

Surgical correction

Radial keratotomy
Radial and transverse keratotomy for myopic astigmatism
  Straight or arcuate transverse
  Radial or semiradial incisions

Epikeratoplasty
  Human donor
  Artificial lenticule
    Collagens
    Collagen-hydrogel copolymers
    Coated hydrogels

Keratomileusis
  Cryolathe
  Planar, nonfreeze
  In situ

Surgical correction—cont'd

Intracorneal lenses
  Hydrogels or copolymers
  High–index of refraction plastics
  Rings

Laser photorefractive keratectomy
  Laser keratomileusis (large area ablation, corneal sculpting, or reprofiling)
  Linear excision (radial, transverse)

Thermokeratoplasty
  Surface
  Intrastromal
  Hot wire laser

Lens extraction
  Clear or cataractous lens
  Low-power intraocular lens implantation
  Anterior chamber intraocular lens in phakic eye

Medications

Atropine or tropicamide to reduce accommodation
Special diets

Eye exercises and hygiene

Bates system of ocular and mental relaxation
Biofeedback neurologic training
Ocular hygiene with good posture and lighting
Decreased amount of near work

*Effectiveness varies greatly among the methods.

---

myopia is important because studies of the stability of refraction after radial keratotomy assume that the baseline refractive error is stable; changes over time are attributed to the changes in the cornea caused by the keratotomy. Interestingly most of the eyes that have 1.00 D or more of change after radial keratotomy show a continued effect of the surgery with continued flattening of the cornea and a continued decrease in the minus power of the refraction (sometimes called progressive hyperopia). This is the opposite direction of the natural progression of the underlying myopia, so the continued effect of radial keratotomy may be underestimated (see Chapter 24, Stability of Refraction After Refractive Keratotomy).

MANAGEMENT OF PHYSIOLOGIC AND INTERMEDIATE MYOPIA

The myriad methods of managing myopia have been reviewed thoroughly by Goss[19]; their detailed discussion is beyond the scope of this textbook. The development of refractive surgical correction of myopia is reviewed in Section II. The box above lists some of the methods used to correct or reduce the progression of myopia, without evaluative comments.

PATHOLOGIC MYOPIA

Because pathologic myopia is not treated by keratotomy, it is not discussed here. The interested reader can consult Curtin's textbook.[13]

UNFINISHED BUSINESS

For any disease entity the fundamental quest is for the cause, on which basis prevention can be designed. The cause of myopia, both simple and pathologic, is unknown, not because of a lack of research efforts, but because the mechanisms remain elusive. Publications on the pathophysiology of myopia fill volumes. Organizations such as the Myopia International Research Foundation, Inc. foster both laboratory and clinical research. Numerous theories have been propounded. Some remain possible, some tenable, and others have been discarded. Among the latest and most intriguing observations is that of David H. Huble, M.D., and Torsten N. Wiesel, M.D., who observed serendipitously while studying the pathogenesis of amblyopia that an eye deprived of vision from birth begins to elongate and become myopic. The basic mechanism for this observation also remains elusive, but it raises the intriguing relationship between nervous tissues and connective tissues. Certainly, large scale, long-term, carefully designed, and adequately funded clinical trials are an essential part of research on myopia, and such trials have been sorely lacking. This certainly seems inappropriate, given the expense and morbidity that myopia creates for the human population.

REFERENCES

1. Abdulla MC and Hamdi M: Applanation ocular tension in myopia and emmetropia, Br J Ophthalmol 1970;54:122.
2. Baldwin WR: A serial study of refractive status in youth, Am J Optom 1957;34:486.
3. Betsch A: Ueber die menschliche Refraktionskurve, Klin Monatsbl Augenheilkd 1929;82:365-379.
4. Blegvad O: Ueber die Progression der Myopie, Klin Monatsbl Augenheilkd 1918;60:155.
5. Brown EVL: Net average yearly changes in refraction in atropinized eyes from birth to beyond middle life, Arch Ophthalmol 1938;19:719-734.
6. Brown EVL and Kronfeld PC: The refraction curve in the US with special reference to the first two decades, Council on Ophthalmology, vol 1, Amsterdam, 1930, F van Rossen.
7. Bucklers M: Changes in refraction during life, Br J Ophthalmol 1953;37:587.
8. Byer NE: Clinical study of lattice degeneration of the retina, Trans Am Acad Ophthalmol Otolaryngol 1965;69:1065-1081.
9. Cambiaggi A: Myopia and retinal detachment, Am J Ophthalmol 1964;58:642-650.
10. Clausen W: Refraktionen des Auges, In Gutt A, editor: Handbuch der Erbkrankheiten, Leipzig, 1938, Thieme.
11. Criswell MH and Goss DA: Myopia development in non-human primates—a literature review, Am J Optom Physiol Optics 1983;60:250-268.
12. Curtin BJ: The pathogenesis of congenital myopia, Arch Ophthalmol 1963;6:166-173.
13. Curtin BJ: The myopias: basic science and clinical management, Philadelphia, 1985, Harper & Row Publishers, Inc.
14. Curtin BJ and Karlin DB: Axial length measurements and fundus changes of the myopic eye, Am J Ophthalmol 1971;71:42-53.
15. Department of International, Economic, and Social Affairs, United Nations: Global estimates and projections of populations by age and sex, 1984.
16. Duke-Elder S and Abrams D: System of ophthalmology. Vol 5. Ophthalmic optics and refraction, St Louis, 1970, The CV Mosby Co.
17. Dzen TT: Refraction in Peking, Natl Med J China 1921;7:206.
17a. Fyodorov SN: Personal communication, March 22, 1988.
18. Goldschmidt E: On the etiology of myopia, Copenhagen, 1968, Munksgaard.
19. Goss DA: Attempts to reduce the rate of increase of myopia in young people—a critical literature review, Am J Optom Physiol Optics 1982;59:828-841.
20. Graham MV and Gray OP: Refraction of premature babies' eyes, Br Med J 1963;12:1453.
21. Hayden R: Development and prevention of myopia at the United States Naval Academy, Arch Ophthalmol 1941;25:539-547.
22. Hermann J: The accommodative requirement of myopia and hyperopia: contact lenses versus spectacles, Int Ophthalmol Clin 1971;11:217.
23. Hermann J and Johnson R: The accommodation requirement in myopia: a comparison of contact lenses and spectacles, Arch Ophthalmol 1966;76:47.
24. Hirsch MJ: Relation of visual acuity to myopia, Arch Ophthalmol 1945;34:418-421.
25. Hirsch MJ: The longitudinal study of refraction, Am J Optom 1964;41:137-141.
26. Hirsch MJ: Predictability of refraction at age 14 on the basis of testing at age 6: interim report from the Ojai longitudinal study of refraction, Am J Optom 1964;41:567-573.
27. Hirsch MJ and Weymouth F: A longitudinal study of refractive state of children during the first six years of school, Am J Optom 1961;38:564-571.
28. Hofstetter HW: Some interrelationships of age, refraction and rate of refractive change, Am J Optom 1954;31:161.

29. Hoyt CS and Billson FA: Monocular axial myopia associated with neonatal eyelid closure in human infants, Am J Ophthalmol 1981;91:197-200.

30. Hyams SW and Neumann E: Peripheral retina in myopia with reference to retinal breaks, Br J Ophthalmol 1969; 53:300-306.

31. Hynes EA: Refractive changes in normal young men, Arch Ophthalmol 1956;56:761-767.

32. Jackson E: Changes in refraction with age, Am J Ophthalmol 1920;3:228.

33. Jackson E: Norms of refraction, JAMA 1932;98:132-137.

34. Joffe TM: Myopic workers, Ophthalmol Bull 1949;28:18.

35. Kamali K and Hamdi M: Relation between applanation tonometry and errors of refraction, Ain Shams Med J 1969;20:235.

36. Karlsson JI: Concordance rates for myopia in twins, Clin Genet 1974;6:142-146.

37. Karlsson JI: Genetic factors in myopia, Acta Genet Med 1974;23:45.

38. Lepard CW: Comparative changes in the error of refraction between fixing and amblyopic eyes during growth and development, Am J Ophthalmol 1975;80:485-490.

39. Lichter PR and Shaffer RN: Iris processes and glaucoma, Am J Ophthalmol 1970;70:905-911.

40. Morgan RW and Munro M: Refractive problems in northern natives, Can J Ophthalmol 1973;8:226-228.

41. Newcomb JR: Refraction methods employed in the Department of Ophthalmology of the Attending Surgeon's Office, US Army, Washington, DC, Am J Ophthalmol 1919;2:326.

41a. Odell LW and Wyzinski P: Radial keratotomy in teenagers, Refractive Corneal Surg 1989;5:315.

42. Otsuka J: Research on the etiology and treatment of myopia, Acta Soc Ophthalmol Jpn: 1967;71(suppl):1-212.

43. Perkins ES: Morbidity from myopia, Sight Sav Rev 1979;49:11-19.

44. Perkins ES and Phelps CD: Open angle glaucoma, ocular hypertension, low-tension glaucoma and refraction, Arch Ophthalmol 1982;100:1464-1467.

45. Rabin J, Van Sluyters RC, and Malach R: Emmetropization: a vision-dependent phenomenon, Invest Ophthalmol Vis Sci 1981;20:561-564.

46. Rasmussen OD: Incidence of myopia in China, Br J Ophthalmol 1936; 20:350-360.

47. von Rotth A: Ueber Augenhefund von Zwillingen, Klin Monatsbl Augenheilkd 1937;98:636.

48. Sato H: Studies of school myopia, Ganko Rinsho Iho 1973;62:123.

49. Sato T: The causes and prevention of acquired myopia, Tokyo, 1957, Kanehara Shuppan.

50. Singh A, Paul SD, and Singh K: A clinical study of the vitreous body (in emmetropia and refractive errors), Orient Arch Ophthalmol 1970;8:11.

51. Smith P: Introduction to a discussion on the diagnosis, prognosis and treatment of pernicious myopia, Ophthalmic Rev 1901;20:331.

52. Sorsby A: Normal refraction in infants and its bearing on development of myopia, London Co Council Rep 1933; 4:55.

53. Sorsby A, Sheridan M, and Leary GA: Refraction and its components in twins, Special Report Series No 303, Medical Research Council, London, 1962, Her Majesty's Stationery Office.

54. Sperduto RD, Seigel D, Roberts J, et al: Prevalence of myopia in the United States, Arch Ophthalmol 1983;101: 405-407.

55. Stenstrom S: Untersuchungen uber die Variation und Kovariation der optischen Elemente des menschlichen Auges, 1946, Am J Optom 1948;25:218 (Translated by D Woolf).

56. Takahashi T: Study of the preventive medicine for myopia, Natl Hyg 1939; 16:66.

57. Tasman IS: Frequency of the various kinds of refractive errors, Am J Ophthalmol 1932;15:1044.

58. US Department Commerce, Bureau of Census: Statistical abstract of the United States, 1988.

59. van Alphen GWHM: On emmetropia and ametropia, New York, 1961, S Carter.

60. Waardenburg PJ: Refraktion und Zwillingsforschung, Klin Monatsbl Augenheilkd 1930;84:593-637.

Corneal Anatomy and Physiology as Applied to Refractive Keratotomy

George O. Waring III

Refractive keratotomy works by altering corneal anatomy to create a new shape—flatter in the center and steeper in the periphery. The incisions sever a graded amount of corneal stroma, allowing the biomechanical forces to produce a gaping of the incisions and repositioning of the uncut corneal tissues. Wound healing holds this new corneal contour, but the wounds are not as strong as the original uncut cornea. If this surgery were carried out on a homogeneous material of known physical properties, such as steel or plastic, the surgeon could accurately predict the surgical outcome. However, the cornea has a nonhomogeneous structure that undergoes not only acute changes in shape immediately after it is incised, but also slower changes in shape because of its viscoelastic properties and the process of wound healing. These complex elements make it difficult to predict the result of refractive keratotomy accurately.

I present here a working concept of the cornea that integrates corneal structure and function and forms a basis for understanding the changes induced by refractive keratotomy. The concept is neither a superficial survey for the beginning ophthalmology student nor a reference source chock-full of quantitative details; each of these is available elsewhere.[39] Rather its purpose is to present a concise qualitative picture of the structure and function of the cornea as it applies to refractive keratotomy. A description of corneal wound healing is presented in Chapter 20, Corneal Wound Healing and Its Pharmacologic Modification after Refractive Keratotomy.

FUNCTIONS OF THE CORNEA

The cornea protects the intraocular contents and refracts light. To accomplish these functions the cornea must maintain its strength and transparency, which is

BACKGROUND AND ACKNOWLEDGMENTS
This chapter is modified from material I have presented elsewhere.[34a,43a] The histology and electron micrographs were provided by Yves Pouliquen, director of ophthalmology at Hotel Dieu Hospital in Paris. The content is drawn from the cited references.

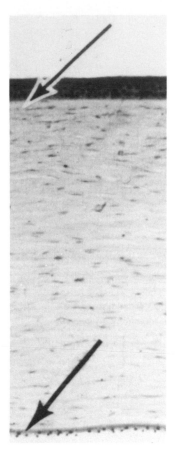

Figure 2-1

Human cornea consists of normal epithelium *(top)*, Bowman's layer *(top arrow)*, stroma *(middle)*, Descemet's membrane *(lower arrow)*, and endothelium *(bottom)*. (H & E; ×80.) (From Rodrigues MM, Waring GO, Hackett J, and Donohoo P: Cornea. In Duane TD and Jaeger EA, editors: Biomedical foundations of ophthalmology, vol 1, Hagerstown, Md, 1982, Harper & Row Publishers, Inc.)

no easy task for an avascular connective tissue. The cornea is 550 μm thick centrally and 700 μm thick peripherally and has a 12 mm diameter horizontally and a 11 mm diameter vertically. For comparison a credit card is about 800 μm thick; a dime is 13 mm in diameter. (See Chapter 15, Surgical Instruments Used in Refractive Keratotomy, for a discussion of corneal thickness.)

The cornea must be strong. Contrary to the layperson's concept that the eyeball is a delicate structure, the corneoscleral connective tissue shell can withstand considerable blunt force (approximately 5 kg/cm^2) before rupturing and can resist lacerating insults, both accidental and surgical.[22] The major structural component of the cornea is the collagenous connective tissue stroma, which is confluent with the sclera at the limbus. The incisions made during refractive keratotomy weaken this structure.

The corneal surface must remain smooth. The tear-air interface forms the first and most powerful refracting surface of the eye, accounting for approximately 48.00 of the 60.00 D (80%) of the eye's total refractive power. Thus the corneal surface must remain smooth and the eyelids must spread the tears uniformly over the epithelium, since the slightest distortion degrades the geometric image received by the retina. The scars resulting from refractive keratotomy create small permanent surface irregularities (irregular astigmatism) that can be seen as slight distortion of the rings on keratographs and are manifest as the stellate epithelial iron line.[30,32] Fortunately these irregularities are outside the central cornea and seem to interfere little with functional visual acuity.

The cornea must remain transparent. It is remarkable that this epithelium-lined connective tissue has a specialized structure and function that maintains functional optical clarity. Any opacity of the cornea, such as the scars from keratotomy wounds, scatters light, both degrading the geometric image and decreasing contrast sensitivity.

One can consider the cornea fancifully as a sandwich dipped in nutritious soup. Two surface layers, the epithelium and the endothelium, contain a central filling, the stroma. All three layers receive nourishment and oxygen from the tears, aqueous humor, and limbic vessels. More precisely the structure of the cornea fits that of many other tissues. The surface epithelium and endothelium rest on basement membranes (the epithelial basement membrane and Descemet's membrane) that lie in turn on a layer of connective tissue (the stroma).[38]

Translating this basic structure into histologic terms (Fig. 2-1), the five-layered stratified squamous epithelium maintains a smooth optical surface and blocks the penetration of water and solutes from the tears into the stroma. In the stroma, proteoglycan molecules hold collagen fibrils in orderly lamellar array to maintain structural strength and optical clarity. To accomplish this the proteoglycans must remain relatively dehydrated. The single layer of endothelium performs this dehydrating function by partially blocking the flow of aqueous humor into the stroma and continuously removing water from the stroma. To nourish the cornea, the tear film conveys oxygen and the aqueous humor provides amino acids, carbohydrates, and lipids.

CORNEAL EPITHELIUM
Functions of the epithelium

The corneal epithelium has the following three major functions[42,47]:
1. Formation of a mechanical barrier to foreign material and microorganisms
2. Creation of a smooth, transparent optical surface to which the tear film can adhere
3. Maintenance of a barrier to the diffusion of water, solutes, and drugs

At the time of keratotomy surgery each of these functions is disrupted. Foreign material can enter the wound, and microorganisms may produce infection.

In addition, the corneal surface and air–tear film interface become irregular and produce the symptoms of glare and blurry vision in the postoperative period. Finally the tears pass readily into the corneal stroma and swell the area adjacent to the incisions with the associated, but transient, excess steepening of the paracentral and peripheral cornea and excess flattening of the central cornea.

Structure of the epithelium

The corneal epithelium is a five- to seven-layer (30 to 50 μm thick) stratified squamous epithelium that is organized in a more orderly fashion than similar epithelia elsewhere in the body—a prerequisite for the formation of a smooth, transparent optical surface (Fig. 2-2).

The epithelium contains three morphologic types of cells—a single layer of columnar basal cells, two layers of wing-shaped polygonal cells, and approximately three layers of superficial, flat squamous cells. It also contains four other types of cells—neurons, melanocytes, modified macrophages called Langerhans' cells that may play a role in the initial processing of antigens, and occasional leukocytes.[34]

The corneal epithelial cells contain organelles, the endoplasmic reticulum and the Golgi apparatus, designed primarily for protein synthesis. Because the epithelium turns over about once a week, there must be high production of structural molecules for this purpose. Mitochondria are sparse, indicating that energy-requiring metabolic processes are less important than production of structural molecules. The large amount of filamentous material in the cytoplasm plays a role in the epithelium's organized structure (cytoskeleton), its attachment functions (tonofilaments), and its role in migration during wound healing (actin filaments).[18]

Epithelial–tear film interaction

The plasma membrane of the epithelial cell is a typical unit membrane that consists of a lipid bilayer containing protein macromolecules. This lipid surface is hydrophobic; as a result the aqueous tear film, left to its own devices, would bead up on the corneal surface like raindrops on a newly waxed car. However, the goblet cells in the conjunctiva and other epithelial cells produce mucin that spreads directly over the epithelial surface and decreases surface tension so that the aqueous component of the tears can spread over and adhere to the epithelial surface and maintain an intact tear film for 20 to 30 seconds between blinks.[20,24,25,31,36] Abnormalities of the mucin layer or the epithelial surface cause the tear film to break up into dry spots rapidly after the resurfacing effect of a blink. This phenomenon can be seen during the early healing of keratotomy wounds when there is some edema and irregularity of the epithelial surface and fluorescein-stained tears flow off the top of the small ridge of the incision. As the surface remodels, this phenomenon disappears and the tears can produce an intact layer over the corneal surface.

Since the preocular tear film is hypertonic to corneal stroma, it has a normal function of osmotically drawing some water out of the stroma. During waking hours the normal evaporation of the tears raises the osmolarity, so more water is drawn out of the cornea; but during sleep when the closed eyelids decrease evaporation, the osmolarity of the tears falls and less fluid is removed from the stroma. This nocturnal stromal swelling is generally not noticed by individuals with normal corneas but can produce persistent stromal edema for a few hours after waking in patients with compromised endothelial function, such as that in Fuchs' endothelial dystrophy and pseudophakic corneal edema. This swelling may be one cause for the diurnal fluctuation in refraction and acuity experienced by some patients after refractive keratotomy. Both the persistent epithelial

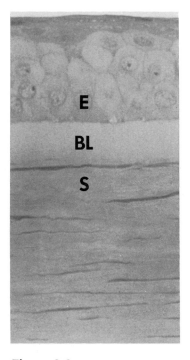

Figure 2-2
Normal anterior human cornea showing five– to six–cell thick epithelium *(E)* with its basal, polygonal, squamous cells; acellular Bowman's layer *(BL);* and anterior stroma *(S).* (Courtesy Yves Pouliquen, MD.)

plug in the wound and the decreased tensile strength of the scar may allow an increased amount of nocturnal stromal swelling in the area of the incision, producing transient flattening of the central cornea. Topical hypertonic agents may decrease corneal edema after refractive keratotomy.

Epithelial squamous cells

The superficial squamous cells have three unique features important in corneal function—adsorption of the tear film, maintenance of a barrier to the flow of water and solutes into the stroma, and provision of a first line of defense against microorganisms.

Spread over the surface of the epithelium is a layer of glycoprotein. This protein-sugar complex probably has two constituents—mucin from the tear film that decreases surface tension and glycolipids and glycoproteins in the plasma membrane that send out branching arms of polymerized sugars over the cell surface and that play a role in the adhesive properties of the cell during wound healing and desquamation. Disruption of these surface molecules may allow increased adherence of microorganisms, especially when associated with gross or surface irregularities. This could be one reason for the occurrence of late, nontraumatic corneal infections in the area of keratotomy scars.[19,37]

The surface of the squamous cells is not itself smooth but contains myriad projections in the form of fingerlike microvilli and ridgelike microplicae. These projections create a corrugated surface that may help stabilize the tear film, increase absorption of metabolites, and increase the amount of plasma membrane available for elongation during migration.

In addition to the usual desmosomal (macula adherens) intercellular junctions, the superficial squamous cells are zippered together by zonulae occludentes—tight junctions—that encircle the cells and adhere the two adjacent plasma membranes. The zonulae occludentes create a formidable barrier that minimizes the flow of fluid, electrolytes, and metabolites from the tears into the stroma and that blocks the penetration of microorganisms except those that can directly parasitize the epithelium, such as herpes simplex virus and *Neisseria gonorrhoeae*. This blockade also prevents the flow of nutrients that might be present in the tear film, so the cornea must obtain most of its nutrition from the aqueous humor. Oxygen, however, can diffuse across this barrier easily, and the tear film is the major source of oxygen for the cornea. The superficial squamous epithelial cells are not a mere passive barrier, since they also contain an active chloride pump that plays a small role in corneal hydration.

The stratified squamous epithelium normally does not produce a surface layer of keratin, but the cells do contain corneal keratins and can produce surface keratin under stress such as vitamin A deficiency.

Polygonal wing cells

Multisided wing cells interdigitate with each other, their plasma membranes meshing like pieces of a jigsaw puzzle. They adhere with large numbers of desmosomal attachments in which cytoplasmic tonofilaments converge on a focal thickened plaque in the plasma membrane, extend across the intercellular space where an additional adhesive substance is present, and attach to the adjacent cell (Fig. 2-3). It is the interdigitation and these desmosomes that produce the tenacious adhesions that allow the epithelium to be distended in bullae or to come off in sheets without disintegrating into individual cells.

It is probably the wing cells that constitute the majority of the epithelial plug in keratotomy incisions (Fig. 2-4).

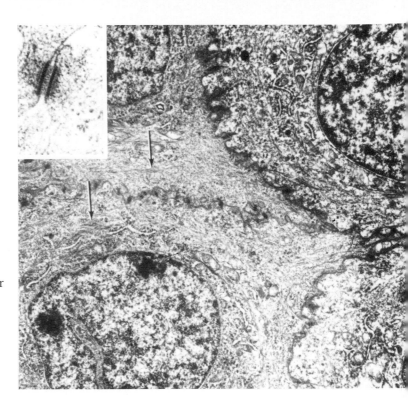

Figure 2-3
Polygonal wing cells of the epithelium exhibit prominent interdigitations and desmosomes. The cytoplasm contains numerous tonofilaments *(arrows)*, rough endoplasmic reticulum, scattered mitochondria, and ribosomes. (×13,000.) Inset shows desmosomal connection between wing cells. (×49,500.) (From Rodrigues MM, Waring GO, Hackett J, and Donohoo P: Cornea. In Duane TD and Jaeger EA, editors: Biomedical foundations of ophthalmology, vol 1, Hagerstown, Md, 1982, Harper & Row Publishers, Inc.)

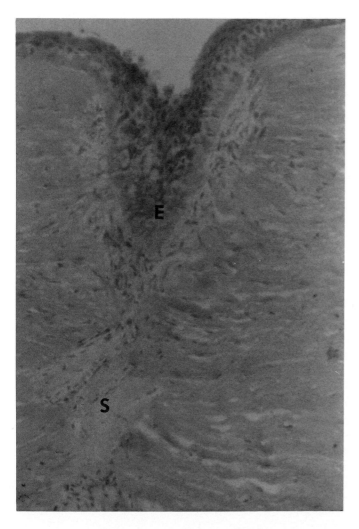

Figure 2-4
Partially healed keratotomy wound shows epithelial plug *(E)* and stromal scarring *(S)* (Mason's trichrome). (Courtesy Yves Pouliquen, MD.)

Basal epithelial cells

Columnar basal cells line up in single file along the basement membrane. Their plasma membranes interdigitate less, and they have fewer desmosomal attachments than wing cells. These cells are responsible for secreting the epithelial basement membrane and forming the hemidesmosomes and attachment complexes. They are also the cells that undergo mitosis and differentiate to form the polygonal and squamous cells.

The basal cells accumulate iron in disorders that produce depressions in the corneal surface. This iron forms the stellate iron line seen in the vast majority of cases after radial keratotomy.[40] Melanocytes are also present within the epithelium, and in pigmented races these melanocytes can sometimes be seen streaming in from the limbus toward the keratotomy incisions (striate melanosis) along with epithelial cells that also contain melanin.

Epithelial basement membrane and attachment complexes

The epithelial cells remain adherent to the cornea through a complex series of attachments that, if abnormal, can lead to recurrent epithelial erosions sometimes associated with epithelial–basement membrane dystrophy. The linkage of molecules and tissues includes the following:

1. Intracytoplasmic microfilaments such as actin
2. An intracytoplasmic glycoprotein, vinculin
3. A transmembrane glycoprotein, integrin
4. Extracellular surface glycoproteins, including fibronectin[28]
5. The hemidesmosome modification of the plasma membrane with its transmembrane microfilaments
6. The epithelial basement membrane comprising its dense layer and its clear layer, to which fibronectin and similar molecules attach and through which the hemidesmosomal microfilaments penetrate
7. Anchoring fibrils and plaques within Bowman's layer (Fig. 2-5)[14]

After a keratotomy incision the epithelium migrates into the incision and fills it with an epithelial plug. Because the epithelium remains present within the incision for months to years, a basement membrane, complete with the hemidesmosomal attachment, is laid down along the wall of the incision. In general the attachment of the epithelium after refractive keratotomy seems normal, and reports of postoperative recurrent erosion are rare.[9]

When the basement membrane becomes abnormally thick and multilayered or grows within the epithelium, it produces the clinical appearance of maps and fingerprints. These have been described in the majority of eyes at one Prospective Evaluation of Radial Keratotomy (PERK) clinical center with changing patterns and gradual decreased prominence over the few months after surgery.[29]

Metabolism of the corneal epithelium

One can conceptualize corneal (and epithelial) metabolism by remembering that the cornea breathes oxygen from the tears and eats nutrients from the aqueous humor.[12] Atmospheric oxygen dissolves in the tear film and diffuses into the cornea across the epithelium. Under normal waking conditions more than enough oxygen is available. The epithelium requires a minimum of 7 to 15 mm Hg partial pressure of oxygen in tears to remain clear, and with the eyes open the partial pressure of oxygen dissolved in tears is about 155 mm Hg. With the eyes closed, oxygen diffuses into the tears from the conjunctival capillaries and still provides an environment of 55 mm Hg partial pressure of oxygen. This oxygen must diffuse across the epithelium, through the stroma, and to the endothelium, even though there is a contribution of oxygen to the posterior cornea from the iris and ciliary body capillaries by way of the aqueous humor.[7,27,35]

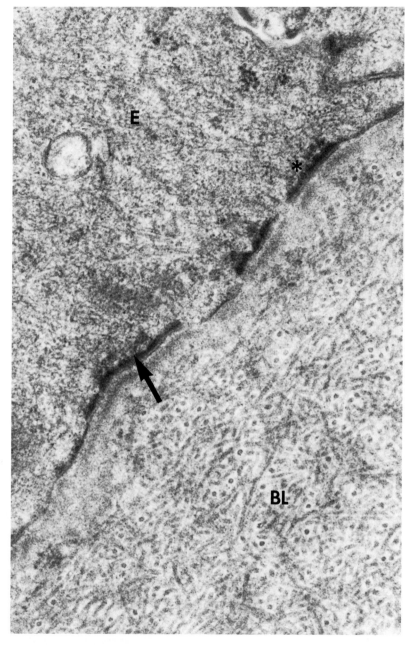

Figure 2-5
Basal epithelial cell cytoplasm *(E)* is packed with microfilaments—some connected to hemidesmosomes *(*)*. Epithelial basement membrane consists of lamina lucida and lamina densa *(arrow)*. Bowman's layer *(BL)*. (×61,500.) (Courtesy Yves Pouliquen, MD.)

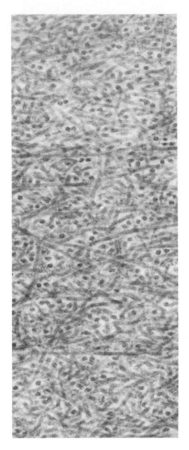

Figure 2-6
The acellular Bowman's layer consists of a feltlike interweaving of short collagen fibrils. (×49,200.) (Courtesy Yves Pouliquen, MD.)

The epithelium uses glucose as a primary source of energy and amino acids as structural building blocks, both of which diffuse from the aqueous humor across the endothelium and stroma. The aqueous origin of the nutrients can be demonstrated clinically by inserting an impermeable membrane, such as a polysulfone intracorneal lens, into the stroma. An impermeable membrane blocks the flow of water and nutrients, gradually causing the epithelium to lose its glycogen stores, slough, and produce an aseptic, necrotic corneal thinning and ulceration. This process can be prevented by drilling holes in the membrane or by using permeable hydrophilic materials that allow passage of nutrients.[5,6]

Under conditions of hypoxia and mild trauma, such as those caused by poorly fitted contact lenses, epithelial glycogen supplies decrease and anaerobic metabolism commences, producing lactic acid that can diffuse into the stroma, raise its osmolality, and have a toxic effect on the endothelium with resulting stromal edema.

Minimal metabolic stress seems to be exerted on the epithelium after refractive keratotomy, and persistent epithelial edema and defects rarely occur.

BOWMAN'S LAYER

Bowman's layer is a compact feltwork of fine, randomly oriented collagen fibrils that lies between the epithelial basement membrane and the cellular stroma (Fig. 2-6). This acellular, 12 μm thick tissue probably helps maintain corneal shape, although the details of its biomechanical properties and its function are unknown. It is not elastic; its poor distensibility is one reason that stromal edema causes the cornea to protrude toward the anterior chamber, creating folds in Descemet's membrane, whereas the anterior cornea maintains its generally normal curvature.

Because Bowman's layer is acellular, it cannot regenerate. In every case of keratotomy, Bowman's layer is permanently cut and does not heal (Fig. 2-7). The cut ends of Bowman's layer assume a variety of configurations—end-to-end approximation, overlapping, and bending down into the incision. The space between the cut ends of Bowman's layer fills with cellular scar tissue that creates a permanent opacity.

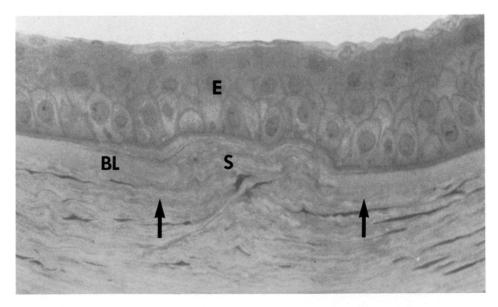

Figure 2-7
In keratotomy the epithelium *(E)* is intact over a break *(between arrows)* in Bowman's layer *(BL)* that is filled by scar tissue *(S)*. (Courtesy Yves Pouliquen, MD.)

CELLULAR CORNEAL STROMA
Structural components of the stroma

Keratocytes (also called corneal stromacytes or fibrocytes) synthesize the extracellular matrix of the stroma. The collagen fibrils are of relatively uniform diameter and are stacked in orderly sheets that form approximately 200 lamellae (Fig. 2-8). Proteoglycans, which have a protein core with glycosaminoglycan side chains, are the molecules that hold the collagen fibrils in an orderly array and contain the water within the stroma.

Cells in the corneal stroma

The predominant cell in the corneal stroma is the keratocyte, a flat cell that lies sandwiched between the collagen lamellae and extends five to seven cell processes out to adjacent keratocytes. Keratocytes are more concentrated within the stroma than commonly thought, as shown by recent tandem scanning microscope and cell marker studies.

The structure of keratocytes resembles that of fibrocytes. Keratocytes have a large nucleus, cytoplasm containing fine filaments, less rough endoplasmic reticulum than an ordinary fibroblast, and few lysosomes. Under stress such as refractive keratotomy the keratocytes probably convert into fibroblasts in the area around the corneal wound, become phagocytic, and secrete the new extracellular matrix that ultimately constitutes the linear scar.

Other cellular components in the stroma include the phagocytic histiocytes that become activated around keratotomy incisions to help clean up and remodel the wound. Polymorphonuclear leukocytes, plasma cells, and lymphocytes also appear in the normal stroma and become much more concentrated around the area of incisions during the early phases of wound healing.

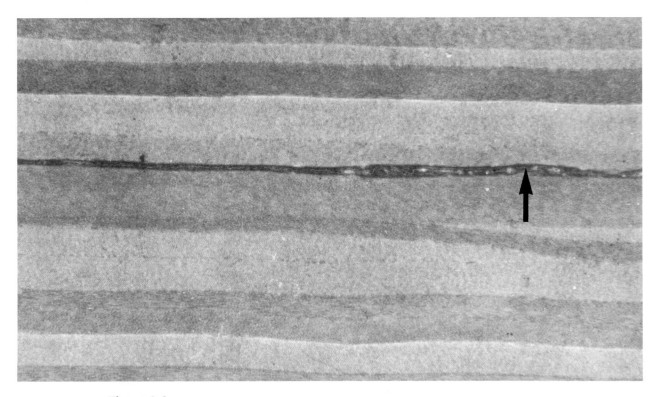

Figure 2-8
A keratocyte *(arrow)* is sandwiched between lamellae within the corneal stroma.
(Courtesy Yves Pouliquen, MD.)

Neurons traverse the stroma from the limbus to terminate as free nerve endings in the epithelium. Their general course is radial, and thus four or eight incisions of radial keratotomy sever only a few of the nerves so that corneal sensation is decreased only minimally. Transverse keratotomy, however, severs the nerves extending across the arc length of the incision, decreasing corneal sensation central to the incision for months to years after surgery. Neurotrophic signs and symptoms have not been described after properly performed refractive keratotomy.

Collagen in the stroma

In terms of refractive keratotomy the most important material in the cornea is the stromal collagen because the collagen fibrils, including Bowman's layer, provide the structural strength and dimensional stability of the cornea. The collagen fibrils apparently extend from limbus to limbus, forming an orderly array with the fibrils of one lamella running in a different direction from those of the adjacent lamellae. In the anterior stroma the lamellae are not as discrete because bundles of fibrils interdigitate from one lamella to another. In the midstroma, the interdigitation becomes less prominent. In the posterior stroma, the lamellae are extremely organized and discrete (Fig. 2-9). This can be observed with the slitlamp microscope; the anterior third of the stroma in humans has a slightly grayer appearance than the posterior two thirds because of more light scattering.

The orientation of the lamellae in the peripheral and limbal cornea was the object of study by several investigators in the earlier part of this century.[1,10,17] Maurice[21] has observed that the methods of studying lamellar structure 50 years ago were rather primitive, and he is not convinced that the identification of a peripheral "ligament" of the cornea is valid either statistically or in terms of its mechanical interpretation.* He notes that there is no biomechanical necessity for the fibrils to exist in a circular pattern at the limbus to maintain the curvature or outline of the cornea. Histologic studies have demonstrated fibrils running circumferentially near the limbus and into the sclera. This configuration may account in part for the thickening of the cornea near the limbus. The fibrils are more likely to extend from one point to another on the limbus, rather than as a circumferential band.

The individual collagen fibrils have a structure similar to collagen fibrils elsewhere in the body.[16] They consist of units of tropocollagen, each containing three protein chains wound together in a helical pattern. The tropocollagen units are assembled into microfibrils that are crosslinked to form the collagen fibrils. The staggered arrangements of the tropocollagen units create the characteristic 64 nm banded pattern seen by transmission electron microscopy. The collagen fibrils are 22 to 32 nm in diameter, with a uniform diameter in the center of the cornea but varying in size near the limbus (Figs. 2-10 and 2-11). The human corneal stroma contains different types of collagen, each distinguished according to the biochemical composition of the three protein chains.[11] The predominant collagen is type I, which is the type present most commonly in connective tissues such as tendons and the dermis of the skin. There is some type III collagen, which becomes much more prominent during wound healing and is present characteristically in tissues that support epithelia. Some type IV collagen, which is characteristic of basement membranes, is present in the stroma. Type VII collagen constitutes the anchoring fibrils of the epithelium.[14]

*References 1,10,11,17,22,32,33.

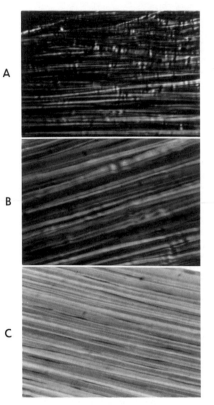

Figure 2-9
Light micrograph uses polarized light and birefringence illumination to demonstrate the lamellar patterns in the corneal stroma. **A,** Anterior stroma shows interdigitating lamellae. **B,** Middle stroma shows more regular lamellar pattern with some interweaving of lamellae. **C,** Posterior stroma shows extremely regular lamellar pattern. (Courtesy Yves Pouliquen, MD.)

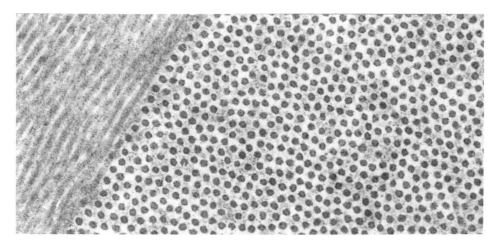

Figure 2-10
In corneal stroma collagen fibrils have a regular arrangement in both cross section and longitudinal section. (Courtesy Yves Pouliquen, MD.)

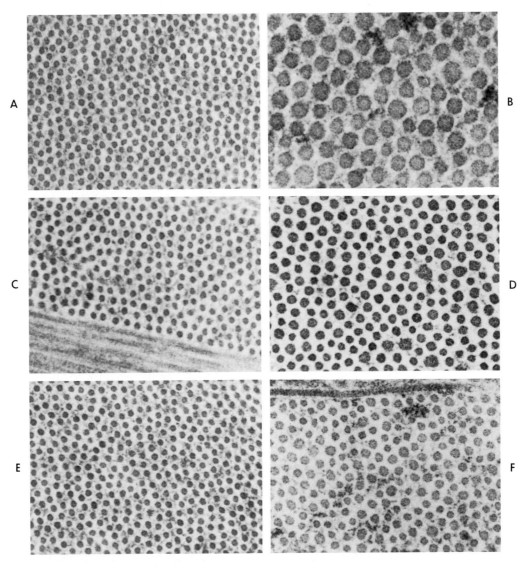

Figure 2-11
Transmission electron micrographs of corneal stroma compare the regular structure of the central corneal fibrils *(left)* to the more variable structure of the peripheral fibrils *(right)*. **A** and **B,** Anterior area of stroma. **C** and **D,** Middle area of stroma. **E** and **F,** Posterior area of stroma. (Courtesy Yves Pouliquen, MD.)

Proteoglycans in the stroma

Unlike other connective tissues, the cornea must remain transparent. Transparency results from the regular architecture of the cornea, which allows light to pass through with minimal disruption. The molecules responsible for maintaining the uniform spacing of the collagen fibrils are the proteoglycans, also referred to as acid mucopolysaccharides. These molecules constitute the central protein core from which glycosaminoglycans extend like bristles from a hairbrush. The glycosaminoglycan molecules are sugars in which repeating disaccharide units form longer polymer chains. These molecules lie between the collagen fibrils and link to the collagen fibrils, holding them apart by a fixed distance of approximately 30 to 60 nm. The exact mechanism by which they accomplish this spacing is unknown, but the glycosaminoglycans are negatively charged, and the repulsive forces within the molecules may be responsible for maintaining this regular structure.

Two glycosaminoglycans are present in the normal human stroma: keratan sulfate, which contains both galactose and glucosamine, and dermatan sulfate (also called chondroitin sulfate B), which contains both galactosamine and glucuronate. These two proteoglycans are attached to different protein cores.

The glycosaminoglycans play an important role in stromal hydration. The normal corneal stroma is approximately 78% water by weight. If more water enters the stroma, as in endothelial dysfunction, the glycosaminoglycan molecules take up the water and swell, increasing corneal thickness. The swelling displaces the collagen fibrils, disrupting their regular alignment so that light is scattered and the stroma appears opaque.

Glycoproteins are also present in the corneal stroma and may aid in communication between cells. Some elastic fibrils occasionally appear in the stroma as well.

Mechanical properties of the cornea

The mechanical properties of the cornea are determined primarily by Bowman's layer and the stromal collagen. Chapter 27, Biomechanics: A Primer for Corneal Surgeons, Chapter 28, A Finite Element Model of Radial Keratotomy Surgery, Chapter 29, Preliminary Computer Simulation of Radial Keratotomy, and Chapter 33, Biomechanics of Transverse Incisions of the Cornea, describe corneal biomechanics, and only a couple of salient points are mentioned here.[22]

The corneal stroma has little elasticity and stretches only by approximately 0.25% in the range of normal intraocular pressure.[22] Therefore the cornea can maintain a reasonably constant shape and curvature. Under normal circumstances the entire thickness of the cornea supports stress from intraocular pressure, but the exact distribution of the tension across the stroma has not been clearly defined. It is certain, however, that when a refractive keratotomy incision is made through Bowman's layer and approximately 90% of the stroma, the remaining 10% of the posterior stroma and Descemet's membrane must support the intraocular pressure. These tissues cannot support the pressure without deformation, and therefore the cornea bows forward paracentrally and peripherally, producing gaping of the incisions and compensatory flattening of the central cornea. Once the structural integrity of the anterior layers of the cornea has been severed by the first few incisions, the forces are taken up by the remaining stroma and the further change in the shape of the cornea is not affected much by additional cuts.

The tensile strength of the corneal stroma is high; blunt injury to the cornea seldom ruptures the globe through the cornea, but rather usually through the thinner sclera near the equator of the globe or around the optic nerve. However, the collagen fibrils severed by keratotomy never heal end-to-end, and the intervening corneal scar, which creates the new configuration of the cornea by filling in and maintaining the gap within the incision, never regains the tensile strength of the normal cornea. Therefore the probability of rupture of the cornea from blunt injury is increased after keratotomy.[3]

Corneal transparency

Light passes undisturbed through materials with uniform density and uniform indexes of refraction.[23] However, when inhomogeneities, such as dust particles in the air of a movie theater, water droplets in the air on a foggy night, or air bubbles in a clear swimming pool, are present, the light is refracted and scattered by the materials because they have a different index of refraction from the air or water surrounding them. This scattering is perceived as haze and opacification of an otherwise clear medium. As visible light passes through the cornea, only approximately 1% is scattered. Thus the cornea is commonly called "transparent," even though the slight light scattering allows the cornea to be seen with the slit-lamp microscope. How is it that the cornea with its relatively inhomogeneous structure can appear as transparent as it does?

A proper explanation quickly involves us in mathematic formulations, but it can be understood in simpler conceptual terms.[26] In the cornea the changes in the index of refraction between the collagen fibrils and the intervening extracellular matrix occur over distances of only 30 to 60 nm (Figs. 2-10 and 2-11). These distances are far less than half the wave length of visible light (200 to 300 nm), so the light makes its way through this structure with minimal disruption. However, when the structure is disturbed, such as by lakes of edematous fluid, the light is scattered and the cornea becomes opaque. The scattered light waves interfere with each other both constructively (in phase) and destructively (out of phase).

One can conceptualize this by considering that the light waves have a limit to their resolution; they cannot detect variations that are less than half their wave length. Two analogies help explain. If one rubs the surface of a finely finished sculpture, it feels very smooth, even though a scanning electron micrograph shows considerable surface irregularity. Similarly a basketball rolling down a driveway is not deflected by small pieces of gravel, but it bounces wildly among potholes. In a like manner, light waves make their way through the normal cornea unable to detect small variations in the indexes of refraction that are present.

Scar tissue that forms within keratotomy wounds has a structure much less regular than the normal corneal stroma, and therefore light scatters from it, making the scars visible. This light scattering is transmitted into the eye and is perceived by patients as glare—either the common starburst pattern around focal lights or sometimes as a diffuse veiling glare that may become disabling. In general the more scars present and the closer they are to the center of the cornea, the greater the light scattering and clinically perceived glare.

CORNEAL ENDOTHELIUM AND DESCEMET'S MEMBRANE
Structure of the endothelium

The corneal endothelium is the most posterior layer of the cornea and comprises approximately 350,000 cells at birth—approximately 3000 cells/mm^2.[43,44] The cells are arranged in a continuous monolayer 4 to 6 μm thick (Fig. 2-12), creating a uniform paving-stone mosaic of closely apposed polygonal cells with an average of six sides, the cells being approximately 20 μm in diameter with a cell surface area of approximately 250 μm^2. The endothelial population is distributed uniformly over the cornea[41] and is generally symmetric in both eyes of

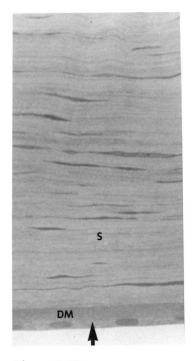

Figure 2-12
The posterior cornea shows the lamellar structure of stroma *(S)*, Descemet's membrane *(DM)*, and monolayer of endothelium *(arrow)*.

an individual. In the peripheral limbal area of the cornea, the cells become progressively irregular as they merge with the trabecular endothelium.

In early years of life endothelial cell densities vary from approximately 2000 to 4000 cells/mm^2, but as the cells age, some die and disappear. Unfortunately, the adult human corneal endothelium does not have the capacity to divide rapidly enough to replace the aging or injured cells, although mitosis of human endothelium has been demonstrated histopathologically and clinically by specular microscopy and tissue culture. When endothelial cells age or become injured, the remaining cells must enlarge, reorganize, and migrate to maintain an intact monolayer. Therefore the morphologic health of the endothelium can be judged by the uniformity of its mosaic pattern, as measured by the following three variables[43]:

1. Cell density—the more cells per square millimeter, the better. Normally the endothelium has 2000 to 3000 cells/mm^2.
2. The coefficient of variation of cell size—the larger the coefficient, the greater the variability in cell size. Normal values for the coefficient are 0.22 to 0.29.
3. The percentage of hexagonal cells—the greater the proportion of hexagonal cells, the more normal the endothelium. Normal percentages of hexagonal cells are 60% to 75%.

The endothelium contains abundant mitochondria specialized for active metabolism. Some rough endoplasmic reticula and Golgi apparatus are present for protein synthesis. The apical, "tight" intercellular junctions are not occluding and therefore allow some leakage of aqueous humor into the stroma (Fig. 2-13); gap junctions are present for intercellular communication. Changes in morphology reflect insults to the endothelium, such as might occur with multiple corneal perforations during refractive keratotomy, but they do not depict endothelial cell function. In fact a cornea may remain clear and compact with as few as 300 to 500 endothelial cells/mm^2, presumably because individual endothelial cells have considerable functional reserve and can develop additional pump sites to control corneal hydration.

Function of the endothelium

The major function of the corneal endothelium is to maintain corneal hydration at a fixed level, preserving corneal transparency. This is accomplished by two mechanisms. The first is the establishment of a semipermeable barrier that keeps most of the aqueous humor out of the cornea, although some of the aqueous humor with its essential nutrients is allowed to diffuse into the cornea through the leaky intercellular junctions. The second mechanism is the active removal of water from the corneal stroma through a sodium-potassium, adenosine triphosphatase–bicarbonate pump located in the lateral plasma membrane of the cell. This pump removes electrolytes that osmotically carry water with them and maintain stromal hydration at a fixed level. Disruption of either the barrier or the pump function allows excess hydration of the stroma, producing stromal edema, thickening, and opacification.[44]

The endothelium and refractive keratotomy collided in the hands of T. Sato and his colleagues, who practiced posterior keratotomy in the 1940s and 1950s, a time when the function of the endothelium was largely unknown (see Chapter 6, Development of Radial Keratotomy in Japan, 1939-1960). Despite 40 radial incisions made in the posterior cornea, the endothelia of relatively young patients were able to recover, reestablish monolayers, and maintain corneal clarity—but for only approximately 20 years. The normal aging process or other insults gradually took their toll and reduced the number of endothelial cells to the point that stromal edema appeared in many cases.

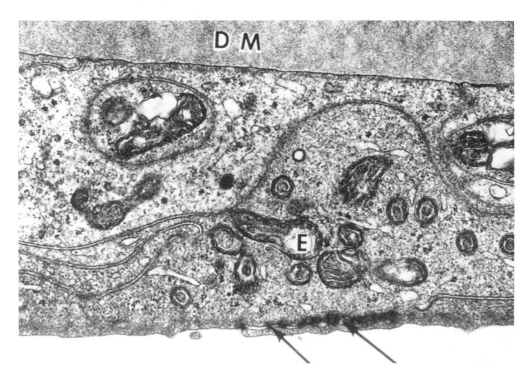

Figure 2-13
Corneal endothelial cells *(E)* are characterized by numerous mitochondria with a longitudinal orientation of cristae and by abundant free ribosomes. Junctional complexes are indicated by arrows. Posterior portion of Descemet's membrane *(DM)* is amorphous (×30,000.) (From Rodrigues MM, Waring GO, Hackett J, and Donohoo P: Cornea. In Duane TD and Jaeger EA, editors: Biomedical foundations of ophthalmology, vol 1, Hagerstown, Md, Harper & Row Publishers, Inc.)

During uncomplicated anterior refractive keratotomy the endothelium may suffer mild damage secondary to stretching of the cornea, but current evidence indicates that it recovers well and maintains a close-to-normal morphology for some years after the surgery. Of course corneal perforations produce transient focal endothelial damage and increased edema in the wound until the barrier and pump functions are reestablished; this reduces the total number of endothelial cells (see Chapter 23, Complications of Refractive Keratotomy).

Descemet's membrane and the posterior collagenous layer

Descemet's membrane, the normal basement membrane of the corneal endothelium, comprises predominantly type IV collagen and glycoproteins, including fibronectin. Descemet's membrane thickens throughout life, being present at birth as a 3 μm thick layer that shows a 110 nm vertically banded pattern on transmission electron microscopy. Throughout life a posterior, homogeneous, nonbanded layer is added, becoming 10 to 12 μm thick in the latter decades.

Descemet's membrane forms the scaffolding on which the endothelial cells spread themselves.[43] The mechanism by which the endothelium attaches to Descemet's membrane is unknown, since no basal attachment complexes are present. The stromal swelling pressure created by the endothelial pump and the fibronectin within Descemet's membrane may both play a role in this attachment.

Descemet's membrane serves as a barrier to the penetration of leukocytes and blood vessels into the corneal stroma and has remarkable tensile strength. Descemet's membrane can remain intact in the absence of the corneal stroma by forming an anteriorly protruding descemetocele; this has occurred in a very deep radial keratotomy wound. Descemet's membrane is elastic. It recoils at the edges of a laceration, such as that produced by a keratotomy perforation, and folds in the face of stromal edema, forming striae.

The injured corneal endothelium produces a new abnormal extracellular matrix as a nonspecific response.[43] This collagenous tissue accumulates posterior to the normal preexisting Descemet's membrane and is called the posterior collagenous layer of the cornea; it has also been designated a retrocorneal fibrous membrane and a thickened Descemet's membrane. Clinically this abnormal tissue appears as a gray sheet on the back of the cornea that may take on discrete forms such as cornea guttata. It is seen in the area of corneal perforations from refractive keratotomy as a focal gray plaque that appears a few months after surgery and persists indefinitely.

CORNEAL THICKNESS

The thickness of the cornea is determined by the amount of tissue and the amount of water present. In fact the thickness of the cornea is directly proportionate to the hydration of the stroma. Since the thickness can be measured accurately by pachometry, one can estimate the stromal hydration and the health of the endothelium.

Measurement of the corneal thickness is a fundamental activity in keratotomy surgery because it forms the basis for setting the length of the knife blade in an attempt to make uniformly deep incisions through approximately 90% of the cornea. Measurement of corneal thickness by optical, ultrasonic, or specular microscopic pachometry is discussed in Chapter 15, Surgical Instruments Used in Refractive Keratotomy.

Figure 2-14
Stress strain curves for cornea and sclera from intact globes of human and rabbit cornea and sclera demonstrate that the rabbit cornea has considerably more elasticity than the human cornea. The rabbit cornea is a poor model for refractive keratotomy surgery. (From Maurice DM: Mechanics of the cornea. In Cavanagh HD, editor: The cornea: transactions of the world congress on the cornea III, New York, 1988, Raven Press.)

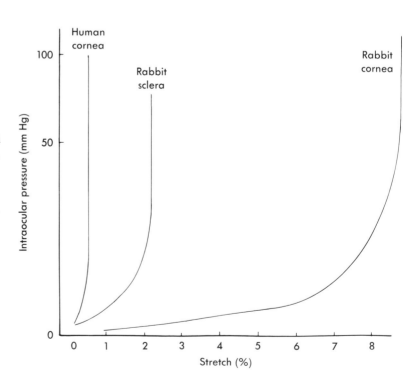

Setting a knife blade at a given length will not necessarily produce an incision of exactly that depth, because of variability in knife blade configuration and sharpness and also because the stromal collagen is relatively resistant to cutting, so some of the posterior collagenous lamellae in the stroma are displaced rather than cut by the knife (see Chapter 17, Atlas of Surgical Techniques of Radial Keratotomy).

SPECIES DIFFERENCES IN CORNEAL STRUCTURE

There is considerable variability among species in the anatomy, physiology, and biomechanical properties of the cornea. For example, Bowman's layer is present only in primate, chicken, and goose corneas, so one might expect the biomechanical properties of these corneas to differ from those without a Bowman's layer. The rabbit cornea is a poor model for keratotomy surgery because it is thinner (300 μm) centrally, does not thicken peripherally, has no Bowman's layer, is more elastic and pliable than human corneas (Fig. 2-14), and heals more rapidly (including the endothelium) than the human cornea. The cat cornea is as thick as the human cornea, but little is known about its response to corneal surgery.[4] Even the monkey cornea seems to have different biomechanical properties, such as being more elastic than the human cornea, with differences among monkey species. This type of variability is one reason why the results of research on laboratory animals cannot be directly translated to human surgery.

UNFINISHED BUSINESS

Understanding the structure of the cornea continues to challenge clinicians and researchers, even though the tissue itself appears reasonably simple. For example, what is the function of Bowman's layer? Is it structural? Is it to separate the epithelium from the keratocytes? Does it play a special role in the maintenance of corneal curvature? The answers to such simple questions have remained elusive. What latitude does the structure and function of the corneal epithelium have? What is the limit of the nutrients it needs from the aqueous humor to remain structurally normal, and how thin can the cornea get (is one layer adequate?) before it ceases to perform its barrier and protective functions?—a question pertinent to those who would place refractive lenticules within the cornea. The structure of the anterior corneal stroma differs from that of the posterior corneal stroma, both in terms of lamellar organization and proteoglycan content. Do these differences play a role in corneal function, and do they have applications to lamellar refractive surgery, or are they vestigial reflections of the ontogeny of the cornea? Is there really a circular ligament around the cornea that plays a role in modulating corneal curvature and shape? How does light get through the cornea with minimal scattering so as to form an acceptable image on the retina, and what are the limits of light scattering within the cornea that are compatible with normal visual acuity and contrast sensitivity? Such questions intrigue any refractive surgeon who creates corneal scars. Fundamental studies on corneal anatomy and biophysics may have practical implications for refractive surgery.

REFERENCES

1. Barraquer C, Gutierrez AM, and Espinosa A: Myopic keratomileusis: short-term results, Refractive Corneal Surg 1989;5:307-313.
2. Becher H and Osterhage KH: Uber die morphologischen und funktionellen Beziehungen zwischen kollagenen und elastischen Fasern in der Sklera des Rilnderauges, Z Ges Anat 1987;101:294-306.
3. Binder PS, Waring GO, Arrowsmith PN, and Wang C: Histopathology of traumatic rupture of the cornea after radial keratotomy, Arch Ophthalmol 1988;106:1584-1590.
4. Climenhaga H, Macdonald JM, McCarey BE, and Waring GO: Effect of diameter and depth on the response to solid polysulfone intracorneal lenses in cats, Arch Ophthalmol 1988;106:818-824.
5. Climenhaga H and McCarey BE: Biocompatibility of polysulfone intracorneal lenses in the cat model abstracted, Invest Ophthalmol Vis Sci 1986;26(suppl):14.
6. Edelhauser HF, Van Horn DL, and Records RE: Cornea and sclera. In Duane TD and Jaeger EA, editors: Biomedical foundations of ophthalmology, vol 2, Hagerstown, Md, 1982, Harper & Row Publishers, Inc, Ch 4.
7. Edelhauser HF, Van Horn DL, and Records RE: Cornea and sclera. In Records RE, editor: Physiology of the human eye and visual system, Hagerstown, Md, 1979, Harper & Row Publishers, Inc, pp 68-97.
8. Fatt I: Gas transmission properties of soft contact lenses. In Ruben M, editor: Soft contact lenses: clinical and applied technology, New York, 1978, John Wiley & Sons, Inc, pp 83-110.
9. Fine BS and Yanoff M: Ocular histology, ed 2, Hagerstown, Md, 1979, Harper & Row Publishers, Inc, pp 161-194.
10. Fischer E: Die konstruktive Anordnung der kollagenen Fasern in der Sklera und den Sehnerven scheiden des Rinderauges, A Ges Anat 1933;101:168-210.
11. Francois J and Victoria-Troncoso V: Disposition of the collagen structures in the corneal stroma, Contact Intraocular Lens Med J 1975;1:13.
12. Friend J: Biochemistry of ocular surface epithelium. In Thoft RA and Friend J, editors: The ocular surface, Boston, 1979, Little, Brown & Co, Inc, pp 73-91.
13. Gipson IK and Keezer L: Effect of cytochalasins and colchicine on the ultrastructure of migrating corneal epithelium, Invest Ophthalmol Vis Sci 1982;22:633-642.
14. Gipson IK, Spurr-Michaud SJ, and Tisdale AS: Anchoring fibrils from a complex network in human and rabbit cornea, Invest Ophthalmol Vis Sci 1987;28:212-220.
15. Hogan MJ, Alvarado JA, and Weddell JE: Histology of the human eye, Philadelphia, 1971, WB Saunders Co, pp 55-180.
16. Klintworth GK: The cornea—structure and macromolecules in health and disease: a review, Am J Pathol 1977;89:718-808.
17. Kokott W: Uber mechanisch-funktionelle Strukturen des Auges, Graefes Arch Ophthalmol 1938;138:424-485.
18. Leibowitz HM: Corneal disorders: clinical diagnosis and management, Philadelphia, 1984, WB Saunders Co.
19. Mandelbaum S et al: Late development of ulcerative keratitis in radial keratotomy scars, Arch Ophthalmol 1986;104:1156-1160.
20. Marquardt R, Stodtmeister R, and Christ TH: Modification of tear film break-up time test for increased reliability. In Holly FJ, editor: The preocular tear film: in health, disease, and contact lens wear, Lubbock, Tex, 1986, Dry Eye Institute, Inc, pp 57-63.
21. Maurice DM: The cornea and stroma. In Davson H, editor: The eye, vol 1B, Orlando, Fla, 1984, Academic Press Inc, pp 1-158.
22. Maurice DM: Mechanics of the cornea. In Cavanagh HD, editor: The cornea: transactions of the world congress on the cornea III, New York, 1988, Raven Press, pp 187-194.
23. McCally RL and Farrell RA: Interaction of light in the cornea: light scattering versus transparency. In Cavanagh HD: The cornea: transactions of the world congress on the cornea III, New York, 1988, Raven Press, pp 165-172.
24. McMonnies CW and Ho A: Marginal dry eye diagnosis: history versus biomicroscopy. In Holly FJ, editor: The preocular tear film: in health, disease, and contact lens wear, Lubbock, Tex, 1986, Dry Eye Institute, Inc, pp 1-40.
25. Mengher LS, Bron AJ, Tonge SR, and Gilbert DJ: Noninvasive assessment of tear film stability. In Holly FJ, editor: The preocular tear film: in health, disease, and contact lens wear, Lubbock, Tex, 1986, Dry Eye Institute, Inc, pp 64-75.
26. Miller D and Benedek G: Intraocular light scattering, Springfield, Ill, 1973, Charles C Thomas, Publisher.
27. Mishima S: Corneal physiology under contact lenses. In Gasset AR and Kaufman HE, editors: Soft contact lens, St Louis, 1972, The CV Mosby Co, pp 19-36.
28. Mosher DF: Physiology of fibronectin, Annu Rev Med 1984;35:561-575.
29. Nelson JD, Williams P, Lindstrom RL, and Doughman DJ: Map-finger-dot changes in the corneal epithelial basement membrane following radial keratotomy, Ophthalmology 1985;92:199-205.
30. Newsome DA, Gross J, and Hassel JR: Human corneal stroma contains 3 distinct collagens, Invest Ophthalmol Vis Sci 1982;22:376-381.
31. Norn MS: Tear film breakup time. A review. In Holly FJ, editor: The preocular tear film: in health, disease, and contact lens wear, Lubbock, Tex, 1986, Dry Eye Institute, Inc, pp 52-56.
32. Polack FM: Morphology of the cornea. I. Study with silver stains, Am J Ophthalmol 1961;51:1051-1056.
33. Pratt-Johnson JA: Studies on the anatomy and pathology of the peripheral cornea, Am J Ophthalmol 1959;47:478.
34. Rodrigues MM, Rowden G, Hackett J, and Bakos I: Langerhans' cells in the normal conjunctiva and peripheral cornea of selected species, Invest Ophthalmol Vis Sci 1981;21:759-765.
34a. Rodrigues MM, Waring GO, Hacket J, and Donohoo P: Cornea. In Tasman W, and Jaeger EA, editors: Duane's biomedical foundations of ophthalmology, vol 1, Philadelphia, JB Lippincott Co, pp 1-13.

35. Roscoe WR and Hill RM: Corneal oxygen demands: a comparison of the open- and closed-eyed environments, Am J Optom Physiol Opt 1980;57:67-69.

36. Seal DV and Mackie IA: The questionably dry eye as a clinical and biochemical entity. In Holly FJ, editor: The preocular tear film: in health, disease, and contact lens wear, Lubbock, Tex, 1986, Dry Eye Institute, Inc, pp 41-51.

37. Shivitz IA and Arrowsmith PN: Delayed keratitis after radial keratotomy, Arch Ophthalmol 1986;104:1153-1155.

38. Spencer WH: Cornea. In Spencer WH, editor: Ophthalmic pathology, ed 3, vol 1, Philadelphia, 1985, WB Saunders Co, pp 229-338.

39. Spencer WH and Kenyon KR: Morphology and pathologic responses of the cornea to disease. In Smolin G and Thoft R, editors: The cornea, ed 2, Boston, 1987, Little, Brown & Co, Inc, pp 63-92.

40. Steinberg EB, Wilson LA, Waring GO, Lynn MJ, and Coles WH: Stellate iron lines in the corneal epithelium after radial keratotomy, Am J Ophthalmol 1984;98:416-421.

41. Sturrock GD, Sherrard ES, and Rice NSC: Specular microscopy of the corneal endothelium, Br J Ophthalmol 1978;62:809-814.

42. Thoft RA and Friend J, editors: The ocular surface, Boston, 1979, Little, Brown & Co, Inc.

43. Waring GO: Posterior collagenous layer of the cornea: ultrastructural classification of abnormal collagenous tissue posterior to Descemet's membrane in 30 cases, Arch Ophthalmol 1982;100:122-134.

43a. Waring GO: Corneal structure and pathophysiology. In Leibowitz HM, editor: Corneal disorders. Clinical diagnosis and management, Philadelphia, 1984, WB Saunders Co, pp 3-28.

44. Waring GO, Bourne WM, Edelhauser HF, and Kenyon KR: The corneal endothelium: normal and pathologic structure and function, Ophthalmology 1982;89:531-590.

45. Waring GO, Lynn MJ, Culbertson W, Laibson PR, Lindstrom RD, McDonald MB, Myers WD, Obstbaum SA, Rowsey JJ, Schanzlin DJ and the PERK Study Group: Three year results in the prospective evaluation of radial keratotomy (PERK) study, Ophthalmology 1987;94:1339-1354.

46. Waring GO, Lynn MJ, Fielding B, Asbell PA, Balyeat HD, Cohen EA, The PERK Study Group, et al: Results of the Prospective Evaluation of Radial Keratotomy (PERK) 4 years after surgery for myopia, JAMA 1990;263:1083-1091.

47. Waring GO and Rodrigues MM: Patterns of pathological response in the cornea, Surv Ophthalmol 1987;31:262-266.

48. Yee RW et al: Changes in normal corneal endothelial cellular pattern as a function of age, Curr Eye Res 1985;4:671-678.

Optics and Topography of Radial Keratotomy

Jack T. Holladay
George O. Waring III

BACKGROUND AND ACKNOWLEDGMENTS

Writing this chapter presented two challenges. The first was to scale the amount of information on optics so that it was neither perfunctorily simple nor confusingly complex. We have tried to present information at a level appropriate for the ophthalmic surgeon who wishes to understand the effect of radial keratotomy on ophthalmic optics. The information available on corneal topography changed dramatically during the writing of this chapter because the whole field of quantitative analysis of keratographs and computerized analysis of videokeratographs evolved. We have attempted to be as current as possible concerning corneal topography.

Many individuals contributed information to this chapter. James Rowsey, M.D., Mr. Roy Monlux, and their colleagues at the PERK Keratography Reading Center at the University of Oklahoma fostered many of the ideas embodied in the analysis of photokeratographs. Stephen Klyce, Ph.D., spawned much of the conceptual basis for videokeratography and clinically relevant representations of corneal topography. Sadeer Hannush, M.D., Stephen Bogan, M.D., and Osama Ibrahim, M.D., provided practical information concerning videokeratography of normal corneas and corneas after refractive keratotomy. Robert Maloney, M.D., contributed information on the mathematical analysis of keratographs and corneal topography. Ms. Linda Curtis provided technical assistance on videokeratography. Computed Anatomy, Inc., provided a Corneal Modeling System and technical support for videokeratography, with distinctive contributions from Mr. Martin Gersten and Dennis Gormley, M.D. The NIDEK Corporation provided a qualitative photokeratoscope from which much information on photokeratoscopy was derived. The Kera Corporation provided a CorneaScope and KeraScanner to foster quantitative aspects of photokeratography, with special contributions from Mr. Jerry Ditto. The EyeSys Corporation provided a computer-assisted videokeratoscope, with special contributions by Lorena Riverall, M.D., Kerry Hagen, M.D., and Joe Wakil, M.D. Other contributions are acknowledged in the text and the figure legends. Some material on the terminology of corneal topography has been previously published.[115]

In this chapter we provide fundamental, clinically relevant information about the effects of radial keratotomy on corneal curvature, optics, and topography.

We discuss both the general principles of the optics of myopia and the basic methods of measuring corneal curvature and topography and then apply these principles to the specific situation of radial keratotomy* (see Chapter 30, Optics and Topography of Corneal Astigmatism).

The desire to measure the refractive power and shape of the human cornea has arisen historically from four clinical imperatives. The first was the need in the mid-1800s to improve the accuracy of refraction. As better methods of clinical refraction and retinoscopy became available, the need for keratometry diminished. The second impetus was the appearance of contact lenses in the 1940s, which made measurement of corneal shape and power a necessity and which created a need both for better keratometers to measure the cornea off-center and for keratography to define the contours of the cornea. Subsequent improvements in contact lens design and the emergence of soft contact lenses have resulted from detailed measurement of corneal shape. The third area was the need to calculate the power of intraocular lenses accurately. The fourth force was the emergence of modern refractive corneal surgery in the 1960s. This is currently an area of intense interest for surgeons wishing to know the effect of surgery on corneal shape and power and whether the original shape of the cornea affects the outcome.

In each of these four phases, the demand for accuracy and precision has increased. This is particularly true in refractive surgery, in which only a 17-μm change in the anterior curvature of the cornea produces a 1-diopter change in ocular refraction.

The optical effects of radial keratotomy seem intuitively simple: the operation weakens the paracentral and peripheral cornea, produces central flattening, decreases the refractive power of the cornea, and reduces the amount of myopia. Behind this basic concept are more complex mechanical and optical factors that help explain the variety of clinical phenomena induced by keratotomy.

THE OPTICS OF MYOPIA
Correlation and component ametropia

Four variables determine the refractive power of the eye: the power of the cornea, the depth of the anterior chamber, the power of the lens, and the axial length of the globe. Each of these factors has a range of normal values distributed in a bell-shaped Gaussian curve for eyes with refractions of approximately +6.00 to −4.00 D. Sorsby[104] has classified the refractive state of the human eye into the following three groups:

1. In *emmetropic* eyes (Fig. 3-1), the four components correlate with each other in such a way that there is minimal refractive error (less than 0.25 D). For example, an eye with a slightly longer globe will have a slightly flatter cornea or a less curved lens.
2. In eyes with *correlation ametropia* (approximately 25% of the population), the values of the four variables mentioned earlier fall in the normal range but are incorrectly correlated, resulting in a refractive error (Fig. 3-2). For example, an eye with an axial length in the upper normal range and a cornea in the steeper range of normal will be myopic.
3. In eyes with *component ametropia* (approximately 3% of the population), one of the four variables lies outside the normal range, producing a more extreme refractive error. In most cases the abnormal component is the ax-

*References 16, 25-27, 31, 81, 89, 96, 101.

ial length. For example, an abnormally long globe with posterior staphyloma will produce high pathologic myopia, regardless of corneal and lens power.

Thus myopic eyes with refractions of −0.50 to −4.00 or −5.00 D generally have normal values for the four elements (correlation ametropia), whereas those with more than 4.00 to 5.00 D of myopia tend to have longer axial lengths (component ametropia), commonly showing a scleral crescent around the optic nerve (intermediate myopia) or a posterior staphyloma (pathologic myopia) (see Chapter 1, Myopia: A Brief Overview).

Role of the cornea in myopia

Infants and children younger than approximately 3 years of age have a corneal curvature and corneal refractive power greater than that of an adult.[43,53,54] Newborns characteristically have a keratometric corneal power greater than 47 D, which declines gradually to the normal adult value of approximately 43.5 to 43.75 D by 3 years of age (Fig. 3-3 and Table 3-1). This makes sense in terms of the correlation of the components of refraction: as the axial length of the globe increases from approximately 18 mm to 23.5 mm during this period of growth, the steep cornea at birth gradually flattens, keeping the image in focus on the retina. From 3 years of age to the early teenage years, the globe continues to elongate slightly, but the corneal curvature seems to remain constant, requiring a decrease in the power of the crystalline lens to maintain emmetropia. If lens power does not decrease, myopia can result.

The central radius of the curvature in the normal cornea has been measured by keratometry in numerous studies. One of the most extensive series, which included over 30,000 patients, was conducted by Senstrom (cited by Clark[19]) in 1948. The mean central radius of curvature was 7.80 mm (43.25 D) with the

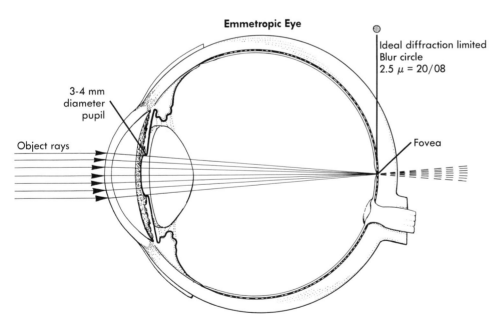

Figure 3-1
In the normal emmetropic eye, images from infinity pass through the pupil and are focused on the fovea to create a small blur circle with a limit of resolution of 2.5 μm, which corresponds to a visual acuity of 20/08. The normal correlation between the refractive power of the cornea, the refractive power of the lens, and the length of the eye results in emmetropia.

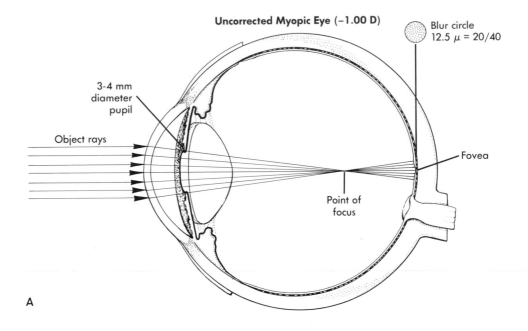

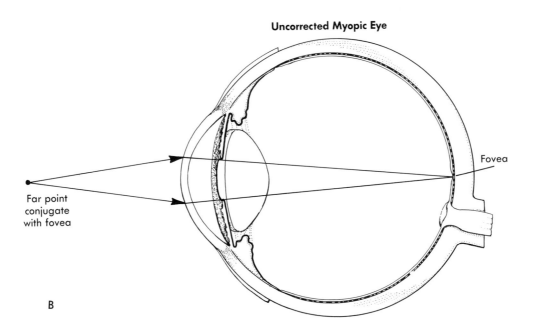

Figure 3-2

Myopic eye. **A,** The uncorrected myopic eye has excessive plus power in either the cornea or the lens or an excessive axial length, so the point of focus falls within the vitreous, creating a large blur circle and decreased uncorrected visual acuity. **B,** When an object is brought closer to the uncorrected myopic eye, there is a point at which it is in focus on the fovea. This point is the far point of the eye. This is the reason that myopic eyes are called "nearsighted," since there is a point near to the eye where objects are in focus.

Spectacle-Corrected Myopic Eye

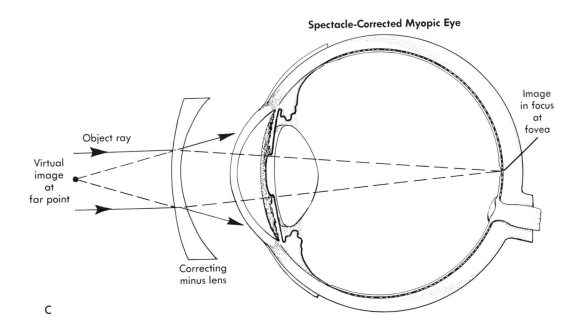

C

Radial Keratotomy–Corrected Myopic Eye

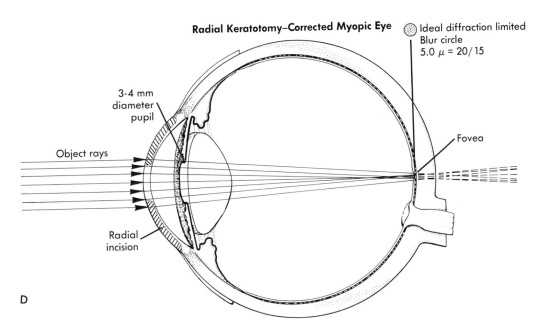

D

Figure 3-2, cont'd
C, A minus power lens, either spectacle or contact, can correct the myopic eye by placing the image of the object at the far point so that it is in focus on the fovea. **D,** Radial keratotomy corrects the myopic eye by decreasing the refractive power of the cornea and ideally placing object rays in focus on the fovea. However, spherical aberrations of the paracentral cornea may bring light rays to focus either in front of or behind the fovea, creating a larger blur circle than that in the emmetropic eye.

range from 9.4 mm (35.7 D) to 6.7 mm (50.2 D). In the PERK study (unpublished data), the mean central corneal power measured by Bausch & Lomb keratotomy before surgery in 435 eyes of patients 21 to 58 years of age with spherical equivalent refractions of −2.00 to −8.00 D was 44.00 D (range, 40.3 to 48.9) (Fig. 3-4). Sorsby[105] measured 408 normal adult corneas and found a mean power of 43.1 D (range, 39.0 to 47.5 D) (Table 3-2).

The question remains: Do myopic eyes have steeper corneas? Most do not. In general, corneal curvature is normal in myopia,[41] although some studies have

Figure 3-3
Keratometry values (mean, SD) plotted with respect to age on logarithmic scale. Negative number represents months of prematurity. Values are from 148 normal eyes of 79 patients. Adult values of approximately 44 D appear around 3 years of age. (From Gordon RA and Donzis PB: Arch Ophthalmol 1985;100:785-789.)

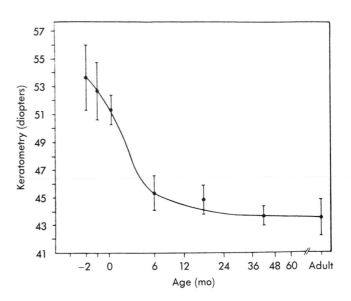

Table 3-1

Variations in Refractive Components of the Human Eye with Growth

Age group (yr)	No. of eyes	Mean ±SD				
		Axial length (mm)	Keratometry (D)*	SRK lens power (D)†	Modified SRK lens power (D)	Refractive error (D)*
30-35 wk‡	11	15.1±0.9	53.6±2.5	31.9±0.5	43.5±3.6	−1.0±0.9
35-39 wk‡	14	16.1±0.6	52.6±1.9	28.4±1.1	36.9±2.4	0.3±1.6
39-41 wk‡	10	16.8±0.6	51.2±1.1	27.7±1.6	34.4±2.3	0.4±1.5
0-1	11	19.2±0.7	45.2±1.3	26.4±0.5	28.7±1.0	0.9±0.9
1-2	8	20.2±0.3	44.9±0.9	25.1±0.5	26.4±0.6	0.3±0.6
2-3	8	21.4±0.1	44.1±0.3	22.5±0.2	23.0±0.4	0.5±0.6
3-4	8	21.8±0.4	43.7±0.5	21.7±0.2	22.1±0.4	0.6±0.2
4-5	5	22.3±0.2	43.2±0.7	20.7±0.5	20.9±0.6	0.7±0.6
5-6	9	22.7±0.9	43.7±0.9	19.4±0.5	19.5±0.5	0.9±1.5
6-7	5	22.9±0.4	43.4±0.6	18.6±0.9	18.7±0.9	1.0±1.1
7-9	10	22.6±1.2	44.2±1.6	19.2±0.5	19.3±0.7	0.6±1.8
10-15	7	23.8±0.7	43.5±0.7	18.9±0.3	18.9±0.6	−0.8±0.9
15-20	6	23.8±0.5	43.5±1.1	18.6±0.5	18.6±0.8	−0.6±1.0
20-36	36	23.6±0.7	43.5±1.2	18.8±0.7	18.8±0.8	−0.5±1.5

From Gordon RA and Donzis PB: Arch Ophthalmol 1985;103:785-789.
*All values are in spherical equivalents.
†*SRK*, Sanders-Retzlaff-Kraff formula.
‡Total gestational age plus age since birth for premature and full-term newborns.

found the cornea to have greater power than normal.[22,105,107] For example, Sorsby[104] found steeper corneas (45 D or greater) in approximately 12% of hyperopic and emmetropic eyes, but found the same conditions in 35% of myopic eyes (Fig. 3-5). Eyes with a refraction of −4.37 to −8.00 D had a mean corneal power of 44.24, statistically significantly steeper (*p* = 0.03) than eyes with a refraction of −2.00 to −3.12 D (mean, 44.01 D) and eyes with a refraction of −3.25 to −4.25 (mean, 43.83 D). It is not possible to draw a direct correlation between the amount of myopia and the curvature of the cornea.[106]

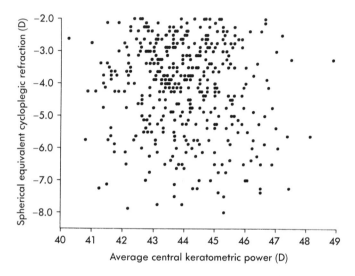

Figure 3-4
Correlation of cycloplegic refractive error and central average keratometric readings for 435 normal eyes in the PERK study. Scattergram demonstrates no correlation between refractive error and keratometric power.

Table 3-2

Range, Mean, and Standard Deviation of the Major Optical Components in 408 Adult Eyes

Ocular refraction (D)	No. of eyes	Corneal power (D) Range	Mean	SD	Lens power (D) Range	Mean	SD	Axial length (mm) Range	Mean	SD
+8.0 to +11.60	4	44.2−45.8	45.1	0.66	21.1−24.7	23.0	1.49	19.2−20.2	19.8	0.45
+6.0 to +7.99	5	39.7−45.1	42.9	2.01	19.0−21.8	20.8	1.07	21.2−22.9	21.7	0.69
+5.0 to +5.99	11	41.1−43.9	42.3	0.98	16.3−25.8	21.0	2.61	21.1−23.3	22.2	0.65
+4.0 to +4.99	11	40.1−45.3	42.4	1.54	19.4−22.7	20.9	1.09	21.4−23.5	22.7	0.60
+3.0 to +3.99	10	38.3−45.1	41.7	1.96	18.5−24.8	21.4	1.72	21.6−24.7	23.2	0.88
+2.0 to +2.99	21	41.2−46.6	43.6	1.55	16.4−24.7	21.3	2.28	21.4−24.5	22.9	0.83
+0.51 to +1.99	127	39.6−45.9	43.0	1.39	16.2−26.1	20.5	1.76	21.7−25.9	23.8	0.80
0.00 to +0.50	107	39.0−47.6	43.1	1.62	15.5−23.9	19.7	1.62	22.3−26.0	24.2	0.85
−0.01 to −0.99	34	39.2−46.5	43.1	1.36	17.5−22.4	19.6	1.40	22.2−26.7	24.5	0.81
−1.0 to −1.99	19	40.6−45.1	43.1	1.39	15.6−23.0	18.7	1.90	23.8−27.2	25.3	0.91
−2.0 to −2.99	16	41.7−46.3	44.2	1.15	17.4−21.4	19.6	1.14	23.9−25.9	24.9	0.52
−3.0 to −3.99	6	41.2−46.2	44.7	1.81	19.6−24.9	21.7	2.10	23.3−26.1	24.6	1.01
−4.0 to −4.99	4	41.2−42.8	42.2	0.70	18.4−20.9	20.0	1.12	26.2−27.1	26.7	0.38
−5.0 to −5.99	5	40.0−45.6	43.4	1.83	19.0−20.8	19.8	0.81	25.8−27.2	26.3	0.73
−6.0 to −6.99	7	41.4−44.4	42.7	1.12	19.6−22.3	20.6	0.96	26.3−27.6	27.1	0.50
−7.0 to −7.99	5	40.7−45.5	43.2	2.09	17.5−20.7	19.7	1.30	26.3−29.7	27.7	1.54
−8.0 to −20.30	16	40.7−46.9	43.2	1.90	18.2−24.3	21.1	1.80	26.2−36.0	31.0	2.77

From Sorsby A, Leary GA, and Richards MJ: Vision Res 1962;2:309.
The series of figures framed in unbroken lines give the essential findings in the five refraction groups with not less than 19 cases. The values on axial length framed in broken lines are clearly outside the range seen in emmetropic eyes.

Larger amounts of corneal astigmatism are associated with high myopia. Curtin[25] found that over 50% of children with congential myopia had corneal astigmatism of 2 D or greater, and other studies are in general agreement with this.[57,80,102,107] Slight thinning of the cornea has been observed in high myopes when compared with normal, although the difference is small, on the order of 10 to 20 μm.[99,113]

Thus the goal of refractive keratotomy is not to flatten a cornea that is abnormally steep, but rather to flatten the central cornea so that its final refractive power fits (correlates) with the power of the lens, the anterior chamber depth, and the axial length of the eye to achieve the desired final refraction. Whether steeper or flatter corneas have a different response to refractive keratotomy remains to be determined (see Chapter 13, Predictability of Refractive Keratotomy).

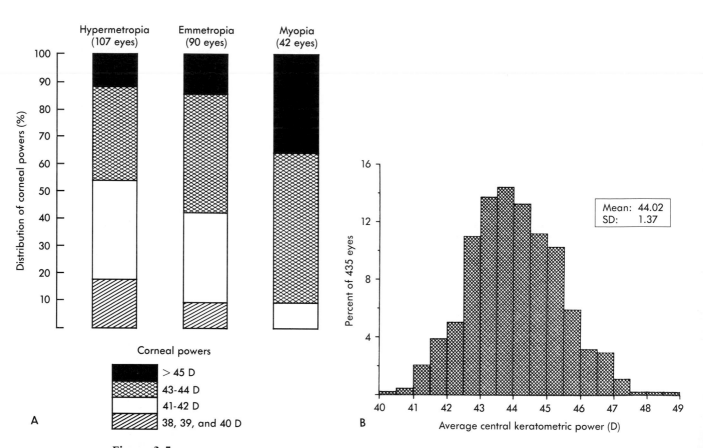

Figure 3-5
Distribution of average central keratometric power. **A,** Comparing hypermetropic, emmetropic, and myopic eyes in the refractive range of +4.00 D to −4.00 D shows more steeper corneas in the myopic group. **B,** For 435 eyes (one eye per patient, ages 21 to 58 years) with a spherical equivalent cycloplegic refraction of between −2.00 D and −8.00 D in the PERK study, the mean and standard deviation were 44.02 ±1.37 D, and the distribution of powers was a normal Gaussian appearance with no recognizable skew toward steeper corneas. (**A** from Soresby A, Benjamin B, Davey JB, et al: Emmetropia and its aberrations, London, 1957, Her Majesty's Stationery Office.)

Optical and surgical correction of myopia

The myopic eye is an eye with too much plus power, so an object at infinity is focused in front of the retina. In addition, the far point of the eye—the point at which an object is located when its image is in focus on the retina—is within 2 meters from the cornea for all eyes more myopic than 0.50 D (as demonstrated by the formula for the focal point of a lens, 1/0.5 D = 2 meters).[26,97] Thus the individual with uncorrected myopia has blurred visual acuity for objects beyond the far point; the greater the myopia is, the more blurred distant objects are for a given pupil size (Fig. 3-6).

Having the far point of the eye within arm's length is an intrinsic advantage to the myope, who always has the option of seeing well at near without optical correction. Indeed, many myopes instinctively remove their spectacles for near work, particularly after the onset of presbyopia.

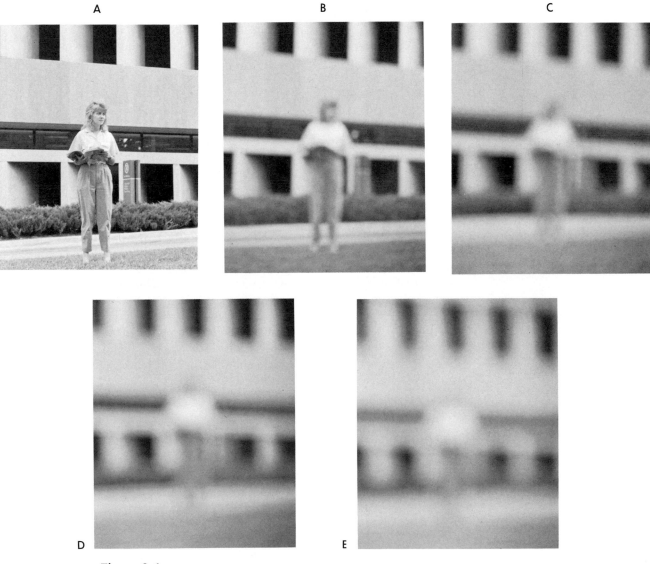

Figure 3-6
Photographic simulation of the visual blur and defocus seen by an individual with uncorrected myopia. **A,** Emmetropic eye. **B,** −1.00 D. **C,** −2.00 D. **D,** −3.00 D. **E,** −4.00 D. (Simulation by Mr. James Gilman.)

Correction of myopia with spectacles or contact lenses requires focusing the image at the far point of the eye (see Fig. 3-2). Such a lens is a minus, or concave, lens that diverges light rays and forms a virtual image in front of the lens, where the far point of the myopic eye is located. Correcting myopia with refractive corneal surgery is a different undertaking; refractive surgery attempts to move the far point of the eye to infinity by eliminating the relative excess plus power inherent in the myopic eye. In radial keratotomy this is done by flattening the cornea to reduce its refractive power.

Discussions of the optics of myopia and its correction with spectacle lenses and contact lenses have been presented by Ruben,[97] Curtin,[26] and Michaels.[81] We emphasize only two or three points about the correction of myopia with lenses.

The correction of myopia with spectacle lenses accrues advantages and disadvantages for the myope. The obvious advantage is bringing distant objects into focus. The disadvantages increase in rough proportion to the strength of the lens. Most myopes begin wearing spectacle lenses in childhood and therefore incorporate the less desirable cosmetic, convenience, and optical disadvantages into their routine of daily living; however, this adaptation varies among individuals.

Among the optical drawbacks of minus spectacle lenses is the minification of the image, placing the spectacle-wearing myope in a "lilliputian world," to borrow Curtin's allusion to Swift's *Gulliver's Travels.* The closer the spectacle lens to the eye (the less the vertex distance), the less the minification. At a vertex of 12 mm there is approximately 2% minification per diopter of spectacle power; for example, a −2.00 D lens produces 4% minification. Contact lenses have about one fourth the minifying effect of spectacles. The thick edges and supporting frames of minus spectacle lenses distort and restrict the peripheral visual field.

Minus lenses also have effects on visual function at near. When the myope's eyes converge for near work, he or she looks through the base-in prisms created by the spectacle lens. The prismatic effect is equal to the distance from the optical center of the lens in centimeters multipled by the dioptric power of the lens (Prentice's rule). This induces an esophoria and decreases the convergence demand at near. The minus lens also augments the range of accommodation for the eye, decreasing the accommodative effort required to maintain the object in focus. Thus the myope who is corrected by a minus lens has advantages for near work because there is less convergence demand and an expanded accommodative range. These are important facts to keep in mind when treating middle-aged patients with radial keratotomy because the corrected myopia will immediately increase the accommodative and convergence requirements for near work, plunging the patient into presbyopic symptoms. Such individuals may not be entirely pleased to find they have replaced their distance lenses with reading glasses. These phenomena are well known in the fitting of contact lenses in prepresbyopic individuals. One way to handle them is to attempt an undercorrection, leaving a residual myopia of −0.50 to −1.00 D.

TERMINOLOGY OF CORNEAL OPTICS AND TOPOGRAPHY

Standardized terminology used in describing corneal optics and topography would clarify communication and reduce confusion in a subject area already complex. We propose conventional terminology here.

Those who feel that dickering over terminology is a waste of time might consider the consequences of unbridled keratospeak as expressed by Dr. Stephen Klyce: "This section is a corneagram for the keratophilic keratosage to better understand the corneomorphy with the keratolithic, keratoantrophic, keratomegalous, keratopendulous, keratophimotic, and schizokeratophreninic corneanomalies using keratographs and keratoglyphs that even the keratopsychotic keratodolt can interpret."

Shape of the cornea—radius of curvature and power

The radius of curvature of the anterior and posterior corneal surfaces and the index of refraction of the surrounding media determine its refractive power (Fig. 3-7). The shorter the radius of curvature, the steeper the arc and the greater the refractive power of its surface.

Conversely, the longer the radius of curvature, the flatter the arc and the less the refractive power of its surface. All keratometers and keratoscopes measure the radius of curvature of the anterior surface of the cornea. Conversion of radius of curvature to corneal power is made according to the relationship: power (P in diopters) = index of refraction of the cornea (n_2) minus the index of refraction of air (n_1 = 1.00) divided by the measured radius of curvature of the cornea (r in meters):

$$P = \frac{n_2 - n_1}{r}$$

Most keratometers use 1.3375 as the index of refraction for the cornea, the so-called keratometric index, even though the real index of refraction of the cornea is 1.376 and the index of refraction of the tear film is 1.336; the reason for this is discussed in the section on keratometry.

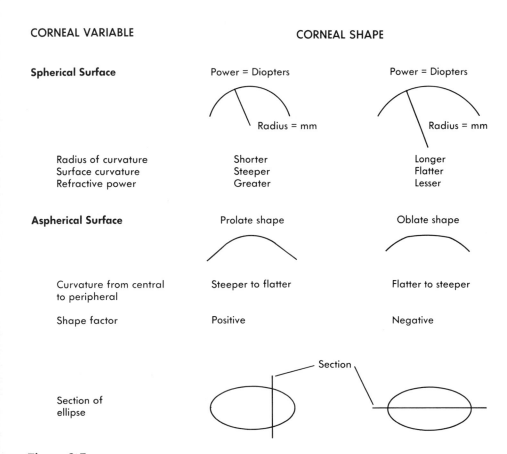

CORNEAL VARIABLE

CORNEAL SHAPE

Spherical Surface

| | Power = Diopters | Power = Diopters |
| Radius = mm | Radius = mm |

Radius of curvature — Shorter — Longer
Surface curvature — Steeper — Flatter
Refractive power — Greater — Lesser

Aspherical Surface — Prolate shape — Oblate shape

Curvature from central to peripheral — Steeper to flatter — Flatter to steeper

Shape factor — Positive — Negative

Section

Section of ellipse

Figure 3-7
Terminology used in describing corneal configurations. The left column indicates the corneal variables described. The right columns present terminology descriptive of the topography of both spherical corneas and aspherical corneas. (From Waring GO: Refract Corneal Surg 1989;5:360-367.)

Corneal asphericity

Since the corneal surface is not spherical, other terms must be used to describe its topography (Fig. 3-7). In general, there are two topographic patterns. The first pattern occurs in most normal eyes: the central cornea is steeper than the paracentral and peripheral cornea. This condition is referred to as a *positive shape factor* (positive because the radius of curvature becomes larger as one moves peripherally) and is also designated as a *prolate shape* (a term taken from the fact that it resembles a section across the steep end of an ellipse). The second topographic pattern occurs rarely in normal eyes but commonly after radial keratotomy: the central cornea is flatter than the paracentral and peripheral cornea, a condition referred to as a *negative shape factor* (negative because the radius of curvature becomes smaller toward the periphery) and also as an *oblate cornea* (because it resembles a section across the flatter side of an ellipse) (see Fig. 3-7).

Anatomic surface zones of the cornea

For practical and functional purposes, we can divide the surface of the cornea into two general regions: the central optical zone and the remainder of the cornea.[82] The optical zone is in the region of the cornea responsible for forming the foveal image. It corresponds to the entrance pupil of the eye projected onto the cornea. The rest of the cornea serves as a mechanical support structure, as a source of cells during normal turnover and repair, and as a refracting lens when the pupil is widely dilated or for off-axis objects in the peripheral visual field.

More conventionally, we recognize four concentric anatomic zones, the exact size of each varying from one eye to another: the central, paracentral, peripheral, and limbal zones (Fig. 3-8). These anatomic zones are useful to designate general locations on the cornea. For example, transverse keratotomies are placed in the paracentral and peripheral cornea; an excimer laser keratomileusis (photorefractive keratectomy) with a 5-mm diameter ablation zone covers the central and part of the paracentral cornea; a 9-mm diameter disc of cornea removed with a microkeratome covers the central, paracentral, and part of the peripheral cornea.

The reference center of these anatomic zones is the *geometric center of the cornea*. This is a different location than the *apex of the cornea* (which is the most anterior point on the cornea at its greatest sagittal height relative to the plane of the iris), the *pupillary axis* (which connects the center of the entrance pupil and the center of curvature of the cornea), the *line of sight,* which connects the fixation point with the center of the entrance pupil, the *visual axis,* which connects the fixation point and the center of the foveola, and the *optical axis,* which is the line perpendicular to the corneal surface that connects the optical centers of the cornea and the lens (see Chapter 16, Centering Corneal Surgical Procedures).

Quibbling over where one anatomic zone stops and another starts is fruitless because the surface contours gradually blend together and because there is variability among eyes.[42,63,90,96]

Central zone. The central zone is approximately 4 mm in diameter and has been called the optical zone, the corneal cap, and the central spherical zone, all terms intended to designate the more spherical, symmetrical, optically important portion of the cornea. It roughly overlies the entrance pupil of the eye. Anatomically, it is not concentric with the pupil, but optically the pupillary axis can be considered at its center.

The central 3 to 4 mm of the cornea is optically more important than the remaining cornea for two reasons. First, it is the largest portion of the cornea that overlies the pupil and refracts rays that form the foveal image; therefore it must be clear. Clinical experience has shown that the central clear zones in refractive keratotomy that are less than 3 mm in diameter are associated with more glare than those larger than 3 mm. This would be expected from the average size pupil. Similarly, Miller and Wolf[83] demonstrated that in corneal grafts, a clear "optical zone" of about 4 mm in diameter was necessary to prevent glare effects. Second, the Stiles-Crawford[38,109] effect states that light rays of equal intensity passing through the pupil are not perceived equally by the retina under photopic conditions. The more peripheral the ray, the less its perceived brightness. If the central ray is perceived as having a brightness of 100%, a ray 1 mm off-center appears 93% as bright, 2 mm off-center 71% as bright, and 3 mm off-center, only 41% as bright. The net result of these two factors, the pupil size and Stiles-Crawford effect,[109] is that the area of the cornea that forms the foveal image is only slightly larger than the pupil diameter of approximately 3 mm. The rays most central in this 3-mm zone are weighted most heavily and are therefore most significant in forming the foveal image. This fact must be included in at-

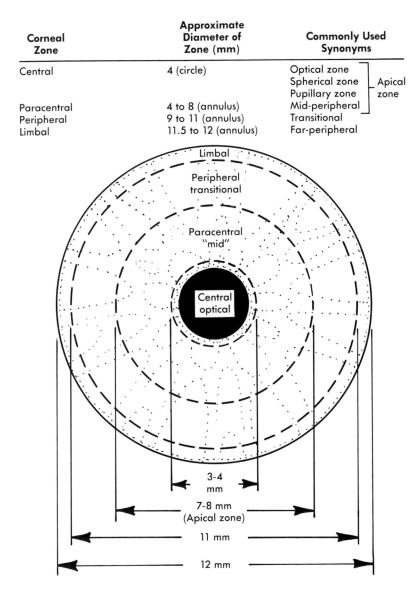

Corneal Zone	Approximate Diameter of Zone (mm)	Commonly Used Synonyms	
Central	4 (circle)	Optical zone Spherical zone Pupillary zone	Apical zone
Paracentral	4 to 8 (annulus)	Mid-peripheral	
Peripheral	9 to 11 (annulus)	Transitional	
Limbal	11.5 to 12 (annulus)	Far-peripheral	

Figure 3-8
Terminology for describing the *anatomic* (not the optical) topographic regions (zones) of the cornea, including the circular central zone and the three concentric annular zones. (From Waring GO: Refract Corneal Surg 1989;5:360-367.)

tempts to correlate topographic measurements of the cornea to visual acuity and visual function. Fortunately, the effective pupil diameter does not exceed 5.4 mm because of the Stiles-Crawford effect; even a 7-mm diameter pupil functions as if it were 5.4 mm in diameter. The central "optical zone" of the cornea must be considered optically more important than the paracentral and peripheral zones.

The term "optical zone" is used with four different meanings in the context of refractive surgery. The first meaning is that just defined, the central more spherical portion of the normal cornea overlying the entrance pupil. The second meaning refers to the portion of a keratomileusis lenticule, epikeratoplasty lenticule, or excimer laser surface ablation that creates the major refractive change; in this context it is possible to decenter the "optical zone." The third meaning is the central uncut clear zone in refractive keratotomy; the term "optical zone" (OZ) is so ingrained in the refractive keratotomy literature that is it not likely to disappear, even though the preferred designation is "clear zone." The fourth meaning of optical zone is the diameter of any circular mark on the cornea, for example, a "7-mm optical zone" used for placement of transverse incisions; in this context, "optical zone" is truly a misnomer and should be replaced by the simple designation "zone" or "zone mark," as in "the transverse incisions were placed at the 7-mm zone."

Paracentral zone. The paracentral, or mid, zone, an annulus from approximately 4 to 7 mm in diameter, is flatter than the central zone but is still generally spherical. The central and paracentral zones together constitute what contact lens fitters call the apical zone. After radial keratotomy, the paracentral zone is where there is a marked change in curvature—the "paracentral knee"—between the new central flatter and the peripheral steeper cornea. Some authors refer to this area as the "midperipheral" cornea, a misnomer because it does not occupy the middle of the periphery.

We must be careful about accurately referring to the area of the cornea that is measured by a keratometer or a keratoscope. Most of these instruments in clinical use measure 2.4 to 3.2 mm outside the central area. As long as the central-paracentral zones are approximately spherical, the clinician can infer the optical properties of the central cornea from keratometric measurements, but when there are distortions, such as those induced by refractive keratotomy, these inferences are less accurate, and a poorer correlation between keratometric and refraction measurements results.

Peripheral zone. The peripheral zone, an annulus approximately 7 to 11 mm in diameter, is the area in which the normal cornea flattens the most and becomes more aspheric. For this reason it has been called the "transitional" zone. Of course, after refractive keratotomy, the main "transition" in corneal curvature occurs in the paracentral zone. During refractive keratotomy the incisions are made in the paracentral and peripheral zone.

Limbal zone. The limbal zone is the rim of the cornea approximately 0.5 mm wide that abuts the sclera. It is usually covered by the limbal vascular arcade. A focal steepening occurs here adjacent to a small furrow known as the scleral sulcus. In general, this area is not incised during refractive keratotomy.

Apex and vertex of the cornea. The terminology identifying the point of greatest curvature, the high spot, and the center of a reflected image (such as a keratoscope image) has given rise to some confusion. This terminology has been clarified by Maloney.[73a] The point of greatest curvature of the cornea is commonly called the corneal apex. In a normal cornea the apex is a bit temporal to the center of the pupil, but after radial keratotomy the apex moves to the paracentral knee, which is the inflection point approximately 3 mm from the center of the clear zone. The vertex of the cornea is the point where the line from the fixation intersects the corneal surface at right angles. This point defines the center of ring 1 on a keratoscope image, such that the light from the first ring travels down the axis of the keratoscope, reflects off the corneal surface, and returns to the keratoscope along the same axis. This is possible only if the corneal surface is perpendicular to the axis of the instrument at the point of reflection. Therefore, this point is called the vertex normal. The corneal vertex does not necessarily coincide with the point of greatest curvature of the cornea (the corneal apex) as illustrated after radial keratotomy. Furthermore, the entrance pupil is not always centered around the corneal vertex; this is well known because in normal eyes the first Purkinje image generally lies nasal to the center of the entrance pupil. In eyes with keratoconus or with eccentric pupils, the disparity between the center of the first ring image and the entrance pupil may be much greater. The important clinical point to remember is that the cornea overlying the entrance pupil determines the image that enters the eye, whether or not that area of cornea contains the apex or vertex of the cornea. This principle is illustrated by the case in the box on pp. 52-53.

Directions on the cornea: meridians and axes

In geography a meridian is a line connecting the north and south poles, designated as latitudinal lines from 0 to 180 degrees east or west of the Greenwich prime meridian (0 degrees) and as longitudinal lines 0 to 90 degrees north and south of the equator. A specific location on the surface of the earth is designated by the intersection of latitudinal and longitudinal lines. In ophthalmology (Fig. 3-9), locations on the surface of the cornea are designated as meridians, lines that span the diameter of the cornea from one point on the limbus to the opposite point. Meridians are designated from 0 to 180 degrees, proceeding counterclockwise for both the right and left eyes.

The term "axis" designates the direction in a cylindrical lens along which there is no power; it is parallel to the focal line. Because clinicians align the axes of cylindrical lenses with meridians on the cornea, it is common practice to substitute the term "axis" for "meridian" when referring to directions on the cornea. Thus clinicians commonly refer to the steep "axis" when they mean steep "meridian," a habit that is unlikely to change. When a clinician says that a cylinder is placed at a certain axis, he or she is simply using a shortened way of saying that the cylinder is placed with its axis in a certain meridian. Such shorthand is acceptable. However, when clinicians refer to the "steep axis" of the cornea, the term "axis" is used incorrectly; the term meridian should be used when referring to the direction of corneal refractive power.

Locating meridians from 0 to 180 degrees is conventional. But, unlike geographers, ophthalmologists have no "north-south" convention to indicate a direction along a given meridian; there are no longitudinal lines to indicate a point along a specific meridian. Therefore clinicians designate locations around the circumference of the cornea in degrees, such as the "225-degree semimeridian."* Another convention is to consider the cornea as the face of clock so that 2:30 indicates the 45-degree semimeridian and 7:30 indicates the 225-degree semimeridian. This clock-hour system is too crude for refractive surgery, which requires more precision. (Where is an incision made at 1:45 o'clock?)

A specific point on the corneal surface is designated by indicating its location in millimeters from the center of the cornea along a semimeridian (Fig. 3-9). For example, at 6 mm along the 225-degree semimeridian the corneal power may be 42.00 D. Thus a transverse incision could be placed at the 6-mm zone centered on and perpendicular to the 225-degree semimeridian (in current jargon, "a T cut at the 6-mm optical zone at 7:30").

---

*The term "semimeridian" is etymologically correct, both components deriving from Latin roots; "hemimeridian" is a Greek-Latin hybrid and therefore less preferable.

Eccentric Corneal Vertex after Myopic Epikeratoplasty

A 24-year-old man with high myopia was referred to the Emory University Eye Center for consideration of myopic epikeratoplasty. He had been unable to tolerate contact lenses. In the left eye, visual acuity was 20/30− with a refraction of −26.00 +3.00 × 70°. Keratometric measurements in the left eye were 46.00 × 175°/47.75 × 85°, with regular mires. He underwent myopic epikeratoplasty with fresh donor tissue prepared with the BKS 1000 instrument. The tissue lens was centered over the pupil. The intended postoperative refraction was emmetropia. The postoperative course was uneventful, and 6 months after the procedure, best-corrected visual acuity was 20/40.

Two years after the procedure, visual acuity LE was 20/40+ with a manifest refraction of −0.25 +2.25 × 120°. Keratometric measurements were 40.25 × 145°/41.00 × 40°. The tissue lens and interface remained clear. Corneal topography was measured with the Corneal Modeling System. The image of the keratoscope rings (Fig. 1) revealed that the first Purkinje image of the fixation light was displaced to the edge of the pupil, and the mires appeared grossly irregular. The color dioptric map, however, revealed a relatively uniform area of marked corneal flattening superonasal to the center of the map (Fig. 2; see insert for color version) overlying the area of the pupil. To confirm the regularity of the cornea overlying the pupil, the patient was instructed to fixate to the left of the fixation light, until the first Purkinje image of the fixation light was approximately centered over the pupil. This resulted in fairly circular keratoscope mires (Fig. 3) and revealed regular corneal topography over the pupil (Fig. 4; see insert for color version) consistent with 20/40+ best-corrected acuity.

In this example, the first Purkinje image of the fixation light was markedly displaced from the center of the pupil, and appeared to lie on the shoulder of the tis-

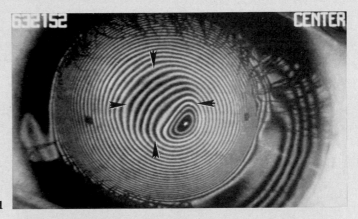

Figure 1

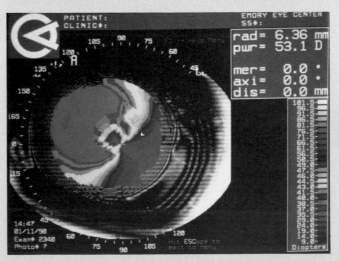

Figure 2

From Maloney RK: Refract Corneal Surg 1990;6:364-372.

Eccentric Corneal Vertex after Myopic Epikeratoplasty—cont'd

sue lens. The shoulder was the thickest part of the myopic tissue lens, and tended to bulge forward because the flange was rotated posteriorly to tuck into the lamellar keratectomy bed. As a result, the point on the cornea closest to the point of fixation could easily lie on the shoulder of the tissue lens; this point was the corneal vertex. This explained why the image of the fixation light lay on the shoulder, instead of nearer to the center of the pupil.

This example also illustrated the importance of location of the pupil in assessing corneal topography. The keratoscope mires appeared grossly distorted (Fig. 1) because they were centered over the shoulder of the tissue lens (the corneal vertex) rather than over the optical zone. The clinician might conclude from casual inspection that severe irregular astigmatism was present. The color dioptric map (Fig. 2) showed relative uniformity of the area over the pupil, but the regularity of the optical zone was best seen by altering the patient's fixation to center the image of the fixation light over the pupil (Figs. 3 and 4).

The location of the pupil explained the disparity between the change in keratometry and the change in refraction induced by the procedure. The change in average keratometric power was only 6.25 D, whereas the change in manifest refraction was 25.38 D. Because the keratometric image centered around the vertex normal, the postoperative keratometry readings were taken on the shoulder of the tissue lens rather than the optical zone. The color dioptric map revealed a curvature of 23.6 D in the center of the optical zone. The difference between 23.6 D postoperatively and the keratometric spherical equivalent of 46.88 D preoperatively was 23.28 D, which was much closer to the measured change in refraction.

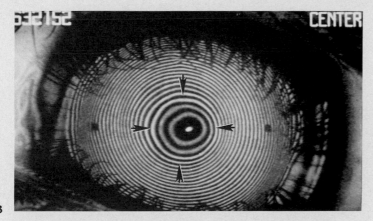

Figure 3

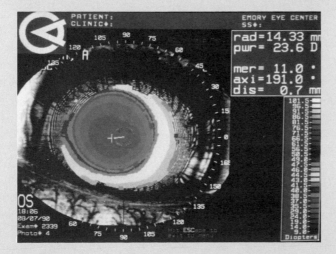

Figure 4

54

Direction of Refractive Power on the Cornea: Meridians and Axes from 0° to 180°

Meridian: Arc across the cornea from limbus to limbus along which corneal power is measured

Axis: Orientation of cylindrical lens where there is no refractive power

Examples of three power meridians or cylindrical axes:

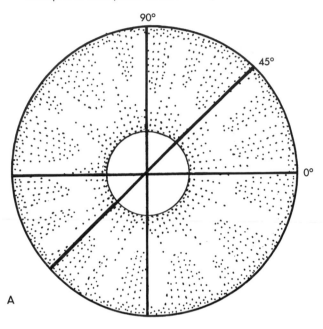

Locations on the Cornea: Semimeridians from 0° to 360° or from 1:00 O'Clock to 12 O'Clock Plus Distance from Center of Cornea

Examples of point locations on three semimeridians

Point **A** is located on the 0°, or 3:00 o'clock, semimeridian at 2 mm from the center. This is on the 4-mm diameter zone mark.

Point **B** is located on the 90°, or 12:00 o'clock, semimeridian at 3.5 mm from the center. This is on the 7-mm diameter zone mark.

Point **C** is located on the 215° semimeridian at 5 mm from the center. This is on the 10-mm diameter zone mark.

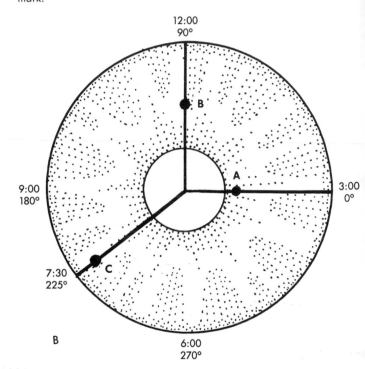

Figure 3-9
Directions and locations on the cornea. **A,** Terminology describing meridional directions on the surface of the cornea and the axes of correcting cylindrical lenses. **B,** Locations of specific points on the cornea are described in terms of the semimeridian along which the point lies and the distance from the geometric center of the cornea. (From Waring GO: Refract Corneal Surg 1989;5:360-367.)

Central corneal curvature, refractive power, and corneal topography

The cornea is the most powerful optical element in the human eye, contributing approximately 74% (43.50 D) of the total 58.6 dioptric power (Fig. 3-10). The cornea is convex anteriorly and concave posteriorly. The nominal anterior central curvature is 7.7 mm, and the posterior central curvature is 6.9 mm, resulting in a positive meniscus lens that is thinner centrally (0.54 mm) than peripherally (0.70 mm). It is bound anteriorly by the preocular tear film and posteriorly by the aqueous humor. The refractive indexes of the tear film and the aqueous humor are virtually the same at 1.336, and the refractive index of the corneal stroma is 1.376.[58] We discuss the keratometric index of refraction (1.3375) in the next section.

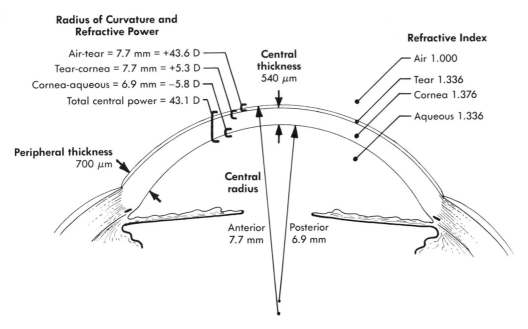

Figure 3-10
Measurements of the human cornea important in refractive surgery.

The total central corneal power of 43.1 D is the sum of the powers of each of the three optical interfaces: air-tear (+43.6 D), tear-cornea (+5.3 D), and cornea-aqueous (−5.8 D). If the curvatures of the anterior and posterior cornea were equal, the tear-corneal surface and the corneal-aqueous surface would have equal and opposite power and would add no net power to the cornea. However, because the posterior surface is 0.6 mm steeper than the anterior surface, the net effect from these two surfaces reduces the total corneal power by 0.5 D less than that in the air-tear film surface.

Topography refers to the shape of a surface, whether it be the surface of the earth or the surface of the cornea, as measured by a variety of methods, including contour lines, stereography, comparison with surfaces of known shape, and mathematical interpolation. The most common representation of a surface is a topographic map on which the relative elevations of the surfaces are delimited by contour lines. (For clarity, we point out that topology is not used to study corneal shape. Topology is a branch of mathematics concerned with the properties of a geometric surface that remain unaltered by deformations. The refractive power of the cornea is not a topologic property because it is altered by deformation of the cornea.)

Terminology of instruments used to measure corneal curvature and topography

Four categories of instruments are currently used to measure anterior corneal curvature: keratometers, keratoscopes, rasterstereography, and interferometers, each measuring a different area of the ocular surface (Table 3-3 and Fig. 3-11).

Keratometers. The original designation by Von Helmholtz in 1853 for an instrument measuring the central corneal curvature was "ophthalmometer," a term still used outside the United States. This is a good example of how colloquial usage can set linguistic standards. "Keratometer" is the trade name of Bausch & Lomb, but like Xerox and Kleenex, the commercial term has taken on a generic use. A keratometer implies manual operation. The term "autokeratom-

Table 3-3

Methods of Analysis and Measurement of Corneal Curvature and Topography

Method	Simple definition	Examples of instruments

Keratoscopy	Qualitative visual inspection of the reflected image	Single rings
		  Flieringa
		  Troutman/Weck
		Multiple rings
		  Flat
		    Placido disc
		    Klein keratoscope
		    Astigmatism Control Enforcer
		  Cone or cylinder
		    VanLuehnan
		    Maloney

Keratometry	Quantitative measurement of radius of curvature of central cornea using two spots approximately 3 mm apart	Central
		  Bausch & Lomb manual
		  Canon automated
		  Terry surgical
		Eccentric
		  Soper topogometer on Bausch & Lomb keratometer
		  Humphrey automated

Photokeratography	Qualitative photographic film picture of reflected mires; can be quantified with computer image analysis	Qualitative
		  Nidek photokeratoscope
		  Kera Corneascope
		Quantitative
		  KeraScanner

Videokeratography	Video picture of reflected mires with on-line quantitative digital image analysis of surface power	Computed Anatomy corneal modeling system EyeSys corneal analysis system
Rasterstereography	Video picture of grid projected onto corneal surface with on-line quantitative digital image analysis of surface elevation	PAR Micro Systems
Interferometry	Use of interference fringes to depict and quantify corneal surface contours	Kerametric corneal topographer

eter" refers to instruments that contain microprocessors and other electromechanical apparatus to record and print out the measurements. The single circular keratometer mire actually covers a 100-μm area of the paracentral cornea. The image is doubled optically so that the two areas lie approximately 3 mm apart. Therefore the keratometer samples a minuscule fraction of the ocular surface—two points on a circle approximately 3 mm in diameter. It assumes that the cornea between these points is spherical. Small mire keratometry can be done with special instruments to bring the two images closer together. Keratometry can be done at any location on the cornea using instruments such as the Soper Topogometer attachment on the Bausch & Lomb keratometer or the American Optical CLC keratometer, neither of which is currently marketed. Both have a fixation light that moves on x-y axes, which allows the patient to fixate eccentrically so that paracentral and peripheral keratometric measurements can be taken.

Keratoscopes and keratographs. The second category of instruments used to measure anterior corneal curvature is the keratoscope,[32] which projects a series of mires (most commonly, concentric rings) onto the surface of the cornea. The concentric ring mires are commonly called Placido rings, but strictly speaking

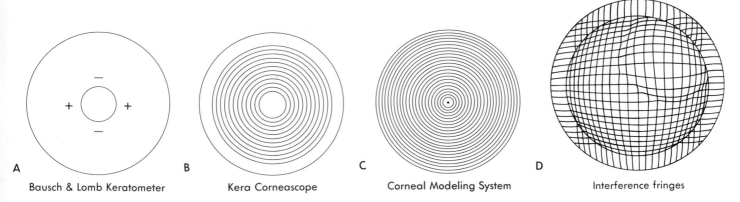

A Bausch & Lomb Keratometer   B Kera Corneascope   C Corneal Modeling System   D Interference fringes

Figure 3-11
Drawing shows the surface area of the cornea covered by mires of Keratometer, Corneascope, Corneal Modeling System, and an interferometer. **A,** The keratometer mires measure only two points approximately 3 mm apart. **B,** The twelve-ring Corneascope mires cover approximately 70% of the surface, omitting the central and peripheral zones. **C,** The Corneal Modeling System covers approximately 95% of surface. **D,** The interference fringes cover the entire cornea and limbus. (**A** to **C** from Hannush SB, Crawford SL, Waring GO, Gemmill MC, Lynn MJ, and Nizam A: Arch Ophthalmol 1989;107:1235-1239.)

that designation should describe only Placido's flat disc with the equally spaced circular black rings. Modern keratoscope rings may be unequally spaced, placed in a concave drum, and internally illuminated.

Keratoscopy is the direct observation of images of mires reflected from the surface of the cornea (Gk., *keras,* cornea + *skopein,* to see). The term is used in the same sense that examination of the ocular fundus with an ophthalmoscope is called ophthalmoscopy. Keratoscopy is a qualitative activity based on visual inspection and interpretation of the shape and spacing of the mires. Numerous types of instruments are used, including simple rings (Flieringa, safety pin), comparators (Hyde, Karichoff), and concentric rings (classical Placido disc, Klein keratoscope, Da-Lur slit-lamp mounted keratoscope). The pattern of the mires is interpreted in the orientation that it is observed, so a distortion of the mires at 12 o'clock indicates a disruption of the cornea superiorly; this is in contrast to conventional keratometers, in which the orientation of the mires is optically inverted 180 degrees, so a distortion of the 12 o'clock mires indicates a disruption in the cornea inferiorly at 6 o'clock.

If a photographic film camera is attached to a keratoscope, the instrument is called a photokeratoscope. If a television camera is attached to the keratoscope, it is called a videokeratoscope. "Corneascope" is the trade name used by Kera Corporation. Some have referred to a keratoscope as a "corneal topographer."[37] Keratoscopes vary greatly in the surface area of the cornea that they image, from the small sampling of a single circular ring to mires that cover the entire surface of the cornea (see Fig. 3-23).

The term "keratography" denotes a record or portrayal of the cornea in the same sense that photography records or portrays its subject. The resulting image is a keratograph. With photographic film, one uses a photokeratoscope to produce a photokeratograph (sometimes called a keratoscope photograph), a process called photokeratography—in the same sense that one uses a photomicroscope to take a photomicrograph, a process called photomicrography, or in the same sense that one does fluorescein angiography. With video recording, one uses a videokeratoscope to produce a videokeratograph, a process called videokeratography.

A keratograph can be interpreted qualitatively or quantitatively. A qualitative interpretation is achieved by visual inspection of the shape and spacing of the mires and has practical value in diagnosing corneal disorders, such as keratoconus, or in adjusting sutures after penetrating keratoplasty. Quantitative keratography is done by assigning numerical coordinate values to points on the mires and describing mathematically the curves that the points form. Because the corneal surface is asymmetrically aspheric, complex formulas and algorithms are required for accurate depiction of its topography. Both photokeratographs and videokeratographs can be interpreted quantitatively with the assistance of a computer that uses image analysis programs and is located either in a separate instrument (as in the Kera and the Nidek systems) or in the keratoscope itself (as in the Computed Anatomy, Visioptic, and EyeSys instruments—all computer-assisted videokeratoscopes).

Rasterstereographs. The third method to measure corneal topography is rasterstereography, which uses a direct image on the corneal surface. It projects a calibrated grid onto the fluorescein-stained tear film, takes a photograph, and uses computer algorithms to analyze the pictures. The geometry of the grid makes it possible to collect a mesh of equally spaced data points, in contrast to the circular ring mires, which provide data from semimeridians that are equal angles apart.[6,7] This creates an elevation map of the cornea.

Interferometers. The fourth type of instrument used to measure corneal topography and curvature is an interferometer, which uses techniques of light-wave interference. The interference fringes can cover the entire anterior ocular surface, not just the cornea. This includes both holography and moiré fringe techniques, but these are not in widespread clinical use because their resolution (a fraction of the wavelength of light) is so high that the eye must be stabilized to an extraordinary degree and the techniques of analysis must be extremely sophisticated.

Principles of keratometry and keratoscopy

Many textbook chapters and research articles describe keratometry and keratoscopy, and it is not our intention here to reiterate the optics, instrument mechanics, or clinical measurement techniques in detail.* We review only the theoretical and practical considerations that apply to refractive keratotomy.

Optical considerations. All keratometric instruments use the anterior corneal surface (that is, the surface of the tear film) as a mirror to reflect an object of known size. They measure the size of the reflected image and compute the radius of curvature and dioptric power of the cornea from that measurement. The basic principle is that a steeper cornea will reflect a smaller image than a flatter cornea (Figs. 3-12 and 3-13). In fact, one could measure corneal power by simply holding a coin of known size in front of the cornea and measuring the size of its reflected image with a ruler. However, three problems obviate this simplistic approach: (1) the distance from the object to the cornea would not be fixed; (2) the minified image reflected from the convex corneal surface would be too small to measure accurately; and (3) the constant microsaccadic eye movements would make the image a moving target. Clearly the inaccuracies of this crude approach are unacceptable.

Keratometers and keratoscopes have design features that compensate for these three problems. First, the instruments place the object a fixed distance from the cornea and allow the examiner to focus the object so that this distance between the object and the image is always constant. Second, a telescopic system of lenses magnifies the image so that it can be measured. Third, a prism-doubling mechanism creates two images that can be overlapped (in keratometers only), which neutralizes the ocular movements, since both images move the

*References 17, 19, 26, 36, 37, 61, 73, 84, 92, 94, 98, 101.

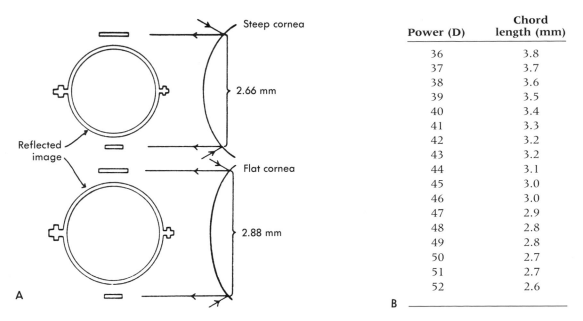

Power (D)	Chord length (mm)
36	3.8
37	3.7
38	3.6
39	3.5
40	3.4
41	3.3
42	3.2
43	3.2
44	3.1
45	3.0
46	3.0
47	2.9
48	2.8
49	2.8
50	2.7
51	2.7
52	2.6

Figure 3-12

The principle for quantifying corneal curvature using keratometers and keratoscopes. **A,** Drawing depicts relationship between corneal steepness, the chord length of the cornea, and the image size from the keratometer. A steeper cornea with a shorter chord length reflects a smaller image. **B,** Table lists minimum chord length necessary between the two mire images for several dioptric powers when measured with the Bausch & Lomb Keratometer. The steeper the cornea is, the closer together are the reflected mires. (From Dabezies OH and Holladay JR. In Dabezies OH, editor: Contact lenses: the CLAO guide to basic science in clinical practice, Orlando, 1987, Grune & Stratton.)

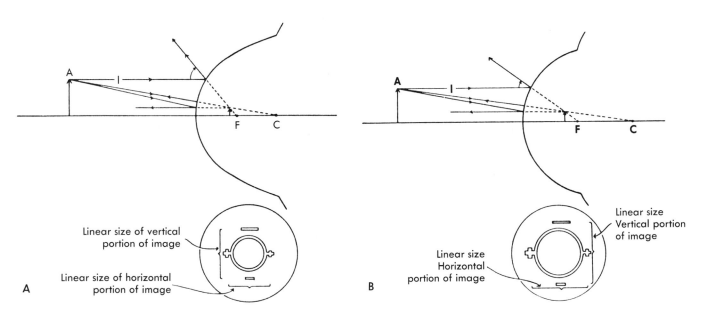

Figure 3-13

Optical ray trace diagrams demonstrate why steeper corneas reflect smaller images. **A,** Ray trace diagram shows that a steep cornea creates a small virtual image. The keratometry mires below are small. **B,** Ray trace diagram shows that a flatter cornea reflects a larger virtual image. The keratometry mires below are larger. (From Dabezies OH and Holladay JR. In Dabezies OH, editor: Contact lenses: The CLAO guide to basic science in clinical practice, Orlando, 1987, Grune & Stratton.)

same amount at any moment. The optical and mechanical details of these instruments are described by other authors.[50,84,110]

Once the size of the image is known, all other variables can be calculated. With most instruments, calculating the radius of corneal curvature assumes the cornea is spherical and the radius proportionate to the size of the reflected image. Once the radius of curvature is known, the refractive power of the cornea can be calculated based on an assumed index of refraction, an assumed corneal thickness, and an assumed radius of posterior corneal curvature.

For detailed analysis of corneal topography, the assumption that the cornea is spherical is inadequate. In fact, the normal corneal surface is asymmetrically aspheric. The amount of asphericity and surface irregularity increases after refractive keratotomy and corneal surgery in corneal disease, such as keratoconus or contact lens warpage. Thus keratometric and standard photokeratographic measurements as carried out in 1990 give useful approximations of corneal power and shape but do not describe it in accurate enough detail for sophisticated optical analysis. This is one of the reasons why there can be clinically meaningful discrepancy among the measurements obtained by keratometry, keratography, refraction, and visual acuity.

Surface area of the cornea measured. Keratometers and most keratoscopes sample only a portion of the corneal surface (see Fig. 3-11). Simple qualitative keratoscopes using a single ring image give information about the area of the cornea beneath the ring. The keratometer measures two 50-micron spots approximately 3 mm apart. A nine-ring photokeratoscope covers approximately 55% of the corneal surface. A 32-ring videokeratoscope covers almost the entire corneal surface. Rasterstereographs and interference fringes cover the entire cornea, limbus, and limbal conjunctiva. Of course, merely imaging the corneal surface is not adequate; the mires must be measured accurately and repeated, from center to limbus. As we state throughout this chapter, not all areas of the cornea are equally important in visual function. The most important area is that overlying the pupil (see Chapter 16, Centering Corneal Surgical Procedures).

The advantages and disadvantages of each of the different types of instruments are discussed in the following sections.

Keratometry—sampling the central cornea

The standard manual keratometers currently used in office practice are not significantly different from the original designs developed in the late 1800s[81] (Fig. 3-14). The instrument has proved itself practical and useful in measuring normal corneas, but it is less useful in measuring the changes induced by refractive corneal surgery.

Keratometric measurement of corneal power. In addition to the assumptions discussed in the preceding section, the calculation of the radius of curvature of the cornea is influenced by several factors: (1) the size of the target mires, (2) the distance of the target mires from the cornea, (3) the separation between the reflected images, and (4) the power of the objective. These factors can vary from one keratometer to another, so for consistent readings the same observer should use the same keratometer with the same eye piece setting for all examinations.

The relationship of the image and object sizes can be approximated by the following keratometer formula used to calculate the radius of curvature:

$$\text{Radius of corneal curvature} = \frac{\text{Distance between target and cornea} \times \text{Image size}}{\text{Target size}}$$

The image size is influenced by the area of the cornea used for the reflection. This area differs considerably among keratometers. For example, Ruben[96] has

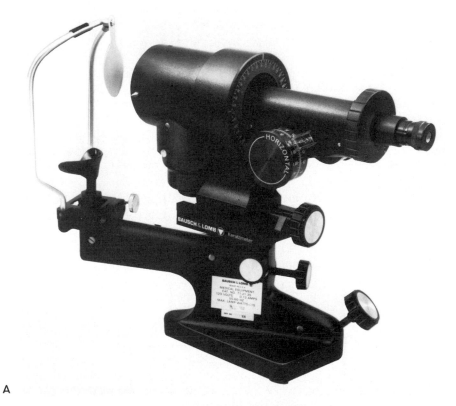

A

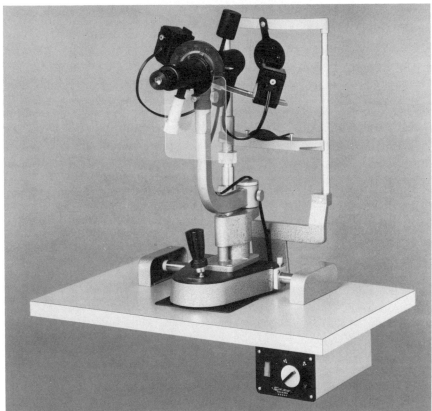

B

Figure 3-14
Two types of manual keratometers. **A,** Bausch & Lomb, which keeps the object size constant. **B,** Haag-Streit-Javal, which varies the size of the object.

demonstrated that the separation between the areas of reflection in different instruments varies from approximately 2.0 to 4.0 mm (Fig. 3-15). Similarly, the size of the area covered by the target itself varies from one instrument to another[65]: Bausch & Lomb, 0.1 mm; Zeiss & Gambs, 0.2 to 0.3 mm; Hagg-Streit, 0.3 to 0.4 mm.

The size and separation of the mires are important after refractive keratotomy because the target is reflected from the edge of a central zone 3 to 4 mm in diameter, where the ends of the incisions cause local variation in aspheric corneal curvature (Fig. 3-15). A keratometer with mires 2 mm apart reads inside the uncut clear zone, but one with mires 4 mm apart reads over the incisions. Thus the size and placement of the reflected mires may induce meaningful changes in measurement.

Once the radius of curvature is calculated on the keratometer, the dioptric power must be calculated according to the following simple spherical refraction surface formula:

$$\text{Power (D)} = \frac{\begin{array}{c}\text{Index of refraction} \\ \text{of cornea (n)}\end{array} - \begin{array}{c}\text{Index of refraction} \\ \text{of air (n}' = 1.00)\end{array}}{\begin{array}{c}\text{Radius of curvature of cornea (r)} \\ \text{in meters}\end{array}} = \frac{n - n'}{r}$$

The important variable here is the number selected as the index of refraction (n) of the cornea. A careful computation of this value requires use of the index of refraction of the three "lenses" that comprise the cornea: cornea-air, 1.336; cornea, 1.376; and cornea-aqueous, 1.336 (see Fig. 3-10). To simplify the calculations, keratometer manufacturers have calculated an assumed "keratometric index of refraction," which is used to convert the radius of curvature to dioptric power on the dial of the keratometer. The keratometric index of refraction is determined by a formula that assumes the thickness of the cornea to be 0.55 mm, the posterior curvature of the cornea to be 1.00 mm steeper than the anterior curvature, and the power for a radius of 7.5 mm to be 45 D. For most keratometers, this index is 1.3375. (It is 1.332 for the Zeiss and 1.336 for the American Optical instruments; the error induced by the different instruments is on the order of 0.2 D.) It is probably more accurate to make calculations about the cornea based on the radius of curvature itself, avoiding all of the assumptions that convert a radius of curvature to dioptric power. This practice is commonly followed by contact lens fitters but not by most ophthalmologists, who prefer to think in terms of dioptric power of the cornea.

Adjusting the parameters of the keratometer is not a revolutionary concept, given the historical fact that the keratometric index of refraction of 1.3375 was selected for the simple assurance that a cornea with a radius of 7.5 mm would have a power of 45 D.

When the cornea remains clinically unaltered and refractive correction is achieved primarily by spectacles, using the standard keratometric index of refraction (1.3375) is clinically valid, so a normal human cornea with a central radius of curvature of 7.7 mm has a power of 43.83. However, this validity is altered when the cornea is altered. For example, when a contact lens is placed on the cornea, it changes the radius of curvature of the air-tear film interface, and therefore the index of refraction of 1.336 for tears can be used for contact lens calculations, so a normal cornea with a radius of 7.7 has a power of 43.63 D. When an estimate for the total corneal power is desired, as for intraocular lens calculations or refractive surgery calculations, an index of 1.332 can be used, so a normal cornea with a radius of 7.7 has a power of 43.11 D. When a surgeon alters the cornea by refractive surgery, the standard assumptions on which the keratometric index of refraction was based are changed. Corneal thickness is decreased (as in keratomileusis) or increased (as in intracorneal

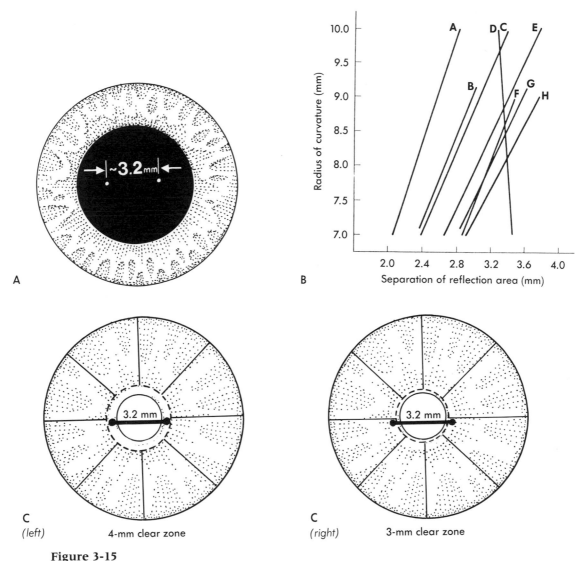

Figure 3-15

Location of keratometry mires image on cornea. **A,** Drawing demonstrates the location of the two mires projected from the keratometer that are approximately 3.2 apart. Keratometer assumes that the cornea is spherical between and outside the mires. **B,** The distance between the two mires is slightly different for eight different keratometers. Comparison of separation distance (mm) for eight different keratometers. *A*, Gambs; *B*, American Optical Company; *C*, Zeiss; *D*, Haag-Streit; *E*, Guilbert-Routit topographical, used conventionally; *F-H*, Bausch & Lomb. **C,** If keratometer mires fall in the uncut central clear zone after radial keratotomy, readings will be minimally disturbed by the scars and paracentral steepening *(left)*. If mires fall at the edge of or outside central clear zone, they will be affected by paracentral steepening and scars and will probably correlate more poorly with measured refraction *(right)*. (**B** from Layman PR: Optician 1987;154:261 and Mandel RB and St. Helen R: Br J Physiol Optom 1971;26:183-197.)

lenses), and these changes in thickness are not uniform across the cornea, so the anterior and posterior surfaces are even less parallel. Furthermore, adding lenticules to the cornea, such as those for epikeratoplasty or intracorneal lenses, alters the index of refraction within the cornea itself. All of these factors alter the accuracy of keratometric measurements after refractive corneal surgery[111] and require adjustments of keratometric readings to fit the clinical circumstance. For example, Arffa and colleagues[5] observed that keratometric measurements can better estimate the actual change in power of the anterior surface of the cornea after epikeratoplasty if the refractive index of the corneal stroma (1.376) is used instead of the keratometric index (1.3375). This makes the change in power of the anterior corneal surface approximately 11% greater (1.376/1.3375 = 1.114). Thus a cornea with a radius of 7.7 mm would have a power of 48.83 D. A similar adjustment could even be made for keratometric power calculations after radial keratotomy, in which the change in refractive power is commonly measured as approximately 0.50 D greater than the change in keratometric power.

Automated keratometers. Since 1980 numerous automated keratometers have become available (Fig. 3-16). These use the same basic principles as the manual keratometers but have smaller targets closer together to better describe the central "optical zone." These instruments have numerous convenience features, including operator-independent readings, digital displays, computation of astigmatism, printout of results, and a video screen for easier centration. Clinical trials comparing manual and automated keratometry show the automated keratometers to be equally or more accurate and reproducible.[34,56,68,112]

The instrument manufactured by Humphrey (Fig. 3-17) combines automated features with the ability to take eccentric measurements, one set of readings be-

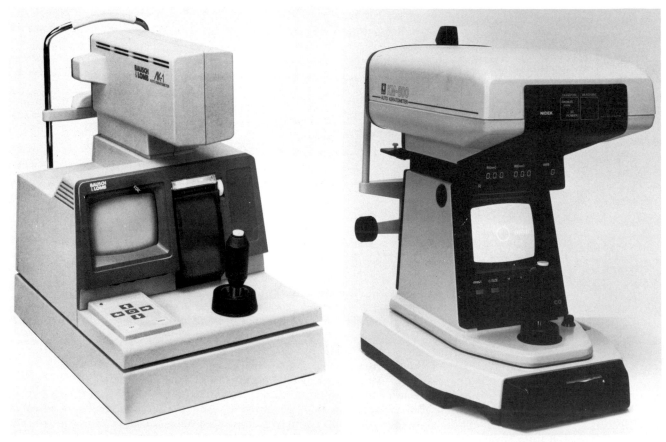

A   B

Figure 3-16
Two autokeratometers. **A,** Bausch & Lomb AK-1. **B,** Nidek KM-800.

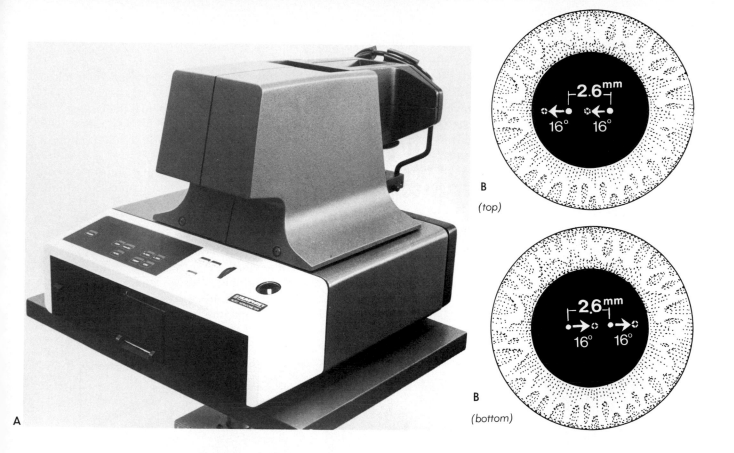

The Humphrey Auto Keratometer Printout

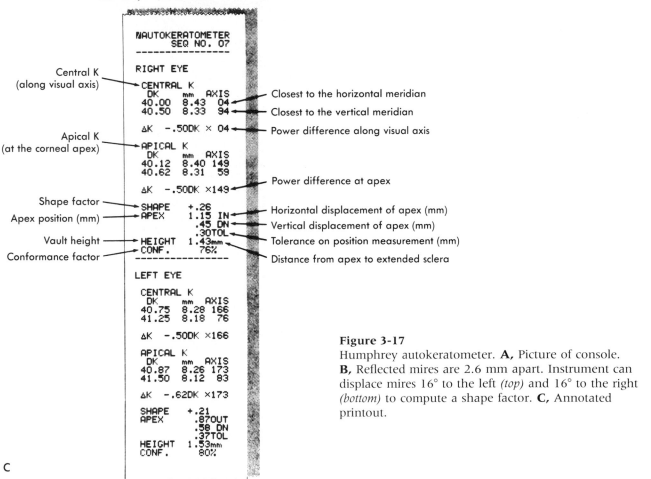

Central K (along visual axis) → CENTRAL K

DK	mm	AXIS
40.00	8.43	04	← Closest to the horizontal meridian
40.50	8.33	94	← Closest to the vertical meridian

ΔK −.50DK × 04 ← Power difference along visual axis

Apical K (at the corneal apex) → APICAL K

DK	mm	AXIS
40.12	8.40	149
40.62	8.31	59

ΔK −.50DK ×149 ← Power difference at apex

Shape factor → SHAPE   +.26 ← Horizontal displacement of apex (mm)
Apex position (mm) → APEX   1.15 IN
    .45 DN ← Vertical displacement of apex (mm)
    .30TOL ← Tolerance on position measurement (mm)
Vault height → HEIGHT 1.43mm ← Distance from apex to extended sclera
Conformance factor → CONF.   76%

LEFT EYE

CENTRAL K

DK	mm	AXIS
40.75	8.28	166
41.25	8.18	76

ΔK −.50DK ×166

APICAL K

DK	mm	AXIS
40.87	8.26	173
41.50	8.12	83

ΔK −.62DK ×173

SHAPE   +.21
APEX   .87OUT
    .58 DN
    .37TOL
HEIGHT 1.53mm
CONF.   80%

Figure 3-17
Humphrey autokeratometer. **A,** Picture of console.
B, Reflected mires are 2.6 mm apart. Instrument can
displace mires 16° to the left *(top)* and 16° to the right
(bottom) to compute a shape factor. **C,** Annotated
printout.

ing taken from the central cornea along the visual axis and a second being taken from the adjacent areas approximately 1.6 mm (16 degrees) on either side. The keratometer computes a shape factor, which would be positive if the cornea flattened paracentrally and negative if the cornea steepened paracentrally. Even with all this sophistication, the instrument samples only a minuscule portion of the corneal surface.

None of the automated keratometers has provided enough information to make them more advantageous after refractive surgery than manual keratometers.

Keratoscopy and keratography: measuring the corneal surface

Principles of keratoscopy. Since 1882 ophthalmologists have been projecting concentric rings onto the surface of the cornea, using the shape of the reflected image to map corneal topography. Conceptually, this is similar to measuring geographic elevations on the surface of the earth, from ocean floor to Himalayan peaks (Fig. 3-18), except that geographic topography deals with surface varia-

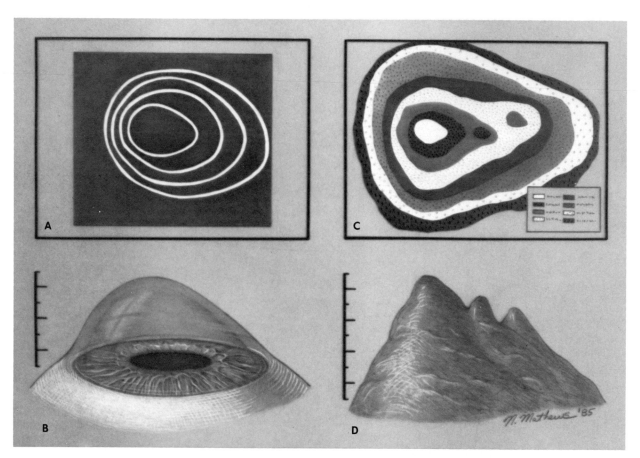

Figure 3-18
The principles of topography are similar for measuring the surface of the cornea, with variations of microns, or the surface of a mountain range, with variations of kilometers. Contour lines are used to depict the elevation and overall topography of the surface. **A** and **B,** In the corneal example, the keratoconus provides produces an asymmetrical protruding cornea with a certain elevation above the iris. The contour lines show that the cornea is steep on the left side of the picture where the lines are close together and flatter on the right side of the picture where the lines are further apart. **C** and **D,** Similar topographic map of a mountain range shows the contour lines of different elevations, for which a scale is provided. (Courtesy R. Doyle Stulting.)

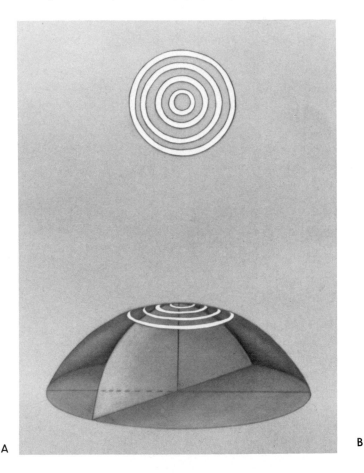

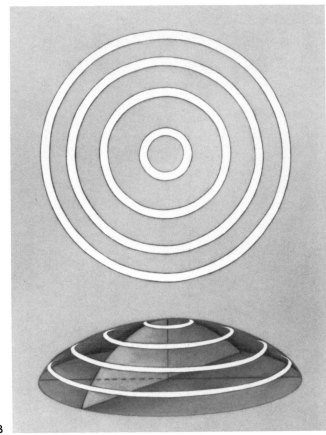

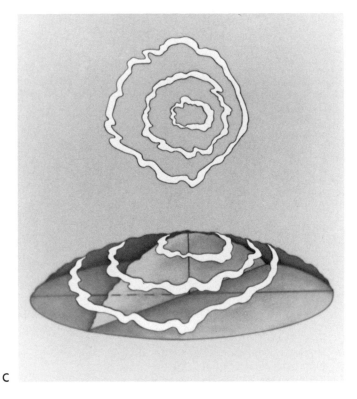

Figure 3-19

Drawings of typical keratographic patterns. **A,** A steep cornea reflects the rings closer together and narrower. **B,** A flat cornea reflects the rings farther apart and wider. **C,** An irregular cornea reflects the rings irregularly, but some topographic patterns can still be discerned, as in this drawing where the cornea is steeper on the right side and flatter on the left. (Courtesy R. Doyle Stulting.)

tions of thousands of meters, whereas corneal topography deals with surface variations of thousands of millimeters.

The qualitative analysis of keratographs using rings borrows the principles of geographic topography maps. A spherical cornea reflects round circles; steeper corneas have narrower circles closer together; flatter corneas have wider circles farther apart (Fig. 3-19). Corneas with regular astigmatism reflect oval mires in the shape of an ellipse, the lines being narrower and closer together in the steeper part of the cornea and wider and farther apart in the flatter part. Corneas with focal irregular astigmatism, such as that seen in the area of a tight corneal transplant suture, have contour lines close together in the steeper area of the cornea. Corneas with diffusely irregular astigmatism reflect rippling lines.

The image of most photokeratoscope rings covers the paracentral cornea, overlapping into the central and peripheral zones but leaving unmeasured the optically important central 2 to 3 mm as well as the peripheral cornea. In gen-

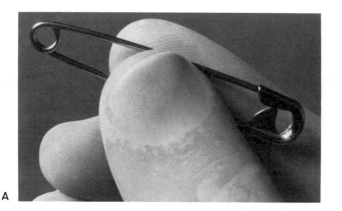

A

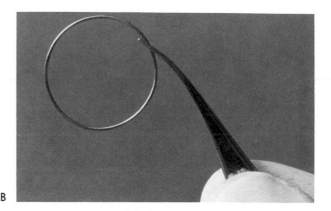

B

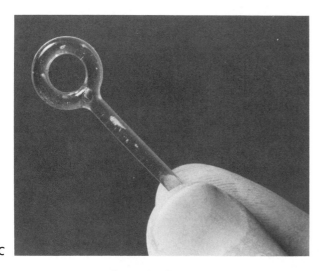

C

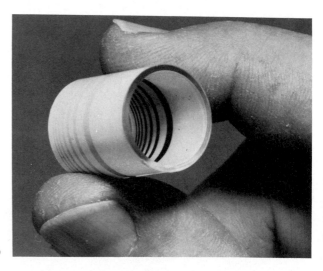

D

Figure 3-20
Examples of qualitative keratoscopes that can be used intraoperatively or clinically. All reflect an image of a circular object. The ovality of the object is proportionate to the amount of astigmatism. **A,** Safety pin. **B,** Flieringa ring. **C,** Barret plastic lolly-pop. **D,** Cylindrical keratoscope. **E,** Maloney conical keratoscope. **F,** Klein hand-held, internally illuminated keratoscope. **G,** Astigmatism control enforcer with applanation tonometer. **H,** Varidot quantitative operating keratometer (patient's view).

eral, the more rings the greater the surface area measured; current photokerato-scopes have 9 to 15 rings. Most of these instruments cover 55% to 75% of the corneal surface. Videokeratoscopes have 15 to 32 rings and cover approximately 60% to 100% of the corneal surface. The area of the corneal surface covered by the rings is inversely proportionate to the radius of curvature of the cornea: the steeper the cornea the less area measured. For example, on a 40-D cornea, the ninth ring of the Corneascope has a chord length of 8.3 mm, whereas the chord length on a 50-D cornea is 6.7 mm.

Qualitative keratoscopy. The numerous instruments available for projecting rings onto the surface of the cornea for qualitative assessment of corneal topography (Fig. 3-20) are useful for inspection of the cornea either in the clinic or operating room to identify gross distortions. They have neither a camera to create a permanent record nor a method to quantify the corneal curvature. The face of the instrument must be parallel to the plane of the iris and perpendicular to

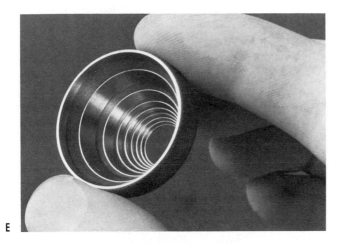

E

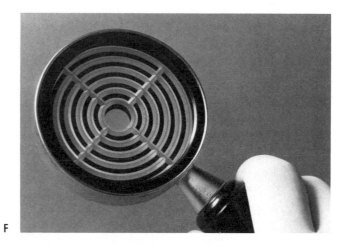

F

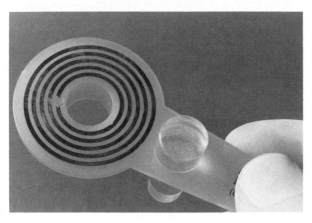

G

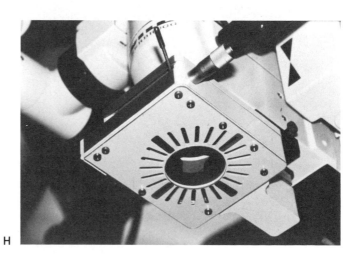

H

Figure 3-20
For legend see opposite page.

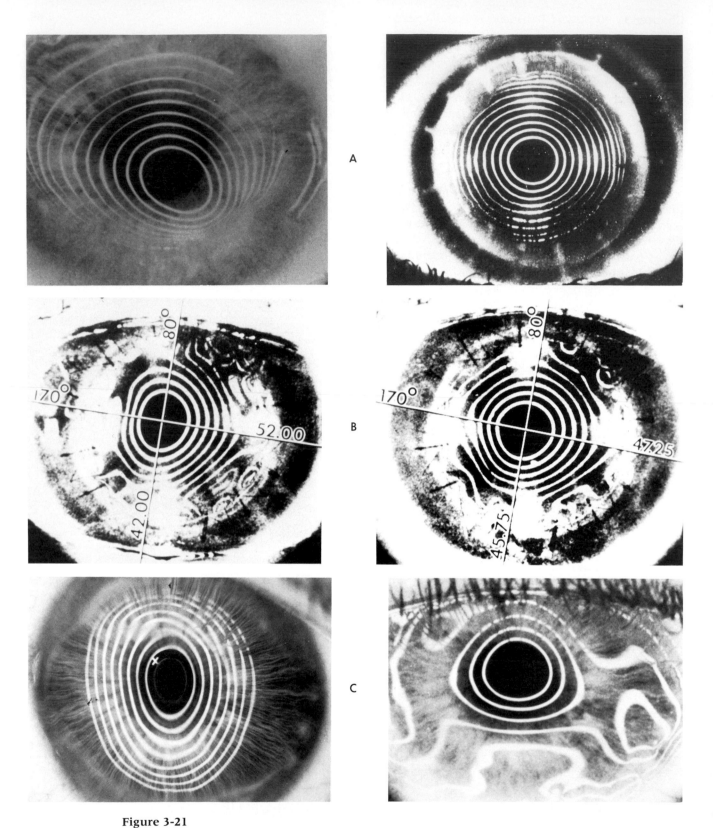

Figure 3-21
Examples of qualitative photokeratography. **A,** Epikeratoplasty for keratoconus. *Left:* Preoperative photokeratograph shows steep mires inferiorly. *Right:* Postoperative photokeratograph shows regular mires after suture removal. Peripheral scar is apparent on keratograph. **B,** Selective suture removal after penetrating keratoplasty. *Left:* Tight suture at 170° creating 10 D of astigmatism. *Right:* Suture removed, reducing astigmatism to 1.50 D. **C,** Terrien's marginal degeneration. *Left:* Before surgery keratography mires are vertically oval as a result of superior and inferior corneal thinning. *Right:* After crescentic resection superiorly, central mires are rounder, but now horizontally oval indicating overcorrection with vertical steepening.

the visual axis. It must be positioned so that the rings are in focus. Both good patient cooperation and a steady examiner's hand are necessary to detect subtleties in surface contours. These instruments help detect gross distortions (more than 3 D) of the cornea, such as in keratoconus or Terrien's marginal degeneration (Fig. 3-21), but they are not very useful in refractive surgery because of the need to quantify subtle changes in corneal shape. Therefore photokeratoscopes and videokeratoscopes have been devised.

Surgical keratoscopes and keratometers. An array of keratoscopes and keratometers is available for use intraoperatively (Table 3-4) to allow the surgeon to adjust the shape of the cornea and leave it in the desired configuration at the end of surgery. Currently no photokeratoscopes or videokeratoscopes are available for commercial use on the operating microscope.

There are three major problems with intraoperative keratoscopy and keratometry. First, it is difficult to obtain a good reflected image from the surface of the cornea during surgery because the surface is irregular, especially after penetrating keratoplasty. Therefore a balanced salt solution or a thin layer of viscoelastic substance must be spread over the surface of the cornea to fill in irregularities. This creates a new surface meniscus, so readings may not be accurate. However, it gives a clear image to detect the relatively large amounts of astigmatism (approximately 3 D or more) that must be present to be seen by qualitative visual inspection. During radial keratotomy, the reflection of mires off the ends of the newly made incisions gives highly variable results, and it is not possible to quantify the changes accurately during operation.

The second problem with intraoperative keratoscopy and keratometry is poor accuracy and reproducibility of measurements. The final problem is that the readings taken during surgery will change postoperatively as corneal edema subsides and wound healing progresses. Intraoperative keratometry may eliminate large amounts of astigmatism in the early postoperative period after cataract extraction or penetrating keratoplasty, but no study has shown it can predict the final postoperative astigmatism.[86]

On the other hand, intraoperative keratoscopy and keratometry can help determine the end point of astigmatism surgery, particularly when adjusting sutures at the conclusion of cataract extraction and penetrating keratoplasty and when performing arcuate transverse relaxing incisions after penetrating keratoplasty, as discussed in Chapter 31, Keratotomy for Astigmatism, and in Chapter 32, Atlas of Astigmatic Keratotomy.

Photokeratoscopes and videokeratoscopes. Creating a permanent photographic or video record of the corneal topography allows more careful qualitative analysis and enables quantitative analysis as well. The steps necessary to provide a properly quantified keratograph include the following[62]:

1. Obtaining a photokeratograph or videokeratograph for permanent analysis
2. Identifying the corneal contours as depicted by the pattern of the circular mires, including image feature recognition, extraction, and capture
3. Accurately analyzing the corneal shape by mathematical description of the topographic data to create a quantified representation of the corneal surface
4. Presenting the corneal topography in a manner that is understandable to clinical users, such as a color-coded contour map
5. Validating and testing the repeatability of the accuracy of the representation

Currently, videokeratoscopes are undergoing considerable development in both analytical computer algorithms and in the design of the clinical instruments. Much of this information is proprietary. Therefore we point out only some of the major features of these instruments.

Table 3-4

Selected Surgical Keratometers

Brand	Class	Compatible microscope	Display	Meridian identified	Accuracy (D)	Cost	Manufacturer
Karickhoff	Qualitative	All	Single ring	No	±2.50*	$54/box of six	Surgidev Corp., Goleta, Calif., (800) 235-5781
Barrett	Qualitative	All	2 bright concentric rings	No	±2.50		Graham Barrett 2 Verdun St., Nedlards, Western Australia, Australia G009 09 389 2811
Van Loehnan	Qualitative	All	7 concentric rings	No	±2.50*	$99/box of six	Jed Med Corp., St. Louis, Mo., (314) 968-0822
Maloney	Qualitative	All	7 concentric rings	No	±2.50*	$135	Jed Med Corp., St. Louis, Mo., (314) 968-0822
A.C.E.	Qualitative	All	5 concentric rings	No	±2.50*	$60	Hi-Line Medical, El Toro, Calif., (800) 524-6007
Troutman	Qualitative	Weck, Zeiss	Single ring	No	±2.50*	$600-$800	Edward Weck Co., Research Triangle Park, NC, (800) 334-8511
Amoils†	Quantitative	Zeiss	Analogue	No	±0.50	$1,950	Keeler Instruments, Broomall, Penn., (800) 223-9044
OV-1†	Quantitative	Zeiss, Wild	Analogue	No	±0.50	$3,750	Ophthalmic Ventures, Norwood, Mass., (800) 426-6713
Terry	Quantitative	Zeiss, Wild	Analogue or Digital	No	±0.25	Digital: $17,750-$18,000; Analogue: $8,000-$8,500	Innomed Corp., Brea, Calif., (714) 990-5740
Varidot‡	Quantitative	All	Analogue	No	±0.10	$8,000	Syscomp Surgical, Dunanville, Tex., (800) 544-4146
Zeiss†‡	Quantitative	Zeiss	Digital	No	±0.25	$13,881 to $14,115	Carl Zeiss, Inc., Thornwood, N.Y., (914) 747-1800
Nidek†	Quantitative	Zeiss, Wild, Topcon	Digital	Yes	±0.50 ±10 degrees	$19,000	Nidek, Inc., Palo Alto, Calif., (800) 223-9044

Modified from Frantz JM, Reidy JJ, and McDonald MB: Refract Corneal Surg 1989;5:409-413.
*Changes of less than 2.50 D are difficult to detect, even by an experienced observer.
†May obstruct view through observer scope.
‡Extends below the microscope toward the surgical field.

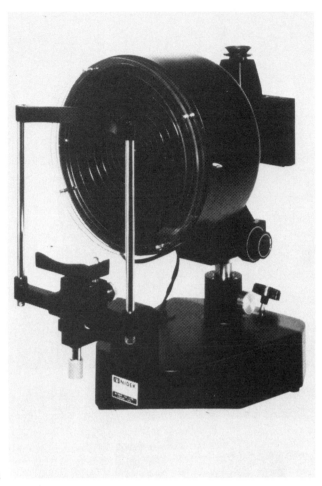

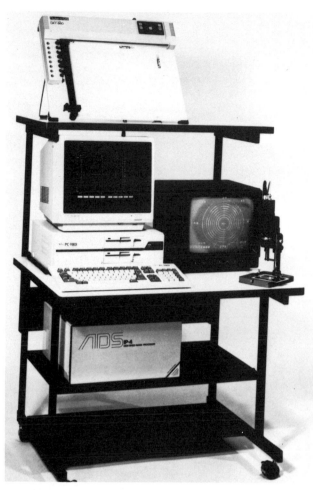

Figure 3-22
Nidek Photokeratography System. **A,** Flat photokeratoscope (PKS 1000) in front of
patient headrest. Polaroid film camera is mounted on back. **B,** Anterior Eye Analysis
System (EAS 1000) demonstrates photokeratograph placed beneath video camera
with image on video screen. Computer console and printer also are shown.

Current photokeratoscopes in clinical use (Figs. 3-22 and 3-23) consist of
small consoles, on the front of which are 9 to 12 internally illuminated rings
projected onto the patient's cornea. The patient's head is placed on a chin rest,
the photokeratoscope is manually centered and focused, and a Polaroid camera
photographs the image with a joy stick. It is somewhat difficult to take reproducible photographs because of problems of focusing and the dimensional instability of the photographic film and paper.

To quantify the photokeratoscope picture, the photograph is placed in an image analyzer that digitizes the circular mires and uses computer programs to
quantify the corneal curvature and power. The computer can produce graphic
representations of the corneal contour.

Rowsey and colleagues[93] tested the accuracy and reproducibility of the Kera-
Corneascope and Kerascanner in the PERK study. In studying the variables that
affect the results, they found the greatest variability was induced by the positioning of a steel ball in front of the instrument and by the personnel who performed
the image scanning of the photographs. Moving the photographs from one posi-

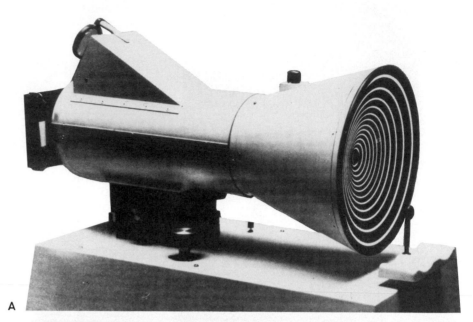

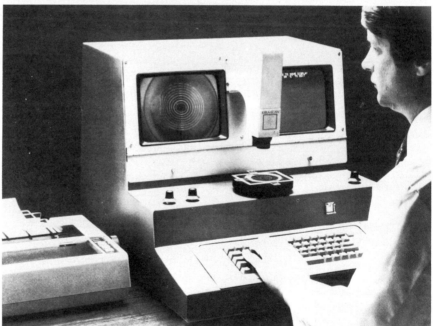

Figure 3-23
Kera Photokeratography System. **A,** Concave, 12-ring photokeratoscope (Corneascope) with Polaroid camera mounted on back and patient chin rest in front. **B,** Image analysis system (KeraScanner) shows photokeratograph placed beneath video camera with image on left video screen and computer console. Right video screen is for graphic presentation. Note printer at left.

tion to another induced a small amount of error. Very little was induced by the photographic process itself. They found that calibration balls could be photographed with a resolution of ±4 microns and that corneal photographs of patients can be repeatedly taken with a variability of ±40 μm.

Videokeratography uses a videokeratoscope that consists of 15 to 32 internally illuminated rings projected onto the cornea, the image of which is recorded with a video camera. The old style analog video cameras with Videcon vacuum tube detectors are inherently unstable, so modern units use digital video cameras that capture images on a semiconductor circuit, guaranteeing dimensional stability and more accurate recording. The digital video image can be quantified directly using mathematical algorithms in computer software. Graphic depiction of the corneal topography can be presented in four ways: as a direct picture of the keratoscope rings, as a color-coded topography map in which different colors are assigned different dioptric power values, as meridional cross sections of the cornea, and as three-dimensional graphic reconstructions.

The instrument in widest clinical use in 1990 is the Computed Anatomy Corneal Modeling System (Fig. 3-24 and Table 3-5). The narrow cone contains 32 rings and is placed inside the orbital rim so that the projected rings cover the entire surface of the cornea. The cone is difficult to use on patients with small orbits or those with deeply recessed eyes. The patient fixates a light centered in the cone while the operator aligns the rings around the patient's fixation point on the cornea with a joy stick. The operator focuses on the corneal surface by overlapping two helium-neon slit beams, which give a somewhat imprecise end point, or by placing a cross within a box. A series of still video images is captured on the screen. Details of the operation of the corneal modeling system have been published.[15,44] The company also markets the updated Topographic Monitoring System.

Proprietary algorithms provide a power measurement and polar coordinates for 256 points on each ring for which there is a clear image. The information is displayed as the corneal topography in a color-coded contour map, different colors corresponding to different radii of curvature and dioptric powers. New programs improve the accuracy and repeatability of the readings. A cursor can be moved on screen to identify the radius of curvature and dioptric power at any point on the corneal surface. The operator may take Polaroid photographs of the pictures displayed on the video screen to place in the patient's record.

The EyeSys Laboratories Corneal Analysis System[65] (Fig. 3-25) uses a planar Placido disc with eight illuminated rings that are projected on the cornea, and the image is captured with a video camera; proprietary algorithms measure at each light-dark interface, thus permitting acquisition of 16 rings. It covers an annulus of 1.5 to 8 mm diameter and can read a range of 9 to 99 D. It also can be measured in radii of curvature (mm). Fixation, as in other systems, has to be perfected, and the zone diameter covered depends on the steepness of the cornea. The display format includes keratometric data, tabular data, contact lens maps, profile graphs, color map functions with comparative isodioptric maps (with a difference map option), data overview, and an optional display of the eye image (see Table 3-5).

The Computerized Corneal Topographer (EH-270)[36] (Fig. 3-26) projects 22 rings on the cornea, covering most of the corneal surface. It produces color-coded, cross-sectional maps of the cornea, which emphasize astigmatism and asphericity along meridians of the cornea in 10-degree steps.

The Nidek videokeratoscope (Fig. 3-27) is a compact console with 15 rings that almost cover the entire corneal surface and are focused by an infrared auto-focusing device. An imaging process computer within the console uses algorithms based on a conocoid curve to produce keratometry readings in the center

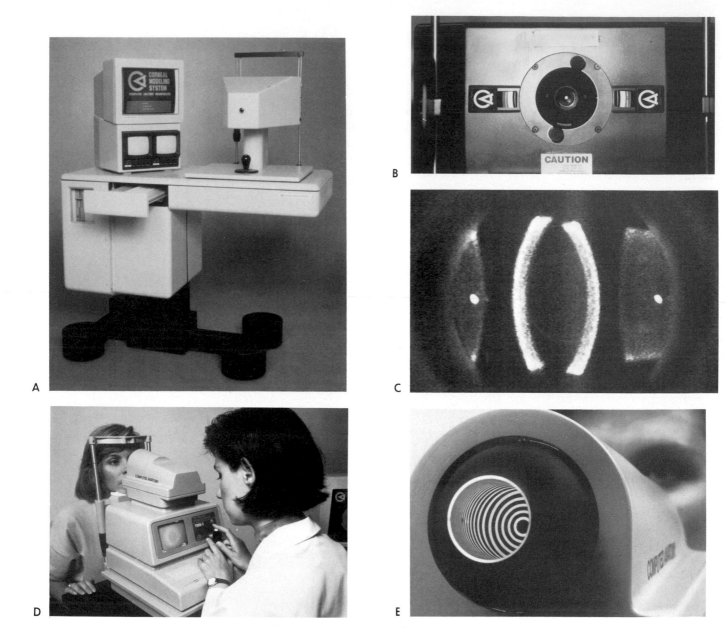

Figure 3-24
A, Computed Anatomy Corneal Modeling System. View from operator's side shows video screen, computer keyboard, and joystick. **B,** View from patient's side shows chin rest and cone containing illuminated rings. The helium-neon slit beams enter either side of the cone. **C,** The two helium-neon slit beams intersect the cornea. When they are overlapped with the front edge of one touching the back edge of the other, the instrument is in focus. The beams also allow digitizing of the anterior and posterior contours of the cornea and the determination of corneal thickness. **D,** The Topographic Modeling System (TMS) is a smaller version that measures topography but not corneal thickness. **E,** The TMS cone contains concentric rings that are projected over most of the corneal surface.

Table 3-5

Specifications for Two Videokeratoscopes (March 1991)*

Components	Computed Anatomy, Inc. Topographic Modeling System	EyeSys Laboratories Corneal Analysis System
IBM AT compatible computer	Yes (386)	Yes (386)
101 key-enhanced keyboard	Yes	Yes
Hard disc drive	Yes	Yes
Floppy disc drive	Yes	Yes
High-resolution CCD video camera	Yes	Yes
Monitors	14″ high-resolution color and 5″ black and white	14″ color monitor
Motorized table	Yes	Yes
Keratoscope	Solid-state light cone; patented	Conical Placido
Optionals		
Change of keratoscope for greater coverage	Yes; requires cone replacement only	No
High-speed computer upgrade	Yes	Yes; to 33 mHz
Polaroid hard copy camera	Yes	Yes
Ink jet color printer	Yes	Yes
Specifications		
No. of rings	25 to 32	8 (16 edges; 360 pts/edge)
Area of coverage	Entire cornea 0.5 to > 11 mm	Entire cornea 0.7 to 9.6 mm at 42.50 D
Focus	Laser range finder	Paired focus light beams
Color map	Shows analyzed area; fail-safe prevents plotting missing or false data; continuous edges; no nose shadow	Circular map; distinct error colors; jagged edges; presence of nose shadow
Proprietary software	Yes	Yes
Pupil detection algorithm	Yes	Yes
Contact lens fitting program	Yes	Yes
Numerical map	Yes	Yes
Profile graph	No	Yes, at 1-degree increments
Normal and absolute scales	Yes	Yes
Selectable scales	Yes	Yes
Map data subtraction	Yes	Yes
Multiple maps	Two to three on screen	Two to four on screen
Diopter range	10 to 100 D	9 to 99 D
Accuracy	±0.2 D	±0.2 D
Processing speed	Variable (> 10 sec)	Variable (> 10 sec)
Base system price	$24,950	$21,500

*The comparisons do not include qualitative features such as (1) user and patient comfort and convenience and (2) display capabilities, which are frequently changed and improved.

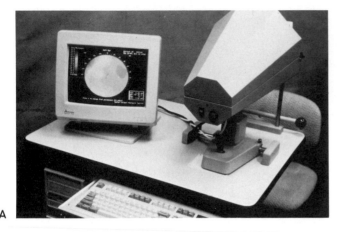

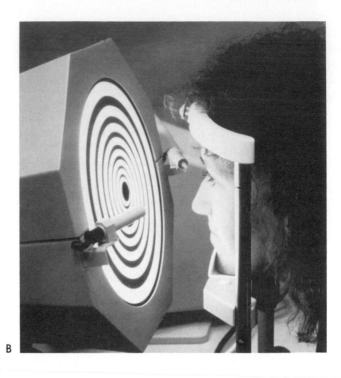

A

B

Figure 3-25

The EyeSys Corneal Analysis system demonstrates the computer housed in the lower left of the instrument along with a keyboard. The display monitor is on the top of the table on the left. The housing for the Placido disc is moved with a joystick. The disc can be either flat or conical, depending on the type of machine used. **A,** View from the examiner's side. **B,** View from the patient's side. The patient's head is placed on a chin rest, and the patient fixates an object in the middle of the Placido rings. Focusing is done by placing two cross-hairs within circles located approximately at the limbus and viewed by the examiner on the monitor.

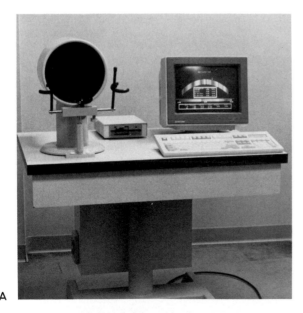

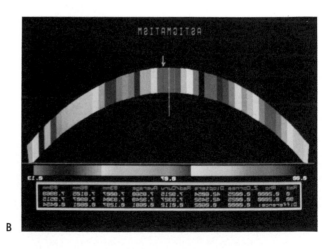

A

B

Figure 3-26

Computerized Corneal Topographer. **A,** Console shows concave keratoscope with patient chin rest, computer disc drive and keyboard, and video display terminal. **B,** Example of printout showing cross section of cornea with astigmatism presented as colors codes, seen here as different shades of gray, black, and white. Numerical tabulation below shows readings at the 0° and 90° meridia and computes the differences for corneal curvature, corneal power, radius of curvature, and the radii at 3-, 6-, and 9-mm zones. (Courtesy S. El Hage.)

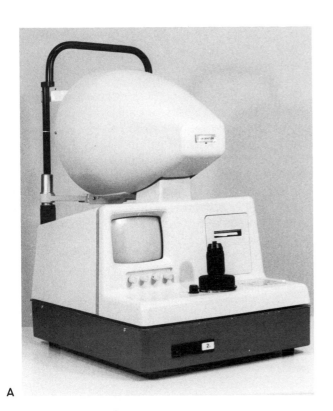
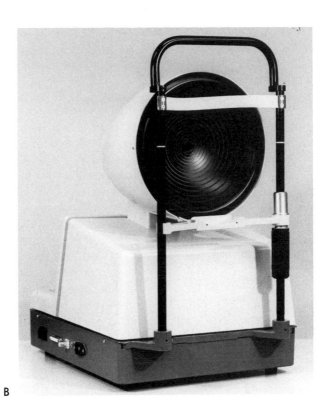

A   B

Figure 3-27
The Nidek SK-2000 videokeratography system consists of a 15-ring faceplate that is
coarsely focused with the joystick, as seen on the small television screen, and then
autofocused by an infrared device. The built-in image processing computer gives radius of curvature readings along eight semimeridians and prints out the values on a
paper printer, with calculations of contact lens fit.

and along eight meridians and has the ability to create wire-mesh graphics and
color-coded maps of corneal power based on the 120 points imaged. The instrument has special algorithms for calculating the fitting of hard and soft contact
lenses.

Taunton Technologies has a digital keratoscope incorporated into its excimer
laser beam delivery.[66] The device consists of a spherical array of 104 light-
emitting diodes. Beams from these reflect from the patient's cornea to an image
analyzer. The stored image is analyzed by proprietary algorithms to determine
the optical power distribution over the central 7 mm of the cornea with an accuracy of 0.3 $\pm$0.15 D.

New instruments, improved analytical algorithms, and increasingly user-
friendly displays are certainly in the future. The integration of videokeratoscopes
with other instruments, such as scanning laser ophthalmoscopes, autorefractors
with regional weighting, and laser corneal surgical instruments, will create advanced diagnostic and therapeutic systems.

Clinical keratography. Taking keratographs appears easy but requires careful
technique. The patient's eye must be open widely to decrease shadows from the
eyelashes and eyelids, the head turned to decrease nose shadows. The patient
must fixate well to center the keratograph. The image of the keratoscope rings
will center around the apex of the cornea (the vertex normal); this location is
not coincident with the line of sight, the geometric center of the cornea, or the
center of the pupil, especially after refractive corneal surgery. The image of the
rings must be properly focused to establish a known distance between the in-

strument and the cornea to serve as a basis for quantitative measurement. The instrument must be accurately calibrated, either internally or by taking a picture of a calibration ruling, such as a Ronchi ruling. The patient should blink just before the photograph to decrease surface-drying artifacts.

Qualitative keratography. The keratograph can be used in qualitative analysis to describe the distortion pattern of the rings. This can help diagnose keratoconus (pear-shaped pattern displaced anteriorly) and can identify tight sutures (indented, D-shaped, or oval mires) during selective suture removal to reduce astigmatism after penetrating keratoplasty. The overall pattern of the rings depicts the amount of astigmatism, both regular and irregular, and is useful clinically in explaining decreased visual acuity when the cornea appears clear, compact, and smooth by slit-lamp microscopy. However, to detect and measure subtler changes in the cornea that occur after refractive keratotomy, accurate and reproducible quantification of the keratographs is necessary.

Quantitative keratography. To quantify the keratograph, the image is digitized manually or by an image analyzer. Manual methods require a digitizing pad to mark specific points at defined locations on each of the mires, an inherently inaccurate and time-consuming procedure.[61] Using photogrammetric or automated image scanning densitometric techniques, the keratographs can be analyzed, as is done in the Kera Corporation Kerascan unit.[90] However, only a limited number of points can be scanned, and the inaccuracies of photographic recording remain. The most accurate and reproducible method in current clinical use for quantifying keratographs is digitizing the video image directly off a frame grabber, which permits storage in computer memory, as is done with modern videokeratoscopes. This allows recording a large number of points, corresponding to the 512 × 512 pixel array on the video image.

Each point is located along a series of defined coordinates (Fig. 3-28), which allows the mathematical formulae and computer algorithms to identify its location and reconstruct the surface. Mires that approximate a circle or straight line are easier to quantify; aspheric or distorted corneal surfaces make it more difficult to create algorithms that quantify the irregularities. In general, measurements of more points on a corneal surface allow a more accurate depiction of the surface because there is less interpolation between the points.

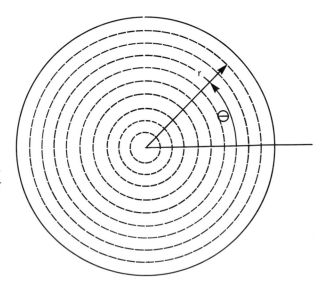

Figure 3-28
The Corneal Modeling System represents the processed keratoscopic data in polar coordinates. Three variables locate each corneal point in space. Theta shows its semi-meridian location. Its distance from the calculated center point is r_s. Its sagittal location, Z (not shown), is determined by proprietary algorithm. The ray tracing programs use these data and the corneal power calculation of each point to make the point-spread function. (From Camp JJ, Maguire LF, Cameron BM, and Robb RA: Am J Ophthalmol 1990;109:379-386.)

Quantifying corneal topography requires complex, refined mathematical equations based on optical principles and the assumptions that the cornea is a sphere or a spherocylinder, or that it has definable aspheric contours. The closer these assumptions approximate the actual shape of the cornea, the more accurate the mathematical reconstruction. As discussed previously, such a quantitative analysis depends on knowing two facts about the reflected image of the rings—their size and their shape. In a previous section, we discussed how the size of the reflected mires is determined by corneal curvature (a smaller radius of curvature with a steeper cornea produces a smaller reflected image), and we emphasized that the distance between the object rings and the corneal surface must be known. Keratometers fix the distance to the cornea through its narrow focus depth, but keratoscopes project target rings that do not lie in the same plane, so the depth of focus must be large enough to allow all the rings to be in focus: it is difficult to know the exact distance between each target ring and the corneal surface, creating less accurate and reproducible measurements. The Corneal Modeling System solves the focusing problem by superimposing two He-Ne laser beams on a cross in a square, which is more accurate.

A more difficult problem to solve, however, is the assumption concerning the shape of the corneal surface. Most algorithms assume the cornea is a sphere, thereby explaining the circular profile of the rings. The assumption is then made that the rings are centered on the sphere and that the circular ring can be used to measure the radius of the corneal curvature along any meridian. Of course this assumption is only an approximation, since the cornea is asymmetrically aspheric. However, it has practical clinical value because the central zone of the cornea approximates the sphere.

The methodology used to quantify the ring images involves measuring short arcs along one of the innermost rings and using the measurements as a starting point to calculate the arc of the second ring, the third ring, and so forth until enough information is available to construct a profile of the cornea along any semimeridian as a series of short-connected arcs.[30] This method produces an estimate of the refractive power of the cornea at each point, since the dioptric power is proportional to 1/radius of curvature of the arc.

Another difficulty in using reflected rings to calculate the corneal profile is the assumption of coplanarity, which postulates that the incident ray of light from the target to the cornea and the reflected ray of light from the cornea back to the keratoscope's imaging lens lie in the same plane as the corneal apex.[30] Of course this assumption is true only if each semimeridian of the cornea has an identical profile, which is not the case. Therefore rays of light reflected from the cornea return to the keratoscope's imaging lens at a skewed angle. To solve the problem of coplanarity of the incident and reflected light rays requires an analysis of the corneal surface in three dimensions.

As quantitative keratography improves, the foregoing simple assumptions will be replaced by those more complex. The ability to measure the distance from the object to the image exactly on the surface of the cornea will improve. The assumption that the cornea is spherical will be replaced by other assumptions using more accurate surfaces, such as ellipses and aspheric surfaces, to describe corneal topography. The power calculations will use ray tracing based on Snell's law of refraction (Fig. 3-29). Details of the mathematics of these approaches are beyond the scope of this text but have been presented elsewhere.*

Once a completely accurate depiction of corneal topography is possible, a daunting problem still remains: the creation of a clinically understandable and useful method of quantifying and classifying the surface. The color-coded maps

*References 21, 30, 34, 37, 61, 76, 114.

of the distribution of dioptric power on the cornea are useful and present information that allows an observer to read the pattern of the cornea and even to detect certain familiar corneal diseases, such as keratoconus. However, if topography is to be used as a basis to predict the response of corneas to refractive surgery, quantify the results of corneal surgery, and correlate with visual function, it is necessary to develop quantitative descriptors of the shape of the cornea, both over the pupil and from limbus to limbus.

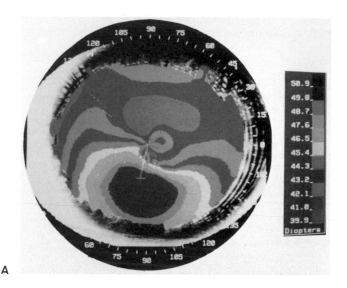

A

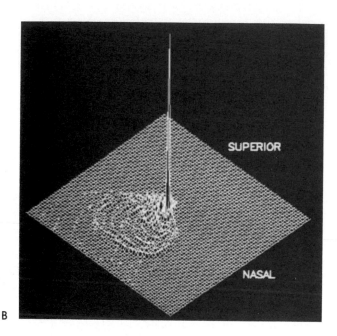

B

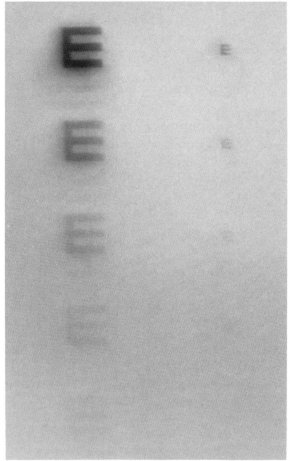

C

Figure 3-29
Computer model of corneal optical performance using ray tracing. **A,** Contour map shown here in different shades of gray, black, and white of patient with keratoconus demonstrates steep area inferior to the center. Best-corrected visual acuity was 20/20 with a −2.50 D sphere. (See insert for color version.) **B,** Computer graphic demonstration of the point spread function derived by ray tracing analysis of the cornea depicted in **A.** A perfect lens system would focus all light at a single point. The keratoconus cornea produces a high amplitude central peak of "good acuity" with a low amplitude asymmetrical peripheral spread that would degrade the image. **C,** Images of Snellen letter E generated by ray tracing analysis for the keratoconus cornea shows that the larger letters (20/80) are resolved to 6.25% contrast with an obvious ghost image that surrounds the lateral and inferior parts of the letter. The smaller image (20/20) is recognizable to 25% contrast. (From Camp JJ, Maguire LF, Cameron BM, and Robb RA: Am J Ophthalmol 1990;109:379-386.)

Comparison of keratometry, photokeratography, and videokeratography

Hannush and colleagues[45,46] have studied the accuracy and repeatability of keratometry, photokeratography, and videokeratography on steel test balls of varying radii of curvature and on normal human eyes. They found that the Bausch & Lomb Keratometer and the Computed Anatomy Corneal Modeling System were more accurate and repeatable than the Kera Corneascope ($p <$ 0.01) (Fig. 3-30). Of the 32 rings projected on the surface of the steel balls by the Corneal Modeling System, rings 2 through 26 on test balls with powers of 39 and 43 D were read accurately and reproducability; the ball with steeper curvature of 50 D gave more variable readings.

On normal human corneas the keratometer read most consistently, the Corneal Modeling System next, and the Corneascope the least (Fig. 3-31). Of the 31 rings projected on the surface of the cornea by the Corneal Modeling System, rings 1 through 27 were read by the software; rings 2 through 20 could be interpreted; and rings 3 through 9 were read with a precision of 0.50 D.

As improved mathematical descriptions of aspheric surfaces and improved computer algorithms to handle the data from keratographs are devised, improved accuracy and precision can be expected from the images produced by keratoscopes.

Corneal modeling: measuring corneal topography and thickness

Although most of the ocular refraction occurs at the tear-air interface, corneal thickness and posterior corneal curvature also play a role in refraction, as discussed previously under keratometry. Current keratometers and keratoscopes make assumptions about corneal thickness and posterior corneal curvature when computing corneal power based on anterior surface measurements. Some instruments also can measure corneal thickness to create a geometric model of the cornea. Three technical approaches have been used to do this: helium-neon laser slit beams on the Computed Anatomy Corneal Modeling System, confocal microscopy on the Heidelberg Instruments Laser Tomographic Scanner, and Scheimpflug photography in an experimental system from IBM in Paris.

The Computed Anatomy system has two helium-neon slit beams that intersect the cornea and serve as a focusing device on current models. The image of these slit beams can be captured on video, allowing measurement of both the anterior and posterior contours of the cornea. Interpolating between multiple slit-beam images creates a graphic model of anterior and posterior corneal surfaces.

The Heidelberg Instruments Laser Tomographic Scanner (Fig. 3-32) uses a laser slit to scan small areas of the cornea. The density of the reflected light is measured by a confocal microscope. Multiple measurements are made over the surface and through the thickness of the cornea, and computer programs construct a model of the cornea.

A third approach has been taken by Hanna and colleagues at IBM in Paris (personal verbal communication, November 1989), where they have used a Scheimpflug camera that provides a light beam with great depth of focus (Fig. 3-33). Multiple slits are projected across the cornea, and the images are stored in a computer and analyzed, measuring the anterior and posterior curvature and thickness. The resulting curves are interpolated and converted to a graphic model of the cornea.

At the time of this writing, all of these modeling instruments are being used experimentally and are undergoing improvement and modification. All share a drawback: they sample only small, selected, cross-sectional areas of the cornea and must interpolate between these small areas based on mathematical assumptions to construct the graphic, quantitative "model" of the cornea.

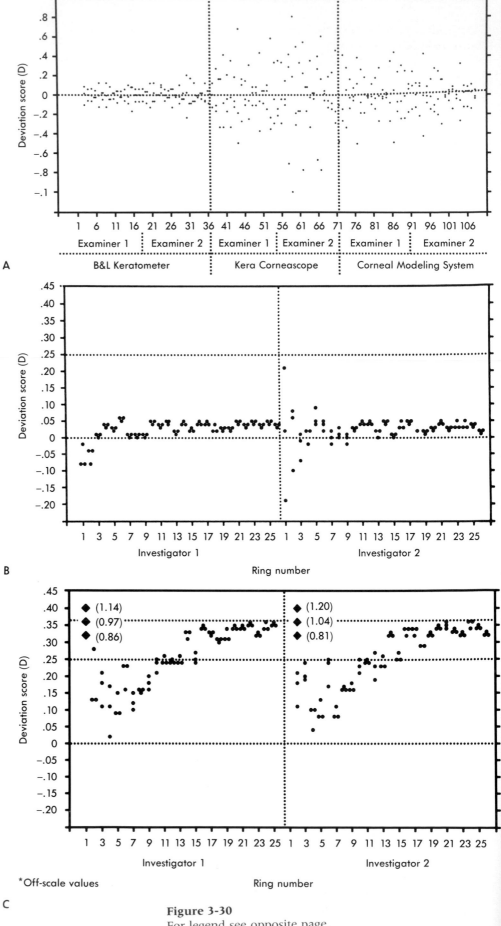

A

B

C

*Off-scale values

Figure 3-30
For legend see opposite page.

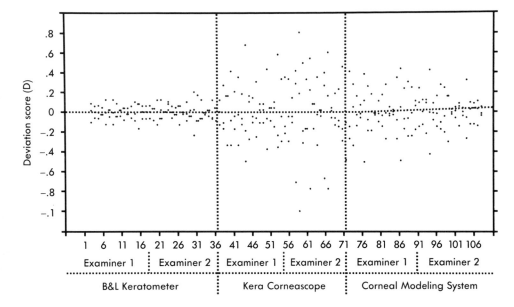

Figure 3-31

Comparison of the reproducibility of measurement at approximately the 3-mm zone by three instruments on 18 normal human corneas. The scattergram shows the deviation from the mean of each of the three measurements made on the cornea by one investigator with each instrument on the vertical axis. The 18 normal eyes, the two investigators (A and B), and the three instruments are indicated across the horizontal axis. The Keratometer was the most reproducible instrument, followed by the Corneal Modeling System and the Corneascope. (From Hannush SB, Crawford SL, Waring GO, Gemmill MC, Lynn MJ, and Nizam A: Arch Ophthalmol 1989;107:1235-1239.)

Figure 3-30

Comparison of accuracy of Keratometer, Corneascope, and Corneal Modeling System on steel test balls. **A,** Scattergram shows comparative accuracy of the three instruments in terms of the deviation score, which is the difference between the actual and measured values as indicated on the y-axis in diopters. Two examiners performed three readings on each of four steel balls (A, 43.00 D; B, 42.52 D; C, 50.14 D; and D, 38.66 D). The Keratometer and Corneal Modeling System were more accurate than the Corneascope. **B,** Accuracy of rings 1 through 26 of Corneal Modeling System. The deviation score indicates the difference between the actual and measured values on the x-axis. On the y-axis our readings are results of readings from rings 1 through 26 by two investigators with three readings taken per ring. Except for ring 1, the deviation scores for the 43.00 D ball were within ±0.1 D. **C,** The readings for rings 1 through 26 of the Corneal Modeling System were less accurate for the 50.14 D ball, particularly rings 13 through 26. (From Hannush SB, Crawford SL, Waring GO, Gemmill MC, Lynn MJ, and Nizam A: Arch Ophthalmol 1989;107:1235-1239.)

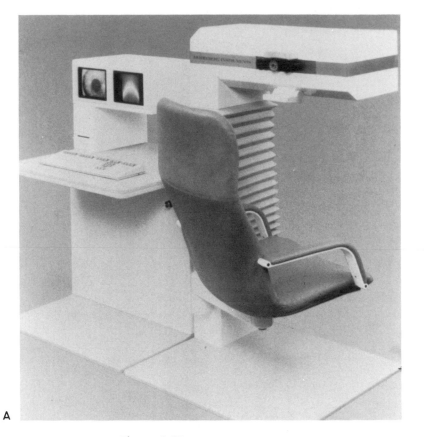

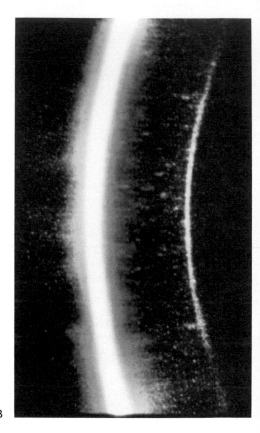

Figure 3-32
Heidelberg Instruments Confocal Laser Slit Corneal Imaging System. **A,** Console consists of computer keyboard, video imaging and display screens, and patient chair with chin rest and eyepiece. **B,** Confocal slit image of the cornea covers approximately a height of 2.5 mm. Multiple images are assembled by computer algorithms to represent the corneal contours. (Courtesy Heidelberg Instruments, Inc.)

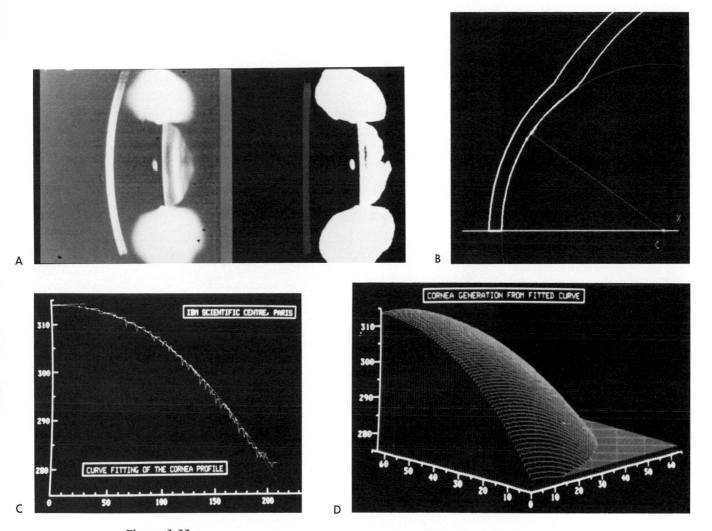

Figure 3-33
IBM—Paris, Hanna Corneal Imaging System and Scheimpflug camera. **A,** The Scheimpflug slit image demonstrates both the cornea and the lens shadows. White areas at top and bottom are reflections from iris *(left)*. The slit image is processed by the computer and smoothed *(right)*. **B,** Computer coordinates create a cross section of the cornea based on the anterior and posterior curvatures. **C,** These curvatures are smoothed and fitted to the corneal profile. **D,** A three-dimensional graphic representation of the cornea results. (Values on axes are arbitrary scale units.) (Courtesy Khalil D. Hanna.)

Rasterstereography: measuring the ocular surface

Rasterstereography (Fig. 3-34) involves projecting a grid of horizontal and vertical parallel lines onto the ocular surface and recording their pattern on the surface with a video camera.[6,7] A stereo photoslit-lamp has been adapted by Arffa and colleagues for this purpose, consisting of two cine-optical elbows mounted on a beam splitter with a fixed angle between the two optical paths. One elbow holds a flash illuminator that projects through an etched grid to create the lines, and the other elbow holds a black and white high resolution video camera that records the image. When viewed at the camera angle, the grid lines are seen deviating in direct proportion to the elevation of the cornea. The lines can be enhanced by staining the tear film with fluorescein and placing a cobalt blue filter in the path of the projected lines and a yellow barrier filter in front of

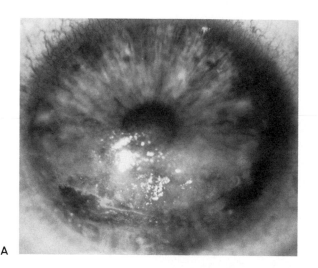

A

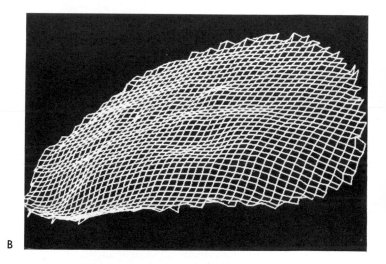

B

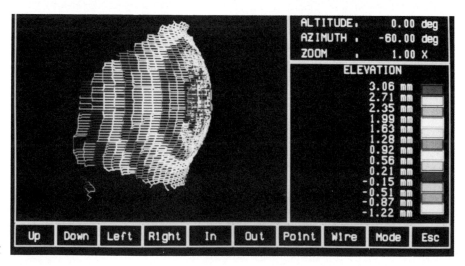

C

Figure 3-34
Corneal topography using rasterstereography. **A,** Clinical photograph of cornea demonstrates inferior exposure keratopathy with irregularity. **B,** Rasterstereography contour of the surface shows inferior irregularity. The inferior portion of the cornea has been rotated forward. **C,** Corneal topography display using rasterstereography shows mesh with color coding on left and color-coded scale demonstrating millimeters of elevation on the right. (From Arffa RC, Warnicki JW, and Rehkopf PG: Refract Corneal Surg 1989;5:414-417.)

the video camera. The image captured by the video camera is sent to an image processor for digitization, storage, calculation of corneal curvatures, and generation of graphic displays.

A two-dimensional matrix that consists of approximately 3000 elevation points is used to create three-dimensional contour plots of the corneal surface and to quantify its radii of curvature. Rasterstereography measures the elevation of the corneal surface directly, rather than calculating its curvature, as is done with keratography. The quantitative graphic representation can be color coded so that each color represents an area of equal elevation of the corneal surface.

At the time of this writing, the clinical evaluation of the PAR Technology rasterstereography system has been limited, and therefore it is unknown whether its ability to depict the surface topography directly is an advantage over localized measurements of corneal curvature using keratography.

Interference fringe techniques: measuring with high resolution

Using two wave fronts of light to cause interference fringes that are projected onto the surface of the cornea can produce extremely accurate measurements, on the order of less than the wavelength of the light that is used. Only preliminary experimental work has been done using this technique because the rigorous demands for stability of the eye are difficult to achieve.

Moiré fringes. Moiré fringes (Fig. 3-35) are a more complex form of surface imaging than rasterstereography, requiring two rulings, or grid patterns, to be projected onto the ocular surface. In those areas where the rulings overlap, an interference fringe pattern forms, with a lower frequency spacing than either of the two grids. This lower frequency pattern creates moiré fringes, so-called because of their resemblance to light passing through the translucent cloth used for draperies and clothing. The moiré fringe pattern can be photographed and analyzed in a manner similar to that described for rasterstereography.

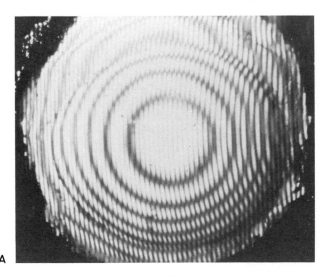
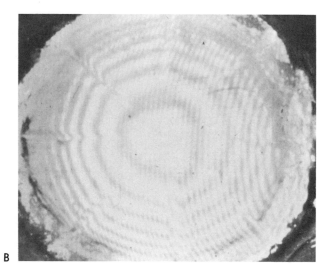

A

B

Figure 3-35
Moiré fringe imaging of surface of human donor eye bank eye. **A,** Normal ocular surface shows regular spacing of fringes. **B,** Fringe pattern immediately after eight-incision radial keratotomy shows less regular spacing and wider spread of fringes centrally, indicating corneal flattening. (Courtesy Raymond P. Vito.)

Holography. A more sophisticated technique to measure corneal topography is holographic interferometry (Fig. 3-36). Holography works by revealing the strain on the ocular surface caused by small stresses, such as the changes in intraocular pressure from the ocular pulse.

A three-dimensional holographic image of the corneal surface is generated while the eye is maintained at a static level of intraocular pressure. Any subsequent variation in intraocular pressure (stress) induces strain in the collagen fibril network, thus deforming the surface contour. Either a second holographic

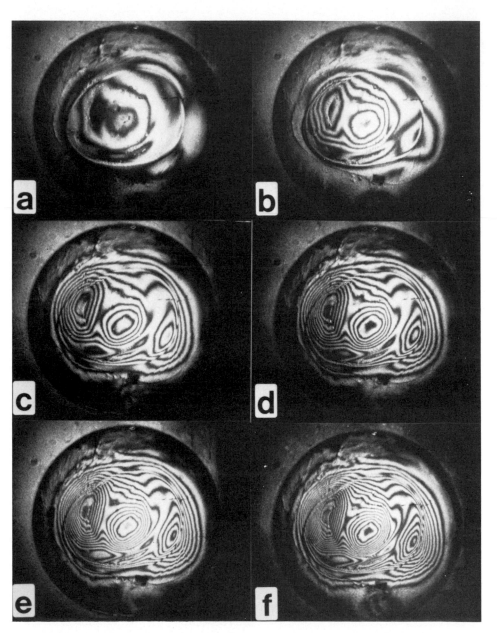

Figure 3-36
Holographic interferometry of a bovine cornea shows changes induced by varying the intraocular pressure. The baseline pressure was 18.0 mm Hg. The change in pressure in each figure was: *a,* 0.0 mm Hg; *b,* 0.1; *c,* 0.2; *d,* 0.5; *e,* 0.9; and *f,* 1.0. As the pressure gradually increased by only 1 mm Hg, the holographic strain pattern changed markedly and the interference fringes became smaller and closer together. Such sensitive measurements may be a benefit to refractive surgery in the future. (Courtesy Michael Smolek.)

image or the light-wave front from the real cornea can be superimposed on the first holographic image. The production of tissue strain is shown by the pattern of bright and dark interference fringes generated by the combined wave fronts. This fringe pattern can be analyzed to determine the surface distention in physical dimensions.

Calkins and colleagues[14] recorded double-exposure holograms of postoperative corneas; the use of the double-exposure method limits analytic interpretation of the fringe pattern. Smolek[103] used a real-time method to derive elasticity coefficients for various locations on enucleated bovine eyes and qualitatively examine strain development in corneas. It is difficult to control motion between the two wave fronts; thus the double-exposure method may work better in vivo, the real-time method better in vitro. A keratoscope that uses holographic technology is being developed by DGH Corporation.

In addition to surface imaging, holography has the potential of measuring corneal wound healing in the living eye. By measuring the changes in stress in the area of a keratotomy wound, holography can reveal the mechanical properties of the wound and compare with those of the unincised adjacent intact cornea. In this way it would be possible to measure the time course and strength of corneal wound healing after refractive keratotomy, which might determine when wound healing is nearly complete. This could be correlated with refractive stability.

Practical considerations about topography instruments

Klyce and colleagues[62] have emphasized the following criteria by which a clinician can judge a corneal topography device:
1. *Utility*—How practical will the instrument be in the purchaser's practice?
2. *Availability*—Is the instrument in production and is there a company that stands behind it to provide service and improvements?
3. *Accuracy*—Does the instrument measure the actual shape of test surfaces and of the cornea? Is information published about the technical design of the device and the mathematical assumptions and computer algorithms used to generate the model of the corneal surface?
4. *Reproducibility*—Does the instrument repeatedly achieve the same readings on the same surface?
5. *Price*—Will the purchaser get a fair value for the final investment?

NORMAL CORNEAL TOPOGRAPHY AND ASPHERIC OPTICS

Studies of corneal topography using keratography emphasize that the cornea is not spherical, not even in the central zone.

Corneal asphericity and asymmetry

The early observations of Sneff in 1864, Von Helmholtz in 1896, and Gullstrand in 1924 documented that beyond the central 3 to 4 mm of the cornea the anterior surface flattens symmetrically in the paracentral and peripheral zones. The refractive power decreases approximately 3 D from the center to the limbal zone. This makes the entire cornea an aspheric, positive meniscus lens (Fig. 3-37) with the advantage of producing a clear retinal image when the pupil is large. If the cornea were completely spherical and the pupil large (greater than 4 mm), the peripheral rays would be refracted anterior to the central rays, forming a blurred retinal image (Fig. 3-38). This undesirable blurred image produced by a spherical surface or lens as a result of a relative excess power peripherally is termed spherical aberration. Cameras commonly use aspheric lenses to decrease spherical aberration, and aspheric condensing lenses are commonly used with the indirect ophthalmoscope. Since the indirect aspheric lens has less power peripherally, similar to the cornea, it produces a clearer aerial image of the retina.

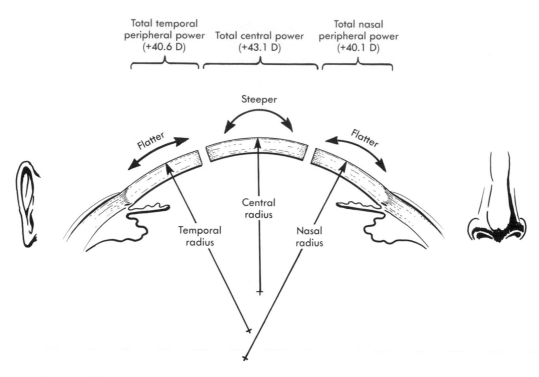

Figure 3-37
The human cornea is aspheric; the central cornea is steeper than the paracentral
and peripheral cornea. The nasal cornea flattens sooner in the paracentral area and
is flatter peripherally than the temporal cornea.

In addition to being aspheric, the corneal surface is radially asymmetric. The
nasal and superior areas begin flattening closer to the center; the temporal and
inferior areas remain steeper farther from the center (Fig. 3-39) (see Chapter 17,
Atlas of Surgical Techniques of Radial Keratotomy). One way to conceive of corneal asphericity is to describe it in terms of sections of a cone. A section through
a cone parallel to its base creates a circle. As the tilt of the sections increases, the
sections become elliptical with a prolate (steep to flat) side and an oblate (flat to
steep) side. Description of the corneal shape in these regular geometric terms is a
simplification (see Fig. 3-7) because the corneal surface is radially asymmetric.[96]

Normal corneal topography

Many other observers have contributed to our early knowledge of corneal topography, including Ludlam,[67] Wittenberg,[116] Mandel,[75] and Edmund.[35]

In 1961 Knoll[63] observed the great variety of topography among individual
corneas as measured by photokeratography and proposed a classification of four
types of normal corneal topography based on photokeratoscopic data. The type
A cornea exhibited semimeridional symmetry and little asphericity; the type B
cornea showed semimeridional symmetry and definite positive asphericity; type
C showed semimeridional asymmetry and little asphericity; and type D showed
semimeridional asymmetry and positive asphericity. Knoll emphasized that the
nasal semimeridians invariably flattened more than the temporal semimeridians.
There is great individual variation in the amount of central to limbal flattening
of the human cornea, making each person's anterior surface configuration almost unique. Using small mire keratometry, Mandel[74] demonstrated the variable curvature from one cornea to another over the central 8 mm.

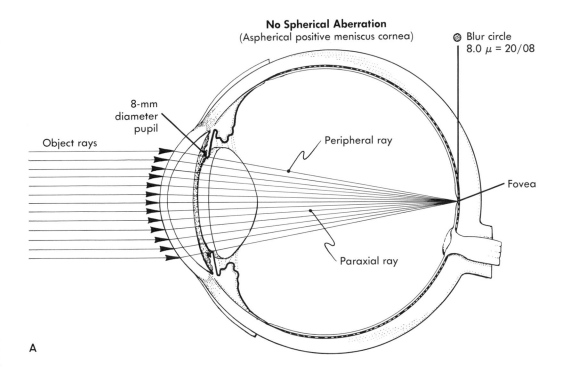

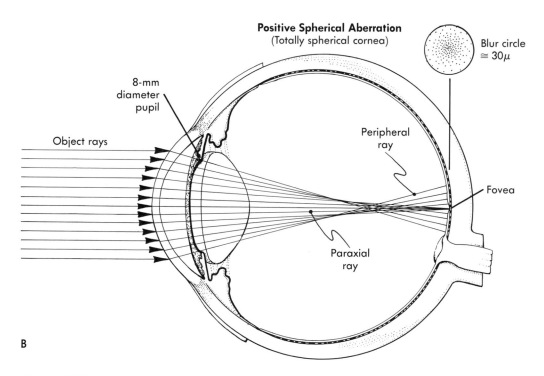

Figure 3-38
Effect of spherical aberration on retinal image. **A,** When there is minimal spherical aberration in the eye as created by an aspheric positive meniscus cornea, the peripheral and paraxial rays come to focus on the fovea creating a small blur circle. **B,** When there is positive spherical aberration in the eye, as would be created by a totally spherical cornea, the paraxial and peripheral rays do not come to a single focal point, but cross in the vitreous and create a large blur circle on the retina.

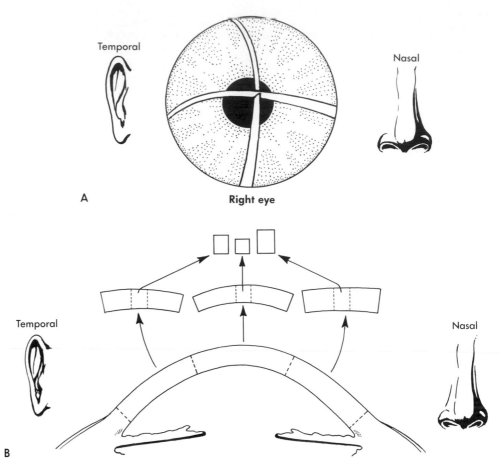

Figure 3-39
A, Normal human cornea is thicker nasally and inferiorly by the rubric NASICK (NASal-thICKer) and TEMPIN (TEMPoral-thINner). **B,** Cross section of the cornea emphasizes that the central cornea is thinnest, the temporal cornea is the next thickest, and the nasal cornea is thickest.

The topography studies of Clark[19] and Kiely[60] have demonstrated that the normal human cornea is not always steeper centrally and flatter peripherally. Clark studied the topography of 164 normal corneas in 82 subjects with a photokeratoscope and found a mean positive asphericity (flattening from center to periphery) of 0.10 mm in the nasal semimeridian and 0.06 mm in the temporal semimeridian. Nearly 10% of Clark's subjects exhibited negative corneal asphericity. Similarly, Kiely and colleagues found that 88.3% of the corneas they studied exhibited flattening from the center to the periphery (positive asphericity), whereas 11.4% showed peripheral steepening (negative asphericity). Kiely also noted that the rate of paracentral corneal flattening was independent of the central curvature, proving the topography of an individual cornea cannot be inferred from simple central keratometric measurements.

In 1981 Doss and colleagues[30] developed mathematical algorithms for calculating corneal radius of curvature and dioptric power from photokeratographs. Derivations of this system were used in the Kera Corneascope and Kerascanner. Rowsey and colleagues[93] demonstrated that the system could read 8- and 10-mm diameter test balls with accuracy, the 90% confidence interval being approximately 0.1 to 0.2 mm wide. Rowsey and colleagues[90] used photokeratog-

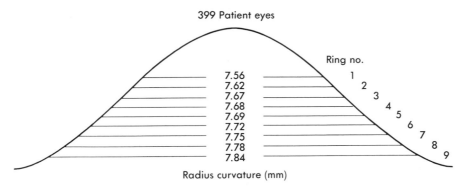

399 Patient eyes

Ring no.

7.56
7.62
7.67
7.68
7.69
7.72
7.75
7.78
7.84

Radius curvature (mm)

Figure 3-40
The gradual increase in radius of curvature from the
paracentral to the peripheral cornea as determined from
nine-ring photokeratoscope pictures of 399 myopic eyes
before surgery in the PERK study. The radii represent an
average of eight data points around each photokeratoscope ring. (From Rowsey JJ, Balyeat HD, Monlux R,
Holladay J, Waring GO, Lynn MJ, and the PERK Study
Group: Ophthalmology 1988;95:322-334.)

raphy to study the corneal topography of 368 myopic eyes before surgery in the
PERK study, documenting the positive aspheric shape over the area measured
(Fig. 3-40). In 1984 Klyce and colleagues[61] introduced a computer-based topographic analysis system that relied on manual digitization of photokeratographs
and could provide high-resolution, graphic representations of corneal topography. In a study of 44 normal corneas from 22 subjects, Dingeldein and co-
workers[28,29] found that the central cornea was not always spherical and demonstrated variations in topographic pattern and central power.

Bogan and colleagues[12] used the Corneal Modeling System to study the topography of 212 normal corneas from 212 individuals 8 to 79 years of age with
a range of spherical equivalent refraction from +5.50 to −8.37 D (mean, −1.04
D). They derived a qualitative system for classifying normal corneal topography
based on patterns identified on color-coded topographic maps (Fig. 3-41). There
were 49 corneas (23%) with a round pattern, 45 (21%) with an oval pattern, 38
(18%) with a symmetric bowtie pattern, 69 (32%) with an asymmetric bowtie
pattern, and 15 (7.0%) with an irregular pattern. In contrast to the findings of
Clark[20] and Knoll,[63] all corneas were steeper centrally and flattened paracentrally and peripherally, that is, they had a prolate shape and a positive shape factor. There were no statistically significant differences among any of the five patterns for age, sex, left or right eye, spherical equivalent refraction, or mean keratometric power. There was not a significant difference in keratometric astigmatism between the round and oval patterns ($p = 0.60$); however, the symmetric
and asymmetric bowtie patterns had more astigmatism (Table 3-6). The bowtie
patterns were significantly different from each other and from the round and
oval patterns ($p \leq 0.0001$), with the symmetric bowtie pattern having the greatest mean astigmatism and the round pattern the least.

Although the patterns identified in this qualitative classification system were
distinctive, the divisions between groups were arbitrary and the variations in
normal corneal topography probably form a continuum (Fig. 3-42).

In a subset of 47 normal corneas, Bogan and colleagues[11] confirmed the radial asymmetry of the normal cornea by finding that the superior and nasal

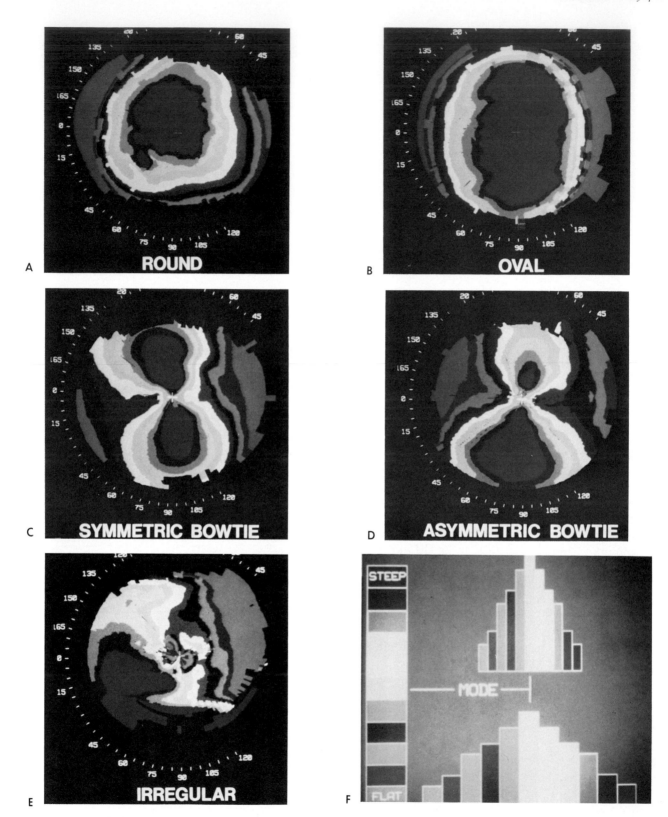

Figure 3-41
Five qualitative patterns of normal corneal topography based on computer-assisted videokeratography using the normalized scale. Criteria for each pattern are listed in the text. **A,** Round. **B,** Oval. **C,** Symmetric bowtie. **D,** Asymmetric bowtie. **E,** Irregular. **F,** In the normalized scale the range of dioptric power represented by each color varies among eyes depending on the degree of corneal asphericity. See insert for color versions of these illustrations. (From Bogan SJ, Waring GO, Ibrahim O, Drews C, and Curtis L: Arch Ophthalmol 1990;108:945-949.)

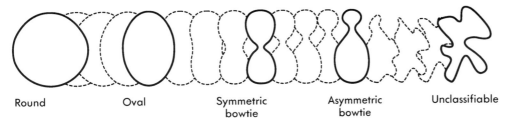

Round   Oval   Symmetric   Asymmetric   Unclassifiable
                       bowtie   bowtie

Figure 3-42
The five patterns recognized in color-coded topographic maps of normal eyes probably form a continuum. (From Bogan SJ, Waring GO, Ibrahim O, Drews C, and Curtis L: Arch Ophthalmol 1990;108:945-949.)

Table 3-6

Relationship of Keratometric and Refractive Astigmatism with Topographic Pattern in 216 Normal Eyes*

Keratographic pattern†	Keratometric astigmatism (D)		Refractive astigmatism (D)	
	Mean ± SD	% ≥ 1.00 D	Mean ± SD	% ≥ 1.00 D
Round	0.47 ±0.34	10	0.28 ±0.39	8
Oval	0.57 ±0.30	20	0.26 ±0.41	7
Symmetric bowtie	1.40 ±0.98	73	1.00 ±1.20	43
Asymmetric bowtie	0.89 ±0.70	41	0.47 ±0.78	19
Irregular	0.64 ±0.53	27	0.53 ±0.51	27

From Bogan SJ, Waring GO, Ibrahim O, Drews C, and Curtis L: Arch Ophthalmol 1990;108:945-949.
*One eye per subject.
†Normalized scale of Corneal Modeling System.

semimeridians flattened faster and to a greater amount from the center to the periphery than the inferior and temporal ones (see Fig. 3-39).

Refractive corneal surgery continues to spur interest in corneal topography for two reasons: to understand the aspheric and multifocal optics created in the cornea by surgery and to use corneal topography as a predictive factor in determining the outcome of surgery. Both of these areas are in their early stages of development.

Influence of pupil size

Applegate and Gansel[1] have emphasized the importance of pupil size in measuring refractive error, visual acuity, and optical quality. (For a detailed discussion, see Chapter 16, Centering Corneal Surgical Procedures.) The optical function of the eye is influenced by the diameter of the pupil, which is the limiting aperture of the optical system, just as the diaphragm is the limiting aperture of a camera. This aperture can influence the quality of the optical image, particularly when the optics are affected by problems such as spherical and chromatic aberrations, defocus from refractive errors, aspheric corneal topography, and the like.

The larger the pupil, the greater the effect of the paracentral and peripheral corneal topography. For example, after radial keratotomy an eye with a 3-mm or smaller diameter pupil receives its image through the uncut central clear zone where the optics of the cornea are reasonably uniform. With a moderately dilated pupil, 4 to 6 mm, the paracentral zone of the cornea will affect the foveal image. Since this portion of the cornea is often steeper than the central zone after radial keratotomy, the effects of the aspheric optics, aberrations from the cornea, and glare from the corneal scars will affect visual function. A widely dilated pupil, 7 to 9 mm, will probably increase these effects (see Chapter 23, Complications of Refractive Keratotomy). Holladay and colleagues[51,52] have correlated refraction, visual acuity, and pupil size in normal eyes based on published data (Fig. 3-43 and Table 3-7).

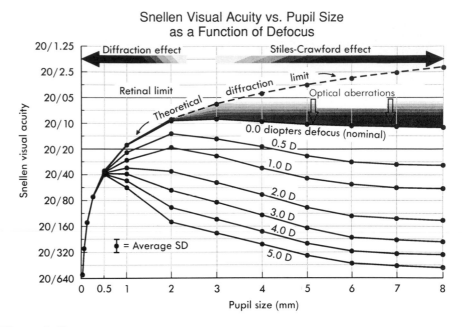

Figure 3-43

The Snellen visual acuity versus pupil diameter as a function of defocus in normal eyes. For pupil diameters less than 0.5 mm, the visual acuity is completely determined by the diffraction limit and is not affected by defocus up to 5 D. Between 0.5 mm and 3.0 mm pupil diameters, the visual acuity is determined by a complex interplay between diffraction, defocus, and optical aberrations. Above 3.0 mm diameters, diffraction is no longer a factor, but the Stiles-Crawford effect becomes a contributing factor. Above 5.4 mm, the additional pupil area has little effect on Snellen visual acuity because of the Stiles-Crawford effect. (From Holladay JT, Lynn MJ, Waring GO, Gemmill MC, Keehn GC, and Fielding B: Arch Ophthalmol 1991;109:70-76.)

Table 3-7

Snellen Visual Acuity as a Function of Pupil Size and Defocus

Defocus (D)	Pupil size (mm)								
	0.5	1.0	2.0	3.0	4.0	5.0	6.0	7.0	8.0
TDL (D)*	20/36	20/18	20/09	20/06	20/04	20/04	20/03	20/03	20/02
0 D	20/36	20/18	20/09	20/09	20/11	20/14	20/17	20/20	20/23
0.5 D	20/36	20/22	20/16	20/18	20/22	20/26	20/31	20/37	20/43
1.0 D	20/36	20/27	20/24	20/26	20/35	20/42	20/51	20/62	20/74
2.0 D	20/37	20/32	20/50	20/63	20/82	20/103	20/126	20/150	20/178
3.0 D	20/38	20/38	20/87	20/115	20/153	20/192	20/230	20/288	20/307
4.0 D	20/39	20/45	20/129	20/185	20/253	20/317	20/360	20/443	20/507
5.0 D	20/40	20/52	20/175	20/258	20/348	20/438	20/526	20/604	20/693

From Holladay JT, Lynn MJ, Waring GO, Gemmill MC, Keehn GC, and Fielding B: Arch Ophthalmol 1991;109:70-76.
*Theoretical diffraction limits in diopters.

Corneal topography and visual function

Some researchers have studied how variations in corneal topography affect ocular image formation and visual function. Of course the cornea has been recognized as the major source of astigmatism, and extensive literature is available on the Stiles-Crawford effect, which observes that light rays entering the central pupil are perceived as brighter than those entering the outer parts of the pupil. However, with the advent of refractive surgery, interest in the effects of topography on visual function has increased, since refractive corneal surgery creates new types of aspheric curves in the cornea that can affect refraction and visual acuity more than normal asphericity.* This has been particularly important after keratomileusis and epikeratoplasty, after which the newly created optical zone can produce multifocal effects and diplopia if decentered from the entrance pupil. Similarly, with radial keratotomy, the central flattening and paracentral steepening are not always uniform, concentric, and centered over the entrance pupil. This topography could create a larger blur circle or a multifocal lens effect, as discussed below.

Knowing the refractive power and the topographic configuration of the cornea is only the first step in understanding the effect of the cornea on visual function. For example, studies of corneal topography have demonstrated that reasonably good Snellen visual acuity of 20/20 to 20/40 is compatible with moderately severe amounts of corneal irregularity.[69-71,117] Thus correlations between corneal topography and image formation within the eye must be found, and this must be further correlated with the psychophysical process of visual perception. Camp and colleagues[15] have attempted to correlate corneal topography with image formation by using a computer program that mimics the function of an optical bench and depicts the effect of distortions of corneal topography on image formation by using point spread functions (see Fig. 3-29). They observed that a perfect lens system would focus all light on a single point in the image plane of best focus, whereas an irregular corneal surface can produce fairly severe amounts of image degradation. Even so, they emphasize that good Snellen visual acuity and contrast sensitivity can persist. The authors call for increased study of the differences between irregular corneas with good optical performance and those with bad optical performance.

To correlate corneal topography and visual acuity, Dingledein and colleagues[29] devised topographic indices. The surface asymmetry index was defined as the centrally weighted summation of differences in corneal power between corresponding points on individual photokeratographs 180 degrees apart (Fig. 3-44); for example, if on ring one the calculated dioptric power at 0 degrees is 44 D and at 180 degrees is 42 D, the value of two is entered into the summation for the whole corneal surface average. For a perfect sphere, the surface asymmetry index would be zero. The authors reviewed 39 photokeratographs of corneas with keratoconus, compound myopic astigmatism, epikeratoplasty, radial keratotomy, and two normal corneas analyzed by manual digitalization. The correlation between the surface asymmetry index and the best spectacle-corrected visual acuity was statistically significant ($R = 0.76$, $p > 0.001$). The authors also found that the centrally weighted average corneal power and the power and location of the steepest and flattest corneal meridians correlated well with standard keratometry measurements (correlation coefficient = 0.98). The weighting of the more central rings is important because they overlie the pupil where the topography affects retinal image formation. The weighting was achieved by taking each keratographic ring and using its surface area as an inverse indicator of its importance (the larger the area the less important the ring).

*References 9, 49, 72, 77, 78, 91, 100.

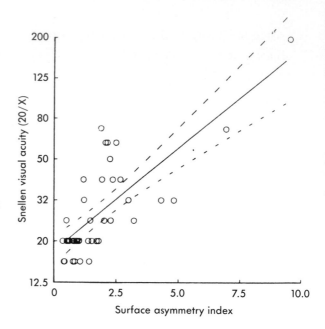

Figure 3-44
Correlation between the Surface Asymmetry Index (in diopters) and the Snellen visual acuity. The solid line represents the best fit of the data determined by linear regression. The dashed curves denote the 95% confidence limits for the slope of the regression line. Numbers on the vertical axis are the denominators of Snellen visual acuity. (From Dingeldein SA, Klyce SD, and Wilson SE: Refract Corneal Surg 1989:5:372-378.)

OPTICS AND CORNEAL TOPOGRAPHY AFTER RADIAL KERATOTOMY

Since the initial experiments of Lans (see Chapter 5, Development of Refractive Keratotomy in the Nineteenth Century), the detailed analysis of Sato (see Chapter 6, Development of Radial Keratotomy in Japan, 1939-1960), and the computations of Fyodorov (see Chapter 7, Development of Refractive Keratotomy in the Soviet Union, 1960-1990), the body of knowledge has gradually increased concerning the mechanism by which anterior partial-thickness incisions change corneal shape. Current concepts are presented in the mathematical models of Seiler,[31] Vito,[27] Hanna,[96] and Au[26] (see Chapters 28, 29, and 33). The analysis of photokeratographs in the PERK study by Rowsey and colleagues,[91] and the study of videokeratographs by McDonnell[77-79] and others[39,72] have elucidated the effect of radial keratotomy on corneal topography. However, this body of information is not synthesized in one place, and reading the papers in succession often results in a blur of information that is difficult to formulate into a cohesive concept. Therefore we summarize here how radial incisions affect corneal topography and optics. A similar analysis of the effect of transverse incisions is presented in Chapter 31, Keratotomy for Astigmatism.

Changes induced in corneal shape by radial keratotomy

Radial incisions made in the paracentral and peripheral cornea alter corneal shape in two phases: the acute phase, which lasts a few days after the incisions are made, and the long-term phase of wound healing, which lasts for years.

Three major premises underlie the mechanism of action of radial incisions. First, the corneal stroma is nondistensible and does not stretch under physiologic conditions; any changes in shape must arise from changes in position of the cornea. Second, the incisions gape open, and displacements of the cornea are necessary to accommodate these gaping wounds. Third, relatively deep incisions are necessary to weaken the cornea and allow it to change shape.

The factors that affect the change in shape include intraocular pressure, swelling of the corneal stroma, pressure from the eyelids, and filling of the gaping wounds with an epithelial plug and stromal scar tissue. The effect contributed by each of these factors is unknown, and in the discussion that follows, we embody all the forces under the term "intraocular pressure." Thus we can state the general concept of the mechanism of action of radial incisions as follows. The partial-thickness (80% to 90% depth) incisions in the paracentral and peripheral cornea create wounds that gape open under the force of intraocular pressure. This gaping is sustained as the wounds are filled acutely with edema, then with an epithelial plug, and finally with scar tissue. The gaping wounds increase the corneal surface area and weaken the cornea so that the paracentral and peripheral areas are displaced anteriorly and steepened, creating a compensatory central posterior displacement and flattening (Fig. 3-45).

The early explanation of Fyodorov,[40] that the mechanism of action was based on the incisions severing the circular limbal ligament of the cornea (ligament of Kokot), has been proven incorrect because incisions confined within the clear cornea have as great an effect. The theory of Ivashina[53] that "the cornea at the central optical zone is stretched as a result of compensatory flattening" also seems incorrect, based on the nondistensibility of the unincised corneal stroma under physiologic conditions. The wound gape model presents the best explanation of the mechanism of action of radial keratotomy. The changes in corneal shape induced by radial keratotomy are summarized in Fig. 3-45.

Text continued on p. 107.

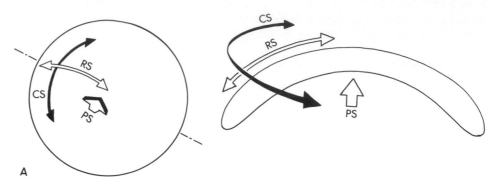

A

Figure 3-45

The sequence of drawings and explanations correlates the surgical, biomechanical, topographic, and optical results of radial keratotomy.

A, Normal stresses in the cornea. The normal cornea maintains a fixed shape determined by the fixed boundary at the limbus and by the stresses within it. A number of stresses have been described; three are illustrated here: the circumferential stress *(CS)* around the cornea, the radial stress *(RS)* along the meridians, and the perpendicular stress *(PS)* across the thickness of the cornea. Under normal circumstances, small changes in the stresses, such as an increase in the perpendicular stress from an increase in intraocular pressure, produce little change in the shape of the cornea because the inelastic collagen fibrils do not deform easily and the high water content makes the cornea virtually incompressible. (Sheer stresses and torsional stresses play little or no role in determining corneal shape.)

Radial Keratotomy

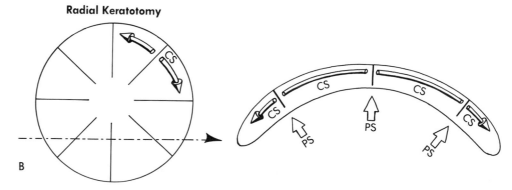

B

B, Effect of radial keratotomy. When partial thickness radial incisions are made in the cornea, the amount of tissue available to support the stresses in the area of the incisions is reduced from a thickness of approximately 0.60 mm to a thickness of approximately 0.06 mm. The stresses impinging on the cornea are redistributed. The circumferential stress *(CS)* and the perpendicular stress *(PS)* are taken up by thinner tissue.

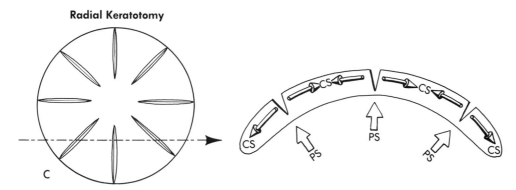

C, Gaping of incisions. This redistribution of the stresses *(PS, CS)* on the cornea produces gaping of the incision wounds, a phenomenon that can be seen on the operating table immediately after surgery.

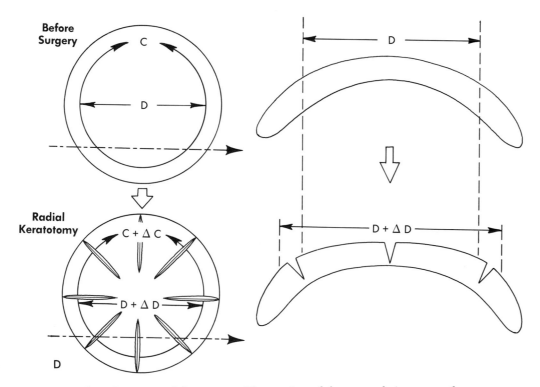

D, Increased surface area of the cornea. The gaping of the wounds increases the outer surface area of the cornea without adding any tissue. This can be visualized by considering a circular zone on the surface of the cornea with a circumference *(C)* and a diameter *(D)*. After radial keratotomy, the gaping of the wounds increases the circumference by an amount ΔC and increases the diameter of the circle by an amount ΔD. The circumference of the circle after surgery now is $C + \Delta C$, and its diameter is $D + \Delta D$.   *Continued.*

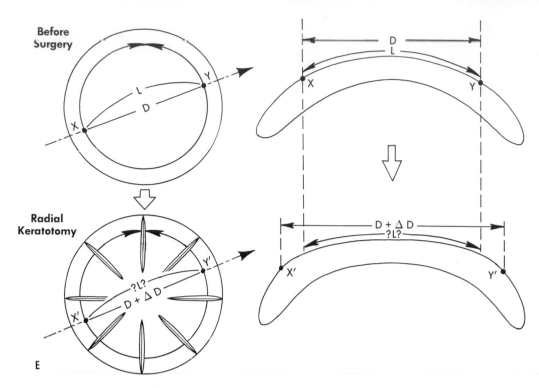

Before Surgery

Radial Keratotomy

E

Figure 3-45, cont'd
E, Problem of uncut tissue. What happens to the tissue that has not been cut? Before surgery the tissue along the arc length *(L)* spanned the distance between two points *X* and *Y* on the circle. After surgery the circle enlarged *(D+ Δ D),* and *X* and *Y* moved anteriorly and farther apart to *X'* and *Y',* but the amount of uncut tissue across *L* remained the same. How does this tissue continue to span the enlarged circle?

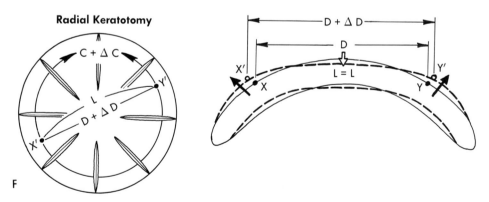

Radial Keratotomy

F

F, The answer to the question in **E** is that the only way the corneal arc *L* can continue to span the increased diameter is for the arc to flatten. The uncut tissue that includes arc *L* and extends from one side of the limbus to the other is fixed and the limbus itself is in a fixed position. The tissue does not stretch radially. No new tissue or tissue space is created along this arc. The original points *X* and *Y* are displaced anteriorly and outward along the new circumference *(C+ Δ C)* at either end of the new diameter *(D+ Δ D)* so that they have a new location at *X'* and *Y'.* The length of the tissue arc *L* remains the same, but the arc itself flattens in order to take up the distance between *X'* and *Y'.* This flattening is accompanied by a compensatory steepening in the peripheral cornea. The entire corneal arc does not flatten; if it did so, the fixed length of tissue along a single meridian from one side of the limbus to the other would have to undergo folding to occupy the overall flatter arc. (In fact, this is the phenomenon that occurs when the normal cornea swells and forces the normal arc of Descemet's membrane into an overall flatter configuration that spans a decreased length from one side of the limbus to the other, creating folds in Descemet's membrane.)

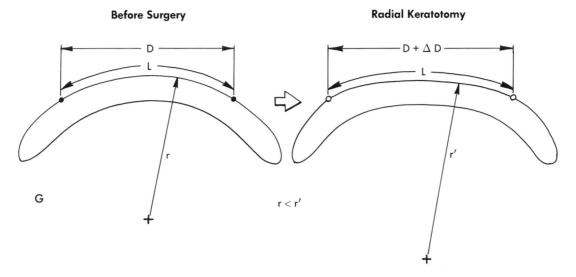

Before Surgery   **Radial Keratotomy**

G, Increased radius of corneal curvature. This induced central flattening changes the radius of curvature of the central cornea from shorter *(r)* to longer *(r′)*.

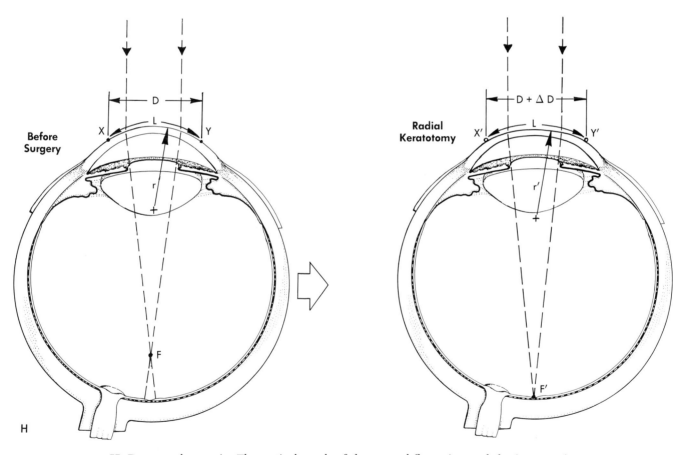

H, Decreased myopia. The optical result of the central flattening and the increase in the radius of curvature is a decrease in the central refractive power of the cornea. In a myopic eye, this pushes the focal point from its location in the vitreous *(F)* back toward the retina *(F′)*. Theoretically, an effective change in refractive power could also result from the posterior axial movement of the central cornea and not from its change of curvature. However, we know that a contact lens moves the effective power of the cornea forward by the thickness of the lens (0.3 mm) and that this difference has no measurable effect on the refraction. Thus, even if the central cornea did move backward by a few tenths of a millimeter, it would not significantly affect the refractive power of the eye.   *Continued.*

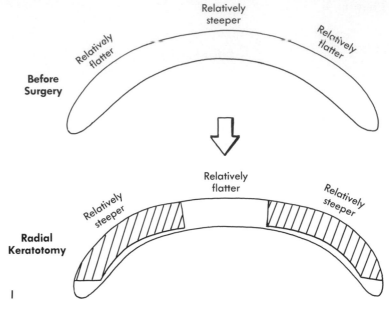

Figure 3-45, cont'd

I, Change in corneal shape and asphericity. A normal cornea before surgery is relatively steeper in the center and becomes flatter paracentrally and peripherally, a prolate shape with a positive shape factor. After radial keratotomy the central cornea is relatively flatter and becomes steeper paracentrally and peripherally, an oblate shape with a negative shape factor.

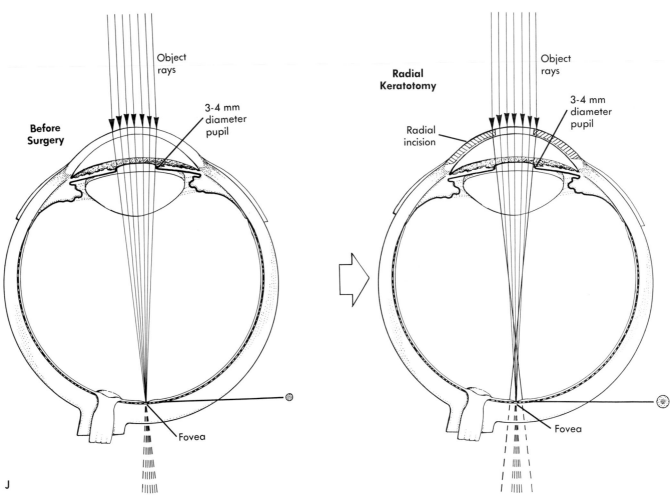

J, Refractive effect of changing corneal asphericity. *Left,* The corrected myopic eye before surgery has an optical system, including an aspheric cornea, that brings light rays to a focal point at the fovea, creating a small blur circle compatible with excellent visual acuity. *Right,* After radial keratotomy the paracentral changes in corneal shape induced by the incisions create more asphericity in the central-paracentral zones, resulting in a larger blur circle on the fovea. Depending on the size and location of the areas of different refractive power, a multifocal effect can be created in the cornea.

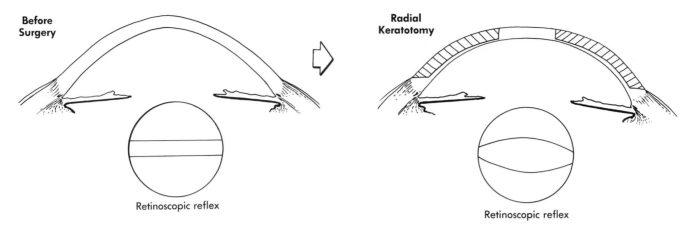

K, Retinoscopic reflex and radial keratotomy. *Left,* In the unoperated myopic eye, the retinoscopic reflex shows a linear streak that gives against motion. *Right,* After satisfactory radial keratotomy, the retinoscopic reflex is wider in the central pupil and narrower near the edge of the pupil because of the paracentral steepening of the cornea, giving an overall scissors motion.

Keratometric measurements after radial keratotomy

After radial keratotomy the central cornea flattens and the keratometric power decreases in almost all eyes (see box below). In general there is a linear relationship between the change in keratometric power and the change in cycloplegic refractive power after radial keratotomy, the refractive change usually 0.50 to 1.00 D greater than the keratometric change[8] (Fig. 3-46). For example, in 398 eyes studied in the PERK study (unpublished data), the change in keratometric and refractive power was within 0.50 D of each other in 40% of eyes; 50% had more than 0.50 D greater change in refractive power than in keratometric power; and 10% had more than 0.50 D greater change in keratometric

---

Topographic Features of the Cornea after Radial Keratotomy

Flattening of central cornea

Oblate configuration
Negative shape factor
Basis for central stellate epithelial iron line

Paracentral and peripheral steepening of the cornea

Paracentral "knee"

Irregularity over incision scars

Basis for stellate iron line
Polygonal pattern on color-coded videokeratographs

Multiple central and paracentral radii of curvature

Multifocal cornea
Central steep zone ("nipple")

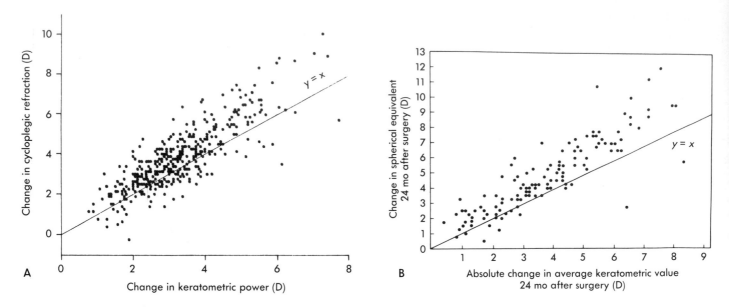

Figure 3-46
Relationship between change in central keratometric power and change in cycloplegic refractive power after radial keratotomy. **A,** For 435 eyes in the PERK study
at 3 years after surgery, the mean refractive change was 0.61 D greater than the
mean change in keratometric power. The relationship can be described by the regression formula: $\Delta SE = 1.11 \times \Delta K + 0.28$, $R^2 = 0.74$, where ΔSE is the change
in spherical equivalent refractive power and ΔK is change in keratometric power.
B, In the series reported by Arrowsmith and Marks at 2 years after surgery, the
change in refractive power was greater than the change in keratometric power for
most eyes. The best linear equation describing a relationship between these two
variables was $\Delta SE = 1.15 \times \Delta K + 0.42$, $R^2 = 0.81$. (**B** from Arrowsmith PN and
Marks RG: Arch Ophthalmol 1987;105:76-80.)

power than refractive power. A wide range of difference was found between refractive and keratometric power changes, from approximately 3 D more change
to 3 D less change in refractive power.

It is instructive to compare the difference between the change in refractive
and keratometric power for the three clear zone diameters in the PERK study.
Although no difference was noted in the average change in refractive and keratometric power in the 4-mm clear zone, the 3.5-mm clear zone group exhibited
a difference of 0.5 D, and the 3.0-mm clear zone group showed a difference of
1.0 D. This increasing disparity with the increasingly small clear zone diameters
probably occurred because the keratometric images on the corneal surface were
reflected from within the 4-mm clear zone; thus both the keratometric readings
and the refraction were coming from approximately the same undisturbed area
of the cornea and therefore exhibited less disparity. In the 3.5- and 3.0-mm diameter clear zones, the keratometric mires were closer to the ends of the incisions where there was a greater change in corneal curvature, so the refraction
was influenced more by the central unincised cornea and the keratometric readings were affected more by the paracentral incised cornea, thereby increasing the
disparity (see Fig. 3-15).

Corneal topography after radial keratotomy

Although Sato in the 1950s and Fyodorov in the 1970s were aware that radial keratotomy induced central corneal flattening and paracentral corneal steepening, the details of these changes in corneal topography have become apparent only with the careful study of keratographs (Fig. 3-47). Some commonly published graphic depictions of the changes in corneal shape exaggerate and oversimplify the reality of topographic changes.

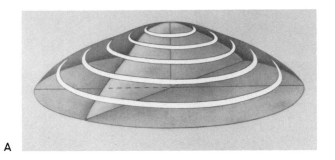

A

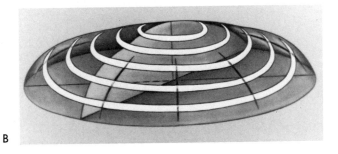

B

C

—— Before radial keratotomy

– – – After radial keratotomy

Figure 3-47

Topographic changes induced by radial keratotomy. **A,** Drawing of normal cornea with circular rings is exaggerated to show the prolate configuration with steeper central and flatter paracentral and peripheral zones. **B,** Drawing demonstrates exaggerated corneal topography after radial keratotomy demonstrating the oblate shape with a flatter central and steeper paracentral and peripheral zones. **C,** Cross-sectional drawing demonstrates the contours of the cornea before and after radial keratotomy to emphasize that the central zone and part of the paracentral zone become flatter while parts of the paracentral and peripheral zones become steeper. (For a detailed explanation, see Fig. 3-45.)

Different types of keratography present different types of information about the cornea after radial keratotomy. We present a series of examples in Figs. 3-48 to 3-52. Fig. 3-48 shows a quantitative analysis of nine-ring photokeratography over 5 years after radial keratotomy using the Corneascope and the Kerascanner; Fig. 3-49 presents the output of the Nidek photokeratoscope, showing contours and graphic representation of the cornea after radial keratotomy; Fig. 3-50 displays the hand-digitized analysis of a Nidek photokeratograph of an unoperated cornea and a cornea after radial keratotomy using the LSU system; Fig. 3-51 illustrates a Computed Anatomy videokeratograph representation of a normal cornea and a cornea after radial keratotomy; and Fig. 3-52 depicts an Eye-Sys videokeratograph and graphic analysis of a cornea after radial keratotomy.

Rowsey and colleagues[91] quantified corneal shape of 368 eyes in the PERK study at baseline and 6 months after radial keratotomy using a nine-ring Corneascope and a KeraScan digitizer that produced radius of curvature values at eight points on each of the nine rings. For analysis, the eight values along a ring were averaged to give the average radius of curvature around the ring. Before surgery the corneas were steeper in the center and gradually flattened toward the periphery. The mean and standard deviation of the average radius of curvature was

Text continued on p. 120.

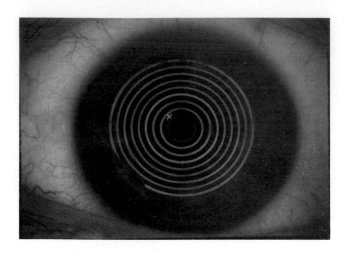

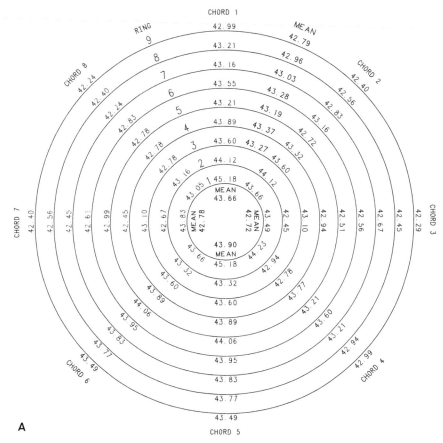

A

Figure 3-48

Quantification of nine-ring photokeratograph at serial times after an eight-incision radial keratotomy with a 3-mm central clear zone. **A,** Preoperative. **B,** 6 months. The mean values within the first ring are those for each of the four cardinal semimeridians. The mean values for rings 3 through 9 represent the average dioptric power around each ring. Each of the other values represents the dioptric power at the intersection of each of the eight radials with each of the nine rings. (Courtesy James Rowsey, MD.)

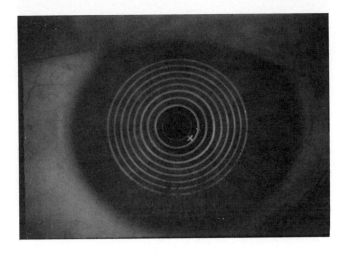

TX HX: 6 MONTHS POST-OP 8 INCISION, 3.0 MM CCZ RADIAL KERATOTOMY

CYCLOPLEGIC REF: -1.25 -1.25 X 180   PHOTO DATE: 6 MONTH   PRINTED: 8/24/87

CONTROL VALUE: 7.96   PHOTO MAG: 4.81   I.R. 1.3375   PERK # 0379   MED REC#

M.D./LOCATION: CHORD ONE IS   90 DEGREES

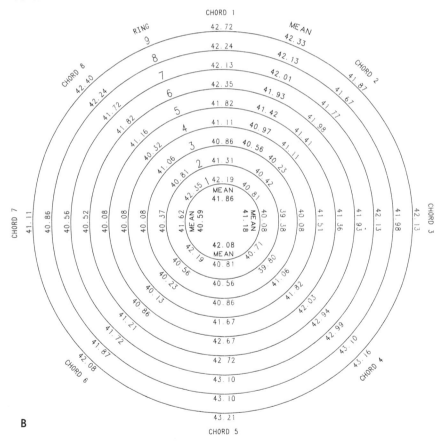

B

Figure 3-48, cont'd
For legend see opposite page. *Continued.*

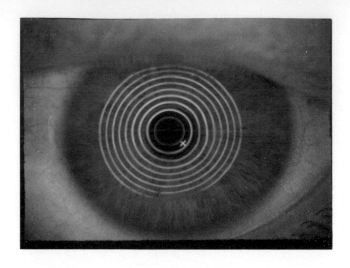

TX HX: 1 YEAR POST-OP 8 INCISION, 3.0 MM CCZ RADIAL KERATOTOMY

CYCLOPLEGIC REF: -0.50 -1.00 X 5   PHOTO DATE: 1 YEAR   PRINTED: 8/24/87

CONTROL VALUE: 7.96   PHOTO MAG: 4.81   I.R.: 1.3375   PERK #: 0379   MED REC#:

M.D./LOCATION: CHORD ONE IS   90 DEGREES

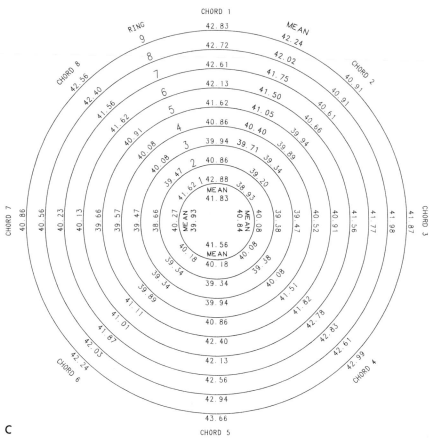

Figure 3-48, cont'd

Quantification of nine-ring photokeratograph at serial times after an eight-incision radial keratotomy with a 3-mm central clear zone. **A,** Preoperative. **B,** 6 months. The mean values within the first ring are those for each of the four cardinal semimeridians. The mean values for rings 3 through 9 represent the average dioptric power around each ring. Each of the other values represents the dioptric power at the intersection of each of the eight radials with each of the nine rings. (Courtesy James Rowsey, MD.)

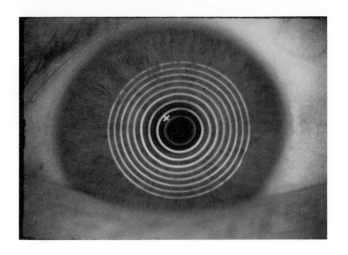

TX HX: 3 YEARS POST-OP 8 INCISION, 3.0 MM CCZ RADIAL KERATOTOMY

CYCLOPLEGIC REF: SPHERE −1.50 X 180   PHOTO DATE: 3 YEAR   PRINTED: 8/24/87

CONTROL VALUE: 7.96   PHOTO MAG: 4.81   I.R. 1.3375   PERK # 0379   MED REC#

M.D./LOCATION: CHORD ONE IS   90 DEGREES

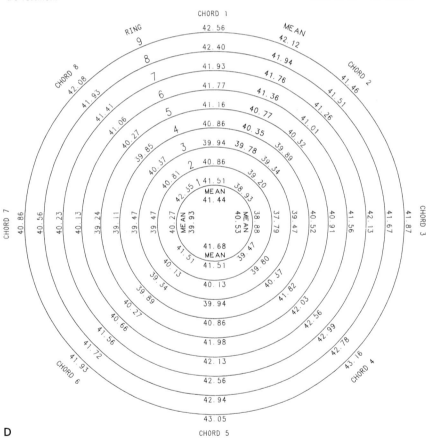

D

Figure 3-48, cont'd
For legend see opposite page.

Right Eye
Unoperated

Left Eye
Radial Keratotomy

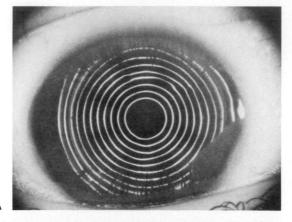

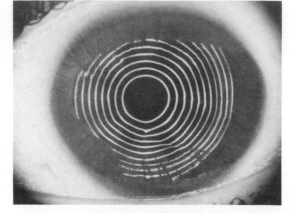

A

B

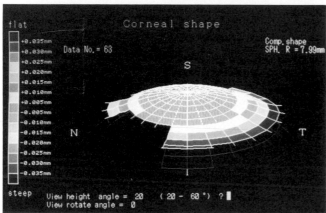

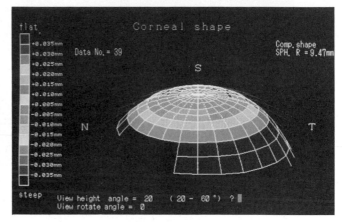

C

D

Figure 3-49

Comparison of keratographs taken with the Nidek photokeratoscope on a patient with an unoperated right cornea and a left cornea that had radial keratotomy.

Keratographs **(A** and **B):** The keratographs demonstrate normal mires in the unoperated eye, and mires with increased diameter of the rings and mild irregular astigmatism in the operated eye.

Color-coded wire mesh diagrams **(C** and **D):** The wire mesh diagrams depict the cornea as compared with a sphere (depicted in the red wire mesh). The color-coded mesh has colors that correspond to the difference in radius of curvature from the central power. In the normal cornea the curvature flattens toward the periphery. After radial keratotomy the cornea steepens toward the periphery. The directions on the cornea are indicated by nasal *(N)*, temporal *(T)*, superior *(S)*, inferior *(I)*. See insert for color versions of these illustrations.

Faceplates **(E** and **F):** The faceplates present the refractive powers along eight meridians around each ring. The unoperated cornea gradually flattens from the center toward the periphery. The cornea after radial keratotomy steepens from the center to the periphery. (Analyses done by Nidek Corporation using the Nidek Photokeratoscope and Keratoanalyzer.)

Corneal profile **(G** and **H):** Profile views of the cornea across the horizontal meridian (0° to 180°) demonstrate in the normal right eye more rapid flattening on the nasal side than the temporal side. The table presents the refractive power (*R*, diopter) across this meridian in both the nasal and temporal directions by ring number and by the distance from the center (mm). The reference curve on the left has a radius of curvature of 7.45 mm; the dotted line demonstrates the contour of the unoperated cornea with its peripheral flattening. After radial keratotomy in the left eye the profile shows the central flattening and paracentral steepening of the cornea, the "knee" being accentuated by the magnified scale. The reference curve at the left has a radius of 8.42 mm that fits the central cornea; the dotted line shows the paracentral steepening in the operated cornea.

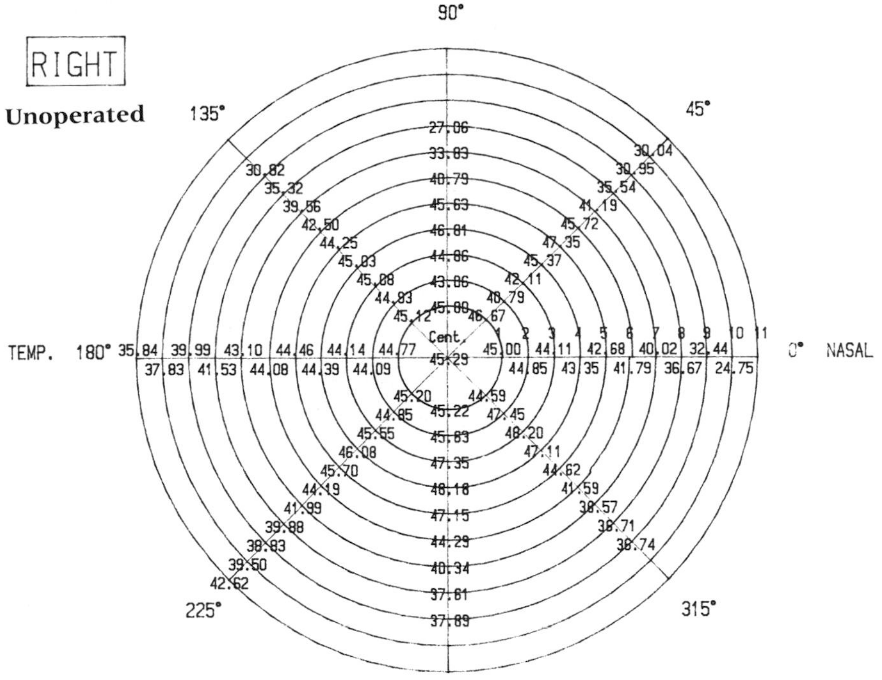

E

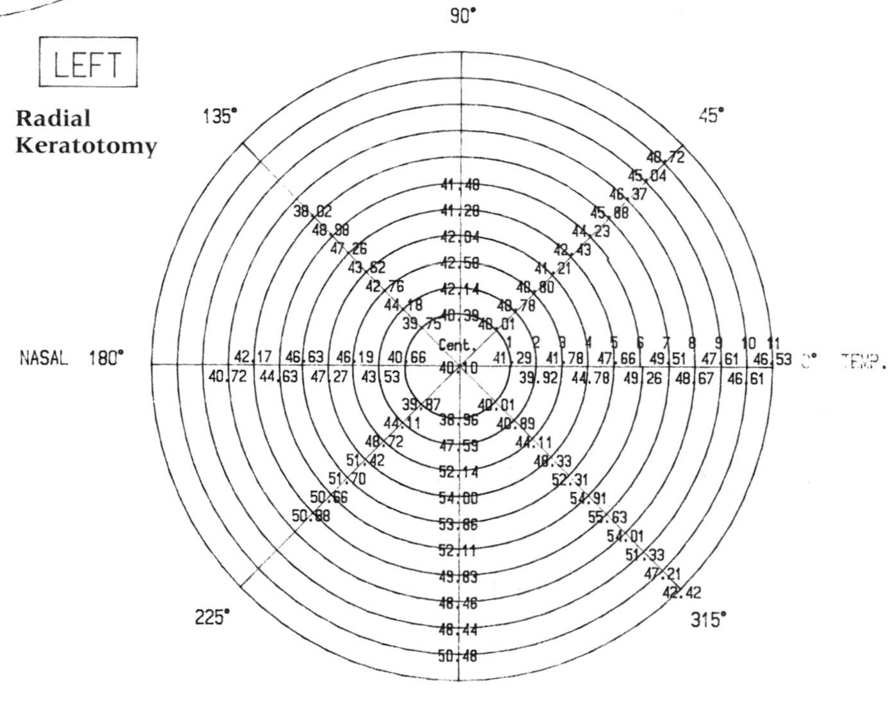

F

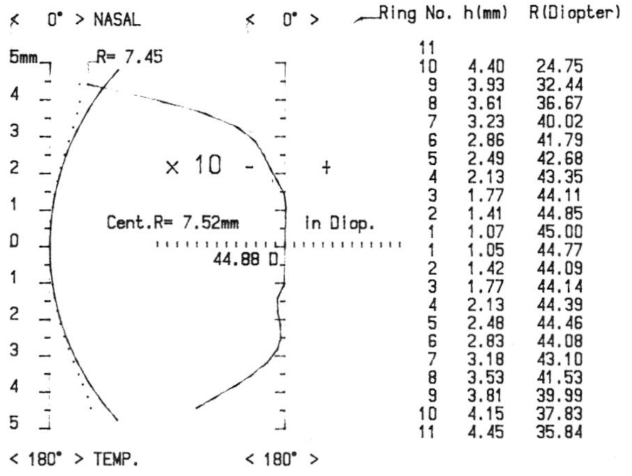

G

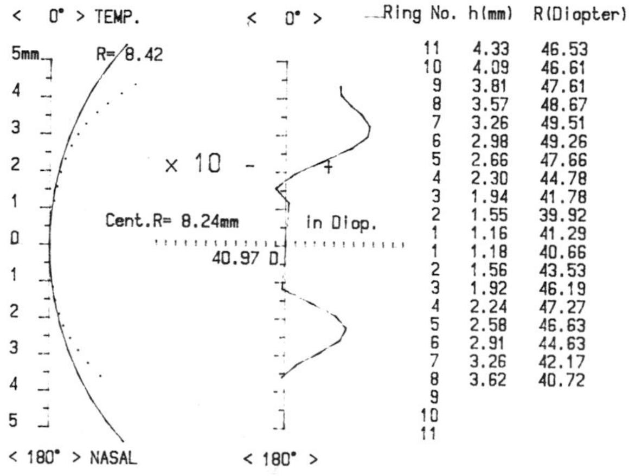

H

Figure 3-49, cont'd
For legend see opposite page.

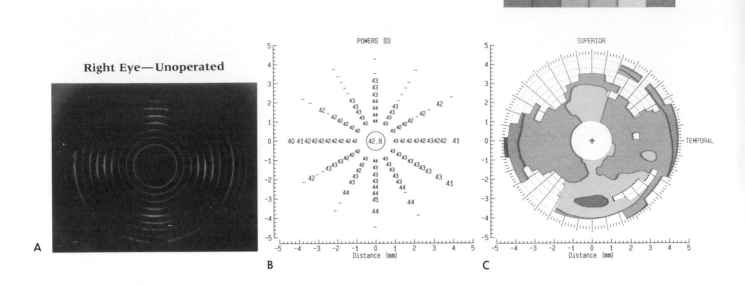

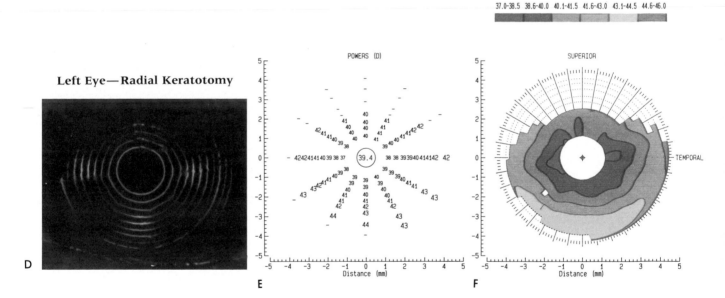

Figure 3-50

Analysis of manually digitized Nidek keratographs as a color-coded map comparing a normal cornea to a cornea after radial keratotomy. The display emphasizes the absence of readings in the central and peripheral cornea as well as the absence from areas where the rings are not imaged.

Keratographs (**A** and **D**): The keratographs show the increased diameter of the rings and the irregular astigmatism after radial keratotomy. *Face Plates* (**B** and **E**): Display of corneal powers across the paracentral zone shows gradual central to peripheral flattening of approximately 1 diopter in the normal cornea and gradual steepening of approximately 4 diopters in operated cornea. *Topographic Map* (**C** and **F**): The color-coded topography maps of the surface have 1.5-diopter intervals between the colors. The map of the unoperated eye (**C**) shows mild astigmatism with the steep meridian vertical (with-the-rule). The postoperative map (**F**) shows the disappearance of that astigmatism and marked flattening of the central cornea. Absent from this keratographic analysis of radial keratotomy is the paracentral "knee." The refractive power gradually increases across the entire paracentral zone, and the entire paracentral cornea is flatter after surgery than before, in contrast to the Nidek analysis and similar to the Kera analysis. See insert for color versions of these illustrations. (Photokeratographs and computer analysis performed by Steven A. Dingeldein and Stephen D. Klyce, Louisiana State University Eye Center, New Orleans, Louisiana.)

Unoperated Eye

Radial Keratotomy

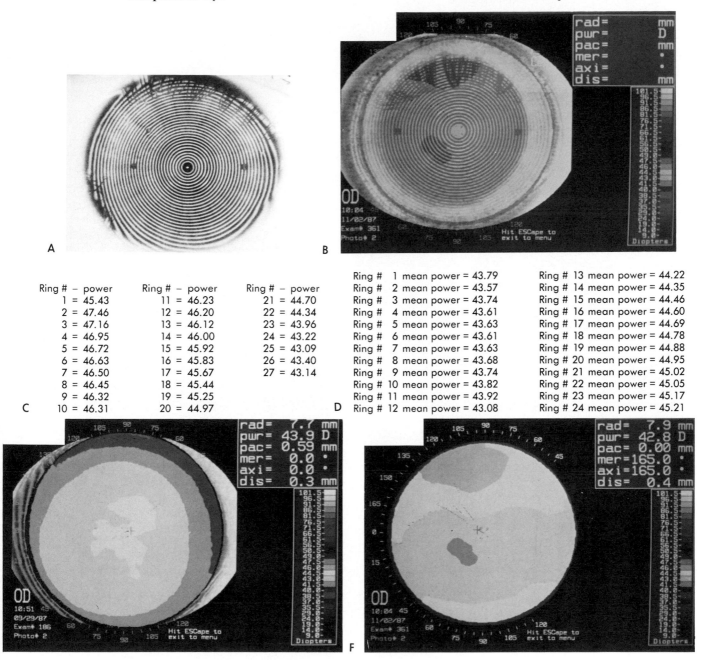

Ring # – power	Ring # – power	Ring # – power
1 = 45.43	11 = 46.23	21 = 44.70
2 = 47.46	12 = 46.20	22 = 44.34
3 = 47.16	13 = 46.12	23 = 43.96
4 = 46.95	14 = 46.00	24 = 43.22
5 = 46.72	15 = 45.92	25 = 43.09
6 = 46.63	16 = 45.83	26 = 43.40
7 = 46.50	17 = 45.67	27 = 43.14
8 = 46.45	18 = 45.44	
9 = 46.32	19 = 45.25	
10 = 46.31	20 = 44.97	

C

Ring # 1 mean power = 43.79	Ring # 13 mean power = 44.22
Ring # 2 mean power = 43.57	Ring # 14 mean power = 44.35
Ring # 3 mean power = 43.74	Ring # 15 mean power = 44.46
Ring # 4 mean power = 43.61	Ring # 16 mean power = 44.60
Ring # 5 mean power = 43.63	Ring # 17 mean power = 44.69
Ring # 6 mean power = 43.61	Ring # 18 mean power = 44.78
Ring # 7 mean power = 43.63	Ring # 19 mean power = 44.88
Ring # 8 mean power = 43.68	Ring # 20 mean power = 44.95
Ring # 9 mean power = 43.74	Ring # 21 mean power = 45.02
Ring # 10 mean power = 43.82	Ring # 22 mean power = 45.05
Ring # 11 mean power = 43.92	Ring # 23 mean power = 45.17
Ring # 12 mean power = 43.08	Ring # 24 mean power = 45.21

D

Figure 3-51

Measurement of corneal topography with the Computed Anatomy Corneal Modeling System, comparing an unoperated normal cornea with a cornea after radial keratotomy.

Keratographs **(A** and **B):** The rings cover the entire surface of the cornea. In the operated eye the rings are superimposed over a color-coded map.

Average ring power **(C** and **D):** Computation of the average power (D) around each of the 24 readable rings shows a gradual flattening of approximately 3.00 D in the normal cornea from central to periphery and a gradual steepening of 1.50 D in the cornea after radial keratotomy (D).

Topographic maps (absolute scale) **(E** and **F):** Color-coded topographic maps using an absolute scale with 1.50-diopter steps between colors show that the unoperated cornea is steeper centrally and flattens approximately 3.00 D from center to periphery. In the eye after radial keratotomy the cornea is flatter centrally and steepens approximately 3.00 D from center to periphery; there is asymmetric astigmatism with-the-rule in which the superior semimeridian is steeper (red) than the inferior part (blue). See insert for color versions of these illustrations.

Continued.

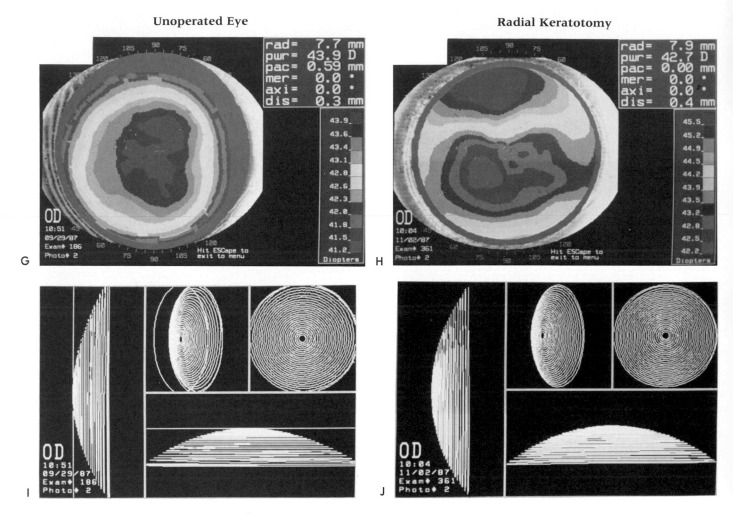

Figure 3-51, cont'd

Color-coded topographic maps (normalized scale) **(G** and **H):** A color-coded topographic map of the surface using a relative color scale with approximately 0.25-diopter steps between colors. The normal cornea shows minimal astigmatism with-the-rule and progressive flattening from center to periphery. In the cornea after radial keratomy the central flatter area has a polygonal configuration, and there is an asymmetric steep area superiorly. See insert for color versions of these illustrations.

Profiles **(I** and **J):** A graphic reconstruction of cross sections of the cornea in the vertical and horizontal meridians. In the normal cornea the cross section demonstrates the more rapid central to peripheral flattening of the nasal side and the persistence of a steeper spherical contour on the temporal side. In the cornea after radial keratotomy the horizontal cross section shows a generally more rounded appearance of the profile as a result of the relative paracentral steepening. In the vertical cross section, the asymmetric astigmatism shown on the color-coded maps is not apparent. (Photographs taken and analyzed by Sadeer Hannush.)

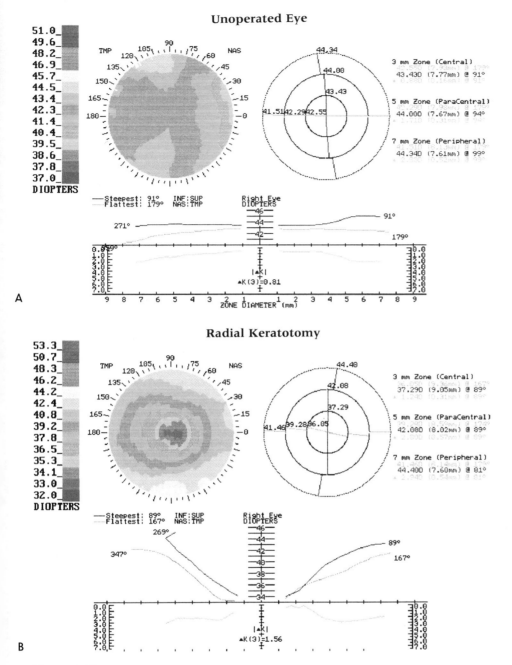

Figure 3-52

Printout for the EyeSys Corneal Analysis System. The system shows a color-coded map with a relative scale to show the distribution of power over the surface of the cornea. Analysis of astigmatism is presented at three different zones, the central, paracentral, and peripheral. Cross-sectional profiles are presented for the steepest and flattest semimeridians nasally and temporally, with a difference to show the amount of astigmatism. **A,** Normal cornea shows the color-coded map steeper centrally and flattening toward the periphery. There is reasonably uniform astigmatism in the three zones. The semimeridional cross-sectional plots show gradual steepening centrally to flattening peripherally with approximately 1 D of astigmatism. **B,** An eye after radial keratotomy shows a flatter central cornea that steepens toward the periphery. The astigmatism map shows approximately 1.75 D of astigmatism in the 3-mm zone and approximately 3.00 D of astigmatism at the 7-mm zone. The semimeridional cross section of the map shows the marked change from the flat center of around 34 D to the steeper paracentral and peripheral zone of about 41 to 42 D. The overall astigmatism is shown as the difference between the steepest and flattest meridians, ranging from approximately 1.00 D centrally to approximately 2.00 to 3.00 D peripherally. See insert for color versions of these illustrations.

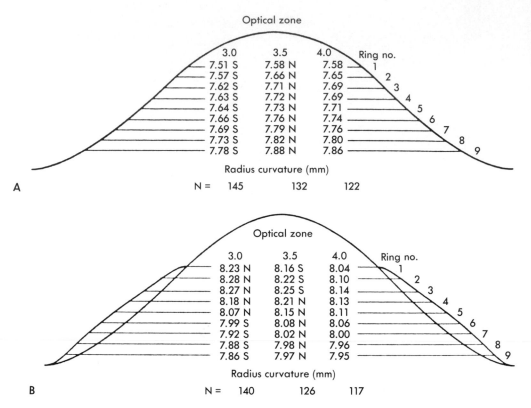

Figure 3-53
Relationship of radius of corneal curvature to refractive power as determined by diameter of optical clear zone. **A,** Before surgery, radius of curvature represents the average of eight readings around each ring. The clear zone 3.0 mm was used for eyes with a refraction of −4.50 to −8.00 D, 3.5 mm for eyes with a refraction of −3.25 to −4.37 D, and 4.0 mm for eyes with a refraction of −2.00 to −3.12 D. The 3.0-mm group with the larger amount of myopia had steeper corneas across all rings than the other two groups. *S,* Significant at $p < 0.01$; *N,* not significant. Number of eyes in each group is indicated below. **B,** After an eight-incision radial keratotomy, the average radii of curvature are flattest for the 3.0-mm population and less flat in the 3.5- and 4.0-mm groups. *S,* Significant difference at the $p < 0.05$ level between columns; *N,* not significant between columns. (From Rowsey JJ, Balyeat HD, Monlux R, Holladay J, Waring GO, Lynn MJ, and PERK Study Group: Ophthalmology 1988;95:322-334.)

7.56 ±0.29 mm at ring one and 7.84 ±0.26 mm at ring nine. The PERK study used three clear zone diameters (3.0, 3.5, and 4.0 mm) depending on the amount of preoperative myopia. Eyes with the highest myopia (3.0-mm clear zone group) had steeper corneas compared with the other two clear zone groups; the mean radius of curvature in this group was approximately 0.1 mm smaller in each of the nine rings (Fig. 3-53). After radial keratotomy surgery the corneas had flattened in all nine rings (Figs. 3-53 and 3-54). However, more flattening occurred in the inner rings and less flattening in the outer rings, so the central cornea was flatter than the paracentral and peripheral cornea. Comparing the three clear zone groups, greater flattening resulted as the clear zone diameter decreased for rings one through four. However, for rings five through nine similar flattening occurred among the clear zone groups.

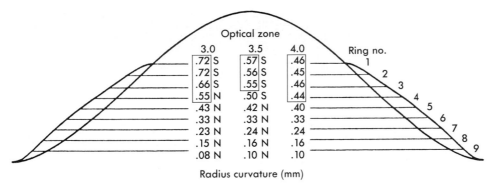

Figure 3-54
The radius of curvature represents the difference between the values preoperative and those 6 months postoperative for each ring. The cornea flattens in all of the rings for all three diameter zone groups. The central cornea flattened more in the eyes with the smaller 3.0-mm optical zone. Pairs of numbers that are significantly different at the $p < 0.01$ level between columns are in the boxes. *S,* Significant at $p < 0.05$ between columns; *N,* not significant. There was a significant difference in flattening of the inner three to four rings in all three optical zones, but the outer five to nine rings were not significantly flatter among the three groups. It is important to remember that the nine-ring keratoscope does not read the central 1 to 2 or the peripheral 2 to 3 mm of the cornea. (From Rowsey JJ, Balyeat HD, Monlux R, Holladay J, Waring GO, Lynn MJ, and PERK Study Group: Ophthalmology 1988;95:322-334.)

Patient age affected the amount of corneal flattening after surgery. In all three clear zone groups, patients less than 30 years of age had 0.1 to 0.3 mm less flattening than patients 40 years of age and older.

Bogan and colleagues[10] used computer-assisted videokeratography to compare the corneal topography of 32 eyes after radial keratotomy with 47 control subjects matched for age and keratometric and refractive powers. The pattern of dioptric power distribution revealed that 60% of the corneas had a polygonal pattern of power distribution, which was not present in normal corneas. The number of points on the polygon was similar to the number of incisions in the cornea, four incisions creating a square, eight incisions creating an octagon, and so forth. Not all of the polygonal patterns were distinct, and some were incomplete or asymmetric (Fig. 3-55). Presumably, the polygonal pattern originates from small focal zones of flattening at the ends of the incisions. The mean range of dioptric power in the 4-mm central area of the cornea overlying a 4-mm standard entrance pupil was 4.8 ±2.4 D after radial keratotomy and only 2.0 ±0.5 D in normal corneas. This twofold increase in the power distribution over the entrance pupil substantiates the concept of a "multifocal cornea" after radial keratotomy.

Analysis of the cross-sectional shape of the cornea showed that approximately 80% were flatter centrally than peripherally after radial keratotomy (oblate shape) with an increase in dioptric power from the center to approximately a zone diameter of 9 mm was 2.8 ±2.2 D, with a sharp inflection zone (the paracentral knee) at a location of approximately 5.5-mm diameter zone. The location of the paracentral knee outside of the pupil suggests that the spherical aberration produced by this would not always affect the optical function of the cornea, since it lies outside the pupil. There was more paracentral and peripheral steepening in the vertical meridian than in the horizontal meridian (Fig. 3-56).

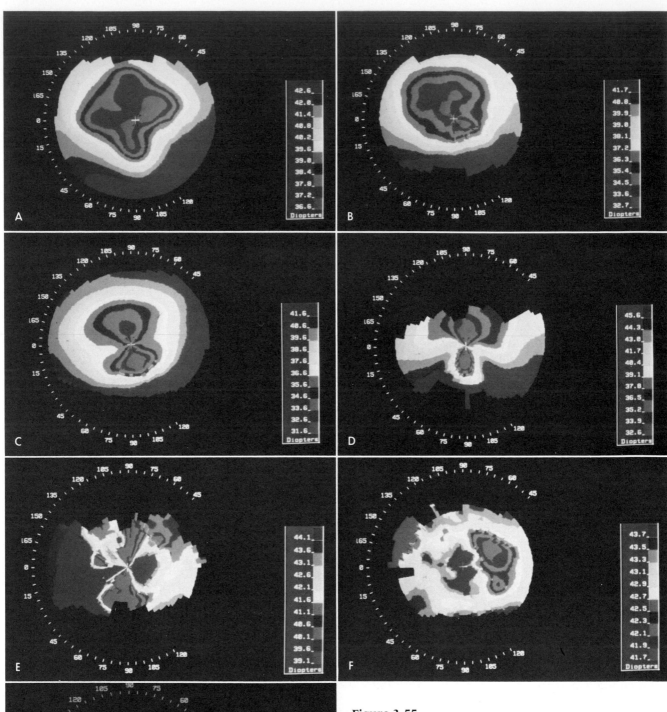

Figure 3-55

Videokeratographs showing patterns of power distribution and cross-sectional shape configurations after radial keratotomy. The polygonal pattern was not seen in normal eyes. **A,** Polygonal pattern, oblate shape. **B,** Round pattern, oblate shape. **C,** Symmetric bowtie pattern, oblate shape. **D,** Asymmetric bowtie pattern, oblate shape. **E,** Bowtie pattern, mixed prolate/oblate shape. **F,** Polygonal pattern, oblate shape. Steep/flat/steep ("nipple") configuration. **G,** Irregular pattern, irregular shape. See insert for color versions of these illustrations. (From Bogan SJ, Maloney RK, Drews C, and Waring GO: Arch Ophthalmol 1991;109:834-841.)

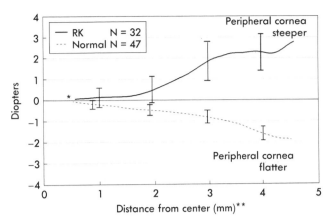

*Average of 0°, 90°, 180°, and 270° semimeridians.
**From corneal image of fixation light.
A   Vertical bars show standard deviation.

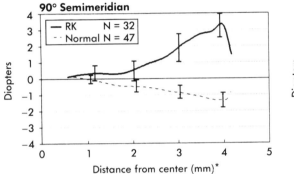

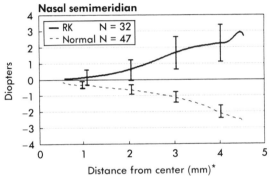

B

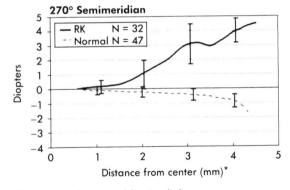

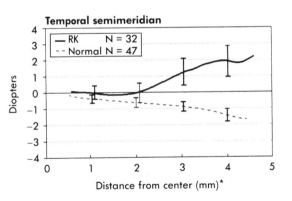

*From corneal image of fixation light.
Vertical bars show standard deviation.

Figure 3-56
Corneal asphericity represented by a plot of the difference in dioptric power between ring 1 and rings 2 through 27. **A,** Average of values for 0°, 90°, 180°, and 270° semimeridians combined. The curves demonstrate that after radial keratotomy the cornea is more aspheric and has a more variable rate of change in dioptric power than normal corneas. **B,** 0°, 90°, 180°, and 270° semimeridians individually. Asymmetry in asphericity among semimeridians is greater after radial keratotomy than in normal eyes. (From Bogan SJ, Maloney RK, Drews C, and Waring GO: Arch Ophthalmol 1991;109:834-841.)

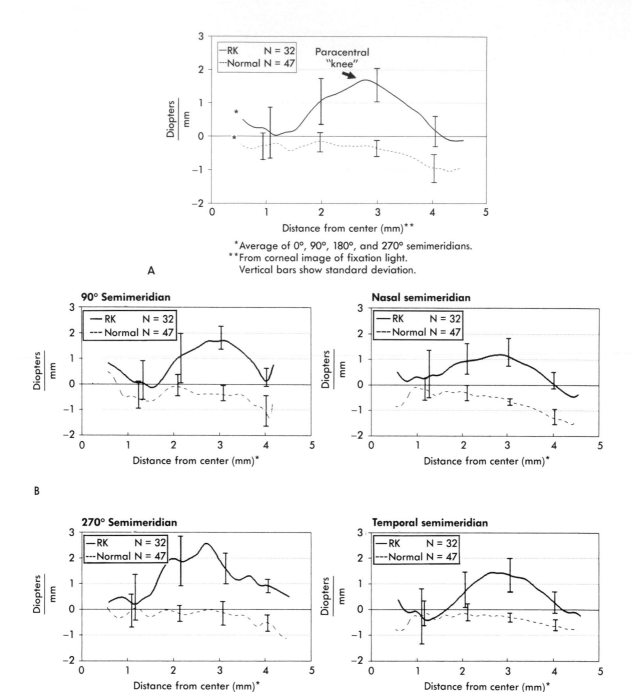

Figure 3-57
Rate of change in corneal dioptric power between ring 1 and rings 2 through 27. **A,**
Average of 0°, 90°, 180°, and 270° semimeridians combined. The curves demonstrate
a sharp inflection zone ("paracentral knee") after radial keratotomy, 2.7 ±0.1 mm
from the center. **B,** 0°, 90°, 180°, and 270° semimeridians individually. Graphs show
asymmetry in the rate of change in corneal power along semimeridians. (From
Bogan SJ, Maloney RK, Drews C, and Waring GO: Arch Ophthalmol 1991;
109:834-841.)

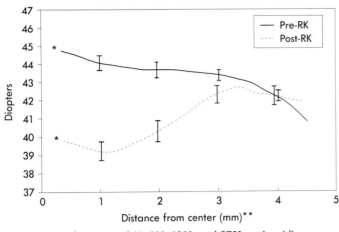

*Average of 0°, 90°, 180°, and 270° semimeridians.
**From corneal image of fixation light.
Vertical bars show standard deviation.

Figure 3-58
Example of corneal asphericity in one eye before and after radial keratotomy shows central flattening and peripheral steepening after radial keratotomy. (From Bogan SJ, Maloney RK, Drews C, and Waring GO: Arch Ophthalmol 1991;109:834-841.)

The paracentral knee was located at the edge of or outside of the normal pupillary diameter of 5.5 to 6.0 mm (Fig. 3-57). The paracentral knee showed more steepening in the vertical meridian than the horizontal meridian. It is possible that the difference between vertical and horizontal meridians reflects the force of the lids moving up and down over the cornea, which might have a compressive effect, producing slightly more change in the vertical meridian. In eight eyes for which both preoperative and postoperative videokeratographs were available, the peripheral cornea was steeper after radial keratotomy than preoperatively (Fig. 3-58), indicating that radial keratotomy does produce a central flattening and a peripheral steepening of the cornea.

RELATIONSHIP OF REFRACTIVE ERROR, VISUAL ACUITY, AND CORNEAL TOPOGRAPHY

The cornea is more aspheric ("multifocal") than normal after radial keratotomy, creating new relationships between uncorrected visual acuity and residual refractive error.

Refractive error and visual acuity in normal eyes

Methods of measuring the refractive error and visual acuity are important and must be defined in any study. Manifest refraction, particularly in myopic individuals, may measure more minus power than is actually present because of accommodation. Accommodation can be controlled by the fogging technique of placing excess plus power before the eye to relax accommodation and gradually adding minus power to neutralize the myopia. Alternatively, mild cycloplegia, such as 0.5% tropicamide (Mydriacyl), can be used to decrease accommodation without producing maximal pupillary dilation. Full cycloplegia associated with a large pupil adequately controls accommodation but will also induce optical aberrations from the paracentral or peripheral cornea that may be irrelevant to daily visual function, although such aberrations might account for nocturnal visual phenomena.

Methods of reporting the refractive error also are important. Expressing the refractive error as the spherical equivalent is a useful shorthand way to deal with many eyes, but it can be misleading. For example, an eye with a refractive error of +0.50 D sphere has the same spherical equivalent as an eye with a refractive error of +2.00 −3.00 × 90°. Clearly, the uncorrected visual acuity of these two

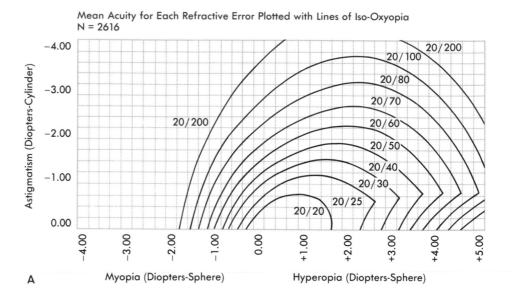

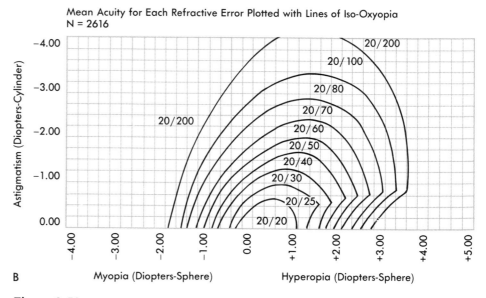

Figure 3-59

Relationship between refractive error and visual acuity. **A,** Age group, 25 to 35 years. **B,** Age group, 45 to 55 years. The spherical portion of the refractive error is represented on the x-axis and the amount of refractive astigmatism on the y-axis. Uncorrected visual acuity is represented between the arching lines. Age has little effect on the relationship between myopia and visual acuity, but a marked effect on the relationship between hyperopia and visual acuity. For hyperopic persons, small amounts of astigmatism (less than 1.00 D) actually improve uncorrected visual acuity. (From Peters HB: Am J Optom and Arch Am Acad Optom 1961;38:194-198.)

"equivalent" refractive errors would not be the same; any study of the correlation between uncorrected visual acuity and refractive error must recognize astigmatism.

Peters[83] studied the relationship between spherical and astigmatic refractive error in normal eyes of patients in different age groups (Fig. 3-59), including 2216 eyes of individuals between 25 and 35 years of age and 2183 eyes of individuals between 45 and 55 years of age. All eyes were structurally normal with a 20/20 or better spectacle-corrected visual acuity. He concluded that visual acuity decreased with increasing amounts of myopia at all ages. In hypermetropic individuals, uncorrected visual acuity decreased progressively with age and the onset of presbyopia. Small amounts of astigmatism, expressed in minus cylinder, improved visual acuity in eyes with higher amounts of hyperopia, but astigmatism greater than 0.75 D decreased visual acuity for all individuals.

Refractive error, visual acuity, and corneal topography after radial keratotomy

Studies of the relationship between refractive error and visual acuity after radial keratotomy have been carried out by the PERK Study Group. In one study,[100] the authors selected all eyes whose residual spherical equivalent cycloplegic refractive error at 1 year was between −3.00 and +3.00 D. The range was selected because all but one eye had an uncorrected visual acuity of 20/200 or better. This group represented 394 of the 435 PERK patients, one eye of each patient, omitting those that had repeated operations. Operated eyes 1 year after radial keratotomy had a better average uncorrected visual acuity (noncycloplegic) than unoperated eyes with similar cycloplegic refractive errors ($p < 0.0001$). Visual acuity without correction after radial keratotomy spanned five to ten Snellen lines within each 0.50- to 1.00-diopter range of refractive error. This was true for both myopic and hyperopic eyes.

A curvilinear relationship existed between the refraction and the uncorrected visual acuity (Fig. 3-60), as described mathematically by the following polynomial regression equation:

$$VA = 55.74 + 5.67 \ (REF) - 3.80 \ (REF^2) - 0.32 \ (REF^3)$$

where *VA* represents the uncorrected visual acuity and *REF* represents the spherical equivalent of the cycloplegic refraction. The constant term 55.74 was the average number of letters seen by an eye that was emmetropic 1 year after radial keratotomy (20/20). The 90% prediction interval of the visual acuity spanned six to seven Snellen lines. For example, the PERK authors were 90% confident that the visual acuity of a patient with a refraction of −2.00 D would be between 20/32 and 20/100, a range of six Snellen lines.

Another way to look at the relationship between visual acuity and refraction is to group the eyes according to visual acuity. Within each level of visual acuity between 20/16 and 20/50, the cycloplegic refractive error spanned 3 to 5 D in the PERK study.

Astigmatism reduced visual acuity in patients with 1.00 D or less of spherical equivalent refractive error, but it had no significant effect on the visual acuity of patients with 1.25 D or more spherical equivalent refraction.

To obtain a more detailed comparison of uncorrected visual acuity before and after radial keratotomy, eyes with a cycloplegic refractive error between −2.00 and −2.50 D were selected; this included 56 eyes before radial keratotomy and 29 eyes 1 year after radial keratotomy. The unoperated eyes had a mean uncorrected, noncycloplegic visual acuity of 20/125 (range, 20/40 to 20/200), whereas the operated eyes in the same range of refraction had a mean uncorrected visual acuity of 20/60 (range, 20/30 to 20/125), an improvement over the unoperated

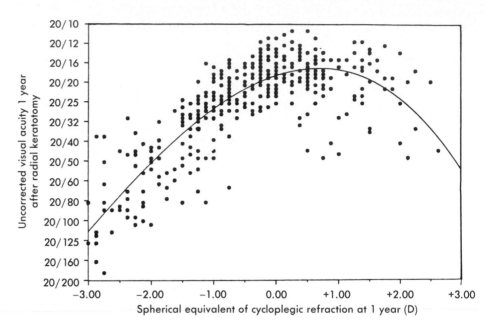

Figure 3-60

Relationship of uncorrected visual acuity after radial keratotomy to spherical equivalent cycloplegic refraction in the PERK study. Scattergram of 394 eyes demonstrates six Snellen line range of acuity that exists for most refractive errors. Curved line represents the following polygonal regression equation relating uncorrected acuity *(VA)* and refractive error *(REF):* $VA = 55.74 + 5.67 (REF) - 3.80 (REF^2) - 0.32 (REF^3)$, for which $R^2 = 0.70$. (From Santos VR, Waring GO, Lynn MJ, et al: Arch Ophthalmol 1987;105:86-92.)

eyes of three Snellen lines. Of the unoperated eyes, 82% had a visual acuity of 20/100 or worse, compared with only 38% of the operated eyes (Figs. 3-61 and 3-62). Clearly, some optical change had occurred in the cornea after radial keratotomy to improve uncorrected visual acuity. Presumably this resulted from a "multifocal" effect of the central and paracentral cornea that was not measured by the cycloplegic refraction alone. Applegate and Jones[3] have offered an interpretation of these findings. Applegate and Jones[3] pointed out that the PERK study compared uncorrected visual acuity in the manifest state, when the pupil was relatively small, with the residual cycloplegic refractive error, when the pupil was dilated allowing the central and the paracentral-peripheral optics of the cornea to affect the result. These authors compared the findings in the PERK study with those in three other studies of refractive error and visual acuity in unoperated eyes (Fig. 3-63) and observed that the uncorrected visual acuities for eyes receiving radial keratotomy in the PERK study were consistently better for any given refractive error than for the unoperated eyes in other studies. They correctly emphasized that the PERK authors should publish data for manifest acuity and manifest refraction using a pupil of equal size for both measurements to give a more realistic relationship between the visual acuity and the refractive error and to better draw conclusions about the effect of radial keratotomy on central corneal optics. When the PERK authors did compare the manifest refraction with the manifest visual acuity (unpublished data), the results were essentially the same as those found for the cycloplegic refraction, and a significant dif-

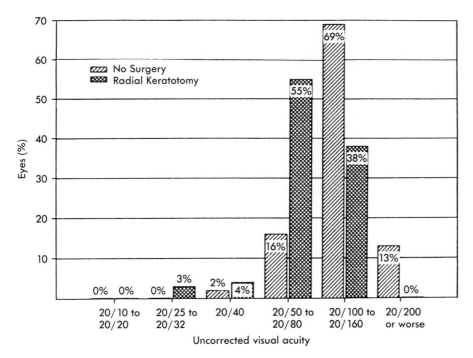

Figure 3-61
Comparison of uncorrected visual acuity for eyes before and after radial keratotomy with spherical equivalent cycloplegic refractive errors between −2.00 and −2.50 D. The uncorrected visual acuity was better in the operated eyes (N = 29) 1 year after radial keratotomy than in the unoperated eyes (N = 56) in the PERK study. (From Santos VR, Waring GO, Lynn MJ, and the PERK Study Group: Arch Ophthalmol 1987;105:86-92.)

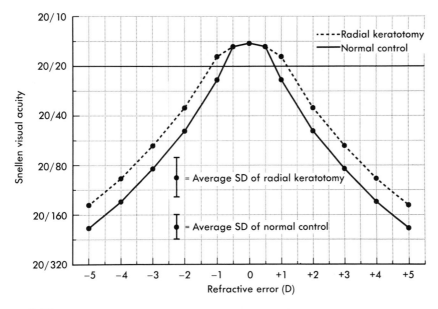

Figure 3-62
Schematic representation of relationship between visual acuity and refractive error and normal eyes and eyes after radial keratotomy. For small refractive errors, normal eyes see better. However, as the refractive error increases, the eyes after radial keratotomy see better. (From Holladay JT, Lynn MJ, Waring GO, Gemmill M, Keehn GC, and Fielding B: Arch Ophthalmol 1991;109:70-76.)

ference remained in the mean uncorrected visual acuity between eyes with a manifest refraction of −2.00 and −2.50 D before and after surgery (Fig. 3-64). The normal pupillary diameter in indirect sunlight outdoors is approximately 3.0 mm (range 1.7 to 3.6) and at night is 5.0 mm (range 3.5 to 6.1) (Table 3-8).

Holladay and colleagues[52] have studied the relationship of visual acuity, refractive error, and pupil size after radial keratotomy, emphasizing that pupil di-

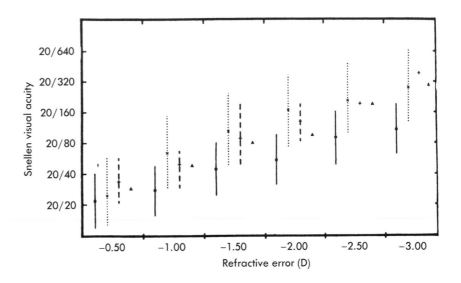

Measurement Parameters in Four Studies of Visual Acuity as Function of Refractive Error

Study	Error bar	Central tendency	VA* as determined by pupil	Refraction
PERK[100]	90% confidence interval	Midpoint of confidence interval	Bailey-Lovie chart: undilated	Cycloplegic
Hirsch[50]	95% confidence interval	Mean	Clason VA meter: undilated	Manifest
Crawford et al.[23]	Range	Mean	AO* chart: undilated	Cycloplegic
Pincus[88]	—	Mean	AO* chart: dilated or undilated†	Cycloplegic or manifest‡

*VA, Visual acuity; AO, American Optical.
†It is unclear from the article whether the acuity was measured before the instillation of the cycloplegic agent.
‡Cycloplegic refractions were performed on individuals under 40 years of age; manifest refractions, on individuals over 40 years of age.

Figure 3-63
Uncorrected visual acuity as a function of refractive error in four different studies. (Measurement parameters for each study are shown in the table.) Solid lines indicate PERK study[100]; dotted lines, Hirsch study[50]; broken lines, study of Crawford et al.[23]; and triangles, Pincus study.[88] Uncorrected visual acuity in the PERK study after radial keratotomy is better for given refractive errors than in the other three studies, in which normal eyes are shown. (From Applegate RA et al: Refract Corneal Surg 1990;6:47-54.)

ameters between 0.5 mm and 3.0 mm create a complex relationship between visual acuity, diffraction, defocus, and optical aberrations. When the pupil diameter is between 3.0 and 5.4 mm, diffraction no longer plays a role, and defocus and optical aberrations are joined by an additional factor, the Stiles-Crawford effect; decreasing the pupil diameter greater than 5.4 mm has little effect on the visual acuity because of the Stiles-Crawford effect. The relationship of visual

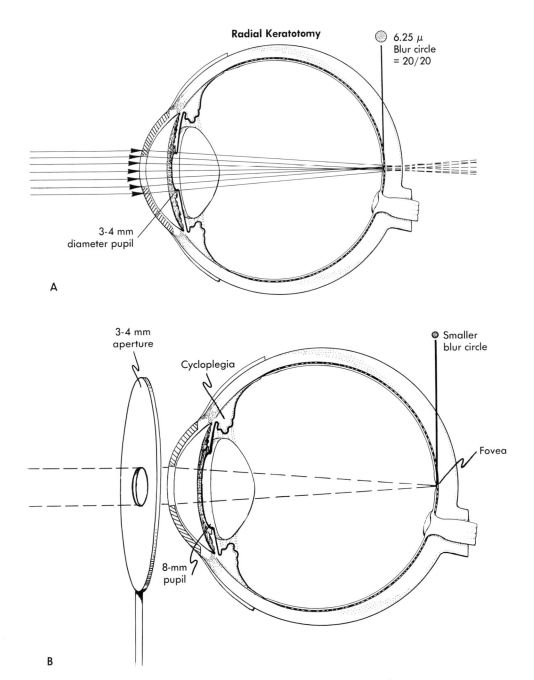

Figure 3-64
Relationship of pupil diameter and visual acuity after radial keratotomy. **A,** The aspheric curvature of the paracentral cornea after radial keratotomy creates a larger than normal blur circle on the fovea. **B,** If the pupil is dilated, the paracentral and peripheral aspheric cornea has a greater effect on the refraction visual acuity. This can be controlled by placing an aperture the size of the normal pupil in front of the eye and refracting through it. Cycloplegia controls accommodation under these circumstances.

Table 3-8

Pupil Diameter (mm) for Patients* 20 to 70 Years of Age under Different Illumination Conditions

Illumination† (ft-candles)	Fixation target	Simulated activity	No. of patients	Mean (SD)	Range
0	Distance	Night driving	37	5.1 (0.7)	3.5-6.1
20	Near	Reading—low illumination	43	3.4 (0.6)	2.2-5.2
80	Near	Reading—high illumination	42	2.8 (0.4)	1.7-3.9
320	Distance	Outdoors—indirect sunlight	43	2.7 (0.4)	1.7-3.6
1000	Distance	Outdoors—direct sunlight	43	2.2 (0.3)	1.5-3.1

Courtesy Douglas Koch, M.D.
*Measured pupil size reduced 14% to account for corneal magnification. Subjects not using topical ocular medication; no history of prior ocular surgery, iritis, severe ocular trauma, or retinal or optic nerve disease.
†Approximate values as registered by light meter.

acuity, defocus (refractive error), and pupil diameter is nonlinear for pupils larger than 0.5 mm. In general, the larger the pupil, the worse the uncorrected visual acuity for a given refractive error (see Table 3-7).

In an attempt to determine the effect of corneal topography on uncorrected visual acuity and refractive error, the authors refracted patients with their pupils under cycloplegia, with their pupils dilated, and then through a fixed aperture the same size as their natural pupil to see what the effect of the paracentral cornea was (see Fig. 3-64). Surprisingly, they found shifts between the aperture refraction and the dilated pupil refraction in both the myopic and hyperopic directions. In a control group, only 9% eyes had a change in refraction with and without the aperture, 7% being in the myopic direction. These results are consistent with previous measurements of the spherical aberration of the human eye, in which the marginal rays of the eyes are focused anterior to the paraxial rays when the pupil is dilated, creating a myopic change in the refraction. Ninety percent of humans have less than 0.50 D of refractive change with normal pupillary dilation. In the radial keratotomy group, 36% had a change in the cycloplegic refraction with a pupil dilated, indicating that radial keratotomy increases the incidence of clinically significant spherical aberration (0.50 D). In the Holladay study,[52] the change in refraction was almost equally split between the myopic (19%) and the hyperopic (17%) directions. These findings help clarify the role of corneal topography after radial keratotomy. The paracentral cornea flattens less than the central cornea, creating a relatively steeper "paracentral knee" (see Fig. 3-57). If this "paracentral knee" were within the effective optical zone of the cornea (the zone less than 5.4 mm diameter), most of the radial keratotomy patients should have a myopic change with pupillary dilation; but this did not happen in the Holladay study. However, if the "paracentral knee" were present at 6 mm or greater, it would have a minimal result on the refraction. Indeed, this is the location of the paracentral knee described by Bogan and colleagues[10] using videokeratographic analysis after radial keratotomy (see Fig. 3-57). Thus the better uncorrected visual acuity and the increase in the incidence of a refractive change with a larger pupil after radial keratotomy indicate that the optical configuration of the cornea following surgery has been changed,

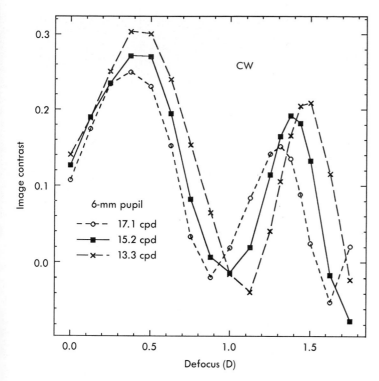

Figure 3-65
The modulation transfer (image contrast/object contrast) as a function of defocus (distance in diopters of the receiving plane in front of the paraxial focus) for a model eye at three spatial frequencies. The eye has 2.00 D of positive longitudinal spherical aberration at the edge of a 6-mm pupil. It has no other aberrations. (From Hemenger RP, Tomlinson A, and McDonnell PJ: Invest Ophthalmol Vis Sci 1990;31:1644-1646.)

so the best-corrected visual acuity is no different than normal, but the uncorrected visual acuity is better. This change in optical configuration of the cornea creates a multifocal effect similar to aspheric multifocal intraocular lenses.

Hemenger and colleagues[48] (Fig. 3-65) have quantified the positive longitudinal spherical aberration (that is, the increase in dioptric powers from the center to the paracentral and peripheral cornea) by measuring the sagittal height for a series of semichord lengths and using a polynomial equation to approximate the corneal shape. They found two separate focal points, the second focus anterior to the first (as we have illustrated in Figs. 3-2 and 3-64). This formed a plausible explanation for the observation that uncorrected visual acuity in patients with residual hyperopia or presbyopia after radial keratotomy is better than expected.

Another approach to analyzing the relationship between topography and visual acuity after radial keratotomy is to consider the central portion of the cornea to be "multifocal." McDonnell and colleagues[78] propounded this hypothesis when they observed on videokeratographs that areas in the central cornea might differ by 2 D or more in refractive power.

Maguire and Bourne[70] also attributed the maintenance of good visual acuity over such a wide range of refractive correction to the multifocal effect. However, because the inferior portion of the corneas of their patients had a much greater range of central to peripheral change than the superior portion, they suggested that the patient may have had subclinical keratoconus before the operation (Fig. 3-66).

Applegate and colleagues[2,4] have reported the use of the aberroscope to study the aberrations induced by the cornea after radial keratotomy. The instrument projects a perfect grid through the pupil onto the retina, and the patient draws the perceived grid, drawing the distortions induced by the ocular media. The authors studied 31 eyes of 17 individuals after radial keratotomy, but only five patients were able to produce drawings of the grid across a large enough corneal

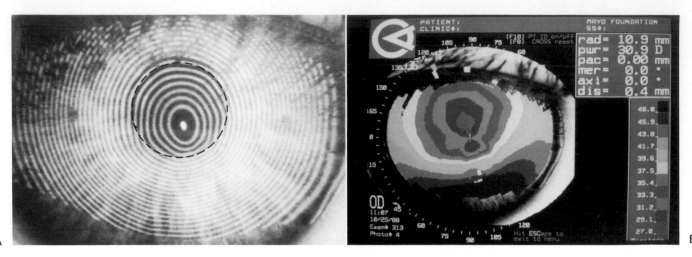

Figure 3-66

Multifocal cornea with possible early keratoconus after radial keratotomy. **A,** Videokeratograph shows rings closer together inferiorly. Note position of entrance pupil *(dotted line).* **B,** Gray-scale contour map demonstrates small area of central power with measurements below 30 D that is surrounded by concentric bands of increasing higher power. There is wide variability in power in the area corresponding to the entrance pupil, creating a "multifocal" cornea and allowing the patient to accept a wide range of refractive corrections. (From Maguire LJ and Bourne WM: Refract Corneal Surg 1989;6:394-397.)

surface to allow analysis. In these five eyes, the aberrations had magnitudes approximately 100 times that of nonoperated eyes, the aberrations diminishing somewhat during the first few months after surgery. The aberroscope pictures showed that dilation of the pupil to 4 to 6 mm decreased the modulation transfer function, indicating that as the image of the grid passed (transferred) through the optics of the eye it was modulated and lost contrast; this occurred more often after radial keratotomy with a dilated pupil than under normal circumstances (Fig. 3-67). This suggests that contrast sensitivity was decreased, a subject discussed in more detail in Chapter 23, Complications of Refractive Keratotomy.

Refraction after radial keratotomy

Rowsey and Ruben[95] have emphasized the problems of refracting patients and prescribing spectacles after radial keratotomy. The major problem is that the retinoscopic reflection is quite different from the simpler linear streak seen preoperatively, since after surgery it shows a scissors motion and a different configuration, often wider in the center and narrower at the edges of the pupil. Thus after full neutralization of the peripheral retinoscopic reflex, there is likely to be residual against motion in the center of the pupil. This probably results from the central flatter area and the paracentral relatively steeper area producing multifocal reflexes (see Fig. 3-45, *K*).

We describe here a step-by-step approach to the refraction of the patient after radial keratotomy.[51]

The retinoscopist must concentrate on the central 3 mm of the reflex, since this area is most important in forming the foveal image. It is sometimes easier to concentrate on this area through an undilated pupil so that the paracentral and peripheral reflexes are not visible and distracting. When the pupil is undilated, however, the problem of accommodation often makes the eye appear exces-

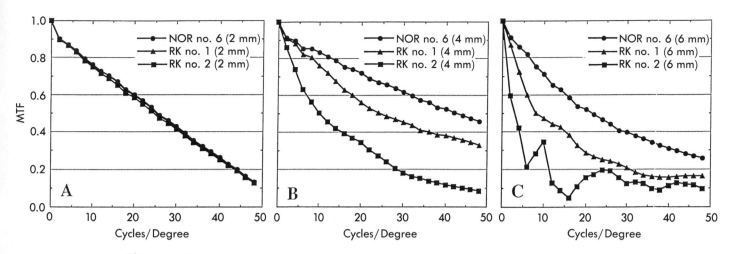

Figure 3-67
Three graphs depict the modulation transfer function *(MTF)* as a function of band width on the horizontal axis for two radial keratotomy patients *(RK #1, RK #2)* and one normal patient *(Nor #6).* **A,** With a 2-mm pupil there is no difference in MTF of the three eyes. **B,** However, as the pupil dilates to 4 mm, MTF of the two radial keratotomy patients drops below that of the normal patient. **C,** This condition continues when the pupil is dilated to 6 mm. This indicates disruption of the quality of the visual image as the incised paracentral cornea comes into play after radial keratotomy. (From Applegate RA and Gansel KA: Refract Corneal Surg 1990;6:47-54.)

sively myopic. The best compromise is to use a weak cycloplegic drug, such as 0.5% tropicamide (Mydriacil) with no sympathomimetic, such as phenylephrine. The pupil size is usually 4 to 5 mm with tropicamide alone, yet adequate cycloplegia is attained.

The patient should first have a dry manifest refraction with no cycloplegic drugs. Fogging techniques must be employed to reduce accommodation to a minimum. Usually this involves simply overplussing the contralateral eye during the manifest refraction. Unfortunately, many patients take much more minus power than their actual refraction requires because of accommodation; since this additional minus can cause miosis of the pupil, the letters appear smaller and darker.

After the dry manifest refraction, the pupil should be dilated using only 0.5% tropicamide (Mydriacil) and the refraction repeated approximately 20 to 30 minutes later. If the pupil becomes very large the final vision may be decreased and the refraction is less useful because of the paracentral cornea's influence on the foveal image. The patient, who may otherwise have been very happy with the visual results, can become discouraged.

To control both accommodation and pupil size, cycloplegia can be induced and a 3- to 4-mm (approximately ⅛ inch) aperture placed in a trial frame and positioned so that the patient achieves the clearest vision (see Fig. 3-64). The patient should be encouraged to move his or her head to find the position yielding the clearest vision.

A smaller aperture should be avoided because the pinhole effect increases the depth of field and makes it difficult for the patient to see differences in lenses as they are presented. A larger aperture may be used, but it should not exceed the diameter of the central clear zone of the radial keratotomy.

The topography of the cornea must be related to optical function. Computerized ray tracing will become increasingly sophisticated and must take into account not only geometric optics of the cornea, but also psychophysical functions of the visual system, such as the effect of rays entering different areas of the pupil and contrast sensitivity functions; the human brain is not an optical bench. There is a need to correlate the optical effects of corneal topography and to differentiate between irregular corneas with good and bad optical performance, for both Snellen visual acuity and contrast sensitivity. The development of spatially integrated autorefractors that can measure the refraction in different areas of the cornea would greatly improve our understanding of the change in corneal optics created by refractive keratotomy. In a few years, clinicians may regard simple keratometry, spherocylindrical refraction, and Snellen visual acuity testing as laughably archaic methods of assessing the optical function of the visual system.

UNFINISHED BUSINESS

Aspheric optics have played a major role in the development of ophthalmology, particularly in instrument design. An improved understanding of the physiologic implications of aspheric optics in the cornea is a challenge for the future of refractive surgery. The first challenge is to measure the corneal curvature, a task currently approached by way of corneal topography with videokeratography. Although the ability to image the entire corneal surface is improving, a method is needed to quantify corneal topography in a clinically meaningful fashion by the development of topographic indices and shape factors, respecting the important fact that the portion of the cornea overlying the entrance pupil of the eye is the most important portion for forming the retinal image. Optical ray tracing must then be done to understand the images created by the aspheric cornea, including multifocal effects and various optical aberrations. Finally, this optical information must be proved clinically relevant by psychophysical testing, since it is well known that a less-than-perfect optical image can be compatible with excellent visual acuity without loss of contrast sensitivity because of retinal and central processing of the image.

On the clinical level the relationships among refraction, corneal topography, central keratometry, visual acuity, and contrast sensitivity need to be clarified and explained, with the overall goal of meaningful clinical assessment of optical and visual function of the cornea, the eye, and the patient. Presently, high-contrast Snellen visual acuity, manifest and cycloplegic refraction, and central keratometry are the mainstays of clinical assessment. Will these be replaced by contrast sensitivity testing, autorefraction, and measurements of corneal topography? Probably so, but not until better methods of practically assimilating these newer techniques into clinical practice emerge.

Increasing this challenge is the radial asymmetry of the cornea. Understanding topography, planning astigmatic surgery, and analyzing the results of refractive procedures in general require thinking in terms of semimeridians, and not simply "the steep and flat axis." This greatly increases the complexity of clinical understanding and the mathematical algorithms necessary to analyze such a complex surface. It takes us beyond the simple idea of a "central spherical cornea," past the concepts of the cornea as an elliptical conic section with oblate and prolate axes, to the reality of an anatomically eccentric, radially asymmetric, aspheric optical surface. How much of this detailed information is truly clinically relevant must be defined. All such definitions must take into account the location and diameter of the entrance pupil of the eye.

REFERENCES

1. Applegate RA and Gansel KA: The importance of pupil size in optical quality measurements following radial keratotomy, Refract Corneal Surg 1990;6:47-54.
2. Applegate RA, Johnson CA, Holland HC, et al: Optical aberrations of the eye following radial keratotomy: initial results, Invest Ophthalmol Vis Sci 1988;29(suppl):280.
3. Applegate RA and Jones DH: Relationship between refractive error and visual acuity in the PERK study, Arch Ophthalmol 1987;105:1478-1479.
4. Applegate RA, Johnson CA, Howland HC, et al: Monochromatic wave-front aberrations following radial keratotomy. In Technical Digest Series: Noninvasive assessment of the visual system, vol 9, Washington, DC, 1989, Optical Society of America, pp 98-102.
5. Arffa RC, Klyce SD, and Busin M: Keratometry and epikeratophakia, J Refract Surg 1986;2:61-64.
6. Arffa RC, Warnicki JW, and Rehkopf PG: Corneal topography using raster-stereography, Eur J Implant Refract Surg 1989;1:45-48.
7. Arffa RC, Warnicki JW, and Rehkopf PG: Corneal topography using raster-stereography, Refract Corneal Surg 1989;5:414-417.
8. Arrowsmith PN and Marks RG: Visual, refractive, and keratometric results of radial keratotomy: a 2-year follow-up, Arch Ophthalmol 1987;105:76-80.
9. Binder PS: Optical problems following refractive surgery, Ophthalmology 1986;93:739-745.
10. Bogan SJ, Maloney RK, Drews C, and Waring GO: Computer-assisted videokeratography of corneal topography after radial keratotomy, Arch Ophthalmol (in press).
11. Bogan SJ, Maloney R, and Waring GO: Computer-assisted analysis of corneal topography after radial keratotomy, Invest Ophthalmol Vis Sci 1990;31:30.
12. Bogan SJ, Waring GO, Ibrahim O, Drews C, and Curtis L: Classification of normal corneal topography based on computer-assisted videokeratography, Arch Ophthalmol 1990;108:945-949.
13. Burk LL, Radjee B, Waring GO, and Stulting RD: The effect of selective suture removal on astigmatism following penetrating keratoplasty, Ophthalmic Surg 1988;19:849-854.
14. Calkins JL, Hochheimer BF, and Stark WJ: Corneal wound healing: holographic stress-test analysis, Invest Ophthalmol Vis Sci 1981;8:322.

15. Camp JJ, Maguire LF, Cameron BM, and Robb RA: A computer model for the evaluation of the effect of corneal topography on optical performance, Am J Ophthalmol 1990;109:379-386.
16. Campbell CJ, Koester CJ, Rittler MC, and Tackaberry RB, editors: Physiological optics, New York, 1974, Harper & Row Publishers, Inc.
17. Carsten E and Jontofte S: The central-peripheral radius of the normal corneal curvature: a photokeratoscopic study, Acta Ophthalmol 1985;63:670-677.
18. Chandler M: Photokeratography using moiré techniques, Appl Optics 1976;15:2694.
19. Clark BAJ: Variations in corneal topography, Aust J Optom 1973;56:140-155.
20. Clark BAJ: Mean topography of normal corneas, Aust J Optom 1974;57:107-114.
21. Cohen KL, Tripoli NK, Pellom AC, Kupper LA, and Fryczkowski AW: A new photogrammetric method for quantifying corneal topography, Invest Ophthalmol Vis Sci 1984;25:323-330.
22. Cooper SN and Docrat YA: Keratometry study in refractive conditions of the eye, particularly with reference to myopia, Proc All India Ophthalmol Soc 1951;12:27.
23. Crawford JS, Shagass C, and Pashby TJ: Relationship between visual acuity and refractive error in myopia, Am J Ophthalmol 1945;28:1220-1225.
24. Curtin BJ: The pathogenesis of congenital myopia, Arch Ophthalmol 1963;69:166.
25. Curtin BJ: The components of refraction and their correction. In The myopias: basic science and clinical management, Philadelphia, 1985, Harper & Row Publishers, Inc, pp 17-37.
26. Curtin BJ: The optical considerations of myopia. In The myopias: basic science and clinical management, Philadelphia, 1985, Harper & Row Publishers, Inc, pp 153-166.
27. Dabezies OH and Holladay JR: Measurement of corneal curvature: keratometer (ophthalmometer). In Dabezies OH, editor: Contact lenses: the CLAO guide to basic science in clinical practice, Orlando, Fla, 1987, Grune & Stratton, Inc.
28. Dingeldein SA and Klyce SD: The topography of normal corneas, Arch Ophthalmol 1989;107:512-518.

29. Dingeldein SA, Klyce SD, and Wilson SE: Quantitative descriptors of corneal shape derived from computer-assisted analysis of photokeratographs, Refract Corneal Surg 1989;5:372-378.
30. Doss JD, Hutson RL, Rowsey JJ, and Brown R: Method for calculation of corneal profile and power distribution, Arch Ophthalmol 1981;91:1261-1265.
31. Duane DT and Jaeger EA: Clinical ophthalmology, vol 1, Philadelphia, 1987, Harper & Row Publishers, Inc.
32. Duke-Elder S and Smith RJH: The foundations of ophthalmology, vol 7, System of ophthalmology, St Louis, 1962, The CV Mosby Co, pp 241-242.
33. Duke-Elder S and Abrams D: Ophthalmic optics and refraction, vol 5, System of ophthalmology, St Louis, 1970, The CV Mosby Co, p 130.
34. Edmund C: The significance of using different methods for analyzing photokeratoscopic data, Acta Ophthalmol 1986;64:97-100.
35. Edmund C and Sjontoft E: The central-peripheral radius of the normal corneal curvature: a photokeratoscopic study, Acta Ophthalmol 1985;63:670-677.
36. El Hage S: A new concept of the corneal topography and its application, Optica Acta 1972;19:431.
37. El Hage S: A computerized corneal topographer for use in refractive surgery, Refract Corneal Surg 1989;5:418-424.
38. Enoch JM: Summated response of the retina to light entering different parts of the pupil, J Optical Soc Am 1958;48:392-406.
39. Fleming JF: Corneal topography and radial keratotomy, J Refract Surg 1986;2:249-254.
40. Fyodorov SN and Durnev VV: Operation of dosaged dissection of corneal circular ligament in cases of myopia of mild degree, Ann Ophthalmol 1979;11:1885-1890.
41. Gardiner PA: Corneal power in myopic children, Br J Ophthalmol 1962;46:138-143.
42. Girard LJ: Nomenclature of corneal contact lenses. In Girard LJ, editor: Corneal contact lenses, St Louis, 1970, The CV Mosby Co, pp 1-4.
43. Gordon RA and Donzis PB: Refractive development of the human eye, Arch Ophthalmol 1984;103:785-789.
44. Gormley DJ, Gersten M, Koplin RS, and Lubkin V: Corneal modeling, Cornea 1988;7:30-35.

45. Hannush SB, Crawford SL, Waring GO, Gemmill MC, Lynn MJ, and Nizam A: Accuracy and precision of keratometry, photokeratoscopy, and corneal modeling on calibrated steel balls, Arch Ophthalmol 1989;107: 1235-1239.

46. Hannush SB, Crawford SL, Waring GO, Gemmill MC, Lynn MJ, and Nizam A: Reproducibility of normal corneal power measurements with a keratometer, photokeratoscope, and video imaging system, Arch Ophthalmol 1990;108:539-544.

47. Harris DJ, Waring GO, and Burk LL: Keratography as a guide to selective suture removal for the reduction of astigmatism after penetrating keratoplasty, Ophthalmology 1989;96: 1597-1607.

48. Hemenger RP, Tomlinson A, and McDonnell PJ: Explanation for good visual acuity in uncorrected residual hyperopia and presbyopia after radial keratotomy, Invest Ophthalmol Vis Sci 1990;31:1644-1646.

49. Henslee SL and Rowsey JJ: New corneal shapes in keratorefractive surgery. Ophthalmology 1983;90:245-250.

50. Hirsh MJ: Relation of visual acuity to myopia, Am J Ophthalmol 1987; 105:86-92.

51. Holladay JT: Optical correction following radial keratotomy. In Current therapy in ophthalmic surgery, Philadelphia, 1989, BC Decker, Inc, pp 68-71.

52. Holladay JT, Lynn MJ, Waring GO, Gemmill MG, Keehn G, and Fielding B: The relationship of visual acuity, refractive error and pupil size after radial keratotomy, Arch Ophthalmol 1991;109:70-76.

53. Inagaki Y: The rapid change of corneal curvature in the neonatal period in infancy, Arch Ophthalmol 1986; 104:1026-1027.

54. Insler MS, Cooper HD, May SE, and Donzis PB: Analysis of corneal thickness and curvature in infants, CLAO J 1987;13:182-184.

55. Ivashina AI: Radial keratotomy as a method of surgical correction of myopia. In Fyodorov SN, editor: Microsurgery of the eye: main aspects, Moscow, 1987, Mir Publishers, pp 46-80.

56. Jarvis VN, Levine R, and Asbell PA: Manual vs. automated keratometry: a comparison, CLAO J 1987;13:235-238.

57. Katel-Block R: Die Beziehunghen Des Hornhaut Astigmatismus zur Myopie, Klin Montasbl Augenheilkd 1906;44:68.

58. Katz M: The human eye as an optical system. In Duane DT and Jaeger EA, editors: Clinical ophthalmology, vol 1, Philadelphia, 1987, Harper & Row Publishers, Inc, pp 1-52.

59. Kawara T: Corneal topography using moiré contour fringes, Appl Optics 1979;18:3675.

60. Kiely PM, Smith G, and Carney LG: Meridional variations of corneal shape, Am J Optom Physiol Opt 1984;61:619-626.

61. Klyce SD: Computer-assisted corneal topography: high-resolution graphic presentation and analysis of keratoscopy, Invest Ophthalmol Vis Sci 1984;25:1426-1436.

62. Klyce SD and Wilson SE: Methods of analysis of corneal topography, Refract Corneal Surg 1989;5:368-371.

63. Knoll HA: Corneal contours in the general population as revealed by the photokeratoscope, Am J Optom 1961;38:389-397.

64. Koch DD, Foulks GN, Moran T, and Wakil JS: The corneal EyeSys system: accuracy analysis and reproducibility of first-generation prototype, Refract Corneal Surg 1989;5:424-429.

65. Layman PR: Measuring corneal areas utilizing keratometry, Optician 1987;154:261.

66. L'Esperance FA, Warner JW, Telfair WB, Yoder PR, and Martin CA: Excimer laser instrumentation and technique for human corneal surgery, Arch Ophthalmol 1989;107:131-139.

67. Ludlam WM, Wittenberg S, and Rosenthal J: Photographic analysis of the ocular dioptric components. Part III. The acquisition, storage, retrieval, and utilization of primary data in photokeratoscopy, Am J Optom 1967;44:276.

68. Lusby FW, Franke JW, and McCaffery JM: Clinical comparison of manual and automated keratometry in a geriatric population, CLAO J 1987; 13:119-121.

69. Maguire LJ: Corneal topography of patients with excellent Snellen visual acuity after epikeratophakia for aphakia, Am J Ophthalmol 1990;109: 162-167.

70. Maguire LJ and Bourne WM: A multifocal lens effect as a complication of radial keratotomy, Refract Corneal Surg 1989;5:394-397.

71. Maguire LJ and Bourne WM: Corneal topography of early keratoconus, Am J Ophthalmol 1989;108: 107-112.

72. Maguire LJ and Bourne WM: Corneal topography of transverse keratotomies for astigmatism after penetrating keratoplasty, Am J Ophthalmol 1989;107:323-330.

73. Maguire LJ, Singer D, and Klyce SDF: Graphic presentation of computer-analyzed keratoscope photographs, Arch Ophthalmol 1987;105: 223-230.

73a. Maloney RK: Corneal topography and optical zone location in photorefractive keratectomy, Refract Corneal Surg 1990;6:364-372.

74. Mandel R: Contact lens practice. Springfield, Ill, 1965, Charles C Thomas, Publisher.

75. Mandel RB and St Helen R: Position and curvature of the corneal apex, Am J Optom 1969;46:25-29.

76. Mandel RB and St Helen R: Mathematical model of corneal contour, Br J Physiol Optom 1971;26:183-197.

77. McDonnell PJ and Garbus J: Corneal topographic changes after radial keratotomy, Ophthalmology 1989;96: 45-59.

78. McDonnell PJ, Garbus J, and Lopez PF: Topographic analysis and visual acuity after radial keratotomy, Am J Ophthalmol 1988;106:692-695.

79. McDonnell PJ, McClusky DJ, and Garbus J: Corneal topography and fluctuating visual acuity after radial keratotomy, Ophthalmology 1989; 96:665-670.

80. Mende E: Statistische Untersuchungen uber die Beziehungen des Hornhautastigmatismus zur Myopie, Klin Monatsbl Augenheilkd 1906;44:26.

81. Michaels DD: Visual optics and refraction, ed 3, St Louis, 1985, The CV Mosby Co.

82. Miller D and Carter J: A proposed new division of corneal functions. In Cavanagh HD, editor: The cornea. Transactions of the World Congress on the Cornea III, New York, 1980, Raven Press, pp 155-158.

83. Miller D and Wolf E: A model for comparing the optical properties of different sized corneal grafts, Am J Ophthalmol 1969;67:724-728.

84. Mohrman R: The keratometer. In Duane TD and Yaeger AE, editors: Clinical ophthalmology, vol 1, Philadelphia, 1987, Harper & Row Publishers, Inc.

85. Nordan LT and Grene RB: The importance of corneal asphericity and irregular astigmatism in refractive surgery, Refract Corneal Surg 1990;6:200-204.

86. Perl T, Binder PS, and Earl K: Post-cataract astigmatism with and without the use of the Terry keratometer, Ophthalmology 1984;91:489-493.

87. Peters HB: The relationship between refractive error and visual acuity at three age levels, Am J Optom and Arch Am Acad Optom 1961;38:194-198.

88. Pincus MH: Unaided visual acuities correlated with refractive errors, Am J Ophthalmol 1946;29:853-858.

89. Refractive and Corneal Surgery: Special issue on corneal topography, 1989;5:359-432.

90. Rowsey JJ: Corneal topography. In Dabezies OH, editor: Contact lenses, Orlando, Fla, 1984, Grune & Stratton, Inc, pp 4.1-4.16.

91. Rowsey JJ, Balyeat HD, Monlux R, Holladay J, Waring GO, Lynn MJ, and PERK Study Group: Prospective Evaluation of Radial Keratotomy: photokeratoscope corneal topography, Ophthalmology 1988;95:322-334.

92. Rowsey JJ and Isaac MS: Corneoscopy in keratorefractive surgery, Cornea 1983;2:133-142.

93. Rowsey JJ, Monlux R, Balyeat HD, Stevens SX, Gelender H, Holladay J, et al: Accuracy and reproducibility of KeraScanner analysis in PERK corneal topography, Curr Eye Res 1989;8:661-674.

94. Rowsey JJ, Reynolds AE, and Brown DR: Corneal topography: Corneascope, Arch Ophthalmol 1981;99:1093-1100.

95. Rowsey JJ and Ruben ML: Refraction problems after refractive surgery, Surv Ophthalmol 1988;32:414-420.

96. Ruben M: Contact lens practice, Baltimore, 1975, Williams & Wilkins, pp 97-129.

97. Ruben ML: Optics for clinicians, ed 3, Gainesville, Fla, 1990, Triad Scientific Publishers.

98. Sampson WG and Soper JW: Keratometry. In Girard LJ, editor: Corneal contact lenses, St Louis, 1970, The CV Mosby Co, pp 65-92.

99. Santoni A: Sullo spessore della cornea in caso di miopia elevata, Rass Ital Ottal 1952;21:219.

100. Santos VR, Waring GO, Lynn MJ, et al: Relationship between refractive error and visual acuity in the Prospective Evaluation of Radial Keratotomy (PERK) study, Arch Ophthalmol 1087;105:86-92.

101. Schanzlin DJ and Robin JB, editors: Corneal topography, New York, Springer-Verlag, Inc (in press).

102. Sccfclder R: Ueber Astigmatismus bei Soldaten nebst Bermerkungen uber die Beziehungen des Astigmatismus zur Myopie, Klin Monatsbl Augenheilkd 1907;45:486.

103. Smolek MK: Analysis of bovine ocular distension via real-time holographic interferometry, doctoral dissertation, Bloomington, Ind, 1986, Indiana University.

104. Sorsby A: Biology of the eye as an optical system. In Duane TD and Jaeger EA, editors: Clinical ophthalmology, vol 1, Philadelphia, 1986, Harper & Row Publishers, Inc, pp 1-17.

105. Sorsby A, Leary GA, and Richards MJ: Correlation ametropia and component ametropia, Vision Res 1962;2:309.

106. Sorsby A, Benjamin B, Davey JB, et al: Emmetropia and its aberrations. Special Report Series No 293, London, 1957, Her Majesty's Stationery Office.

107. Steiger A: Ueber Beziehungen Zwichen Myopie und Astigmatismus, Z Augenheilkd 1908;20:97.

108. Steiger A: Die Entstehung der Spharischen Efraktionen des Menschlichen Auges, Berlin, 1913, S Karger.

109. Stiles WS and Crawford BH: Luminous efficiency of rays entering eye pupil at different points, Proc Roy Soc Lond 1933;112:428-450.

110. Stone J: Keratometry. In Ruben M, editor: Contact lens practice, Baltimore, 1975, Williams & Wilkins, pp 104-129.

111. Swinger CA and Barker BA: Prospective evaluation of myopic keratomileusis, Ophthalmology 1984;91:785-792.

112. Tate GW, Safir A, and Mills SZ: Accuracy and reproducibility of keratometric readings, CLAO J 1987;13:50-58.

113. Tokoro T, Hayashi K, Muto M, et al: Central corneal thickness in high myopia, Folia Ophthalmol Jpn 1976;27:610.

114. Wang J, Rice DA, and Klyce SD: A new reconstruction algorithm for improvement of corneal topographical analysis, Refract Corneal Surg 1989;5:379-387.

115. Waring GO: Making sense of keratospeak. II. Proposed conventional terminology for corneal topography, Refract Corn Surg 1989;5:362-367.

116. Wittenbeg S and Ludlam WM: Derivation of a system for analyzing the corneal surface from photokeratoscope data, J Opt Soc Am 1966;56:1612-1618.

117. Wyzinski P and O'Dell L: Subjective and objective findings after radial keratotomy, Ophthalmology 1989;96:1608-1611.

Development of Refractive Keratotomy

BACKGROUND AND ACKNOWLEDGMENTS

Keratotomy for myopia and astigmatism has developed during the past century in three major phases (see the table on p. 143 and the figure on p. 144). In the first phase surgeons in Europe and the United States defined the principles of keratotomy in the late 1800s. In the second phase surgeons in Japan detailed the effects of anterior and posterior keratotomy in the 1940s and 1950s. And in the third phase ophthalmologists in the Soviet Union, the United States, Europe, and Latin America refined modern refractive keratotomy between 1976 and the present. To place this information in perspective, we summarize the development of refractive keratotomy in this section, purposely presenting in detail its scientific and social development, including clinical rediscoveries and political conflict.

The history of keratotomy is replete with rediscoveries of previously known principles. For example, the eighteenth century European surgeons and Sato and his colleagues knew well that a transverse corneal incision flattens the meridian perpendicular to it and steepens the meridian parallel to it and that intersecting incisions create problems in wound healing. These facts were apparently lost during the development of keratotomy in the Soviet Union, but were rediscovered by surgeons in the Americas. Similarly Sato demonstrated that a circular keratotomy steepened the central cornea, and yet a few U.S. surgeons in the 1980s propounded its use with radial incisions to decrease myopia, only to find it ineffective and to have colleagues advocate it once again in the form of a hexagonal keratotomy for the treatment of hyperopia.

Keratotomy has not evolved in a clinical and laboratory vacuum. Social forces propelled it forward; World War II motivated Japanese researchers, and medical entrepreneurism drove some Americans.

We have acknowledged the contributions of many individuals, but the accuracy of such acknowledgment is obscured by the fragmentary record, the fact that published observations may not reflect the actual time the contribution was made, and the problem that ideas conceived by one individual may be published by another. It is relatively easy to acknowledge the major contributors early in the development of radial keratotomy, but in more recent years—particularly in the United States—many innovative and diligent individuals have contributed simultaneously to our body of knowledge, so it is difficult to cite the originator of each contribution.

Highlights in the Development of Keratotomy for Myopia and Astigmatism

Date	Individual	Country	Contribution
1885	H. Schiøtz	Norway	Performed transverse keratotomy for astigmatism
1886-1896	W.H. Bates E. Faber J. Luciola	United States Netherlands Italy	Performed transverse keratotomy for astigmatism
1898	L.J. Lans	Netherlands	Described principles of transverse and radial keratotomy in laboratory
1939-1955	T. Sato K. Akiyama	Japan	Established principles of transverse and radial keratotomy in rabbits and man; poor results with posterior keratotomy
1960s	M.P. Pureskin	Soviet Union	Confirmed poor results with Sato's anteroposterior incisions
1970s	V.S. Beliayev M.K. Tin V.F. Utkin F.S. Yenaleyev	Soviet Union	Studied anterior keratotomy with variable number of incisions
1972-present	S.V. Fyodorov V.V. Durnev	Soviet Union	Included multiple ocular variables, including smaller clear zones, to tailor keratotomy for each patient
1978-1980	L.D. Bores W.D. Myers J. Cowden	United States	Started keratotomy in the United States; added centrifugal and deepening incisions
1980-present	Many individual surgeons	United States	Improved surgical instruments and techniques
1980s	L.A. Ruiz R.L. Lindstrom	Colombia United States	Developed and refined combined radial and transverse incisions for astigmatism
1980-1995	G.O. Waring and the Prospective Evaluation of Radial Keratotomy (PERK) Study Group	United States	Conducted a monitored, prospective trial of radial keratotomy
1983	S.D. Trokel R. Srinivasan	United States	Described excimer laser for refractive keratectomy
1985	T. Seiler	Germany	Performed transverse excimer laser keratectomy for astigmatism

144

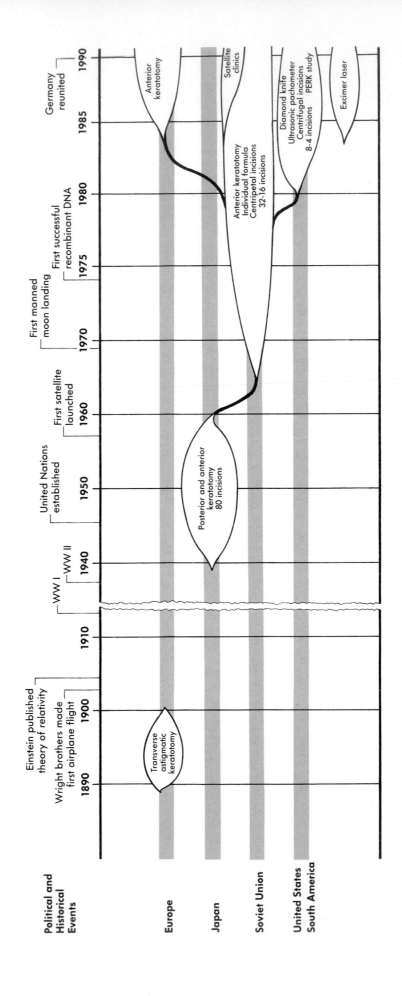

Development and Classification of Refractive Surgical Procedures

George O. Waring III

The increasing interest in refractive corneal surgery, especially in keratotomy for myopia and astigmatism, places new pressure on ophthalmic practitioners. Most ask, "Should I incorporate refractive surgery into my practice? If so, should I offer my patients keratotomy or some type of refractive keratoplasty? What specific techniques should I study? How do I use these techniques on an individual patient?" We need reliable sources of information to answer these questions.

SOURCES OF INFORMATION ABOUT REFRACTIVE SURGERY
Colloquial sources

Authority often guides our decisions: "Professor Renown does the flapjack refractive procedure and says it works great. I think I'll do what he does." But such authority can prove fragile, unworthy, and misleading. Custom may be the basis for our decisions: "I would never operate on a normal eye just to get rid of glasses and contact lenses." But custom can stand in the way of progress. Personal experience is a powerful guide: "I have done three zippy keratotomies; they turned out fine. And I know a doctor who has done 10,000 with outstand-

BACKGROUND AND ACKNOWLEDGMENTS
Refractive keratotomy is but one of a dozen or so refractive corneal surgical procedures, almost all of which are in various stages of evolution and development in the early 1990s. This chapter presents a brief survey of these alternative surgical techniques and emphasizes the process of their development and evaluation. The material has been published previously.[118,119] The classification of surgical procedures was first presented as an article in the *Archives of Ophthalmology* entitled "Making Sense of Keratospeak."[117] The material on the development of refractive surgery was presented as the first Lans Distinguished Refractive Surgery Lecture before the International Society of Refractive Keratoplasty in 1987[120] and was subsequently published in the *Journal of Refractive Surgery* (now *Refractive and Corneal Surgery*).[116] I thank Susanne Gardner, D. Pharm., for valuable concepts and suggestions concerning the paradigms presented here.

An Early Controlled Clinical Trial

A controlled clinical trial is not a new approach to clinical experimentation. In the mid-eighteenth century when British sailors lived in the squalid holds of the queen's ships for months at a time, more of them died from the ravages of scurvy than from the assaults of combat. None of the remedies proposed during the previous two centuries of global exploration and naval warfare had erased this scourge, so in 1747 Dr. James Lind decided to test the different treatments with head-to-head comparisons. Descending to H.M.S. *Salisbury's* dank infirmary, he "took twelve patients in the scurvy, on board the *Salisbury* at sea. Their cases were as similar as I could have them. . . . They lay together in one place in the forehold, and had one common diet, water gruel sweetened with sugar in the morning, fresh mutton broth often times for dinner; and for supper, barley and raisins, rice and currants, sago and wine, or the like." In addition to this standard diet, Lind divided the sailors into six groups of two and treated the groups in six different ways as follows:

1. One quart of cider daily
2. 25 drops of *elixir vitriol* three times a day plus a vitriol gargle
3. Two spoonfuls of vinegar three times a day with vinegar gargle
4. Half a pint of seawater daily
5. Two oranges and one lemon daily (treatment lasted only 6 days because of limited supply)
6. A combination of garlic, mustard seed, horseradish, balsam of Peru, gum myrrh, and barley water with cream of tartar daily.

"The consequence was that the most sudden and visible good effects were perceived from the use of oranges and lemons; one of those who had taken them, being at the end of 6 days fit for duty. . . . The other was best recovered of any in his condition."[13,59]

Lind's embryonic randomized controlled clinical trial had three interesting characteristics. The treatments tested were not new. Indeed, 150 years previously the Dutch had known that citrus fruits and juices were of benefit to sailors on long voyages, but this knowledge had never been properly tested. In addition, Lind's approach was prospective, purposeful, and free of apparent bias in favor of one treatment over the other. Finally Lind's lifesaving observations were not accepted during his lifetime; the British navy delayed 40 years before adding lemon juice to seamen's rations.

---

ing results." But personal experience is often a euphemism for individual bias and self-aggrandizement. Many of us rely on intuition and common sense: "It seems quite obvious to me that using a Focus-All corneal implant should be the most effective procedure." But it was also quite obvious for centuries that the sun revolved around the earth. We may turn to published studies for guidance: "I'll read the literature and do what the data indicate." Unfortunately, clinical studies may be done shoddily and the results may be interpreted improperly. Some studies hide behind the guise of a "prospective trial," which just means the investigators thought of doing the study before they actually did it, or of a "controlled trial," which just means the investigators studied two different procedures.

Since all of these approaches to clinical decision making in refractive surgery—authority, custom, personal experience, common sense, and informal studies—have substantial weaknesses, where can ophthalmic surgeons turn for definitive information?

Formal trials

Objective, verifiable information is most likely to come from laboratory and clinical studies that include methods of reducing investigator bias, clearly defined techniques of surgery and examination, and statistical analysis of the data with impartial interpretation of the results—in other words, from formal trials. The most powerful of these methods of investigation, the randomized controlled clinical trial, which is illustrated in the box above, has been developed in the past few decades. This technique has affected medical practice as powerfully as the invention of the microscope[101] because it allows us to see clinical phenomena not visible by other means.

Need for formal clinical trials

The history of medicine is replete with popular methods of therapy later found to be ineffective, unnecessary, or unsafe. The most long-lived and widespread treatment of this kind was bloodletting, used to palliate a variety of ailments for more than 2000 years

(400 BC to 1950). Another popular operation was adenotonsillectomy performed for decades in up to 50% of children.[82] Adenotonsillectomy was generally abandoned, though, not because the surgery was ineffective or because there were widespread complications, but because the operation was simply unnecessary.[83] More recently jejunoileal bypasses for morbid obesity were performed on thousands of patients, and although they resulted in weight loss and an improved outlook for these individuals, they were abandoned because late complications appeared, including renal damage, colonic ulceration, osteomalacia, and hepatic fibrosis.[25,44] Today randomized controlled trials have raised serious questions about whether coronary artery bypass surgery and extracranial-intracranial arterial bypass surgery are more effective than medical therapy in specific groups of patients.[29] These trials have supported single preventive measures such as the use of aspirin in the primary prevention of myocardial infarction.[85]

Popularity alone is an inadequate guide to medical and surgical therapy, refractive surgery included.

The more common diseases are the ones most in need of randomized controlled trials but are the last ones to be tested with such a trial because of the existence of so many accepted forms of therapy. For example, in 1987 the National Cancer Institute held a consensus conference on prostate cancer.[51] The consensus panel was so hobbled by the lack of solid information that it ended up making only the blandest of statements. The chairman lamented, "We are dealing with the situation where data have been accumulated, but they are difficult to compare, and we don't have randomized controlled trials to help us. We can only offer vague guidelines." For that reason, he said, the goal of the consensus statement was to "stimulate the government to support randomized control clinical trials and to stimulate responsible members of the medical community to support such trials and to enter patients." The panel wanted clinical researchers to "accept a uniform method for data reporting and statistical analyses that will allow meaningful comparisons of treatment results reported by various disciplines."

The message is clear enough. To prevent a similar informational quagmire in refractive surgery, we must conduct formal trials and, when the time is appropriate, randomized controlled comparisons of various refractive surgical techniques.

Current controlled clinical trials

During the past half century, diligent physicians, epidemiologists, and biostatisticians have refined clinical testing to the point that it is codified in textbooks, such as Meinert's *Clinical Trials,*[79] Silverman's *Human Experimentation,*[101] and Shapiro and Louis' *Clinical Trials,*[98] debated in meetings of the Society for Clinical Trials, and refined in the monthly journal *Controlled Clinical Trials* (600 Windhurst Ave., Baltimore, MD 21210).

Ophthalmic researchers have conducted numerous randomized controlled clinical trials, but none have been conducted in refractive surgery.[118] Why not? The answer becomes apparent when we examine the different stages in the development and evaluation of keratotomy and other refractive surgical procedures.

STAGES IN THE DEVELOPMENT AND EVALUATION OF KERATOTOMY

No surgical procedure is immediately ready for testing in a randomized controlled trial. All surgical procedures develop through arduous gestation, difficult birth, and awkward adolescence before they are mature enough for sophisticated testing. I have conceptualized this continuum of development in the following five stages (Fig. 4-1, Table 4-1):

1. Initial creativity[106]
2. Trial-and-error refinement[7]
3. Informal testing
4. Formal trial[14]
5. Randomized controlled clinical trial[79,98,101]

Each of these five steps is valuable; each plays a distinctive role; each builds on its predecessors; and each finds its value independent of the social role of its progenitor. Truth knows no social boundaries, and important contributions to refractive surgery come from all quarters—students, residents, postdoctoral fellows, private practitioners, full-time academic faculty, and researchers in industry. Indeed no single individual or research group can achieve excellence in activities along this entire spectrum. Rather all researchers find their niches and contribute where their talents allow, cooperating with colleagues of different skills to congeal the partial truths about refractive surgery into a useful whole. Individuals with different personalities play different roles along the spectrum. Those more romantically inclined gravitate toward the freedom of fancy and conception that is part of the creative-refinement phases. Those of a more classical temperament gravitate to the formality that characterizes clinical trials.

Progress through the five stages also makes it easier for us to identify the truth by controlling natural bias and confounding clinical variables and by ferreting out

Table 4-1

Five Stages in the Development and Evaluation of Refractive Surgical Techniques

Stage	Initial creativity	Trial-and-error refinement	Informal testing	Formal trial	Randomized controlled clinical trial
Characteristics	New ideas; changes in the existing order; new relationships	Unstructured exploration of many alternatives with frequent changes based on a few cases	Series of cases studied under the nonstandardized conditions	Series of cases studied according to strict prospective protocol	Concurrent comparison of of treatments according to strict prospective protocol
Common response from ophthalmologists	Opposition from established authority; welcomed by those seeking new information	Interest proportionate to the enthusiasm of investigators and to the amount of publicity	Uncertainty about the place of the procedure in office practice	Opposition from those with vested interests; welcomed by those seeking definitive information	Response same as formal trial
Study population	Isolated cases	Few selected cases	Case series selected by pragmatic availability	Consecutive case series assembled according to defined entry criteria; one eye per patient reported	Eyes or patients randomized to concurrent treatment groups
Surgical protocol	None	Variable	Multiple techniques	Standardized and replicable	Concurrent comparison of standardized procedures
Clinical examination conditions	None	Office practice	Office practice	Standardized	Standardized
Support personnel	None	Few	Colleagues and office staff	External monitors, study coordinators, and independent examiners	Same
Follow-up	None	Quick	Short-term; many patients lost	Long-term; few patients lost and all patients accounted for	Same
Analysis of results	None	Descriptive	Arithmetic	Statistical by statistician	Statistical by statistician, masked
Timing of analysis	Immediate	Retrospective	Retrospective or prospective	Prospective	Prospective

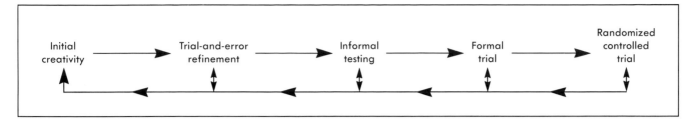

Figure 4-1
Feedback loops in development and evaluation of refractive surgery emphasize importance of all five phases. From any point in the continuum, one may move forward to the next stage or drop back to a previous stage. Leaping ahead past a phase may lead to premature claims of success. (From Waring GO: J Refract Surg 1987; 3:142-157.)

Table 4-2

Pitfalls in Stopping the Development and Evaluation of Refractive Surgery at Each Stage

Initial creativity	Trial-and-error refinement	Informal testing	Formal trial	Randomized controlled clinical trial
Produces only ideas and isolated experiences with no change in practice	Inherent errors propagated with premature dissemination of observations	Information not definitive, so confusion persists and new practice is based on authority and personal experience	Limited scope without innovation; no concurrent comparison group	Limited scope without innovation

fraudulent information purveyed by *Betrayers of the Truth.*[18]

In this chapter I characterize briefly each of the five stages in development (Table 4-1). The chapter emphasizes the role each plays along the continuum, illustrates each stage with examples from refractive surgery, and indicates the pitfalls of stopping the developmental process at each stage (Table 4-2).

Initial creativity

Characteristics. The creative act establishes new relationships, finds new connections, juxtaposes things in a way not previously conceived. Our conception of what is possible expands. The creation of a new idea or observation in medicine is a rare event, but when it occurs, it changes the existing order in medicine. The iconoclasm inherent in creative ideas, for example, operating on a structurally normal eye to change its refractive state, invariably upsets standards. Few creative individuals have escaped the wrath of their colleagues, although those with the ability to demon-

strate the truth of their contentions are often venerated in the end. Such has been the experience of José Barraquer in Bogota, Colombia, who introduced the term "refractive keratoplasty" in 1949,[9] was ostracized from organized ophthalmology in the 1950s, and is now honored as the modern father of refractive keratoplasty.

Another common thread in creativity has been characterized elegantly by James Austin in *Chase, Chance and Creativity.*[7] The box on p. 150 addresses the occurrence of chance observations that often lead astute people to draw new conclusions, just because they were lucky, because they had prepared themselves thoroughly in their fields, or because they happened to be in the right place at the right time. Such was the experience of William Bates, a New York ophthalmologist who observed in the 1890s that some patients with peripheral surgical or traumatic corneal scars developed flattening of the cornea in the meridian that intersected the scar. This chance, astute observation led him to suggest transverse keratotomy for

Chase, Chance and Creativity

Medical research is no clear, blue, inorganic crystal which grows symmetrically and predictably in solution. Instead, it is a live, organic growth, a wild vine winding in and around an intellectual trellis. It ventures a tendril here, thrusts out a leaf there, proliferates in odd directions, rarely bursts into bloom. It draws sustenance both from tangible earthly sources and, seemingly, from thin air.

Discovery is pluralistic. It springs from a dynamic interplay between one's own life-style and that of other persons, between intuition and reason, between the conventional scientific method and chance in all its forms. The more diversity there is among these elements the more unique is the resulting creative product. Random elements, seemingly incongruous, can be drawn together and fused only when the personal life-style of one individual interacts with chance. Some kinds of chance happen, others are stirred up, discerned, or instigated.

A moment of creative inspiration is rare. It has both a long incubation period and, if it is to prove fruitful, a lengthy subsequent development. We find that the creative experience in science begins with an unconventional person, of abilities both diverse and contrasting, who is well-grounded and receptive in his professional field. He not only prefers but needs novelty, for he is bored if not disenchanted by a physiological status quo. He has grown up to be a questioning, "adverbial man" whose curiosity is piqued to solve problems for more reasons than he is aware of. His search incorporates some elements of the primitive chase, brings all his senses to a peak, and sweeps him up in a tangle of stimulating ideas. Soon, however, his progress is blocked, and he may appear to have abandoned a fruitless struggle. But preconsciously, his mind probes and scans for clues throughout all his sources of information and experience, rapidly discerning those that will fit, neatly discarding the others. He keeps on going.

Often, through an accident that has a distinctive personal flavor, he will finally stumble on a fresh clue. At a conscious level, the clue might appear irrelevant, but it immediately opens up wide avenues of useful information. He suddenly finds himself in a state of enhanced awareness. His thoughts steer themselves at lightning speed to a new conscious insight. The new solution is vivid and intensely satisfying both intellectually and emotionally. His visual recollection of the moment is usually indelible. The "moment" may be a major flash of insight, or it may be an attenuated "spark", or a related series of faint glimmers spread out over months or years.

In broad perspective, we see in the way the two sides of his brain create one solution an analogy with the love-hate, tug-of-war going on between romanticism and rationalism since the dawn of man. The struggle is resolved when the two sides join forces in their common cause and go off reunited hand in hand.

For, with a fresh insight, the investigator's work has just begun. He fashions his inspired ideas into a testable hypothesis, then laboriously creates a series of increasingly rigorous experiments to prove or disprove it. Persisting in these experiments through trial and error, he ultimately meanders into an entirely new set of problems. He leans forward once more, staying in motion, and his chase, his search, his quest begins anew.

From Austin JH: Chase, chance and creativity, New York, 1978, Columbia University Press, pp 189-190.

---

the treatment of astigmatism.[11] Similarly T. Sato, another ophthalmologist, got the idea of posterior keratotomy to treat astigmatism when he observed two patients with keratoconus who developed acute breaks in Descemet's membrane (corneal hydrops) followed by gradual central flattening of the cornea as the breaks healed with scarring.[92]

A modern example of the creative application of existing technology occurred when R. Srinivasan, Ph.D., the developer of excimer lasers to etch polymers in microcircuits by ablative photodecomposition, joined with Stephen Trokel, M.D., in New York in 1983 to demonstrate that excimer lasers could also ablate corneal tissue with exquisite accuracy.[109]

Pitfalls. The major pitfall of stopping the developmental process during the initial creativity stage is that the ideas—no matter how revolutionary and constructive they are—do not develop into clinically useful techniques. This problem is illustrated well by the ingenious work of L.J. Lans, who worked in Leiden, Netherlands, in the 1890s and demonstrated in rabbits the basic principles of radial keratotomy. He published his results as a doctoral dissertation,[57] but after graduating, he entered a private ophthalmology practice and allowed his innovative observations in refractive corneal surgery to languish in the dust of history.[120]

Trial-and-error refinement

Characteristics. In the stage of trial-and-error refinement investigators try many variants of their new ideas and techniques. Short follow-up provides quick feedback. Activity is intense and full of promise. Enthusiasm soars.

A hallmark of trial-and-error refinement is active exchange of information among researchers and clinicians, which is an especially important activity, since the quality of experience is often colloquial, unstructured, anecdotal, and preliminary. Study groups, satellite sessions at major meetings, brief preceptorships with surgeons developing new techniques, individual lectures, and personal communications constitute this network[63] that allows individuals to refine their techniques more quickly. Anecdotal case reports record these experiences.

Quick refinement characterized the work of Bernard McCarey and colleagues in Atlanta who tried to change corneal curvature by implanting hydrogel intracorneal lenses in stromal pockets. They rapidly observed that they had to sever all the anterior stromal collagen fibrils with microkeratome and place the hydrogel lens beneath the lenticule (alloplastic keratophakia) to alter the curvature.[12,43,72]

Trial-and-error refinements have played a dominant role in the clinical and laboratory development of patterns of keratotomy for astigmatism. The trial-and-error refinement process demonstrated the inadequacy of multiple parallel incisions in the steep axis, longer incisions in the steep axis (oval optical zone), transverse incisions intersecting radial incisions, and four or five transverse incisions in trapezoidal keratotomy (Ruiz procedure), and led to the demonstrations by Richard Lindstrom, Spencer Thornton, and others that one or two transverse incisions in the steep axis are effective.[46,108]

The stage of refinement also includes new applications of previous ideas, such as two modifications of Barraquer's cryolathe keratomileusis, one by Theodore Werblin and Herbert Kaufman in New Orleans in 1980 in the form of the simpler onlay epikeratoplasty,[48] and the other by Jorge Krumeich in Bocum, West Germany, and Casimer Swinger in New York in the form of nonfreeze, planar keratomileusis.[54,105]

A current example of trial-and-error refinement is the development of polysulfone intracorneal lenses, in humans by Peter Choyce in London[21,50] and in laboratory animals by the collaborative group of Stephen Lane, Richard Lindstrom, Perry Binder, Bernard McCarey, and George Waring.[55] Solid polysulfone lenses produced stromal lipid deposits and anterior stromal thinning in many eyes, prompting the use of fenestrated implants, a technique previously used in the 1950s.[103]

Pitfalls. Development may stop in the stage of refinement for many reasons. The new techniques may simply be ineffective, as discovered in 1986 by James Rowsey in Oklahoma City during his development of microwave thermokeratoplasty.[88] Sometimes more effective methods of management appear, as happened when contact lenses were introduced in Japan in the late 1950s and Sato stopped performing anterior and posterior keratotomy. Sometimes investigators become

discouraged by failure and their inability to identify the right factors to create success, as occurred when P. Siva Reddy attempted radial keratotomy with shallow incisions and found an inadequate effect.[102] Under these circumstances, researchers revert to the earlier stage and tap their creative resources.

The biggest danger in the stage of refinement may occur when premature claims of success—especially claims coupled with intense promotion—rocket a procedure into the next stage of extensive informal clinical testing.

For example, even though Sato and Akiyama invested almost 15 years in extensive refinement of anterior and posterior keratotomy in the laboratory and the clinic, they fell into the trap of premature claims of success in the treatment of myopia based on treatment of only 32 eyes followed for an average of 7 weeks (see Chapter 6, Development of Radial Keratotomy in Japan, 1939-1960).

A more recent illustration of premature claims of success during trial-and-error refinement occurred when circular keratotomy was touted as a supplement to radial incisions in treating myopia, a claim made on the basis of 13 cases followed for less than 3 weeks each.[35] Even though the author called for "double-blind controlled studies" to determine the effectiveness of adding the circular keratotomy, some unfortunate patients were treated in this manner on the basis of the preliminary claims that were published by the well-known authority before a longer follow-up had demonstrated the lack of effectiveness and the complications. This illustrates one drawback of publishing the proceedings of meetings in non–peer-reviewed, privately produced booklets. Stephen Lock discussed this problem in his 1985 analysis, *A Difficult Balance: Editorial Peer Review in Medicine.*[63]

Too often, unwary surgeons make their patients unknowing experimental subjects by trying new techniques that are in this rudimentary stage of development. I have seen this happen in patients with the implantation of toxic hydrogel intracorneal lenses, hexagonal keratotomy for hyperopia, thermokeratoplasty for keratoconus, and intersecting transverse and radial keratotomies for astigmatism.

Informal testing

Characteristics. An apparently successful refinement of a procedure spurs the investigation to broader clinical or laboratory testing, usually in the form of a case series. Often the innovator trains a group of surgeons in the basics of the procedure, and they operate on a series of patients available in their practices, using different instruments and contributing further refinements of the technique. Preoperative and postoperative examinations are usually done as routine office practice. An observational data base develops.

Initial results on a few of the patients are presented after only a few months of follow-up. A series of papers and presentations appear with longer follow-up on increasing numbers of patients and with new variations of surgical technique. Analysis of the data is generally arithmetic, consisting of percentage results, minimum and maximum range, and calculation of means and standard deviations.

One of the strengths of informal testing is that it is flexible. The absence of a rigid protocol allows it to accommodate changing technology. The techniques used by the surgeon may be more realistic. Patients have rapid access because of minimal screening and therefore may be more representative of the general population because entry criteria are not so strict as with formal testing and because compliance is more representative of everyday life, rather than of the more artificial setting of a strictly controlled trial.

The most extensive informal testing has been with radial keratotomy. Reports include small anecdotal series,[42] summaries of larger numbers of cases,[33] more thorough reports of cases done with an informal protocol,[45] and reports of hundreds of cases done by an individual surgeon.[99,100]

Fruitful informal testing of radial keratotomy resulted from the Analysis of Radial Keratotomy (ARK) Study Group,[89] established by Donald Sanders and his collaborators in the United States.

An example of commercially sponsored informal testing was the nationwide clinical study of epikeratophakia directed by Marguerite McDonald and Herbert Kaufman of New Orleans. Hundreds of investigators were trained in 2-day laboratory courses, and it was required that results of all procedures performed be reported to the sponsoring company, which compiled and analyzed the data with the subsequent assistance of an independent data analyst.[49,74-76]

Relaxing incisions and wedge resections for the reduction of astigmatism after penetrating keratoplasty were conceived by Richard Troutman in New York and Jay Krachmer in Iowa City and have been tested informally for the past decade.[62,67,110]

Pitfalls. Weaknesses of the informal observational data base include the following:

1. The strong influence of patient and physician bias because of poorly controlled conditions, making conclusions less meaningful
2. Incomplete data collection
3. Changes over time in techniques and patient selection, so information gained early in the series may be quite different from that gained later in the series

There are three reasons for stopping the development of a refractive surgical procedure at informal testing. The procedure may be found to be inadequate, so the investigators either abandon it or return to the stage of refinement, as did physicians researching intersecting keratotomies to correct astigmatism. In addition, resources may not be available for completing the testing and reporting the results, as occurred with the National Radial Keratotomy Study Group[16] and the Keratorefractive Society Radial Keratotomy Registry.[95]

Finally the results of informal testing may be deemed good enough, so formal trials are not undertaken and the procedure is absorbed into clinical practice. This is often a mistake because it leaves practitioners and patients without definitive, verifiable, objective information. The situation becomes even more confusing when oral presentations are enthusiastically reported by ophthalmic newspapers in stories that some readers mindlessly regard as the equivalent of (or substitutes for) articles in peer-reviewed journals and that some physicians cite as "publications." The resulting uncertainty—fueled by conflicting claims, commercial pressures, and limited personal experience—leads to practices based on the flimsy foundations of authority, custom, intuition, and flawed reports.

Cautious, critical skepticism—not unrestrained therapeutic exuberance—should characterize the informal testing stage.

Formal trials

Characteristics. A formal trial is a case series studied according to a well-defined protocol written in advance and adhered to throughout the trial.

All activities are structured to identify and control the factors known to affect the outcome, to reduce controllable variables to a minimum, and to exclude the biases of the surgeon, other investigators, and the patient.[79] The formal trial is simply a series of cases studied without a randomized control group according to the principles of modern clinical investigation. The criteria for selecting participants are strictly defined; the number of patients needed is determined in advance; surgical and examination techniques are standardized; data are collected on specially designed forms and managed with a computer; all patients (one eye of each patient) are accounted for within a specified time interval in each report; and data are analyzed by a biostatistician.

Hlatky and colleagues[43] have recently observed that clinical decisions are most secure when they are based on findings from several large randomized clinical trials. But relevant randomization trial data are often unavailable. Information from formal observational trials is more commonly available. Hlatky and colleagues have demonstrated that analyses using clinical data bases provide useful information because statistical methods can adequately correct for the lack of randomization. To do this they compare the findings of three major randomized clinical trials of coronary bypass surgery with predictions of multivariable statistical regression models derived from observational formal clinical trials. Specifically the regression model predictions agreed well with the randomized trial in terms of survival rates. Thus carefully performed analyses of observational data can complement the results of randomized trials.

The most formal clinical trial of refractive surgery has been the National Eye Institute–funded Prospective Evaluation of Radial Keratotomy (PERK) Study, a multicenter clinical trial of a single technique of radial keratotomy.[65,122-124] There have been semiformal evaluations of keratomileusis[81,104] in which authors used a standardized surgical technique on a consecutive group of patients with some standardization of clinical examination techniques.

Pitfalls. Since there is no concomitant control group, the investigators must try some other way to identify factors that affect the outcome. One approach is to use regression analysis, which is a sort of mathematic substitute for randomizing patients to concomitant treatment groups.

The danger of stopping development and evaluation here is that a formal trial gives information about only one refractive surgical procedure without direct comparison with other procedures intended to treat populations with a similar anomaly. The practitioner is left to shuffle through the literature and lectures, comparing the results of different quality studies of different techniques, trying to select the one that seems best.

The formal trial also restricts innovation because variations from the protocol are not acceptable. This emphasizes the importance of all five stages in the developmental continuum (Fig. 4-1). A formal trial uncovers deficiencies that should propel creative investigators back to refine techniques further.

Randomized controlled clinical trial

Characteristics. The randomized controlled clinical trial is currently the most sophisticated tool for clinical investigation, comprising all the features of a formal trial with one major difference—the study population is randomized to different refractive surgical procedures done concurrently, allowing a head-to-head comparison of the strengths and weaknesses of each.[31,79] Ideally the two procedures are done on one eye each of the same patient. Many randomized trials compare treatment of one eye with no treatment of the other eye in each patient, for example, the diabetic retinopathy study that demonstrated photocoagulation was more effective than no treatment.[27] In refractive surgery a no-treatment control group is inappropriate because spontaneous reduction and rapid progression of refractive errors seldom occur.

To date there have been no successful randomized controlled clinical trials of refractive surgery because the subspecialty is still proceeding along the continuum of development and has not reached the stage where such trials are appropriate. Table 4-3 lists some possible randomized clinical trials of refractive surgery.

Pitfalls. The most common reason for stopping evaluation of a surgical procedure at the stage of a randomized controlled trial is that one procedure is proved superior to another, as occurred in the senile macular degeneration study when argon laser photocoagulation demonstrated a clear therapeutic advantage over no treatment before the trial was completed.[66]

Table 4-3

Possible Randomized Controlled Trials of Refractive Surgery*

Ametropia	Procedure 1	Procedure 2
Moderate to high myopia	Keratomileusis	Epikeratoplasty
Moderate to high myopia	Cryolathe keratomileusis	Nonfreeze keratomileusis
Lower myopia	Radial keratotomy	Laser keratomileusis
Aphakia	Epikeratoplasty or hyperopic keratomileusis	Secondary intraocular lens implantation
Aphakia	Epikeratoplasty or hyperopic keratomileusis	Intracorneal lens
Keratoconus	Penetrating keratoplasty	Epikeratoplasty

*Two eyes of each patient with symmetric ametropia randomized between procedures 1 and 2.

Because randomized controlled trials are complex and expensive, another pitfall is starting without adequate resources. This occurred in a prospective randomized controlled trial of penetrating keratoplasty and epikeratoplasty in the treatment of keratoconus. The study was well designed with good entry criteria, standardized data forms, and well-trained surgeons using similar surgical techniques. The trial failed to provide a definitive answer, however, because of poor patient recruitment and poor patient follow-up, two problems that could have been eliminated by the provision of clinical coordinators and monitors.[77]

A major danger of stopping development and evaluation at this stage is the failure of the trial to spark insight, foster creative ideas, and lead to further refinements and informal testing, thus completing the feedback loop (Fig. 4-1).

Different characteristics along the continuum of development

The box below illustrates the different qualities of each stage in the continuum of refractive surgery. By appreciating these different qualities, researchers are less likely to misinterpret the type of investigative activity that occurs along the way. Earlier stages on the developmental continuum of refractive surgery are more subjective, fueled by intuition and speculation, whereas later stages are more objective and produce information with a higher probability of accuracy. Earlier stages are more random and less efficient, but the process becomes more directed and precise in later stages. Creativity, refinement, and informal testing produce personal observations commonly introduced with the phrase "in my experience," whereas formal and controlled trials produce verifiable data. Investigators in the early stages of development have the free-

dom to try new things, but in the later stages they must work within a rigid protocol. Activities are simpler in the early stages when a few individuals concentrate on one or two new ideas; things invariably become more complex in the later stages because formal testing involves more participants attempting to control more variables. The early stages are cheaper, and the later stages are more expensive.

Clinical use of the five developmental stages

One reason to identify and describe the five developmental stages is to help investigators and clinicians interpret oral and published information about refractive surgery. If researchers can identify where along the continuum the information lies, they will be more apt to use it properly in clinical practice. However, not all ophthalmologists interpret the results of a trial the same way. For example, the 90% confidence interval of approximately 3.50 D for predicting the outcome of radial keratotomy was interpreted by Arrowsmith and Marks[5] as "predictable" but by the PERK group[65] as "unpredictable." Individual practitioners and patients ultimately have to make up their own minds.

Rate of progress along the continuum of development

Even in the age of information explosion and instant replays, progress along the continuum of development does not occur rapidly, but it can be accelerated by employing the methods of formal trials as early as is practical during development. This minimizes the amount of physician time, investment money, and patient risk spent proving the efficacy and safety of a refractive surgery technique and clearly defines its role in patient care. The arrival at the stage of formal trials can be thwarted by mistakes and blun-

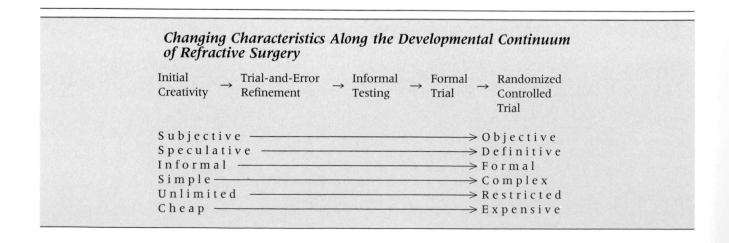

Changing Characteristics Along the Developmental Continuum of Refractive Surgery

Initial Creativity → Trial-and-Error Refinement → Informal Testing → Formal Trial → Randomized Controlled Trial

Subjective ————————————————→ Objective
Speculative ———————————————→ Definitive
Informal ——————————————————→ Formal
Simple —————————————————————→ Complex
Unlimited ———————————————————→ Restricted
Cheap ————————————————————————→ Expensive

ders that send the inventive investigator and curious clinician scurrying back to earlier stages where they refine observations and verify data (Fig. 4-1). Or just as one technique becomes ready for formal study, a new procedure appears and the process begins again.

Advances in refractive surgery have proceeded at a slow and measured pace. Keratotomy has the longest legacy,[114-116] spanning a century of multinational development and evaluation by Norwegian, Dutch, Japanese, Soviet, Indian, and American investigators.[57,123] Thermokeratoplasty for keratoconus kept pace from 1884,[28] but despite the creative efforts of many individuals in refining and testing this procedure, no effective thermokeratoplasty technique exists today. Fifteen years passed between Barraquer's coining the term "refractive keratoplasty" in 1949 and the publication of his first article on keratomileusis for the correction of myopia in 1964.[8] Another 20 years lapsed before the first semiformal trial in 1984.[104]

For more than 30 years investigators have sought a safe, effective plastic intracorneal lens.[70] Research to achieve this goal is still in the informal trial stage.

As long as the medical establishment allows the rate of development of refractive surgery to be determined by the natural, undirected flow of clinical observations or by the mad dash to be first to use the newest techniques without finishing a thorough evaluation of the older ones, ophthalmologists will practice in a fog of confusion and uncertainty—a fog that will lift slowly and at great cost. In the quest for faster access to the newest and best forms of refractive surgery, researchers must remember the advice of workers in fireworks factories: "It is better to curse the darkness than to light the wrong candle."[101]

STAGES OF DEVELOPMENT IN THE LABORATORY

During laboratory investigation, refractive surgery passes through the same five stages with some clear advantages—conditions are more controlled; there is more latitude for trial and error; distinctions between possibly useful and completely ineffective surgical techniques appear more quickly; and there is no danger to humans.

There are the following limitations to laboratory evaluation:

1. Animal corneas (even monkey corneas with a Bowman's layer) do not behave exactly like the human cornea. Once more is known about the biomechanical properties of the cornea in different species, we may understand why.
2. Anesthetized animals cannot fixate; therefore it is difficult to measure corneal curvature and refraction because it is difficult to center a keratometer, keratoscope, and retinoscope on an animal's eye.
3. Because animals give no verbal response, measurement of visual acuity, glare, and satisfaction is difficult.

These limitations and the fact that laboratory work is expensive, time consuming, and not in the purview of most practicing ophthalmologists should never be excuses for premature experiments on humans.

Computer simulation may shorten the time required for laboratory and clinical development. This is discussed in Chapter 29, Preliminary Computer Simulation of Radial Keratotomy.

In refractive surgery research, researchers must accurately measure the refractive and topographic changes induced in the cornea. In addition, subjective response is helpful in judging the clarity, quality, and meaning of the refractive change. These requirements make the study of refractive surgical procedures in laboratory animals difficult because the animals cannot fixate, making keratometry and keratography difficult. Instruments with reliable alignment and systems such as the laser scanning ophthalmoscope combined with video keratography should be developed. Of course animals cannot give a subjective response. Thus at a certain level of development, experimentation on humans is required.

Slit-lamp microscopy and photography, as well as corneal thickness measurements, can be done on most laboratory animals without difficulty. The most valuable aspect of laboratory animals is the ability to design clinical trials with control of different variables and experimental circumstances that would be inappropriate in humans. Sequential removal of animal corneas in eyes for histopathologic, ultrastructural, and immunohistochemical studies is an important part of understanding the cornea's response to refractive surgery.

Unfortunately, little is known about comparative biomechanics and biophysics of human and animal corneas, but there is little doubt that as one proceeds up the phylogenetic tree toward humans, higher-animal corneas behave more like human corneas, making nonhuman primates the best experimental models.

Small mammals

Laboratory animals such as mice, rats, and the like have corneas that are too small for the study of refractive surgical procedures.

Rabbits

The rabbit is the classical laboratory experimental animal for ocular research because the animals are inexpensive to purchase and maintain and easy to handle and because there is a large rabbit data base in the ophthalmic literature. Rabbits are useful in studies of refractive surgical procedures in early trial-and-error refinements, such as excimer laser keratomileusis, to document the epithelial and subepithelial response to the ablation. In the study of intracorneal lenses, the rabbit represents a challenging test system because the cornea is reactive, so an intracorneal lens that allows rabbit corneas to remain intact is likely to allow monkey and human corneas to remain intact.

The rabbit has many drawbacks as an experimental animal for refractive corneal surgery. The rabbit cornea is thinner, floppier, and more elastic than the human cornea and lacks a Bowman's layer, so procedures that depend on corneal biomechanics cannot be accurately tested. The rabbit cornea heals much more readily than the human cornea and vascularizes more readily, so that responses of stromal wound healing cannot be well studied. This is particularly true of the corneal endothelium, which heals readily in rabbits with considerable mitotic activity, unlike that in the adult human. Rabbits blink infrequently, making epikeratoplasties more difficult to evaluate. Refraction cannot be tested accurately in rabbits.

Cats

Cats are more expensive than rabbits. They must be put to sleep to be examined. Less clinical information is available about the cat eye and cornea than the rabbit eye and cornea.

The cat cornea is thicker than the rabbit cornea and also has biomechanical properties that seem to resemble those of the human more closely. Cat eyes have no Bowman's layer, however. The cat endothelium seems to heal more similarly to the human than to the rabbit. Refraction in cats cannot be measured reliably, particularly because of the bright reflections from the tapetum.

Useful experiments in intracorneal lens research, comparing fenestrated with nonfenestrated polysulfone lenses, have been carried out in cats. The nonfenestrated lenses produce lipid degeneration and fatty necrosis similar to that seen in the human, but more intense. Cat corneas seem to vascularize more rapidly than do human corneas.

The cat has been used for some studies of corneal transplantation.

Dogs

Dogs cost more to purchase and maintain. They are rarely used in corneal research.

Monkeys

Monkeys are quite expensive to purchase and maintain. A primate center is required, and their use is regulated heavily. Corneal examination can only be done with the monkey anesthetized. The monkey cornea is structurally similar to the human cornea, with a Bowman's layer and an endothelium that seems less likely to replicate. The biomechanical properties of the monkey cornea are not identical to those of the human, the monkey cornea being smaller, steeper, more pliable, and more reactive to insult.

Differences among monkey species may be important. For example, when polysulfone intracorneal lenses were placed in baboon corneas, a marked inflammatory response occurred,[25] but when similar lenses from the same manufacturer were placed in rhesus monkeys, the corneas remained uninflamed.

Research on monkey corneas has been done for radial keratotomy, implantation of intracorneal lenses, epikeratoplasty, excimer laser surgery, and corneal transplantation.

It is possible to test monkeys' refraction but difficult to do so reliably, the variability among observations often being more than 1.00 D and larger than the minimal acceptable variability that would be tolerated for humans. Similarly it is difficult to get repeatedly reliable keratometry or keratography results.

Blind human eyes

Patients with eyes that are blind from retinal or optic nerve disease or eyes that are scheduled for enucleation for disorders such as choroidal melanoma are often willing to allow experimentation as long as they are assured of no untoward effects. This has been done with the development of excimer laser surgery. This allows the study of both clinical response and, after enucleation or biopsy, study of wound healing. In unsighted eyes reliable refractive measurements are difficult because of the lack of patient fixation.

Sighted human eyes with ocular pathology

Patients with high amounts of pathologic myopia or with aphakia, especially those with macular degeneration, might benefit from a refractive correction and can be reasonable subjects for refinement or refractive corneal surgical procedures. Chances for better corneal and refractive measurements would improve in this population.

Ametropic sighted human eyes

The ultimate test for the effectiveness, safety, stability, predictability, and modifiability of refractive surgical procedures is their use in normal ametropic human eyes. This involves the stages of clinical development discussed early in this chapter.

SURVEY OF REFRACTIVE CORNEAL SURGICAL PROCEDURES

To put refractive keratotomy in perspective, I present here a brief survey of refractive corneal surgery (Fig. 4-2). Details are available in the sources referenced. The box on p. 159 classifies refractive surgical techniques; all of them change the anterior corneal curvature except one—polysulfone high−index of refraction intracorneal lenses. Table 4-4 presents my opinion about how far along the developmental spectrum 11 of these procedures have progressed. All of them have been through the stages of initial creativity and trial-and-error refinement. The box presents the results of some procedures as reported in selected articles, using simple minimal criteria for comparison.[121]

Keratomileusis

Keratomileusis is the term derived by José Barraquer from the Greek words that mean "carving or chiseling the cornea." Although the term was first applied to Barraquer's cryolathe techniques, I think it can be used as a more generic term to indicate all of the lamellar refractive corneal surgical procedures that remove a portion of the patient's corneal stroma to effect the refractive change (Fig. 4-3). Cryolathe keratomileusis (Fig. 4-4) has been refined on thousands of patients since the 1960s with improved control of the multiple variables that affect the outcome, as contained in the now-standardized Barraquer techniques and computer programs. Four small, consecutive, semiformal series have been reported.[10,10a,69,81,104]

Nonfreeze, planar keratomileusis is emerging from the phase of trial-and-error refinement, which produced a new microkeratotome and the cutting bench that replaced the cryolathe, and is entering informal clinical testing as the instruments and the shape of the dies used to mold the tissue improve.[53,54,105]

In situ keratomileusis is a variant in which a plano lenticule of cornea is removed and then a plano layer of stroma is resected from the bed with the microkeratome to create the refractive change. Little information has been published on this technique, which is in the trial-and-error stage.

Table 4-4

Position of 11 Refractive Corneal Surgical Procedures in the Five Stages of Development and Evaluation in 1990

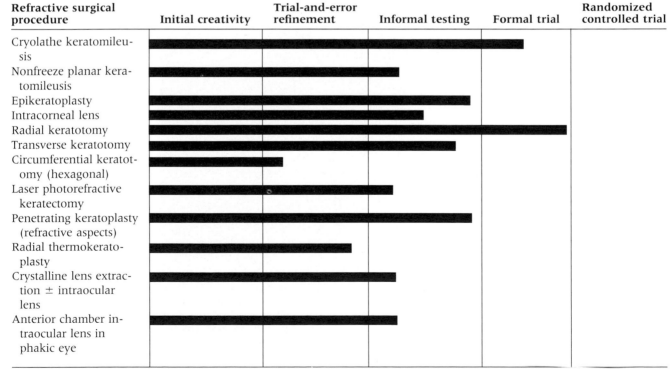

Revised from J Refract Surg 1987;3:142-157.

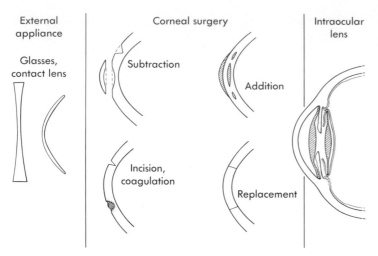

Glasses,
contact lens

Subtraction

Addition

Incision,
coagulation

Replacement

Figure 4-2
Composite drawings illustrate the different methods of correcting refractive errors. External appliances such as glasses and contact lenses are the most commonly used methods. Refractive corneal surgery involves numerous techniques, including those that subtract tissue (keratomileusis and wedge resection), add tissue (such as epikeratoplasty and intracorneal lenses and rings), incise corneal (radial and transverse keratotomy), coagulate the cornea (thermokeratoplasty), and replace the cornea (such as penetrating keratoplasty). Replacement of an intraocular lens in the anterior or posterior chamber is routine after cataract surgery and under experimental evaluation for correction of phakic refractive errors. A complete classification of refractive corneal surgical procedures is presented in the box on p. 159.

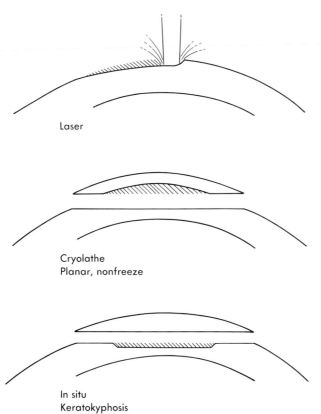

Laser

Cryolathe
Planar, nonfreeze

In situ
Keratokyphosis

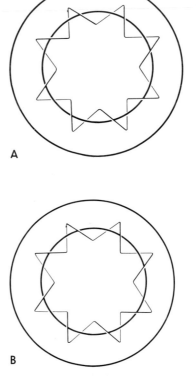

A

B

Figure 4-3
The term "keratomileusis" means carving the cornea and applies to all techniques of lamellar refractive keratoplasty that remove corneal stroma to change the anterior curvature of the cornea, including laser ablation of the anterior cornea, cryolathe or planar nonfreeze carving of an anterior corneal disc, and excision of material from the posterior stromal bed as in in situ keratomileusis and keratokyphosis. Of course, a laser could also be used to remove tissue from the excised disc or the lamellar bed.

Figure 4-4
A, Keratomileusis for myopia involves excision of a lamellar disc of the patient's cornea with a microkeratome, carving of the disc on a cryolathe or die to form a concave lenticule, and suturing the lenticule back onto the cornea. This flattens the central corneal curvature and decreases the refractive power. **B,** Keratomileusis for aphakia involves a similar process using a convex lenticule that steepens the corneal curvature and increases refractive power. (From Waring GO: Arch Ophthalmol 1985;103:1472-1477.)

Classification of Refractive Corneal Surgery Techniques

Lamellar

Keratomileusis with microkeratotome for myopia, hyperopia, aphakia (Fig. 4-4)

Barraquer microkeratome excision and cryolathe carving of lenticule

Nonfreeze, planar, microkeratome carving of lenticule on mold (BKS 1000 instrument, Krumeich)

Keratokyphosis—microkeratome with mold carving of lamellar bed* (Hofmann)

In situ with excision of tissue from lamellar bed with microkeratome (Ruiz)

Excimer laser excision of lenticule and/or ablation of stromal bed

Epikeratoplasty (Fig. 4-5)

Human donor lenticule

Cryolathe; lyophilization (Kaufman, McDonald) or preservative tissue culture medium

Nonfreeze, planar, microkeratome (Krumeich)

Refractive change

Lenticule with power: myopia, hyperopia, aphakia, and astigmatism* (Fig. 4-5, A, B)

Lenticule without power: keratoconus (Fig. 4-5, C)

Synthetic lenticule (collagen, hydrogel, etc.)* (Fig. 4-5, D)

Intracorneal lens (keratophakia) (Fig. 4-6)

Human donor for hyperopia and aphakia (Barraquer)

Hydrogel for aphakia, myopia, and hyperopia (McCarey et al.) (Fig. 4-6, A)

Fenestrated polysulfone* for aphakia, myopia, and hyperopia (Lane, Lindstrom) (Fig. 4-6, B)

Intracorneal ring* for myopia, hyperopia, and aphakia (Flemming) (Fig. 4-6, C)

Lamellar keratoplasty (Fig. 4-7)

Central for keratoconus

Peripheral for marginal thinning

Lamellar keratotomy for hyperopia

Keratotomy

Radial for myopia (Fig. 4-8, A)

Transverse (straight or arcuate) ± radial for astigmatism (many patterns) (Fig. 4-9)

Naturally occurring astigmatism

After penetrating keratoplasty (Fig. 4-8, B), cataract extraction, refractive keratotomy

Circumferential (hexagonal, circular) for hyperopia or astigmatism (Fig. 4-6, B)

Keratectomy—manual (Fig. 4-11)

Crescentic (wedge resection) for astigmatism after penetrating keratoplasty (Fig. 4-13)

Crescentic lamellar for marginal thinning (Fig. 4-11)

Laser photorefractive keratectomy (Fig. 4-10)

Photorefractive keratectomy (large area ablation, reprofiling, sculpting) for myopia, hyperopia, aphakia (Trokel) (Fig. 4-3)

Transverse linear keratectomy for astigmatism (Seiler)

Radial linear keratectomy for myopia

Intrastromal photodisruption or heating for myopia*

Penetrating keratoplasty and cataract surgery (refractive aspects) (Fig. 4-14)

Incision techniques to reduce astigmatism

Wound closure techniques to reduce astigmatism

Suture placement

Selective removal or adjustment of sutures

Cataract extraction with intraocular lens implantation

Endocapsular cataract extraction with refilling of capsular bag to preserve accommodation*

Intraocular lens refractive surgery

Clear lens extraction with intraocular lens for high myopia

Anterior chamber intraocular lens in phakic eye for myopia

Sutures in cornea

Purse-string intrastromal suture to correct hyperopia

Corneal tuck to correct astigmatism

Thermokeratoplasty

Central heat probe or microwave* for keratoconus (Fig. 4-15, A)

Radial peripheral intrastromal thermocoagulation for hyperopia (Fyodorov) (Fig. 4-15, B)

Modified from Waring GO: The changing status of radial keratotomy. I. J Refract Surg 1:81, 1985, and Waring GO: The changing status of radial keratotomy. II. J Refract Surg 1:119, 1985. Used with permission.
*Procedures not now in clinical use.

Epikeratoplasty

Epikeratoplasty (epikeratophakia) (Fig. 4-5) has undergone considerable trial-and-error refinement since its inception in 1980. Pressed tissue has replaced hydrated tissue; commercial preparation of the lenticules has replaced preparation in a university laboratory; scraping has replaced alcohol for epithelial removal; buttons oversized 1.5 mm are preferred to those oversized 0.5 mm; lamellar undermining has been added; circular keratotomy has replaced the circular keratectomy; techniques of cryolathing have improved; designs of the lenticules continue to change; storage of lenticules in preservative media is being studied as a substitute for lyophilization; and nonfreeze preparation of lenticules with the microkera-

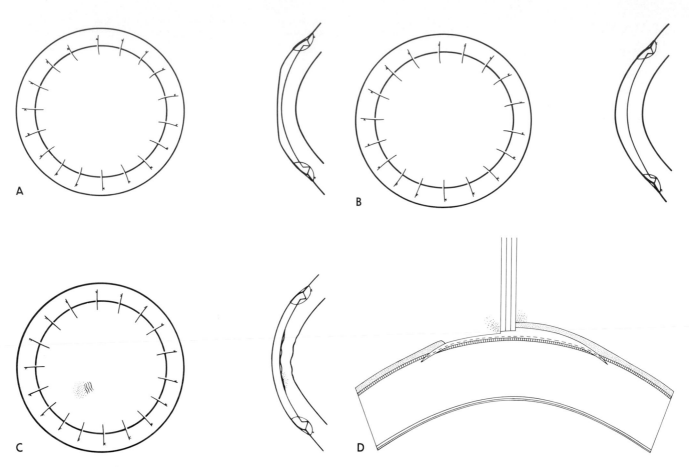

Figure 4-5

A, Epikeratoplasty for myopia involves the removal of a lamellar disc from a donor cornea, carving it on a cryolathe or die to form the concave lenticule, placing it on the surface of de-epithelialized recipient cornea, and suturing it into a peripheral circumferential groove or incision. This flattens the central corneal curvature and decreases refractive power. **B,** Epikeratoplasty for aphakia involves a similar process using a convex donor lenticule that steepens the corneal curvature, increasing refractive power. **C,** Epikeratoplasty for keratoconus employs a donor lenticule without power to flatten the cornea and diminish myopia and irregular astigmatism. **D,** Laser adjustable synthetic epikeratoplasty. A synthetic epikeratoplasty lenticule (clear in this figure) has been placed onto the surface of Bowman's layer and into a peripheral circular keratotomy. The epithelium has grown over the epikeratoplasty lenticule. If the curvature of the lenticule is not that desired, a laser is used to recarve the lenticule into a new shape. This has the advantage of repeated adjustability, the absence of wound healing, since the lenticule contains no cells, and potential replacability, since the lenticule can be removed and replaced. (From Waring GO: Arch Ophthalmol 1985;103:1472-1477.)

tome refractive bench of Krumeich has developed. The commercially sponsored, multicenter, nationwide study of lyophilized epikeratoplasty is a well-supervised program of informal testing.[74,75,112] In 1990 the U.S. Food and Drug Administration (FDA) issued regulatory guidelines for epikeratoplasty. The guidelines emphasized the usefulness of epikeratoplasty in aphakic young children who were contact lens intolerant, because no reasonable alternative existed for correcting the aphakia. Aphakic epikeratoplasty is contraindicated in infants younger than approximately 1 year of age. In adult aphakics epikeratoplasty is indicated when the placement of a secondary intraocular lens implant is not appropriate. In keratoconus, where a plano lenticule is used to flatten the cone for improved contact lens fitting, the procedure is indicated when there is minimal corneal scarring and a penetrating keratoplasty is thought to be inappropriate. Myopic epikeratoplasty was retained on core investigative status by the FDA, prompting the cessation of the commercial manufacture of the lenticules and reducing their availability to one or two centers in the United States. The major problems with myopic epikeratoplasty were the gradual loss of effect in some patients with poor predictability of refractive outcome.[36,37,80,96]

Since only approximately 40,000 human corneas annually are judged by eye banks to be not usable for penetrating keratoplasty, these are potentially available for epikeratoplasty. This is a small fraction of the people with ametropia who might benefit from epikeratoplasty, and thus research in synthetic epikeratoplasty is going forward, having reached a level of trial-and-error refinement in laboratory animals. Lenticules made of type IV or type I collagen, collagen-hydrogel polymers, and coated hydrogels have been developed, but successful transition to clinical trials requires overcoming the following three challenges:

1. Adequate attachment of the lenticule to Bowman's layer with lamellar pocket keratotomy, adhesives, or laser welding
2. Adequate and permanent epithelialization
3. Absence of erosion or melting of the lenticule

Keith Thompson and colleagues have suggested combining synthetic epikeratoplasty with excimer laser surface ablation to create a laser-adjustable synthetic epikeratoplasty (LASE), an idea that is still in the initial creative stage (Fig. 4-5, *D*).[107]

Intracorneal lenses

After José Barraquer creatively suggested the use of artificial intracorneal lenses (glass and plastic), he shifted his attention to the use of a human donor lenticule placed in the bed of a microkeratome excision (keratophakia) (Fig. 4-6). However, the complexity of that operation led to its replacement with modern synthetic intracorneal lenses.[71] Hydrogel intracorneal lenses are now being evaluated in informal clinical trials in humans, having the advantage of biocompatibility but the disadvantage of requiring a microkeratome excision to make a lamellar bed. High−index of refraction polysulfone plastic lenses have the advantage of requiring only a pocket lamellar dissection in the cornea for implantation, but the lenses must be fenestrated to allow nutrients from the aqueous humor to reach the anterior cornea. This technique is undergoing trial-and-error refinement.[22,56,84]

Intracorneal rings can be placed in a lamellar microkeratome bed or threaded into a peripheral tunnel, avoiding the central cornea and theoretically allowing adjustment of the tension on the ring to modify the refractive error postoperatively[32] (Fig. 4-6).

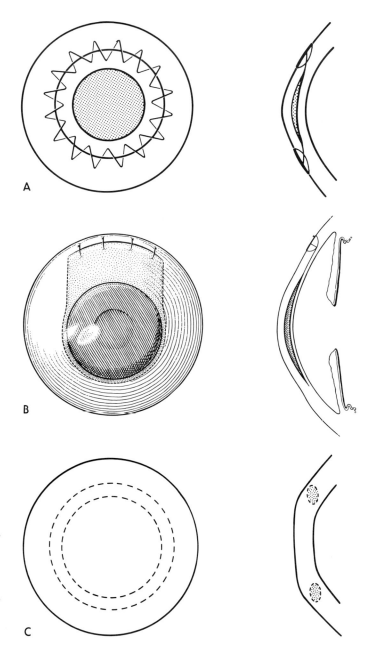

Figure 4-6

Keratophakia involves the placement of a lenticule within the corneal stroma to change the refraction of the cornea. **A,** If the lenticule is designed to change the curvature of the anterior surface of cornea, excision of a lamellar disc of cornea with a microkeratome is necessary. Then the lenticule of a human donor cornea or hydrogel material is placed in the lamellar bed and the disc of the recipient cornea is resutured into its original position. **B,** If the donor lenticule has a different index of refraction, thereby changing the refraction of the cornea, it can be placed in a deep lamellar pocket. **C,** Developing technology involves the use of intracorneal rings placed in the peripheral cornea, reducing the hazard of placing a lenticule in the visual axis. (From Waring GO: Arch Ophthalmol 1985;103:1472-1477.)

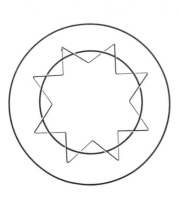
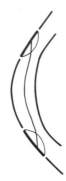

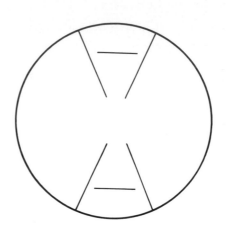
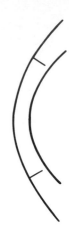

Figure 4-7
Lamellar keratoplasty can be done to reinforce and to flatten ectatic corneas, as in advanced keratoconus and keratoglobus, thus decreasing the myopia inherent in these disorders. A deep lamellar keratotomy allows anterior bowing of the thin remaining stromal bed, thus decreasing hyperopia; the lamellar disc is sutured back in place over the steepened cornea.

Figure 4-9
Keratotomy for astigmatism involves transverse incisions made in the steep meridian that do not intersect other incisions. The incisions flatten the steep meridian and steepen the flat meridian.

Lamellar keratoplasty

Although a plano lamellar keratoplasty lenticule is usually placed for tectonic and reinforcement purposes and not for refractive correction it can play a role as a refractive surgical technique. For example, in eyes with advanced keratoconus or keratoglobus, a lamellar keratoplasty may be carried out to both reinforce and flatten the cornea (Fig. 4-7). Hanna and colleagues[40] have described a method of using the microkeratome on both the donor and the host for lamellar keratoplasty.

Radial keratotomy for myopia

Radial keratotomy for myopia (Fig. 4-8) is the most thoroughly studied refractive surgical procedure, having made its way through the first four stages of development and evaluation, including the formal PERK trial.* Details are presented throughout this book.

Keratotomy for astigmatism

Approximately a dozen patterns of keratotomy to correct astigmatism have muddled through a decade of trial-and-error refinement. Current evidence supports the original concepts in the 1890s that transverse (tangential, "T") incisions made perpendicular to the steep meridian are the most effective (Fig. 4-9),[60,61,108] as described in Chapter 31, Keratotomy for Astigmatism, and Chapter 32, Atlas of Astigmatic Keratotomy. Current informal clinical testing is helping define other

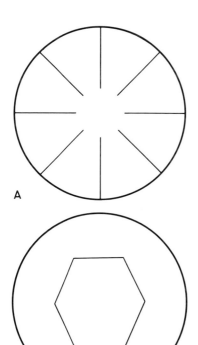
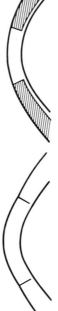

Figure 4-8
A, Radial keratotomy for myopia involves equally spaced radial incisions made deeply into the corneal stroma to flatten the central part of the cornea and decrease its refractive power. **B,** Circumferential keratotomy (hexagonal keratotomy) for the management of hyperopia is undergoing trial-and-error refinement. (From Waring GO: Arch Ophthalmol 1985;103:1472-1477.)

*References 1, 6, 17, 26, 33, 35, 42, 65, 89-91, 93, 94, 99, 100, 102, 114-116, 123, 124.

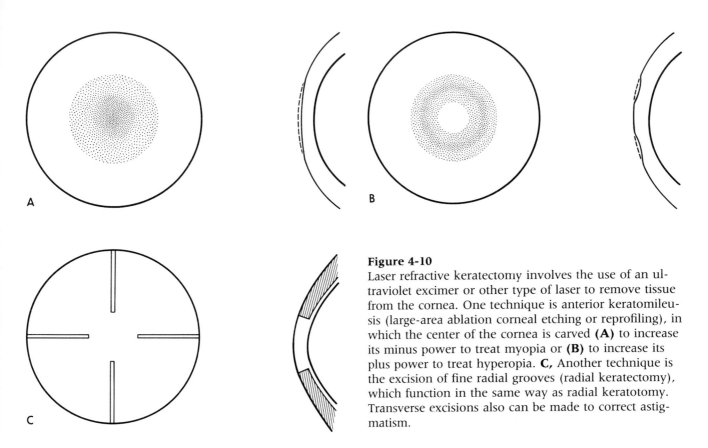

Figure 4-10
Laser refractive keratectomy involves the use of an ultraviolet excimer or other type of laser to remove tissue from the cornea. One technique is anterior keratomileusis (large-area ablation corneal etching or reprofiling), in which the center of the cornea is carved **(A)** to increase its minus power to treat myopia or **(B)** to increase its plus power to treat hyperopia. **C,** Another technique is the excision of fine radial grooves (radial keratectomy), which function in the same way as radial keratotomy. Transverse excisions also can be made to correct astigmatism.

variables, such as the effect of combined radial and transverse incisions, curved versus straight transverse incisions, the most effective number of transverse incisions, the use of keratography as a guide for placement of the incisions, and intraoperative keratoscopy and keratometry to titrate the amount of surgery. It is time for selected techniques to enter formal trials, as has been proposed in the Prospective Evaluation of Astigmatic Keratotomy (PEAK) study.

Circumferential keratotomy for hyperopia

Circumferential keratotomy is now undergoing slow trial-and-error refinement as hexagonal keratotomy to reduce hyperopia (Fig. 4-8, *B*).[125] Current techniques avoid connecting the six incisions. One variant technique uses a second set of six transverse incisions outside the apexes of the original set (hexagonal-T).[34]

Laser photorefractive keratectomy

Excimer laser corneal surgery is discussed in detail in Chapter 19, Laser Corneal Surgery. It was introduced in 1983 by Trokel and Srinivasan[109] as a potential replacement for radial keratotomy, on the theory that the linear excisions made by the laser would be more accurate and reproducible than manual incisions made with a diamond knife. However, since both types of incisions require extensive wound healing, the use of lasers for linear keratectomy has taken second place to the development of laser use for laser keratomileusis (large-area ablation, reprofiling, and sculpting) (Fig. 4-10). The techniques are currently undergoing refinement in both laboratory and human experiments under FDA control. This high-tech approach to corneal surgery requires a 193-nm argon fluoride excimer laser, a homogeneous beam, an appropriate mask system to shape the beam, including fixed apertures, diaphragms, moving slits, ablatable masks, and axicon lenses, a delivery system that can transmit the beam to the cornea with minimal loss of energy and homogeneity, and a method of stabilizing the eye during ablation. Many of these technical factors have been controlled to the point that a predictable ablation to correct myopia and hyperopia can be achieved, but the problems of wound healing still plague this technique, with mild subepithelial fibroplasia producing corneal haze and modifying the refractive effect by filling in the ablated zone. Other types of lasers (for example, hydrogen fluoride, holmium YAG, and Nd:YLF) are being developed for intrastromal surgery.

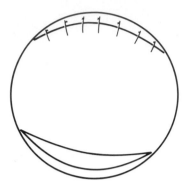
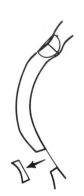

Figure 4-11
Crescentic lamellar keratectomy can help manage thinning disorders of the peripheral part of the cornea by strengthening thin areas and steepening the flat meridian of the central part of the cornea. (From Waring GO: Arch Ophthalmol 1985;103:1472-1477.)

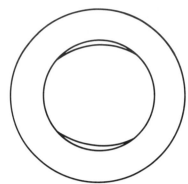
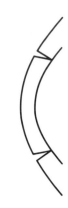

Figure 4-12
Arcuate keratotomy (relaxing incision) in penetrating keratoplasty consists of deep incisions across the steepest meridian in scar or donor (but not host) tissue to flatten that meridian and reduce astigmatism. (From Waring GO: Arch Ophthalmol 1985;103:1472-1477.)

Crescentic lamellar keratectomy

Removal of a banana-shaped crescent of peripheral cornea (Fig. 4-11) can help manage peripheral thinning disorders such as Terrien's marginal degeneration or pellucid marginal degeneration. The technique described by Caldwell[20] needs clinical verification by other observers. The resection of a wedge of tissue from the wound of a penetrating keratoplasty in the flat semimeridian can help reduce high astigmatism, a technique that is in the stage of informal clinical testing.

Penetrating keratoplasty

The refractive aspects of penetrating keratoplasty and cataract surgery have been refined informally for decades. Efforts to prevent astigmatism have focused on making symmetric uniform wounds and on suturing techniques that distribute the tension uniformly. These efforts have reduced the amount of postoperative astigmatism in cataract surgery,[47] but there has been less success in penetrating keratoplasty. Management of astigmatism after surgery has involved selective removal of interrupted sutures or adjustment of running sutures,[78] techniques now being tested informally with the use of keratography after penetrating keratoplasty,[41,52] and techniques of arcuate (Fig. 4-12) and trapezoidal relaxing incisions and of wedge resections (Fig. 4-13).

Calculation of the proper power of an intraocular lens implanted during penetrating keratoplasty (Fig. 4-14) is challenging and in need of refinement because the postoperative corneal power cannot be predicted accurately.[23] Many surgeons use their own average

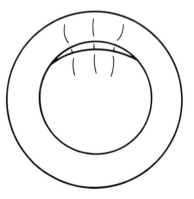
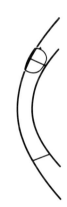

Figure 4-13
Crescentic wedge resection can reduce astigmatism in penetrating keratoplasty by removing a piece of tissue from corneal scar in the flat meridian and resuturing the wound together, which steepens that meridian and increases the refractive power of the cornea. (From Waring GO: Arch Ophthalmol 1985;103:1472-1477.)

postkeratoplasty keratometry power and the preoperative axial length of the patient's eye to calculate the intraocular lens power.

Thermokeratoplasty

Thermokeratoplasty in the management of keratoconus (Fig. 4-15, *A*) has bounced back and forth between refinement and informal testing for a century.

Attempts in the 1970s to use a flat thermoprobe to reduce keratoconus and facilitate the fitting of contact lenses resulted in excessive corneal complications and was abandoned.[2,3] More recent attempts to use microwave thermokeratoplasty to treat keratoconus were proved ineffective.[87]

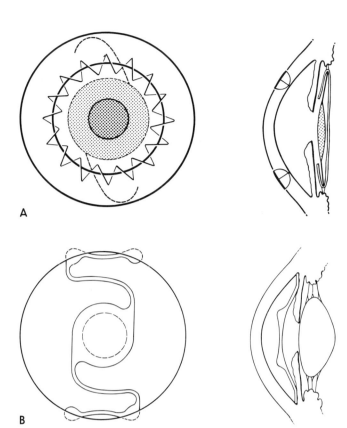

Figure 4-14
A, In penetrating keratoplasty, residual astigmatism can be diminished by careful attention to wound configuration, suture pattern, and trephination. In eyes that contain an intraocular lens, the spherical power of the corneal graft should correlate appropriately with that of the intraocular lens and with the axial length of the globe to achieve the desired final refraction. **B,** Placement of a vaulted, open-loop anterior chamber intraocular lens in a phakic eye to correct myopia raises questions about the long-term development of damage to the angle with glaucoma, endothelial damage with rubbing of the eye, and possible cataract formation in the clear crystalline lens. (From Waring GO: Arch Ophthalmol 1985; 103:1472-1477.)

Figure 4-15
In thermokeratoplasty, controlled application of heat into the stroma can shrink and scar stromal collagen. **A,** Central surface thermokeratoplasty involves the application of heat to the surface to shrink underlying collagen and reduce ectasia of the cornea in keratoconus. **B,** Radial intrastromal thermokeratoplasty shrinks the peripheral and paracentral stromal collagen, producing a central steepening of the cornea to treat hyperopia. (From Waring GO: Arch Ophthalmol 1985;103:1472-1477.)

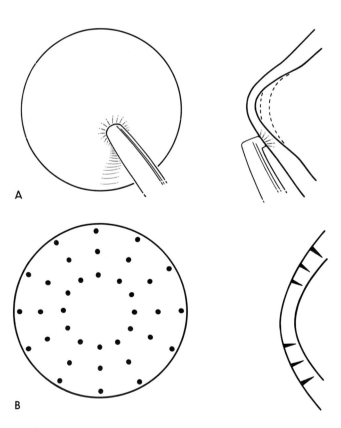

Since 1982 Fyodorov and colleagues have used peripheral intrastromal thermocoagulation (radial thermokeratoplasty) to treat hyperopia and presbyopia (Fig. 4-15, *B*).

The instrument Fyodorov and colleagues use comprises a motorized handle with footplates and a small needle that penetrates the corneal stroma momentarily and applies heat within the stroma, shrinking the collagen in that area. Applications are made in eight to 12 radial rays around the cornea with three to four burns per ray. Peripheral arcuate burns can be made to decrease astigmatism. The result of the peripheral shrinking of the stromal collagen produces central corneal steepening for the correction of hyperopia. Although the technique has been done on a few thousand cases in the Soviet Union with reported success, the procedure is undergoing slow trial-and-error refinement in the United States with reports of varying results.[30]

Crystalline lens and intraocular lens surgery

The most commonly performed ophthalmic surgery in the United States is cataract extraction, and well over 90% of these operations have the placement of an intraocular lens to correct the aphakia. This is refractive surgery, since the power of the intraocular

UNFINISHED BUSINESS

The task of developing refractive corneal surgery has occupied ophthalmologists for almost 100 years, with a sustained effort over the past 50 years. New techniques will continue to evolve; before 1983 no one had thought of using an excimer laser to reshape the corneal surface. The task of finding a surgical procedure that can replace glasses and contact lenses because it is truly effective, safe, predictable, adjustable, reversible, and affordable is truly unfinished business. My personal prejudice is toward techniques in which corneal wound healing does not play an important role in determining the refractive outcome. Thus I think techniques that use synthetic materials, such as intracorneal lenses and synthetic epikeratoplasty, have the greatest potential, although they are far from practical clinical realization in 1990.

Honest, standardized comparison of the multiple refractive surgical techniques is sorely needed. An individual surgeon's enthusiasm over a particular technique will provide the personal impetus and collective leadership to further refine and test the technique. However, that enthusiasm should not be allowed to bias the collection and analysis of data or the presentation of results in a way that would mislead other ophthalmologists and interested patients; this would delay the overall advance of refractive surgery while other investigators invest time and effort to verify the results. Critical caution, not unrestrained enthusiasm, should characterize the assessment of refractive surgical techniques. If a particular technique emerges as clearly superior there will be plenty of time for exultation, as well as fame and profit.

Both the ophthalmologist and the patient—as consumers of information—face the unfinished business of assessing information, in the popular media, at professional meetings, and in the published professional literature. Keeping in mind the simple five-stage paradigm presented in this chapter will help these individuals decide where along the spectrum of development a particular procedure has progressed.

The task of comparing numerous refractive surgical techniques is complex. Individual surgeons who can master more than one technique will be in the best position to make such a comparison. Adhering to conventional standards of reporting results will make comparison among different studies by different surgeons easier. The new techniques of metaanalysis will help assess the overall effectiveness and safety of a technique as presented by numerous investigators.

lens must be calculated based on preoperative formulas and refined preoperatively based on the needs of the patient. This is a good example of a surgical technique reaching virtual universal acceptance while progressing through only the phase of informal clinical testing, including FDA trials.[47]

Extraction of a clear crystalline lens was introduced to treat high myopia in the nineteenth century, and its current refinement as an extracapsular technique with posterior chamber lens implantation is now undergoing informal testing. Although the technique can be done with minimal technical complications, the incidence of retinal detachment seems to be higher in myopes, especially those with axial elongation.[113]

The insertion of intraocular lenses into phakic eyes to correct refractive errors, particularly myopia, was attempted in the 1950s by Joaquin Barraquer, but the design of the lenses was so poor that severe complications resulted and the technique was abandoned. Now with more refined styles of open-loop, flexible, vaulted, finely polished, anterior chamber intraocular lenses, informal clinical trials of phakic anterior chamber intraocular lenses for the correction of myopia are under way (Fig. 4-14, *B*).

REFERENCES

1. Akiyama K, Tanaka M, and Kanai A: Problems arising from Sato's radial keratotomy procedure in Japan, CLAO J 1984;10:179-184.

2. Aquavella JA, Smith RS, and Shaw EL: Alterations in corneal morphology following thermokeratoplasty, Arch Ophthalmol 1976;94:2082-2085.

3. Arentson JJ, Rodrigues MM, and Laibson PR: Histopathologic changes after thermokeratoplasty for keratoconus, Invest Ophthalmol Vis Sci 1977;16:32-38.

4. Aron-Rosa DS, Boerner CF, Bath P, et al: Corneal wound healing after excimer laser keratotomy in a human eye, Am J Ophthalmol 1987;103:454-464.

5. Arrowsmith PN and Marks RG: Evaluating the predictability of radial keratotomy, Ophthalmology 1985;92:331-338.

6. Arrowsmith PN and Marks RG: Visual, refractive, and keratometric results of radial keratotomy: a two-year follow-up, Arch Ophthalmol 1987;105:76-80.

7. Austin JH: Chase, chance, and creativity, New York, 1978, Columbia University Press.

8. Barraquer JI: Keratomileusis for the correction of myopia, Arch Soc Am Oftal Optom 1964;5:27-48.

9. Barraquer JI: Basis of refractive keratoplasty, Arch Soc Am Oftal Optom 1967;6:21-68.

10. Barraquer JI: Cirugia refractiva de la cornea, Bogota, Colombia, 1989, Institute Barraquer de America, Ophthalmology 1981;88:701-708.

10a. Barraquer JI, Gutierrez AM, and Espinosa A: Myopic keratomileusis: short-term results, Refract Corneal Surg 1989;5:307.

11. Bates WH: A suggestion of an operation to correct astigmatism, Arch Ophthalmol 1984;23:9-13.

12. Beekhuis WH, McCarey BE, Waring GO, et al: Hydrogel keratophakia: a microkeratome dissection in the monkey model, Br J Ophthalmol 1986;70:192-198.

13. Bender GA and Tom RA: Great moments in medicine, Detroit, 1966, Northwood Institute Press, pp 124-130.

14. Bernard C. An introduction to the study of experimental medicine, New York, 1949, Henry Schuman, Inc (Translated by H.C. Greene).

15. Binder PS: Selective suture removal can reduce post keratoplasty astigmatism, Ophthalmology 1985;92:1412-1416.

16. Bores L: Purpose, protocol, and goals of the National Radial Keratotomy Study Group. In Schachar RA, Levy NS, and Schachar L, editors: Radial keratotomy, Dennison, Tex, 1980, LAL Publishing, pp 21-23.

17. Bores LD: Historical review and clinical results of radial keratotomy. In Binder PS, editor: Refractive corneal surgery, the correction of aphakia, hyperopia, and myopia, Int Ophthalmol Clin 1983;23:93-118.

18. Broad W and Wade N: Betrayers of the truth, New York, 1982, Simon & Schuster, Inc.

19. Burk LL, Redjaee B, Stulting RD, et al: Changes in astigmatism after removal of individual sutures in penetrating keratoplasty, Invest Ophthalmol Vis Sci 1986;27(suppl):92.

20. Caldwell DR, Insler MS, Boutros G, et al: Primary surgical repair of severe peripheral marginal ectasia in Terrien's marginal degeneration, Am J Ophthalmol 1984;97:332-336.

21. Choyce DP: The correction of refractive errors with polysulfone corneal inlays: a new frontier to be explored? Trans Ophthalmol Soc UK 1985;104:332-342.

22. Climenhaga H, Macdonald JM, McCarey BE, and Waring GO: Effect of diameter and depth on the response to solid polysulfone intracorneal lenses in cats, Arch Ophthalmol (in press).

23. Crawford GJ, Stulting RD, Waring GO, et al: The triple procedure: analysis of outcome, refraction, and intraocular lens power calculation, Ophthalmology 1986;93:817-824.

24. Danish Obesity Project: Randomized trial of jejunoileal bypass versus medical treatment in morbid obesity, Lancet 1979;2:1255-1257.

25. Deg JK and Binder PS: Histopathology and clinical behavior of polysulfone intracorneal implants in the baboon model, Ophthalmology 1988;95:506-515.

26. Deitz MR, Sanders DR, and Raanan MG: A consecutive series (1982-1985) of radial keratotomies performed with the diamond blade, Am J Ophthalmol 1987;103:417-422.

27. Diabetic Retinopathy Study Research Group: Photocoagulation treatment of proliferative diabetic retinopathy: the second report of the Diabetic Retinopathy Study findings, Ophthalmology 1978;85:82-105.

28. Duke-Elder S: System of ophthalmology, St Louis, 1962, The CV Mosby Co., p 740.

29. EC/IC Bypass Study Group: Failure of extracranial-intracranial arterial bypass to reduce the risk of ischemic stroke: results of an international randomized trial, N Engl J Med 1985;313:1191-1200.28a.

30. Feldman ST, Ellis W, Frucht-Pery J, Chayet A, Brown SI: Regression of effect following radial thermokeratoplasty in humans, Refractive Corneal Surg 1989;5:288-291.

31. Ferris FL: Evaluation of medical data: role of clinical trials, Ophthalmology 1986;93:964-966.

32. Fleming JF, Reynolds AE, Kilmer L, et al: The intrastromal corneal ring: two cases in rabbits, J Refract Surg 1987;3:227-232.

33. Fyodorov SN and Agranovsky AA: Long-term results of anterior radial keratotomy, J Ocular Ther Surg 1982;1:217-223.

34. Gilbert ML, Friedlander M, Aiello JP, and Granet N: Hexagonal keratotomy in human cadaver eyes, J Refractive Surg 1988;4:12-14.

35. Gills JP: Trephination in combination with radial keratotomy for myopia. In Schachar RA, Levy NS, and Schachar L, editors: Radial keratotomy, Dennison, Tex, 1980, LAL Publishing, pp 91-100.

36. Goosey JD, Prager TC, Goosey CB, Allison ME, and Marvelli TL: Stability of refraction during 2 years after myopic epikeratoplasty, Refractive Corneal Surg 1990;6:4-10.

37. Goosey JD, Prager TC, Goosey CB, and Martin DL: 1 year follow-up of epikeratoplasty for myopia, J Cataract Refract Surg 1990;16:21-30.

38. Goosey JD, Prager TC, Vidaurri LJ, et al: Myopic epikeratophakia performed with and without an annular keratectomy, Invest Ophthalmol Vis Sci 1987;28(suppl):275.

39. Hanna KD, Chastang JC, Agfar L, Samson J, Pouliquen Y, and Waring GO: Scanning slit delivery system, J Cataract Refract Surg 1989;15:390-396.

40. Hanna KD, David T, and Pouliquen Y: Lamellar keratoplasty with the Barraquer microkeratome, Refractive Corneal Surg (in press).

41. Harris DJ, Waring GO, and Burk L: Keratography as a guide to selective suture removal for the reduction of astigmatism after penetrating keratoplasty, 1989;96:1957.

42. Hecht SD and Jamara RJ: Prospective evaluation of radial keratotomy using the Fyodorov formula: preliminary report, Ann Ophthalmol 1982; 14:319-330.

43. Hlatky MA, Califf RM, Harrell FE, Lee KL, Marx PB, Pryor DB: Comparison of predictions based on observational data with the results of randomized controlled clinical trials of coronary artery bypass surgery, J Am Coll Cardiol 1988;11:237-245.

44. Hocking MP, Duerson MC, O'Leary P, et al: Jejunoileal bypass for morbid obesity: late follow-up in 100 cases, N Engl J Med 1983;308:995-999.

45. Hoffer K, Darin J, Petit T, et al: Three year experience with radial keratotomy: the UCLA study, Ophthalmology 1983;90:627-636.

46. Hofmann RF: The surgical correction of idiopathic astigmatism. In Sanders DR, Hofmann RF, and Salz JJ, editors: Refractive corneal surgery, Thorofare, NJ, 1986, Slack, Inc., pp 21-289.

47. Jaffe NS: Postoperative corneal astigmatism. In Jaffe NS, editor: Cataract surgery and its complications, ed 3, St Louis, 1984, The CV Mosby Co., pp 111-127

48. Kaufman HE: The correction of aphakia, Am J Ophthalmol 1980;89:1-10.

49. Kaufman HE: Refractive surgery, Am J Ophthalmol 1987;103:355-357 (editorial).

50. Kirkness CM, Steele ADM, and Garner A: Polysulfone corneal inlays: adverse reactions; a preliminary report, Trans Ophthalmol Soc UK 1985; 104:343-350.

51. Kolata G: Prostate cancer consensus hampered by lack of data, Science 1987;236:1626-1627.

52. Kozarsky AM and Waring GO: Photokeratoscopy in the management of astigmatism following keratoplasty, Dev Ophthalmol 1985;11:91-98.

53. Krumeich Jorg H: The planar non-freeze lamellar refractive keratoplasty techniques: non-freeze keratomileusis and non-freeze epikeratophakia. In Boyd BF, editor: Highlights of ophthalmology refractive surgery with the masters, vol 2, Coral Gables, Fla, 1987, Highlights of Ophthalmology, pp 122-136.

54. Krumeich JH and Swinger CA: Non-freeze epikeratophakia for the correction of myopia, Am J Ophthalmol 1987;103:397-403.

55. Lane SL, Cameron JD, Lindstrom RL, et al: Polysulfone corneal lenses, J Cataract Refract Surg 1986;12:50-60.

56. Lane SS, Lindstrom RL, Cameron JD, et al: Fenestrated intracorneal lenses, Invest Ophthalmol Vis Sci 1987; 28(suppl):276.

57. Lans LJ: Experimentelle Untersuchungen uber Entstehung von Astigmatissus durch nicht-perforirende Corneawunden, Albrecht Von Graefes Arch Ophthalmol 1898;45:117-152.

58. Lieurance RC, Patel AC, Wan WL, et al: Excimer laser cut lenticules for epikeratophakia, Am J Ophthalmol 1987;103:475-476.

59. Lind J: A treatise on the scurvy, ed 3, London, 1772, Crowden. In Classics of medicine library, Birmingham, Ala, 1980, Gryphon Editions.

60. Lindquist TD, Rubenstein, Hofmann RF, et al: Astigmatic keratotomy. In Sanders DR, editor: Radial keratotomy: surgical techniques, Thorofare, NJ, 1986, Slack Inc., pp 119-129.

61. Lindquist TD, Rubenstein JB, Rice SW, et al: Trapezoidal astigmatic keratotomy, Arch Ophthalmol 1986; 104:1534-1539.

62. Lindstrom RL and Lavery GW: Correction of post-keratoplasty astigmatism. In Sanders DR, Hofmann RF, and Salz JJ, editors: Refractive corneal surgery, Thorofare, NJ, 1986, Slack, Inc., pp 215-240.

63. Lock S: A difficult balance: editorial peer review in medicine, London, 1985, The Nuffield Provincial Hospitals Trust.

64. Loertscher H, Mandelbaum S, Parrish RK, et al: Preliminary report on corneal incisions created by a hydrogen fluoride laser, Am J Ophthalmol 1986;102:217-221.

65. Lynn MJ, Waring GO, Sperduto RD, et al: Factors affecting outcome and predictability of radial keratotomy in the PERK Study, Arch Ophthalmol 1987;105:42-51.

66. Macular Photocoagulation Study Group: Argon laser photocoagulation for senile macular degeneration, results of a randomized clinical trial, Arch Ophthalmol 1982;100:912-918.

67. Mandel MR, Shapiro MB, and Krachmer JH: Relaxing incisions with augmentation sutures for the correction of postkeratoplasty astigmatism, Am J Ophthalmol 1987; 103:441-447.

68. Marshall J, Trokel S, Rothery S, et al: Photoablative reprofiling of the cornea using an excimer laser: photorefractive keratectomy, Lasers Ophthalmol 1986;1:21-25.

69. Maxwell WA: Myopic keratomileusis: initial results and myopic keratomileusis combined with other procedures, J Cataract Refract Surg 1987;13:518-523.

70. McCarey BE: Alloplastic refractive keratoplasty. In Sanders DR, Hofmann RF, and Salz JJ, editors: Refractive corneal surgery, Thorofare, NJ, 1986, Slack, Inc., 529-548.

71. McCarey BE: Current status of refractive surgery with synthetic intracorneal lenses: Barraquer lecture, Refractive Corneal Surg 1990;6:40-46.

72. McCarey BE, van Rij G, Beekhuis WH, et al: Hydrogel keratophakia: a freehand pocket dissection in the monkey model, Br J Ophthalmol 1986;70:188-191.

73. McDonald MB, Beuerman R, Falzoni W, et al: Refractive surgery with the excimer laser, Am J Ophthalmol 1987;103:469-472.

74. McDonald MB, Kaufman HE, Aquavella JV, et al: The nationwide study of epikeratophakia for aphakia in adults, Am J Ophthalmol 1987; 103:358-365.

75. McDonald MB, Kaufman HE, Aquavella JV, et al: The nationwide study of epikeratophakia for myopia, Am J Ophthalmol 1987;103:375-383.

76. McDonald MB, Kaufman HE, Durrie DS, et al: Epikeratophakia for keratoconus: the nationwide study, Arch Ophthalmol 1986;104:1294-1300.

77. McDonald MB, Safir A, Waring GO, et al: A preliminary comparative study of epikeratophakia or penetrating keratoplasty for keratoconus, Am J Ophthalmol 1987;103:467-468.

78. McNeill JI and Wessels IF: Adjustment of single continuous suture to control astigmatism after penetrating keratoplasty, Refractive Corneal Surg 1989;5:216-221.

79. Meinert CL: Clinical trials: design, conduct, and analysis, New York, 1986, Oxford University Press.

80. Neumann AC, McCarty G, and Sanders DR: Delayed regression of effect in myopic epikeratophakia vs. myopic keratomileusis for high myopia, Refractive Corneal Surg 1989; 5:161-166.

81. Nordan LT and Fallor MK: Myopic keratomileusis: 74 consecutive nonamblyopic cases with one year of follow-up, J Refract Surg 1986; 2:124-128.

82. Oydhouse N: A controlled study of adenotonsillectomy, Lancet 1969; 2:931-932.

83. Paradise JL: Clinical trials of tonsillectomy and adenoidectomy: limitations of existing studies and a current effort to evaluate efficacy, South Med J 1976;69:1049-1053.

84. Pettit D, McCarey BE, McDonald MB, et al: Refractive results of hyperopic hydrogel intracorneal lens implantation in primate eyes, Invest Ophthalmol Vis Sci 1987;28 (suppl):276.

85. Preliminary Report: Findings from the aspirin component of the ongoing physicians' health study, N Engl J Med 1988;318:262-264.

86. Puliafito CS, Steinert RF, Deutsch TF, et al: Excimer laser ablation of the cornea and lens: experimental studies, Ophthalmology 1985;92:741-748.

87. Rowsey JJ: Electrosurgical keratoplasty: update and retraction, Invest Ophthalmol Vis Sci 1987;28(suppl): 224.

88. Rowsey JJ and Doss JD: Preliminary report of Los Alamos keratoplasty techniques, Ophthalmology 1981; 88:755-760.

89. Sanders DR: Radial keratotomy, Thorofare, NJ, 1984, Slack, Inc.

90. Sanders DR, Hoffmann RF, and Salz JJ: Refractive corneal surgery, Thorofare, NJ, 1986, Slack, Inc.

91. Sanders DR et al: Radial keratotomy: surgical techniques, Thorofare, NJ, 1986, Slack, Inc.

92. Sato T: Treatment of conical corneal incision of Descemet's membrane, Acta Soc Ophthalmol Jpn 1939; 43:544-555.

93. Sato T, Akiyama K, and Shibata H: A new surgical approach to myopia, Am J Ophthalmol 1953;36:823-829.

94. Sawelson H and Marks RG: Three-year results of radial keratotomy, Arch Ophthalmol 1987;105:81-85.

95. Schachar RA, Levy NS, and Schachar L, editors: Radial keratotomy, Dennison, Tex, 1980, LAL Publishing.

96. Schlichtemeier WR and Arbegast KD: Long-term loss of effect of epikeratophakia, J Refract Surg 1987; 3:46-49.

97. Seiler T, Berlin MS, Bende T, and Trokel S: Excimer laser keratectomy for correction of astigmatism, Am J Ophthalmol 1988;105:117-120.

98. Shapiro SH and Louis TA: Clinical trials: issues and approaches, New York, 1983, Marcel Dekker, Inc.

99. Sheppard DD: Radial keratotomy: analysis of efficacy and predictability in 1058 consecutive cases. I. Efficacy, J Cataract Refract Surg 1986;12:632-650.

100. Sheppard DD: Radial keratotomy: analysis of efficacy and predictability in 1058 consecutive cases. II. Predictability, J Cataract Refract Surg 1987; 13:32-34.

101. Silverman WA: Human experimentation: a guided step into the unknown, New York, 1985, Oxford University Press.

102. Siva Reddy P and Ranga Reddy P: Anterior keratotomy, Ophthalmic Surg 1980;11:765-767.

103. Stone W: Study of patency of openings in corneas anterior to intralamellar plastic artificial disc, Am J Ophthalmol 1955;39:185-196.

104. Swinger CA and Barker BA: Prospective evaluation of myopic keratomileusis, Ophthalmology 1984;91:785-792.

105. Swinger CA, Krumeich JH, and Cassiday D: Planar lamellar refractive keratoplasty, J Refract Surg 1986; 2:17-25.

106. Taylor CW and Barron F: Scientific creativity: its recognition in development, New York, 1963, John Wiley & Sons, Inc.

107. Thompson K, Hanna K, and Waring G: Emerging technologies for refractive surgery: laser adjustable synthetic epikeratoplasty, Refract Corneal Surg 1989;5:46-52.

108. Thornton SP: Graded non-intersecting transverse incisions for correction of idiopathic astigmatism. In Sanders DR, editor: Radial keratotomy: surgical techniques, Thorofare, NJ, 1986, Slack, Inc., pp 91-103.

109. Trokel SL, Srinivasan R, and Braren B: Excimer laser surgery of the cornea, Am J Ophthalmol 1983;96:710-715.

110. Troutman RC: Microsurgery of the anterior segment of the eye, vol 2, St Louis, 1977, The CV Mosby Co., p 286.

111. Troutman RC and Gaster RN: Surgical advances and results of keratoconus, Am J Ophthalmol 1980;90:131-136.

112. Varnell R, McDonald M, and Kaufman H: Myopic epikeratophakia performed without keratectomy in human patients, Invest Ophthalmol Vis Sci 1987;28(suppl):275.

113. Verzella F: Microsurgery of the lens in high myopia for optical purposes, Am Intra-ocular Implant Soc I 1985; 11:65-69.

114. Waring GO: The changing status of radial keratotomy for myopia. I. J Refract Surg 1985;1:81-86.

115. Waring GO: The changing status of radial keratotomy for myopia. II. J Refract Surg 1985;1:119-137.

116. Waring GO: History of radial keratotomy. In Sanders DR, Hofmann RF, and Salz J, editors: Refractive corneal surgery, Thorofare, NJ, 1986, Slack, Inc., pp 3-14.

117. Waring GO: Making sense of keratospeak: a classification or refractive corneal surgery, Arch Ophthalmol 1986;103:1472-1477.

118. Waring GO: Development and evaluation of refractive surgical procedures. Part I. Five stages in the continuum of development, J Refract Surg 1987;3:142-157.

119. Waring GO: Development and evaluation of refractive surgical procedures. Part II. Practical implementation of formal clinical trials, J Refract Surg 1987;3:173-184.

120. Waring GO: Lans distinguished refractive surgery lecture, J Refract Surg 1987;3:140-141.

121. Waring GO: Conventional standards for reporting results of refractive surgery, Refract Corneal Surg 1989; 5:285-290.

122. Waring GO, Lynn MS, Culbertson W, Laibson PR, Lindstrom RL, McDonald MB, Myers WD, Obstbaum SA, Rowsey JJ, Schanzlin DJ, and the PERK Study Group: Three year results of the Prospective Evaluation of Radial Keratotomy (PERK) Study, Ophthalmology 1987;94:1339-1354.

123. Waring GO, Lynn MJ, Fielding B, Asbell PA, Balyeat HD, Cohen EA, and the PERK Study Group: Results of the Prospective Evaluation of Radial Keratotomy (PERK) Study 4 years after surgery for myopia, JAMA 1990;263:1083-1097.

124. Waring GO, Lynn MJ, Gelender H, et al: Results of the Prospective Evaluation of Radial Keratotomy (PERK) Study one year after surgery, Ophthalmology 1985;92:177-198.

125. Yamashita T, Schneider ME, Fuerst DJ, et al: Hexagonal keratotomy reduces hyperopia after radial keratotomy in rabbits, J Refract Surg 1986;2:261-264.

Development of Refractive Keratotomy in the Nineteenth Century

Bernd H. Schimmelpfennig
George O. Waring III

Ferreting out the true origins of an operation that is more than a century old is like peeling an onion—each early description seems to lead to another predecessor. Identifying who performed the first refractive procedure and when is almost impossible, not only because the true originators may not have published their work, but also because the century-old documents are not easily accessible.

OPTICS AND REFRACTIVE SURGERY

It can be said safely, however, that refractive surgery would not have appeared without refined knowledge of the optical principles underlying refractive errors, principles that were clearly defined in the mid-nineteenth century. In 1864, Cornelieus Donders, from Utrecht, Netherlands, published the first modern treatise, *On the Anomalies of Accommodation and Refraction of the Eye.*[5] Donders systematically described the optical and clinical aspects of refractive errors, making the information digestible for clinicians.

In discussing the myriad treatments proposed for myopia, Donders caustically dismissed surgical methods:

The cure of myopia belongs to the pia vota. The more our knowledge of the basis of this anomaly has been established, the more certainly does any expectation in that direction appear to be destroyed, even with respect to the future. So long as it was thought that the cause of myopia might be found in increased convexity of the cornea, the endeavour to restore the later, by pressure, to its normal curvature (Purkinje and Ruete) appeared perhaps not altogether to be rejected; but the idea, that the extended, attenuated, atrophic membranes in myopia, might be brought back to their natural condition is

BACKGROUND AND ACKNOWLEDGMENTS
Numerous individuals provided information, photographs, and translations of writings concerning early work in keratotomy for Chapter 5. Among them are Harold Henkes, Rotterdam, Netherlands; Claire C. Kok-van Alphen (deceased), Leiden, Netherlands; Theo Seiler, Berlin, Germany; Gabriel van Rij, Groningen, Netherlands; Hennie J. Volker-Dieben, Leiden, Netherlands.

simply absurd. We should not even be able to approve of the practice of those, who, in order to compensate for the excessive length of the visual axis, endeavoured to bring the arching of the cornea below the normal.

Treatment is, alas, partly a matter of fashion. Thus discharging the aqueous humour from the anterior chamber of the eye, is now the order of the day. Some have even spoken of applying this method in myopia. If it be intended thereby to make the cornea flatter, the object will not be attained in this way.

We formerly lived under the rule of the myotomists. Rendered rash by ignorance, some have actually employed their operation for the relief of myopia, and have even persuaded themselves that they had thus accomplished a cure.

Lastly, the removal of the crystalline lens has also been suggested. When in a case of highly myopic structure of the eye, a lens affected with cataract has been successfully extracted, and a nearly emmetropic condition has been obtained, the operator has been exposed to the temptation of endeavouring, by the abstraction of a normal lens, to remove the myopia. A patient, who was an amateur in dioptrics, endeavoured to induce me to perform this operation! But I need not say, that such a momentous undertaking, doubly dangerous where a myopic eye and a transparent lens are concerned, without that, even in the most favourable case, any real advantage is to be expected, would exhibit culpable rashness.[5]

He concluded that spectacles were the most effective mode of management. Similarly in his thorough discussion and classification of astigmatism, Donders proposed spectacles as a useful, although imperfect, method of correction; he did not address any other modalities.

In the German edition of his 1866 book, Donders ironically teased French ophthalmologists by mentioning Emile Javal who, at the German ophthalmologic meeting in 1865, "saved" his French countrymen from being looked on as being completely ignorant about corneal astigmatism by pointing out that two French academicians had worn cylindric glasses for more than 10 years.

Not all early attempts to manage nearsightedness were based on optical or surgical principles; folk medicine had its day, as exemplified by the spring-mounted mallet that was suspended over the eye in an eye cup and used to pound the cornea flat through closed eyelids (Fig. 5-1).

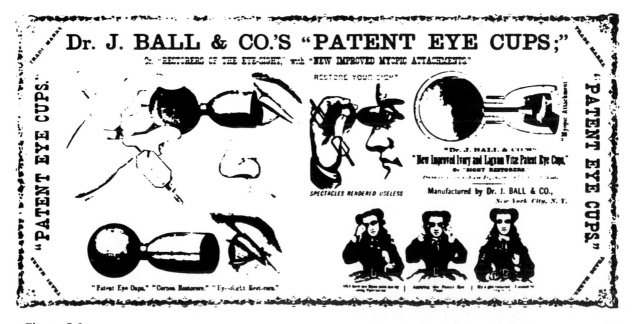

Figure 5-1
Advertisement by Dr. J. Ball shows a mid-nineteenth century method of flattening the cornea to treat myopia. Ball's patent eye cup was a small spring-mounted mallet that pounded the cornea flat through closed eyelids. "It restores your eyesight and renders spectacles useless!"

EARLY CLINICAL KERATOTOMY FOR ASTIGMATISM

In the 1850s Albrecht von Graefe in Berlin described his new surgical technique of cataract extraction by means of an *ab externo* excision at the limbus using his special knife.[20] This was not only the birth of modern cataract surgery, but also the genesis of a century-long epidemic of surgically induced corneal astigmatism. An early detailed report on this problem was published in 1869 by v. Reuss and Woinow,[18] residents at the University Eye Department in Vienna. Woinow, originally from Moscow, had studied with the physicist von Helmholtz in Heidelberg. They measured the preoperative and postoperative astigmatism in 31 eyes with the Helmholtz keratometer; in 21 of these eyes they found an increase in astigmatism after surgery caused by flattening of the vertical corneal meridian. In 1877 Weiss[21] reported astigmatic changes after cataract extraction and found the curvature of the vertical axis decreased and that of the horizontal axis increased—changes he attributed to the forward displacement of the corneal flap because of the intraocular pressure, which caused the vertical axis to approach a straight line. So the management of high astigmatism became a real clinical challenge.

Schiøtz, Bates, Faber, and Lucciola, four nineteenth century clinicians, used intuition and serendipitous observations to form the foundation for keratotomy in the treatment of astigmatism.

The first ophthalmic surgeon to report keratotomy to treat astigmatism seems to be Hjalmar August Schiøtz in Norway in 1885. In a terse case history,[16] he describes a 33-year-old patient, A.S. Maurer, who developed 19.50 D of astigmatism after cataract surgery, the vertical meridian being the steepest. Schiøtz used a Graefe's knife 4 months postoperatively to make a 3.5 mm *ab interno* incision at the upper limbus, reducing the astigmatism to 7.00 D by 5 months after the keratotomy. His approach foreshadowed the posterior keratotomy described by Sato 60 years later and the more modern "relaxing incision."

In New York City William H. Bates observed six patients independently in his practice with peripheral surgical or traumatic corneal scars who developed flattening of the cornea in the meridian that intersected the scar, with no change in the meridian 90 degrees away. This led Bates to suggest an operation for astigmatism in 1894: "Incisions of the cornea are made at right angles to the most convex meridian. The amount of correction can be regulated by the number, depth, and location of the incisions."[1] Unfortunately, Bates did not capitalize on his observations, but rather dropped out of sight for a decade.[9] When he reemerged, the eccentric physician had turned his attention to the unorthodox theory of attributing all refractive errors to eye strain that resulted from an "abnormal condition of the mind." This led Bates to create a series of exercises—both physical and mental—to restore normal vision, as described in his book published by the Central Fixation Publishing Company in 1920, "The Cure of Imperfect Sight by Treatment Without Glasses,"[2] a book that has been plagiarized and popularized, attracting adherents no less famous than Aldous Huxley.[11] The Bates method of treating refractive errors remains popular to this day, with exercises such as palming, swaying, and the application of small weights to the eyelids to assist in strengthening exercises.[4]

E. Faber, a Dutchman, acknowledged the occupational needs of some patients for keratotomy by using anterior transverse keratotomy in 1895 to treat a 19-year-old man who had been rejected by medical authorities of the Royal Military Academy because his refractive error of $+0.75\ -1.50 \times 30°$ gave him a visual acuity of 20/60.[7] The highly motivated young man was prepared to undergo any new treatment, and although Faber had never heard of someone performing an operation to correct astigmatism, he thought the circumstances justified a try. He made a 6 mm long, full-thickness incision at the corneoscleral limbus at axis 120°, using a lance. The refractive error was $+0.75\ -0.75 \times 120°$ 3 weeks after

Figure 5-2
Leendert Jan Lans, the Dutch ophthalmologist who made the first systematic study of refractive surgery and defined the basic principles of keratotomy in the laboratory. (Courtesy Harold Henkes, M.D., Rotterdam.)

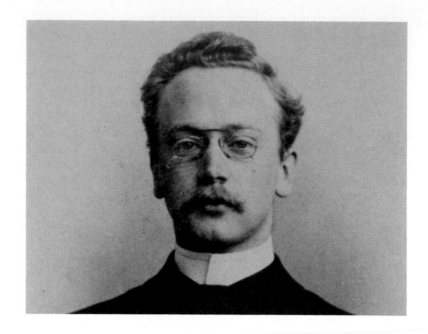

surgery, and the young man passed his medical test with a visual acuity of 20/25. Faber cautioned that the predictability of outcome would be difficult in such cases.

While these three surgeons described full-thickness transverse corneal incisions, J. Lucciola, working in Turin, Italy, published an early article that dealt more thoroughly with astigmatism after surgery. In the article Lucciola speculated about the cause of this astigmatism, including the influence of muscle action, intraocular pressure, type and location of the incisions, thickness of the scar tissue, and corneal perforations.[15] In 1896 he reported 10 cases of nonperforating corneal incisions made to flatten the steep meridian.

EARLY LABORATORY STUDY OF KERATOTOMY

The first systematic experiments performed in the laboratory to study corneal incisions and excisions were done by Leendert Jan Lans (Fig. 5-2). Lans was born in 1869 in Delft, Netherlands, and graduated cum laude from the University of Leiden in 1897, earning a doctor's degree with defense of a thesis titled "Experimental Studies of the Treatment of Astigmatism with Non-perforating Corneal Incisions."[14] Lans was aware of the early clinical experiences of Schiøtz, Bates, Faber, and Lucciola and set out to improve surgical techniques by systematic experimentation in rabbits, using patterns of keratotomy, keratectomy, and thermal cautery to create astigmatism.

The results of Lans' studies defined the following basic principles of radial keratotomy:
1. Nonperforating incisions parallel to the limbus result in bulging of the peripheral cornea and simultaneous flattening of the central cornea in that meridian (Fig. 5-3).
2. The scar formation that occurs during wound healing produces additional corneal flattening (Fig. 5-4).
3. Flattening in the meridian perpendicular to the incision is associated with steepening in the opposite meridian (Fig. 5-5).
4. Radial corneal wounds made with the galvanocautery produce peripheral steepening and central flattening in the meridian parallel to the wounds (Fig. 5-6).
5. Deeper incisions have a greater effect.

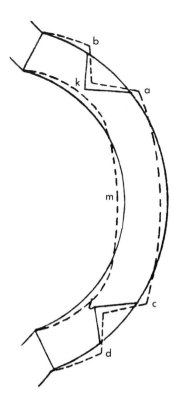

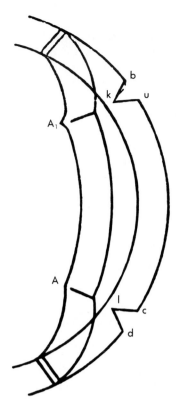

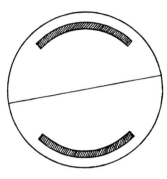

Figure 5-3
Lans' drawing illustrates the peripheral bulging and central flattening induced by partial-thickness corneal incisions parallel to the limbus.

Figure 5-4
Lans' illustration demonstrates that scarring of keratotomy wounds produces further flattening of the central cornea.

Figure 5-5
Lans' illustration of arcuate incisions parallel to the limbus; flattening occurred in the corneal meridian perpendicular to them.

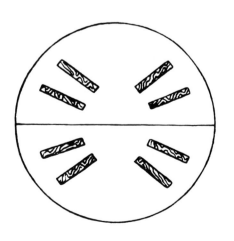

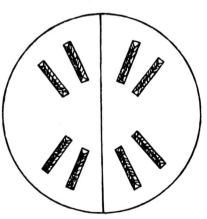

Figure 5-6
Lans' illustration of radial wounds that flattened the central cornea, especially along the meridian parallel to the wounds.

After receiving his degree, Lans studied with Snellen in Utrecht, Netherlands, maintaining his interest in astigmatism. Snellen defined with-the-rule and against-the-rule astigmatism but did not propose surgery for the problem.[17] From 1899 to 1903 Lans practiced general clinical ophthalmology in Dordrecht, Netherlands, a small town south of Rotterdam, where he became successful and respected and pursued his fanatic love of swimming and sailing. In 1904 he moved to Arnhem, Netherlands, where he founded the first medical committee for health care in schools and helped establish the Society for the Prevention of Tuberculosis. His election as the president of the Netherlands Ophthalmological Society in 1908 reflected his prominence, and he continued as a socially active person until he died in 1941 in his hometown of Delft, mourned by the medical profession and his patients alike. In 1987 Lans was honored by the International Society of Refractive Keratoplasty, which established the annual Distinguished Refractive Surgical Lecture in his name.

EARLY TWENTIETH CENTURY: A LATENT PERIOD

Despite the published clinical and experimental descriptions of surgery to correct astigmatism, the ophthalmic community turned its back on refractive surgery and concerned itself with structural problems after cataract surgery—wound closure, infections, and iris incarceration—ignoring the problems of astigmatism. For example, H. Knapp in New York City reported a series of 800 cataract extractions in 1884 without mentioning postoperative astigmatism.[13]

Even though there was little interest in astigmatism and its surgical correction, the early twentieth century saw the persistent introduction of techniques to treat myopia. Removing the clear crystalline lens in people with high myopia, an idea introduced 200 years before in the Netherlands by Boerhaave,[3] condemned by Donders in the Netherlands, and propagated by Fukala in Austria,[8] continued to find proponents such as Elschnig[6] from Prague, even though the results were poor and the operation fell out of favor. Clear crystalline lens extraction to treat high myopia was revived by Franco Verzella in Bologna, Italy, in the late 1980s using extracapsular techniques with the implantation of a posterior chamber intraocular lens.[19]

In 1911 Holth[10] suggested shortening the sclera to diminish the axial length of the globe in people with high myopia, taking a hint from scleral shortening procedures in the treatment of retinal detachment. Variations of this operation have developed in the 1980s.

And the cornea was not ignored. Inonye[12] in Japan in 1922 used a firm rubber band to compress and subsequently flatten the cornea. His patients were young women and Navy officers with small amounts of myopia. Inonye claimed that his patients had stable, good uncorrected vision for many years, although the largest decrease in myopia he could induce was 0.75 D.

Another Japanese, Tsutomu Sato, would later become the standard bearer for refractive corneal surgery.

UNFINISHED BUSINESS

How can there be unfinished business concerning history? It's a matter of accurate documentation and appreciation. We should continue to unearth the early manuscripts, in whatever language, that concern refractive corneal surgery, not only to acknowledge those who conceived of and even implemented these techniques a century or more ago, but also to benefit from their experience as part of the human knowledge base on which we are all building. This responsibility falls largely to nationals fluent in the languages of our surgical progenitors.

REFERENCES

1. Bates WH: A suggestion of an operation to correct astigmatism, Arch Ophthalmol 1894;23:9-13.
2. Bates WH: The cure of imperfect sight by treatment without glasses, New York, 1920, Central Fixation Publishing Co.
3. Boerhaave H: Praelectiones publicae de morbis oculorum, thesis, Goettingen, 1746, Gottingae, apud a. von den hoeck.
4. Brookings WC: Vision without glasses, Minneapolis, 1978, Visual Techniques, Inc.
5. Donders FC: On the anomalies of accommodation and refraction of the eye, London, 1864, New Syndenham Society, pp 415-417. (Translated by William Daniel Moore.)
6. Elschnig H: Ueber die Extraktion der durchsichtigen Linse bei hochgradiger Myopie, Arch f Augenheilk 1928; 98:312-321.
7. Faber E: Operative Behandeling von astigmatisme, Nederl Tijdschr v Geneesk 1895;31:495-496.
8. Fukala F: Operative Behandlung der hochstgradigen Myopie durch Aphakie, Archiv Fur Ophthalmologie 1890; 36:230.
9. Gardner M: Fads and fallacies in the name of science, New York, 1957, Dover Publications.
10. Holth S: Neue operative Behandlung der Netzhautablosung und der hochgradigen Myopie (Trepanatio sclerae praeaequatorialis), Ber Deutsch Ophthalmol Ges 1911;37:293.
11. Huxley AL: The art of seeing, New York, 1942, Harper & Brothers Publishers.
12. Inonye T: Ueber die Korrektion von leichter Myopie durch neue Behandlung mit Gummidruckverband, Archiv Fur Ophthalmologie 1922;110:337.
13. Knapp H: Bericht uber ein achtes Hundert Staarextractionen, nebst Bermerkungen, Arch f Augenheilk 1884; 13:150.
14. Lans LJ: Experimentelle Untersuchungen uber Entstehung von Astigmatismus durch nicht-perforirende Corneawunden, Archiv Fur Ophthalmologie 1898;45:117-152.
15. Lucciola J: Traitement chirurgical de l'astigmatisme, Arch d'Ophthalmol 1896;16:630.
16. Schiøtz H: Ein Fall von hochgradigem Hornhautastigmatismus nach Starextraction, Besserung auf operativem Wege, Arch f Augenheilk 1885;15:178-181.
17. Snellen H: Die richtung der Hauptmeridiane des astigmatischen Auges, Archiv Fur Ophthalmologie 1869;15:199-207.
18. v Reuss und Woinow M: Ophthalmometrische Studien, thesis, Wien, 1869, Wilhelm Braumuller.
19. Verzella F: Microsurgery of the lens in high myopia for optical purposes, Cataract 1984;2:28.
20. von Graefe A: Ueber die lineare Extraction des Linsenstaares, Archiv Fur Ophthalmologie 1855;1:219.
21. Weiss L: Ueber den nach dem Weber'schen Hohlschnitt entstehenden Cornealastigmatismus und die Ursache des nach Extractionen entstehenden Astigmatismus uberhaupt, Arch f Augenheilk u Ohrenheilk 1877;6:58.

Development of Radial Keratotomy in Japan, 1939-1960

Koichiro Akiyama

Hirohiko Shibata

Atsushi Kanai

Shuichi Akiyama

Tatsuo Yamaguchi

Akira Nakajima

George O. Waring III

There is no identifiable link between the experience of ophthalmic surgeons with keratotomy in the late eighteenth and early nineteenth centuries and the development of modern keratotomy in Japan in the 1940s and 1950s. Modern surgery for myopia was initiated by the original ideas and experiments of the late Professor Tsutomu Sato of Juntendo University, Tokyo. Dr. Akiyama gives a personal portrait of Sato in the box on pp. 180-182.

DEVELOPMENT OF ANTERIOR-POSTERIOR KERATOTOMY

Professor Sato was an astute clinician who drew lessons from his observations. In fact he observed that spontaneous breaks in Descemet's membrane in keratoconus produced flattening of the cornea as the breaks healed. This provided hints for his idea of posterior corneal incisions.[24] Sato drew further analogies from naturally occurring disease, observing that deep scleritis with scarring in the posterior cornea produced flattening of the cornea with increased hyperopia and that surface corneal ulceration and scarring sometimes gave rise to kerectasis and increased myopia. He observed that the flattening induced by an

BACKGROUND AND ACKNOWLEDGMENTS

This chapter was written by Koichiro Akiyama, M.D., and his colleagues. Dr. Akiyama supervised much of the animal and human surgery done with Professor Tsutomu Sato and therefore has detailed the development of radial keratotomy in Japan from firsthand recollection and experience. Dr. Akiyama died May 22, 1989, after completing this work. I am sorry he did not live to see it in print. He is mourned and missed by friends and colleagues around the world. The original manuscript for this chapter was well over 100 pages. I have revised and condensed it considerably to fit the space available for this book and take responsibility for the final rendering. A. Momose also contributed historical information in his unpublished manuscript, "History of Radial Keratotomy in Japan and Long-Term Results of Prof. Sato's Operation."

Professor Tsutomu Sato—a Personal Portrait

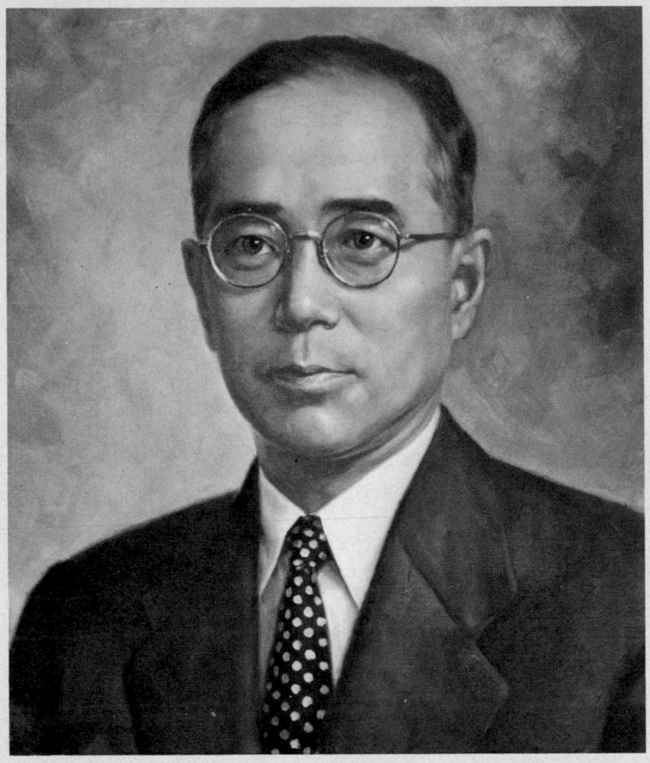

Figure 6-1
Portrait of Professor Tutomu Sato painted by S. Fukuhara in 1960.

Tsutomu Sato was born the third son of Susumu Sato, a surgeon who had studied in Berlin and was the third generation heir to the Sato family, which founded and owned Juntendo University Hospital in Tokyo. This is one of the oldest occidental-style hospitals in Japan, having assimilated Dutch and German medicine. Sato's two elder brothers were professors of internal medicine at the university.

Sato (Fig. 6-1) graduated from Tohoku University and joined the ophthalmologic staff of Tokyo University in 1932, where his academic advisor, Professor S. Ishihara, who invented the test charts for colour blindness, got him interested in the study of ocular refractions. At that time Professor Sato didn't know that his future as a scientist would be devoted to the study of the surgical treatment of myopia and astigmatism. He did, however, marry Professor Ishihara's daughter and rose quickly to the rank of full professor. The years 1933 to 1936 marked the turning point in Professor Sato's life. It was during this period that he got the idea of making posterior corneal incisions for the treatment of keratoconus.

Strangely and ironically it was World War II with its devastation that provided an opportunity for one of God's gifts of healing to be given to mankind—a cure for myopia. Professor Sato was a patriot and a believer in Shintoism. He was seriously concerned about the well-being of his nation and wanted to offer his knowledge and skill for her service. He felt the urgent need to eradicate myopia so that Japan's military power would be strengthened. His ardent desire to control myopia even made him lift his self-imposed ban on writing a book during his lifetime (he had always thought himself unworthy of writing one). The book, *The Cause and Prevention of Myopia*, was written in simple words for the general public.[23] In this book

Professor Sato emphasized that hundreds of young Japanese soldiers who had myopia could not become fighter pilots and good marksmen. The greater the number of soldiers with myopia, the weaker the military power of the nation.

Sato also pointed out that heredity was not the primary cause of myopia in most cases and that it was actually the environment, including the use of "kenji"—Chinese characters—in the Japanese language. He was so convinced of this that he invented his own Romanized style of writing Japanese and strongly recommended its public acceptance, an almost sacrilegious act in Japan at that time. Now this must have been very shocking to most Japanese people, giving the impression that he was a raving mad scientist. Yet this story reveals how much Professor Sato loved his country. Indeed the patriotism in Professor Sato was the major motivation, incentive, and source of energy for his work from 1940 to 1955.

I can remember the time when the members of Professor Sato's research team gathered on the second floor of our friend's house near Juntendo University, where medical facilities had been partially destroyed by bombings, to listen to the news of Japan's defeat and the Potsdam Declaration over the radio. Wiping away his tears, Professor Sato walked out into a burnt field in front of the shops. Facing the Imperial Palace he bowed deeply and shouted, "Long live the emperor." Then he turned to us and said, "Let us now gather our spirits and strength and work for the rebuilding of our country." He devoted all his energy to the attainment of this goal. In the misery of postwar Japan, Professor Sato was truly a distinguished leader.

Professor Sato was in every way a classic example of a Japanese medical professor, balancing his insatiable desire to pursue new developments in every field of knowledge with his belief in Shintoism and his deep understanding and love of traditional Japanese esthetics.

His house reflected his life-style. A large house by Japanese standards, it was divided equally into two portions that were almost identical; one portion was his residence where he ate and slept and the other portion was his study where he spent most of his time when not at the university. Members of his staff often had to stay overnight at his house and would often sleep in the same room. Many noted that before going to sleep, Professor Sato would extract one volume from a huge set of encyclopedias on the shelf and start reading it. We were astounded to find that the professor knew everything in the books from A to Z because he had memorized them. He literally slept with the encyclopedia!

He received an infinite amount of love and support from his wife and family—but in the Japanese style. His wife was always with him in his study. She sat not too far behind him, usually knitting or doing some other quiet activity. Her presence was demanded; she was not to be heard; she spoke only when spoken to. This may sound harsh to occidental ears, but in terms of the Japanese customs and culture of the time, their relationship mirrored that intangible bond of personal love and devotion. This was expressed clearly in the very words of Mrs. Sato on the day after her husband's death, "In my silence I was with him all the time."

Bonsai and horticulture were Professor Sato's hobbies. He personally attended his large garden where he cared for plants of the four seasons. He was fond of discussing his hobby with colleagues around the world.

Professor Sato won the love and admiration of his disciples at Juntendo University. He instructed and directed his staff like a good father, but was also a man of immediate action. His instructions were to be carried out instantly. A split second delay would ensure a loud barking from his lips. When it came to tutoring, however, he was a gentle and patient teacher. He taught his disciples the meaning of dedication and showed them what medical research should really be.

The staff at the University called him "our old man, our daddy" and indeed sometimes treated him like a family member, as one spine-chilling story illustrates. Rabbits were used for animal experiments, but the experiments were to be done in the rooms with the rabbit pens, since animals were banned from the medical staff building. Nevertheless, the staff often smuggled rabbits in and out of the building past the security guard so that they could work in better quarters. With the rabbit

Continued.

Professor Tsutomu Sato—a Personal Portrait—cont'd

wrapped in a blanket, a staff member would sweat and pray past the guard, hoping the rabbit would not become wild and start shrieking. Injecting anesthetics intravenously in the rabbits' ears killed some of them and the problem of how to dispose of the dead rabbits was a challenge. One staff member had a brilliant idea—why not eat them? Food was scarce. No one was sure it was safe to eat the meat because of the overdose of anesthetics. Who would try first? The staff reached a silent accord and that evening presented Professor Sato with finely prepared rabbit meat that he ate with sukiyaki. Sato's workers all spent a sleepless night and were at the university earlier than usual the next morning, silent in their anxiety. Much to their genuine relief, Professor Sato strolled into the room with a bright smile and said, "Thank you for that wonderful meat. It was just delicious." We were blessed with the assurance of a continual supply of meat in the future.

Professor Sato was not immune to the anxieties that affect all lecturers, as apparent from a notation in his diary on June 21, 1954, concerning a lecture at the Ophthalmological Conference of Vienna.

Prof. Linder, who was famous for his surgery of retinal detachment and had written outstanding textbooks on ophthalmology, came to pick me up at the airport. I had imagined Dr. Linder to be a person of grand and dignified stature, but was happy and relieved to find that he was small and not the least overpowering. He was such an amiable person. At 9:30 AM I was suddenly asked to take the morning lecture all alone because Professor Paufique of Leone was absent. This was impossible! I cannot even control the speed of delivery of my talks in Japanese, not to mention German. I decided to speak as clearly and slowly as possible to stretch it out and finally finished my lecture. When I walked out of the conference hall with the feeling of doom, Professor Lohlein, a reputed stern critic among academic circles, approached me and said, "Very good talk. I could understand you very well."

Professor Sato was a sensitive man, as shown in his diary entry the next day.

I had noticed a slight shadow of sadness when I first met Professor Linder. As our conversation became more intimate, he confirmed that my impressions were correct. He told me that he had lost two of his three sons in the war and that communication was bleak and difficult between Vienna and his wife's home in Moscow.

During his clinical and research career two main factors supported Professor Sato. The first was the philosophy of Juntendo University, which always fostered a liberal spirit of research, encouraging the development of new methods and new ideas. The second factor was his many talented, devoted collaborators and assistants. Their work in the laboratory and the clinic culminated in reports on surgery for myopia and astigmatism in the Japanese, American, and German literature in the 1950s.

After Professor Sato died from a myocardial infarction on June 9, 1960, at 58 years of age, his corneas were transplanted into two male patients by Drs. A. Nakajima and Y. Kogure. Through these corneas he is still living with us today.

injury to Descemet's membrane, such as birth injury or hydrops in keratoconus, was greater than that induced by an injury to Bowman's layer, suggesting that surgery on the posterior cornea would be more effective than surgery on the anterior cornea.

The first clue came in 1933 when Sato was examining a female patient with keratoconus who had suddenly lost her vision on awaking from an afternoon nap. She had dense central corneal edema and a rupture of Descemet's membrane. Knowing little about these cases at the time, Sato administered no treatment, and to his surprise the cornea cleared during the next 3 months and returned almost to its normal shape, the patient's vision returning to 20/25.

This observation was reinforced 3 years later on August 24, 1936, by a 20-year-old patient with keratoconus who had come from the United States for treatment of acute hydrops in the right eye. As the involved eye healed, vision improved and the shape of the cornea became more normal; in contrast, progressive keratoconus without breaks in Descemet's membrane developed in the left eye.

Altogether, Sato studied 22 cases of hydrops in keratoconus and deduced that it must be technically possible to treat keratoconus by making an artificial rupture of the endothelium and Descemet's membrane from the posterior corneal surface. He modified a de Lapersonne's knife, designing an angled, sharp tip that could be introduced into the anterior chamber through the limbus; the knife came to be known as "Sato's knife." He did posterior keratotomy in 10 eyes of eight keratoconus patients, reporting his observations in his first paper on kera-

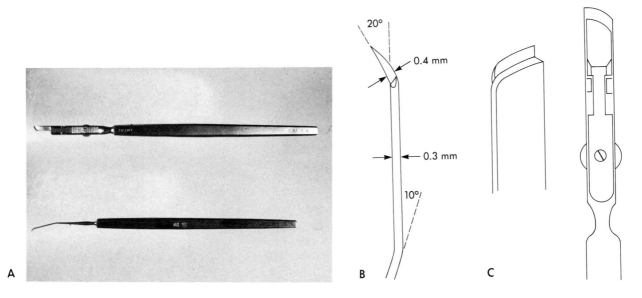

Figure 6-2
The knives used for anterior and posterior half-corneal incisions. **A,** Okamura's trachoma knife used for anterior keratotomy *(above)* and Sato's corneal knife used for posterior keratotomy *(below)*. **B,** Sato's corneal knife underwent numerous design changes, generally aimed at making it finer and refining the angle of the blade and handle. The length of the blade was 2.5 mm. **C,** Okamura's trachoma knife, originally designed for scraping the superior tarsus, was redesigned with a thinner blade and a guard to limit the depth of the anterior corneal incisions. The length of the blade could be adjusted by turning the round screw. (**A** courtesy of Minoru Tanaka, M.D.; **B** and **C** from Sato T, Akiyama K, and Shibata H: Am J Ophthalmol 1953;36:823.)

totomy in 1939.[19] He embodied this event in the aphorism, "The discovery and development of new techniques begin with the close observation of the patient's illness."

In the 1930s there were no effective treatments for keratoconus. Chemical and thermal cautery of the cone, lensectomy, creation of an ectopic or slit-shaped pupil, lowering intraocular pressure by paracentesis or cyclodialysis, and excision of the apex of the cone had all been tried. By contrast a posterior keratotomy seemed simple and effective, and Professor Sato operated on some 200 keratoconus cases between 1938 and 1943.

Under the instructions and exacting demands of Professor Sato, Mr. S. Umeda employed his ingenuity and dexterity to refine the special corneal knife, which was given the honorable name "Japan" (Fig. 6-2). This new knife, made of high-quality steel, cut Descemet's membrane "very smoothly and effortlessly"; the feel of it was a pleasure. Without it Sato could not have achieved what he did. Since numerous other clinics in Japan adopted Sato's method, he established a quality control system of the corneal knives under Mutsuo Komori, who issued certificates to those that met the strict requirements.

Every day Sato and his staff performed careful operations on rabbits. The staff members took turns for nightly shifts and worked around the clock. Their efforts were rewarded with great success. And with the accumulation of sufficient data from the animal experiments, as summarized in the following paragraphs, Sato decided to apply his anteroposterior keratotomy technique to humans.

He assigned Hirohiko Shibata, M.D., the task of evaluating the effects of astigmatic surgery and Dr. Akiyama the task of assessing the effects of myopic surgery. Pathologic studies of animal and human corneas were conducted by Mutsuo Komori, M.D.

In 1943 the staff began experimental studies on radial and tangential incisions in rabbits to correct astigmatism. In the late 1940s anterior incisions were added to enhance the effect of the posterior incisions. At the same time Dr. José Barraquer was developing his concepts of lamellar refractive keratoplasty in Bogota, Colombia (see box on p. 186).

Sato pursued methods of treatment beyond keratotomy, including contact lenses. In 1925 Ishiwaru brought glass contact lenses from Germany, and Professor Sato had an interest in them in the 1930s. In 1951 Sato assigned Hisao Magatani, M.D., to study contact lenses and in 1952 founded the Association of Japanese Contact Lens Research (currently the Japan Contact Lens Society) with Professors N. Kunitomo of Nihon University and Mutso Kajiure of Fukushimz University and Y. Mizutani, M.D.

Myopic surgery was performed most frequently in the early 1950s (Fig. 6-3). The surgeons would operate on one patient after another. If the aqueous humor leaked despite the many precautions that were taken, the doctors would immediately stop, operate on the next patient on the neighboring table, and then return to the first patient to complete the operation.

Other surgeons compiled their own series of cases. For example, Professor Ahira Nakijima, an assistant professor under Sato, reported the results of 60 eyes in 40 patients on whom he operated.[16] Few ophthalmologists outside Juntendo tried the procedure. The ophthalmic surgeons at Juntendo University operated on 861 eyes up to 1959.[4]

This decade of creative work produced numerous publications,* two of which stand out as important summaries of Professor Sato's work. One, published in the *American Journal of Ophthalmology* in 1953,[29] described Sato's experience with anterior and posterior half incisions in 32 eyes, with the conclusion that "this new surgical approach is a proven, safe method which definitely cures or

*References 1-4, 10-13, 16, 17, 19-22, 24-27, 29-32.

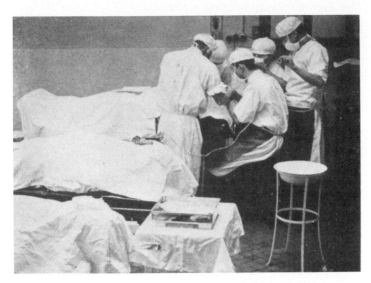

Figure 6-3
Professor Sato standing at the back, watching Professor Nakajima and his three assistants performing radial keratotomy. The two patients in the forefront had been treated with surgical antiseptics, covered with drapes, and were awaiting their turn.

adequately alleviates over 95% of all cases of myopia in Japan. Emmetropia is a professional necessity for many myopes, and this may be accomplished by the method described." This claim was eventually disproved. The second paper published in *Klinische Monatsblater für Augenheilkunde* in 1955[28] detailed seven different operations for astigmatism.

In the mid-1950s Sato visited Asia, Europe, and the United States, attending congresses and giving lectures. Despite Sato's numerous lectures, surgical demonstrations, and publications on the subject, the response of the ophthalmic community to his keratotomy surgery was one of general disinterest. Sato never manufactured his high-quality corneal knife for export even though he observed that the similarly designed knives in Germany and the United States were of poor quality.

The increasing popularity of contact lenses around the world in the 1950s shifted the emphasis of treatment of myopia and astigmatism from surgical correction to optical correction. In addition, Sato began to sense that the corneal endothelium was important. Corneal transplantation was becoming popular worldwide, and it was becoming apparent that the endothelium played an important role in the survival of a corneal graft. Throughout his life Sato had focused his interest on Descemet's membrane as important in keratotomy and gave the endothelium little thought in relationship to keratotomy. He died unaware of the long-range complications of corneal edema.

Interestingly Svyataslav Fyodorov from the Soviet Union visited Japan shortly after Professor Sato's death in 1960. The two men had never met. Fyodorov lectured on radial keratotomy and exchanged information with Akiyama, returning to the Soviet Union to perform Sato's operation on a few clients, but he had poor results.

As far as we know, the only person who opposed Professor Sato's surgical treatment of myopia and astigmatism was Professor Jin Otsuka of the Tokyo Medical and Dental University. Professor Otsuka had been skeptical and predicted that the operation would produce irregular astigmatism and glare but did not anticipate corneal edema.

In 1965, 5 years after Professor Sato's death, Jiro Inoue, M.D., of Tokyo University reported bullous keratopathy that developed in a patient 12 years after the Sato procedure for myopia was performed on him. Of course no one at the time the procedures were being performed could have possibly foreseen the development of bullous keratopathy from endothelial damage, since no one at that time knew the function of the endothelium in preserving corneal clarity.

Lamellar Refractive Keratoplasty of José Barraquer

It is an interesting historical parallel that while Sato was refining the different patterns of keratotomy during the 1940s, José Barraquer, working in Bogota, Colombia, began developing lamellar refractive keratoplasty. His experience with persistent ametropia after penetrating keratoplasty led him to use oversized donor corneal buttons to make the cornea steeper, which decreased hyperopia in aphakic eyes, and to use smaller donor buttons to flatten the cornea, which decreased coexisting myopia.

His real interest in refractive keratoplasty started in 1949 when he proposed autokeratoplasty for the modification of naturally occurring ametropia. The first operation he suggested on humans to treat myopia was the excision of a 3 mm wide ring of cornea—an approach that had been tried by Sato (see Fig. 6-19). Barraquer went one step further than Sato; he did a central lamellar dissection, removing the remaining central anterior half of the cornea, performing a paracentesis to deflate the anterior chamber, and resuturing the smaller central corneal disc into the original bed. This flattened the cornea and decreased myopia (Fig. 6-4).[5,6]

Barraquer established the entire field of lamellar refractive keratoplasty including keratomileusis, keratophakia, and intracorneal lenses.[7,8]

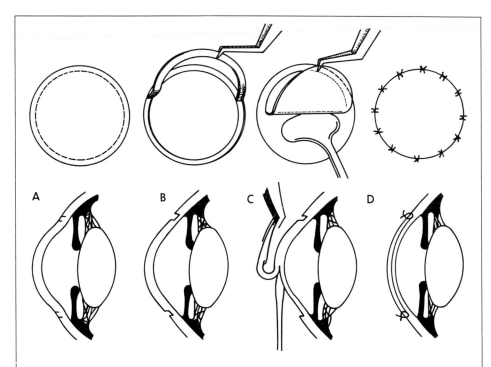

Figure 6-4
Early lamellar refractive keratoplasty technique of José Barraquer. **A,** Parallel 10 and 11 mm partial-thickness trephine incisions. **B,** Excision of a lamellar circular strip of cornea. **C,** Lamellar dissection of the remaining central cornea. **D,** Resuturing of the corneal disc to flatten cornea and reduce myopia. (From Barraquer JI: Queratoplastia refractiva, vol 1, Bogota, Colombia, 1970, Instituto Barraquer de America.)

As the number of cases of corneal edema increased, every member of Professor Sato's research team expressed sincere regret at having made these patients suffer such a fate. Their intentions had been good and noble. None of the disciples of Professor Sato took over his study of the surgical treatment of myopia and astigmatism, in part because of the advent of contact lenses, in part because of the appearance of the delayed corneal edema, and in part because of the memory of the war and the excessive and oppressive spirit of nationalism that drove Professor Sato in his work. All the members of Sato's staff and research team expressed the sincere desire to practice the healing profession of ophthalmology for the health and love of all people and to promote peace on this small planet.

The shock caused by consequences of Professor Sato's operation lingered for decades in the Japanese ophthalmologic profession and fueled the controversy about anterior radial keratotomy when it reemerged in the early 1980s. Akira Momose started anterior radial keratotomy in Japan in 1981 against considerable opposition. By 1986 approximately 10 ophthalmologists were performing keratotomy in Japan. Momose has observed[15] that radial keratotomy has been approved for payment under the government health insurance system in Japan since Sato's days. The surgical fee is currently fixed at approximately 5900 yen ($50 U.S.), which creates a strong financial disincentive for Japanese ophthalmic surgeons to perform radial keratotomy.

ANTERIOR AND POSTERIOR KERATOTOMY IN RABBITS

The vigor with which Sato attacked the problems of refractive surgery was typified in the laboratory experiments in rabbits that were carried out between 1940 and 1950. The variety of incision patterns, the careful attempts at measuring refraction in rabbits, and the duration of follow-up are all testimony to the care taken in exploring this new type of surgery and attempting to establish principles and techniques that could be applied to humans.

We report here the experiments exactly as they were carried out, without regard to the validity of the technical details. Some of the underlying concepts in these experiments were not well grounded, particularly the use of posterior incisions through the endothelium. Nevertheless, the experiments established principles of keratotomy surgery that remain valid today. Sato's contributions are listed in the box on p. 218.

General laboratory methods

The keratotomy operations were performed on one eye of each rabbit under topical anesthesia with loupe magnification. General anesthesia was reserved for those rabbits requiring more difficult surgical techniques. The eye that was not operated on served as a control.

The following three methods were used to mark the location of the incisions:

1. Pieces of gray human hair were placed on the cornea along the line that the incision was to be made (Fig. 6-5).
2. Sutures were placed at the limbus to mark the direction of the incisions.
3. Black dye was dotted onto the surface of the cornea to indicate the pattern of the incisions.

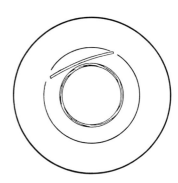

Figure 6-5
Sato preferred to mark the 6-mm central clear zone and the location of tangential incisions for astigmatism with gray human hairs because they kept their shape during the operation and were easily visible against the dark iris or pupil. One presumes they were also available at a moment's notice. (Sato T: Am J Ophthalmol 1953;36:463.)

Incisions into the posterior cornea were made with Sato's knife (Fig. 6-2). During the operation it was not possible to visually confirm the depth of the incision, but experience enabled the surgeon to know and feel how deeply the cut was made. Anterior corneal incisions were made with a guarded Okamura knife (Fig. 6-2), generally set at 0.6 mm.

The quality of the knives varied greatly, the blades being made of carbon steel and having been used many different times. A fresh sharp blade would cut quickly and deeply into the posterior cornea, producing a smooth incision, but a dull blade would tear Descemet's membrane and rip it loose from the posterior surface, sometimes in small pieces and sometimes in sheets. Dull knives cut shallow incisions, whereas an especially sharp knife might perforate the cornea. In general, the sharper the knife, the smoother and deeper the cut and the greater the effect.

Retinoscopy of the rabbit eye to detect the induced refractive change was extremely difficult, and all of the workers were aware of the inaccuracy inherent in this method. Cases in which measurements were impossible to make were omitted. In general the magnitude of the changes in refraction induced by the surgery were large enough to be easily detected by retinoscopy and were indicative of the efficacy of the operations. In all cases the corneas were also examined by Placido's keratoscope to determine the amount of irregular astigmatism. The observation periods ranged from 28 to 436 days.

The results of each pattern are summarized in a series of figures that show a drawing of the incisions, a description of the surgical technique, the change in refraction in the 90 degree and 180 degree meridians at the end of follow-up, and the conclusions concerning the technique (Figs. 6-6 to 6-22).

Immediately after the posterior incisions were made, an edematous corneal opacity appeared. It gradually cleared after 2 to 3 weeks, leaving translucent scars. In general, the rabbit corneas healed well and the amount of residual nebular opacity was proportionate to the amount of surgery performed. The simple posterior linear tangential or radial cuts left faint opacities in the cornea visible only with a slit-lamp microscope, but the multiple parallel tangential cuts and the lamellar resections left large dense scars.

The rabbits were usually observed for 3 to 6 months (some up to 1 year) after surgery. In general the effect of the posterior corneal incisions stabilized by a few weeks after surgery and remained more or less stable throughout the follow-up course. In contrast the effect of the anterior incisions gradually diminished over time. The combined anterior and posterior incisions maintained their effect.

Placido's keratoscope images demonstrated in many cases a peripheral irregular astigmatism in the region of the incisions, both posterior and anterior, but in all cases where the central cornea remained uncut there were only regular astigmatisms and smooth surfaces.

This laboratory experience, using 10 or more patterns of corneal incisions on more than 70 rabbit eyes followed for up to 1 year, demonstrated the feasibility of keratotomy to permanently alter the refractive power of the cornea. This effectiveness and the virtual absence of postoperative complications led Sato to deem the surgery acceptable for humans.

Text continued on p. 197.

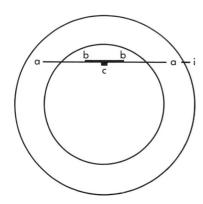

Number of rabbit eyes =   7
Average change at 90° = + 2.29 D
Average change at 180° = − 1.07 D
Average net astigmatism induced =   3.20 D

Figure 6-6
Single tangential posterior half-corneal incision for astigmatism in rabbits. (From Akiyama K: Acta Soc Ophthalmol Jpn 1952;56:1142.)

Surgical Technique
The corneal knife was inserted at point *i* and used to cut the posterior cornea along line *a-a*. Repeated cuts were sometimes made in the same central area along the segment *b-b*. An intentional perforation at the central point *c* was made in some cases.

Conclusion
These incisions produced marked central flattening of the cornea (increase in hyperopia) along the meridian perpendicular to the incision line and slight steepening (increase in myopia) in the corneal meridian parallel to the incision.

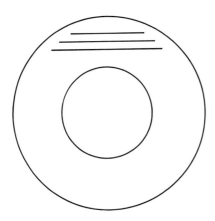

Number of rabbit eyes =   10
Average change at 90° = + 5.38 D
Average change at 180° = − 1.25 D
Average net astigmatism induced =   4.70 D

Figure 6-7
Multiple parallel tangential posterior half-corneal incisions for astigmatism in rabbits. (From Akiyama K: Acta Soc Ophthalmol Jpn 1952;56:1142.)

Surgical Technique
Two to 10 parallel incisions were used to enhance the effect of the single linear incision.

Conclusion
Marked flattening was induced in the meridian perpendicular to the incisions with some steepening in the meridian parallel to the incisions. Too many incisions resulted in a large corneal opacity that could be tinted with dye. The operation could be performed in two or three stages.

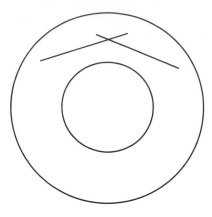

Number of rabbit eyes =   4
Average change at 90° =   + 0.75 D
Average change at 180° =   − 2.00 D
Average net astigmatism induced =   2.70 D

Figure 6-8
Crossed posterior half-corneal incision for astigmatism in rabbits. (From Akiyama K: Acta Soc Ophthalmol Jpn 1952;56:1142.)

Surgical Technique
Two slanting tangential incisions that intersected each other were made. The knife blade sometimes got stuck at the crossing point, making the second incision extremely difficult and sometimes peeling off Descemet's membrane.

Conclusion
The amount of astigmatism change was less than expected, and the surgical technique was too complex to be practical.

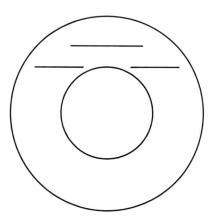

Number of rabbit eyes =   2
Average change at 90° =   + 2.75 D
Average change at 180° =   + 0.25 D
Average net astigmatism induced =   2.50 D

Figure 6-9
Staircase posterior half-tangential corneal incision for astigmatism in rabbits. (From Akiyama K: Acta Soc Ophthalmol Jpn 1952;56:1142.)

Surgical Technique
Three parallel, staggered, nonintersecting linear incisions were made in the posterior cornea.

Conclusion
The amount of astigmatism change was less than expected, and the difficulty in making precise parallel incisions made this an impractical technique.

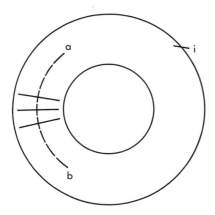

Number of rabbit eyes = 7
Average change at 90° = + 0.93 D
Average change at 180° = + 3.29 D
Average net astigmatism induced = 2.40 D

Figure 6-10
Radial posterior half-corneal incisions for astigmatism in rabbits. (From Akiyama K: Acta Soc Ophthalmol Jpn 1952;56:1142.)

Surgical Technique
Sato's corneal knife was inserted in the limbus at *i* and passed across the anterior chamber. Six incisions were made within 90 degrees of each other (from *a* to *b*), cutting from the limbus to the pupillary margin. The radial incisions were easier to make than the tangential incisions.

Conclusion
The cornea flattened (increase in hyperopia) parallel to the meridians of the incision lines. Slight flattening (increase in hyperopia) was also produced along the meridian at right angles to the incision lines. Therefore this method was considered for the correction of human compound myopic astigmatism.

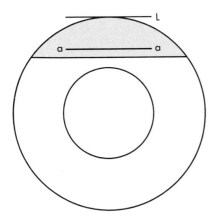

Number of rabbit eyes = 8
Average change at 90° = + 4.81 D
Average change at 180° = − 0.81 D
Average net astigmatism induced = 4.50 D

Figure 6-11
Lamellar dissection combined with tangential posterior half-corneal incision for astigmatism in rabbits. (From Akiyama K: Acta Soc Ophthalmol Jpn 1952; 56:1142.)

Surgical Technique
This operation was designed to simulate the cases of rupture of Descemet's membrane caused by the use of forceps during birth, a circumstance that produces severe astigmatism. An incision was made at limbus *(L)* and a lamellar dissection made with a spatula into the stroma covering the upper third of the cornea. Using Sato's knife, an incision was made in the posterior half of the cornea entering the anterior chamber *(a-a)*. The aqueous humour leaked out, and the anterior chamber shallowed.

Conclusion
Marked flattening of the cornea was produced along the meridians at right angles to the incision line, and a slight steepening of the cornea was produced in the meridians parallel to the incision line. The operation was more effective than the simple linear posterior half corneal incision.

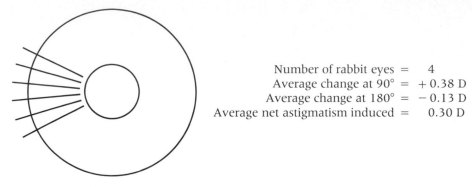

Number of rabbit eyes =   4
Average change at 90° = + 0.38 D
Average change at 180° = − 0.13 D
Average net astigmatism induced =   0.30 D

Figure 6-12
Anterior radial half-corneal incisions for astigmatism in rabbits. (From Akiyama K: Acta Soc Ophthalmol Jpn 1952;56:1142.)

Surgical Technique
The purpose of this technique was to compare the effectiveness of anterior half corneal incisions with the posterior ones. Eight to 12 radial incisions were made with the guarded Okamura knife within a 90-degree section of the cornea, cutting from near the pupillary margin out to the limbus, the opposite direction than that used for the posterior radial incisions.

Conclusion
A smaller amount of astigmatism was induced than with posterior incisions, and the change gradually disappeared over 5 weeks.

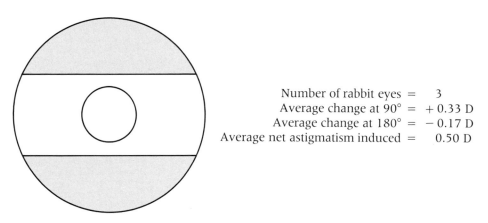

Number of rabbit eyes =   3
Average change at 90° = + 0.33 D
Average change at 180° = − 0.17 D
Average net astigmatism induced =   0.50 D

Figure 6-13
Lamellar anterior corneal resection for astigmatism in rabbits. (From Akiyama K: Acta Soc Ophthalmol Jpn 1952;56:1142.)

Surgical Technique
Because the anterior corneal incisions did not produce satisfactory change in refractive power, the technique of extensive resection of anterior layers of the cornea was tried. A limbal incision was made and a lamellar corneal dissection carried out across the upper third and lower third of the cornea, the anterior flap being resected. The surface was allowed to heal spontaneously or was covered with a conjunctival flap.

Conclusion
A high amount of astigmatism was temporarily introduced, but almost all of it disappeared by 1 month.

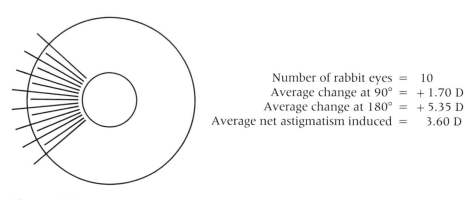

Number of rabbit eyes =   10
Average change at 90° = + 1.70 D
Average change at 180° = + 5.35 D
Average net astigmatism induced =   3.60 D

Figure 6-14
Radial anterior and posterior half-corneal incisions for astigmatism in rabbits.
(From Akiyama K: Acta Soc Ophthalmol Jpn 1952;56:1142.)

Surgical Technique
This was a combination of the techniques depicted in Figs. 6-10 and 6-12, using three to eight radial posterior indicisions followed by five to fifteen radial anterior incisions.

Conclusion
Marked flattening was produced in the meridian parallel to the incision line, the amount being greater than that produced by posterior half-corneal incisions alone. A slight flattening of the cornea occurred along the meridian at right angles to the incision line.

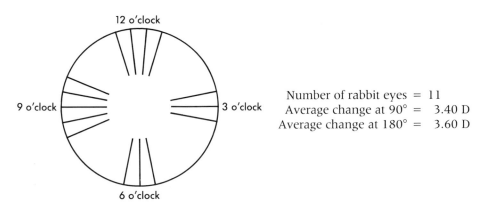

Number of rabbit eyes = 11
Average change at 90° = 3.40 D
Average change at 180° = 3.60 D

Figure 6-15
Radial posterior half-corneal incisions for myopia in rabbits. (From Akiyama K: Acta Soc Ophthalmol Jpn 1952;56:1142.)

Surgical Technique
The Sato knife was inserted through the limbus, extended across the anterior chamber, and five to seven radial incisions were made from the limbus to the 5-mm circular central zone outlined by the gray hair. This procedure was repeated in each of four quadrants for a total of 32 to 55 incisions.

Conclusion
The cornea flattened in all meridians.

第8圖　放射線狀角膜表面切開，（鞏膜切らず，）

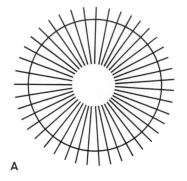

Anterior Corneal Incision
without Incision in Sclera

Number of rabbit eyes =   5
Average change at 90° = +1.60 D
Average change at 180° = +1.60 D

A

第9圖　放射線狀角膜輪部切開

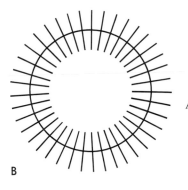

Corneal Limbal Incision

Number of rabbit eyes =   3
Average change at 90° = +1.50 D
Average change at 180° = +1.50 D

B

第10圖　放射線狀角膜鞏膜表面切開

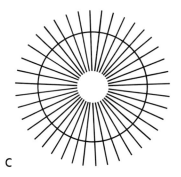

Anterior Corneoscleral Incision

Number of rabbit eyes =   7
Average change at 90° = +1.00 D
Average change at 180° = +1.25 D

C

Figure 6-16
Radial anterior half-corneal incisions for myopia in rabbits. **A,** Without incising sclera. **B,** With incision of limbus. **C,** With incision of sclera. (From Akiyama K: Acta Soc Ophthalmol Jpn 1952;56:1142.)

Surgical Technique
Fifty to 60 anterior radial incisions were made in three patterns: (1) stopping in clear cornea, (2) just across limbus, or (3) into sclera. The surgeon attempted to achieve an adequate depth without perforation.

Conclusion
There was an overall flattening of the cornea with little difference among the three techniques, although incisions far into sclera seemed to decrease the effect. The anterior radial incisions were not as effective as posterior radial incisions.

第13圖　放射線狀角膜表裏兩面切開

短線は後面切開　　長線は表面切開　　第14圖　放射線狀角膜鞏膜表裏兩面切開

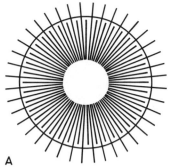
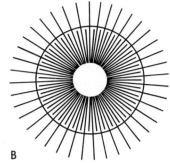

A　B

Number of rabbit eyes = 4
Average change at 90° = 8.50 D
Average change at 180° = 8.00 D

Figure 6-17
Radial anterior and posterior half-corneal incisions for myopia in rabbits. **A,** Anterior incisions extended to the limbus. **B,** Anterior incisions extended into the sclera. (From Akiyama K: Acta Soc Ophthalmol Jpn 1952;56:1142.)

Surgical Technique
The knife was inserted into the limbus, extended across the anterior chamber, and a series of radial incisions were made. Five to ten incisions per quadrant were made for a total of 20 to 40 incisions. Then the anterior radial incisions were made, approximately another 10 per quadrant for a total of 40. The incisions extended into the clear cornea (Fig. 6-17, *A*) or out into the sclera (Fig. 6-17, *B*).

Conclusion
The combined anterior and posterior incisions were more effective than either one alone and were most effective when all the incisions were successfully made. If astigmatism occurred, additional incisions could be made in the steep meridian of astigmatism, either anteriorly or posteriorly.

第3圖．シボリ型角膜後面切開の順序

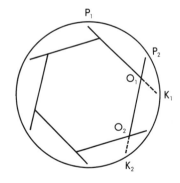

Number of rabbit eyes = 10
Average change at 90° = + 18.00 to − 12.00 D
Average change at 180° = + 6.00 to − 15.00 D

Figure 6-18
Diaphragm posterior corneal incision for hyperopia in rabbits. (From Akiyama K: Acta Soc Ophthalmol Jpn 1952;56:1142.)

Surgical Technique
The knife was inserted at the limbus $(K_1$ and $K_2)$ and extended across a chord length of approximately 60 degrees. The knife was pulled back making a long tangential incision $(P_1$-K_1 and P_2-$K_2)$. This procedure was repeated six to nine times, the incisions overlapping each other $(O_1$ and $O_2)$ and in the end encircling the pupillary zone in the shape resembling the diaphragm of the iris of a camera.

Conclusion
A general steepening of the cornea (myopization) occurred, but the results were variable, with the induction of large amounts of astigmatism in some cases. The technical difficulty of the procedure and the highly variable results made this an undesirable technique.

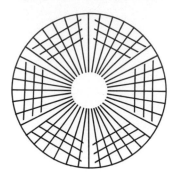

第15圖　龜甲型角膜表面切開

Figure 6-19
Tortoise shell—shaped anterior incisions with radial posterior incisions. (From Akiyama K: Acta Soc Ophthalmol Jpn 1952;56:1142.)

Surgical Technique
Forty radial incisions were made in the posterior cornea, and then groups of three tangential incisions were made in the anterior surface at right angles to the posterior incisions, covering the circumference of the peripheral cornea.

Conclusion
The corneal apex flattened, but a staphyloma developed, increasing the minus power.

Figure 6-20
Circular superficial anterior keratectomy for myopia in rabbits. (From Akiyama K: Acta Soc Ophthalmol Jpn 1952;56:1142.)

Surgical Technique
A 3 mm wide paracentral trephination was made into the stroma, and a circular strip of anterior cornea was excised.

Conclusion
A central protrusion of the cornea resulted, and marked pannus occurred. No refractive results could be obtained.

第 11 圖　角膜表層切除（輪狀）

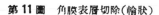
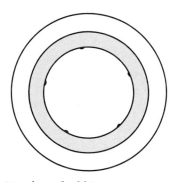

Number of rabbit eyes = 17
Average change at 90° = − 7.3 D
Average change at 180° = − 6.8 D

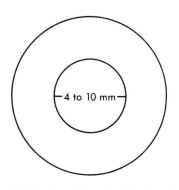

-4 to 10 mm-

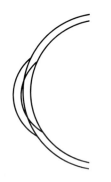

第17圖　角膜管錐術施行後の角膜模型圖

Figure 6-21
Circular full-thickness trephination of cornea in rabbits. (From Akiyama K: Acta Soc Ophthalmol Jpn 1952;56:1142.)

Surgical Technique
A motor-driven trephine with a diameter from 4 to 10 mm was used to make a uniform incision completely through the cornea, the corneal disc being left in its position and the anterior chamber deepening the following day.

Conclusion
The trephined corneal disc bulged forward and increased the minus power of the refraction (increase in myopia), the smaller diameter trephines having the greater effect. This may be effective in the treatment of hypermetropia.

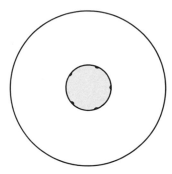

第12圖　角膜表層切除（瞳孔領）

Figure 6-22
Central superficial keratectomy for myopia in rabbits. (From Akiyama K: Acta Soc Ophthalmol Jpn 1952;56:1142.)

Surgical Technique
A central 3- to 4-mm, partial thickness, circular trephine incision was made and a superficial keratotomy performed with a spatula. This was designed to flatten the central cornea.

Conclusion
The procedure was followed by pannus formation, and no refractive results could be obtained.

ANTERIOR AND POSTERIOR KERATOTOMY IN HUMANS

A high prevalence of myopia in Japan was another factor that spurred the development of keratotomy.[9,18] The prevalence of myopia is higher in Japan than in occidental countries. Estimates in 1985 demonstrate that myopia occurs in 21.3% of Japanese and hyperopia in 2.7% of Japanese.[18] Interestingly the major reason given by Sato's patients for having radial keratotomy was "recommendation of physician" (Table 6-1), a reminder of the powerful role a physician can play in the decisions of a patient.

Table 6-1

Subjective Responses of Patients Approximately 20 to 30 Years after Sato's Keratotomy

Reason for having surgery	Number of patients	Satisfaction with result		
		Yes	No	No answer
Occupational	8	4	3	1
Cosmetic	4	1	3	0
Recommendation of physician	28	10	6	12
TOTALS	40	15	12	13

General surgical plan

Surgery was done on an outpatient basis generally under retrobulbar and topical anesthesia with loupe magnification and the previously described knives (Fig. 6-2). The refraction was the basis for surgery, including the refractive measurement of astigmatism.

The central 5 to 6 mm uncut clear zone was outlined with a gray human hair, although alternative materials such as fishing line, rabbit hair, the hair of a horse's tail, and sewing thread were also used. Longer, more complex procedures involved corneal irrigation, which made the surface markers move. Therefore in these cases small dots of dye were placed on the epithelium to guide the surgery. Because the location of the tangential incisions was extremely important for astigmatism correction, a short hair was placed in a linear fashion across the meridian of the steepest astigmatism in the area beneath which the tangential incision was to be made.

One can only marvel at the surgical skill required to use these metal knife blades—without an operating microscope—for making 40 incisions in the pos-

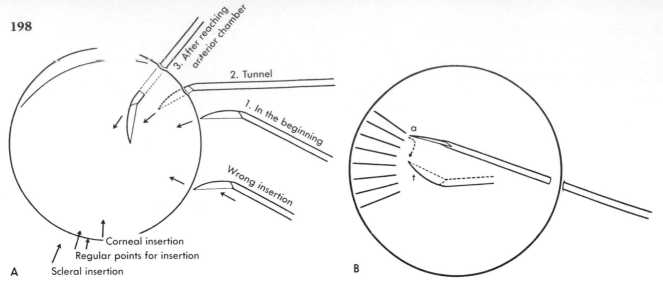

3. After reaching anterior chamber

2. Tunnel

1. In the beginning

Wrong insertion

Corneal insertion

Regular points for insertion

Scleral insertion

A

a

t

B

Figure 6-23

Technique of posterior keratotomy. **A,** With the knife blade parallel to the surface of the iris and perpendicular to the limbus *(1),* the surgeon implanted the tip of the knife blade in the corneal limbus opposite the area to be incised and tunneled it into the stroma for approximately 2 mm *(2).* The shaft of the knife was swung away from the limbus and the point of the blade pushed into the anterior chamber *(3).* The surgeon advanced the knife in a series of short movements across the anterior chamber, without rotating the blade tip toward the lens or toward the cornea, to the opposite limbus. The three possible entries are indicated at the bottom of the drawing. **B,** The blade was stabbed into the posterior cornea, and the surgeon drew the knife blade back toward the entry wound, cutting the posterior cornea to the edge of the overlying 6-mm circled gray hair. The surgeon attempted to cut as deeply as possible into the stroma without perforating the anterior cornea. When the incision was complete, the blade was rotated so that it was parallel to the iris again (as shown with the arrow) and special care was taken to remove the tip from the cornea, so as not to damage the cornea further as the knife was pushed forward again for the next incision. Throughout these maneuvers, the surgeon neither lifted up nor pushed down on the incision wound, so no aqueous humor escaped and the anterior chamber remained deep. The knife was left in the anterior chamber until the completion of all of the incisions in a given quadrant and was then flattened and carefully withdrawn from the anterior chamber without striking the lens. The surgeon then reinserted the knife through the limbus opposite the area where the next series of incisions was to be made; this procedure was followed until all transverse or radial incisions were completed. (From Akiyama K: Acta Soc Ophthalmol Jpn 1955;797-853.)

terior cornea through four different limbal stab wounds without flattening of the anterior chamber and then following these by 40 or more anterior radial incisions, carefully placed between the posterior ones. To fixate the eye, Sato placed a suture beneath the superior and inferior rectus muscle or grasped the anterior bulbar conjunctiva with two pairs of fixation forceps. It was necessary to have good control of the globe and torque it in different directions to gain the right angle for the knife in the anterior chamber.

Sato had no nomograms for calibrating his procedures. He was aware of the following basic principles:

1. The amount of correction is increased by longer incisions. The closer the incision is made to the center of the cornea, the greater is the effect.

2. It is extremely important to cut a very deep incision, and therefore, when indicated, incisions were recut two or three times, sometimes to perforation.

3. In general the more incisions made, the greater the effect, but Sato did not quantify this carefully.

Fig. 6-23 details Sato's technique for posterior incisions.

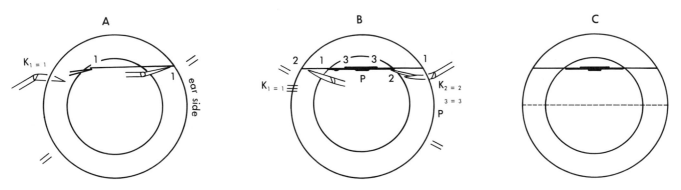

Figure 6-24
Tangential posterior corneal incisions for astigmatism in humans. **A,** Parallel lines at 2 and 8 o'clock positions indicate fixation forceps. A knife was inserted through the temporal limbus, extended across the anterior chamber, and then pulled back creating a 5- to 6-mm incision *(1-1),* approximately 3 mm from the limbus and tangential to the pupil margin. **B,** The knife was withdrawn and reinserted from the temporal corneal limbus to make a second incision *(2-2)* parallel with and intersecting the first. With the knife still held in the anterior chamber, a deepening incision was made *(3-3)* until a central 1- to 2-mm perforation *(P)* occurred. **C,** The completed incision is parallel to the flat meridian of the cornea. (From Akiyama K: Acta Soc Ophthalmol Jpn 1955;797-853.)

Tangential posterior half-corneal incision for astigmatism

The tangential posterior half-corneal incision for astigmatism was indicated for myopic astigmatism with the rule, the steepest axis being at 90 degrees (Fig. 6-24). Care was taken not to cut the pupillary region of the cornea. The operation left a faint linear keratoleukoma that was covered by the upper eyelid. The size of the scar was related to the number of incisions.

In a series of 15 eyes treated with a single tangential incision 5 mm long placed tangent to a 6-mm clear zone, the reduction in astigmatism ranged from none to 4.75 D (mean reduction was 2.50 D). In all cases the meridian perpendicular to the incision became flatter by 1.00 to 4.75 D (mean amount of flattening was −1.90 D). The meridian parallel to the incision behaved more erratically, becoming flatter in four eyes, remaining the same in three eyes, and becoming steeper in eight eyes by 0.25 to 1.75 D. This suggested a "coupling effect" of transverse incisions that flatten the steep meridian and steepen the flat meridian.[27]

Anteroposterior corneal incisions for astigmatism

Anteroposterior corneal incisions for astigmatism are indicated for myopic astigmatism against the rule with the steep meridian at 180 degrees, when incisions must be carried out parallel to the palpebral fissure (Fig. 6-25). In a series of eight eyes with posterior radial incisions alone, the mean reduction of astigmatism was 1.90 D, with a maximum reduction of astigmatism of 4.75 D. In a series of 29 eyes with anterior and posterior incisions, the mean effect was 2.30 D, with a maximum effect of 6.00 D. The resultant keratoleukoma in the palpebral fissure was minimal and resorbed within 1 or 2 months, so it was not noticeable in the light.

A tangential incision for myopic astigmatism against the rule was technically more difficult to perform, and the scar remained visible in the palpebral fissure, scattering light.

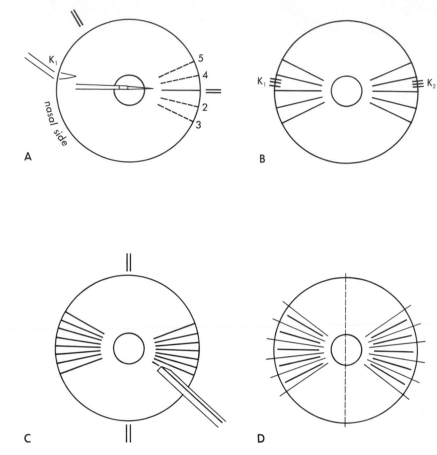

Figure 6-25

Radial anterior and posterior half-corneal incisions for astigmatism in humans.
A, Parallel lines at 11 o'clock and 3 o'clock positions indicate fixation forceps. Sato's corneal knife was inserted at the nasal limbus *(K₁),* extended across the anterior chamber, rotated with the point toward the cornea, and pulled centrally to
make five deep radial incisions extending from the limbus to the 5- to 6-mm clear
zone mark. **B,** The knife was withdrawn, reintroduced at *K₂,* and used to make five
incisions nasally. **C,** The Okamura knife was used to make a series of deep radial
anterior half-corneal incisions between the posterior incisions, both nasally and
temporally. **D,** Completed operation shows the anterior and posterior incisions in
between each other and the orientation of the incisions perpendicular to the steep
axis of the cornea. (From Akiyama K: Acta Soc Ophthalmol Jpn 1955;59:797-
853.)

Comb-type posterior corneal incision for astigmatism

The comb-type posterior corneal incision for astigmatism was indicated in
moderate myopic astigmatism with the rule (Fig. 6-26). Care was taken to ensure that the end point of each line of incision was exactly on, and never beyond, the line of the tangent type incision and that the corneal tissue on the pupillary side of the tangential line was not turned up by the tip of the knife. The
surgeon could reverse the sequence of incisions, performing the tangential incision (without perforation) before the comb.

In 31 cases of astigmatism of this type there was a mean reduction in astigmatism of 2.40 D, with a maximum effect of 4.25 D.

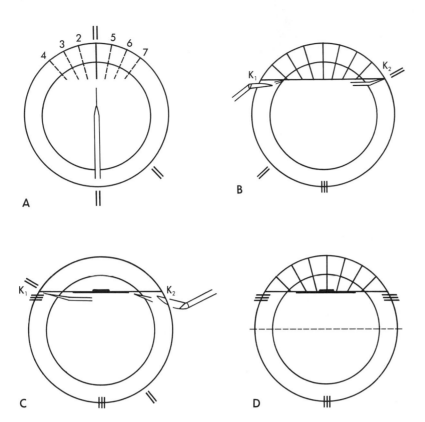

Figure 6-26
Comb-type posterior corneal incisions for astigmatism in humans. **A,** Parallel lines
indicate fixation forceps. Sato's corneal knife was introduced into the anterior
chamber inferiorly and used to make a series of widely spaced, deep posterior corneal incisions across the superior cornea. **B,** The knife was introduced at K_1, extended across the anterior chamber, and used to join the tips of the incisions with a
tangential incision. **C,** The knife was removed and reintroduced at K_2 to make a
second deepening transverse incision that was further deepened centrally to perforation. **D,** The completed comb-type pattern is parallel to the flat axis of the cornea. (From Akiyama K: Acta Soc Ophthalmol Jpn 1955;59:797-853.)

In eyes with a large amount of astigmatism, a comb pattern of posterior incisions made in an aggressive manner could be supplemented with a radial anteroposterior incision in the lower part of the cornea (Fig. 6-27). In a series of 15
cases using this combination, the mean reduction in astigmatism was 4.10 D
with a maximum effect of 8.50 D.

Corneal interlayer separation and posterior tangential incision for high astigmatism

With corneal interlayer separation and posterior tangential incision for high
astigmatism, a limbal-based conjunctival flap was made followed by a lamellar
stab incision approximately 1 mm wide at the limbus. A flat spatula was introduced through the incision, and a lamellar dissection was carried out. Then a
Graefe's knife was introduced into the lamellar dissection to incise the posterior
layers of the cornea into the anterior chamber, making a tangential incision of
approximately 3 mm perpendicular to the 90 degree meridian. The conjunctival
flap was closed over the dissection.

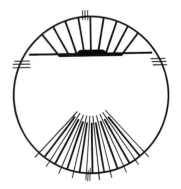

Figure 6-27
Combined comb-type poste-
rior corneal incisions and anteroposterior radial corneal
incisions for astigmatism in
humans. (From Akiyama K:
Acta Soc Ophthalmol Jpn
1955;59:797-853.)

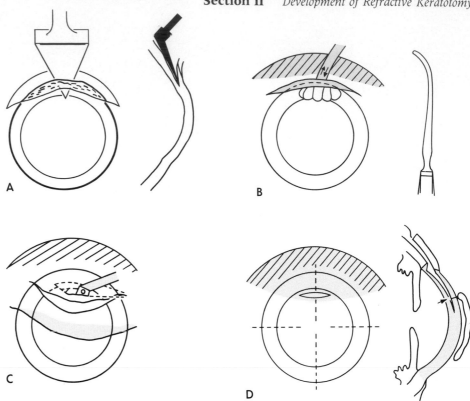

Figure 6-28
Corneal interlayer separation and posterior tangential incision for high astigmatism.
A, After forming a limbal based conjunctival flap, the surgeon inserted a triangular
blade into the superior stroma. **B,** A spatula was used for lamellar dissection about
3 mm in from the limbus. **C,** Graefe's knife was used to make a full-thickness tangential incision in the bed of the lamellar dissection. **D,** Completed operation
shows lamellar dissection and posterior corneal incision *(arrow)*. (From Akiyama K:
Acta Soc Ophthalmol Jpn 1955;59:797-853.)

The operation (Fig. 6-28) was indicated in mixed or hyperopic astigmatism,
since it often resulted in moderate increase in hyperopia in the vertical meridian
passing through the center of the incision and a marked increase in myopia
along the horizontal meridian parallel with the incision. In 18 eyes the average
reduction in astigmatism was 4.20 D, and 10.00 D was the maximum reduction
in astigmatism.

The cornea in the dissected region became transparent; the only visible nebula, if any, appeared along the line of incision made by the linear knife. The operation caused transient pannus formation in some eyes.

Radial posterior incisions for myopia

Sato performed a limited number of radial posterior incisions for myopia,
generally finding this technique ineffective and later combining it with anterior
incisions.

In general the operation involved six groups of approximately five radial posterior incisions (Fig. 6-29). Too deep an incision in the anterior chamber angle
caused bleeding. The cuts were at right angles to the surface of the cornea so
that the incisions were not oblique, minimizing the visible scar. Stabbing the
cornea at a number of sites helped ensure that the incisions were at right angles
to the corneal surface. Entering in only four or five different directions did not
allow for free movement of the knife. After the procedure was completed, the
knife was gently removed from the anterior chamber.

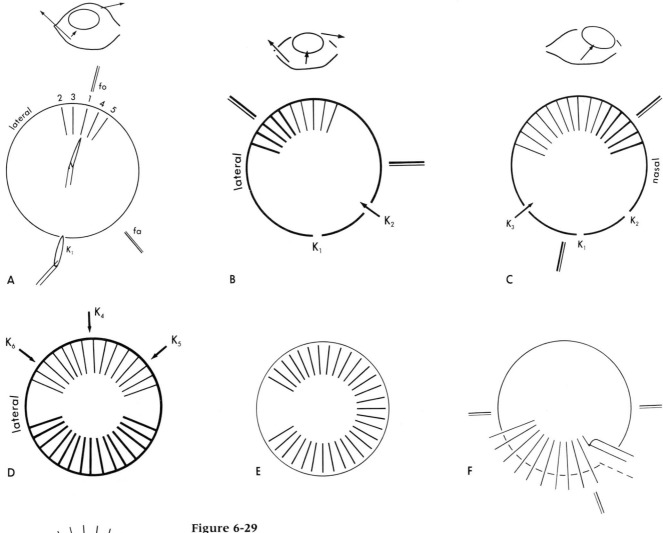

Figure 6-29
Sequence for performing radial anterior and posterior half-corneal incisions for myopia in humans. **A,** Parallel lines at the 12:30 and 4 o'clock positions indicate fixation sites. Pupil was constricted. Sato's corneal knife was inserted at the inferior limbus (K_1) and used to make five radial posterior incisions. **B,** The knife was reinserted at K_2 and used to make five more incisions. **C,** The knife inserted at K_3 made five more incisions. **D,** The inferior array of incisions was made through entry points K_4, K_5, and K_6. **E,** The sequence was completed with the final incisions in the region of the 3 o'clock axis. **F** and **G,** The anterior half-corneal radial incisions were made with the Okamura knife between the posterior incisions, extending 1 to 2 mm in the sclera. (From Akiyama K: Acta Soc Ophthalmol Jpn 1955;59:797-853.)

The limbal wounds of the cornea produced a fall in intraocular pressure. When the knife was removed from the anterior chamber, the assistant pressed the wound of the limbus with a scoop to help prevent the aqueous humor from leaking. With a well-made knife, six perforations of the cornea per operation were by no means difficult to make. If the anterior chamber became more shallow than expected in the course of the operation, it was advisable to postpone the next sequence of maneuvers for 30 minutes to a few hours, during which time the anterior chamber became deep enough for the operation again. One advantage to this operation was that it caused virtually no irritation.

Akiyama[1] studied 35 eyes that had posterior radial corneal incisions for myopia. Preoperative refraction ranged from −1.75 D to −12.00 D, 28 of the eyes ranging from −3.00 D to −9.00 D. The eyes were followed for a mean of 8 weeks (range was 14 to 138 days). There was an average decrease in myopia of 1.25 D (the range was +1.00 D to −4.50 D). Of the eyes, 51% had less than 1.00 D decrease in myopia and 42% had a decrease in myopia of 1.00 D to 2.00 D. The surgeons concluded, "This method of operation is appropriate for people with a light case of myopia, below 2.00 D, who needed to meet their professional qualifications."

Radial anterior and posterior corneal incisions for myopia

A large decrease in myopia could be expected only when the posterior incisions were combined with a series of anterior half corneal incisions (Figs. 6-29 and 6-30).

A

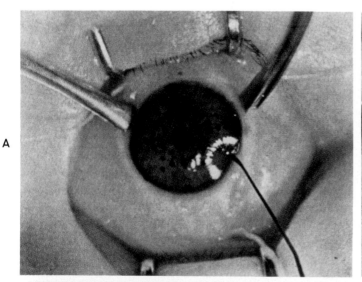
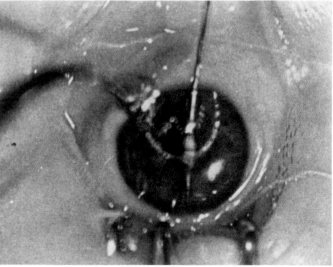

C

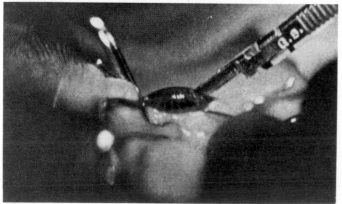

Figure 6-30
Intraoperative photographs of Sato's radial anterior and posterior half-corneal incisions for myopia. **A,** Fixation forceps were applied at 10 o'clock and 2 o'clock positions. Spots of dye on the surface outlined the 5 to 6 mm clear zone and the orientation of the radial quadrants. Sato's corneal knife was inserted at the limbus at 4 o'clock. **B,** Corneal knife inserted in anterior chamber at 12 o'clock position created radial posterior incisions inferiorly. **C,** Lateral view shows Okamura knife making anterior half-corneal radial incisions. (From Akiyama K: Acta Soc Ophthalmol Jpn 1955;59:797-853.)

General surgical technique for combining radial anterior and posterior corneal incisions. Approximately 40 radial incisions were made centrifugally, like the ribs of an umbrella, with a 5 mm pupillary clear region of the cornea. The cornea was cut as forcibly and deeply as possible throughout with the blade pressed heavily. A 1 or 2 mm incision in the extralimbal sclera was also made because no satisfactory effect could be achieved with an anterior half incision if it left the entire sclera intact. Individual incisions measured 4 or 5 mm in length.

For increased effect the anterior half incisions of an anteroposterior operation were extended 4 or 5 mm into the sclera, that is, up to near the equator; this is referred to as an anteroposterior corneoscleral incision (Fig. 6-31). No special pretreatment of the conjunctiva was required for the corneoscleral incision. No separate results of this specific technique were reported.

Preliminary results. Sato's major report of the technique of combining radial anterior and posterior corneal incisions in English was published in the *American Journal of Ophthalmology* in 1953. He reported a series of 32 eyes with preoperative myopia ranging from 2.50 D to 15.00 D (patients' mean myopia was 10.00 D). Patients had anterior and posterior keratotomy, with variations of the technique made according to the amounts of myopia and astigmatism, with a follow-up of 3 to 19 weeks (mean follow-up was 7 weeks). The reduction in myopia ranged from 0.50 D to 7.00 D (mean reduction in myopia was 3.00 D), leaving residual refractions ranging from +1.00 D to −13.00 D.[29]

Final results. A larger series of 177 eyes that received radial anterior and posterior keratotomy by Sato and Akiyama between 1951 and 1953 was carefully analyzed in the Japanese literature in 1955.[3] No systematic preoperative surgical plan was followed, but rather an attempt was made to vary the number of cuts, the depth of cuts, and the length of cuts to achieve the best outcome. The surgeons used approximately 35 posterior (range was 18 to 60) and 35 anterior (the range was 18 to 47) incisions. Incisions were made shallow, medium, or deep into the cornea, but a careful study showed considerable variability in the depth among incisions. The diameter of the central clear zone averaged 6 mm (range was 4 to 8 mm). Incisions were made across the limbus into the sclera in eyes with larger amounts of myopia.

Preoperative refractions ranged from −2.00 to −16.00 D. The patients were followed for a mean of 3 months (range of the follow-ups was 4 to 365 days). Fig. 6-32 shows a scattergram comparing the preoperative refraction with the change in refraction.

The majority of eyes experienced a decrease in myopia from none to 5.00 D (Fig. 6-33). Of the 177 eyes, 74 (42%) had a final refraction between −1.00 and +1.00 D; nine eyes (5%) were overcorrected, and 94 eyes (53%) were undercorrected. An increase in astigmatism of 1.00 D or more occurred in 9% of the eyes; 83 eyes (47%) saw 20/40 or better uncorrected at the time of the last examination. A loss of best corrected visual acuity occurred in nine eyes (5%) 8 weeks or more after surgery.

Factors that affected outcome. Akiyama studied the patient variables that affected outcome and found that age (patients ranged from 17 to 32 years of age), patient sex, and preoperative central keratometry measurements did not affect outcome and that there was no difference in the right and left eyes in terms of outcome. In studying the effect of surgical variables on the outcome, Akiyama found that more than 35 posterior incisions and more than 40 anterior incisions gave an increased effect of approximately 1.00 D when compared with the effect of fewer than this number of incisions. Deeper posterior incisions increased the effect of the surgery, but this was not true of anterior incisions in which no relationship between the depth of the anterior incision and the change in refraction appeared. The diameter of the central clear zone ranged from 4 to 8 mm

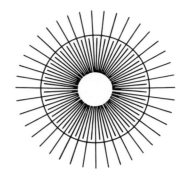

第14圖　放射線狀角膜鞏膜表裏兩面切開

Figure 6-31
Anterior half incisions extended 4 to 5 mm into the sclera, called anteroposterior, corneoscleral incisions. (From Akiyama K: Acta Soc Ophthalmol Jpn 1955;59:797-853.)

Subjective measurement: the relationship of preoperative myopia, postoperative induced refraction, and the number of cases

Preoperative myopia (D) \ Induced refraction (D)	0	0.5	1.0	1.5	2.0	2.5	3.0	3.5	4.0	4.5	5.0	5.5	6.0	6.5	7.0	7.5	8.0	8.5	9.0	9.5	10.0	10.5	11.0	11.5	12.0	12.5	13.0	13.5	14.0
9.0															1				1										
8.5																													
8.0																							1						1
7.5																									1				1
7.0																													
6.5								8					3	2	5														
6.0																													
5.5											3	1	2						1				1						
5.0												1		1			1				1								1
4.5								2	6		1	2	2																
4.0					1		5	2	1		3	2	3	2	2				1		1								
3.5				3	5	7	1		2		2		2	1															
3.0					1	1	4	1	1		4	1	2	2	2		1				1			1					
2.5			1	1			2					2	1		1														
2.0					5		1		4		5	2			1						1		1						
1.5			1	1		1			1		2						1												
1.0					1				1		3			1	2														
0.5		1							1																				
0	1	1																											
Average change		0.5	0.5	1.1	1.5	2.2	2.3	3.2	2.7	3.5	2.9	2.8	3.9	3.8	4.4		2.8		6.3		3.5		5.8	3.5	7.0				6.1

Figure 6-32   For legend see opposite page.

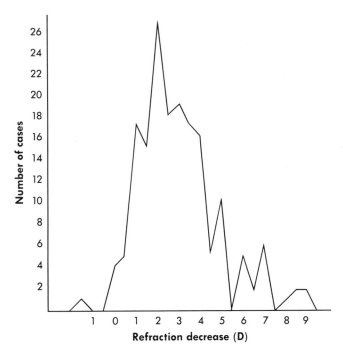

Figure 6-33
Graph indicates the change in refraction, plotting the number of eyes (y-axis) that had a given decrease in refraction (x-axis). The vast majority of eyes had a decrease in refraction between 1.00 D and 4.00 D. (From Akiyama K: Acta Soc Ophthalmol Jpn 1955;59:797-853.)

both anteriorly and posteriorly, and no differences could be found in the effect of larger or smaller clear zone diameters. Incisions across the limbus into the sclera were not associated with a greater effect.

Stability of results and complications. The analysis of stability was not thorough, but the surgeons observed a gradual loss of initial effect over 4 to 8 weeks after surgery and an unstable visual acuity until about 3 months after surgery, after which things were generally stable with "slight fluctuations." Discussion of complications in terms of perforation rate, severity and persistence of glare, postoperative infections, and the like never occurred.

Akiyama concluded optimistically that anterior and posterior keratotomy decreased myopia but called for development of methods that would make it possible to make more incisions more deeply.

Comparison with current findings. Some of Sato and Akiyama's following findings differ from current data.

1. Patient age had no effect. Current data demonstrate that keratotomy has a greater effect in older patients.

Figure 6-32
Scattergram comparing the preoperative amount of myopia on the x-axis with the change in refraction on the y-axis. The diagonal solid line represents eyes in which the outcome was emmetropia. The numbers within the two dotted lines indicate eyes that have a refractive error between ±1.00 D. The average values across the bottom of the x-axis are the average final outcome for each preoperative refractive group. The scattergram shows that approximately half of the eyes were undercorrected by more than 1.00 D and that the remaining half were within approximately 1.00 D of emmetropia. Few eyes were overcorrected. (From Akiyama K: Acta Soc Ophthalmol Jpn 1955;59:797-853.)

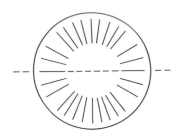

Figure 6-34
Placement of radial half-corneal posterior incisions for compound myopic astigmatism. The incisions in the quadrants along the meridian of steepest corneal curvature were deeper, longer, and more numerous than those in the quadrants along the flatter meridian *(broken line)*. (From Akiyama K: Acta Soc Ophthalmol Jpn 1955;59:797-853.)

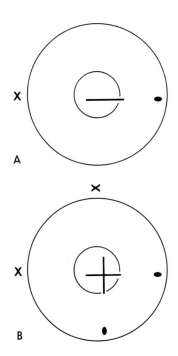

Figure 6-35
Central posterior half-corneal incisions for keratoconus. **A,** Transverse incision made under apex of cone. **B,** Additional crossing incision made in second stage of operation. The *X's* and dots mark the direction of the incision and the point of entry of the knife. (From Sato T: Am J Ophthalmol 1950;33:943-948.)

2. The diameter of the central clear zone had little effect on outcome of keratotomy. Current data indicate that a smaller diameter clear zone has a greater effect. It may be that the clear zones of 6 mm or more diameter were outside the range where differences in the effect of clear zone diameter could be detected.

3. More incisions had a greater effect. Current data indicate that more than eight incisions add little to the effect of the procedure.

Akira Nakajima adopted Sato's surgical techniques and performed anterior and posterior radial keratotomy on 60 eyes over 3 years. The outcome was similar. Although almost all eyes had a reduction in myopia (average effect was 1.25 D), only approximately 50% achieved a refraction of less than −2.00 D with an uncorrected visual acuity of 20/25 or better. He concluded that patients with lower amounts of myopia had a more successful outcome. The major complication he recognized was the induction of mild astigmatism.[16]

Radial incisions for myopic astigmatism

In cases with compound myopic astigmatism, radial incisions were spaced with more incisions clustered in the steeper meridian than in the flatter meridian in the hope of eliminating the astigmatic component (Fig. 6-34). In a series of 25 cases, Sato was able to flatten the steep meridian by an average of 3.90 D (range was 1.50 D to 8.00 D).

Central posterior keratotomy for keratoconus

A transverse posterior incision 3 to 4 mm long was made in the thin apex of the cone to treat keratoconus (Fig. 6-35). If a corneal perforation occurred, the incision was extended quickly to complete it before the anterior chamber shallowed. If a second crossing incision was used, it was done a few days later.

The incision in Descemet's membrane spread open by itself and became spindle shaped within 1 minute. A crosswise incision created a diamond-shaped or kite-shaped rupture of Descemet's membrane. An opacity appeared the day after surgery around the incision, but most of the edema was absorbed in several weeks, leaving only a narrow nebula.

No results for keratoconus were reported.

Clinical course after posterior keratotomy

There was mild pain after posterior keratotomy. Hyperemia subsided in 2 to 6 weeks, depending on the number of incisions in the sclera. Fluorescein staining of the incisions disappeared within 1 week. The corneal edema gradually subsided.

In the early postoperative course there were two different patterns of changes in refraction. A marked increase in hyperopia, which became less prominent over a few weeks, occurred immediately. The hypermetropic effect was modest initially but became more pronounced over a few weeks, presumably because of ciliary spasm. It took at least 2 to 3 months until the refractive power was stabilized, and then the refraction tended to remain stable for at least 1 year.

The largest correction achieved was 20.00 D in the principal meridian, but it gradually fell to 10.50 D in 2 months and remained at that level.

The surgery also increased astigmatism, particularly when the placement of incisions was asymmetric. This occurred most often when a quadrant of posterior incisions could not be completed because the anterior chamber became shallow. This usually occurred superiorly or inferiorly because the vertical radial incisions were more difficult than the horizontal ones.

Once the cornea was healed, residual astigmatism could be reduced by further incisions, especially if the cornea was steepest in the vertical meridian. Sato was an advocate of repeated operations to try to achieve the desired result.

Sato's hypothetical biomechanical explanation of the effect of corneal incisions

Sato's curious mind was not satisfied with simply observing effects of this surgery. He sought to explain them in what today would be called biomechanical terms. In translating his work, we have left the terminology similar to his original language, rather than using more contemporary terms. The hypotheses were spelled out by Akiyama in his doctoral dissertation[15] to explain the mechanism responsible for the dynamic structure of the cornea.

Apart from all external forces or conditions outside the cornea, the shape of the cornea itself is maintained by the presence of omnidirectional forces of tension within the cornea. These omnidirectional forces can be analytically divided into two kinds of perpendicularly opposing tensions—radial and circular (Fig. 6-36). The radial type of posterior corneal incisions removed the circular tension

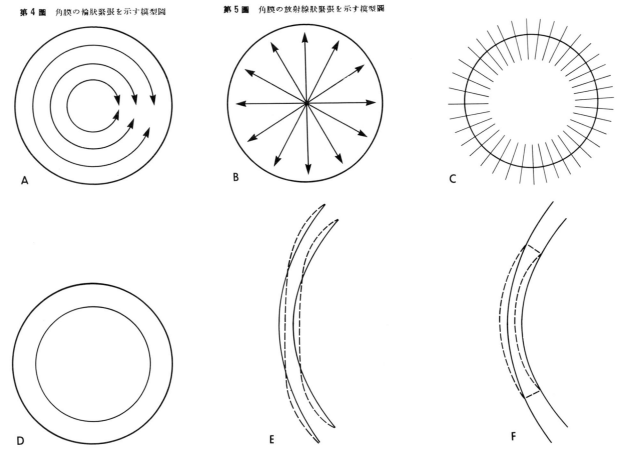

Figure 6-36
Sato's biomechanical concepts of the mechanism of action of corneal incisions. There are two inherent tensions in the cornea, radial **(A)** and circular **(B).** Radial incisions **(C)** interrupt the circular tension but not the radial tension, whereas circular or diaphragm incisions **(D)** interrupt the radial but not the circular tension. Therefore the radial incisions allow an increase in the circumference of the cornea in the area incised, producing an anterior bulging and steepening in the incised area, with a compensatory flattening of the central area **(E)** because the radial tension is still intact. On the other hand, diaphragm or circular incisions allow protrusion of the central cornea because the radial tension has been disrupted, producing a central steepening of the cornea **(F).** (From Akiyama K: Acta Soc Ophthalmol Jpn 1955;59:797-853.)

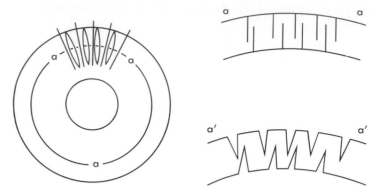

Figure 6-37
Mechanism of action of combined radial anterior and posterior half-corneal incisions. The posterior incisions *(open ellipses)* and anterior incisions *(lines)* release the circular tension and allow the circumference of the cornea *(a-a)* to increase *(a'-a')*. (From Akiyama K: Acta Soc Ophthalmol Jpn 1955;59:797-853.)

(Fig. 6-37); the diaphragm pattern posterior corneal incisions and full-thickness trephine incisions removed the radial tension. The results of laboratory experiments showed that the basic principle for changing the shape of the cornea was to use incisions to reduce the amount of radial or circular tension inherent in the cornea and to control the amount of tension that remains.

There was a striking difference between the shapes of the cornea after radial posterior corneal incisions and diaphragm pattern posterior corneal incisions; the radial incisions increased hyperopia (to treat myopia); the diaphragm incisions increased myopia (to treat hyperopia).

The resultant structural change made the cornea markedly less resistant than before to a tension or bending moment perpendicular to the incision, while keeping the cornea normally resistant to a force parallel with the incision.

In the vicinity of the wounds made by radial incisions, protrusion of the cornea occurred because of the release of the circular tension naturally and inherently present in the corneal fibers but without the release of the forces of radial tension. These facts led us to the assumption that the severing of Descemet's membrane might be of critical importance because it may play a major role in maintaining the necessary amount of tension that enables the cornea to retain its natural shape. The sudden release of tension in and around the incised areas of Descemet's membrane triggered the stretching of the entire incised surface of the cornea in a circumferential direction. This caused the forward protrusion of the incised surface without stretching the cornea in the radial meridians because the corneal fibrils in this direction were not affected. The central pupillary area of the cornea therefore flattened in compensation for the protrusion of the peripheral incised area (Fig. 6-37).

In contrast the circular diaphragm incision released the tension in a radial direction, so the corneal meridians were elongated and a forward protrusion of the cornea inside the area of the wound occurred. The depth of the anterior chamber increased, the radius of the cornea diminished, and the refractive power increased, inducing myopia. The closer the circular diaphragm incision was to the center of the cornea, the more anterior a protrusion was produced, sometimes protruding far enough to resemble keratoconus. These changes in surface shape could be seen macroscopically with a naked eye, particularly when viewed in oblique illumination. They could also be observed using Placido's disk.

For two reasons Sato thought posterior corneal incisions were more effective than anterior ones. The first was that Descemet's membrane was the chief source

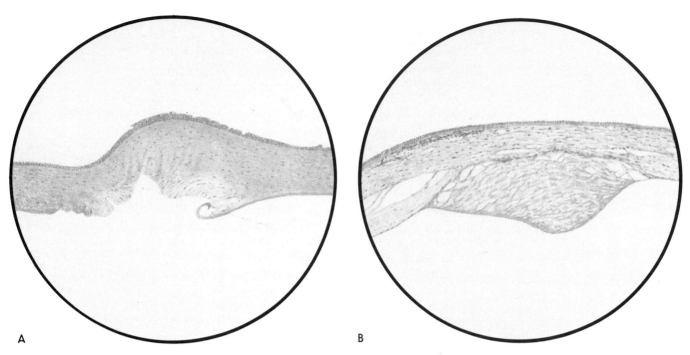

A   B

Figure 6-38
Histologic sections of posterior corneal incisions in rabbits. **A,** Acutely, Descemet's membrane retracted and coiled toward the stroma, and the incised stroma retracted and became edematous. **B,** Twenty days after surgery, the posterior wound was filled with a focal plug of scar tissue that held the wound open and produced the effect of the surgery. (From Akiyama K: Acta Soc Ophthalmol Jpn 1955;59:797-853.)

of the inherent corneal tension necessary to maintain the natural shape of the cornea. The second was the difference in the healing between anterior and posterior layers, the anterior wounds healing quickly but the posterior wounds healing slowly because of the retraction of the severed ends of Descemet's membrane that never healed. Therefore the addition of anterior radial incisions was introduced, with the caution not to cross the incisions because crossed incisions produced more prominent corneal scars.

Moreover, laboratory experiments established that incisions severing almost all the corneal fibrils were the most effective. That is, combined anterior and posterior radial incisions could be extremely effective in reducing myopia, whereas anterior incisions alone were only slightly effective and posterior incisions alone were only moderately effective. In the rabbit studies the radial posterior incisions induced an average of 4.00 D of hyperopia as compared with 8.50 D with anterior incisions plus posterior incisions. Similarly, full-thickness corneal trephination induced more myopia than the partial-thickness diaphragm pattern posterior incisions.

Histologic examination of the posterior corneal incisions helped support these mechanical hypotheses (Fig. 6-38). The thickening of the cornea initially was caused by edema of the stroma and a defect of the endothelium. As healing progressed, scar tissue filled in the wound, separating the cut ends of Descemet's membrane and bulging into the anterior chamber. No white blood cell infiltration occurred unless there was an infection or an anterior iris adhesion; this was probably why no permanent dense leukoma occurred. A separate, newly regenerated Descemet's membrane appeared and covered the retrocorneal connective tissue but did not close the wound enough to return the cornea to its former shape.

Long-term follow-up in humans

The total number of patients who had anterior and posterior radial keratotomy is unknown. Of the 681 eyes that were operated on at Juntendo University, 170 eyes in 103 patients have been followed up to March 1986. No information was available on the other 511 eyes. Of these 103 patients, 99 returned with a history of decreased visual acuity. A questionnaire was answered by 40 of these patients. The most common reason given for having this surgery was recommendation of the physician (see Table 6-1). Surprisingly, approximately one third of these patients expressed satisfaction with the operation despite the appearance of corneal edema.

The visual acuity and refraction could be measured on 59 eyes that had been followed for 10 years or more after surgery; 51 eyes were myopic and eight eyes were hyperopic. The average spherical equivalent was -2.55 D. Eight eyes had a refractive error within 1.00 D of emmetropia, and 34 eyes had a refractive error of -2.00 D or more. The average astigmatism was 1.04 D, 27 eyes showing an astigmatism of 1.00 D or less. The maximum astigmatism was 4.50 D.

Of the 170 eyes that were followed up, 121 (71%) developed bullous keratopathy and 49 eyes (29%) retained clear corneas (Fig. 6-39). Data on the time of onset of bullous keratopathy were available in 92 eyes. These patients received their surgery between 14 years of age and approximately 40 years of age. The average onset of corneal edema was around 43 years of age for the patients younger than 30 years of age. The average time between surgery and the onset of corneal edema was 20 years (range was 15 to 25 years).

Clinically the symptoms of hyperemia, blurred vision, and pain that were usually worse in the morning became more severe and gradually total corneal edema developed. The appearance of the cornea at the slit-lamp microscope was one of diffuse corneal edema with opacities of the posterior corneal surface that had the appearance of a thickened Descemet's membrane protruding into the anterior chamber, particularly in the region of the peripheral incisions. Some areas of scrolled, dislocated, and distorted Descemet's membrane were seen. Epithelial edema varied from diffuse bedewing to large bullae (Figs. 6-40 to 6-42). In patients who had single posterior corneal incisions for astigmatism edema developed in the area of the superior incision, but usually not inferiorly.

Table 6-2 reports the status of 96 eyes as of March 1986—44 of the eyes underwent penetrating keratoplasty, 16 of them successfully, and 27 eyes had an opaque graft, 17 after the first operation, 8 after the second operation, and 2 after the third operation.

Table 6-2

Status of 96 Eyes That Had Anteroposterior Radial Keratotomy Between Approximately 1945 and 1955 as of March 1987

Status of eyes	No. of eyes
Clear corneas	34
Opaque corneas	61
Successful keratoplasty	16
Failed keratoplasty	27
Refused keratoplasty	10
Awaiting keratoplasty	8
No data	1
TOTAL	96

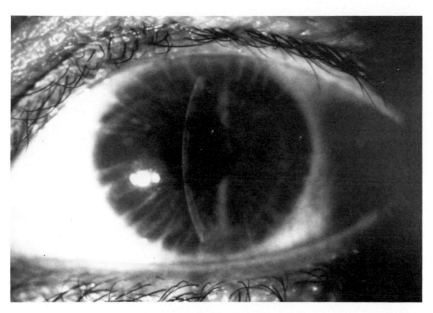

Figure 6-39
Clear central cornea many years after anterior and posterior half-corneal incisions for myopia. Incision scars are visible extending across the limbus. (Courtesy Minoru Tanaka, M.D.)

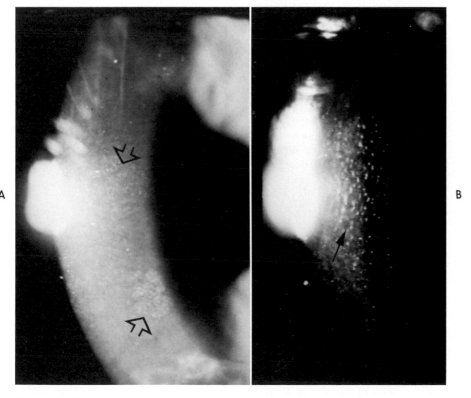

Figure 6-40
Posterior collagenous layer induced by interior half-corneal incisions. **A,** Early appearance of posterior collagenous layer, a gray "thickening" of Descemet's membrane *(arrows).* **B,** Specular reflection reveals cornea guttata in the central cornea *(arrow).* (From Yamaguchi T, Kanai A, Tanaka M, et al: Am J Ophthalmol 1982; 93:602.)

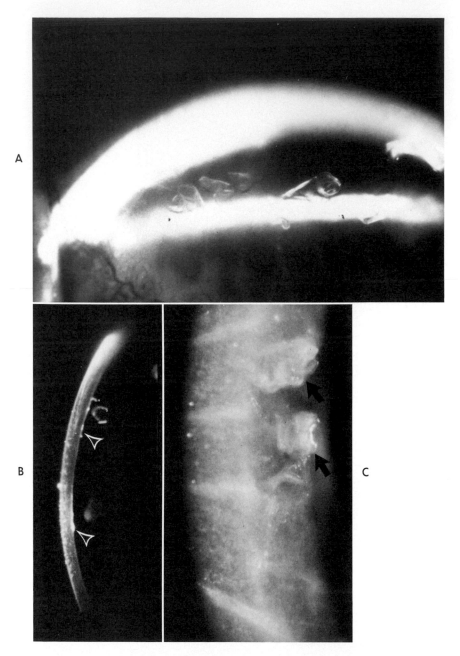

Figure 6-41
Clinical appearance of Descemet's membrane many years after radial posterior half-corneal incisions for myopia. **A,** Wide slit shows scrolls and curls of Descemet's membrane in retroillumination. **B,** Focal thickening and protuberances of Descemet's membrane *(arrows)* show in narrow slit view. **C,** Broad slit beam shows plaques of thickened Descemet's membrane and retrocorneal membrane at end of incisions *(arrows)*. (**A** courtesy Minoru Tanaka, M.D. **B** and **C** from Yamaguchi T, Kanai A, Tanaka M, et al: Am J Ophthalmol 1982;93:602.)

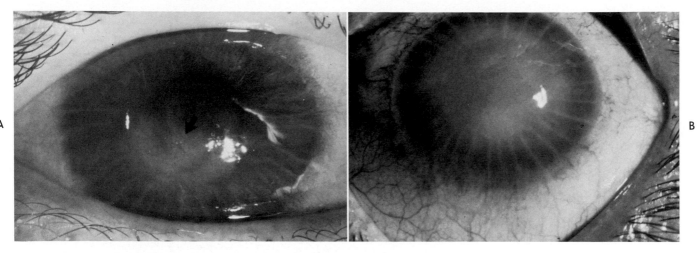

Figure 6-42
Corneal edema after anterior and posterior half-corneal incisions for myopia.
A, Partial edema in lower half of cornea. **B,** Total corneal edema. (**A** from Ya-maguchi T, Kanai A, Tanaka M, et al: Am J Ophthalmol 1982;93:602; **B** courtesy O. Itoi, M.D.)

Momose has studied specular microscopy of the endothelium in 9 eyes of 5 patients examined 10 to 20 years after surgery around the time of the onset of corneal edema.[32] (Momose A. History of radial keratotomy in Japan and long-term results of Prof. Sato's operation. Personal, written communication, September 1987). The endothelial cell density ranged from 600 to 800 cells/mm^2 (normal density is 2500 cells/mm^2) and the percentage of hexagonal cells ranged from 3% to 9% (normal percentage of hexagonal cells is 85%). Clearly the gradual attrition of endothelial cells was the cause for the corneal edema.

The results of penetrating keratoplasty were much worse than that obtained in bullous keratopathy caused by other diseases. This was theoretically attributed to the extensive damage to the host peripheral corneal endothelium, requiring the donor endothelium to attempt to recover the posterior cornea, depleting its reserve to the point of developing edema in the graft.

Histopathologic findings

Corneal buttons were obtained at the time of penetrating keratoplasty and were examined with light and electron microscopy.[12,13,30] There were epithelial edema and subepithelial bullae (Fig. 6-43). The basal epithelial cells extended projections into the subepithelial region. Bowman's layer was often absent and was replaced by electron-dense material. The keratocyte showed highly dense cytoplasm and scattered collagen fibrils around them. Descemet's membrane was generally thickened and was curled near the incision, with folds and extensions protruding into the anterior chamber (Fig. 6-44, *A*). In some areas no endothelial cells were present and secondary cornea guttata appeared (Fig. 6-44, *B*). A posterior collagenous layer was present, containing widely spaced material with a periodicity of 50 and 100 nm. Flat, fibroblast-like endothelial cells containing prominent filaments and few organelles were present on the posterior surface (Fig. 6-45).

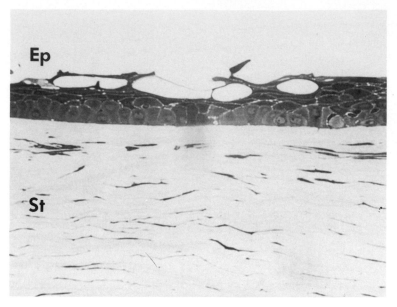

Figure 6-43
Light micrograph of anterior cornea after anterior-posterior half-corneal incisions for myopia demonstrates epithelial bullae *(Ep)*. Bowman's layer is replaced by acellular connective tissue. Stroma *(St)* is hypercellular and edematous (Yamaguchi blue, ×150). (From Yamaguchi T, Kanai A, Tanaka M, et al: Am J Ophthalmol 1982;93:604.)

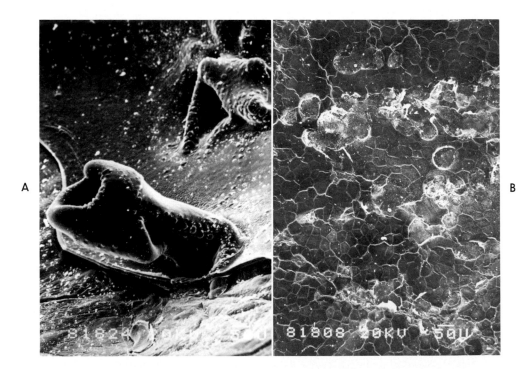

Figure 6-44
A, Scanning electron micrograph of a cornea after posterior keratotomy shows region near edge of corneal button removed at penetrating keratoplasty. Areas of elevated and curled Descemet's membrane protrude into the anterior chamber. No endothelial cells are present (×150). **B,** Scanning electron micrograph from the center of a corneal button removed for corneal edema after anteroposterior keratotomy shows irregularity of the size and shape of the endothelial cells, although the monolayer is confluent (×150). (Courtesy Atsushi Kanai, M.D.)

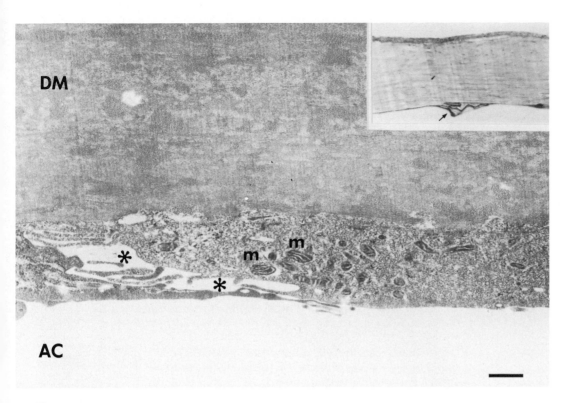

Figure 6-45

Transmission electron micrograph of posterior cornea after Sato's operation for myopia. Inset shows wrinkled, duplicated Descemet's membrane in the area of a posterior radial incision *(arrow)*. Main figure demonstrates thickened Descemet's membrane *(DM)* with the deposit of a posterior collagenous layer consisting of fine collagen fibrils in an amorphous matrix. Flattened fibroblastic endothelial cells contain few organelles but prominent filaments and many mitochondria *(m)*. The intercellular spaces *(*)* are distended. *AC,* Anterior chamber. (From Yamaguchi T, Kanai A, Tanaka M, et al: Am J Ophthalmol 1982;93:605.)

ANTERIOR AND POSTERIOR KERATOTOMY IN MONKEYS

To study the effects of anterior and posterior keratotomy in a more modern setting, Yamaguchi and colleagues[33] performed anterior and posterior radial keratotomy, as well as modern anterior radial keratotomy on monkeys, and followed them for 1 year. Overall the anterior and posterior keratotomy produced a greater refractive change than the anterior keratotomy alone. Specular microscopy demonstrated that anterior and posterior keratotomy produced 16.4% average central endothelial cell loss, whereas the isolated anterior radial keratotomy produced a 10% cell loss at 1 year after surgery.

Contributions of Prof. T. Sato to Keratotomy Surgery

The laboratory experiments on rabbits and clinical trials in humans by Sato and his team reinforced the findings of Lans and established the following basic principles of modern keratotomy for astigmatic and spherical refractive errors:

1. The effect of the keratotomy increases with greater depth, number, and length of the incisions.
2. Transverse incisions in the cornea flatten the meridian perpendicular to the incision and slightly steepen the meridian parallel to the incision.
3. The effect of transverse incisions decreases with their distance from the center of the cornea.
4. Radial incisions placed in one axis or meridian flatten the meridian parallel to them and slightly flatten the meridian perpendicular to them.
5. Circular incisions steepen the central cornea.
6. Posterior incisions flatten the cornea more than anterior incisions.
7. Biomechanical principles explain that radial and transverse incisions release "circular tension" within the cornea, allowing a gaping of the cornea in the area of the incisions with relative steepening in that area and relative flattening centrally, inducing hyperopia. Circular incisions reduce "radial tension" in the cornea, allowing the central cornea to protrude forward and steepen, inducing myopia.
8. The incisions create irregular astigmatism in the peripheral area where they are made but leave a regular surface in the central uncut zone.
9. Crossed incisions create larger scars and should be avoided.

With hindsight we can see that the following errors were made by Sato and his colleagues:

1. The posterior incisions damaged the corneal endothelium, producing late corneal edema in the human eyes. This was not detected in rabbits because the rabbit endothelium has a regenerative capacity far superior to that of humans and because the follow-up was less than 1 year. At the time of these experiments the biology of the endothelium was unknown.
2. The rabbit is generally considered a poor model for refractive surgery because of the absence of Bowman's layer and the great flexibility of the cornea, and therefore it is remarkable that Sato's team could deduce as much valid information from the rabbit as they did. The direct transfer to man of laboratory information that was gained from the study of rabbits would not be done now.
3. Sato found anterior incisions alone generally ineffective, but they are commonly used today. The clear zone diameter of 5 to 6 mm that was designed to keep the incisions outside the pupil was too large. The Okamura trachoma knife, even as modified by Sato, was probably not sharp enough to cut deeply enough into the cornea to create consistent incisions, especially in a soft eye after six limbal stab wounds.
4. Sato's experimental design in humans was flawed, comprising too few cases followed for too short a time. He fell into the common error of premature enthusiastic promulgation of his surgical techniques. (See Chapter 4, Development and Classification of Refractive Surgical Procedures.)

Thus Sato and his team established the potential benefit of refractive corneal surgery and described the basic keratotomy patterns that were effective. It would remain for Soviet surgeons in the 1970s to modify these principles by reducing the diameter of the clear zone and using variations in surgical technique tailored for the individual eye, innovations that would improve the predictability of outcome.

UNFINISHED BUSINESS

The major unfinished business regarding the contributions of professor Sato and his colleagues is proper acknowledgment. All too much emphasis has been placed on the fact that incisions made in the endothelium produce late corneal edema, eclipsing the enormous breadth of laboratory and clinical information that resulted from these experiments. It is our intention that this chapter partially completes this unfinished business.

REFERENCES

1. Akiyama K: Study of surgical treatment for myopia. I. Posterior corneal incisions, Acta Soc Ophthalmol Jpn 1952; 56:1142-1150 (in Japanese).
2. Akiyama K: Study of surgical treatment for myopia. II. Animal experiment, Acta Soc Ophthalmol Jpn 1955;59:294-312 (in Japanese).
3. Akiyama K: The surgical treatment for myopia. III. Anterior and posterior incision, Acta Soc Ophthalmol Jpn 1955; 59:797-853 (in Japanese).
4. Akiyama K, Tanaka M, Kanai A, and Nakajima A: Problems arising from Sato's radial keratotomy procedure in Japan, CLAO J 1984;10:179-184.
5. Barraquer JI: Queratoplastia refractiva, Est E Infor Oftal 1949;2:10.
6. Barraquer JI: Refractive keratoplastic, preliminary information. In Barraquer JI, editor: Queratoplastia refractiva (Recopilacion de reimpresos), vol 1, Bogota, Colombia, 1970, Instituto Barraquer de America.
7. Barraquer JI: Queratomileusis y queratofaquia, Bogota, Colombia, 1980, Instituto Barraquer de America.
8. Barraquer JI: Keratomileusis for myopia and aphakia, Ophthalmology 1981; 88:701-708.
9. Curtain BJ: The myopias, Philadelphia, 1985, Harper & Row Publishers, Inc.
10. Funahashi M, Yoshida M, Kanai A, Niwa Y, Komatsu S, Itoi M, and Nakajima A: A case of bullous keratopathy after antero-posterior incision of the cornea for myopia, Folia Ophthalmol Jpn 1973;24:19-23 (in Japanese).
11. Inoue J: A case of bullous keratopathy developed 12 years after the operation of myopia, Jpn Rev Clin Ophthalmol 1965;59:38-40 (in Japanese).

12. Kanai A, Tanaka M, Ishii R, and Nakajima A: Bullous keratopathy after anterior-posterior radial keratotomy for myopia and astigmatism, Am J Ophthalmol 1982;93:600-606.
13. Kanai A, Yamaguchi T, Yajima Y, Funahashi M, and Nakajima A: The fine structure of bullous keratopathy after anteroposterior incision of the cornea for myopia, Folia Ophthalmol Jpn 1979;30:841-849 (in Japanese).
14. Momose A: Personal communication, September 1987.
15. Momose A: Radial keratotomy in Japan, J Refract Surg 1987;3:117.
16. Nakajima A: Effects of antero-posterior incision of cornea on myopia, Jpn J Clin Ophthalmol 1965;14:1943-1946 (in Japanese).
17. Nakamura M and Mikawa T: Degeneration of corneal epithelium seen after the operation for myopia, Jpn Rev Clin Ophthalmol 1971;65:26-29 (in Japanese).
18. Okamoto E: RK in Japan, J Refract Surg 1987;3:62.
19. Sato T: Treatment of conical cornea (incision of Descemet's membrane), Acta Soc Ophthalmol Jpn 1939;43:544-555.
20. Sato T: Ueber eine Operationsmethode zur Behandlung des Keratocornus (Descemetspaltung), Klin Monatsble Augenheilkd 1941;107:234-238.
21. Sato T: Crosswise incisions of Descemet's membrane for the treatment of advanced keratoconus, Acta Soc Ophthalmol Jpn 1942;46:469-470.
22. Sato T: Experimental study on surgical correction of astigmatism, Juntendo Kenkyukai-zasshi 1943;589:37-39 (in Japanese).
23. Sato T: The cause and prevention of myopia, Tokyo Kosei no Nippon Sha, 1944.

24. Sato T: Posterior incision of the cornea: surgical treatment for conical cornea and astigmatism, Am J Ophthalmol 1950;33:943-948.
25. Sato T: Experimental study of posterior half-corneal incisions for myopia, Acta Soc Ophthalmol Jpn 1951;55:219-224 (in Japanese).
26. Sato T: Experimental study of anterior and posterior half-corneal incisions for myopia, Jpn J Clin Ophthalmol 1952; 6:209-211 (in Japanese).
27. Sato T: Posterior half-incision of the cornea for astigmatism: operative procedures and results of the improved tangent method, Am J Ophthalmol 1953;36:462-466.
28. Sato T: Die operative behandlung des astigmatismus, Klin Monatsbl Augenheilkd 1955;126:16-31.
29. Sato T, Akiyama K, and Shibata H: A new surgical approach to myopia, Am J Ophthalmol 1953;36:823-829.
30. Sato T and Komori M: Histological finding of posterior corneal incisions, Acta Soc Ophthalmol Jpn 1953; 57:710-712 (in Japanese).
31. Sato T, Shibata H, and Akiyama K: Anterior and posterior half-corneal incisions for myopia, results in human eyes, Acta Soc Ophthalmol Jpn 1952; 56:1137-1140.
32. Tanaka M, Ishii R, Yamaguchi T, Kanai A, and Nakajima A: Bullous keratopathy after the operation for myopia, Acta Soc Ophthalmol Jpn 1980;84:2068-2074.
33. Yamaguchi T, Asbell PA, Ostrick M, Safir A, Kissling GE, and Kaufman HE: Endothelial damage in monkeys after radial keratotomy performed with a diamond knife, Arch Ophthalmol 1984; 102:765-769.

Development of Refractive Keratotomy in the Soviet Union, 1960-1990

George O. Waring III

As the contributions of Sato and his colleagues to the development of keratotomy wilted and died in Japan, they took root and blossomed in the Soviet Union. Although Sato never traveled to the Soviet Union, ophthalmologists there attempted to replicate his procedure, gradually modifying it to become the modern anterior refractive keratotomy.

SATO'S ANTERIOR AND POSTERIOR KERATOTOMY IN THE SOVIET UNION

In 1960 shortly after Sato's death Svyatoslav Fyodorov, M.D., attended the Japanese Ophthalmological Society Conference in Niigata, Japan. After the conference Fyodorov tried Sato's technique in four cases of myopia and two cases of astigmatism but found it difficult to place the full number of posterior incisions without flattening the anterior chamber. Other Soviet ophthalmologists tried different techniques of keratotomy, but Fyodorov's insight and persistence produced the modern concepts and techniques of anterior radial keratotomy.

BACKGROUND AND ACKNOWLEDGMENTS

I was unable to entice a Soviet ophthalmologist to write a firsthand account of the development of radial keratotomy in the Soviet Union, despite invitation and cajolery in person, by letter, by cable, and by emissary. Therefore I have written this chapter based on published literature and interviews with Svyatoslav Fyodorov and Sergei Avetisov; Koichiro Akiyama provided further background information and reprints. I have drawn information on the early development of radial keratotomy in the Soviet Union from A.I. Ivashina's chapter[17a] in S.N. Fyodorov's book, *Microsurgery of the Eye: Main Aspects*, published in 1987. I have also drawn from the experience of John Kiser III, who related his experiences with Fyodorov in his book, *Communist Entrepreneurs* (New York, 1989, Franklin Watts, Inc.) and Sergei Vlasov's adulatory biography of Fyodorov called *Svyatoslav Fyodorov: Just a Magician Who Gives Back Sight* (Moscow, 1988, Norosti Press Agency Publishing House). Helena Fedukowica assiduously translated numerous Russian articles, as did Victor Zhelezniak, and I greatly appreciate their contribution. Some of the background was derived from my visit to Dr. Fyodorov's clinic in April 1980.

Sato's results were duplicated in rabbits by M.P. Pureskin, who worked in the department of M.M. Krasnov in Moscow.[27] In 1967 Pureskin and Krasnov published results of a series of 70 operations; nine groups of experiments were performed using the following different patterns:

1. Anterior radial
2. Posterior radial of 3, 4, and 5 mm length
3. Posterior transverse of 5, 6, and 8 mm length at different clear zones
4. Combined anterior and posterior incisions

Their conclusions were identical to Sato's. Anterior radial incisions were not very effective, and posterior incisions were necessary for the desired effect. In addition, there was a relationship in the change in curvature between the incised and nonincised meridians in astigmatic surgery. Radial incisions flattened the meridian parallel to the incisions more than the meridian 90 degrees away, and transverse incisions flattened the meridian perpendicular to them but slightly steepened the meridian 90 degrees away. Finally, the Soviets concluded that the effect of the surgery was contingent on the length, distance from the limbus, and depth of the transverse incisions.

ANTERIOR KERATOTOMY IN THE SOVIET UNION

As in Japan during World War II, the military played an important role in the development of anterior keratotomy in the Soviet Union. Much of the early surgery in the Soviet Union was performed on soldiers.

In 1969 F.S. Yenaleyev, a military ophthalmologist, changed Sato's techniques and performed only anterior radial keratotomy in 426 eyes of 231 patients between 1969 and 1977. He selected patients with less than 12.00 D of simple (nonpathologic) myopia and varied the number of incisions, using 24 incisions in 290 eyes, 12 incisions in 50 eyes, 8 incisions in 30 eyes, and 4 incisions in 56 eyes. The surgical technique included retrobulbar anesthesia and cutting from the center to the periphery with either a scalpel blade or razor blade in a blade breaker, set at a length of 0.5 mm. He followed 80% (342) of the eyes for at least 6 months and found an average correction of 3.00 to 4.00 D with stability in approximately 73% of the eyes, the remainder showing continued progression of myopia that offset the effect of the surgery.[33]

M Kio Tin, working in the department of V.S. Belyaeve, used the combination of scleral slings around the posterior pole to record the progression of high myopia and subsequent anterior radial keratotomy to treat the residual myopia. He basically followed Sato's

approach, using a 6-mm diameter central clear zone, short incisions 2 to 3 mm long, making up to 32 incisions in the peripheral cornea with a razor blade fragment following marks made with a template. Improvement in uncorrected visual acuity was insignificant. The effect of treatment on 60 patients was 1.0 to 3.0 D in 63% of the eyes.[18,19]

V.F. Utkin, another military ophthalmologist working in Riazan, used a freehand razor blade with no central marker to perform surgery on 34 eyes of 24 individuals, mostly soldiers. He made 16 to 32 short incisions with a large central clear zone and with a fixed depth of 0.5 to 0.6 mm. The number of incisions varied. He obtained only a small change in the myopia, with an effect of 1.2 to 2.8 D of correction that stabilized approximately 3 months after surgery. Utkin noted that if the length and depth of the incisions were constant, the effect of the operation depended on the number of incisions.[32]

Yenaliev (1979) used a curved crystalline cystotome or razor blade fragment adjusted to a fixed depth of 0.5 mm and made short peripheral incisions with a large diameter central clear zone in 178 patients with mild to moderate myopia. He observed 110 of these patients for 1 year postoperatively, noting that the myopia returned to the initial amount in 26.5%. He obtained his best results in the patients with myopia from 3.0 to 3.5 D.

Mamikonyan and colleagues (1980) and Grusha and colleagues (1981) took a different approach at the All-Union Institute of Eye Diseases. They used a four-incision anterior radial keratotomy with a large diameter clear zone and then applied pressure through the eyelids by means of a special plate, an operation they called orthokeratotomy. They proposed to weaken the cornea with the incisions and then to use the back of the eyelid as a conformer to press the cornea into the new desired flatter shape. They reported small groups of patients with the maximal effect of 3.5 D, and this approach was abandoned.

During the 1970s, Fyodorov and colleagues changed the fundamental approach to anterior refractive keratotomy by attempting to customize the operation for each individual.

FYODOROV'S INDIVIDUALIZED ANTERIOR RADIAL KERATOTOMY

Important contributions to modern anterior refractive keratotomy were made during the 1970s and 1980s by S.N. Fyodorov and his colleagues in Moscow (Figs. 7-1 and 7-2). Born in 1929 and educated in the Soviet Union, "Slava," as his friends call him, has struggled against the bureaucracy and reticence

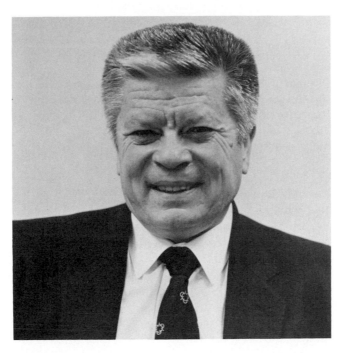

Figure 7-1
Svyatoslav N. Fyodorov, champion of modern anterior
radial keratotomy. (Photographed in 1983.)

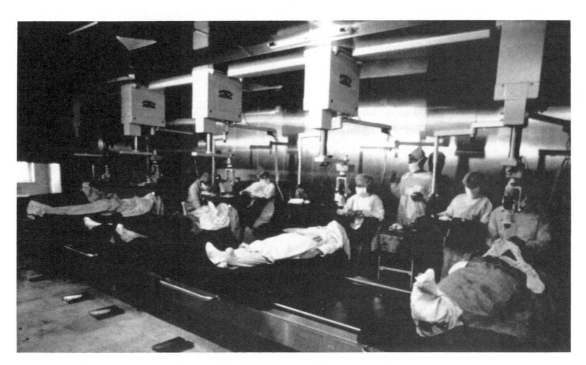

Figure 7-2
"Assembly line" surgical suite in Moscow consists of conveyer belt that moves patients past
multiple stations (photographed in 1989). At each station a physician or technician performs
one part of the operation. The arrangement is more efficient than moving patients in and out of
a single room. The system resembles Sato's arrangement of multiple tables in one room and the
approach used in cataract camps for decades.

of the Soviet medical establishment since the early 1950s, when he attempted to duplicate Ridley's concepts of implanting an intraocular lens after cataract surgery. His indomitable energy and unquenchable optimism have propelled him into world prominence as a physician-businessman and into political prominence as a member of the Soviet Presidium. The box on pp. 226-228 chronicles my 1980 trip to Fyodorov's institute and adds some recent observations.

Optical clear zone diameter

Working in Fyodorov's institute in the early 1970s, Dr. Valerie Durnev observed that lengthening the anterior keratotomy incisions by making the diameter of the central clear zone as small as 3 mm increased the effect of keratotomy—an observation confirmed in a series of 150 rabbits.

In the rabbit experiments 32 incisions 4.5 to 6 mm long were made with a razor blade, using a clear zone of 3 to 5 mm and a depth of about 90% of corneal thickness. Histochemical studies showed normal wound healing with fibrin and epithelial plugs and the reappearance of mucopolysaccharides. Wound healing appeared complete by 3 months after surgery, leaving a focal scar without degeneration.[4] The majority of nerve fibers were not damaged, and those that were cut regenerated in about 3 months, either through or parallel to the scar.[5] After 1 year the rabbits demonstrated persistent flattening of the retinal cornea.

Durnev placed contact lenses with an opaque periphery and clear center on patients to determine the effect of smaller central clear zones, and found that a 3-mm clear zone was acceptable but that a smaller clear zone reduced the visual acuity.[7]

Biomechanics of keratotomy

Durnev and Fyodorov carried forward the ideas of Sato concerning the mechanism of effect of radial keratotomy. They stated the incisions interrupted the "circular tension" and conceptualized this in anatomic terms as the peripheral circular ligament of the cornea.[20,25,26] Using a photokeratoscope in humans, the Soviet researchers observed that the peripheral corneal curvature steepened and the central corneal curvature flattened after radial keratotomy. They attributed this to severing of the circular deep ligament around cornea, allowing the intraocular pressure to push the cornea forward and steepen it peripherally with passive compensatory flattening centrally (Fig. 7-3). The authors emphasized this theoretic mechanism in the title of their first article in English, "Operation of Dosaged Dissection of the Corneal Circular Ligament in Cases of Myopia Mild Degree."[10]

Durnev and Fyodorov were also aware that the rigidity and elastic qualities of the cornea were important and varied from one person to another.

Subsequent experience and modern biomechanical analysis supports the basic concept of Sato and Fyodorov but shifts the emphasis to the paracentral—not the peripheral—portion of the incision. Indeed the incisions can stop inside the corneal limbus and achieve approximately the same effect as those extending into the sclera.[24]

Individualized prediction formula

Fyodorov's goal was to remove the art from keratotomy and devise a mathematic formula that used anatomic and mechanical parameters of the cornea to accurately calculate the results in each individual case. He used geometric calculations (Fig. 7-3) to demonstrate that the amount of flattening of the central cornea was proportionate to the preoperative diameter of the cornea, which would make the incisions longer, and inversely proportionate to the preoperative radius of curvature, which would make the central optical zone smaller and cause steeper corneas to flatten more than flatter corneas. In addition, clinical experience was showing that corneas with a greater preoperative rigidity showed a greater change in refraction. Finally the investigators were aware of the asphericity of the cornea, in which the peripheral cornea gradually flattens. To allow for this, they computed a coefficient called the "clinical coefficient," which was given a value of 1.54. Later this was reinterpreted as the "practical coefficient for the surgeon" to allow for variations in surgical technique—especially depth of incision.

All of these considerations came together in a geometrically derived formula designed to predict the change in refraction.[11] (Fig. 7-3, *E*).

Currently, there is evidence that greater intraocular pressure, greater patient age, and greater uniform depth of the incision enhance the effect of keratotomy surgery. More detailed study of these variables would await American surgeons.

The effect of the number of incisions was studied in patients, Durnev observing the change in corneal power was the same with 16 incisions (2.78 D ± 0.19 D) as with 32 incisions (2.79 D ± 0.03 D), so the number of incisions was fixed at 16 for early cases.[6]

Clinical results

Fyodorov started performing surgery in humans in 1974 using a freehand razor blade fragment in a blade holder, checking the depth of the incision with a depth gauge, and deepening the incisions as needed.

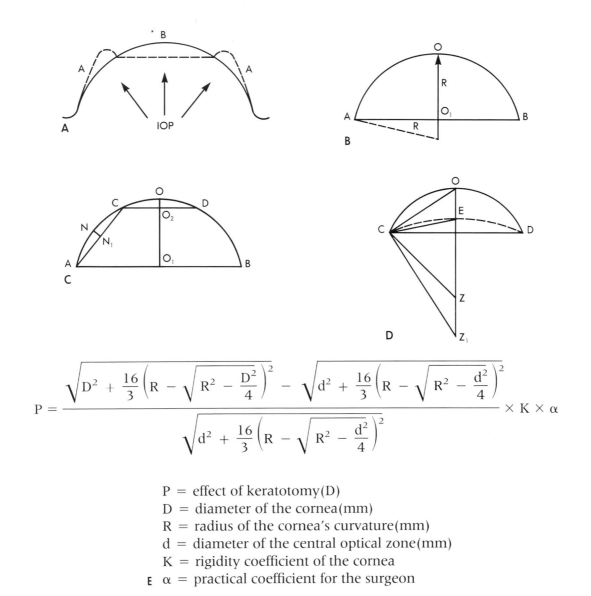

$$P = \frac{\sqrt{D^2 + \frac{16}{3}\left(R - \sqrt{R^2 - \frac{D^2}{4}}\right)^2} - \sqrt{d^2 + \frac{16}{3}\left(R - \sqrt{R^2 - \frac{d^2}{4}}\right)^2}}{\sqrt{d^2 + \frac{16}{3}\left(R - \sqrt{R^2 - \frac{d^2}{4}}\right)^2}} \times K \times \alpha$$

P = effect of keratotomy(D)
D = diameter of the cornea(mm)
R = radius of the cornea's curvature(mm)
d = diameter of the central optical zone(mm)
K = rigidity coefficient of the cornea
α = practical coefficient for the surgeon

Figure 7-3
Geometric calculations based on anatomic measurements of cornea formed basis for Fyodorov-Durnev formula designed to calculate outcome of radial keratotomy for individual cases. **A,** Change in corneal profile after radial keratotomy shows anterior displacement and steepening of incised portion of cornea with posterior displacement and flattening of central cornea under influence of intraocular pressure. **B,** Profile of the cornea before radial keratotomy. **C,** Profile of the cornea after radial keratotomy with incisions made from A to C and the central optical zone (CD) flattening from O to O_2. Length of arc ANC was thought to increase, and length of the arc COD was thought to decrease. **D,** Shortening of arc COD was associated with a lengthening of radius of curvature and decrease in refractive power of cornea. **E,** Geometrically derived formula to predict the change in refraction. (From Fyodorov SN, Ivashina AI, Klimova TL, and Kolmanovskii SA: Surgery for anomalies in ocular refraction, Moscow, 1981, Moscow Research Institute for Ocular Microsurgery, Ministry of Health.)

Slava Fyodorov: A Personal Portrait

The intense interest in radial keratotomy in the United States in 1979 and 1980 triggered a stampede of ophthalmologists traveling to Moscow to learn the technique from its champion, Slava Fyodorov. I was no exception.

While planning for a multicenter trial of radial keratotomy, I found it difficult to collect verifiable information about the results of the thousands of cases that had reportedly been done in the Soviet Union. Therefore I set off for Moscow to observe the work of Fyodorov and to determine the results in his patients 4 to 5 years after surgery. In 1980 visas for travel to the Soviet Union were not easy to get, but through the persuasive efforts of three individuals who had traveled frequently to Moscow—Drs. Leo Bores, Miles Galen, and Stephen Obstbaum—I was able to get a visa on short notice. Traveling alone, I savored the spartan conditions aboard Aeroflot and arrived at 3 AM in the deserted, stadium-sized Moscow air terminal. After the customs agents relieved me of my books on the history and political structure of the Soviet Union, I shuffled outside through the patches of melting spring snow and mud and climbed into a black limousine. At the hotel just off Red Square, my natural American suspicions made me cringe under the scrutiny of the floor matron as I dragged my bags to the room.

The next morning I sped across Moscow in the black limousine driven by Fyodorov's personal driver who had had radial keratotomy performed on both eyes—I hoped successfully. After a 1-hour drive through the bleak Moscow suburbs, we penetrated a pristine forest and arrived at Fyodorov's dacha (country home), which resembled a small Swiss chalet with adjacent barns. Resplendent in a fur coat, Fyodorov greeted me with a warm "zdrahsstyĕh" (a hearty hello), introduced me to his charming wife, and began to prepare his two favorite horses for an afternoon ride. As we galloped over the countryside, plunging through the still-deep snow, I fully expected Yuri Zhivago to come dashing through the trees with the Red Guards in pursuit. An accomplished and stalwart horseman despite his artificial leg, Fyodorov led me through forest and across farmland to a small home occupied by the people who managed his land. The candles and fire warmed the dank interior, our host's cordiality warmed my heart, and the afternoon vodka and bread warmed my body. The conversation, all in Russian, was punctuated by international smiles, nods, and backslapping.

Things were not always so cushy for Slava. Born into a military family in 1927, Fyodorov's ambitions to become a pilot were encouraged by acceptance in a flying academy at age 16 and quickly crushed when he was running to catch a trolley car and was dragged under the tram, resulting in the loss of one leg. With characteristic determination, he turned to a career in medicine, gravitating toward ophthalmology because of his interest in photography. He observes philosophically now that the loss of his leg may have been one of the best things that happened to him. After receiving his medical degree from the institute in Rostov, Fyodorov took a job at a small eye institute in the town of Cheboksary, where he caught Harold Ridley's vision of implanting an artificial lens in the eye after cataract surgery. Since such lenses were unavailable, Fyodorov proceeded to manufacture the lenses in his kitchen and to implant them experimentally in rabbits. In approximately 1956 he performed his first intraocular lens implant in a schoolgirl with a reportedly successful result, which elicited an outcry of protest from the Moscow medical establishment and the fickle officials at Cheboksary. Doggedly, Fyodorov persuaded the Deputy Minister of Health in Moscow to support his work, but local authorities provided only further delays, spurring Fyodorov's move to a hospital in remote Arkhangel on the White Sea. Here he encountered multiple failures in the development of intraocular lenses but was able to find a skilled craftsman in Leningrad who produced technically superior lenses that became successful. In 1967 he moved to Moscow to oversee the construction of a new hospital, No. 81, which was to become the now enormous Moscow Research Institute of Eye Microsurgery.

At the Institute I spent a week observing surgery, examining patients, running computer formulas, comparing the predicted results with the clinically documented outcome and giving lectures. There was no apparent preselection of patients, and I was able to observe both good and bad results with unrestricted freedom. As we discussed the shallow incisions, the multiple inclusions within the scars, and the lack of correlation between predicted and achieved results, Fyodorov's irrepressible optimism smothered any concern with the refrain, "All is beautiful." I enjoyed the cordiality and camaraderie of my Soviet counterparts. Our pleasant friendship increased as each day passed, culminating in the midafternoon break, where I learned to handle the successive vodka toasts by gulping down handfuls of bread before the jiggers were filled.

Although Fyodorov's interest in refractive keratotomy stemmed from the work of Sato, he is fond of relating a chance observation that spurred him to more active research. In about 1972 he treated Boris Petrov, a 16-year-old boy who was hit in his glasses during a schoolyard fight, sustaining multiple lacerations in his cornea. As the lacerations healed, Petrov's preexisting myopia diminished, leaving an uncorrected visual acuity of 20/30. Fyodorov remarked, "We began to think that if a boy without any ophthalmic knowledge can treat myopia with his fist, maybe with our more sophisticated laser beams and radio-frequency probes and computers we could also treat myopia."[8] I was reminded of the similar chance observations of Bates, Faber, and Sato.

Fyodorov is also fond of telling his response to Woody Allen's movie *Sleeper,* in which the hero awakes from a frozen sleep in the twenty-second century with a pair of thick spectacles on and sees everyone else wearing glasses too. Fyodorov thought it incongruous that people would still wear such simple spectacles to achieve good vision in the postmodern world. He pursued the goal of a permanent cure for myopia.

Throughout my visit I received a full dose of Fyodorov's admirable philosophy: improve ophthalmic surgical technology by taking the art out of medicine; the artist will create a different result every time, even under the same conditions. Fyodorov's goal is to reduce variability from one patient to another and to increase the predictability of outcome for each individual. The best quality eye care should be provided for the largest number of patients in the most efficient and cost-effective manner.

Fyodorov has bucked not only the medical establishment but also the economic establishment. His basic philosophy that people who work harder should live better was certainly at odds with the tenets of communism in the 1970s. Nevertheless, Fyodorov has taken a distinctively entrepreneurial approach to fostering the growth of his institute and eye care in the Soviet Union. Indeed, he proposed a system of earning money for his institute based on the number of patients treated, all employees benefitting on a per-production basis through an incentive fund and a benefits fund based on the profits. Under this incentive program, if the hospital can use state funds and perform the procedure for less and increase volume as well, the savings stay within the institute. This quasi-capitalist philosophy that lay at the root of the success of Fyodorov's institute in the mid-1980s provided a foretaste of the sweeping economic reforms throughout the Soviet Union instituted by Mikhail Gorbachev in the late 1980s.

While visiting Fyodorov, I met some English-speaking Muscovites at the ballet and the circus, who greatly desired my Western goods and currency; I declined their offers. One affable couple invited me to their home but refused to call me at the hotel or pick me up there, stating that the rooms were bugged and under constant surveillance and that they would be punished if found with a foreign visitor. Thus, trembling, I slipped out of the hotel after dark and walked a few blocks to our prearranged meeting place in an alley behind a post office. Slouched low in the backseat of their car, I remained concealed until given the high sign to sneak up the stairs to their one-room apartment, where we chatted until sunrise about the differing sociopolitical styles of the Eastern and Western worlds.

What a contrast to circumstances in 1990, under the philosophies of glasnost

Continued.

Slava Fyodorov: A Personal Portrait—cont'd

and perestroika, where hundreds of thousands of Muscovites parade the streets with banners demanding democracy. And where is Fyodorov? In the thick of things! Taking advantage of the new political order in the Soviet Union, Fyodorov has been elected to the Presidium. A master at handling the media, Fyodorov travels with a public relations staff who have the knack of thrusting him into the public eye. He has garnered a spotlight of adulation on the usually critical *60 Minutes* news show in the United States and had his picture on the front page of the *International Herald Tribune* as an activist politician. What does he have in store for the 1990s?

Fyodorov's search for controllable high quality has led him to use assembly line techniques for surgery, techniques that acknowledge that the surgeon is essential in only 10% of the operating time, a percentage, however, that determines 90% of the results. Fyodorov harnessed concepts of efficient production with high quality control by placing patients on a series of stretchers that move from one station to another, personnel at the early stations performing preparatory parts of the operation, the surgeon completing the most important, and personnel at the latter stations completing the case (see Fig. 7-2). Such standardized techniques are the basis for Fyodorov's plans to establish branches throughout the Soviet Union, and indeed throughout the world. His institute has now become a complex that will soon comprise eye centers in 12 cities from Khabarovsk in eastern Siberia to Krasnodar in the Crimea, and thereafter franchised clinics all around the world. Already, Fyodorov is seeking locations in the Middle East and has created a cruise-hospital ship on which, under opulent conditions, patients can receive eye surgery and enjoy a pleasant cruise at the same time. And of course the doors are open in Moscow, where enterprising travel agents offer week-long packages that combine surgery at Fyodorov's institute with sightseeing in Moscow and Leningrad. Fyodorov exports not only surgery but also the technical innovations of his institute. The Fyodorov Sputnik intraocular lens was exported around the world until newer designs supplanted it. Through licensing agreements with Bausch and Lomb in the United States, he has made available absorbable collagen contact lenses as well as sets of surgical instruments.

I left Moscow in 1980 gratified, more knowledgeable about the realities of radial keratotomy. I was buoyed by Fyodorov's vision and enthusiasm but cautioned by his claims of superior results. Fyodorov has reported some 99% good results after refractive keratotomy and has stated that no more than one or two complications have occurred in tens of thousands of cases. Such results, which are so remarkably different from those achieved by other well-trained surgeons around the world, demand critical evaluation and assessment, even though they come from the mouth of one of the acknowledged masters of modern ophthalmology.

He stated he specifically refrained from reporting his early results so that he could have a reasonable follow-up on many patients. Crystal blades were first used in 1978, and a special set of marking instruments and guarded knives was made in 1979. Surgeons used four to sixteen incisions with blades set to a length of 450 to 750 μm. The first comprehensive report of his surgeries appeared in 1979[10] and was followed by a second paper with a longer follow-up in 1982.[9] The results of the 1982 paper are presented and discussed in Chapter 23, Complications of Refractive Keratotomy.

Throughout his oral and written presentations Fyodorov has remained enthusiastically optimistic about keratotomy for myopia and astigmatism, extolling its virtues and minimizing its drawbacks. His results have supported his enthusiasm: 100% of 230 eyes with baseline refractions of -1.00 to -6.00 D, achieving a final refraction within ± 0.50 D of emmetropia 1.5 years after surgery.[9] No other surgeons have been able to replicate these extraordinary results.

Fyodorov and Ivashina reported good results in the management of myopic anisometropia, performing refractive keratotomy on the more myopic eye.[12]

Although many American surgeons credit Fyodorov as the source of their approach to surgical planning for refractive keratotomy, few have reported studies specifically using his formula. Hecht[16] used a modification of the Fyodorov formula in 17 eyes with refractions between −2.00 and −7.50 D; three eyes had reoperations. In the study, Hecht and Jamara excluded one diabetic patient who had a much greater result than expected and one myope with a preoperative refraction of −12.50 D. For the 16 remaining eyes they found a correlation coefficient of 0.77 ($p < 0.001$) between the predicted value and the outcome, a reasonable result. Arrowsmith and Marks[2] used the Fyodorov formula, but with numerous modifications, such as the addition of deepening incisions.

Subsequent studies of human refractive keratotomy have supported some of Fyodorov's postulates but not others. Three studies of human cases using regression analyses[1,23,29] have found an effect of the smaller clear zone (longer incisions), but not of corneal diameter, corneal curvature, or ocular rigidity. Details of the factors that affect outcome are described in Chapter 26, Summary of Factors That Affect the Outcome of Refractive Keratotomy. All surgeons agree that a "practical coefficient" should be used to adjust any formula for surgeons, techniques, and instruments.

Surgery for astigmatism

Like Sato, Fyodorov and his colleagues developed numerous patterns of incisions to correct astigmatism (Fig. 7-4). The principle was to flatten the steep corneal meridian by placing more radial incisions, longer radial incisions, or intersecting transverse and radial incisions there. Although all the patterns were somewhat effective, none is used currently. The placement of grouped radial incisions in the steep corneal meridian or of longer incisions in the steep corneal meridian has been found to be generally unpredictable and ineffective. Intersecting radial and transverse incisions create problems in wound healing.[17] Astigmatism surgery is discussed in Chapters 31 and 32, Keratotomy for Astigmatism, and Atlas of Astigmatic Keratotomy, respectively.

Surgical instruments and technique

Fyodorov introduced a number of surgical instruments to facilitate refractive keratotomy. His first 1600 cases were performed with a freehand metal blade. In the late 1970s he introduced a micrometer knife that advanced the blade a fixed amount past the flat footplate to better control the depth of the incision and to allow for more precise deepening of incisions (Fig. 7-5). The blade was calibrated on a ruler-style gauge block (Fig. 7-6). Fyodorov also introduced circular,

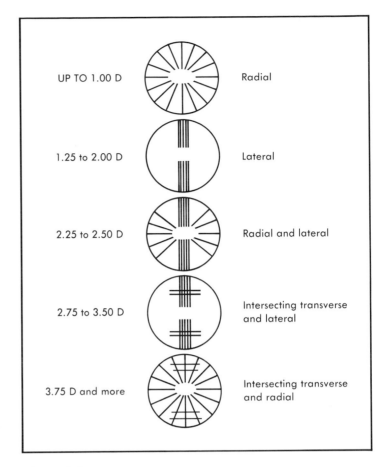

Figure 7-4

Patterns of astigmatism surgery recommended by Fyodorov with amount of astigmatism they were intended to correct *(left)* and type of incision *(right)*. None of the patterns illustrated is currently in use. (From Fyodorov SN: Surgical correction of myopia and astigmatism. In Schachar RA, Levy NS, and Schachar L, editors: Keratorefraction, Denison, Tex, 1980, LAL Publishing.)

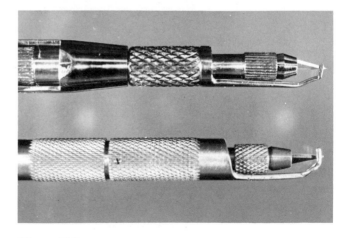

Figure 7-5

Early Fyodorov micrometer knife with metal blade placed in chuck and angled ski-style footplates. (Courtesy Johnny Deen, MD.)

clear-zone markers and radial markers to guide the placement of the incisions (Fig. 7-7).

The Soviet technique of refractive keratotomy used in the late 1970s was a crude progenitor of the more refined techniques in current use worldwide (Fig. 7-8). Central corneal thickness was measured by optical pachometry, and the method of determining the length of the knife blade is not described in Fyodorov's papers. The knife had a razor blade fragment held in the end of a blade holder—at first freehand and later of calibrated length. Fixation was achieved with conventional forceps. Markers for the central clear zone and the radial incisions served as guides. Incisions were made centripetally from the limbus toward the clear zone, starting in the scleral limbus so that each incision filled with blood. The 16 incisions were minimally irrigated, so postoperatively many were studded with yellowish pearls of blood products or epithelial inclusions. Soviet and American innovation rapidly refined the procedure in the early 1980s (see Chapter 17, Atlas of Surgical Techniques of Radial Keratotomy).

At the time of this writing, Fyodorov, Ivashina, and their colleagues continue to refine the procedure with specific goals in mind: (1) destruction of the structure of the corneal collagen with lasers or radio frequencies, (2) intraoperative monitoring of the effect of surgery, (3) an automated knife that advances the blade based on measured corneal thickness during surgery, and (4) robotic surgeons. Fyodorov's institute now uses a stage-by-stage method of surgery on a fully automated conveyor system begun in 1984 (Fig. 7-2).

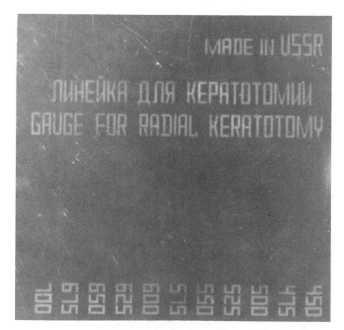

Figure 7-6
Ruler-style gauge block for calibrating knife blade length. (Courtesy Johnny Deen, MD.)

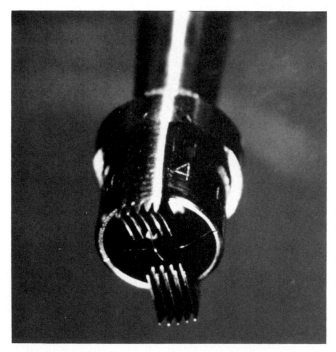

Figure 7-7
Corneal marker for parallel radial incisions to correct astigmatism—the "L" procedure. (Courtesy Johnny Deen, MD.)

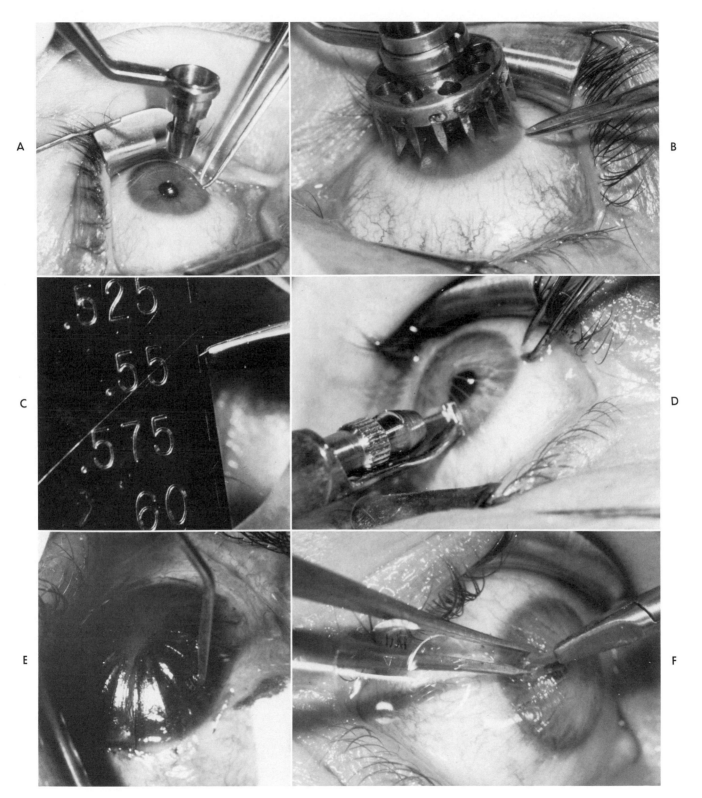

Figure 7-8
Russian technique of radial keratotomy as practiced in the early 1980s. **A,** Marking central clear zone. **B,** Marking location of 16 radial incisions. **C,** Setting length of razor blade fragment. **D,** Making incisions from limbus toward center with single-point fixation using Fyodorov micrometer knife. **E,** Checking depth of incision with dip stick. **F,** Freehand deepening of wound with razor blade and wound spreader. (Courtesy Herbert Gould, MD.)

Radial Keratotomy—A Question of Ethics?

It has been long since known that an incision in the cornea or heating of the cornea with diathermy can result in a change of its radius and thus change the refractive power of the eye.

In the Soviet Union the Russian eye surgeon Professor S. Fyodorov has modified a technique with radial incisions in the cornea and achieved a certain control of the refractive change. This method has gained a considerable interest all over the world, and the technique has been used in many countries for more than five years. In the Western world the debate on whether this kind of surgery is ethical or not has hit the headlines. To perform deep incisions in a normal, healthy cornea in order to change the refraction of the eye so that spectacles can be omitted has to be weighed against the risks of the operation.

All of us who have been working with patients wearing contact lenses know the enormous change and relief these patients experience not having to use their spectacles any more. For many patients it is an unexpected and sometimes very positive reaction. Beyond doubt a great number of people would make not only economical but also physical sacrifices to be able to get rid of their glasses. The question arises whether an ophthalmologist could recommend this kind of surgery to reach the goal or not. About three years ago the Swedish ophthalmologists reached a consensus to abandon this kind of surgery. With the result of the US PERK study and the experiences from other countries as a background, one can still not come to another conclusion than the one that was drawn three years ago. However, some of the Swedish doctors seem to have changed their minds, and some are positive to start performing radial keratotomies. Knowing the tremendous suffering some patients experience when wearing glasses or contact lenses one may ask: can we really refuse the patients this kind of surgery? . . .

We have now experiences from patients who, more or less against their eye doctors' will, have gone through operations of this kind. Despite the results nearly all of these patients are happy with their operations. In Sweden, a travel bureau has started to arrange trips to Moscow for patients who wish to be operated upon by the most experienced surgeon in this special field, Professor S. Fyodorov. I doubt that the satisfaction will be the same with these patients who accept the offer from a travel agency, pay the fee and remember the promises of good results that were advertised. If these results are not achieved, I have a feeling that the claims will amount to a considerable number. Up to now we have seen a number of complications, and this puts an extra load on the hospital facilities. I wonder if this is right?

Colleagues are encouraged to go to Moscow in order to learn the technique. In this context I would like to cite a letter to the editor of the Times (London) from November 25, 1985:

More than meets eye

From Mr. D.P. Choyce

Sir, Peter Kellner, in an article on September 11, praised the Moscow Institute for Eye Microsurgery, under its director, Professor Svyatoslav Fyodorov. There is another side of Professor Fyodorov's activities of which Mr. Kellner appears to be unaware.

What happens when a Western ophthalmologist wishes to go to Moscow to learn from the master? He has to sign an agreement with Licensintorg, the licensing bureau. I have a copy in front of me. The salient features are these:

1. The tuition fees, payable in advance in US dollars, range from US dollars 920 for three days to US dollars 5,680 for one month, in a group; 30 per cent more if the instruction takes place on a one-to-one basis.

2. He must use the correct trademark; he must use Fyodorov's instruments, artificial lenses and surgical techniques. He must make no changes to any of these.

3. He must report his results every year and if his success rate falls below 80 per cent he automatically loses the franchise.

4. He is allowed to do 50 operations "for free"; thereafter he must pay a 5 per cent royalty on every operation he performs to the agency, again in US dollars. He has to agree to open his practice accounts at least once a year to an auditor appointed by the agency to enable it to keep a check on his earnings.

5. He is not allowed to instruct others in the techniques he will have learned in Moscow.

6. The agreement runs for seven years.

7. Should there be any disagreement between the parties the dispute will be referred to the Foreign Trade Arbitration Commission at the All-Union Chamber of Commerce and Industry, Moscow, whose decision shall be binding on both signatories.

Altogether a very remarkable document, about as far removed as possible from the ethics enshrined in the Hippocratic oath upon which Western medicine is based. It is ironic that it takes a citizen of the USSR to think up something which is unacceptable to his colleagues in capitalist countries.

Yours faithfully,

D. P. Choyce (Past President, International Intraocular
Implant Club and United Kingdom Intraocular Implant Society)

I agree with Mr. Choyce that there certainly are different ways of how to interpret the Hippocratic oath in different parts of the world. . . .

From Tengroth B: Acta Ophthalmol 1987;65:1.

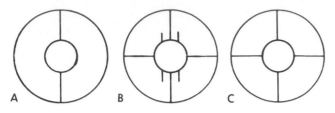

Figure 7-9
Patterns of keratotomy surgery suggested by Avetisov in 1982. **A,** Correction of mixed astigmatism, steep meridian 90°. **B,** Correction of compound myopic astigmatism. **C,** Four-incision radial keratotomy. (From Avetisov SE: Ophthalmol News 1982;6:37.)

REPORTS OF AVETISOV AND KRASNOV

After an initial disappointing experience with keratotomy,[21] workers in the department of M.M. Krasnov rekindled their interest in keratotomy in the early 1980s. S.E. Avetisov published a series of articles on anterior keratotomy, which he called orthokeratotomy, observing little damage to the cornea and no decrease in contrast sensitivity after the surgery. They used four-incision radial keratotomy in 1982 and devised patterned methods for the correction of astigmatism (Fig. 7-9). They postulated that the mechanism of the operation included the compressive effect of the eyelids and suggested that silicone contact lenses might enhance the effect of the surgery.[3,14,15,22]

ANTERIOR REFRACTIVE KERATOTOMY IN THE EAST

In approximately 1978 Fyodorov visited Hyderabad, India, where he taught anterior keratotomy to P. Siva Reddy and P. Ranga Reddy, who performed the surgery on 200 myopic eyes with disappointing results.[31] Because they used a razor blade and cut only superficially into the cornea,[30] the results were similar to those of Sato's anterior keratotomy—transient. Reddy observed that the operation was easy to perform and that there were almost no complications except for photophobia, but that the flattening of the central cornea with the dramatic improvement in visual acuity lasted for only a few weeks and left a residual myopia in all cases. A longer term follow-up of 70% of these eyes from 2 to 5 years showed that only 6.5% could see 20/40 or better uncorrected. Reddy concluded that the operation had not been refined enough to be useful.[28]

Fyodorov also demonstrated keratotomy in Poland, Czechoslovakia, Syria, and Japan, but apparently little interest resulted.

ANTERIOR REFRACTIVE KERATOTOMY IN THE WEST

Fyodorov actively exported anterior keratotomy to the United States, but the start was slow. He visited the United States a number of times in the mid- and late 1970s to speak about his iris-fixated Sputnik intraocular lens, popularizing it in the Northeast. He also extolled the virtues of keratotomy, but, like Sato, he found only American indifference. However, once the news media began to describe the "pinwheel surgery that lets you throw away your glasses," the eruption of interest created an unprecedented surgical, ethical, and socioeconomic upheaval in American ophthalmology. Fyodorov's approach to teaching and exporting keratotomy continues to spawn controversy in Europe. The box on pp. 232 and 233 contains an excerpt from a 1987 editorial published in *Acta Ophthalmologica.*

UNFINISHED BUSINESS

Some ophthalmic surgeons in the Soviet Union perform a high volume of refractive corneal surgery. However, they do not report their results for consecutive series of eyes done with specified techniques. Thus a substantive body of knowledge is not available to the ophthalmic profession, which is left with either brief retrospective reports or oral presentations as their source of information to make judgments about these surgical techniques. I encourage our Soviet colleagues—as well as those in other countries who are able to use newer refractive surgical techniques in clinical trials earlier than we can in the United States—to follow the precepts of prospective clinical trials and to report consecutive series of eyes as they study new techniques.

REFERENCES

1. Arrowsmith PN and Marks RG: Evaluating the predictability of radial keratotomy, Ophthalmology 1985; 92:331-338.

2. Arrowsmith PN, Sanders DR, and Marks RG: Visual, refractive, and keratometric results of radial keratotomy, Arch Ophthalmol 1983; 101:873-881.

3. Avetisov SE, Ermakov NV, Mamikonyan VR, et al: Condition of the cornea after orthokeratotomy, Ophthalmol News 1981;1:25-27.

4. Bargov CH and Durnev VB: Morphological study of corneal tissue after multiple non-perforating incisions. In Fyodorov SN, editor: Surgery for anomalies in ocular refraction, Moscow, 1981, The Moscow Research Institute for Ocular Microsurgery, pp 6-10.

5. Bargov CH, Durnev VB, and Jasenko IA: The condition of nerve fibrils after anterior keratotomy. In Fyodorov SN, editor: Surgery for anomalies in ocular refraction, Moscow, 1981, The Moscow Research Institute for Ocular Microsurgery, pp 11-12.

6. Durnev VV: Characteristics of surgical correction of myopia after 16 and 32 peripheral anterior non-perforating incisions. In Fyodorov SN, editor: Surgery for anomalies in ocular refraction, Moscow, 1981, The Moscow Research Institute for Ocular Microsurgery, pp 33-35.

7. Durnev VV and Ivashina AI: Possibility of maximal elongation of incisions in anterior keratotomy. In Fyodorov SN, editor: Surgery for anomalies in ocular refraction, Moscow, 1981, The Moscow Research Institute for Ocular Microsurgery, pp 19-22.

8. Fyodorov SN: Surgical correction of myopia and astigmatism. In Schachar RA et al, editors: Keratorefraction, Denison, Tex, 1980, LAL Publishing, pp 141-172.

9. Fyodorov SN and Agranovsky AA: Long-term results of anterior radial keratotomy, J Ocular Therapy Surg 1982;1:217-223.

10. Fyodorov SN and Durnev VV: Operation of dosaged dissection of corneal circular ligament in cases of myopia of mild degree, Ann Ophthalmol 1979; 11:1185-1190.

11. Fyodorov SN, Durnev VV, Ivashina AI, and Gudechkov VB: Calculation method of effectiveness of anterior keratotomy in surgical correction of myopia. In Fyodorov SN, editor: Surgery for anomalies in ocular refraction, Moscow, 1981, The Moscow Research Institute for Ocular Microsurgery, pp 114-121.

12. Fyodorov SN, Ivashina AI, Fedchenko OT, et al: Surgical correction of myopic anisometropia by anterior keratotomy, Vestn Oftalmol 1984;1:15-19.

13. Fyodorov SN, Veklich OK, and Kursova TP: Radial keratotomy in rehabilitation of pilots. In Fyodorov SN, editor: Surgery for anomalies in ocular refraction, Moscow, 1981, The Moscow Research Institute for Ocular Microsurgery, pp 39-42.

14. Grusha OV, Avetisov SE, and Mamikonyan VR: Experience in applying silicone contact lenses after anterior keratotomies, Ophthalmol News 1981;4:13-14.

15. Grusha OV, Avetisov SE, and Mamikonyan VR: On the mechanism of the cornea flattening as a result of nonperforating incisions of its frontal part, Ophthalmol News 1981;1:36-38.

16. Hecht SD and Jamara RJ: Prospective evaluation of radial keratotomy using the Fyodorov formula: preliminary report, Ann Ophthalmol 1982;14:319-328.

17. Hofmann RF: The surgical correction of idiopathic astigmatism. In Sanders DR et al, editors: Refractive corneal surgery, Thorofare, NJ, 1986, Slack Inc, pp 241-290.

17a. Ivashina AI: Radial keratotomy as a method of surgical correction of myopia. In Fyodorov SN, editor: Microsurgery of the eye: main aspects, Moscow, 1987, Mir Publishers.

18. Kio Tin M: Scleral keratoplasty in the treatment of progressive myopia, Arch Ophthalmol USSR 1970;3:24.

19. Kio Tin M: Scleralplasty in the treatment of progressing myopia, Ann Ophthalmol USSR 1976;3:24-27.

20. Kokott W: Uber mechanisch—funktionelle Strukturen des Auges, Von Graefes Arch Ophthalmol 1938; 138:424-485.

21. Krasnov MM: First experience of surgical correction of myopia and aphakia by the refractive keratoplasty method, Vestn Oftalmol 1970;2:24-28.

22. Krasnov MM, Avetisov SE, Makashova NV, et al: Orthokeratotomy and frequency-contrast characteristics of the eye. Ophthalmol News 1984; 6:27-30.

23. Lynn MJ, Waring GO, Sperduto RD, and the PERK Study Group: Factors affecting outcome and predictability of radial keratotomy in the PERK study, Arch Ophthalmol 1987;105:42-51.

24. O'Donnell FE: Short incision radial keratotomy: a comparative study in rabbits, J Refract Surg 1987;3:102-103.

25. Polack FM: Morphology of the cornea. I. Study with silver stains, Am J Ophthalmol 1961;51:1051-1056.

26. Pratt-Johnson JA: Studies on the anatomy and pathology of the peripheral cornea, Am J Ophthalmol 1959; 47:478.

27. Pureskin MP: A change in the curvature of cornea by subjecting it to anterior and posterior non-perforating incisions, Ann Ophthalmol USSR 1967; 6:16-22.

28. Ranga Reddy P: Anterior keratotomy follow-up results, Indian J Ophthalmol 1983;31:888-889.

29. Sanders D, Deitz M, and Gallagher D: Factors affecting predictability of radial keratotomy, Ophthalmology 1985; 92:1237-1243.

30. Siva Reddy P: Personal communication, 1981.

31. Siva Reddy P and Ranga Reddy P: Anterior keratotomy, Ophthalmic Surg 1980;11:765-767.

32. Utkin VF: Non-perforating peripheral radial keratotomy in treating spherical and aspherical myopia, Ann Ophthalmol USSR 1979;2:21-24.

33. Yenaleyev FS: Experience in surgical treatment of myopia, Ann Ophthalmol USSR 1979;3:52-55.

Development of Refractive Keratotomy in the United States, 1978-1990

George O. Waring III

In contrast to the development of refractive keratotomy in Japan and the Soviet Union, which centered largely on two prominent individuals, its development in the United States from 1978 to the present has been a convoluted jumble of social, economic, political, and scientific forces—a paradigm of modern medicine.

Social: Refractive keratotomy was introduced to the United States largely through the mass media, creating intense public interest.

Economic: A few entrepreneurial ophthalmologists competed for the potential millions of dollars in fees. Management firms established refractive kerato-

BACKGROUND AND ACKNOWLEDGMENTS

This summary of the development of refractive keratotomy in the United States is based on both my personal experience and published information. I have been interested in radial keratotomy since I saw Dr. Leo Bores do a case at Wayne State University in October 1979. Shortly thereafter Bores visited the ophthalmology department at Emory University; he was a visiting lecturer as part of a proposal from Wayne State University for a collaborative clinical trial, which was never implemented. I was a panelist at the first meeting of the Keratorefractive Society in November 1979, served on the society's Patient Examination Committee, and presented a paper at the November 1980 meeting before resigning. I attended the organizational meeting of the National Radial Keratotomy Study Group in late 1979 and was a core investigator for a short time before voluntarily leaving the group. In April 1980 I studied refractive keratotomy with S.N. Fyodorov in Moscow (see Chapter 7, Development of Refractive Keratotomy in the Soviet Union, 1960-1990). In March 1980 and May 1980 I chaired two workshops on refractive keratotomy.[36] Since September 1980, I have been director of the Prospective Evaluation of Radial Keratotomy (PERK) study. I attended the planning meeting of the Analysis of Radial Keratotomy (ARK) Study Group as a consultant in November 1981. Based on these experiences and my personal refractive surgery practice I present my point of view on the development of refractive keratotomy in the United States from these seminal meetings to the present. The opinions of others may differ from mine. This chapter has been previously published in abridged form.[37]

tomy–oriented practices around the country. Optimistic advertising and direct public sales created the most intense commercialization of ophthalmic surgery in the history of the profession.

Political: Numerous organizations that were centered on refractive keratoplasty in general and refractive keratotomy in particular sprang up; relations between these organizations were more acrimonious and litigious than cooperative.

Scientific: Laboratory investigation and clinical modification of the techniques continued in the hands of individual surgeons and collaborative groups.

By the mid-1980s much of the fuss had died down, but the social, economic, political, and scientific elements smoldered along.

INTRODUCTION OF REFRACTIVE KERATOTOMY IN THE UNITED STATES

Ophthalmologists in the United States shunned the early advances of refractive keratotomy. Sato's visit to American universities in 1953 generated little interest, which was a fortunate turn of events in view of the later severe complications with Sato's approach. Imagine Sato's tour occurring in the 1980s. What a flurry of activity and what consequences might have sprung from his enthusiastic portrayal of 15 years of experience with keratotomy.

Fyodorov had extensive contact with ophthalmologists in the United States during the 1970s as his iris-fixated Sputnik lens was introduced into clinical use. But even those early adventuresome implant surgeons were indifferent to his reports and demonstrations of successful refractive keratotomy.

In 1976 Bores traveled from Detroit to Moscow to observe intraocular implant surgery at Fyodorov's institute. During that visit he examined patients who had had refractive keratotomies performed, observed that their myopia had largely disappeared, and proceeded to do a series of six cases with Fyodorov. Returning to the United States, Bores too found indifference among his colleagues when he described the surgery, a reception that was no warmer when Fyodorov lectured at the Kresge Eye Institute of Wayne State University in Detroit in the fall of 1976.

In 1977 Bores returned to Moscow and observed persistent reduction in myopia in patients on whom he performed refractive keratotomy. He did the first refractive keratotomy operation in the United States in November 1978 at the Kresge Eye Institute and proposed a multicenter clinical trial. Bores triggered coverage of the operation by the popular press, which rocketed refractive keratotomy into national view.

Ophthalmologists scurried to study refractive keratotomy and express their opinions about it. Study groups were established, and courses were given; some physicians appeared in the news, extolling or denigrating the procedure; few remained neutral. Some practitioners reoriented their offices and clinical activity, staking their future on refractive keratotomy.

REFRACTIVE KERATOTOMY ORGANIZATIONS

Perhaps the best understanding of the first decade of refractive keratotomy in the United States emerges from a review of the ophthalmic organizations active in promoting or evaluating the procedure—the National Radial Keratotomy Study Group, the Keratorefractive Society, the National Eye Institute, the Prospective Evaluation of Radial Keratotomy (PERK) Study, the Analysis of Radial Keratotomy (ARK) Study Group, and the International Society of Refractive Keratoplasty.

The National Radial Keratotomy Study Group

In 1979 John W. Cowden of Wayne State University collaborated with Bores and William Myers to write a protocol for a nationwide collaborative study of refractive keratotomy that was to involve five university departments of ophthalmology (Wayne State University, Emory University, the University of Maryland, the University of California at Los Angeles, and the University of Arizona) and the Bethany Medical Center in Kansas City. The philosophy of the study was strict—"independent data verification, both preoperatively and postoperatively was mandatory by a surgeon other than the operating surgeon. As a matter of fact, performance of the surgery would disqualify the surgeon from data collection. At six month intervals, the patients were to be seen by a third physician who had never seen them before. . . . In this way we hope to prevent bias from entering the basic studies that were undertaken."[8] The proposed study was never implemented, but the early findings of the Wayne State University group were published.[9]

In late 1979 Bores moved to Santa Fe, New Mexico where he established the National Radial Keratotomy Study Group, comprising approximately 25 ophthalmologists in the "core group" and an ever-increasing number of "adjunct" investigators who took Bores's courses. A press release in early 1980 said that "the operation must be performed under carefully controlled circumstances. Our organization is prepared to train only qualified microsurgeons, who will be required to follow the investigative protocol and report their data to the national group. Only by carefully studying the surgery can we be assured of its safety and efficacy."

The study group met and wrestled with the early

vagaries of the operative procedure, making recommendations for changes in surgical technique, including centrifugal rather than centripetal incisions, use of peripheral deepening incisions, avoiding performing refractive keratotomy on patients with flat corneas, and rejection of Fyodorov's formula, and created data sheets that the investigators were to complete and submit for analysis. Although many ophthalmologists compiled information, the group gradually dissolved without publishing collaborative results.

Bores, apparently feeling unjustly passed over and restricted by events surrounding refractive keratotomy, joined another ophthalmologist and a small group of patients in 1982 and filed a class-action, antitrust lawsuit against 35 members of the National Advisory Eye Council, the National Eye Institute, the American Academy of Ophthalmology, and the PERK study. The suit was settled in a no-fault, out-of-court action (see Chapter 9, Radial Keratotomy on Trial: New Surgical Procedures and the Antitrust Laws).

The Keratorefractive Society

In 1979 a more popularist approach to refractive keratotomy caught the fancy of ophthalmologists in the form of the Keratorefractive Society, a group begun by two brothers, Ronald and Les Schachar, physicians from Denison, Texas. The society was "founded for the express purpose of disseminating and facilitating the exchange of information concerning refractive alterations of the cornea and their surgical correction. It serves as a repository for clinical data obtained under protocol by its members for purposes of analysis and professional evaluation."[32]

The Keratorefractive Society wished to draw on the insights, skills, and experience of all ophthalmologists interested in refractive surgery and espoused the following libertarian philosophy: "The society firmly believes that no single subgroup of surgeons should be the exclusive evaluator of any single procedure. It defends the right of any well-trained and responsible ophthalmologist to undertake clinical investigations under a well-defined protocol with due regard for his patients' informed consent and rights."[32] This come one–come all approach was immensely popular, and the first meeting of the society during the American Academy of Ophthalmology meeting in November 1979 packed the hotel ballroom and extended late into the evening; it was electric and full of excitement and confusion created by this newly popular operation.

At this and subsequent meetings, the presentations were recorded and the slides were photographed—both being published verbatim in a series of proceedings without editing by the authors.[30-33] These volumes make fascinating reading and preserve the sincere struggle of ophthalmologists to make keratotomy an effective, safe, and predictable operation. They also capture the flavor of the political fighting that characterized the times. Annual meetings of the Keratorefractive Society continued to be held through the late 1980s.

The society worked diligently to capture the information and experience in refractive keratotomy that had accumulated in the ophthalmic community. The cornerstone of this effort was a registry. Citing the experience of registries in other areas of medicine, the society created data forms and encouraged ophthalmologists to fill them out and send them to a central location for compilation and analysis. No results have ever been published in the ophthalmic literature from the registry, although a press release in November 1984 described a study of "63,000 patients out of 103,000 compiled by 2,000 members of the Keratorefractive Society."[20]

In an attempt to get the American Academy of Ophthalmology to view refractive keratotomy more favorably, the Keratorefractive Society encouraged the establishment of an ad hoc committee to review the records in the registry. The committee was formed and apparently received some 5000 case records, but the study was never completed.[1]

The National Radial Keratotomy Study Group and the Keratorefractive Society pooled their respective protocols and submitted them as a grant proposal to the National Institutes of Health for a study called Collective Logical Evaluation of Radial Keratotomy (CLERK). The protocol called for 16 surgeons, each of whom had performed more than 100 refractive keratotomies and each to provide data on every eye on which refractive keratotomy was performed, with a minimum of 1 year follow-up. Apparently the CLERK study was approved but not funded.[19]

The basic philosophy of the society turned out to be its major weakness. All ophthalmologists with any experience or opinion about refractive keratotomy were encouraged to present papers at the meetings. All were encouraged to submit data to the registry. Every person could have a say. Quality control was minimal. Because of this, many members resigned, particularly because the society became politically active in its opposition to formal studies of refractive keratotomy.

Some members complained angrily that organized ophthalmology had conspired to prevent them from speaking at national meetings, had blocked their publications in major journals, had interfered with their private practice of keratotomy, and had induced insurance companies not to pay for the procedure. These feelings led a handful of ophthalmologists, R. Schachar, D. Leslie, L. Schachar, N. Stahl, J. Zellman, T. Farkas, H. Bruckner, and G. Simon, to file an antitrust lawsuit in the name of the Keratorefractive Society against selected members of the Board of Directors of the American Academy of Ophthalmology in 1984, accusing them of restraint of trade in refractive keratotomy. A jury cleared the academy of the allegations in May 1988, and a court of appeals upheld the verdict (see Chapter 9, Radial Keratotomy on Trial: New Surgical Procedures and the Antitrust Laws).

The National Eye Institute and the Prospective Evaluation of Radial Keratotomy (PERK) Study

In the late 1970s, before refractive keratotomy hit the American scene, there was an emerging interest in the lamellar refractive keratoplasty techniques of Dr. José Barraquer, resulting in some grant applications to the National Eye Institute (NEI). In early 1979 The National Advisory Eye Council, which serves as the principal advisory body on vision research to the US Secretary of Health and Human Services and to the National Eye Institute, recommended guidelines for the study of refractive keratoplasty.[3] The following guidelines were included in the recommendations[3]:

1. Refractive keratoplasty as a clinical procedure is experimental.
2. Animal experiments which employ this surgical technique should be encouraged.
3. No clinical research employed for refractive keratoplasty should be supported by the National Eye Institute (NEI) until the results of animal research can be evaluated.

   However, the NEI should attempt to gather follow-up data from ophthalmologists on patients who have already undergone this procedure.

By 1980 the intense interest in refractive keratotomy pressured the council to update its opinion, and on May 29, 1980, it issued the following resolution in a position paper:

1. As the principal advisory body to the National Eye Institute, the Federal government's chief source of support for vision research, the National Advisory Eye Council would like to express grave concern about potential widespread adoption of an operation intended to correct nearsightedness, a common condition that can be easily and safely corrected by the use of eyeglasses or contact lenses. The operation, called radial keratotomy, has received widespread publicity during the last year. It involves cutting the cornea with a series of deep incisions that extend from the sclera toward, but not into, the center of the cornea. The incisions are intended to be deep enough to weaken the tissue so that internal eye pressure causes the edge of the cornea to bulge slightly, thereby flattening the central portion of the cornea which improves focusing. The incisions result in permanent corneal scars.
2. The Council considers radial keratotomy to be an experimental procedure because it has not been subjected to adequate scientific evaluation in animals and humans. Recent reports of radial keratotomy from foreign countries and the United States provide an inadequate basis on which to assure the procedure's safety.
3. The Council calls for carefully controlled research on radial keratotomy to determine the effectiveness of the procedure, safety, long-term and short-term side effects, and the best surgical technique. The need for research on radial keratotomy and other forms of surgical correction of refractive errors (myopia, presbyopia, astigmatism) was recognized by the Council in a statement published in the journal "Investigative Ophthalmology and Visual Science" in August, 1979. Until the results of such research are obtained and fully evaluated by the ophthalmological community, the Council urges restraint on the part of both patients and eye surgeons.
4. The Council therefore urges that the National Eye Institute take whatever measures are necessary to encourage animal research on radial keratotomy while limiting clinical research to controlled clinical trials conducted by responsible investigators.
5. The Council strongly urges that its views on the subject of radial keratotomy as expressed in this resolution be announced to the general public, as well as to health care professionals.

Response of the press and the profession was vigorous (Fig. 8-1). The American Academy of Ophthalmology adopted the position of the council, an action that would later spawn antitrust lawsuits, and the International Society of Refractive Keratoplasty adopted the academy's position as well.

In late 1979 there was only one article in the English-language ophthalmic periodical literature presenting results of refractive keratotomy; Fyodorov was published in the *Annals of Ophthalmology*.[15] Clearly the operation was then developing by trial and error, and the proposed informal approaches to studying it were unlikely to yield objective, verifiable information. Therefore to explore more formal methods of studying refractive keratotomy, a group of approximately 15 academic ophthalmologists, including some who had done refractive keratotomy and some who had visited Fyodorov in Moscow, met in March 1980 for a 1-day workshop. This meeting, held in an airport hotel, has been characterized by some as a secret, conspiratorial plot to control the dissemination of keratotomy in the United States. The participants published the following conclusions[38]:

1. Radial keratotomy is a form of refractive keratoplasty that has the potential to reduce myopia in some individuals. The procedure at this time is experimental.

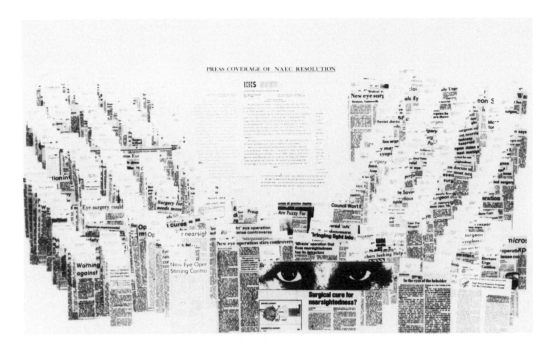

Figure 8-1
Collage of newspaper articles reflects the public interest in the National Advisory Eye Council's statement on radial keratotomy. (Courtesy of Marsha Corbett.)

(The National Advisory Eye Council, Washington, D.C., has also stated that refractive keratoplasty performed on humans is an experimental procedure.)

2. Although the operation can reduce myopia, it is unknown which patients will benefit most from the procedure. The final shape of the cornea, the final refractive error, and the final unaided visual acuity are not predictable.

3. The effect of the operation on the cornea and the eye after many years is unknown.

4. The operation should be performed under an investigational protocol that has been approved by a hospital institutional review board.

5. The operation is best performed under conditions of optimal safety for the patient, including good illumination and magnification with an operating microscope, sterile technique, and immobilization of the globe by retrobulbar anesthesia.

6. Nonsurgical alternatives, such as extended-wear soft contact lenses, may reduce the need for surgery. The Food and Drug Administration should approve extended-wear soft contact lenses for cosmetic use as soon as the data warrant.

Hindsight identifies two glaring errors in these conclusions—the recommendation of retrobulbar anesthesia and the assumption that extended-wear soft contact lenses for cosmetic use would be safer than surgery, an assumption that has been challenged by the emergence of microbial keratitis associated with extended-wear soft contact lenses.[22,34,36]

Many more ophthalmologists attended a second workshop during the Association for Research in Vision and Ophthalmology meeting in May 1980 and created a protocol for a prospective, monitored, multicenter clinical trial that would later become the Prospective Evaluation of Radial Keratotomy (PERK) Study.

In July 1980, 12 requests for grants with the same manual of procedures were submitted to the National Eye Institute where they were reviewed by a Vision Program ad hoc committee. By early 1981, 10 were funded with a caveat by the reviewers[40]:

A difficulty lies in the fact that, ideally, this is not the study that should be done at this point in time. There should be years of research with different animal models to determine safety, efficacy and variations that might produce better results. Here, the human being is really used as the basic research tool in looking at radial keratotomy. This is conscionable only because of the fact that if a small clinical study is not completed now, even greater pressure will exist for the use of the procedure untried and without any knowledge of how safe and efficacious it might be. . . . There is probably no study contemplated now that might have a greater impact on a larger number of patients than this one.

The box on pp. 242-244 lists the investigators in the PERK Study Group. The design of and rationale for the PERK study have been published.

Unfortunately, the desire of ophthalmologists in the National Radial Keratotomy Study Group, the Kera-

The Prospective Evaluation of Radial Keratotomy (PERK)

Coordinating Centers
Clinical Coordinating Center

Emory University, Department of Ophthalmology, Atlanta: George O. Waring III, MD, national director and principal investigator; Ceretha S. Cartwright, DrPh (1980-89), and John T. Carter, PhD (1980-89), national coordinators.

Biostatistical Coordinating Center

Emory University, Department of Biostatistics and Epidemiology, Atlanta: Steven D. Moffit, PhD (1980-83), Michael J. Lynn, MS, Michael H. Kutner, PhD, Brooke Fielding, MS, and Azhar Nizam, MS, principal investigators; Portia Griffin, data coordinator.

Clinical Centers
Emory University, Departent of Ophthalmology, Atlanta

George O. Waring III, MD, principal investigator; H. Dwight Cavanagh, MD, William H. Coles, MD, and Louis A. Wilson, MD, investigators: Eugene Steinberg, LDO, COT (1981-1986), and Mary Gemmill CO, COMT, clinical coordinators.

Louisiana State University Eye Center, New Orleans

Marguerite McDonald, MD, principal investigator; Aran Safir, MD, ; Herbert E. Kaufman, MD, Rise Ochsher, MD, Bruce A. Barron, MD, Joseph A. Baldone, MD, John Lindberg, MD, and Rudy Franklin, MD, investigators; Mike Ostrick, OD (1981-1982), and Deborah Poloson, LDO, CT (1982-1989), clinical coordinators.

University of Miami, Bascom Palmer Eye Institute, Miami

Sidney Mandelbaum, MD, William Culbertson, MD, Henry Gelender, MD, principal investigators; Richard K. Forster, MD, investigator; Teresa Obeso (1981-1983), Mary Anne Edwards (1981-1983), and Millie Espinal, clinical coordinators.

University of Minnesota, Department of Ophthalmology, Minneapolis

Richard L. Lindstrom, MD, and Donald J. Doughman, MD, principal investigators; J. Daniel Nelson, MD, and Douglas Cameron, MD, investigators; Patricia Williams, COT, clinical coordinator.

Mount Sinai School of Medicine, Department of Ophthalmology, New York

Stephen A. Obstbaum, MD, principal investigator; Penny Asbell, MD, Steve M. Podos, MD, Michael J. Newton, MD, and George Pardos, MD, investigators; Norma Justin, COA, clinical coordinator.

University of Oklahoma, McGee Eye Institute, Oklahoma City

J. James Rowsey, MD, principal investigator; Hal D. Balyeat, MD, James C. Hays, MD, and Wayne F. March, MD, investigators; Beth Kuns (1981-1982), Douglas Corley (1982), Becky Hewett, COA (1982-1983), Jack Whiteside, COT (1983-1984), and Janie Shofner, COA, clinical coordinators.

University of Southern California, Estelle Doheny Eye Foundation, Los Angeles

David J. Schanzlin, MD, and Ronald E. Smith, MD, principal investigators; James J. Salz, MD, Douglas L. Steel, MD, and Richard A. Villasenor, MD, investigators; Jan Reinig, LVN (1981-1984), and Jenny Garbus, COT (1981-1989), clinical coordinators.

William Beaumont Eye Clinic, Royal Oak, Michigan

William D. Myers, MD, principal investigator; Robert C. Arends, MD, John W. Cowden, MD, Robert L. Stephenson, MD, Paul Fecko, MD, Jerry Roust, MD, William T. Sallee, MD, and Henry Spiro, MD, investigators; Vicki Roszka-Duggan CO, COMT, clinical coordinator.

Wills Eye Hospital, Philadelphia

Peter R. Laibson, MD, principal investigator; Juan J. Arentsen, MD, Michael A. Naidoff, MD, and Elisabeth Cohen, MD, investigators; Nubia Richman, CO, clinical coordinator.

Reading Centers
Keratography Reading Center

University of Oklahoma, Oklahoma City. J. James Rowsey, MD.

Specular Photomicroscopy Reading Center

Emory University, Atlanta. George O. Waring III, MD.

Psychometric Center

University of California at Los Angeles, School of Public Health, Los Angeles. Linda B. Bourque, PhD.

Clinic Monitoring Group

Jay H. Krachmer, MD, Department of Ophthalmology, University of Iowa, chairperson; James P. McCulley, MD, Department of Ophthalmology, Southwestern Medical School; Walter J. Stark, MD, Wilmer Eye Institute, Johns Hopkins Hospital.

Data and Safety Monitoring Board

Richard A. Thoft, MD, Eye and Ear Hospital, Pittsburgh, chairperson; James V. Aquavella, MD, University of Rochester; Jules L. Baum, MD, Tufts Medical School; Robert J. Hardy, PhD, University of Texas School of Public Health; Jay H. Krachmer, MD, University of Iowa; Robert D. Sperduto, MD, National Eye Institute; Joel Sugar, MD, Illinois Eye and Ear Infirmary; James Ware, PhD, Harvard School of Public Health; George O. Waring III, MD, Emory University; Steven D. Moffitt, PhD, and Michael J. Lynn, MS, Emory University; Aran Safir, MD, University of Connecticut Health Center.

National Eye Institute

Robert D. Sperduto, MD, scientific project officer; Ralph J. Helmsen, PhD, administrative project officer.

Prospective Evaluation of Radial Keratotomy (PERK) Study Investigators

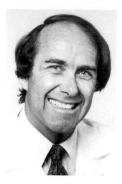

**George O.
Waring III, MD**

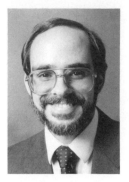

**Michael J.
Lynn, MS**

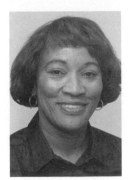

**Ceretha S.
Cartwright, DrPH**

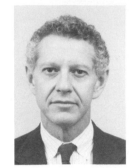

**Richard A.
Thoft, MD**

Left to right

**William Culbertson, MD
Jay H. Krachmer, MD
Peter R. Laibson, MD**

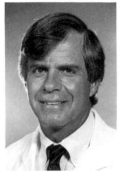
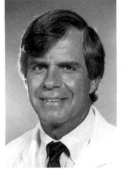
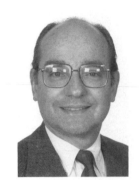

Left to right

**Richard L. Lindstrom, MD
Marguerite McDonald, MD
William D. Myers, MD**

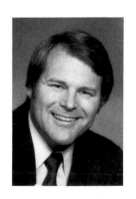
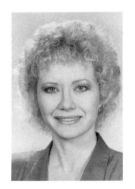
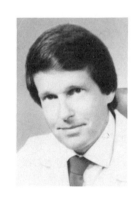

Left to right

**Stephen A. Obstbaum, MD
J. James Rowsey, MD
David J. Schanzlin, MD**

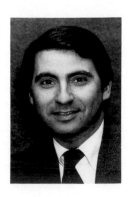
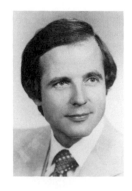
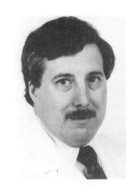

Telegram Aimed at Blocking the PERK Study

Western Union Mailgram 05/07/81

Senator Jesse Helms
Senate Office Bldg.
Washington, DC 10510

Honorable Senator Helms,

The National Eye Institute has recently funded, for 2.4 million dollars, a Prospective Evaluation of Radial Keratotomy (PERK) under grant numbers: EY37611, EY37511, EY37521, EY3752, EY3753, EY3755, EY3756, EY3764, EY3765, EY3767. This study has been undertaken for the past 2½ years and is ongoing in the private sector at no cost to the government. This grant represents unnecessary duplication and waste of government spending and funding of the 2.4 million dollars and should be withdrawn immediately and applied to more worthy eye research. Your prompt attention to this unwarranted allocation of government funds is needed.

Ronald A. Schachar, MD, Ph.D., F.A.C.S.
Secretary of the Keratorefractive Society;
Adjunct Professor, Department of Physics,
University of Texas at Arlington,
Arlington, Texas;
Director of Texoma Eye Institute
Denison, Texas

torefractive Society, the National Eye Institute, and the PERK Study Group to find the truth about refractive keratotomy turned into a political struggle that led to an interesting scenario in the spring of 1981.

Ronald Schachar, on behalf of the Keratorefractive Society, mounted a campaign to prevent the implementation of the PERK study. Through telegrams (refer to the box above) and letters he lobbied federal congressional officials to stop the PERK study. Taking up the charge was U.S. Representative Eugene Johnston, a Republican from North Carolina who had had an apparently successful refractive keratotomy and accused the National Eye Institute of "reinventing the wheel" by funding a study of an operation that had already been proved safe and effective. In response the National Eye Institute convened a panel of ophthalmologists and biostatisticians to review the information collected by the Keratorefractive Society, the National Radial Keratotomy Study Group, and others. Oral presentations and panel discussions were followed by submission of written data for evaluation.

A reporter captured the scene[35]:

A modern day medicine show surged into the usually composed National Institutes of Health campus Thursday, sending forth an array of claims, confessions, and cajolery in

behalf of refractive keratotomy. . . . A Washington public relations firm fired off a news release heralding a government versus private doctor battle over the new surgery and announcing the 'confrontation' would come Thursday afternoon. The NEI quickly countered, holding a news conference Thursday morning during which Carl Kupfer, M.D., NEI Director, outlined the skepticism toward the experimental procedure and the protocol behind the 5 year, 2.4 million dollar PERK study. The medicine wagon ascended that afternoon, driven by keratotomists Ronald Schachar, William Myers, and Leo Bores. They had varied and telling support from a seeing-is-believing North Carolina congressman, a Canadian statistician who compared eye surgery to hip replacement, a boisterous lawyer accusing the medical-research establishment of cover-up, and a dozen very satisfied patients reading 20/15 to 20/40 from an illuminated eye chart.

Neither the Keratorefractive Society nor the National Radial Keratotomy Study Group presented or submitted data. Data were submitted by a few individual ophthalmologists. All of the information was reviewed by the panel, which concluded, "Although their data exceeded requirements for medical and surgical practice purposes, they nonetheless were grossly inadequate for a critical and comprehensive evaluation of the safety and efficacy of refractive keratotomy.

Their data do not answer questions to be addressed by the PERK study. Consequently, it is appropriate that the NEI proceed with plans to support a clinical trial of refractive keratotomy."[8,26,40]

The critics of the PERK study pointed out that only five of the approximately 28 investigators had experience with refractive keratotomy, so William Myers and John Cowden, two ophthalmologists with extensive experience with refractive keratotomy, and three of their associates joined the study. This balanced the PERK investigators to include 12 full-time university professors (29%), 18 geographic, full-time practitioners (44%), and 11 full-time private practitioners (27%).

The American Academy of Ophthalmology also issued the following statement about the PERK study: "The Academy believes that this clinical trial is necessary to validate the predictability of this surgical procedure, its safety and its short-term and long-term effects. Using individual surgical experiences to answer questions of safety and efficacy of a new surgical procedure does not serve to protect the health and well-being of our nation's citizens."[2] This support would later be construed as conspiratorial antitrust activity (Chapter 9, Radial Keratotomy on Trial: New Surgical Procedures and the Antitrust Laws).

The PERK study was funded and implemented. The most difficult aspect of establishing the PERK study was deciding on a surgical protocol. The investigators consulted Fyodorov, Bores, Deitz, Myers, and others who had experience with refractive keratotomy, seeking a consensus about the most useful, standardized procedure. They decided on eight incisions with the diameter of the clear zone based on the spherical equivalent of the refractive error. Interestingly the effect of age on the outcome was not appreciated at that time.

The standard instruments used for refractive keratotomy in 1980 were optical pachometry, metal-bladed knives, and ruler-style gauge blocks. To take advantage of improved technology, the PERK investigators called a moratorium on starting the study so that they could incorporate ultrasonic pachometers, diamond-bladed micrometer knives, and a ridge-style gauge block with a knife cradle—all advances that improved the accuracy and precision of the surgery.

By 1990, members of the PERK Study Group, had published more than 55 articles and abstracts, including the 4-year results published in the *Journal of the American Medical Association*[39] in February 1990.

Analysis of Radial Keratotomy (ARK) Study

Even though thousands of refractive keratotomies had been performed in the United States by 1981, it was difficult to extract data from those procedures that would satisfy critical observers. Therefore Donald Sanders visited the offices of several ophthalmologists who performed refractive keratotomy and in November 1981 started a "high-quality, scientifically rigorous" study involving three private surgeons and two university-based biostatisticians, receiving a National Eye Institute grant to initiate the Analysis of Radial Keratotomy (ARK) Study.[22] The collaboration has proved fruitful, resulting in a series of papers with intermediate term follow-up data.[4-7,10-13,24,25,27-29]

Although the ARK group disbanded in 1983 over disputes concerning commercial aspects of predictability software packages, all of the members have continued to publish useful and meaningful results from their individual practices, emphasizing the value of ongoing collaboration between clinicians and statisticians.[6,13,29]

International Society of Refractive Keratoplasty (ISRK)

The International Society of Refractive Keratoplasty was originally established in the mid-1970s as a study group for the Barraquer lamellar refractive surgical procedures. The society grew gradually and was formally incorporated by Miles Friedlander, Richard Troutman, and Jose Barraquer in November 1979 "to promote, aid, encourage, and foster scientific research, study, and investigation of refractive surgery, as well as the education and dissemination of knowledge in relation to refractive surgery." The society meets twice yearly, usually collaboratively with other societies and often internationally.

The society was not drawn directly into the refractive keratotomy fray, but instead opted for a broader perspective in refractive surgery, offering courses and programs balanced among keratomileusis, epikeratoplasty, and refractive keratotomy, with the later introduction of courses and programs on intracorneal lenses and laser refractive surgery.

The society sponsors a journal, *Refractive and Corneal Surgery*,[16] a peer-reviewed publication first published in 1985 as the *Journal of Refractive Surgery*.

Other professional organizations

In the late 1980s numerous refractive surgical societies were formed throughout the world, on both national and regional lines. For example, the European Refractive Surgical Society, has joined the International Society of Refractive Keratoplasty in sponsoring *Refractive and Corneal Surgery.*

Many cataract and intraocular lens societies sought to broaden their scope by including refractive surgery in their programs. For example, in 1986 the American

Intraocular Implant Society changed its name to the American Society of Cataract and Refractive Surgery. In 1987 the European Intraocular Implant Council christened the *European Journal of Implant and Refractive Surgery*, and the *International Intraocular Implant and Refractive Surgery Journal* also appeared in the late 1980s.

OPHTHALMIC PRACTITIONERS AND THE PUBLIC

Outside the arena of organized societies and study groups, ophthalmic practitioners and nearsighted patients in the early 1980s faced an onslaught of information about refractive keratotomy in the professional and popular press. The public seemed to respond reflexly to whoever was making the most noise with the most interesting story. The upbeat coverage focused on the import of high technology from the Soviet Union and often featured a local practitioner doing his first or second procedure. For example, in 1983 *Family Circle* magazine carried an article in its "True Life Drama" section entitled, "Lee Teste's Private Miracle," in which a 30-year-old woman acquired "perfect vision" from refractive keratotomy just in time to get married without her glasses. *Los Angeles Times* headlines reflected the atmosphere: "Eye Surgery Pitch—Is it Hype or Hope?"[17]

This intense publicity generated a stampede of inquiries from eager myopes pressing their ophthalmologists for the new operation. The beleaguered practitioners responded in different ways. The majority (over 90%) took a wait-and-see attitude, most resisting the idea of performing surgery on a structurally normal eye. A few rushed to Moscow or took regional courses, performing at least one or two cases, responding to the increased competitive pressures with the feeling, "I missed out on phaco, I missed out IOLs, I ain't missin' out on RK." A handful made refractive keratotomy a major part of their practice, renaming their office an "institute," developing outpatient surgical centers, and launching marketing campaigns.

In this climate, conflicts arose, pitting the enthusiastic innovators against the conservative skeptics (see Chapter 4, Development and Classification of Refractive Surgical Procedures).

The enthusiasts claimed that their personal experience and extensive practices would unravel the mysteries of radial keratotomy and that opposition from their colleagues, institutional review boards, and state ophthalmologic societies were politically and economically motivated.

The conservative majority feared that the procedure was being evaluated in the marketplace rather in the laboratory and the clinic, so it was in danger of becoming popular before it could be adequately tested according to peer-reviewed scientific standards. They reacted to protect the public interest and customary practice by publicly urging restraint. A few state ophthalmologic societies passed resolutions defining the criteria under which refractive keratotomy should be performed, a pattern emulated by hospitals and institutional review boards. In their zeal to prevent damage from the keratotomy wildfire, some authorities created unrealistic constraints, such as the Arizona hospital that stipulated that only a PERK investigator working on the PERK protocol could perform refractive keratotomy; there was no PERK center in Arizona.[21]

Average practitioners were also concerned that avaricious keratotomists would launch a marketing blitz, not only duping the unwary public with an unestablished operation, but also drawing patients away from the average practitioners' practices with unfounded claims.[31] Articulate expressions of this opinion appeared, including the editorials by Dr. George Weinstein and Dr. Byron Demorest (see the boxes on pp. 248 and 249).

The economic force was powerful, the arithmetic simple. Approximately 10 million myopes in the United States were potential candidates for refractive keratotomy. At $1500 per eye, this represented a $30 billion market, or approximately $2 million for each of the 15,000 ophthalmologists in the United States. An ophthalmologist who might do five refractive keratotomies on both Tuesday and Thursday mornings each week would add three quarters of a million dollars to his annual income (500 eyes × $1500). At a time when cost containment in medicine was a major economic issue, some wondered how a fee of $1500 was set for an operation that took less than 15 minutes.

As expected, competition increased. The *Los Angeles Times* headlined, "Medical Price War Erupts Over Controversial Eye Surgery. The competition for radial keratotomy business in Phoenix drops the cost from $1500 to $495."[18] Other ophthalmologists took to the courts to get their due. For example, the antitrust lawsuits filed by Bores, Schachar, and their colleagues claimed that the defendants interfered with "interstate commerce in refractive keratotomy." One suit was filed for $75 million (triple damages). (See Chapter 9.)

Some have characterized the uproar as a struggle between academic professors and private practitioners, a classic town-gown conflict. Nothing could be further from the truth. Most university eye departments were not interested in refractive keratotomy. The PERK and ARK studies were collaborations among individuals in both university and private practice. The struggle fol-

The Buccaneer Eye Surgeon

It seemed to start with phaco-emulsification, although it surely had been around a long time before that. Phaco-emulsification, though, did appear to release on the American scene a large number of previously unheard of eye surgeons whose excellent technical skills and business acumen remain untinged by traditional medical ethics. The trend continued with the introduction of intraocular lens implants, and has now been further extended with radial keratotomy. The phenomenon certainly must be one of the most talked about (and least written about) in the modern ophthalmic era.

What have been the common factors during each of these episodes? Firstly, each has developed around a new technical advance whose merits, while controversial, appear promising. Secondly, the printed and electronic media have been the means for introducing information about the new technique not only to the public at large, but to the medical profession. But the third, and by far the most important, ingredient in this familiar formula is the buccaneer eye surgeon who is willing to turn the potentially useful but still unproven surgical procedure into personal profit. None of us are unaware that a large number of such individuals become wealthy, unashamedly advertising their high-priced services to attract the gullible consumer, the patient.

There is nothing evil about phaco-emulsification, intraocular lens implantation or radial keratotomy per se. But those who perform these operations to plunder the public are the shame of ophthalmology. Let us not remain silent about them. Our society has made the task more difficult by tying the hands of medical societies and state licensure boards with "restraint of trade" regulations and legal precedents. But no one, not the Federal Trade Commission nor the attorneys who are so readily available to represent all forms of scoundrels, need tell us what we know to be true. The ethics of the medical profession are based on the interests of the patient, not those of the physician. The buccaneer eye surgeons are not our folk heroes. They should be exposed to the public for what they are.

George W. Weinstein, MD
Editor, *Ophthalmic Surgery*
From Weinstein G: Ophthalmic Surg 1980;11:831.

---

lowed another classic pattern: the conflict between enthusiastic innovators anxious to promulgate their new procedure and traditional conservatives more concerned about public health and the integrity of the profession. In fact, the major opposition to the rampant spread of refractive keratotomy came from the grass-roots, private practicing ophthalmologists.

Many ophthalmologists sought to balance the interests of the innovators, the average practitioner, and the public. Most agreed that refractive keratotomy should be fairly tested and should be available to well-informed patients who desired it. Consensus would not come easily.

An example of the effort put forth to achieve these goals occurred in Georgia, where the state ophthalmological society, a university, and a private hospital created a community-based study of refractive keratotomy. A committee of private practitioners directed the study, which consisted of a practical prospective protocol, a laboratory training course attended by many ophthalmologists, and provision of both equipment and a technician-coordinator by the hospital. The protocol stipulated a standardized surgical technique to be performed without charge to the patient and routine, fee-for-service, follow-up care in the surgeon's office. After a year of planning and implementation, only four cases had been done; the study was abandoned.

The American Academy of Ophthalmology, representing most of the practicing ophthalmologists in the United States, made numerous attempts to provide leadership by clarifying questions about refractive keratotomy for both practitioners and the public. In 1981 the academy did a simple and logical thing; it endorsed the statement issued by the National Advisory Eye Council that designated refractive keratotomy experimental. In 1983 the academy issued its own

They Are Not My Colleagues

Entrepreneurs, advertisers, buccaneers, cataract cowboys—call them what you will—they have all had an unsettling impact on the field of ophthalmology. They have been accused by Congressman Claude Pepper of "fraud—waste—and abuse," and they have been targeted by the Inspector General's Office of HCFA for their "aberrant practice patterns." This is not ophthalmology's finest hour. While bringing the wrath of the government and third-party payers down on all of us, they complain that organized ophthalmology has not worked hard enough politically to defend their fees and practice patterns.

They escape peer review and are suspect of performing unneeded surgery. They "seine the waters" with cruising buses, vans and limos, picking up trusting elderly patients who have suffered visual loss. They advertise in newspapers and on radio and TV, aggrandizing their own abilities and the ease and low risks of surgery.

They rarely participate in collegial activities for professional growth through continuing education. Some of their foundations charge substantial fees to teach technique. They usually do not volunteer to teach, even though others gave up time and income to teach them. They look upon each patient as a financial opportunity, not as a person to be helped. They abdicate postoperative care to poorly trained ancillary personnel, to assure a source of referral for greater personal gain.

They rely on the high esteem that most ophthalmologists have earned from their patients, yet they destroy the very foundations that have allowed us to gain this respect. Their antics and their high incomes bring criticism of all ophthalmologists from physicians in other fields of practice.

Relentlessly and aggressively, they compete for patients with all ophthalmologists while laughing at the codes of ethics and professionalism that most of us support. They serve as poor role models for physicians in training, yet their financial successes tantalizingly encourage greed and avarice that should be suppressed by caring physicians.

They are no longer my colleagues. They have crossed the line into a method and mode of practice that I cannot support. They do not believe in my ethical code, my ideals, or my approach to patients.

The government has declared that they are responsible for the high costs of medical care, for unnecessary surgery and for poor quality. Any governmental intervention to correct this will penalize all of us, and they who have carelessly brought down the wrath of Congress on all of ophthalmology will cry the loudest as they accuse the rest of us for not defending their right to bill and practice as they wish.

They are no longer my colleagues, and it is time to let them know.

Byron Demorest, MD
Past President, American Academy of Ophthalmology

From Demorest B: Argus 1987;10:4.

terse statement about refractive keratotomy, labeling the procedure investigational and calling for a cautious evaluation. By 1985 considerable information was available about the procedure, and the academy's Ad Hoc Committee on Ophthalmic Procedures Assessment assembled a panel of eight experts to prepare a consensus document on refractive keratotomy. The document was intended to review the published information about the procedure and provide a summary that would be more useful than the terse, one-page, 1983 statement. During approximately 18 months, the panel gradually expanded to 17 members, as proponents and opponents of refractive keratotomy lobbied to add supporters of their point of view. By 1987 the group, which had revised the document many times, was hopelessly bogged down in rancorous debate, nit-picking obstructionism, and reactionary bickering. No consensus could be reached, and the deliberations ended in stalemate, leaving the outdated 1983 statement as the official academy position in 1985. In 1988 the committee asked the panel to self-select a smaller group of 10 participants, who successfully produced the document (presented in Appendix B, Position Statements on Radial Keratotomy), which was approved by the Academy Board of Directors on September 10, 1988.

In the latter half of the 1980s, two forces calmed the debate over keratotomy and reduced its popularity. The first was the publication of studies from the PERK group, the ARK group, and other investigators, which took a lot of the mystery out of refractive keratotomy and statistically defined its safety, efficacy, predictability, and stability. The second was reduced insurance coverage. Most insurance companies steadfastly refused to pay for refractive keratotomy, many of them hiding behind the skirts of the Academy's 1983 "investigational" statement. Malpractice premiums increased for keratotomy surgeons, some carriers refusing to extend any coverage for the operation. This combination of scientific data, decreased economic incentive, and increased risk lowered the enthusiasm among ophthalmologists and the public alike.

By the late 1980s keratotomy had emerged from the fire storm of publicity and politics with both strengths and weaknesses and had settled into the more rational world of alternative medical procedures, waiting for further improvements.

CLINICAL DEVELOPMENT OF KERATOTOMY

The clinical and scientific development of keratotomy in the United States involved the experience, insights, and studies of dozens of ophthalmologists working rapidly in an unstructured setting. It is difficult to identify which people were responsible for which innovations and advances.

Table 8-1 emphasizes the major clinical developments in keratotomy that occurred in the United States between the late 1970s and the late 1980s. Continued efforts to improve the surgical technique fostered a proliferation of new surgical instruments. Figures 8-2 through 8-12 portray some of the instruments that evolved during this developmental period but are not in current use. Current practices are described in other chapters.

Text continued on p. 256.

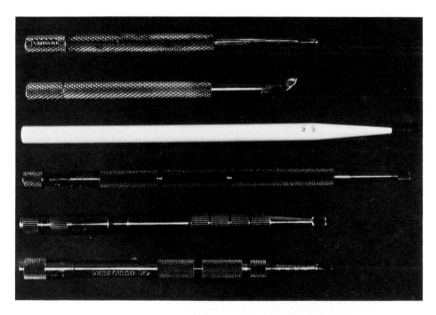

Figure 8-2
Array of knives used during the early development of refractive keratotomy. From bottom to top: straight-pointed blade breaker, angled flat-tipped blade breaker, fixed length disposable blade, diamond knife advanced in steps, diamond knife with screw advance without calibration, and early diamond micrometer knife.

Figure 8-3
Metal blades used for refractive keratotomy. **A,** Carbon steel Feather razor blade and pre-prepared stainless steel blade. **B,** Angled flat-tipped razor blade holder with razor blade fragment in tip.

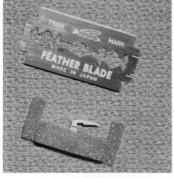

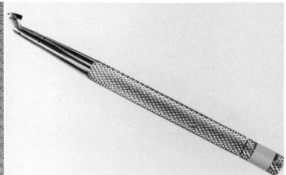

A   B

Table 8-1

Developments in Radial and Astigmatic Keratotomy Between 1978 and 1990 in the United States

	General procedures in the late 1970s	General procedures in the early 1990s
General range of myopia	−2.00 to −12.00 D	−1.50 to −6.00 D
Anesthesia	Retrobulbar	Topical, peribulbar
Pupil	Dilated	Natural
Central mark	Corneal light reflection	Center of pupil
Diameter of clear zone	3 to 5 mm	3 to 4.5 mm
Clear zone marker	Calipers	Circular marker
Fixation device	Single prong forceps	Double prong forceps, compression ring
Knife blade	Razor blade	Diamond, vertical blade
Knife handle	Blade breaker	Micrometer
Footplates	Narrow	Broad
Gauge block	Grooved edge	Raised edge, micrometer microscope
Number of incisions	16	8 or 4
Most important part of incision	Peripheral	Paracentral
Direction of incisions	Centrifugal	Centripetal
Peripheral end of incisions	In sclera	In cornea
Astigmatism incisions	Grouped refractive, intersecting straight transverse	Nonintersecting transverse, arcuate
Achieved depth of incision	75%	90%
Incision depth gauge	Yes	No
Repeated keratotomy	Recut in same scars	Cut between incisions, open and deepen incisions
Postoperative patching	Yes	No
Major patient characteristics used to determine surgical plan	Amount of myopia, corneal thickness, corneal curvature, corneal diameter, ocular rigidity	Amount of myopia, corneal thickness, patient age

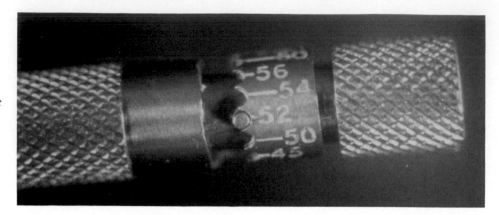

Figure 8-4
Early diamond-bladed knife with step-advance in increments of about 0.02 mm.

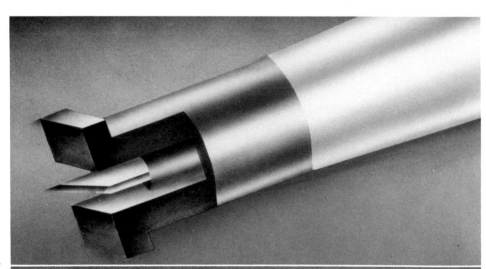

Figure 8-5
Early footplate design for diamond-bladed knives. **A,** "Pontoon" footplate coated with teflon for better gliding (1980). **B,** Narrow, squared-off design (1982). (Courtesy of Spencer Thornton, M.D.)

A

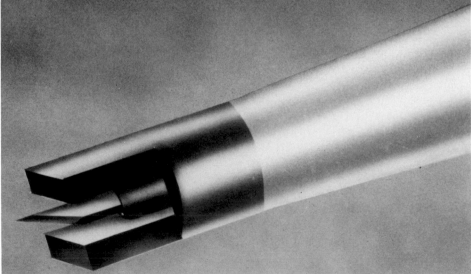

B

A   B

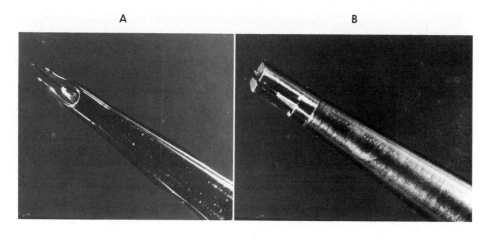

Figure 8-6
Early footplate designs.
A, Very narrow footplates that tended to fall into the wound. **B,** Very wide footplates that obscured the view of the blade.

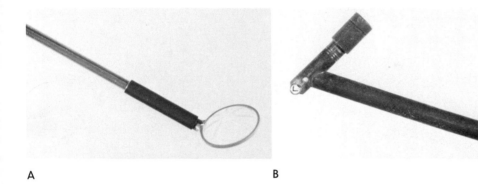

A   B

Figure 8-7
Template system for radial keratotomy designed by David MacIntyre, M.D.
A, Plastic template with radial grooves is placed over the cornea. **B,** Diamond-bladed knife glides through the groove to make the incision of calibrated depth.

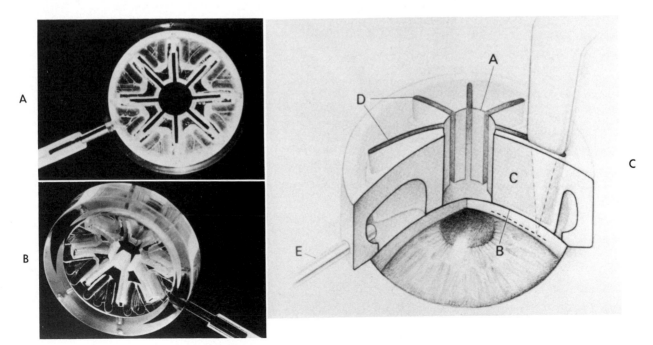

Figure 8-8
Suction-template system reported by Steven Kramer, M.D. **A,** Superior surface of suction template with radial grooves to guide knife. **B,** Inferior surface of suction template with radial grooves to guide knife. **C,** Diagram illustrates *A,* central opening for visual axis, *B,* curved base, *C,* solid struts, *D,* radially oriented slits, and *E,* suction source. (From Kramer SG: Ophthalmol Surg 1981;12:561-566.)

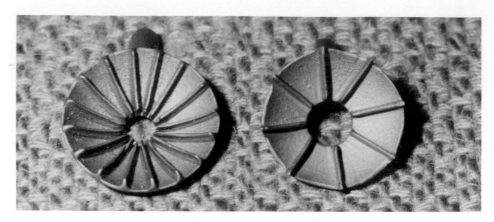

Figure 8-9
Early radial "pizza cutter" markers with 16 *(left)* and 8 *(right)* lines.

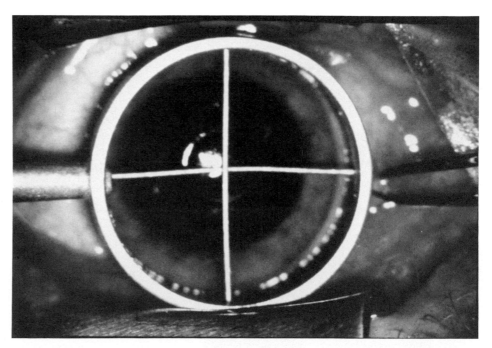

Figure 8-10
Eleven mm diameter marker that was used to make all incisions the same length by locating the peripheral end of the incision. When centered around the center mark, the marker overlapped the limbus eccentrically, so it was seldom used.

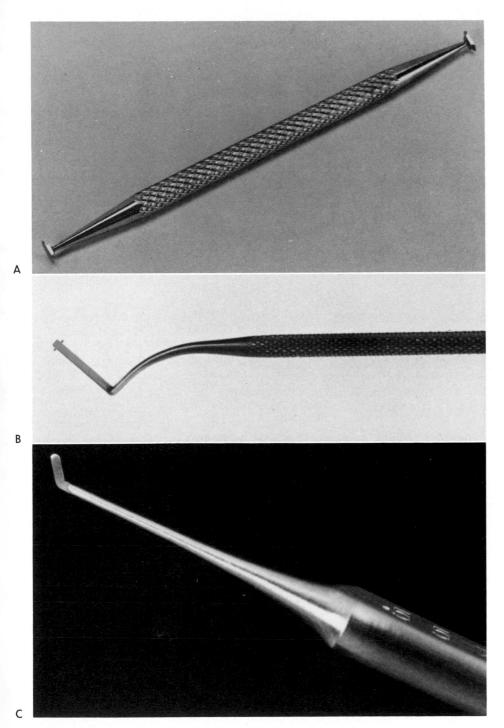

Figure 8-11
Depth gauge "dipsticks" used to measure the depth of the incision. These instruments were inaccurate and impractical because of the corneal edema around the incision, the displacement of the deep stroma, and the requirement for micron accuracy. **A,** Shepard style. **B,** Neumann style. **C,** Deitz style.

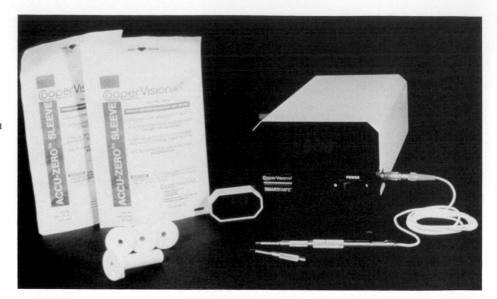

Figure 8-12
Cooper "smart knife" used a helium-neon laser beam to measure the length of the knife blade. (Courtesy of Cooper Vision.)

DEVELOPMENT OF KERATOTOMY OUTSIDE THE UNITED STATES

In general, public and professional interest in keratotomy moved more slowly outside the United States, largely because of the absence of physician advertising, free-market, financial incentives, and the generally more conservative attitude toward medical innovation.

The pattern was similar in many countries. Individual ophthalmologists interested in keratotomy would study outside their country and then return to offer the procedure as part of their practice. The established ophthalmic community often scorned and criticized these bold individualists.

By 1990 keratotomy was being done by some ophthalmologists throughout Canada, South America, Europe, and the United Kingdom. Fewer ophthalmologists offered the operation in Africa, Asia, and the Middle East.

UNFINISHED BUSINESS

The major need from surgeons who do refractive keratotomy in the United States is for well-designed prospective trials of contemporary surgical techniques, including specifically published surgical planning algorithms, four-incision cases, centripetal incisions, and the like.

REFERENCES

1. Abelson M and Ganley J: The American Academy of Ophthalmology and radial keratotomy. In Schachar RA, Levy NS, and Schachar L, editors: Refractive keratoplasty, Denison, Tex, 1983, LAL Publishing, pp 152-155.
2. American Academy of Ophthalmology: Statement on radial keratotomy, June 10, 1981.
3. Announcement: National Advisory Eye Council meetings. Refractive Keratoplasty, Invest Ophthalmol Vis Sci 1979;18:882.
4. Arrowsmith PN and Marks RF: Visual, radial, and keratometric results of radial keratotomy: one year follow-up, Arch Ophthalmol 1984;102:1612-1617.
5. Arrowsmith PN and Marks RF: Evaluating the predictability of radial keratotomy, Ophthalmology 1985;92:331-338.
6. Arrowsmith PN and Marks RF: Visual, radial, and keratometric results of radial keratotomy: a two-year follow-up, Arch Ophthalmol 1989;107:506-510.
7. Arrowsmith PN, Sanders DR, and Marks RG: Visual, radial, and keratometric results of radial keratotomy, Arch Ophthalmol 1983; 101:873-881.
8. Bores L: Purpose, protocol and goals of the National Radial Keratotomy Study Group. In Schachar RA, Levy NS, and Schachar L, editors: Radial keratotomy, Denison, Tex, 1983, LAL Publishing, pp 21-23.
9. Bores LD, Myers W, and Cowden J: Radial keratotomy: an analysis of the American experience, Ann Ophthalmol 1981;13:941-948.
10. Deitz MR and Sanders DR: Progressive hyperopia with long-term follow-up of radial keratotomy, Arch Ophthalmol 1985;103:782-784.
11. Deitz MR, Sanders DR, and Marks RF: Radial keratotomy: an overview of the Kansas City study, Ophthalmology 1984;91:467-478.
12. Deitz MR, Sanders DR, and Raanan MG: Progressive hyperopia in radial keratotomy: long-term follow-up of diamond knife and metal blade series, Ophthalmology 1986;93:1284-1289.

13. Deitz MR, Sanders DR, and Raanan MG: A consecutive series (1982-1985) of radial keratotomies performed with the diamond blade. II. Am J Ophthalmol 1987;103:417-422.
14. Demorest B: They are not my colleagues, Argus 1987;10(7):4.
15. Fyodorov SN and Durnev VV: Operation of dosaged dissection of corneal circular ligament in cases of myopia of mild degree, Ann Ophthalmol 1979;11:1885-1890.
16. Refractive and Corneal Surgery, (originally Journal of Refractive Surgery), Slack, Inc., 6900 Grove Road, Thorofare, NJ 08086.
17. LA Times, March 3, 1985.
18. LA Times, February 9, 1986.
19. Levy NS: CLERK. In Schachar RA, Levy NS, and Schachar L, editors: Refractive keratoplasty, Denison, Tex, 1983, LAL Publishing, pp 139-140.
20. Omaha World Herald, "Surgery to Treat Nearsightedness 'Safe and Effective,' Survey Says" November 12, 1984.
21. Pallin S: Arizona and radial keratotomy. In Schachar RA, Levy NS, and Schachar L, editors: Refractive keratoplasty, Denison, Tex, 1983, LAL Publishing, pp 149-151.
22. Poggio EC, Glynn RJ, Schein OD, Saddon JM, Shannon MJ, and Scardino VA et al: Incidence of ulcerative keratitis among users of daily-wear and extended-wear soft contact lenses, NEJM 1989;321:779-783.
23. Sanders D, editor: Radial keratotomy, Thorofare, NJ, 1984, Slack, Inc.
24. Sanders DR, Deitz MR, and Gallagher D: Factors affecting predictability of radial keratotomy, Ophthalmology 1985;92:1237-1243.
25. Sanders D, Deitz M, Lindstrom R, and Salz J: Computer-aided radial keratotomy predictability programs: comparison of DRS and AMark formulas, J Refract Surg 1986;2:119-123.
26. Sanders D, Marks RG, Deitz MR, Sawelson H, and Arrowsmith PN: Evolution of the ARK study. In Sanders D, editor: Radial keratotomy, Thorofare, NJ, 1984, Slack, Inc, pp 3-6.

27. Sanders DR, Retzlaff J, and Deitz MR: Deitz-Retzlaff-Sanders (DRS) formulas: determination of radial keratotomy surgical parameters, J Refract Surg 1985;1:75-79.
28. Sawelson H and Marks RF: Two-year results of radial keratotomy, Arch Ophthalmol 1985;103:505-510.
29. Sawelson H and Marks RF: Five-year results of radial keratotomy, Refractive Corneal Surg 1989;5:8-20.
30. Schachar RA, Levy NS, and Schachar L: Keratorefraction, Denison, Tex, 1980, LAL Publishing.
31. Schachar RA, Levy NS, and Schachar L: Radial keratotomy, Denison, Tex, 1980, LAL Publishing.
32. Schachar RA, Levy NS, and Schachar L: Refractive modulation of the cornea, Denison, Tex, 1981, LAL Publishing.
33. Schachar RA, Levy NS, and Schachar L: Refractive keratoplasty, Denison, Tex, 1983, LAL Publishing.
34. Schein OD, Glynn RJ, Poggio EC, Saddon JM, and Kenyon KR: Relative risk of ulcerative keratitis among users of daily-wear and extended-wear soft contact lenses: a case control study, N Engl J Med 1989;321:773-778.
35. Sonnebone C: Washington report, Washington, DC, 1981, American Academy of Ophthalmology.
36. Stenson S: Contact lenses and corneal infection, Arch Ophthalmol 1986; 104:1287 (editorial).
37. Waring GO: Radial keratotomy in the United States: the turbulent decade, J Refract Surg 1988;4:204-208.
38. Waring GO and Krachmer J: Conclusions from the workshop on radial keratotomy for myopia, Arch Ophthalmol 1980;98:1377.
39. Waring GO, Lynn MJ, Fielding B, Asbell PA, Balyeat HD, Cohen EA, et al, and the PERK Study Group: Results of the Prospective Evaluation of Radial Keratotomy (PERK) study 4 years after surgery for myopia, JAMA 1990; 263:1083-1091.
40. Waring GO, Moffitt SD, Gelender H, et al: Rationale for and design of the National Eye Institute Prospective Evaluation of Radial Keratotomy (PERK) study, Ophthalmology 1983;90:40-58.
41. Weinstein G: The buccaneer eye surgeon, Ophthalmic Surg 1980;11:831.

Radial Keratotomy on Trial: New Surgical Procedures and the Antitrust Laws*

William S. Duffey, Jr.

In the United States the introduction of radial keratotomy to ophthalmologists' arsenal of available surgical procedures sparked criticism and controversy. There were ophthalmologists who wanted to disseminate this simple and lucrative new surgical technique immediately and without further study. On the other hand, some ophthalmologists sought to investigate the surgery thoroughly by subjecting the procedure to the close and careful scrutiny of an extensive, peer-reviewed clinical trial. This latter group of surgeons urged that the surgery not be performed generally until additional objective information about it was available.

The debate between these two groups of physicians was heated. Those who encouraged the proliferation of the procedure claimed that the ophthalmologists who urged caution were ignoring existing data and were acting simply to control the operation for their own benefit. Those who urged caution countered by claiming that the procedure was proliferating before it was adequately tested. Ophthalmologists who urged caution also claimed that some ophthalmologists

---

*In this chapter the term "radial" is used to include keratotomy for myopia and astigmatism (refractive keratotomy).

BACKGROUND AND ACKNOWLEDGMENTS

Any billion dollar undertaking, especially one that generates public attention, is likely to engender disputes and litigation. Refractive keratotomy qualifies on all counts. Lawsuits concerning refractive keratotomy have pitted doctor against doctor, patient against doctor, doctor against businessman, professional organizations against the government, patients against insurance companies, employees against employers; it's as if the operation were a legal lightening rod. The lawsuits with the highest stakes have been the two antitrust actions described in this chapter by William S. Duffey, Jr., a partner in the law firm of King & Spalding in Atlanta, Georgia. Duffey was a member of the defense team that represented the defendants in the *Vest v. Waring* litigation described in this chapter. The context within which these lawsuits arose has been described in Chapter 8, Development of Refractive Keratotomy in the United States, 1978-1990. Mr. Duffey goes beyond a review of the two legal cases to discuss the overall matter of antitrust laws that apply to new medical and surgical procedures, information that will be of interest to a broad spectrum of readers.

were misrepresenting the operation and its prospects for success to the public.

The dispute transcended debate when Drs. Leo Bores, Robert Marmer, and a handful of their patients instituted a class-action lawsuit in February 1982 against certain physicians involved in the Prospective Evaluation of Radial Keratotomy (PERK) study, members of the Board of Directors of the American Academy of Ophthalmology, members of the National Advisory Eye Council, officials of the National Eye Institute, and the National Eye Institute itself. The major accusation was that the defendants conspired to restrain performance of radial keratotomy in violation of federal antitrust laws.

Dr. Ronald A. Schachar and several other ophthalmologists filed a case against the American Academy of Ophthalmology and its directors 2 years later. This second lawsuit involved antitrust allegations that were essentially the same as Bores and Marmer's allegations. During the course of these two cases, proponents and opponents of radial keratotomy battled over the propriety of the conduct of those ophthalmologists who urged caution in performing radial keratotomy and who sought to scrutinize the unfettered proliferation of the procedure in the United States. Although this litigation provides some guidance regarding the propriety of ophthalmologists who perform radial keratotomy, it has not resolved the issue of such conduct entirely.

In this chapter we not only review these two cases, but also provide a general framework for use in analyzing potential antitrust implications of conduct intended to affect the introduction and practice of new surgical procedures.

SHERMAN ANTITRUST ACT AND TWO RADIAL KERATOTOMY CASES

The central focus of *Vest v. Waring,*[1] or the *Vest* case, brought by Bores and Marmer and *Schachar v. The American Academy of Ophthalmology, Inc.,*[2] or the *Schachar* case, are alleged violations of the federal antitrust laws.* Although the plaintiff groups in both cases also

---

*The *Vest* and *Schachar* cases are the two principal cases brought against those who opposed the proliferation of radial keratotomy in this country. It should, however, be noted that in October 1980, Lloyd Vest brought an action against Dr. George O. Waring, The Georgia Society of Ophthalmology and Emory University in the Superior Court of DeKalb County, Georgia, claiming that these defendants had conspired to prohibit Dr. Marmer from performing radial keratotomy on Mr. Vest's second eye. Mr. Vest alleged, under state law, that the defendants had tortiously interfered with the contractual relationship between Mr. Vest and Dr. Marmer. Dr. Marmer eventually performed the procedure on Mr. Vest's second eye. Thereafter, Mr. Vest offered to settle the case for $15,000. The defendants rejected the settlement offer. The suit was eventually dismissed by Mr. Vest.

claimed violations of various state and common laws, the federal antitrust claims dominated. Therefore this discussion is limited to the plaintiffs' federal antitrust allegations. To understand those claims, a summary review of Sections 1 and 2 of the Sherman Act is appropriate.

CONSPIRACIES AND MONOPOLIES— A CURSORY REVIEW

Section 1 of the Sherman Act generally proscribes collective conduct to restrain competition. Section 1 specifically provides the following:

Every contract, combination . . . or conspiracy, in restraint of trade or commerce among the several States . . . is declared to be illegal.[3]

This section, however, prohibits only "unreasonable" restraints of trade.[4] The elements of a Section 1 violation therefore are the following:

1. Concerted action among a group of persons
2. An unreasonable restraint of trade
3. An effect on interstate commerce

Section 2 of the Sherman Act[5] prohibits conduct aimed at monopolization. An antitrust plaintiff must prove the following two factors to establish a Section 2 monopolization claim:

1. The defendant had monopoly power in a relevant product and geographic market.[6]
2. The defendant willfully acquired or maintained its monopoly power in such market.[7]

In simplistic terms a Section 1 case focuses on whether there has been concerted action that unreasonably restrained trade. A Section 2 case focuses on whether a monopoly was willfully acquired or maintained.

TWO RADIAL KERATOTOMY ANTITRUST LAWSUITS

A brief history of the *Vest* and *Schachar* cases clarifies the manner in which the plaintiffs in these cases constructed their antitrust allegations.

Vest v. Waring

On February 19, 1982, Dr. Leo D. Bores, Dr. Robert H. Marmer, and seven of their patients, including Lloyd Vest, filed an action in the U.S. District Court for the Northern District of Georgia against 36 defendants. The defendants fell into the three following basic groups:

1. Twenty ophthalmologists who were involved in the PERK study—the physician defendants
2. Three members of the National Advisory Eye Council (NAEC), two National Eye Institute

(NEI) officials, and the NEI itself—the federal defendants

3. The members of the Board of Directors of the American Academy of Ophthalmology, Inc. (AAO)—the AAO defendants

Plaintiffs alleged that the defendants had violated the federal antitrust laws by restraining the availability of radial keratotomy in various geographic regions of the United States.* The plaintiffs brought their case as individuals and on behalf of various unnamed persons that the plaintiffs contended had similar claims against the defendants. The named plaintiffs claimed they were entitled to represent the following four classes of people:

1. Patients who wanted radial keratotomy but whose insurance carriers refused to cover the procedure because it had been characterized by the defendants as "experimental."

2. Patients whose insurance companies refused to pay for or offered to pay only a nominal sum for radial keratotomy that had been performed.

3. Patients on whom radial keratotomy had been performed but who experienced a delay in obtaining the procedure.

4. Ophthalmologists who were denied the opportunity to perform the operation.[8]

Antitrust claims were alleged under Sections 1 and 2 of the Sherman Act. The plaintiffs alleged under Section 1 that the defendants had conspired to restrain trade by engaging in a national group boycott of radial keratotomy.[9] The plaintiffs alleged under Section 2 that the defendants had attempted to monopolize and control the dissemination of radial keratotomy to the medical community and the public.[10] Plaintiffs further alleged state law claims that defendants had tortiously interfered with contracts that patients had with ophthalmologists to perform radial keratotomy.[11]

Plaintiffs claimed actual damages in the amount of $26 million, which, they contended, should be tripled under the antitrust laws.† In short, plaintiffs sought approximately $78 million in recovery for the alleged antitrust violations.[12]

In July 1982 the defendants moved for dismissal of the case on various grounds. The court ruled on these motions May 31, 1983.[13] In that ruling the court dis-

missed the federal defendants from the lawsuit on the grounds that they were protected by the doctrine of governmental immunity. The court also dismissed the AAO defendants and six of the physician defendants on the grounds either that the court did not have personal jurisdiction over them or that venue was not proper in the Northern District of Georgia.* Accordingly after the order was issued, only 11 physicians remained as defendants.

Several weeks after the court's May 1983 order, the parties in the *Vest* case began discussing the possibility of settling the litigation. Those discussions were monitored by R.A. Schachar and certain other members of the Keratorefractive Society.

Schachar v. The American Academy of Ophthalmology, Inc.

While the plaintiffs and defendants in the *Vest* case were engaged in active settlement negotiations, Dr. Ronald A. Schachar, eight other ophthalmologists (Drs. Doyle Leslie, Les Schachar, Norman O. Stahl, Jerry Zelman, Tibor Farkas, Howard Bruckner, and George Simon), and the Keratorefractive Society, of which Dr. Schachar was then secretary, considered filing their own lawsuit to challenge certain activities of the AAO concerning radial keratotomy. An action was ultimately brought against the AAO and three members of its board of directors on June 6, 1984, in the U.S. District Court in Chicago.[14] Like the *Vest* case, the suit brought by Schachar and the other plaintiffs was brought under Sections 1 and 2 of the Sherman Act. Plaintiffs also alleged state law claims similar to those alleged by plaintiffs in the *Vest* case. Twelve of the physician defendants in the *Vest* case were named as "co-conspirators" in the complaint filed in Chicago, although they were not named as defendants in the litigation.[15]†

The allegations of misconduct against the AAO, the three members of its Board of Directors, and the identified co-conspirators were similar to the allegations in the *Vest* case. The plaintiffs in the *Schachar* case generally alleged that the defendants and their co-conspirators had instituted a "national boycott and refusal to deal intended to ban, prohibit and restrain the individual plaintiffs—ophthalmologists engaged in private practice—from further performing the [radial keratotomy] surgery. . . ."[16]

---

*Plaintiffs also made allegations against the defendants under state law.
†Damages are trebled under the antitrust law. That is, actual damages that are proved by an antitrust plaintiff are tripled and awarded to the plaintiff. The possibility of a treble damage award is intended to discourage antitrust violations.

*Before the ruling the plaintiffs voluntarily dismissed three of the physician defendants.
†After the suit was filed, the *Schachar* plaintiffs asked the court for permission to name three of the 12 physicians as "defendants" rather than nonparty "co-conspirators." The court refused to add these physician defendants as parties on the grounds that the court did not have jurisdiction or venue over them.

Resolution of the Vest and Schachar cases

The *Vest* case was settled in May 1985 for $250,000. At that time Dr. George O. Waring III issued a statement describing the generally favorable results achieved in the PERK clinical trial. The reason given by the defendants for settling the case was that paying a small amount of money and issuing a conciliatory statement was preferable to the continued payment of expensive legal fees and the onerous commitment of time that would have been required by protracted litigation.

The defendants in the *Schachar* case initially attempted to resolve the claims in that case by filing a motion for summary judgment in which they requested the court to dismiss all plaintiffs' claims without a trial. The summary judgment motion was denied and the case was tried for 4 weeks until late April 1988. On May 3, 1988, the jury returned a verdict in favor of the defendants. In reaching their decision, the jury found that the two individual defendants, Norton and Spivey, had not engaged in an antitrust conspiracy to monopolize the radial keratotomy procedure. Although the jury found that the AAO had engaged in a conspiracy to restrain the procedure, the jury determined that the restraint in which the AAO had engaged was reasonable and therefore not illegal. Since the jury members did not find that any of the defendants had violated antitrust laws, they were not required to consider plaintiffs' alleged damages. The plaintiffs' motion for another trial of the case was denied (see box at right).

On March 3, 1989 the final chapter was written in the *Schachar* case when the United States Court of Appeals for the Seventh Circuit decided the plaintiffs' appeal from the judgment that was entered in the trial court in favor of the defendants. In affirming the trial court's decision, the Court of Appeals characterized the *Schachar* litigation as one involving a claim that the AAO had violated the antitrust laws by "attaching the label 'experimental' to radial keratotomy."[65] The Court noted, however, that none of the plaintiffs in the action maintained "that the Academy prevented him from doing what he wished or imposed sanctions on those who facilitated" the performance of radial keratotomy.[66] The Court pointed out the following[67]:

All the Academy did is state as its position that radial keratotomy was "experimental" and issue a press release with a call for research. It did not require its members to desist from performing the operation or associating with those who do. It did not expel or discipline or even scowl at members who performed radial keratotomies. It did not induce hospitals to withhold permission to perform the procedure, or insurers to withhold payment; it has no authority over hospitals, insurers, state medical societies or licensing boards, and other persons who might be able to govern the performance of surgery.

Motion for New Trial in RK Suit is Denied

BULLETIN. . . A motion for a new trial in the multi-million dollar restraint of trade lawsuit brought against the Academy by eight ophthalmologists was denied by U.S. District Court Judge Harry D. Leinenweber, June 20.

The plaintiffs, Ronald A. Schachar, MD, Denison, TX; Doyle Leslie, MD, Austin, TX; Les Schachar, MD, Norman O. Stahl, MD, Garden City, NY; Jerry Zelman, MD, Miami Beach; Howard Bruckner, MD, Augusta, GA; George Simon, MD, Concord, CA and Stanley Grandon, MD, Dearborn, MI, had sued the Academy and Drs. Bruce E. Spivey and Edward Norton for alleged violations of the Sherman Anti-Trust Act and alleged that a conspiracy existed to restrain the practice of radial keratotomy.

A federal district court jury, May 3, cleared the Academy and Drs. Spivey and Norton of wrongdoing. The plaintiffs were seeking $11 million in damages to be trebled under anti-trust laws bringing their total claim to nearly $36 million.

The plaintiffs' lawsuit arose, in part, from the Academy's endorsement in 1980 of the resolution issued by the National Advisory Eye Council that radial keratotomy had not been subjected to adequate scientific evaluation and should be considered an experimental procedure.

From Motion for new trial in RK suit is denied, ARGUS 1988; 12:(7)1.

The full opinion is presented in the box on pp. 264 and 265.

Finding that the AAO had not, and apparently could not, restrain performance of the procedure, the Court held that the AAO had not violated the antitrust laws. The Court stated "this case should not have gone to the jury; indeed it should not have gone to trial."[68]

ALLEGED ANTITRUST CONSPIRACY IN RADIAL KERATOTOMY

In the *Vest* and *Schachar* cases the plaintiffs alleged that defendants engaged in three general types of concerted conduct that they contend provided a basis for their antitrust claims. These categories of conduct include the following:

1. The "branding of radial keratotomy as 'experimental' "
2. The publication of pronouncements and the encouragement of national and governmental organizations to issue statements that branded radial keratotomy "experimental" and encouraged ophthalmologists to refrain from performing radial keratotomy until it could be studied further.
3. Attempts by certain of the defendants to encourage state and local ophthalmologic societies to

pass policy statements branding radial keratotomy "experimental" and to discourage performance of the operation.[17]

"Concerted action"

The plaintiffs in *Vest* and *Schachar* claimed that defendants conspired, or acted in concert, in the conduct described above. Plaintiffs, however, did not complain about defendants' scientific investigation of radial keratotomy as a surgical procedure. In fact, in *Vest* the plaintiffs stated, "In no way do plaintiffs . . . suggest that *participation* in the PERK study is the 'wrong' upon which this action is predicated."[18] Later they stated, "Plaintiffs wish to dispel the notion that the pursuit of scientific research and 'good' medicine have anything to do with this suit. Indeed, to the extent the PERK Study is directed to these efforts, plaintiffs wholeheartedly support the individuals responsible."[19]

Similarly, the plaintiffs in the *Schachar* case did not criticize the scientific purposes of the PERK study. Although they alleged that the study was improperly used to restrain trade,[20] the focus of their allegations was on the defendants' conduct outside of the scientific investigation of PERK.

The PERK study, however, became a convenient vehicle for identifying individuals alleged to have engaged in wrongful conduct outside the study. For example, the physicians who participated in the PERK study were identified as the core group of alleged conspirators.[21] The plaintiffs in *Vest* and *Schachar*, by establishing a relationship of one or more of the physician defendants to the NAEC, the NEI, and the AAO, brought these organizations into the allegations of conspiracy. For example, the *Schachar* plaintiffs claimed that the physician defendants used their influence at the NAEC and the AAO to obtain resolutions falsely labeling radial keratotomy as "experimental." This labeling, the *Schachar* plaintiffs claimed, ensured that insurance companies would not reimburse patients for the procedure.[22]

The *Schachar* plaintiffs claimed that the AAO joined the conspiracy when the organization passed its resolution in 1981 endorsing the characterization of radial keratotomy as experimental. They claimed and attempted to prove the following at trial:

The Academy, without proper qualifications and based on insufficient or no data, certified radial keratotomy an *experimental* surgical procedure. It then distributed its position on radial keratotomy to its members, the public, and virtually every health insurance company in the United States. Due to the influence of the Defendants and other co-conspirators acting in concert, coupled with the Academy's prestige and reputation, the dissemination of these statements chilled the market for radial keratotomy, prevented thousands of individuals from having the operation, caused many others not to examine the merits of radial keratotomy, and damaged Plaintiffs.[23]

A similar tactic was used in the *Vest* case to include the NAEC as a member of the co-conspirator group. Plaintiffs connected the NAEC with the physician defendants by noting that three members of the NAEC were employed by institutions connected with the PERK study.[24] The *Vest* plaintiffs referred to this as a "very cozy relationship."[25]

In both the *Vest* and *Schachar* cases, the plaintiffs claimed that the defendants engaged in concerted action to suppress and restrain the practice of radial keratotomy. They alleged that the conduct of the defendants made the surgery unavailable to patients because insurance companies refused to pay for it and that the restraint on insurance coverage resulting from the activities of the defendants reduced the number of patients who sought or inquired about the procedure. The plaintiffs alleged that this adversely affected the practices of the plaintiff ophthalmologists. The antitrust case was constructed by tracing, chronologically, the activities of the defendants inside and outside the PERK study in an effort to show that these activities restrained performance of radial keratotomy.

The plaintiffs claimed that the alleged conspiracy to suppress and restrain the practice of radial keratotomy began with a meeting called "Workshop on Radial Keratotomy" conducted on March 15, 1980, near the Atlanta airport. Plaintiffs claimed that this meeting, which was attended by physicians, most of whom later became PERK participants, was more than a meeting to discuss a possible scientific investigation of radial keratotomy. The plaintiffs in the *Schachar* case characterized the meeting as secret.[26]

To support their claim that the airport meeting was called to discuss matters other than a scientific study of a new surgery, the plaintiffs in the *Schachar* case relied, among other things, on certain handwritten notes that they claimed showed that "socio-political and economic aspects of the study" were an agenda item for the meeting and other notes that contained a comment apparently made during the meeting that radial keratotomy had the potential to be a $67 million per year procedure.[27]

The most significant event that plaintiffs claimed occurred at the meeting was the decision of the meeting participants to issue a policy statement to characterize the status of the radial keratotomy procedure. Plaintiffs claimed that the procedure was initially characterized as investigational but that this designation was later changed to experimental. The statement was published in the *Archives of Ophthalmology*,[28] and the plaintiffs claimed that this was intended to disseminate the designation widely so that interest in the surgery would be chilled.

These March 15, 1980, "facts" were cited to support the plaintiffs' contention that the defendants rec-

The Opinion of the United States Court of Appeals For the Seventh Circuit in the Schachar Case

No. 88-2398
Ronald A. Schachar, *et al.*,

Plaintiffs-Appellants,

v.

American Academy of Ophthalmology, Inc.,
et al.,

Defendants-Appellees.

Appeal from the United States District Court
for the Northern District of Illinois, Eastern Division.
No. 84 C 4770—**Harry D. Leinenweber,** *Judge.*

Argued February 6, 1989—Decided March 3, 1989

Before Bauer, *Chief Judge,* and Easterbrook and Manion, *Circuit Judges.*

Easterbrook, *Circuit Judge.* There can be no restraint of trade without a restraint. That truism decides this case, in which eight ophthalmologists contend that the American Academy of Ophthalmology violated the antitrust laws by attaching the label "experimental" to radial keratotomy, a surgical procedure for correcting nearsightedness.

Nearsightedness (myopia) occurs when the cornea of the eye does not focus light on the retina. A thick cornea bends light excessively, so the focal point falls short of the vision receptors. Glasses and contact lenses correct the problem by introducing an offsetting distortion; the net effect of the series of lenses is a proper focal point. Radial keratotomy corrects the problem surgically. The ophthalmologist makes shallow incisions along radii of the cornea; as the cornea heals it becomes flatter, and vision improves.

Svyatoslav Fyodorov of the Soviet Union devised radial keratotomy in 1973. American physicians, including some of the plaintiffs, started performing the operation in 1978. Even the most promising medical developments often turn out to have drawbacks, whose nature and magnitude should be determined. Many who have undergone radial keratotomy report improvement in their eyesight (sometimes so much change that they become farsighted). What are the long-run consequences? Most persons' visual acuity slowly changes with time. Does the eyesight of those who have had this operation change in different ways? Might the invasive procedure weaken the eye in a way that creates problems of a different kind? A surgical procedure used in Japan in the 1950s caused "corneal decompensation" about 10 years later, a serious condition leading to blindness (avoidable with corneal transplants). Radial keratotomy is different, but once burned twice shy.

In January 1979 the National Advisory Eye Council, the principal advisory body to the National Eye Institute (part of the National Institutes of Health) called refractive keratoplasty (a group of surgical procedures that includes radial keratotomy) "experimental." In 1980 it applied this term to radial keratotomy specifically, calling on the profession to use restraint until more research could be done. As the federal government does not regulate surgi-

cal procedures, this was all a federal body could do. In June 1980 the board of directors of the American Academy of Ophthalmology—the largest association of ophthalmologists, with more than 9,400 members—endorsed the Eye Council's position. It issued a press release urging "patients, ophthalmologists and hospitals to approach [radial keratotomy] with caution until additional research is completed."

This suit under §1 of the Sherman Act, 15 U.S.C. §1, contends that the press release issued in 1980 was the upshot of a conspiracy among the Academy's members in restraint of trade. After a month of trial, the jury disagreed. The plaintiffs press objections to the jury instructions, including the district judge's puzzling refusal to define a product market even though the first question in any rule of reason case is market power. *Ball Memorial Hospital, Inc. v. Mutual Hospital Insurance, Inc.,* 784 F.2d 1325, 1334-37 (7th Cir. 1986); *Polk Bros., Inc. v. Forest City Enterprises, Inc.,* 776 F.2d 185, 191 (7th Cir. 1985). (The plaintiffs concede that the Academy's conduct should be assessed under the rule of reason.) Mulling over the jury instructions would be pointless, however, for this case should not have gone to the jury; indeed it should not have gone to trial. *All* the Academy did is state as its position that radial keratotomy was "experimental" and issue a press release with a call for research. It did not require its members to desist from performing the operation or associating with those who do. It did not expel or discipline or even scowl at members who performed radial keratotomies. It did not induce hospitals to withhold permission to perform the procedure, or insurers, state medical societies or licensing boards, and other persons who might be able to govern the performance of surgery.

Plaintiffs concede that the Academy did not attempt to coordinate activities with these groups, actors independent of the Academy. Cf. *Business Electronics Corp. v. Sharp Electronics Corp.,* 108 S. Ct. 1515 (1988); *Zinser v. Rose,* No. 88-1789 (7th Cir. Feb. 15, 1989), slip op. 5. Although plaintiffs believe that the Academy's prestige influenced others' conduct, plaintiffs also concede that after the Academy's press release in 1980 hospitals still allowed them to perform radial keratotomies and many insurers reimbursed them for that work. In 1982 plaintiff Doyle Leslie performed 1,181 radial keratotomies; in 1983 he performed 1,314. Other plaintiffs performed fewer, and all believe that the demand for their services would have been greater if the Academy had not thrown its weight behind the position that their bread-and-butter was "experimental", but none maintains that the Academy prevented him from doing what he wished or imposed sanctions on those who facilitated the work. This uncontested fact required the district court to grant the Academy's motion for summary judgment and on this alternative ground we affirm the judgment in the Academy's favor.

From Refract Corneal Surg 1989;5:143-145.

Antitrust law is about consumers' welfare and the efficient organization of production. It condemns reductions in output that drive up prices as consumers bid for the remaining supply. *NCAA v. University of Oklahoma*, 468 U.S. 85, 103-07 (1984); *Broadcast Music, Inc. v. CBS, Inc.*, 441 U.S. 1, 19-20 (1979); *Indiana Grocery, Inc. v. Super Valu Stores, Inc.*, No. 88-1625 (7th Cir. Jan. 6, 1989), slip op. 6-8; *Premier Electrical Construction Co. v. National Electrical Contractors Ass'n, Inc.*, 814 F.2d 358, 368-71 (7th Cir. 1987). In a market with thousands of providers—that is, in the market for ophthalmological services—what any one producer does cannot curtail output; someone else will step in. See *Indiana Grocery* and *Ball Memorial*. Other trade association cases, such as *National Society of Professional Engineers, Inc. V. United States*, 435 U.S. 679 (1978); *Wilk v. American Medical Association*, 719 F.2d 207 (7th Cir. 1983); *Moore v. Boating Industry Associations*, 819 F.2d 693 (7th Cir. 1987); *Hydrolevel Corp. v. American Society of Mechanical Engineers*, 635 F.2d 118, 124-27 (2d Cir. 1980), affirmed on other grounds, 456 U.S. 556 (1982); and *Indiana Head, Inc. v. Allied Tube & Conduit Corp.*, 817 F.2d 938, 946-47 (2d Cir. 1987), affirmed on other grounds, 108 S. Ct. 1931, 1936 n.3 (1988), involved enforcement devices. Perhaps members boycotted those who fell out of step (as in *Professional Engineers*), or perhaps the producers agreed "not to manufacture, distribute, or purchase certain types of products," as in *Allied Tube*, 108 S. Ct. at 1937. These enforcement mechanisms are the "restraints" of trade. Without them there is only uncoordinated individual action, the essence of competition.

Ophthalmologists are each others' rivals for custom. They offer competing procedures to cope with myopia—some surgical, some optical (glasses plus contact lenses of many kinds: hard, soft, extended wear). Plaintiffs say that the Academy is in the grip of professors and practitioners who favor conservative treatment, forever calling for more research (the better to justify the academics' requests for grants); plaintiffs portray themselves as the progressives, disdaining the Academy's fuddy-duddies in order to put the latest knowledge to work. Warfare among suppliers and their different products *is* competition. Antitrust law does not compel your competitor to praise your product or sponsor your work. To require cooperation or friendliness among rivals is to undercut the intellectual foundations of antitrust law. *Indiana Grocery*, slip op. 6-8; *Ball Memorial*, 784 F.2d at 1338-39. Unless one group of suppliers diminishes another's ability to peddle its wares (technically, reduces rivals' elasticity of supply), there is not even the beginning of an antitrust case, no reason to investigate further to determine whether the restraint is "reasonable."

Consolidated Metal Products, Inc. v. American Petroleum Institute, 846 F.2d 284 (5th Cir. 1988), holds that when a trade association provides information (there, gives a seal of approval) but does not constrain others to follow its recommendations, it does not violate the antitrust laws. See also *Clamp-All Corp. v. Cast Iron Soil Pipe Institute*, 851 F.2d 478, 486-89 (1st Cir. 1988). We agree. An organization's towering reputation does not reduce its freedom to speak out. Speech informed, hence affected, demand for radial keratotomy, but the plaintiffs had no entitlement to consumers' favor. The Academy's declaration affected only the demand side of the market, and then only by appealing to consumers' (and third-party payors') better judgment. If such statements should be false or misleading or incomplete or just plain mistaken, the remedy is not antitrust litigation but more speech—the marketplace of ideas.

Plaintiffs' "smoking guns" show how far this case strayed from the point of antitrust law. Plaintiffs observe that the Academy never before had called a surgical procedure "experimental"; that it acted on the recommendation of the Eye Banks Committee, which they view as unfit to render advice about the topic (after 1982 the Academy gave the subject to a different committee); that the Academy's president in 1980 admitted that he wanted to stop the "proliferation" of radial keratotomy (one would expect no less if he thought the procedure should be treated as "experimental"). Then there is the crowning insult: in 1981 the Academy's president called plaintiff Ronald Schachar "impudent and idiotic" for "demanding that I answer a series of eight or nine questions which he had seen fit to put to me," "despite [plaintiffs say] having had . . . Dr. Schachar's chief of surgery at the University of Chicago tell him that Dr. Schachar was among the very brightest students he had every taught." We may assume that professors at the University of Chicago are infallible judges of talent and that bright ophthalmologists have flawless judgment; what this bickering has to do with the Sherman Act is a mystery. Animosity, even if rephrased as "anticompetitive intent," is not illegal without anticompetitive effects. *Moore*, 819 F.2d at 696 (reversing a verdict because the instructions told the jury that purpose *or* effect supported a finding for the plaintiff); *Olympia Equipment Leasing Co. v. Western Union Telegraph Co.*, 797 F.2d 370, 379-80 (7th Cir. 1986); *Ball Memorial*, 784 F.2d at 1338-40; *Barry Wright Corp. v. ITT Grinnell Corp.*, 724 F.2d 227, 232 (1st Cir. 1983); Philip E. Areeda, 7 *Antitrust Law* ¶1506 (1986).

Plaintiffs' fundamental position, stated in its reply brief, is that: "Issuing such a statement [calling radial keratotomy "experimental"] carried with it an obligation to the public, ophthalmologists, and third party payors to have studied the procedure and reached a considered opinion." Putting to one side the conundrum that once you have "studied" something it is no longer "experimental"—that the declaration of "experimental" status logically precedes the gathering of information—we do not perceive what this has to do with antitrust. See *Indiana Grocery*, slip op. 7 (the Sherman Act "does not reach conduct that is only unfair, impolite, or unethical"). The Sherman Act is not a code of medical ethics or methodology, and whether radial keratotomy *is* "experimental" is a medical rather than a legal question.

AFFIRMED

ognized radial keratotomy as a lucrative new procedure and as a result were motivated to institute a "national boycott and refusal to deal intended to ban, prohibit and restrain the individual plaintiffs-ophthalmologists engaged in private practice from further performing the [radial keratotomy] surgery until defendants and their co-conspirators, university professors and private practitioners who directly compete with plaintiffs, could gain an economic advantage and exploit the procedure to their own economic and professional benefit."[29]

The defendants' view of the "concerted action" alleged

In the *Schachar* case the defendants' version of the purpose of the workshop held near the Atlanta airport and subsequent activities inside and outside PERK were entirely different from the views expressed by the plaintiffs. The defendants noted that after 1978 numerous ophthalmologists in the United States were instructed in radial keratotomy surgery and an increasing number of the procedures was being performed, even though there were few studies of the surgery published in professional journals.[30] Those ophthalmologists who sought to proliferate the surgery widely publicized it in newspaper, magazine, and television advertisements as a "safe and effective method of correcting nearsightedness."[31]

The nature of this advertising alarmed the physician defendants. They believed that it distorted the predictability and reliability of the operation and misled the public. Moreover, "since eyeglasses and contact lenses were available as safe and inexpensive means of correcting myopia," the defendant doctors felt it was sensible to test the claims being made by the proponents of the operation.[32]

The defendants' basic concern was that "no in-depth scientific peer-reviewed study of the procedure had been conducted" in this country and the "safety and efficacy of the surgery were therefore unknown."[33] They argued that it was their professional duty and responsibility to state their opinion on the procedure, to study the procedure in a clinical trial conducted in the United States, and to urge doctors to exercise caution in performing the procedure until its safety and efficacy were established.

The physician defendants noted that Bores, a named plaintiff in the *Vest* case, shared these concerns.[34] Bores had formed a group known as the National Radial Keratotomy Study Group to study the surgery and its results. A press release issued by Bores's study group in 1980 urged caution in the development of radial keratotomy, stating that "only by carefully studying the surgery can we be assured of its

safety and efficacy."[35] G.O. Waring was originally a member of the Bores group. Waring, however, withdrew because the Bores study was not conducted under the formal scientific standards that he believed were necessary for a study as important as that of radial keratotomy.

After discussing with other ophthalmologists the possibility of conducting a rigorous clinical trial of radial keratotomy, Waring held the Atlanta workshop in March 1980 to discuss a possible study of the surgery. His intention was to enlist several ophthalmologists who had experience with radial keratotomy and others affiliated with noted academic institutions to participate in the study. All the physicians invited to attend the workshop held teaching appointments at highly regarded medical schools and had the clinical and practical experience necessary to conduct a formal clinical trial. The support staff and support facilities necessary to control, collect, and analyze the data derived from the study of radial keratotomy were readily available at the institutions with which the workshop participants were affiliated.[36]

Approximately 14 noted corneal specialists from across the country attended the Atlanta workshop. Those who attended were teaching physicians with strong research backgrounds. The attendees agreed that additional scientific study of radial keratotomy was needed to determine the safety and efficacy of the procedure. The nature of the operation, the chance for its widespread and immediate proliferation, and its uncertainty urged the workshop participants to begin a study of the procedure as soon as possible.[37]

The ophthalmologists who attended the workshop agreed to request a grant from the NEI to fund a clinical study of the operation. They also issued a general statement about radial keratotomy, including its designation as an experimental procedure.[38]

Defendants conducted meetings subsequent to the workshop. These meetings were held in conjunction with other ophthalmologic functions and were open to interested ophthalmologists. The purpose of these subsequent meetings was to organize and advance the clinical study proposed to be conducted and which would later become known as the Prospective Evaluation of Radial Keratotomy, or PERK.

The defendants specifically denied that they intended to conduct the study to monopolize the performance of the procedure. On the contrary, in the *Vest* case the defendants noted that the PERK study was designed to limit the surgeons participating in the study to performing the procedure within the study. For example, the PERK protocol specified that the investigators were not allowed to practice radial keratotomy outside of the study while doing surgery for the study. In addition, the physicians who performed the procedure in PERK and those who did the postoperative examinations were not financially compensated from patient fees or grant moneys.[39]

THE "EXPERIMENTAL" DESIGNATION

The *Schachar* plaintiffs claimed that there is an important distinction between designating a surgical procedure as "experimental" and designating it as "investigational." This distinction, plaintiffs claimed, was known to the physician defendants, the NAEC, and the AAO. They further claimed that these defendants intentionally designated radial keratotomy as experimental in the early 1980s knowing that this designation would influence insurance carriers to refuse coverage for the procedure. Plaintiffs contended that this would result in limited availability of the procedure, thus damaging patients and physicians nationwide.[40]

The *Vest* plaintiffs claimed that, in medicine, experimental is defined as "medical knowledge derived from laboratory experiments with animals."[41] In medicine, investigational is defined as "medical knowledge derived from performing a surgical procedure on human beings in accordance with a standardized regimen known as a 'protocol,'" they claimed.[42] To conclude their argument, plaintiffs claimed that "third party payers reimburse physicians for 'investigational' procedures, but frequently do not cover 'experimental' procedures."[43]

The defendants' view of the "experimental" designation

The defendants strongly disputed that there is any meaningful clinical distinction between the characterization of a surgical procedure as experimental or investigational. They disputed that their designation of radial keratotomy as experimental in and of itself had any effect on insurance coverage for the procedure. They denied that their issuance of a statement characterizing the procedures as experimental was intended to influence insurance coverage in any way. In fact, many insurance companies classify procedures as "experimental-investigational."

The defendants contended instead that insurance companies determined, pursuant to the written provisions of the various insurance policies that existed when radial keratotomy was introduced in the United States, whether radial keratotomy was a reimbursable procedure under the provisions of such policies.[44]

Defendants contended that the 1979 NAEC statement labeling refractive keratoplasty as experimental, which was published before radial keratotomy became an issue among ophthalmologists, provided a historical precedent for the designation of radial keratotomy

as experimental[45] and that it was proper to use the 1979 NAEC statement as a model for the statements on radial keratotomy issued by the radial keratotomy workshop participants, the NAEC, and AAO.[46]

The designation of radial keratotomy as experimental was thought by defendants to be accurate and necessary to impress on the medical community and the public that the procedure had not been studied enough to establish its safety and efficacy. The defendants asserted that it was their duty and obligation to label the procedure experimental, as it was the duty and responsibility of the NAEC and the AAO, in the interest of millions of myopes, to issue formal statements expressing their opinion of the surgery. Indeed, the AAO specifically contended in the unsuccessful summary judgment motion it filed in the *Schachar* case that the First Amendment to the United States Constitution protects the AAO and its directors' right to express their opinions and reservations about radial keratotomy freely.[47]

Although little formal discovery was taken on the experimental versus investigational designation issue in the *Vest* case, several depositions of third-party payors were conducted in the *Schachar* case to determine whether the designation of radial keratotomy as experimental affected insurance coverage for the surgery.[48] The AAO claimed at trial that an "overwhelming majority of these [insurance company] representatives stated that they drew no distinction between 'experimental' and 'investigational' in making their decision on whether to pay for surgical procedures."[49] They further claimed that there is "no unity or pattern on coverage of radial keratotomy" by insurers.[50] The facts apparently are that "different third party payors covered or declined to cover radial keratotomy at different times for different reasons."[51]*

The information and authority available on the issue of the appropriate characterization of new medical technologies and surgical procedures is scant. There is, however, recent information that refutes the experimental-investigational distinction sought to be established in the subject cases. For example, a widely respected book on clinical trials published in 1985, *Human Experimentation: A Guided Step into the Unknown,* discredited the argument that experiments are not performed on humans.[52] An authoritative textbook published in 1986, *Clinical Trials: Design, Conduct and Analysis,* defines a clinical trial as a "planned *experiment* designed to assess the efficacy of a treatment

---

*Some had decided not to cover radial keratotomy before the Academy issued any statement; some decided to cover radial keratotomy after the Academy's statement called it experimental; others covered it initially and do not now; and some companies amended their policies to exclude coverage specifically.

in man."[53] These sources, specifically the definition in the latter work, contradict the experimental-investigational distinction that the *Vest* and *Schachar* plaintiffs attempted to create. Indeed, the PERK study, like early clinical studies of artificial hearts, is a planned experiment of a treatment on humans to assess the safety and efficacy of radial keratotomy.

A survey of reported court decisions did not disclose any case regarding insurance coverage for radial keratotomy and whether an experimental or investigational label, in and of itself, affected insurance coverage. Furthermore, no case was discovered that discussed a distinction between experimental and investigational in an insurance-coverage context or otherwise.

There was, however, one case that generally discussed an experimental surgical procedure in the context of insurance coverage. In *Zuckerberg v. Blue Cross and Blue Shield,*[54] the plaintiff brought an action against Blue Cross and Blue Shield for reimbursement for an innovative form of cancer therapy received by the decedent in Tijuana, Mexico.[55] The therapy consisted of a "dietary regimen consisting of large numbers of organically grown fruits and vegetables and their juices, together with certain medications, digestive aids and vitamins."[56] The decedent's insurance policy contained a provision that excluded coverage for any procedure that "is experimental in the sense that its effectiveness is not generally recognized."[57] The court in *Zuckerberg* found that the cancer treatment administered to the decedent was not an effective treatment for cancer and therefore was not covered by the policy.

In *Zuckerberg* the court simply interpreted the language in an insurance contract that contained an exclusion for procedures that were not generally recognized.[58] The *Zuckerberg* court correctly considered the question of insurance coverage based on the provisions of the insurance policy issued to the plaintiff in that case. The *Zuckerberg* case, however, can be considered from an antitrust perspective.

In *Zuckerberg* the insurance policy provision at issue stated that coverage is provided only for procedures that are "generally recognized."[59] The question remains whether it is common in the insurance industry to tie insurance coverage for a medical procedure to the acceptance of that procedure in the medical community. If that approach to coverage is common in the industry and if it was known to the defendants in *Vest* and *Schachar,* the claim could be made that the defendants knew of this industry standard and by engaging in the conduct alleged by plaintiffs intended to prohibit the "general recognition" of radial keratotomy to influence insurance coverage. Although such a claim

would be difficult to prove, It could raise an issue regarding the intent of the defendants. If an issue of intent were raised, the defendants would likely be required to show that their conduct was intended to protect the public health and that there was a sufficient and reasonable basis for designating the procedure as experimental. In fact, this was an issue tried in the *Schachar* case.

Call for "restraint"

The most direct evidence used by plaintiffs to illustrate the defendants' alleged intention to restrain the proliferation of radial keratotomy was the defendants' efforts to persuade various local, state, and national ophthalmologic societies to pass resolutions to restrict performance of the procedure. The *Vest* plaintiffs put it succinctly: "The gravamen of the Complaint is that the Defendants have agreed among themselves to effect a moratorium on the ophthalmic procedure known as radial keratotomy insofar as surgeons engaged in private practice of ophthalmology are concerned."[60]

The *Schachar* plaintiffs made and attempted to prove the same claim. They alleged that the defendants "embarked on a national campaign to pressure various state and local medical societies, governmental agencies, hospital staffs, and third-party payors into declaring a 'moratorium' on radial keratotomy until the self-appointed . . . university group could 'study' the matter."[61]

The plaintiffs then cited a string of events that took place entirely outside the PERK study. They claimed that these events show defendants intended to restrict performance of the procedure. The plaintiffs made the following allegations:

1. Defendants urged the Georgia Ophthalmological Society to pass a resolution endorsing the conclusions of the PERK defendants and to place a temporary ban on the surgery outside the study proposed to be conducted by the defendants.
2. Defendants urged the NAEC to issue a statement declaring radial keratotomy to be an experimental procedure and called for performance of a carefully controlled clinical trial of the procedure.
3. Defendants urged the New Mexico Ophthalmological Society in June 1980 to adopt the Defendants' characterization of the operation as "experimental" and urged a moratorium on the performance of such operation until the procedure was further studied.
4. Defendants urged the AAO in June and July of 1980 to designate the procedure as "experimental" and urged that it not be performed until the defendant physicians' study was completed.

5. Defendants supported the efforts of physicians in Delaware, Virginia, Kentucky, and Tennessee to have the radial keratotomy procedure deemed experimental and a moratorium placed on performance of the surgery.[62]

The plaintiffs used these examples of activities outside of PERK for two purposes. They used them to support their claim that the defendants' characterization of radial keratotomy as experimental was part of the defendants' plan to restrict the performance of the operation or at least to discourage the increasing use of the procedure, and second, to support their claim that the defendants tried to tie restraint of the procedure to the completion of the study. The plaintiffs contended that this supports their theory that the defendants intended to restrain performance of the procedure, allowing themselves to become the noted experts in radial keratotomy through the PERK study.

The defendants denied these claims. They claimed also that they limited the expression of their opinions to publications and forums that were directed at or comprised medical professionals. In the defendants' view, they were simply expressing their medical opinion that the procedure had not been sufficiently studied to warrant widespread use.

The defendants argued that it was necessary to urge restrained use of radial keratotomy to counter the argument of those ophthalmologists who urged widespread proliferation of the procedure without further study. The defendants contended that statements urging caution in the performance of the procedure were a reasonable and responsible way to discourage the rapid proliferation of the procedure until it could be clinically studied in the United States. Defendants emphatically denied that their attempts to restrain performance of the procedure were unreasonable or in any way illegal.

The alleged section 2 monopoly

The plaintiffs in *Vest* and *Schachar* also alleged a claim against the defendants based on Section 2 of the Sherman Act: that defendants acquired or attempted to acquire a nationwide monopoly over the radial keratotomy procedure."[63] The plaintiffs relied on the same conduct and the same arguments on which they relied to support their Section 1 claim.

The Section 2 offense alleged in *Vest* and *Schachar* was not a significant basis on which plaintiffs proceeded in either case. Although the offense remained in the *Vest* case at the time the case was settled, the emphasis in *Vest* was on the plaintiffs' Section 1 claim. This was also true in the *Schachar* case. Indeed, the plaintiffs in *Schachar* abandoned their Section 2 claim.[64]

It is unlikely that a Section 2 claim could be successfully pursued. For example, the evidence developed in the *Vest* case established that by July 1982, thousands of radial keratotomy procedures had been performed by dozens of ophthalmologists across the country. This statistic strongly suggests that there was no monopoly. The evidence in the *Schachar* case indicated that Schachar himself performed as many as 1040 radial keratotomies from 1980 to 1986 and has a practice that is substantially dedicated to the performance of this procedure. Some individual surgeons have done more than 10,000 operations. In 1982 the Keratorefractive Society distributed a news release surveying approximately 63,000 radial keratotomy cases. The PERK physicians, meanwhile, restricted themselves to doing fewer than 500 cases in 1982-1983. A small minority of the PERK surgeons have gone on to practice radial keratotomy extensively.

The verdict of the jury and the opinion of the Court of Appeals in favor of the defendants (see box on pp. 264-265) set important precedent in the field of antitrust law.

The Court acknowledged the plaintiffs' contention that the dispute between members of the ophthalmic community regarding radial keratotomy was heated. The Court, however, dismissed the plaintiffs' view that their more conservative colleagues had wrongfully and illegally advanced their arguments against radial keratotomy. The Court observed that the fundamental purpose of the antitrust laws is to encourage competition emphasizing that "[w]arfare among suppliers and their different products *is* competition."[69] The Court observed further that "[a]ntitrust law does not compel your competitor to praise your product or sponsor your work. To require cooperation or friendliness among rivals is to undercut the intellectual foundations of antitrust law."[70]

In short, the Court of Appeals in *Schachar* viewed the strong disagreement among ophthalmologists regarding radial keratotomy as healthy competition which, in the absence of any restraint, was not illegal. Accordingly, the opinion should provide some comfort to those who wish to express openly their reservations or criticisms about radial keratotomy or any other new surgical procedure. Some ophthalmologists have, however, read the Court of Appeals decision in *Schachar* more broadly. They view the decision as announcing wholesale approval of any action to investigate or control the proliferation of any new surgical procedure, the safety and efficacy of which they believe may not have been established adequately. The opinion does not stand for this broad proposition. To the contrary, the opinion is peppered with provisos indicating that it is the Seventh Circuit's view that where expression of opinion is coupled with action to restrain the performance of a service, the antitrust laws will apply. Indeed, the court clearly indicated that where action is taken, or "enforcement mechanisms" are employed to restrain trade, a person is at risk under the antitrust laws.[71]

PERMISSIBLE CONDUCT: CAN A LINE BE DRAWN?

A review of the *Vest* and *Schachar* cases illustrates the existence of a fundamental problem in the medical community in matters involving the introduction and practice of new surgical procedures. Medical devices and drugs are subject to substantial regulation by the Food and Drug Administration. Surgical procedures, however, are not subject to federal or state control. New surgical procedures that must be performed on an inpatient basis are regulated only to the extent that hospitals require that the procedure be performed by surgeons with staff privileges pursuant to approval by hospital review boards. Procedures that can be performed on an outpatient basis are not subject even to this type of scrutiny.

Since surgical procedures are not the subject of governmental regulation and instead are intended to be regulated by the medical community, the question arises as a result of the *Vest* and *Schachar* cases regarding the extent to which physicians can scrutinize the practice of new surgical procedures without running afoul of the antitrust laws. This difficult question is resolved differently depending on a person's philosophic view. On one hand, there are doctors and members of the public who contend that new medical procedures should be freely introduced in the United States as long as the following holds true:

1. There is some scientific basis that tends to support the safety and efficacy of the procedure.
2. The patient is fully informed of any risks associated with the procedure.
3. The patient consents to those risks.

Other physicians and members of the public believe that new surgical procedures should not be practiced widely in this country until the safety and efficacy of the procedures are established by scientific evaluation. There is, of course, a broad continuum of views between these two extremes.

Conduct that restrains the performance of new surgical procedures will be increasingly subject to antitrust review. Indeed, it has been said that the *Vest* and *Schachar* cases have made "many in the medical technology assessment community apprehensive about their exposure to antitrust suits."[72] The basis for this concern is as follows:

Given the tremendous financial effect that a decision in technology assessment may have, and the potential for securing a treble damage award under the antitrust laws, it is indeed not surprising that those who believe they have been unfairly affected by such a decision may seek recourse in antitrust litigation.[73]

All professions, including the medical profession, are subject to antitrust laws.[74] As long as the antitrust laws apply, physicians must be aware that any conduct that restrains or appears to restrain trade may well result in an antitrust claim. This is demonstrated by the 1987 injunction against the American Medical Association (AMA) resulting from a long-standing feud between the AMA and chiropractors. New medical technologies that are often perceived as a potential source of new income for the medical community are obviously prone to such charges.

The *Vest* and *Schachar* cases teach that the issues involved in scrutinizing and criticizing new surgical procedures and techniques are economic, as well as medical. A person who engages in conduct that limits the availability of a surgical procedure may be subject to claims that the conduct was economically, not medically, motivated. This may in turn result in a claim that the conduct illegally restrained trade in violation of U.S. antitrust laws.* The *Vest* and *Schachar* cases also teach that an antitrust claim will most likely be brought under Section 1 of the Sherman Act against people who engage in conduct that limits the availability of a surgical procedure.[75]

Section 1 and the "rule of reason"

Conduct alleged to violate Section 1 of the Sherman Act is ordinarily judged according to the "rule of reason" unless the conduct constitutes one of the special types of conduct that are deemed illegal per se.† (See the box on p. 271.) The rule of reason as applied under Section 1 of the antitrust laws prohibits:

all contracts or acts which were unreasonably restrictive of competitive conditions, either from the nature or character of the contract or where the surrounding circumstances were such as to justify the conclusion that they had not the legitimate purpose of reasonably forwarding personal interest and developing trade "but rather had been intended" to bring about the evils, such as enhancement of prices, which were considered to be against public policy.[76]

---

*The conduct may also be subject to claims that it violated state unfair trade practice laws and other state regulatory and common law.
†There are certain types of conduct that are not subject to the "rule of reason" and are illegal per se. Illegal conduct includes "price fixing, production restrictions, division of market between competitors, concerted refusal to deal and boycotts, and patent licensing on condition that unpatented materials be used in connection with the patented device." Callmann at § 4.20 (4th ed. 1987).

Excerpt from Antitrust Enforcement and the Medical Profession: No Special Treatment

Clear violations of the antitrust laws occur when otherwise competing professionals agree to do something, or to refrain from doing something, that blocks the free operation of the competitive process without any plausible promise of economic benefits for consumers. Such activity neither involves the creation of any real efficiencies—it does not provide something that consumers want at less cost than could be done through independent action—nor offers some new "product" that would otherwise be unavailable. Instead, it is activity that just eliminates competition, raises price, reduces the quantity of services provided, and thus reaps increased profits for physicians. When this is the case, it makes no difference whether the enriched doctors line their pockets with these profits or use them to increase the quality of care. "Naked" agreements of this kind—to fix prices, to allocate territories, or to boycott competing health-care providers—are unlawful regardless of their purpose and effect.

From Department of Justice: Remarks of Charles F. Rule before the interim meeting of The American Medical Association House of Delegates, Dallas, December 6, 1988.

To determine whether conduct violates the "rule of reason" a court must do the following[77]:

ordinarily consider the facts peculiar to the business to which the restraint is applied; its condition before and after the restraint was imposed; the nature of the restraint and its effect, actual or probable. The history of the restraint, the evil believed to exist, the reason for adopting the particular remedy, the purpose or end sought to be attained, are all relevant facts.

What is reasonable depends on the characteristics of an industry. It is clear, however, that "courts take into consideration that the health care industry is different from other industries."[78] As a result, conduct to scrutinize the introduction and proliferation of new surgical procedures that is challenged on the grounds that it violates the antitrust laws is reviewed according to the standards, principles, and tenets applicable to the health care industry.[79]

The risk analysis: a basic "rule of reason" approach

Physicians or other people who consider engaging in conduct to restrict the introduction of a new surgical procedure—whether by critical opposition or clinical testing—must determine whether such scrutiny is necessary and, if so, must determine the risk that an antitrust claim will be filed if they engage in the restrictive conduct. This consideration involves weighing the medical considerations regarding the procedure and their effect on the public and the profession against the potential economic effect on physicians and patients if the procedure is scrutinized and thus restricted. This balancing of medical need versus economic effect is essentially a rule of reason analysis. That is, the reasonableness of a person's conduct depends on whether the medical need for scrutiny outweighs any restraint on the performance or availability of the procedure.

Furthermore, Section 1 restrains concerted, not individual, activity. If physicians act individually and are not involved with others who may be seeking the same end, their exposure is reduced.

Medical considerations in applying the rule of reason

Medical considerations in applying the rule of reason focus on the medical need for the new procedure and the risks associated with the surgery. The following are relevant questions:

1. Is there a significant risk of injury or complication associated with the new surgery?
2. Are alternatives to the new surgery available and, if so, do such alternative treatments involve less risk of injury or complication than the new procedure?
3. Is the new procedure necessary to treat an injury, disease, or other malady, or is it cosmetic or elective?
4. Has the new surgical procedure been extensively studied according to research practices and procedures that apply in the United States to determine its safety and efficacy?
5. Have the safety and efficacy of the procedure been established?
6. Is there sufficient medical information available to allow medical professionals and their patients to make an informed choice regarding the appropriateness of the new procedure?
7. Can the new procedure be performed on an outpatient basis?
8. If the new procedure must be performed on an inpatient basis, are there established protocols for the performance of the surgery?
9. Is special training required to perform the new surgery and, if so, is such training available and competent?
10. Are special surgical instruments necessary to perform the new procedure and, if so, are they available, safe, and effective?

An analysis of these medical considerations may well lead to the conclusion that the safety and efficacy of the procedure have already been sufficiently established or that there are already sufficient procedures in place to scrutinize the performance of the surgery. For example, a new surgical procedure of relatively low risk that is being studied in an adequate clinical trial and is being performed outside the clinical trial according to acceptable medical protocols may not require further scrutiny. If this conclusion is reached, it is unlikely that a person would want to test or oppose the procedure further and run the risk of an antitrust claim even if the risk is slight.

A more difficult question arises when an analysis of these medical considerations indicates that further testing or critical opposition of the new procedure is necessary. The decision whether to engage in such conduct requires an analysis of various economic considerations to assess the risk that an antitrust claim will be filed.

ECONOMIC CONSIDERATIONS

There are several economic factors that are relevant to any analysis to determine the risk of an antitrust claim being filed associated with conduct to scrutinize a new surgical procedure. The following are relevant considerations:

1. What is the size of the patient population on which the surgery may be performed?
2. Is the new procedure of a type that allows a physician to charge a large surgical fee?
3. How large is the group of physicians interested in performing the new surgery?
4. If the procedure can be performed on an outpatient basis, what is the estimated cost to purchase the equipment and instruments and to hire the personnel necessary to perform the surgery?
5. Is the new surgery likely to be covered by medical insurance?
6. What is the level of physician and patient interest in the surgery?

For example, the risk that an antitrust claim will be filed is increased if the procedure has a known or predictable risk of injury or complication, commands a large surgical fee, and has a high potential physician and public interest. The risk of an antitrust claim being filed is lower if the surgery is highly specialized, the risk of complication is high, the potential patient population is small, and the initial economic investment is large. Put another way, procedures that are considered lucrative to medical professionals are most likely to produce antitrust claims if the conduct of others limits the availability of the procedure. The risk of an antitrust claim is lowest where there is limited interest in and application for the procedure and the potential patient population is small.

The relative risk of an antitrust claim will, of course, depend on the circumstances surrounding the introduction and practice of each new procedure. Indeed, antitrust exposure must be analyzed on a case-by-case basis. Antitrust exposure can arise under a variety of circumstances if the elements of an offense can be proved. For example, in *Richards v. Canine Eye Registration Foundation*[80] the Ninth Circuit Court of Appeals upheld a finding of antitrust liability against a group of veterinarians who filed an antitrust counterclaim in a lawsuit. The court, in affirming the antitrust judgment, found that the filing of the antitrust claim was concerted activity intended to restrain trade and that the filing of the suit alone constituted an antitrust offense.[81]

PRACTICAL CONSIDERATIONS

A rule of reason case that is not resolved by a settlement of the issues must be resolved by a jury or bench trial. A person who decides to criticize or test a new procedure must therefore assess the risk of an antitrust action and must understand the magnitude of the cost, expense, and time commitment that will be required to defend against an antitrust claim—even one that is not well founded.

The time and money required to defend an antitrust case is often large. Discovery in antitrust litigation frequently is intense and can be lengthy. Trial preparation and the trial itself are expensive. The time required to defend against antitrust allegations is often onerous. The *Schachar* case is a classic example. Although the result for the defendants was favorable, the case was in litigation for 4 years before it was tried. The trial lasted more than 3 weeks and the defendants' aggregate litigation expenses through trial were nearly $1 million. In short, antitrust litigation is expensive and time consuming.

ALTERNATIVES AND THEIR RELATIVE RISKS

The person who assesses the risk of an antitrust claim by analyzing the relevant medical and economic considerations, who understands the potential time and cost required to assert an effective antitrust defense, and who, nonetheless, decides to challenge the introduction and proliferation of a new surgical procedure, must next decide on the types of conduct in which to engage. A variety of questions, including the following questions, arise regarding the available alternatives.

1. Should the person express his or her opinion or reservations about the procedure and should it be done orally, in writing, or both?
2. Should the opinion or reservation be expressed privately or should it be expressed as a joint statement?
3. Should the opinion be for dissemination only to other physicians or should it be disseminated to the public at large?
4. Should professional medical organizations be lobbied to pass resolutions or prepare position papers regarding the status of the procedure?
5. Should the procedure be characterized as experimental or investigational or should some other label be used?
6. Should the opinion or reservation about the procedure be given to review boards or other professional groups?
7. Should the procedure be studied in the laboratory or clinic and, if so, by whom?

The answers are different for each new surgery. It is therefore impossible to state what conduct is and is not allowable. Indeed, concrete guidelines should not be established, and the type and scope of conduct should instead be judged on a case by case basis.

There are, however, some basic concepts that can be stated, which may limit physicians' antitrust exposure in those cases where they think that critical opposition or more extensive testing is necessary for the good of the public. A word of caution—these parameters are not given as criteria that will protect the physician from antitrust liability. They are merely general guidelines.

Clinical and laboratory studies

As the *Vest* and *Schachar* cases point out and as common sense dictates, the scientific study of a surgical procedure alone is not an antitrust violation. Unless the study is a sham or used only to cast doubt on the safety or efficacy of a procedure, it is highly unlikely a study itself will be viewed as a violation of the Sherman Act violation. Indeed, "many researchers believe that, under ideal circumstances, safety or effectiveness information is best obtained by a randomized, controlled clinical trial, such as the large-scale evaluations that are typically supported by the National Institutes of Health."[82] Simply put, the scientific study of a new, uncertain surgical procedure is relatively safe from an antitrust claim.

Personal opinions

The expression of a personal opinion that is based on a scientific assessment of the procedure is also relatively safe conduct. A physician who "merely publi-

cizes an opinion about the safety or efficacy of a procedure or device, without conferring with others . . . ," is unlikely to pose a risk of antitrust litigation.[83] The antitrust risk, however, in expressing a personal opinion may increase in certain circumstances. For example, the physician who expresses a personal opinion regarding the safety and efficacy of a new procedure and who is otherwise not acting with others toward a common goal is less likely to be criticized than the physician who joins with others in publishing an opinion that is intended to restrict the use and practice of the procedure. Similarly, an opinion expressed by the head of an influential national professional medical association is more likely to provoke an antitrust charge than an opinion expressed by a practicing physician who does not wield the same degree of influence. In all cases where the opinion expressed could economically affect physicians or those who seek the benefit of the procedure, the risk of antitrust litigation is increased.

Lobbying against technology

Any voluntary effort to encourage others to prohibit the use or performance of a new form of surgery will likely result in close antitrust scrutiny. For example, a group of individuals in a professional society who take action to pass policies or resolutions to prohibit or restrict the use or practice of a new procedure will invite antitrust review. There is less antitrust risk to the physician who requests a professional organization or entity to evaluate the procedure independently and objectively, provided there is a sufficient and legitimate medical basis to request such an evaluation.

The risk of antitrust litigation appears highest where a physician or group of physicians develops an opinion about the procedure and then requests an organization to embrace and disseminate the opinion. The safest course of action is for the physician simply to request that the procedure be reviewed but not participate in the process of determining the association's position on the surgery.

A person who requests a governmental agency to take action regarding new surgical procedures may be protected from an antitrust claim. The *Noerr-Pennington* doctrine protects group solicitation of governmental bodies even if such activity is to request that trade be restrained.[84] The antitrust immunity established by the *Noerr-Pennington* doctrine applies to "businesses and other associations when they join together to petition legislative bodies, administrative agencies, or courts of action that may have anticompetitive efforts."[85]* A solicitation campaign that is "ostensibly directed toward influencing governmental ac-

*See footnote on p. 274.

tion, [and] is a mere sham to cover what is . . . nothing more than an attempt to interfere directly with the business relationships of a competitor" will not be protected under the doctrine.[86]

Conduct to petition governmental bodies, by itself, is probably immune from antitrust liability if it is undertaken based on valid medical concerns and not simply to influence or interfere with business relationships. Any conduct outside petitioning efforts to caution against performance of the procedures may well be used by those who advocate the procedure to support a claim that the petitioning conduct was a sham to cover a restraint of trade.

Requests to a professional organization

The risk of antitrust litigation is greatly diminished where a professional association or organization is requested to review and take a position on a medical technology in accordance with established procedures. For example, use of a medical society's established mechanism for the assessment of new surgical procedures will be less likely to evoke antitrust scrutiny than a request that the technology be reviewed outside of the regularly enacted methods.

An example is the AAO's ad hoc Ophthalmic Procedures Assessment Committee. This committee invites a panel of experts to prepare a consensus document describing the current state of knowledge about new procedures. The panel consists of proponents and critics of the procedure. The resulting document, such as one assessing radial keratotomy,[87] must be reviewed by the Academy's Board of Directors before approval and release. A similar mechanism exists in the American Medical Association's Diagnostic and Therapeutic Technology Assessment (DATTA) program. In this program, unsettled medical questions are presented to a panel of individuals who have particular expertise on the subject at issue. The panel members consider the issue assigned to them, and the AMA thereafter prepares a document summarizing the responses of the panel members, as has occurred with radial keratotomy (see Appendix B for the AAO and AMA statements).[88]

These mechanisms are designed to present to professionals and the public a balanced picture of the pros and cons of a procedure. Unfortunately, approaches of this type are often slow and cumbersome. Indeed,

panels may not be able to reach a consensus, resulting in no opinion or a divided opinion being issued. Furthermore, if the document is negative and is cited by insurance companies as a reason for not paying for the procedure, the risk of an antitrust claim arises.

Any request for extraordinary consideration of a technology will likely be viewed by proponents of the technology as an attempt to limit the availability of the technology to them and their patients. Associations and professional organizations may want to give consideration to enacting standard procedures for review of surgical procedures rather than deal with them on an *ad hoc* basis.

Criticism of individuals who advocate the use of the new procedure

The quickest and surest way to encourage persons to consider antitrust litigation is to attack personally the physicians who seek to practice the procedure. In that regard, any request for the review and assessment of a surgical procedure should be directed at the technology itself and not at those who seek to use or practice it.

For example, during discovery in the *Vest* and *Schachar* cases, the attorneys for the plaintiffs asked numerous questions about the designation of some ophthalmic surgeons as "buccaneers," which was defined by one ophthalmologist as those who use surgery to plunder the public for profit (see Chapter 8, Development of Refractive Keratotomy in the United States, 1978-1990). It was clear that plaintiffs resented such name calling, and this resentment fueled the litigation.

Communications with insurance companies

Communications with insurance companies to influence insurance coverage for new surgical procedures creates significant potential for an antitrust claim. Such conduct, if successful, has a direct economic impact on reimbursement for the procedure. The communication to an insurance company of a person's view regarding the acceptability of a new procedure is strongly discouraged. The risk of an antitrust claim, however, is reduced where a physician at the request of an insurance company simply provides factual information for the insurance company's use in determining whether it will provide insurance coverage for a procedure. For example, the antitrust risk is small if a physician provides an insurance company with information about the number of radial keratotomy procedures the ophthalmologist has performed, the visual acuity of patients before and after the procedure, the types of complications experienced, and whether the physician intends to perform the procedure in the future.

---

*(Refers to p. 273) The defendants in *Schachar* rely on the *Wilk* case. The defendants contend: "Even if plaintiffs do intend to allege that the Academy somehow participated in the PERK study or influenced the NAEC to issue its statement, the *Noerr-Pennington* doctrine would immunize such conduct from antitrust liability." The court agreed with this argument and an instruction to this effect was given to the jury at trial.

An ophthalmologist should not express to an insurance company an opinion whether a procedure is or is not generally accepted or practiced. Decisions regarding whether a procedure is generally acceptable or whether it should be covered by applicable insurance policies should be left to insurance companies and their attorneys and medical staffs.

THE FUNDAMENTAL ISSUE: CAN IT BE RESOLVED?

A review of the *Vest* and *Schachar* cases and the current absence of governmental regulation of surgical procedures in this country presents a unique and challenging dilemma to practicing physicians. Any resolution of this dilemma will be influenced to a large extent by the federal antitrust laws. Physicians know that there is no governmental body with power to regulate the introduction or practice of new surgical procedures in this country and that medical professionals must regulate themselves in this area. Self-regulation, however, requires physician action when the safety and efficacy of a procedure are in doubt. Such action will likely restrain performance of the procedure to some extent and thus will always be susceptible to an antitrust claim.

This situation has caused some to consider whether to limit the exposure to antitrust claims by subjecting surgical procedures to greater governmental and institutional regulation. For example, some have suggested that the Food and Drug Administration take jurisdiction over the introduction and performance of surgical procedures in the United States. This option is unlikely to gain broad support from physicians. Similarly, the performance of surgical procedures could be subject to the regulation of state medical authorities, as is medical licensing, although this too is unlikely to engender physician support. Nonetheless, the enactment of federal and state legislation to review the introduction of new surgical procedures in the United States would help insulate physicians from potential antitrust liability by giving them greater freedom to request government scrutiny and regulation.

Many physicians are concerned about colleagues who use and encourage the use of every new and innovative technique regardless of the amount of study and research that has been done on the procedure. These physicians perhaps are most responsible for causing their experienced colleagues to call for restraint and control of or a halt to the performance of new procedures rather than simply allowing continued practice of the procedure according to a strict protocol until studies are completed to determine the usefulness and effectiveness of the procedure.

Physicians who believe that proliferation of an un-tested surgical procedure is being encouraged by doctors who are deficient in their technical medical skills should request that action be taken under established peer-review procedures and state board policies to investigate the competency of the physicians in question. This plan of action, however, is pursued infrequently for two reasons. First it is difficult for professionals to subject other professionals to disciplinary action or to review and scrutinize the professional competence of a colleague actively when such action may jeopardize the colleague's practice. These review procedures are also susceptible to claims, under the antitrust laws, that the review is motivated by illegal, anticompetitive interests rather than honestly held medical concern based on available medical evidence.

The United States Supreme Court in *Patrick v. Burget*[89] affirmed the application of the federal antitrust laws to peer-review proceedings. In *Patrick*, an Astoria, Oregon, physician alleged antitrust claims under Sections 1 and 2 of the Sherman Act against his former partners in an Astoria medical clinic. The plaintiff doctor alleged, among other things, that the defendant physicians had wrongfully instituted a hospital peer-review proceeding against him in an effort to terminate his hospital privileges at the only hospital in Astoria. The plaintiff claimed that the peer-review proceeding was instituted and prosecuted to "reduce competition from [the plaintiff]."[90] The plaintiff doctor prevailed at trial and was awarded $650,000 in actual damages which, under the antitrust laws, were trebled for a total damage award of almost $2 million.[91]

The Supreme Court ultimately heard this case to decide whether the peer-review proceedings, and thus the defendants' conduct, were so actively supervised by state government that they were immune from antitrust scrutiny. In holding that the proceedings and conduct were subject to antitrust review, the Court stated that antitrust immunity will extend to peer-review proceedings only where "state officials have and exercise power to review *particular* anticompetitive acts of private parties and disapprove those that fail to accord with state policy" (emphasis added).[92] Put another way, the State must have authority and must actually exercise "ultimate authority over private privilege determinations."[93] The Supreme Court rejected the defendants' claim that "effective peer review is essential to the provision of quality medical care and that any threat of antitrust liability will prevent physicians from participating openly and actively in peer-review proceedings."[94] The Court observed that this argument "essentially challenges the wisdom of applying the antitrust laws to the sphere of medical care, and as such is properly directed to the legislative branch," not the courts.[95]

Nevertheless, the use of these available review procedures is a practical and effective method to protect the public from unscrupulous physicians and may ultimately lead to the removal of unqualified physicians from the medical profession.

Another mechanism available to the medical profession to oversee the introduction of new surgical procedures in hospitals is the use of institutional review boards and the award of staff privileges. The institutional review board of a hospital must approve the performance of investigational or experimental procedures. The regulatory muscle of such boards, however, varies enormously. Some simply rubber-stamp requests, whereas others are effective review bodies. If a board allows the performance of a new procedure, further control can be exercised by carefully granting staff privileges to each physician performing the surgery in the hospital on a per-procedure basis. Of course, these review procedures do not apply in outpatient surgical centers, where a large amount of ophthalmic surgery is now done.

The consideration of the extent to which physicians should or will be allowed to scrutinize new procedures must be considered in the context of the public's need for accurate information about new surgical techniques. Health care is in transition in the United States, moving from the staid world of professionalism to an environment of increased competition where business interests are deemed equally important as professional concerns. The public is bombarded with health reports on television, by vigorous advertising from hospitals and practitioners, and by articles on the latest high-technology medical breakthroughs. Physicians-turned-business-people compete for patent rights, high-volume practices, and the public eye. At the same time, the government struggles to control health care costs. All of this could lead to diminished concern for patient welfare.

In the current health care environment, patients are left to their own resources more and more when making health care choices. The best way to help patients make informed health care decisions is to provide them with as many facts as possible. For example, the Health Care Financing Administration (HCFA) encourages the publication of hospital death rates as a measure of the quality of care. Similarly universities and consumer organizations, such as Consumer's Union, publish consumer-oriented health care periodicals. Still another approach is that taken by the AAO Procedure Assessment Committee, which reviews and publishes information regarding new procedures. All of these approaches provide factual and objective information on which consumers of health care services can make educated health care decisions.

Simply stated, physicians must face the fundamental but difficult issue of how to deal with the introduction of new surgical techniques in the United States and how to educate the public about the risks and benefits of such new techniques so that their choices about the procedure are informed ones. Unless the profession takes responsible action to accommodate the interests of those who seek to introduce and use new and innovative surgical procedures and the interests of those who require close scrutinization and control of the introduction of the same procedures, physicians will continue to litigate their challenges to each other's conduct. The manner in which new surgical techniques will be introduced in the United States and made available to the public should be left to the medical profession, not to attorneys and the courts.

UNFINISHED BUSINESS

Antitrust law as applied to medical practice in the 1980s to 1990s is undergoing considerable scrutiny, as physicians and attorneys seek to balance medicine's responsibility to monitor and control the behavior and activities of physicians against the individual physician's right to practice in a manner that he or she sees fit. Numerous decisions have been handed down in favor of individual physicians where organized medicine, such as hospital review boards, local or state societies, and so forth have attempted to exclude physicians from practice. Most of these decisions are based on the premise that such exclusionary rulings are anticompetitive.

On the other hand, there are cases in which attempts to use antitrust law to prosecute individuals for alleged anticompetitive behavior have not been successful, as occurred in the Schachar case discussed in this chapter.

REFERENCES

1. *Vest v Waring*, 565 F. Supp. 674 (ND Ga 1983).
2. *Schachar v American Academy of Ophthalmology, Inc*, F Supp (ND Ill 1984).
3. 15 U.S.C. § 1 (1982).
4. 1 Callmann, *Unfair Competition, Trademarks and Monopolies* § 4.20 at 104-106 (4th ed. 1981) (hereinafter "Callmann").
5. 15 U.S.C. § 2 (1982).
6. *American Key Corp. v. Cole National Corp.*, 762 F.2d 1569, 1579 (11th Cir. 1985).
7. *United States v. Grinnell*, 384 U.S. 563, 570-71 (1966).
8. Complaint, *Vest v. Waring* (hereinafter the "Vest Complaint"), ¶¶13-15.
9. *Id.* ¶35.
10. *Id.* ¶¶36-51.
11. *Id.* at ¶¶52-54.
12. *Id.* ¶57 and Prayer for Relief ¶3.
13. *Vest v. Waring*, 565 F. Supp. 674 (N.D. Ga. 1983).
14. Complaint, *Schachar v. AAO*. The complaint was amended on March 22, 1985 (the "Schachar Amended Complaint").
15. Schachar Amended Complaint ¶¶22-32.
16. *Id.* ¶67.
17. Vest Complaint ¶¶25-34, Schachar Amended Complaint ¶¶71-74.
18. Plaintiffs' Brief in Response to PERK Defendants' Joint Motion for Summary Judgment, *Vest v. Waring* (hereinafter "Response Brief") at 1, fn. 1.
19. *Id.* at 2.
20. Schachar Amended Complaint, ¶ 71
21. *Id.* ¶¶ 22-30.
22. *Id.* ¶ 71(t).
23. Plaintiffs' Memorandum in Opposition to Defendants' Motion for Summary Judgment, (Plaintiffs' Memorandum) at 4.
24. Response Brief at 7.
25. *Id.*
26. Schachar Amended Complaint, ¶ 54.
27. Response Brief at 12.
28. Krachmer J and Waring GO: Conclusions from the workshop on radial keratotomy for myopia, Arch Ophthalmol 1980;98:1377.
29. Schachar Amended Complaint, ¶ 67.
30. Brief of PERK Defendants In Support of Their Joint Motion for Summary Judgment, *Vest v. Waring*, dated August 12, 1987 (hereinafter "Defendants' Joint Brief") at 4.
31. *Id.*
32. *Id.* at 5-6.
33. *Id.* at 6.
34. *Id.* at 9.
35. *Id.*
36. *Id.*
37. *Id.* at 7-8.
38. *Supra* n.32, *Id.* at 9.
39. Protocol, Prospective Evaluation of Radial Keratotomy.
40. Schachar Amended Complaint, ¶ 71 (b-f).
41. Vest Complaint, ¶ 27, Response Brief at 13.
42. *Id.*
43. *Id.* ¶ 28, Response Brief at 13.
44. Defendants' Memorandum in Support of Motion for Summary Judgment, *Schachar v. AAO*, dated February 2, 1987 ("Defendants' Memorandum") at 12-14.
45. Defendants' Joint Brief at 9.
46. *Id.*
47. Defendants' Memorandum at 2, 18-27.
48. *Id.* at 13.
49. *Id.*
50. *Id.*
51. *Id.*
52. Silverman W: Human experimentation: a guided step into the unknown, London, 1985, Oxford University Press.
53. Meinert CL: Clinical trials: design, conduct and analysis, New York, 1986, Oxford University Press at 3 (emphasis added).
54. 487 N.Y.S. 2d 595 (N.Y. Sup. Ct. 1985) 59. Id. at 597.
55. *Id.* at 597.
56. *Id.* at 599.
57. *Id.*
58. *Id.*
59. *Id.*
60. Response Brief at 1.
61. Schachar Complaint, ¶ 67(b).
62. Vest Complaint, ¶¶ 30(a)-30(c).
63. Vest Complaint, ¶ 22, Schachar Complaint, ¶ 81.
64. Conversation with James B. Lynch, counsel for the AAO.
65. *Schachar v. American Academy of Ophthalmology*, 870 F.2d 397 (7th Cir. 1989).
66. *Id.* at 399.
67. *Id.* at 398.
68. *Id.*
69. *Id.* at 399.
70. *Id.*
71. *Id.*
72. Rose M and Leibenluff R: Antitrust implications of medical technology assessment, N Engl J Med 1985;314:1490 (hereinafter "Antitrust Implications") citing Norman C: Clinical trials stirs legal battle, Science 1985;227:1316-1318.
73. *Id.*
74. *National Society of Professional Engineers v. United States*, 435 U.S. 679 (1978).
75. *Antitrust Implications* at 1491.
76. Callmann at § 4.20 citing *Standard Oil Co. of New Jersey v. United States*, 221 U.S. 1 (1910).
77. *Id.*
78. Antitrust Implications at 904.
79. Callmann at § 4.20.
80. 783 F.2d 1329 (9th Cir. 1986).
81. *Id.* at 1333.
82. Finkelstein S, Isaccson K, and Frisekopf J: The process of evaluating medical technologies for third-party coverage, J Health Care Technol 1984;1:90.
83. Antitrust Implications at 1492.
84. Callmann at ¶3.08.
85. *Wilk v. American Medical Assn.*, 719 F.2d 207, 229 (7th Cir. 1983), cert. denied, 467 U.S. 1210 (1984).
86. *Id.* citing *Eastern Railroad Presidents Conference v. Noerr Motor Freight, Inc.*, 365 U.S. 127 at 144.
87. American Academy of Ophthalmology: Ophthalmic procedures assessment: radial keratotomy for myopia, Ophthalmology 1989;96:671-687.
88. Diagnostic and Therapeutic Technology Assessment (DATTA): Radial keratotomy for simple myopia, JAMA 1988; 260:264.
89. *Patrick v. Burget*, 486 U.S. 94 (1988).
90. *Id.* at 98.
91. *Id.*
92. *Id.* at 101.
93. *Id.* at 102.
94. *Id.* at 105.
95. *Id.*

Patient Selection and Planning for Refractive Keratotomy

Patient Educational Materials for Refractive Keratotomy

Pamela Edwards Klein

Jan A. Markowitz

Patient education is the process that bridges the gap between health information and health practice and motivates patients to act on this information. By addressing patients on an intellectual, psychologic, and social level, the educational process can increase their ability to make informed decisions concerning their well-being. Ultimately, patient education should enable the individual to use the health care delivery system to meet their personal needs effectively.

Patient education is a relatively new concept in medicine. In the nineteenth century as medical knowledge increased there was a move away from home remedies and folk cures toward greater acceptance of physicians. As medical practice became more scientific, physicians assumed authoritative roles in making patient health-care decisions. With increasing dependence on medical intervention, patients often accepted their doctors' recommendations without asking many questions.

During the latter half of the twentieth century practitioners emphasized the development of educational programs to change attitudes and modify behavior to reduce the risk of developing chronic diseases. Technologic advances in mass communications and the growth of the consumer movement have advanced greater patient participation in health care.

As patients' responsibility for their own health care has grown, so have their legal rights. The early twentieth century marked the first time physicians were required by law to obtain informed consent before performing medical proce-

BACKGROUND AND ACKNOWLEDGMENTS
Ms. Klein and Dr. Markowitz have drawn on their own training and resources as patient educators and clinical trial administrators in evaluating existing patient education materials on refractive keratotomy and recommending standards for such materials. We are indebted to the contributions made by physicians who forwarded copies of their refractive keratotomy information materials for evaluation. We are also indebted to the companies and offices that provided refractive keratotomy literature and video presentations.

dures. It then became physicians' legal responsibility to ensure that their patients understood the purposes and risks of the recommended procedures.

Initially physicians feared that by informing patients of potential risks, acceptance of treatment would be discouraged. However, well-informed patients are more qualified to assess the possible risks and benefits than are uninformed patients.[14] Increased education may lead to increased compliance with medical regimens,[21] which in turn leads to a greater chance of a successful outcome. In addition, patient education can serve as a bulwark against malpractice suits and the rising costs of malpractice insurance. A well-informed patient who agrees to a procedure with the knowledge and understanding of potential risks and benefits is less likely to enter into malpractice suits hastily in the event of a poor outcome.

ROLE OF MASS MEDIA IN HEALTH EDUCATION

In recent decades patients have become better informed about health care and medical technology. In large part this is a result of the impact of mass media, particularly television, on American society. The public encounters health reports on the national news, health programs, cable television channels, health magazines and newsletters; some of these are designed to promote a particular interest or point of view. There are more than 85 million homes in the United States and 98% of them have a television.[2] On the average, these televisions are in use for about 6 hours a day.[16] It has been estimated that by the time children enter kindergarten they have each spent more time in front of a television than they will devote to earning an undergraduate college degree.[13] Altogether the average American devotes about 2600 hours a year to television, radio, newspaper, magazines, and other forms of spectator entertainment.[13] Consequently the American public has come to rely on the mass media as a prime source of medical information.[7,12,26]

Planned and unplanned information

The role of mass media in coveraged health issues can be divided into planned and unplanned forms.[8] The unplanned forms are those in which health issues are represented incidentally to the main story or purpose of the program or article. Unplanned forms of coverage of health issues by the media include entertainment, such as situation comedies, TV dramas, and movies, news, and current affairs. In all of these forms, even the news, the primary objective is to offer a good story and not necessarily to achieve health education goals. In planned forms of coverage of health issues, the concept of a "good story" is combined with a sense of responsibility to inform the public on a particular issue. Planned forms include documentaries and special features in both print and electronic media. The main difference between these forms and, for example, a news story is that the planned forms are generally more detailed and able to present different perspectives on the issues. Educational television and health promotion compaigns, such as those sponsored by the American Cancer Society, are also considered planned forms of media coverage.

The mass media play an important role in creating a social and cultural climate of opinion on health issues no matter if the media are used purposely to influence health-related decisions or if health issues are covered incidentally. If a character in a popular prime-time soap opera undergoes a new surgical procedure, the presentation of the character's experience can influence the public's perceptions of the procedure. Because much of the public's health information is obtained incidentally, through popular TV shows, advertising, and news briefs, there has been concern about the amount of "health miseducation" to which

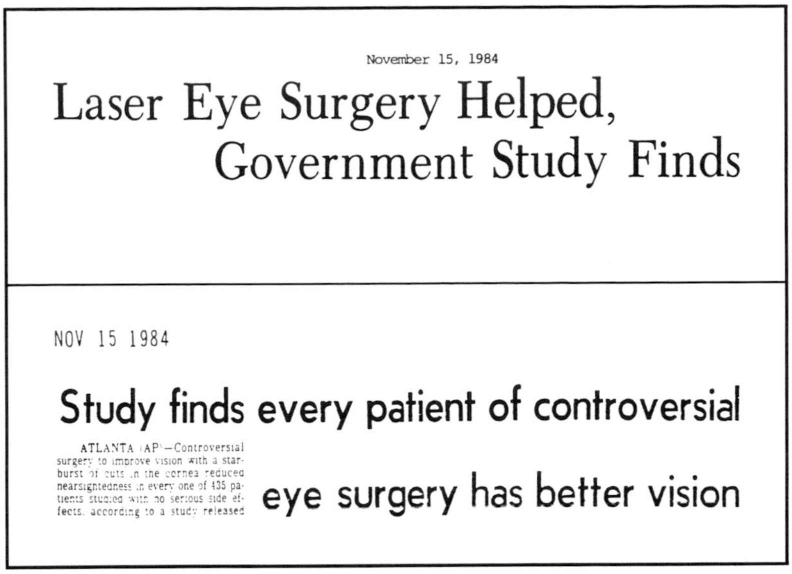

November 15, 1984

Laser Eye Surgery Helped,
Government Study Finds

NOV 15 1984

Study finds every patient of controversial eye surgery has better vision

ATLANTA (AP)—Controversial surgery to improve vision with a starburst of cuts in the cornea reduced nearsightedness in every one of 435 patients studied with no serious side effects, according to a study released

Figure 10-1
Headlines can be misleading or frankly inaccurate, as these headlines from newspaper articles on the PERK study illustrate.

the public is exposed. A Detroit study found that during a typical 130-hour week of television broadcasting, only 7.2% of total broadcast time was devoted to health information. Only 30% of this time offered useful information, and 70% of the health material was inaccurate, misleading, or both.[22]

Sometimes public misperceptions originate from the prominence given a story by the media rather than from the content of the story. For example, in 1983 two reports suggesting a link between cancer and oral contraceptives were published simultaneously in *Lancet*. A week before the *Lancet* reports another study was published suggesting a protective effect of the pill. The reports suggesting the negative effect of the pill were the topic of 195 articles in the national and local press in the United Kingdom, whereas the report suggesting a protective effect received one mention in the national press.[25]

Media excitement was generated when the Prospective Evaluation of Radial Keratotomy (PERK) study results were released in 1984. The headlines overwhelmingly chronicled radial keratotomy as "safe and effective." Although these headlines were misleading at the very least, some were frankly inaccurate (Fig. 10-1). People who only skimmed the headlines might draw the conclusion that PERK had conclusively demonstrated that radial keratotomy was a generally approved and accepted procedure.

Advertising health care

Another source of medical information is advertising. It has been only in recent years, after rulings by the U.S. Supreme Court and actions by the Federal Trade Commission, that physicians have begun to advertise their services. The medical community's attitude toward physician advertising varies.[6,17] Generally advertisements by physicians can be grouped into three categories—informative, educational, and laudatory.[20] Informative advertisements include business cards, telephone directory listings, building signs, and patient information handbooks. Educational advertising includes sponsorship of health fairs, screenings, or seminars, distribution of educational or health-related literature, and publication of health columns or letters to the editor. In contrast, laudatory forms of advertisements claim superiority of service, uniqueness of facilities, exclusivity of therapies, or other similar statements that may be unverifiable or misleading (Fig. 10-2). Informative and educational forms of advertising have gained acceptability among many physicians. However, laudatory forms of advertisement have caused much concern and debate. Although medical societies cannot prevent their members from advertising, some groups, such as the American Academy of Ophthalmology (AAO), have suggested standards for the physician in communicating with the public. The AAO's opinion on advertising is presented in the box on p. 286.

Concern about advertising is understandable. By their nature, all advertisements simplify and all simplification contains potential deception. However, laudatory forms of advertising, the main purpose of which is to sell a product or service rather than to inform, may be more likely to mislead. We reviewed re-

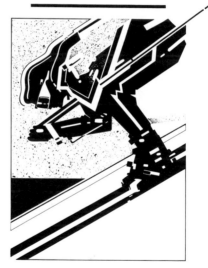

RADIAL KERATOTOMY
$495 per eye

Radial Keratotomy, the procedure for
the correction of nearsightedness
and astigmatism, is a safe and
effective alternative to glasses.
We invite you to our office for a free
RK evaluation.
Please call our office for an
A   appointment.

Figure 10-2
Advertisements for radial keratotomy that we consider undesirable. **A,** In the opinion of the American Academy of Ophthalmology, inappropriate usage of the terms "safe" and "effective" is objectionable, since it can be misleading to the reader.

Continued.

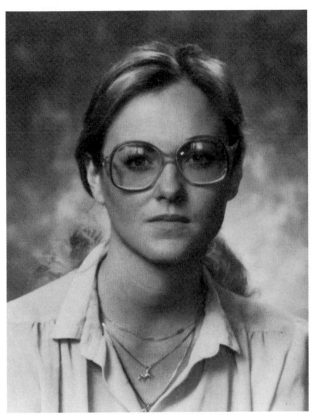
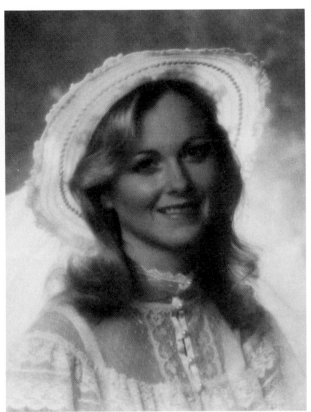

The patient before radial keratotomy surgery at the Center, wearing glasses for nearsightedness.

The same young woman after a 10-minute office surgery on each eye with local anesthesia. She no longer needs glasses.

B

Figure 10-2, cont'd
B, Use of comparisons such as this in advertisements glamorizes the surgery and may lead to unjustified patient expectations.

Advisory Opinion of the Code of Ethics

American Academy of Ophthalmology

Rule 13. Communications to the public. Communications to the public must be accurate. They must not convey false, untrue, deceptive, or misleading information through statements, testimonials, photographs, graphics or other means. They must not omit material information without which the communications would be deceptive. Communications must not appeal to an individual's anxiety in an excessive or unfair way; and they must not create unjustified expectations of results. If communications refer to benefits or other attributes of ophthalmic procedures that involve significant risks, realistic assessments of their safety and efficacy must also be included, as well as the availability of alternatives and, where necessary to avoid deception, descriptions and/or assessments of the benefits or other attributes of those alternatives. Communications must not misrepresent an ophthalmologist's credentials, training, experience or ability, and must not contain material claims of superiority that cannot be substantiated. If a communication results from payment by an ophthalmologist, this must be disclosed unless the nature, format or medium makes it apparent.

From American Academy of Ophthalmology Ethics Committee: Advisory Opinion, 85-86, San Francisco, 1985, The Academy.

---

fractive keratotomy advertisements from across the country, and some illustrate reasons for physician concern and could be viewed as objectionable under the AAO's Rule of Ethics 13. Many glamorize refractive keratotomy and could create an unjustified expectation of improved athletic performance or social grace following the procedure. In several advertisements the physician placing the advertisement makes unsubstantiated claims of being a leader in the field, a pioneer in the procedure, or one of the first to have performed refractive keratotomy. Although some of the advertisements we reviewed state that not everyone is a candidate for refractive keratotomy, none mention any of the risks. Use of terms such as "painless" and "safe," as appear in many of the advertisements, was addressed by the AAO Ethics Committee in September 1985.[1] They found "the term 'painless' with respect to an ophthalmic surgical procedure is really not very accurate, and may be deceptive. Claims that such techniques are 'painless' seem more likely to deceive patients than to assist them in making reasoned decisions about surgery." And in reference to the term "safe," the AAO stated, "Simply using a phrase such as 'safe' is likely to deceive prospective patients by implying an absolute or binary ('safe' vs 'unsafe') standard, when in fact the 'safety' of a surgical procedure is necessarily a qualified concept. The failure to qualify the claim is particularly objectionable since a variety of phrases could easily be employed to communicate the safety/risk relationship (e.g., 'relatively safe,' 'safe for most patients,' or 'among the safer types of surgery')." Lastly, some advertisements stated that the procedure was found safe and effective by the PERK study. This statement is false, since PERK made no such general conclusions.

Of course, not all physician advertising, or even all refractive keratotomy advertising, is objectionable. However, some patients may be unable to interpret and evaluate medical advertising accurately. As more physicians advertise, those who were once opposed to or reluctant to advertise may feel compelled to do so. The continued increase in physician advertising requires vigilance by the medical profession and care by patients—*caveat emptor,* buyer beware.

PHYSICIAN'S ROLE AS INFORMATION PROVIDER
Realistic patient expectations

Each patient brings an individual base of medical knowledge, much gained through the mass media, to his or her physician's office. Because of the attention given to refractive keratotomy by mass media, patients' medical knowledge probably includes a preconceived opinion of refractive keratotomy that may be based on facts, misinformation, or both. This knowledge base affects patients' acceptance of the refractive keratotomy information presented by the physician as well as their experience as refractive keratotomy patients.

Before presenting any formal information on refractive keratotomy, physicians should determine the extent and substance of the patient's knowledge of refractive keratotomy. This can be done informally in conversation with the patient or formally by administering a brief true-false or multiple choice questionnaire. This is to determine any misconceptions or unrealistic expectations about the procedure so that they can be addressed.

How physicians view their role as an information provider determines not only what information they disclose, but also the manner in which the disclosure is made. The interpretation of both legal and ethical obligations to their patients influences this role. Although legal standards may guide physicians in determining what information is given, ethical views have greater effect on the manner in which information is conveyed. At times, physicians' attitudes toward a procedure can be conveyed subtly, as suggested by the covers of their patient information brochures (Fig. 10-3).

A well-informed patient is especially important in refractive keratotomy. Refractive keratotomy is controversial in that it is an elective procedure for which well-established nonsurgical alternatives exist. Although many studies have indicated satisfactory short-term and intermediate results,[4,9,15] it will be many years before adequate information is collected to determine long-term consequences of this procedure. Therefore the patient must understand that long-term success cannot be guaranteed. In addition, the patient must understand that refractive keratotomy cannot correct myopia with the accuracy and predictability of glasses and contact lenses. Therefore realistic expectations are a most important prerequisite for surgery because they may influence patient satisfaction positively even if the final result is less than perfect uncorrected visual acuity. Only the patient can decide if the benefits outweigh the risks.

Within the office setting the physician ideally provides information about surgical procedures by providing educational materials and obtaining informed consent. Merely presenting a patient with a consent form does not constitute an acceptable patient education program.

Patient education

Education is a dynamic process. Studies of learning behavior have shown that retention can be enhanced by repeated exposure to the subject matter. Especially important to the facilitation of learning is the presentation of the material in various forms.[5] Providing information in a variety of forms, printed, audiovisual, or both, increases the likelihood that a patient will understand the information. Many ophthalmologists who perform refractive keratotomy have come to rely on video presentations and patient information booklets to supplement the informed consent process. Some materials are available commercially, whereas others have been developed by individual ophthalmologists. The commercially produced materials are usually general. As an alternative, ophthalmologists have developed materials specifically tailored to their practices and reflecting their personal philosophies.

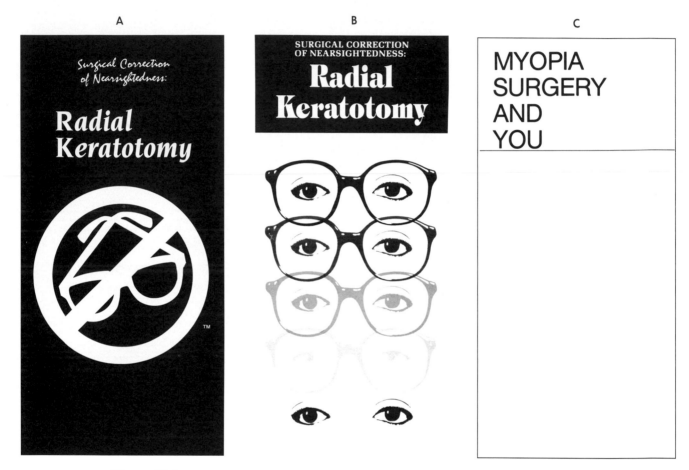

Figure 10-3

Brochure covers suggesting physician attitudes. **A,** "No glasses" sign suggests hard sell. **B,** Fading glasses appeal to patients' desires. **C,** Simple cover suggests no-nonsense information. (**A** courtesy Richard Villasenor, MD, North Valley Eye Center, Mission Hills, Calif; **B,** courtesy Andrew O. Lewicky, MD, Chicago Eye Institute, Chicago.)

INFORMATIONAL MATERIALS FOR REFRACTIVE KERATOTOMY PATIENTS

Refractive keratotomy informational materials, regardless of their source and type, should all address the following topics and issues:

1. Myopia and astigmatism
2. Basic anatomy of the eye and how it functions
3. Clinical evaluation procedures
4. Surgical procedure
5. Postoperative care and precautions
6. Benefits
7. Predictability of result
8. Risks and complications
9. Alternatives to refractive keratotomy
10. Patient selection criteria

In addition to these minimum standards, ideal information booklets should also include the following:

1. Table of contents
2. Glossary/definition of terms
3. History and development of refractive keratotomy
4. Pertinent illustrations, photos, or both
5. Commonly asked patient questions
6. Surgeon's address and telephone number
7. Surgeon's training and experience specific to the procedure
8. References

Information and emphasis in written materials, video presentations, and informal consent documents should be consistent.

The effectiveness of video presentations depends on content and production, as well as the office setting available for viewing. The following criteria are suggested with regard to content and production:

1. The information presented should be consistent with that given in any information booklet and informed consent document.
2. The information should be presented clearly and at an educational level appropriate to the majority of patients.
3. Length of the video presentation should be reasonably brief to maintain patients' attention and to reduce risk of information overload.
4. Featuring the local physician or a physician with national recognition in the video presentation may enhance patient interest and identification.
5. The presentation should be available in a size compatible with most home video cassettes, that is, VHS. This gives the patient the option to view it at home with family.

The viewing area can be an important ingredient to maximize the effectiveness of the presentation. The viewing location should allow for privacy and be large enough to accommodate more than one person. The ophthalmologist should encourage any family members or friends accompanying the patient to also view the presentation. In addition, paper and pencil should be provided so that the patient and friends can write any comments or questions for later discussions with the ophthalmologist. Giving the patient a brief true/false test before viewing the video and then readministering the test afterwards can provide a rough assessment of the patient's understanding of the procedure. This can also serve as a springboard for further discussion before obtaining informed consent, addressing those specific areas of confusion or misunderstanding. However, just because the patient does well on a posttest does not necessarily mean the patient has a complete, accurate understanding of the procedure. The physician should still review the major points, especially risks, with the patient and give him or her the opportunity to ask further questions. Many commercial video presentations include pretest and posttest forms.

INFORMED CONSENT

Patient education is the first component of the informed consent process. It should be consistent with what is later presented in the consent statement. A patient can truly give informed consent only after being fully educated in an unbiased manner. The patient's legal right to education is implied as part of the consent process. However, the extent and importance of this education is determined by the physician.

Informed consent is in the form of a legal document and is the final stage of negotiation between a physician and patient. Informed consent is commonly seen as having two components—informing (or educating) and consenting.[11] Informed consent occurs when a patient understands a test or procedure and is willing to undergo it. This disclosure must be made regardless of whether the patient specifically requests the information and must include all available forms of treatment, including nontreatment. Although physicians have a legal duty to obtain consent, the nature of their disclosures is still at the discretion of the individual physician. To this end the physician assumes the role of the patient's advocate, protecting the patient's legal and moral rights.[10] The informed consent process can be viewed as beneficial to patients by protecting their rights and beneficial to the physician by sharing the decision-making process and its consequent responsibilities. (See Chapter 11, Refractive Keratotomy, the Law of Informed Consent, and Medical Malpractice.)

REVIEW OF AVAILABLE REFRACTIVE KERATOTOMY PATIENT MATERIALS

We surveyed educational materials prepared for potential refractive keratotomy patients. Ophthalmologists throughout the United States who perform refractive keratotomy were contacted and requested to submit copies of the informational materials they supply their patients. Fourteen informational booklets and five video presentations were submitted.

Informational booklets

Of the 14 informational booklets, 12 were developed by ophthalmologists; two were developed by commercial communications organizations. The booklets were evaluated independently by two reviewers and compared with the ideal standard for refractive keratotomy patient information booklets that was outlined earlier. The results are presented in Tables 10-1 and 10-2.

Overall the quality of the booklets was good, although no one booklet contained every point from the ideal set of standards. All booklets included a description of myopia, an explanation of the surgical procedure, and details of postoperative care and precautions. All but one booklet (93%) provided a description of the basic anatomy and function of the eye. The box on p. 292 illustrates how informational material can be simplified for patients.

Risks were at least mentioned in every booklet, but the degree to which they were addressed varied greatly. This concerned us because we feel that risk is probably the single most important issue to be discussed. The discussion of risks is always a sensitive subject. Many surgeons are concerned that if they tell the patient "too much" then the patient will be afraid to have the surgery. However, since refractive keratotomy is an elective procedure and the decision for surgery can be made only by the patient, it is unjust not to ensure that the associated risks are clearly and completely outlined. Only 57% of the booklets mentioned the alternatives to refractive keratotomy (Table 10-1). Since the alternatives, glasses or contact lenses, present minimal medical risks, a clear understanding of the alternatives is necessary to the decision-making process.

Many booklets and video presentations minimized the seriousness of the refractive keratotomy procedure. It would be easy for a patient to form the opin-

Table 10-1

Evaluation of Refractive Keratotomy Information Booklets: Minimal Standards for Content

	Number	Percentage
Description of myopia	14	100
Anatomy of the eye	13	93
Preoperative evaluation procedures	8	57
Explanation of surgical procedure	14	100
Postoperative care	14	100
Benefits of refractive keratotomy	10	71
Risks		
Mentioned but not specified	3	21
Postoperative complications	11	79
Unpredictable outcome	8	57
Use of corrective lens may still be needed	7	50
Possible need for reading glasses in 20/20 patients	4	29
Long-term results unknown	5	36
Possible loss of eye	6	43
Other	6	43
Alternatives to refractive keratotomy	8	57
Patient criteria		
Realistic expectations	5	36
Stable refraction	5	36
Free of residual, recurrent, or active ocular disease	6	43
Best results in mild to moderate myopia	7	50
Best corrected visual acuity such that there is a reasonable chance of useful improvement in uncorrected visual acuity	1	7
Not recommended for one-eyed patients	1	7
Total number of booklets	14	

Table 10-2

Evaluation of Refractive Keratotomy Informational Booklets: Inclusions beyond the Minimal Standard

	Number	Percentage
Format		
Table of contents	2	14
Glossary or definition of terms	5	31
Illustrations and diagrams	14	100
Photographs	6	43
Use of color within brochure	9	64
Note pages	0	0
Content		
Commonly asked questions	3	21
Physician address or telephone number	12	86
Background information on physician	4	29
References	2	14
History and development of refractive keratotomy procedure	10	71
Total number of booklets	14	

Examples of Technical and Simple Explanations

Technical explanation of myopia

In a myopic (nearsighted) eye, parallel rays of light are focused in front of the retina, producing a blurred image. This can be caused by either excessive curvature of the cornea or the shape of the eye itself.

Simple explanation of myopia

In myopia (nearsightedness) objects seen in the distance appear blurry. The blurred vision occurs because light rays cannot focus properly on the back of the eye (the retina). This can be caused when the cornea, the clear tissue on the front of the eye, is too curved or steep or when the eye is too long.

Technical explanation of nighttime glare

Two useful treatments for nighttime glare include using 0.5% pilocarpine at dusk and over-minusing the patient's spectacles by 1.00 D.

Simple explanation of nighttime glare

Some refractive keratotomy patients have problems with glare at night. This can be helped by using an eye drop to make the pupil smaller at night and slightly changing the prescription of patients' glasses.

---

ion that refractive keratotomy is a simple procedure because it does not take long to perform, it is an outpatient procedure, it is usually done under topical anesthesia, and in some cases patients do not need to remove their street clothes. It should be made clear to patients that there is a chance that they may lose their sight because of an infection or may be left with irregular astigmatism that is uncorrectable by glasses or contact lenses. A minority of materials stressed that the results of the operation are less predictable than desired, even in the hands of the most skilled ophthalmologist.

A few booklets contained frankly misleading statements such as the following:

Some doctors have expressed concern about possible long-term effects of refractive surgery. However, corneal transplants—performed on a worldwide basis for some 30 years—have proved to be safe and free from long-term side effects. Since refractive surgery deals exclusively with the cornea, just as corneal transplants do, there is no reason to suspect refractive surgery will have any long-term effects either.

Since approximately 15% of all corneal transplants fail, and since astigmatism, spherical ametropia, delayed microbial keratitis, recurrence of disease, and traumatic dehiscence occur in technically successful clear grafts, it is wrong to imply that they are free from long-term effects. Even if corneal transplants were 100% successful, it would be misleading to imply that the same results would be expected for a different corneal surgical procedure being performed in a different patient population. Care should be taken to explain that not only are the long-term results unknown, but also the short-term results cannot be guaranteed. The PERK study found that approximately 20% of their patients have an uncorrected visual acuity worse than 20/40 1 year after surgery.[24]

Readability and complexity of content are major factors in patients' comprehension of materials. Printed materials are not helpful if they cannot be understood. The box above illustrates this. Furthermore not all patients can read at the level at which they completed their formal education.[19] In the reviewed booklets the reading levels, as determined using the SMOG Grading Formula,[3] ranged from eleventh grade through four years of college, which is beyond the comprehension level of many patients. Most booklets would benefit from readability testing so that they could be appropriately revised before printing. There are many available readability formulas. One of the simplest is the SMOG Grading Formula (see box on p. 294).

Out of necessity most medically related patient materials contain a certain amount of technical language; these terms must be clearly explained to increase patient comprehension. Only 31% of the booklets reviewed provided definition of terms and none included a glossary. One booklet did provide an excellent phonetic pronunciation guide, for example, "refractive keratotomy (ri-frak-tiv ker-a-tot-a-me)."

In most of the reviewed booklets, the quality of the diagrams could be improved. Some diagrams were not labeled, which may lead to some misunderstanding. Most booklets used cross-sectional diagrams of the eye, which are confusing to the average patient (Fig. 10-4.) If such diagrams are used, it is suggested that they

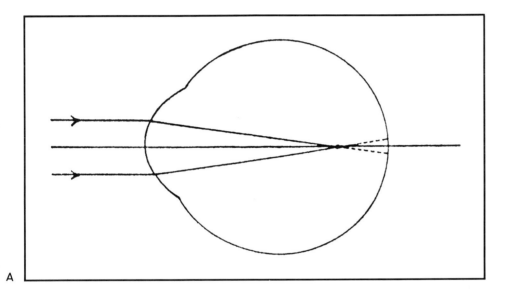

A

Figure 10-4
A, Cross-sectional diagrams can be confusing, especially when unlabeled. **B,** A good example of how to illustrate the anatomy of the eye to a patient. The cross section of the eye is presented within the diagram of the head to provide spatial orientation. The structures are clearly labeled.

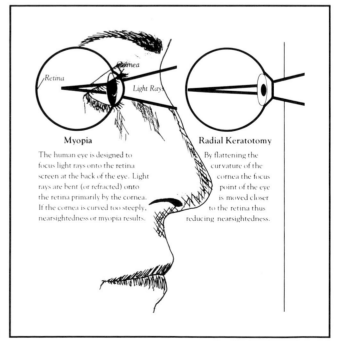

Myopia

The human eye is designed to focus light rays onto the retina screen at the back of the eye. Light rays are bent (or refracted) onto the retina primarily by the cornea. If the cornea is curved too steeply, nearsightedness or myopia results.

Radial Keratotomy

By flattening the curvature of the cornea the focus point of the eye is moved closer to the retina thus reducing nearsightedness.

B

The SMOG Readability Formula

To calculate the SMOG reading grade level, begin with the entire written work that is being assessed, and follow these four steps:

1. Count off 10 consecutive sentences near the beginning, middle, and end of the text.
2. From this sample of 30 sentences, circle all of the words containing three or more syllables (polysyllabic), including repetitions of the same word, and total the number of words circled.
3. Estimate the square root of the total number of polysyllabic words counted. This is done by finding the nearest perfect square, and taking its square root.
4. Finally, add 3 to the square root. This number gives the SMOG grade, or the reading grade level that a person must have reached if he or she is to fully understand the text being assessed.

A few additional guidelines will help to clarify these directions.

- A sentence is defined as a string of words punctuated with a period (.), an exclamation point (!) or a question mark (?).
- Hyphenated words are considered one word.
- Numbers that are written out should also be considered. If numbers are not written out, they should be pronounced to determine whether they are polysyllabic.
- Proper nouns should also be counted if they are polysyllabic.
- Abbreviations should be spelled out to determine whether they are polysyllabic.

Not all pamphlets, fact sheets, or other printed materials contain 30 sentences. To test a text that has fewer than 30 sentences:

1. Count all the polysyllabic words in the text.
2. Count the number of sentences.

3. Find the average number of polysyllabic words per sentence using the following formula:

$$\text{Average} = \frac{\text{Total number of polysyllabic words}}{\text{Total number of sentences}}$$

4. Multiply that average by the difference of 30 and the number of sentences in the text.
5. Add that product to the total number of polysyllabic words.
6. Find the square root of that sum and add 3.

Perhaps the quickest way to administer the SMOG grading test is by using the SMOG conversion table. Simply count the number of polysyllabic words in your chain of 30 sentences and look up the approximate grade level on the chart.

SMOG conversion table*

Total polysyllabic word counts	Approximate grade level (+ 1.5 grades)
0 to 2	4
3 to 6	5
7 to 12	6
13 to 20	7
21 to 30	8
31 to 42	9
43 to 56	10
57 to 72	11
73 to 90	12
91 to 110	13
111 to 132	14
133 to 156	15
157 to 182	16
183 to 210	17
211 to 240	18

*Developed by McGraw HC: Office of Educational Research, Baltimore County Schools, Towson, Maryland.

be presented within the profile of the head to provide additional orientation. The diagram should be at least be labeled with such things as front view and side view. All diagrams and charts should be kept as simple as possible.

Informational video presentations

Five informational video presentations were available for review. Three were produced commercially and two were produced by medical institutions. Results of the review are in Table 10-3. With the exception of one that was institutionally produced, the presentations were quite similar to each other and addressed the major issues. One presentation was judged inadequate because it was brief (7 minutes) and nonspecific, addressing only the eye's anatomy, a description of the disease, a brief explanation of the surgical procedure, and a very limited discussion of risks or complications. This presentation is not included in the remainder of the discussion.

In an effort to maintain the patients' attention, the remaining four video presentations were short, ranging from 11 to 38 minutes. Two of the four were

Table 10-3

Evaluation of Refractive Keratotomy Video Presentations

Content	Master Tape Ventures, Inc.	Milner-Velnick, Inc.	Video Med, Inc.	Neumann Eye Institute	The Eye Institute of Utah
Length (minutes)	38	11	27	13	7
Tape design	V	M	M	V	V
Anatomy of the eye	+	+	+	+	+
Description of myopia	+	+	+	+	+
Explanation of surgical procedure	+	+	+	+	+
Reference to scientific literature or national studies	−	−	−	−	+
Alternatives to refractive keratotomy	+	+	+	+	−
Patient interviews	+	+	+	−	−
Written test for patients	+	−	−	+	−
Risks and complications					
Unpredictable outcome	+	−	−	+	+
Glare or starburst	+	+	+	+	+
Increased sensitivity to light	+	+	+	−	−
Vision may fluctuate	+	+	+	+	−
Vision may decrease	+	+	−	+	−
Possibly still need corrective lenses	+	+	+	+	−
Infection	+	+	+	+	−
Possible loss of eye	+	+	−	−	−
Benefits					
Avoid need for glasses	+	+	+	+	−
Self-image	−	−	−	+	−

+ Part of presentation.
−Not part of presentation.
V, VHS; *M*, U-Matic.

available in VHS, and two were on ¾-inch U-Matic tape. (Video presentations are now released by some companies.) All video presentations offered concise and clear presentations on the anatomy of the eye, description of myopia and astigmatism, presurgery evaluation, and description of the actual surgical procedures. Although not every risk or adverse side effect was discussed, each video presentation did represent the major risks and side effects. Two of the presentations specifically mentioned that because of time limitations, not all risks were discussed and specifically recommended that patients ask their ophthalmologists for more information. The alternatives of glasses and contact lenses were mentioned briefly by each. All four presentations make introductory statements that refractive keratotomy will possibly reduce the need for glasses, but only one specifically stated that patients should avoid surgery if they were comfortable with glasses. Overall not enough emphasis is placed on the fact that refractive keratotomy is an elective procedure with effective noninvasive alternatives.

Immediately following the informational presentation, two of the presentations offered a short series of true/false questions to evaluate the patients' under-

Guide to Developing Educational Materials

Health educators have devoted much attention to designing methods for increasing the effectiveness of patient education materials.[3,18,23] To communicate effectively in print, the following issues should be addressed: legibility, readability, organization, content, and presentation. The following guidelines are offered to assist the physician in developing print materials:

Legibility   Letters and symbols are arranged on the page to facilitate speed and accuracy of reading.

- Use an easily readable type size. Anything smaller than 10-point type may encourage the reader to skip over the text. A larger type size is recommended for patients with poor vision.
- Avoid making lines of type too long or too short. A line length of 50 to 70 characters is recommended for efficient reading.
- Avoid printing words in all capitals. Lowercase type is read more easily.
- Use a pleasing typeface. Most commonly used typefaces are legible with the exception of those that are ornate or not proportionally spaced.

Readability   Content can be understood or comprehended by the target audience.

- Write at an appropriate educational level for the average reader. Pretest the material using a readability formula.
- Use concise sentences.
- Avoid polysyllabic (words of three or more syllables) whenever possible.
- When technical language must be used, a parenthetic definition or a glossary should be included.

Organization   Content and structure of the text is arranged to facilitate comprehension and learning.

- Use headings and subheadings. This may aid recall, search, and retrieval of information.
- Use highlighting techniques such as boldface, italics, or underlining to emphasize important words and ideas.

- Provide an introduction stating the purpose of the material to orient the reader.
- Use one idea per paragraph to emphasize each concept.
- Use examples to clarify ideas to which the reader may not have been exposed.

Content   Comprehensive yet concise presentation of the facts to enable the patient to make an informed choice.

- Do not overwhelm the patient with facts and figures. The patient may be less likely to read long or information-dense literature.
- Maintain an objective balance between the benefits and the risks of any procedures or therapies.
- Do not minimize possible complications.
- Address patient concerns or misconceptions.
- Avoid using unsubstantiated or unverifiable statements and patient testimonials—provide the facts.

Presentation   Pleasing format and visuals can direct attention to the material and aid in comprehension and retention of messages.

- Using white space in the margins and around the sections can increase reading ease and draw attention to important points.
- Use of color, photographs, and illustrations can create interest, emphasize or clarify an idea, and improve organization. Place appropriate visuals such as charts, photos, and graphics next to the related ideas in the text. Keep diagrams and charts simple. Complex visuals can confuse or be misinterpreted.

Many of the guidelines presented above could also be applied to the development of educational video presentations. Most professional producers can offer technical advice for presentation and reaching the target audience. The physician may be most important in ensuring that the points addressed in the contents of an informational guide are incorporated into any video presentation specifically developed for one's practice.

---

standing. These questions help ophthalmologists identify issues patients did not understand and give ophthalmologists an opportunity to review those topics with their patients. Of course answering all test questions correctly does not ensure the patient's complete understanding. In most instances the video presentations contained answers to all the questions. It is still the physician's obligation to assess the patient's understanding through direct one-on-one discussions.

Actual patient interviews were incorporated in three of the four presentations, including brief comments throughout the informational presentation to emphasize specific points of interest. Two presentations, from Master Tape Ventures, Inc. and Video Med, Inc. (Table 10-3), dedicated 24 and 14 minutes respectively to patient interviews. Although the patients represented different viewpoints on specific questions, they all recommended refractive keratotomy. In all the presentations, there was *not one person* who recommended not undergoing the procedure.

In summary, the video presentations were an excellent complement to the informational booklets. Although the artistic quality was better and more original in those that were commercially produced, the content in all was satisfactory. The commercial presentations are available for previewing before ordering. Since they are similar, ophthalmologists are recommended to review each to determine which best meets their individual situations. However, neither the booklet nor video presentations should replace direct interaction with the ophthalmologist. They should serve to reinforce patient discussions. The box on p. 296 provides guidelines on developing educational materials.

CONCLUSION

At one time patient educational materials might have been considered no more than a courtesy that was useful only to promote public relations. However, the role of patients and physicians within the health care system is changing. Patients have become consumer advocates. Many do not just want information concerning their health and medical care, they expect it. With patients sharing greater responsibility for decisions that affect their health care, physicians are becoming not just health care providers, but patient advocates as well. Patient education programs and materials play an important part in the physician-patient relationship of shared health-decision responsibilities. Advertising by physicians should remain informational and educational, avoiding subtly deceptive or misleading statements and exaggerated claims of superiority of the physician's procedure. Advertisements should specify the risks of a procedure.

UNFINISHED BUSINESS

As individuals seeking health care make the transition from passive patients to active consumers, the medical profession carries the increased responsibility of communicating more clearly with individual patients and with the public in general about the preventive and therapeutic options available to them. The elective nature of refractive keratotomy mandates explicit, clear explanations that honestly communicate the benefits and drawbacks of the surgery. Improved written and visual information prepared by individual practitioners, commercial firms, or ophthalmic organizations should improve in quality and directness. Advertising is antithetical to honest communication, and ophthalmology should critically assess the advertising of refractive keratotomy, and through authorized means, such as the American Academy of Ophthalmology ethics code, insist that such advertising meet the standards of the profession.

REFERENCES

1. American Academy of Ophthalmology Ethics Committee: Advertising claims containing certain potentially misleading phrases, Advisory Opinion 85-86, San Francisco, 1985, The Academy.
2. Arbitron Ratings/TV, Universe Estimate Summary, 1983-1984, p. 3.
3. Bader LA: The SMOG Grading Readability Formula, Unpublished paper. Michigan State University.
4. Deitz MR, Sanders DR, and Marks RS: Radial keratotomy: an overview of the Kansas City study, Ophthalmology 1984;91:467-477.
5. DuBois NF, Alverson GF, and Staley RK: Educational psychology and instructional decisions, Homewood, Ill, 1979, The Dorsey Press.
6. Folland ST: Advertising by physicians: behaviors and attitudes, Medical Care 1987;25:311-326.
7. Ford AS and Ford WS: The need for cooperative health education: some survey findings, Int J Health Education 1981;24:83-84.
8. Haslam C: Communication and cooperation between media and health professionals. In Leather DS, Hastings GB, O'Reilly K, and Davies JK, editors: Health education and the media. II. Oxford, England, 1986, Pergamon Press.
9. Hoffer KJ, Darin JJ, Pettit TH et al: Three years experience with radial keratotomy: the UCLA study, Ophthalmology 1983;90:627-636.
10. Lazes PM: The handbook of health education, Germantown, Md, 1979, Aspen Systems Corporation.
11. Levine RJ: Ethics and regulation of clinical research, ed 2, Baltimore-Munich, 1986, Urban & Schwarzenberg.
12. Lieberman Research, Inc.: A basic study of public attitudes toward cancer and cancer tests. Study conducted for the American Cancer Society, New York, February, 1980.
13. Manoff RK: Social marketing: new imperative for public health, New York, 1985, Praeger Publishers.
14. Marshall CC: Toward an educated health consumer, US Department of Health, Education and Welfare, Publication No. (NIH) 77-81, Bethesda, Md, 1977.
15. Nirankari VS, Katzen LE, Karesh JW, et al: Ongoing prospective clinical study of radial keratotomy, Ophthalmology 1983;90:637-641.
16. NTI/NAD (Neilsen Target Information/National Audience Delivery), 11/82; 2/83; 5/83; 7/83.
17. Porter S: Physician advertising: What is legal? What is ethical? What is acceptable? Ohio State Med J 1984;86:437-439.
18. Pretesting in health communications: US Department of Health and Human Services, NIH Publication No. 84-1493, Washington, DC, 1984, US Government Printing Office.
19. Redman BK: Teaching tools: printed and nonprinted materials. In Redman BK, editor: The process of patient education, ed 6, St Louis, 1988, The CV Mosby Co.
20. Rodning CB and Dacso CC: A physician/advertising ethos, Am J Med 1987;82:1209-1212.
21. Rosenthal AR, Zimmerman JF, and Tanner J: Educating the glaucoma patient, Br J Ophthalmol 1983;67:814-817.
22. Smith FA, Geoffrey T, Zuehlke DA, Lowinger P, and Nghiem TL: Health information during a week of television, N Engl J Med 1974;286:516-520.
23. Stewart A: The design of print for health education—principles for communication. In Leather DS, Hastings GB, O'Reilly K, and Davies JK, editors: Health education and the media. II. Oxford, 1986, Pergamon Press.
24. Waring GO, Lynn MJ, Gelendes H, et al: Results of the Prospective Evaluation of Radial Keratotomy (PERK) study one year after surgery, Ophthalmology 1985;92:177-198.
25. Wellings K: Help or hype: an analysis of the media coverage of the 1983 "Pill Scare." In Leather DS, Hastings GB, O'Reilly K, and Davies JK, editors: Health education and the media II, Oxford, 1986, Pergamon Press.
26. Wright WR: Mass media as sources of medical information, J Commun 1974;25:171-173.

Refractive Keratotomy, the Law of Informed Consent, and Medical Malpractice

William S. Duffey, Jr.
Michael P. Kennedy

We discuss two medical-legal aspects of refractive keratotomy in this chapter, detailing the criteria for adequate informed patient consent and surveying and reviewing briefly some aspects of medical malpractice lawsuits and medical malpractice insurance as related to refractive keratotomy.

A physician is obligated to obtain a patient's consent before a medical or surgical procedure is performed. Although the obligation of obtaining a patient's consent is generally recognized by physicians, obtaining this consent has become more complex in recent years. This increased complexity is caused in large part by the public's heightened awareness of the prerogative to be informed fully of the nature of and risks associated with proposed medical treatment. Patients today recognize their right to participate in medical decisions and accordingly have demanded that their physician provide them with information that they deem necessary to make informed medical judgments.

BACKGROUND AND ACKNOWLEDGMENTS

I have invited two attorneys to write this chapter on informed consent because I thought a formal presentation of this approach would be more substantive for readers of this book than a standard colloquial recitation presented by a physician. William S. Duffey, Jr., is a partner with the law firm of King & Spalding in Atlanta, Georgia, and Michael P. Kennedy is an Associate General Counsel at Medaphis Corporation, Atlanta, Georgia. They are familiar with radial keratotomy, specifically because they participated in the legal defense of George O. Waring III, M.D., and Emory University in the *Vest v. Waring* lawsuit, described in Chapter 9, Refractive Keratotomy on Trial: New Surgical Procedures and the Antitrust Laws. We also summarize the work of Jerry Bettman, M.D., reporting his review of a series of malpractice lawsuits concerning refractive keratotomy. The complications of refractive keratotomy are reviewed in detail in Chapter 23, Complications of Refractive Keratotomy, and the criteria for patient education, part of informed consent, are reviewed in Chapter 10, Patient Educational Materials for Refractive Keratotomy.

Almost all jurisdictions,[1] either through judicial decisions or by statute, require physicians to obtain informed consent from their patients. Whether the consent solicited from a patient is informed depends on the quantity and quality of the information given to a patient. Indeed, many medical malpractice claims today arise from allegations that a patient did not really understand the risks of a procedure because the attending physician failed to provide sufficient information to obtain a truly informed consent.

The scope of information that must be disclosed to obtain a patient's informed consent is not always clear. The question presents particular difficulty when a medical or surgical procedure, for example, refractive keratotomy, is relatively new and the long-range benefits and risks of the procedure are uncertain. In this chapter, we do not identify all the potential informed-consent issues that must be addressed before a procedure such as refractive keratotomy is performed. We attempt, however, to discuss the law of consent generally and to provide some guidance concerning what should be disclosed to a patient who is considering undergoing refractive keratotomy.

LAW OF MEDICAL CONSENT
Law of consent

The law generally requires a physician to obtain a patient's consent before a medical procedure is performed. This right is recognized under traditional legal principles that make the unlawful, nonconsensual application of force by one person to the body of another a tortious battery. In other words, a physician who fails to obtain a patient's consent to treatment may be found to have committed a tort and could be responsible for any damages the patient alleges to have suffered. In a landmark decision in the area of medical consent, Justice Cardozo recognized patients' right to determine what is done to them. Justice Cardozo stated the following[2]:

Every human being of adult years and sound mind has a right to determine what shall be done with his own body, and a surgeon who performs an operation without his patient's consent commits an assault for which he is liable to damages.

Tort claims have been successfully asserted against physicians who performed medical or surgical procedures on a patient without the patient's consent,[3] against physicians who performed procedures that exceeded the scope of a patient's consent,[4] and against physicians who performed procedures different from those to which a patient consented.[5] Although most of the cases involving issues of consent today are based on claims that the consent obtained was not informed,

cases still arise in which a physician is held liable for failing altogether to obtain consent.

The likelihood of a lawsuit based on a failure to obtain consent to refractive keratotomy is remote. Because refractive keratotomy is elective surgery, it is unlikely that a physician would fail completely to obtain the patient's consent. A lawsuit based on lack of consent, however, could result if a physician exceeded the scope of the consent given by the patient. For example, if a patient consented to performance of an eight-incision procedure but an unsuccessful or marginally successful 32-incision procedure was performed, the patient could claim that the physician exceeded the scope of the consent.

Law of informed consent

The law of informed consent is based on the proposition that a physician must provide patients with sufficient facts and information so that they can make an intelligent and informed choice about the proposed treatment. The following is true according to the law of informed consent[6]:

A physician violates his duty to his patient and subjects himself to liability if he withholds any facts which are necessary to form the basis of an intelligent consent by the patient to the proposed treatment.

Although the failure to obtain consent is viewed as a battery,[7] the failure to obtain an informed consent is generally viewed as negligence.[8] Courts are increasingly reluctant to recognize a cause of action for battery in informed consent cases because a physician seldom intends to harm a patient.[9] Courts are also reluctant to apply the battery theory because of the potential for punitive damages. Accordingly courts prefer to consider informed consent cases under a negligence standard in which physicians are subject to punitive damages only if their conduct is grossly negligent or willful.

OBTAINING INFORMED CONSENT
Standards for informed consent

It is often difficult to define the information that must be communicated to a patient to allow a truly informed consent to a medical treatment or surgical procedure. A physician, however, is required generally to disclose the following information:

1. The nature of the proposed treatment
2. The risks, consequences, and expected benefits of the treatment
3. An explanation of reasonable alternatives to the treatment
4. The risks to the patient if treatment is not provided[10]

Two standards apply in considering the information that must be given to a patient. The "professional" standard requires a physician to disclose information that a reasonable medical practitioner in the medical community would disclose. The "reasonable-patient," or "lay," standard requires a physician to disclose information that a reasonable person in the patient's position would consider important or material in deciding whether to undergo the proposed treatment.

The professional standard first emerged as the standard in determining whether a physician provided a patient with sufficient information to give informed consent. The Kansas Supreme Court defined the professional standard as follows[11]:

The duty of the physician to disclose . . . is limited to those disclosures which a reasonable medical practitioner would make under the same or similar circumstances. How the physician may best discharge his obligation to the patient in this difficult situation involves primarily a question of medical judgment. So long as the disclosure is sufficient to assure an informed consent, the physician's choice of plausible courses should not be called into question if it appears, all circumstances considered, that the physician was motivated only by the patient's best therapeutic interests and he proceeded as competent medical men would have done in a similar situation.

The professional standard applies in many jurisdictions today.[12]

The modern trend, however, is to apply the reasonable-patient standard in determining whether a patient has given informed consent to treatment. The "reasonable patient" standard was established by the District of Columbia Circuit Court in 1972. This court stated that "true consent to what happens to one's self is the informed exercise of a choice, and that entails an opportunity to evaluate knowledgeably the options available and the risks attended upon each."[13] The reasonable-patient standard therefore focuses on the information needed by an average, reasonable patient rather than what a medical professional would ordinarily disclose to a patient.[14]

Under the reasonable-patient standard a physician may be liable for negligently failing to obtain a patient's informed consent if a court finds that a patient did not receive sufficient material information to allow an informed decision whether to accept the proposed treatment.[15] Materiality has been defined as "that which the physician knows or should know would be regarded as significant by a reasonable person in the patient's position when deciding to accept or reject the recommended procedure."[16] Furthermore, "to be material, a fact must also be one that is not commonly appreciated . . . ."[17]

At least one jurisdiction takes a more subjective approach that concentrates on the information needs of the particular patient. In that jurisdiction it is not enough to show that the information communicated would be sufficient for the "average" patient to make an informed choice. The test is whether the physician provided sufficient information so that the particular patient in question was able to make an informed decision.[18]

What information to communicate

Under either the professional standard or the reasonable-patient standard, certain basic information must be communicated by the physician to the patient. The diagnosis of the patient's condition and the nature and purpose of any proposed treatment should be explained in terms that the patient can reasonably be expected to understand. In the case of refractive keratotomy, the nature of myopia and the manner in which the procedure corrects myopia must be explained in a comprehensible manner.

In addition, physicians should disclose the significant risks that they know or should know are inherent in the proposed treatment.[19] Although all risks may not be required to be disclosed, the more complex and serious the procedure and the risks associated with it, the greater the physician's obligation is to explain the risks. In refractive keratotomy this includes estimates of the chances of perforation of the cornea, overcorrection and undercorrection of visual acuity, loss of corrected visual acuity, glare, fluctuating vision, and an unstable result. Consequently where the risk of injury is high or where the injury that may result is significant, the risk should be disclosed and explained.[20] If the injury that may result is serious, such as keratitis, cataract, endophthalmitis, and traumatic rupture of the globe, the risks should be disclosed even if its probability of occurrence is low.[21]

Obviously where routine procedures are involved, the physician's disclosure obligation is less stringent. One court, however, has ruled that even when simple and routine procedures are involved, a physician is required to inform the patient of the risks of refusing to undergo the treatment[22]; few such risks exist for refractive keratotomy candidates with simple myopia.

A patient should also be informed of reasonable alternatives to the treatment being proposed by the physician. Failure to disclose information about treatment alternatives may result in a finding that the consent given was not informed.[23] In the case of refractive keratotomy this includes a discussion of the relative risks and predictability of vision with glasses and contact lenses, as well as the nature and risks of other refractive surgical procedures such as epikeratoplasty and keratomileusis. Patients' prognosis in the absence of treatment should also be disclosed so that they will have sufficient information to consider the available treatment alternatives. Patients should also be able to compare treatments, with all the risks, with the continued wearing of glasses or contact lenses if refractive keratotomy is not elected.

Consent for new procedures

A physician is under a greater obligation to disclose information to a patient where the procedure involved is new or experimental-investigational. Since 1971, federal guidelines and regulations have regulated experimental research on human beings funded by the U.S. Department of Health and Human Services.[24] Those federal regulations include strict informed-consent requirements for experimental research.[25] The Food and Drug Administration also extensively regulates the manner in which experimental medical devices and drugs are used.[26] Although these federal regulations do not apply to the introduction and practice of new surgical procedures, it is indicated that physicians are obligated to provide full disclosure of the risks associated with new or experimental surgery.[27] A physician is also required to explain to a patient that a proposed surgical procedure is new or experimental[28] and to inform the patient fully of the foreseeable consequences of the treatment and any uncertainty of or known or projected risks associated with the new or experimental procedure.[29]

Refractive keratotomy was considered an experimental-investigational procedure in the late 1970s and early 1980s by the National Advisory Eye Council, the American Academy of Ophthalmology, the PERK Study Group, the International Society of Refractive Keratoplasty, and many ophthalmic surgeons.[30] During that time many surgeons took special care to explain to prospective patients what was and was not known about the procedure. By the late 1980s enough definitive information was known about refractive keratotomy that the experimental-investigational designation was generally removed. However, the absence of well-established standards for the acceptability of refractive keratotomy, the elective nature of the procedure, and the fact that the operation is done by only approximately 10% of ophthalmologists in the United States and that much ambiguous, misleading, or inaccurate information has been disseminated in news and advertising media all suggest that ophthalmologists should be particularly careful to inform patients of relevant information known about refractive keratotomy.[31]

FORM OF CONSENT

Consent can be express or implied. Express consent is ordinarily obtained through oral or written communications with the patient. In the absence of express consent a patient's consent to a procedure or treatment may be implied through the conduct of the patient, such as submitting to a procedure after having discussed the procedure with the treating physician. In all cases the consent need only be informed and voluntarily given.

Although consent in writing is not required,[32] it is usually obtained. This prevents having to prove that a patient's consent was obtained orally or that consent was implied through a patient's conduct. In some jurisdictions a written consent is at least *prima facie* evidence that an effective consent was obtained in the absence of evidence that it was secured by misrepresentation or fraud.[33]

A written consent that purports to insulate a physician from liability is not effective if the consent form used by the physician does not provide adequate information to establish that the consent given was informed. For example, if a consent form is too technical for the patient to understand or if the form does not describe adequately the proposed treatment and potential risks, the consent may be determined to be inadequate.[34] Written consents obtained from people who cannot comprehend their actions are likewise ineffective.[35]

REFRACTIVE KERATOTOMY AND INFORMED CONSENT: OBSERVATIONS AND RECOMMENDATIONS

Refractive keratotomy is a relatively new surgical procedure in the United States, and the risks and benefits associated with it are still being fully determined. Consequently the performance of refractive keratotomy may lead to a higher incidence of malpractice actions based on patient claims that a treating physician failed to obtain informed consent.[36] Physicians who perform refractive keratotomy can reduce the risk of a malpractice claim based on lack of informed consent by developing and implementing a comprehensive informed consent policy.

Informed consent policies, however, must be based on the statutory or case law that exists in the jurisdiction where a physician practices. In developing an informed consent policy, physicians should be guided by two key informed consent principles—disclosure and documentation.

Disclosure

The physician should be responsible for obtaining the informed consent of a patient. The responsibility should *not* be delegated to nurses, other persons in the physician's office, or the staff at the hospital where the physician practices. A physician should directly discuss with the patient all aspects of the procedure, all risks and implications associated with the surgery, and the full range of possible results. It is useful to use informational brochures and videotapes that demonstrate how the procedure is performed and to provide the patient with any other written information concerning the surgery that the physician believes is accurate (see Chapter 10, Patient Educational Materials for Refractive Keratotomy).

In the case of refractive keratotomy, physicians should prepare a written informational checklist that outlines refractive keratotomy in simple, understandable terms. This checklist should be used by the physician when discussing the procedure with a patient. Among other things, the checklist should remind the physician to do the following:

1. Provide information about the patient's diagnosis
2. Describe the nature and purpose of the proposed refractive keratotomy surgery
3. Disclose the risks and benefits of the surgery
4. State the available alternatives to the surgery, including not having the surgery

Because refractive keratotomy is an elective procedure, a physician should disclose to a patient, fully and in detail, the risks and benefits of the surgery. Patients should be told the following:

1. Complications may cause blindness.
2. The cornea may be scarred so much that vision is reduced.
3. Glare may occur.
4. It may still be necessary to wear eyeglasses or contact lenses after surgery.
5. Patients may not be able to wear contact lenses because of the incisions made in their corneas.

Physicians should also inform patients of the uncertainty of the long-range outcome of the procedure. The patient should be told there is a possibility that, as a result of the operation, the refraction may gradually change in the direction of farsightedness and that other eye surgery such as cataract extraction may be more difficult to perform. The patient should also be told that the use of reading glasses may be required sooner than if refractive keratotomy had not been performed.

A physician can further reduce the risk of a malpractice action based on lack of informed consent by providing patients with sufficient time to understand and digest the information provided about the surgery. Even when a patient desires to have the procedure done as soon as possible, it is in the physician's and patient's best interest to provide sufficient time between discussions and disclosures about the surgery

and performance of the procedure to allow the patient to review and analyze the surgery and its risks and benefits. Although the time required to digest information varies from patient to patient, at least several days should be allotted to allow a patient to consider and evaluate the information.

A thorough, straightforward, empathetic explanation by ophthalmologists does not mean their patients will remember what they are told. A study of 100 patients with retinal detachment disclosed interesting results. Each of these 100 patients was given standardized informed consent information before retinal reattachment surgery. After surgery, 97% of the patients recalled the thorough presurgery discussion. However, only 23% remembered the surgical risks that were described. The study further revealed that when patients failed to remember information given to them before the surgery, more than half of them denied that the information had even been discussed. Those who conducted the study concluded that patients primarily retain information that supports their decision to have the surgery.[36] It is important therefore to document what the patient is told.

Documentation

Informed consent documentation should begin at the initial consultation between the physician and the patient. The physician should note on the patient's chart or medical record the date and substance of all communications with the patient about the procedure. Each time a physician provides additional oral, written, or videotaped information to the patient, it should be noted in the patient's medical record and a copy of the information should be put with the chart if possible.

The most important documentation is the informed consent form signed by the patient before the procedure is performed. The written consent form is particularly important for a new, developing procedure such as refractive keratotomy. Because the consent form will, in most cases, be the focus of any malpractice litigation based on an alleged lack of informed consent, the form should contain a thorough, comprehensive presentation of all relevant information about the procedure, its risks, results, and complications, and alternatives to the surgery. Refractive keratotomy patients should be required to acknowledge specifically in writing that they are aware that some unforeseeable risks are associated with the procedure and may not become apparent for years.

A sample consent form is provided in the box on p. 304. It is for informational purposes only. It should not be relied on by physicians in practice until it is reviewed and, if necessary, revised by a lawyer to conform to the law of informed consent in the jurisdiction

Special Authorization and Consent to Refractive Keratotomy Surgery, Including Administration of Anesthetics

Name of Patient: _____ Date: _____ Time: _____

Cross out any provisions that do not apply or are not approved by the patient:

1. *Patient's condition.* I understand from my physician, Dr. _____, that the diagnosis of my condition is as follows: _____
_____

2. *Recommended procedure; alternatives.* Dr. _____ explained to me alternative courses of treatment for my condition, including _____
_____.
After discussing my condition and the alternative treatments for it with Dr. _____
I have decided that I wish to have refractive and/or transverse keratotomy surgery, which consists of the following: (Describe procedure in lay language)
_____
_____.
I hereby authorize Dr. _____ and such assistants as may be selected by him (her) to perform the refractive keratotomy surgery described above.

3. *Risks and consequences.* In addition to the usual risks of surgical or medical procedures (for example, infection, cardiac arrest), I have also been made aware of special risks and consequences that are associated with the refractive keratotomy procedure, including the following: (List major risks associated with refractive keratotomy)
_____
_____.

4. *Uncertainty of future consequences.* I have been informed by Dr. _____ that there may be possible short-term or long-term risks associated with the refractive keratotomy procedure that are currently unforeseeable and unknown. These unforeseeable and unknown risks may adversely affect my eyesight immediately after performance of the refractive keratotomy procedure and in the future, and I authorize the performance of the refractive keratotomy procedure with that knowledge.

5. *Extension of procedure.* Dr. _____ explained to me that during the course of the refractive keratotomy procedure, unforeseen conditions may be revealed that necessitate an extension of the original procedure or performance of a procedure different from the refractive keratotomy procedure. I therefore authorize and request that the above-named physician and his (her) assistant or assistants perform such surgical and medical procedures as are necessary and desirable in the exercise of their professional judgment. The authority granted under this paragraph 5 shall extend to treating all conditions that require treatment and that are not known to my physician at the time the refractive keratotomy procedure is commenced.

6. *Anesthesia.* I hereby authorize the administration of customary and appropriate anesthesia, in connection with the refractive keratotomy procedure, by or under the supervision of Dr. _____. I understand that the anesthesia to be used in my case is _____,
which will be administered in the following form: _____.
I have been advised that, although there are alternative methods of anesthesia, the above type and method is preferable in my case because: _____
_____.
I have been advised, and I understand, that there are always special risks involved in the administration of anesthesia. These risks include:

7. *Explanation and questions.* I have discussed with Dr. _____ my condition, the refractive keratotomy procedure, alternative procedures and the known risks associated with the refractive keratotomy procedure and the fact that currently unknown and unforeseeable risks associated with the refractive keratotomy procedure may exist. I have also had full opportunity to ask questions concerning my condition, the refractive keratotomy procedure, treatment alternatives, and associated risks. The questions I have asked concerning the refractive keratotomy procedure have been answered to my satisfaction. I understand that the explanation which I have received may not be exhaustive and all inclusive and that other more remote and unknown risks may be involved. However, the information that I have received is sufficient for me to consent to and to authorize the refractive keratotomy procedure. I, therefore, hereby authorize performance of the refractive keratotomy procedure on me and I give this consent of my own free will.

8. *No guarantee.* I hereby state that no guarantees or assurances have been made to me concerning the results of the refractive keratotomy procedure. I have fully and completely read this document, I fully understand and comprehend this document and acknowledge that all blanks and spaces have been filled in before my signing.

Patient's signature: _____

Witness: _____

where the form is proposed to be used. Informed consent forms are legal and informational documents. They should therefore be developed with the assistance of an attorney familiar with the law of informed consent.

A consent form should not be used as a substitute for direct communication with the patient. A signed consent form where there has not been any communication between the physician and patient may be given only little, if any, weight in a malpractice action.

STUDY OF MALPRACTICE CASES INVOLVING REFRACTIVE KERATOTOMY

Bettman[36] has reported the results of his study of medicolegal claims regarding refractive keratotomy. He described the context in which malpractice lawsuits over radial keratotomy often arise:

A typical prospective patient was first made aware of refractive keratotomy through the news media, often the television. This was frequently a glowing account, and the risks of the procedure were not mentioned. The next step usually involved contact with the surgeon who performed a large volume of refractive keratotomies. This surgeon often advertised extensively, which is why the patient decided to go to him. The patient was usually given or sent a brochure of 10 to 12 pages that also presented a glowing account and contained a small paragraph with a general statement that complications might occur with any surgical procedure. During the third step the patient was given an appointment with this surgeon's office. Either on entry or shortly before the refractive keratotomy the patient was presented with a printed informed consent form that usually contained an adequate discussion of the risks as well as the benefits. The patient was asked to read and sign this document. However, at this stage the patient had already been convinced that the risks

---

Table 11-1

Summary of Complaints in 25 Medicolegal Claims

Type of complaint	Number of complaints*
Complaints regarding informed consent	25
Informed consent as the chief complaint	13
Poorer vision postoperatively than preoperatively	13
Vision substantially lost	4
Marked problems with glare	12
Persistent wildly fluctuating vision	10
Inability to wear contact lenses postoperatively	7
Inability to work	6
Inability to drive after refractive keratotomy	5
Postoperative presbyopia	4
Problems with retrobulbar injection	4
Perforation of globe	1
Optic atrophy	3
Significant undercorrection	4
Myopia (-10.00 D, -14.00 D, -4.50 D, -4.00 D)	
Significant overcorrection	3
Hyperopia ($+11.00$ D, $+6.00$ D, $+5.25$ D)	
Scarred cornea necessitating operation	3
Transplant	1
Keratomileusis	1
Surgery pending	1
Patient came only for new spectacles	2
Cataracts (1 from perforation, 1 from steroids)	2
Bilateral procedures on same day	2
Pilot could not fly after refractive keratotomy	2

From Bettman JW: Medicolegal claims concerning refractive keratoplasty. In Schwab I, editor: Refractive keratoplasty, New York, 1987, Churchill-Livingstone.
*Total is more than 25 because some patients had more than one complaint.

were minimal. He looked upon the document as he would upon a hospital admission form, which he signed as a perfunctory event. The usual patient had already decided that he wanted the procedure done because of the previous glowing accounts and thought that he should sign this because the surgeon's office asked him to. Even though he had read the entire document, insufficient attention was paid to it.

The review of 25 medicolegal claims made regarding refractive keratotomy surgery revealed interesting results (Table 11-1). All patients complained that informed consent had been inadequate and this was the chief complaint of about half of the responding complaintants. About half claimed they had poorer vision after surgery than they did before surgery, and about half complained about problems with glare. Four claims were made about damage to the eye or optic nerve from retrobulbar anesthesia, a complication not directly related to the keratotomy procedure itself and one that is avoided by most surgeons who use either topical or peribulbar anesthesia. Two patients complained that they consulted the doctor only for new spectacles, but ended up having refractive keratotomy. Two patients sued because they had both eyes operated on the same day. Two aspiring pilots sued because they could not be pilots after refractive keratotomy. Many patients had multiple complaints on which they based their lawsuits. In one case a librarian claimed that she consulted her ophthalmologist for new contact lenses, was encouraged to have refractive keratotomy, and developed glare and irregular astigmatism after two operations on each eye. She complained that she had to stop her work because of complications from the procedure.

CONCLUSION

The failure to obtain the informed consent of a patient before performing a new, elective surgical procedure such as refractive keratotomy can have significant economic and legal consequences. An ophthalmologist can, however, protect against these consequences by doing the following:

1. Developing with the assistance of an attorney an informed consent policy that ensures patient understanding of the surgical risks and benefits
2. Employing proper procedures for obtaining and recording the patient's informed consent
3. Avoiding cases with questionable indications, such as cases in which a patient's occupation is at risk if an unfavorable result occurs or in which an elderly patient may experience a large overcorrection
4. Avoiding performance of the procedure on patients with unrealistic expectations, such as patients who are convinced that the procedure is simple and almost always has perfect results
5. Having a responsive and empathetic office staff who will pay attention to individual patients and their problems and complaints
6. Maintaining meticulous clinical records
7. Consulting with other ophthalmologists in the event that problems arise in an individual case
8. Maintaining adequate insurance coverage.[36]

The employment of such reasonable informed-consent policies and patient-management procedures is an effective way to insulate a physician from claims that a patient was not fully and reasonably informed of the nature, risks, and effects of an elected procedure or treatment.

UNFINISHED BUSINESS

The major piece of unfinished business in the area of informed consent occurs on a daily basis—the requirement for the surgeon to communicate honestly the risks and benefits to each individual patient, adhering to the basic principles of risk reduction. Refractive surgeons and ophthalmic political organizations should critically assess the apparently capricious restrictions and exorbitant fees being levied by malpractice insurance carriers on surgeons who do refractive surgery. The safety record of refractive keratotomy should pave the way for its inclusion under standard ophthalmic surgical procedures in liability insurance.

REFERENCES

1. For statutes, *see, e.g.,* ALASKA STAT. § 09.55.556(a) (1983); ARK. CODE ANN. § 16-114-206 (1987); DEL. CODE ANN. tit. 18, § 6852 (Michie Supp. 1986); FLA. STAT. ANN. § 768.46 (West 1986); IDAHO CODE § 39-4301 (1985); KY. REV. STAT. ANN. § 304.40-320 (Michie/Bobbs-Merrill 1981); LA. REV. STAT. ANN. § 1299.40 (West 1976); ME. REV. STAT. ANN. tit. 24, § 2905(1) (West Supp. 1987); NEV. REV. STAT. § 41A.110 (1986); N.Y. PUB. HEALTH LAW § 2805-d (McKinney Supp. 1988); N.C. GEN. STAT. § 90-21.13 (1985); OR. REV. STAT. § 677.097 (1987); 40 PA. CONS. STAT. ANN. § 1301.103 (West Supp. 1987); TENN. CODE ANN. § 29-26-118 (1976); TEX. REV. CIV. STAT. ANN. art. 4590i; § 6.05 (West Supp. 1988); VT. STAT. ANN. tit. 12, § 1909 (Equity Supp. 1987); WASH. REV. CODE ANN. § 7.70.050(1)(a) (West Supp. 1988); GEORGIA SENATE BILL 367 (to be codified at GEORGIA CODE ANN. § 31-9-6.1).
   For cases, *see e.g., Cobbs v. Grant,* 8 Cal. 3d 229, 104 Cal. Rptr. 505, 502 P.2d 1 (1972) reh'g denied 1989 Cal. A pp Lexis 1126 (1989); *Crain v. Allison,* 443 A.2d 558 (D.C. 1982); *Harnish v. Children's Hosp. Medical Center,* 387 Mass. 152, 439 N.E.2d 240 (1982); *Lincoln v. Gupta,* 142 Mich. App. 615, 370 N.W.2d 312 (1985); *Congrove v. Holmes,* 37 Ohio Misc. 95, 66 Ohio Ops. 2d 295, 308 N.E.2d 765 (1973).
2. *Schloendorff v. Soc'y of N.Y. Hosp.,* 211 N.Y. 125, 105 N.E. 92, 93 (1914) overruled on other grounds, *Bing v. Thunig* 2 N.Y.2d 656, 143 N.E.2d 3, 163 N.Y.S.2d 3 (1957).
3. *Pugsley v. Privette,* 220 Va. 892, 263 S.E.2d 69 (1980). (Physician liable for battery for removing patient's ovaries after patient revoked her consent.)
4. *Gray v. Grunnagle,* 423 Pa. 144, 223 A.2d 663 (1966).
5. *Moser v. Stallings,* 387 N.W.2d 599 (Iowa 1986).
6. *Salgo v. Leland Stanford, Jr. Univ. Bd. of Trustees,* 154 Cal. App. 2d 560, 578, 317 P.2d 170, 181 (1957).
7. *Pugsley v. Privette,* 220 Va. 892, 263 S.E.2d 69 (1980), *Cobbs v. Grant,* 8 Cal. 3d 229, 104 Cal. Rptr. 505, 502 P.2d 1 (Cal. 1972). (Physician may be liable for battery where he has performed an operation to which the patient has not consented.)

8. *Cobbs v. Grant,* 8 Cal. 3d 229, 104 Cal. Rptr. 505, 502 P.2d 1 (1972); *Revord v. Russell* 401 N.E.2d 763 (Ind. Ct. App. 1980).
9. *Twitchell v. MacKay,* 78 A.D.2d 125, 434 N.Y.S.2d 516 (1980). (Failure to obtain informed consent is not an antisocial act within the meaning of traditional intentional tort theory.)
10. *Canterbury v. Spence,* 464 F.2d 772 (D.C. Cir. 1972), *cert. denied,* 409 U.S. 1064 (1972).
11. *Natanson v. Kline,* 186 Kan. 393, 350 P.2d 1093 (1960), clarified 187 Kan. 186, 354 P.2d 670 (1960).
12. *See, e.g.,* 18 DEL. CODE ANN. § 6852(a)(2); FLA. STAT. ANN. § 768.46; HAWAII REV. STAT. § 671-3; N.C. GEN. STAT. § 90-21.13; TENN. CODE ANN. § 29-21-118; GEORGIA SENATE BILL 367 (to be codified at GEORGIA CODE ANN. § 31-9-6.1)
13. *Canterbury v. Spence,* 464 F.2d 772 (D.C. Cir. 1972); *cert. denied,* 409 U.S. 1064.
14. *Id.; Cobbs v. Grant,* 8 Cal. 3d 229, 104 Cal. Rptr. 505, 502 P.2d at 11 (1972). ("[T]he patient's right of self-decision is the measure of the physician's duty to reveal. That right can be effectively exercised only if the patient possesses adequate information to enable an intelligent choice.")
15. *Canterbury v. Spence,* 464 F.2d 772 (D.C. Cir. 1972), *cert. denied,* 409 U.S. 1064 (1972); *Cobbs v. Grant* 8 Cal. 3d 229, 104 Cal. Rptr 505, 502 P.2d 1 (1972).
16. *Truman v. Thomas,* 27 Cal. 3d 285, 165 Cal. Rptr. 308, 611 P.2d 902 (1980).
17. *Id.*
18. *Scott v. Bradford,* 606 P.2d 554 (Okla. 1979). Patients that inquire about refractive keratotomy tend to be well-educated males with good economic standing who, one can assume, would want a complete explanation of the procedure, its risks, and potential outcomes. Under the "particular patient" standard a physician performing refractive keratotomy would be held to a high standard of disclosure.
19. *Sard v. Hardy,* 281 Md. 432, 379, A.2d 1014 (1977).
20. *Harwell v. Pittman,* 428 So.2d 1049 (La. App. 1983), *cert. denied,* 434 So.2d 1092 (1983), *reh'g denied,* 436 So.2d 570 (1983).
21. *Cobbs v. Grant,* 8 Cal. 3d 229, 104 Cal. Rptr 505, 502 P.2d 1 (1972), *Hartke v. McKelway,* 707 F.2d 1544 (D.C. Cir. 1983), *cert. denied,* 464 U.S. 983 (1983).

22. *Truman v. Thomas,* 27 Cal. 3d 285, 165 Cal. Rptr. 308, 611 P.2d 902 (1980). (Court ruled that a physician's duty to disclose includes the responsibility to inform the patient of the risks of refusing to undergo a Pap smear test that he recommended.)
23. *Sard v. Hardy,* 281 Md. 432, 379 A.2d 1014 (1977); *Holt v. Nelson,* 11 Wash. App. 230, 523 P.2d 211 (1974).
24. 45 C.F.R. § 46.101 *et seq.* (1987).
25. 45 C.F.R. § 46.116 (1987).
26. 21 C.F.R. § 50.1 *et seq.* (1987).
27. *See, e.g., Estrada v. Jaques,* 70 N.C. App. 627, 321 S.E.2d 240 (1984); *Ahern v. Veterans Admin.* 537 F.2d 1098 (10th Cir. 1976).
28. *Estrada v. Jacques,* 70 N.C. App. 627, 321 S.E.2d 240 (1984).
29. *Id.*
30. This designation lead, in part, to the two antitrust lawsuits discussed in Chapter 9. Radial Keratotomy on Trial: New Surgical Procedures and the Antitrust Laws.
31. See Chapter 10, Patient Educational Materials for Refractive Keratotomy.
32. *Patterson v. Van Wiel,* 91 N.M. 100, 570 P.2d 931 (Ct. App. 1977), *cert. denied,* 569 P.2d 413 (1977).
33. See, *e.g.,* FLA. STAT ANN. § 768.46(4) (West 1986) (written consent "conclusively presumed" valid); N.C. GEN. STAT § 90-21.13(b) (1985) (rebuttable presumption of validity in absence of evidence that consent was obtained by "fraud, deception or misrepresentation of a material fact.") Georgia Senate Bill 367 (to be codified at GEORGIA CODE ANN § 31-9-6.1) (rebuttable presumption of validity).
34. *Sauro v. Shea,* 257 Pa. Super. 87, 390 A.2d 259 (1978). (Physician liable for death of patient when he failed to warn patient of potential fatal risk of anesthesia even though patient signed a consent form.)
35. *Aponte v. United States,* 582 F. Supp. 65 (D.P.R. 1984) (consent by mentally incompetent patient invalid).
36. Bettman JW: Medicolegal claims concerning refractive keratoplasty. In Schwab I, editor: Refractive keratoplasty, New York, 1987, Churchill-Livingstone.

Examination and Selection of Patients for Refractive Keratotomy

George O. Waring III

In this chapter I present guidelines intended to help ophthalmologists decide which patients are good candidates for refractive keratotomy. Against the back- who seek refractive keratotomy and their motivation. I then specify the preoperative clinical examinations and examine their role in patient selection and surgical planning. This information is synthesized in a discussion of individual patient consultation. The chapter ends with a discussion of the planning of surgery on the second eye and a brief discussion of the economic aspects of refractive keratotomy.

PHILOSOPHIC ATTITUDES THAT AFFECT PATIENT SELECTION

There are specific aspects of refractive keratotomy surgery that make the criteria for patient selection different from the classical criteria for ocular surgery.

BACKGROUND AND ACKNOWLEDGMENTS

Most of the information in this chapter is drawn from my personal experience with patients in the PERK study and in my private practice. The opinions in this chapter reflect predominantly my own point of view, which may differ from that of other conscientious ophthalmologists. The editorial by Michael Dietz, "Radial Keratotomy, Cosmetic or Functional" (J Refract Surg 1986;2:152-153), articulates clearly some of the ideas surrounding patient motivation and selection. The psychometric studies of Bourque and colleagues and of Powers and colleagues (as discussed in the text) form a more objective basis for our assessment of the motivation and characteristics of patients seeking refractive keratotomy. Governmental, organizational, and industrial standards concerning employment of patients who have had refractive keratotomy and other forms of refractive surgery may change based on the attitudes and opinions of the policy-makers and the scientific information generated by the ophthalmic community. The methods of patient examination could fill another textbook. Most of the information on examination techniques is available in other textbooks and articles. I have selected here only those aspects that are directly pertinent to refractive keratotomy and have organized them in a practical way.

Elective surgery

Because spectacles and contact lenses are generally available and socially acceptable in industrialized nations, although quality varies from country to country, people with physiologic and intermediate myopia can readily achieve complete optical correction. Therefore refractive keratotomy is elective surgery for both the patient and the surgeon because the surgery is not necessary to achieve functional emmetropia. This distinguishes myopic patients from patients with progressive cataracts or uncontrolled glaucoma who will ultimately go blind if appropriate surgery is not performed. That refractive keratotomy is elective makes the criteria for success more stringent, since to be considered successful, refractive keratotomy must result in as much or more comfort and visual acuity as could be achieved with spectacles or contact lenses.

Structurally normal eye

As discussed in Chapter 1, Myopia: A Brief Overview, eyes with simple myopia are structurally normal and eyes with intermediate myopia may have mild increased axial length with tessellation of the fundus and formation of a myopic crescent around the optic disc. This distinguishes keratotomy surgery from surgery on eyes with potentially blinding anatomic abnormalities such as retinal detachment, vitreous hemorrhage, or cataract formation. It also increases the risk/benefit ratio because there is more to lose from a complication.

Patient as partner

A new medical ethics has emerged in the past 20 years as part of the egalitarian rights revolution with its rights for minorities, women, students, homosexuals, elderly people, and inevitably patients. The new medical ethics is less concerned with traditional Hippocratic values of having clinicians do what they think will benefit patients and is more concerned with considering patients as partners in medical decisions, an ethical approach developed by Vetach in his book, *The Patient as Partner.*[47]

Many ophthalmologists consider patients who seek refractive keratotomy somewhat nutty or deviant and feel their job is to discourage the surgery, rather than to regard the patients' inquiries as legitimate expressions of personal goals and concerns. However, ophthalmologists no longer have the luxury of "telling" myopes whether they should have refractive keratotomy, but rather are constrained to discuss in detail the risks and benefits of the operation, not only mechanically eliciting informed consent, but also emphatically addressing each patient's attitudes, questions, and needs.

Most myopes seeking refractive keratotomy are in their social and economic prime of life with good educations and adequate incomes, so they are more likely to evaluate information critically and to participate actively in decisions about surgery. A well-trained ophthalmologist can perform refractive keratotomy on a well-informed, consenting patient without being ethically compromised, even if the ophthalmologist would not have the operation personally.

Quality of life

Under any circumstance persons with refractive errors want normal uncorrected visual acuity, and the socioeconomic trends in the United States in the 1990s accentuate this wish. At a time characterized by low unemployment, rising incomes, "me-generation" attitudes, yuppie, two-income families, an acquisitional philosophy of life, and increasing emphasis on health and fitness, it comes as no surprise that myopes try to improve the quality of their life by seeking elective surgery to eliminate the need for glasses or contact lenses. Thus ophthalmologists must expand their clinical goals beyond the time-honored calling of preventing and curing blindness to the subtler task of improving the quality of their patients' visual function as they do with intraocular lens implants in the management of aphakia.

Commercialized medicine

Refractive keratotomy is one of the first surgical procedures to be sold directly to the public (see Chapter 10, Patient Educational Materials for Refractive Keratotomy). Advertisements on billboards and in electronic and print media, seminars designed more to sell than to educate, and extensive coverage of refractive keratotomy by the press all have a direct effect on nearsighted individuals, now designated as health-care consumers. Indeed the coverage of the latest advancements in medicine and ophthalmology (including refractive keratotomy) by the news media may make inquiring patients better informed about the newest operation than the general eye care professional whom they are consulting. Thus many patients are health-care shoppers, responding to the forces of the marketplace and often arriving with unrealistic expectations about refractive keratotomy.

All of these factors make consulting with a potential refractive keratotomy patient a challenge. The inquisitive myope consumes more consultation time, makes more demands, is more likely to seek second opinions, and requires a more personalized empathetic explanation of the surgery than the patient with advanced cataracts who must have a fairly standardized operation if he or she is to regain acceptable visual function.

DEMOGRAPHIC CHARACTERISTICS AND MOTIVATIONS OF CANDIDATES FOR REFRACTIVE KERATOTOMY

Two studies have specifically addressed the demographic characteristics and motivations of patients seeking refractive keratotomy, each based on questionnaires administered to refractive keratotomy patients[6,30] Bourque and colleagues[6] had 307 PERK candidates, who were taking the baseline screening examination, answer 140 questions on a formal psychometric questionnaire that had already been field-tested. The questionnaire was administered before patients discussed refractive keratotomy with any of the PERK study staff and without help or coaching from any staff member; in this way the researchers attempted to determine as realistically as possible the patient's own attitudes. Another 369 individuals who had surgery were tested to determine their motivations after the surgery had been completed. Powers and colleagues[30] mailed a questionnaire to 101 individuals who had had refractive keratotomy; 87% responded.

Demographic characteristics

Sperduto and colleagues[44] analyzed the Health and Nutrition Examination Survey (HANES) data and found that the typical myope in the United States is likely to be white, earn more than $10,000 a year, and have finished high school at least. The average patient in the PERK study fit this profile.[6] Bourque and colleagues found that patients seeking refractive keratotomy ranged in age from 18 and 44 years. The number of males and females was similar, refuting the notion that the more cosmetically conscious women seek this surgery. The vast majority of patients were white. Socioeconomic status was generally high, 85% of the PERK patients having some post–high school education, 36% reporting annual incomes of $20,000 or more, and in the Powers study[30] 51% reporting a professional, or white-collar, occupation. (For details on the demography of myopia, see Chapter 1, Myopia: A Brief Overview, and Curtin's textbook, *The Myopias.*[9])

Self-perceived visual ability

In both the PERK and the Powers studies almost 100% of patients wore eyeglasses or contact lenses most of the time. Dislikes about these optical devices far outweighed likes. Contact lenses seemed to be more acceptable to patients than glasses, even though the majority wore glasses. In the PERK study, most of the women (94%) and almost half of the men (48%) had tried contact lenses and 60% had stopped wearing them.

Patients in the PERK study thought they were more visually disabled than a comparable set of myopes in the Rand Health Survey study (Table 12-1).

Psychologic characteristics

Bourque and colleagues compared the psychologic profiles of PERK patients and a similar group of myopes from the Rand Health Insurance experiment. PERK patients were less likely to be anxious or depressed or to function poorly in their social lives or jobs than were Rand patients. There was no indication of psychologic abnormality or high risk taking among the PERK patients (Table 12-2). Powers found moderate levels of self-esteem on the Cooper self-esteem inventory. The mean level was 74.4, the range was 51 to 95, and the possible range was 25 to 100. Almost all the patients (97%) reported stable marriages and occupations over the previous year. When refractive keratotomy was first introduced in the United States, some ophthalmologists thought that patients

---

Table 12-1

Comparison of Perceived Visual Ability

	Myopes (%)	
Perceived visual ability	PERK study* (N = 307)	Rand study* (N = 429)
Vision with lenses is about the same or better than others their age	91	90
Some pain in eyes during the past 3 mo†	15	21
Some worry about eyesight during the past 3 mo†	57	33
Eye problems have caused some restriction in activity during the past 3 mo†	47	13

From Bourque LB, Rubenstein R, Cosand B, Waring GO, and the PERK Study Group: Arch Ophthalmol 1984;102:1187-1192.
*PERK indicates National Eye Institute Prospective Evaluation of Radial Keratotomy; Rand study, Rand Health Insurance Experiment.
†χ^2 between PERK and Rand study groups is significant at $P < .05$.

Table 12-2

Comparison of Psychosocial Characteristics

	Myopes (%)	
Psychosocial variable	PERK study* (N = 307)	Rand study* (N = 429)
Personal life in past month was happy†	92	75
Little or no loneliness in past month†	87	76
No depression in last month†	37	22
No nervousness in last month†	61	41
Cheerful all or most of the time in the past month†	85	68
Little or no worry in the last month†	88	73
Visit with friends at least once a week†	67	50
Have been in excellent health the last month†	93	43
Avg. no. of close friends	8	9

From Bourque LB, Rubenstein R, Cosand B, Waring GO, and the PERK Study Group: Arch Ophthalmol 1984;102:1187-1192.
*PERK indicates National Eye Institute Prospective Evaluation of Radial Keratotomy; Rand study indicates Rand Health Insurance Experiment.
†χ^2 between PERK and Rand study groups is significant at $P < .05$.

seeking this surgery were likely to be chronically dissatisfied, unbalanced, high risk takers who responded to public hype for the latest health fad. Both the Bourque[6] and Powers[30] studies proved this stereotype wrong.

Patient motivation for surgery

Both the Bourque (Table 12-3) and the Powers studies documented patients' stated motivations for having refractive keratotomy.

Independence from optical devices. There is no question that the most common motivation for patients to have refractive keratotomy is to see well without having to depend on spectacles or contact lenses. This should come as no surprise. Even though glasses and contact lenses are ubiquitous in industrialized societies, almost one third of adults younger than 50 years of age use them, and almost 100% of individuals older than 50 years of age use them to correct presbyopia, they are still bothersome prosthetic devices that most wearers would gladly discard in favor of a truly reliable surgical correction of ametropia.

This attitude expresses the innate desire of most humans to have their bodily functions work naturally without prosthetic aids. Simply stated, most ametropes would rather be emmetropes, or minimally myopic. As Curtin observes, "The willingness with which many myopic patients have undergone expensive or potentially dangerous regimens merely to reduce their myopia or to obtain flashes of clear unaided vision is eloquent testimony to their distaste for visual aids of

Table 12-3

Single, Most Important Reason PERK* Patients Report for Having Surgery (N = 369†)

Reason for having surgery	PERK surgery cases (%)		
	Female	Male	Total
Not to be dependent on eyeglasses or contact lenses	73	58	65
Occupation	3	10	6
To see well all the time	6	6	6
Comfort or convenience of not having to wear eyeglasses or contact lenses	7	3	5
Sports	3	7	5
Cosmetic purposes	3	2	3
To have greater freedom of movement	1	6	3
To be more self-confident	—	2	1
All else (spread over eight other categories)	4	6	6

From Bourque LB, Rubenstein R, Cosand B, Waring GO, and the PERK Study Group: Arch Ophthalmol 1984;102:1187-1192.
*PERK indicates National Eye Institute Prospective Evaluation of Radial Keratotomy.
†Data presented are all consecutive cases who have had surgery to date.

any sort."[9] The strongest evidence of this motivation is the enormous number of individuals who have used the Bates methods of eye exercise and visual training and the immense popular reaction of the American public to the widespread publicity about keratotomy in the early 1980s. (See Chapter 5, Development of Refractive Keratotomy in the Nineteenth Century.)

Interestingly, and unfortunately, many ophthalmologists denigrate this motivation as a misguided attitude on the patient's part. These physicians' reprehensible lack of understanding simply denies the patient's reality and the practitioner's duty to counsel patients fairly about refractive keratotomy surgery.

Both the Bourque and Powers studies document this motivation. In the PERK study, the vast majority of the candidates (71%) stated that their single most important reason for having surgery was "not to be dependent on eyeglasses or contact lenses" or "to see well all of the time." In the Powers study, improving vision was the second most important reason. More than 60% of the PERK study patients stated that the only advantage of eyeglasses is that they allow a person to see better. The PERK patients' dislike of lenses had two interrelated dimensions. The first aspect was a fear of being unable to see if the lenses were lost. "What happens if I am caught in a burning building, a bad storm, or an accident and lose my eyeglasses or contact lenses? How can I encounter life-threatening obstacles with poor vision?" Many patients referred to fear of breaking eyeglasses (45%), having eyeglasses fall off (60%), losing eyeglasses (39%) or contact lenses (74%), being dependent on eyeglasses (84%) or contact lenses (38%), and being without them in an emergency (60%). The second motivating aspect, which relates to the dislike of lenses, was the inconvenience of corrective lenses. PERK patients said eyeglasses distort vision (39%), hurt the nose and ears (75%), cost too much (34%), are inconvenient to clean (41%), get scratched (3%), and interfere with participation in sports (60%). Similarly, those PERK patients who wore contact lenses said the lenses were costly (46%), difficult to care for (50%), and inconvenient to put in (65%). There is no way to distinguish clearly between feelings of fear and those of general inconvenience as motivators for surgery. For most PERK patients, the two motivations were highly related. Similarly Powers and colleagues found that avoiding the inconveniences of glasses and improving vision were the two most important motivating factors mentioned by patients.

Parallels can be made to other aspects of medicine and surgery, where prosthetic devices can be eliminated by surgery, such as leg braces by artificial joints, and hearing aids by middle ear surgery. Permanent correction of a physiologic disorder is preferable to temporary prosthetic palliation.

Occupation, sports, and appearance. Both the Bourque and the Powers studies identified as minor motivating factors a desire for improved cosmetic appearance, improved job performance, and increased convenience in sports. This is important because some ophthalmologists feel that a patient must have a "legitimate" reason for justifying keratotomy surgery—a reason related to job or essential physical activity. Most patients disagree.

Occupation. Occupational factors have played an important role in the development of refractive keratotomy. One of Sato's motivations was to improve the visual function of Japanese pilots in World War II. (See Chapter 6, Development of Radial Keratotomy in Japan, 1939-1960.) In the late 1950s, Nakajima reported that of 40 patients who had anteroposterior keratotomy, 19 were chosen for professional reasons (military, sailors, transportation, mining), 11 for anisometropia, and 10 for cosmetic purposes.[28]

One of the early series of cases reported by Fyodorov[16] was on Soviet pilots (see Chapter 7, Development of Refractive Keratotomy in the Soviet Union, 1960-1990). The authors observed that 5% to 8% of pilots are disqualified every year because of refractive errors, half of them caused by myopia. Eight pilots who had experience in flying for 8 to 20 years received radial keratotomy so that they would not be disqualified. The pilots were allowed to fly 3 to 5 months after surgery. Of 13 eyes, 11 were within ± 1 D of emmetropia, and two had residual myopia of approximately 2 D. Investigation of the pilots under low-oxygen and high-oxygen conditions demonstrated no changes in visual acuity after the surgery. Observation of the pilots during take-off and landing with supersonic planes showed the absence of unstable vision. The authors conclude that radial keratotomy can save the careers of highly qualified flight personnel and retain good visual performance. As might be expected, not all agree. Volkov,[49] in discussing the medical indications for radial keratotomy in the Soviet Union, concludes that there are no special professional indications.

Occupational goals can be extremely important for some individuals; young men and women who want to be police officers, airplane pilots, or professional stage performers (particularly dancers) may view corrective lenses as an impediment to achieving their professional goals. When considering refractive keratotomy for occupational purposes, the surgeon and the patient must know before surgery the visual acuity requirements of the employer, usually having them stated in writing. Recommendations change as information concerning refractive surgery accumulates (see box below). For example, as of 1988 the United States Air Force requires 20/20 uncorrected visual acuity in both eyes for prospective pilots. In addition, any individual who has had radial keratotomy is specifically disallowed from entering U.S. Air Force flight training programs. Because $1 million are invested to train combat-ready pilots fully for a 20-year career, the

---

Policies of Governmental Agencies Concerning Refractive Surgery

There is no consistent policy among federal, state, and local agencies and private businesses concerning employment of individuals who have had refractive keratotomy. We reproduce here the rulings of the United States Air Force and the Commonwealth of Virginia as examples.

The Department of the Air Force issued the following ruling concerning refractive surgery in 1985:

1. As stated in AFR 160-43 History of Corneal Refractive Surgery Disqualifying for Enlistment, USAF personnel already on reserve or active duty who electively undergo corneal refractive surgery in the civilian sector may be retained on duty if thorough evaluation by Air Force ophthalmologists confirm that there are no significant complications and the individual's postoperative vision meets the qualification standards for his/her career field.

2. Flying personnel who undergo corneal refractive surgery will be medically disqualified for flying duty.

3. Radial keratotomy or elective corneal refractive surgery will not be performed by Air Force ophthalmologists on any active duty or reserve forces military personnel.

Recommendations for standards or employees who have radial keratotomy were formulated by the Commonwealth of Virginia in December 1987:

We will accept applicants for medical group I (fire, police, and sheriff) who have had radial keratotomy if: One year has elapsed since surgery. The operative side is healed well. The individual can pass the visual requirements for the type of medical group I job for which he/she is applying on two successive days. The applicant denies any interfering glare at night when looking at lights.

Air Force goes to extreme lengths to screen out any ocular pathologic conditions that may preclude a full flying career (Air Force regulation 160-43).[46] The Federal Bureau of Investigation has a similar policy.

The motivation for some job candidates is high enough that they have refractive keratotomy privately, omit that fact from their application for employment, lie during interviews, and make it through a physical examination without the operation being detected, their uncorrected visual acuity being good enough to qualify for the position. Others file administrative appeals or lawsuits to secure jobs despite exclusionary rules.

Interestingly many of the occupations for which people seek radial keratotomy put people at greater risk of ocular injury. These occupations include the armed forces, law enforcement, and professional athletics. Since radial keratotomy weakens the cornea, this should be clearly explained to potential candidates.

Sports. Although only 5% of PERK candidates identified sports specifically as a motivating factor for having radial keratotomy, the modern emphasis on fitness makes the inconvenience of wearing optical correction during sporting activities something that affects many athletes, both professional and amateur. Anyone who has lost his or her glasses or contacts while involved in a high-risk sport, such as kayaking a remote white-water river, understands this motivation instantly.

Appearance. Because refractive keratotomy affects the primary function of the eye—the creation of an optical image on the retina—it is intrinsically functional and not cosmetic surgery. However, patients may elect to have refractive keratotomy for cosmetic reasons, although few do so. A small percentage of the patients in the Powers study and 3% of the PERK candidates listed improved appearance or cosmetic purposes as their primary motivation.

Overall patient motivation

Patient motivation is a subjective factor, and most patients have more than one motivation in mind when choosing refractive keratotomy as they do when choosing to wear contact lenses. When PERK candidates talked positively about contact lenses, they most frequently mentioned that contact lenses look better than spectacles (81%), allow easier participation in sports (79%), and improve vision (62%).

The analysis of Powers and colleagues[30] of the subjective factors determining postoperative satisfaction supports the view that improved vision is more important than other factors. Regression analysis for patient satisfaction identified two factors as most important in determining satisfaction with radial keratotomy—improvement in vision and quality of uncorrected vision after surgery. These two factors accounted for 72.8% of the factors most important in determining satisfaction. The remaining 8% of factors determining satisfaction were preoperative desire for change in appearance, the cost of the surgery, and the absence of pain following the first operation for those patients who had surgery on the second eye. When a more detailed multiple regression analysis of patient satisfaction was done, including only variables relevant to vision and appearance, satisfaction was strongly related to perceived improvement in vision and to freedom from having to wear spectacles; the variables related to appearance did not enter into the equation as predictors of satisfaction. Powers and colleagues concluded, "It seems that change in appearance, though welcome by patients as a by-product of radial keratotomy surgery, was not the major factor in deciding to undergo surgery nor in gauging the outcome." Similarly, a separate report from the PERK study by Bourque and colleagues[5] created a Satisfaction Index from a postoperative questionnaire and found this index highly correlated with uncorrected visual acuity and residual refractive error.

PREOPERATIVE CLINICAL EXAMINATIONS

In this section, I discuss the pragmatic aspects of clinical examination of candidates for refractive keratotomy without detailed description of the equipment or methods of a proper ophthalmic examination. The examinations are discussed in the approximate order of their importance to patient selection and not in the order in which they would be done during routine clinical practice.

Refraction

Role of refraction in patient selection. The refractive error is usually the first item used to screen patients. Those with myopia less than 1.00 to 1.50 D and greater than 10.00 D are promptly eliminated from consideration, as are patients with hypermetropia. The amount of myopia in patients on whom a surgeon is willing to perform radial keratotomy varies greatly. Published data indicate the best results occur in individuals with myopia between 1.50 and 6.00 D (see Chapter 21, Published Results of Refractive Keratotomy). In patients who have less than 1.50 D of myopia, the danger for overcorrection is usually enough to obviate surgery. In patients who have more than 6.00 D of myopia, there is decreased probability of an acceptable result.

Some surgeons choose to operate on patients with up to 10.00 to 12.00 D of myopia. Salz[35] reviewed six studies of patients who had baseline refractions between −6.00 and −10.00 to −12.00 D and found that roughly 45% of the eyes fell within ±1.00 D of emmetropia (the range was 18% to 62%) and approximately 50% of the eyes were able to see 20/40 or better uncorrected (the range was 38% to 68%). Thus the cutoff values for refraction in keratotomy vary considerably from one surgeon to another.

Cycloplegic and manifest refractions. Both manifest and cycloplegic refractions should be measured, but the cycloplegic refraction should be the basis for calculating surgical plan and for comparing preoperative and postoperative results. The manifest refraction, even using good fogging techniques, tends to overestimate the amount of myopia because of increased accommodation. As Table 12-4 demonstrates, approximately one of four eyes has 0.50 D or more myopia on the manifest refraction than on the cycloplegic refraction. The baseline refraction in the PERK study showed that the manifest refraction measured an average of 0.25 D more myopia (the range was −1.88 to +1.00 D). Thus designing a surgical plan on the basis of the manifest refraction is more likely to cause overcorrection.

Table 12-4

Difference Between Manifest and Cycloplegic Refraction of the Same Eyes in the PERK Study*

		Percentage of eyes showing difference	
Direction of difference	**Amount of difference (D)**	**At baseline (%) (N = 435)**	**At four years postoperatively (N = 332)**
Manifest	1.00 to 1.87	2.8%	10.5%
more myopic	0.50 to 0.87	24.6%	27.1%
Difference	<0.50	70.8%	59.3%
Cycloplegic	0.50 to 0.87	1.6%	2.7%
more myopic	1.00	0.2%	0.3%

*Refractions done by certified PERK coordinator-technicians and verified independently by an ophthalmologist investigator. Manifest done by fogging technique. Cycloplegic done 30 minutes after two doses of 1% cyclopentolate.

Some surgeons use the manifest refraction, realizing that it usually overestimates the amount of myopia by less than 1 D and wishing to avoid the disadvantages of cycloplegia, including the increased time and work in the physician's office and the bothersome loss of accommodation for a few hours for the patient. Abnormal retinoscopic reflexes may signal the examiner to search more diligently for early keratoconus, early nuclear sclerosis, or slight dislocation of the lens. Methods of measuring refraction are described in standard textbooks.[12,24]

Comparison of preoperative and postoperative refraction. Because it is impossible to know exactly how much accommodation is being controlled during a manifest refraction, the cycloplegic refraction must be used for both preoperative and postoperative refractions to measure the results of the surgery accurately. However, as discussed in Chapter 3, Optics and Topography of Radial Keratotomy, the cycloplegic refraction has the postoperative disadvantage of dilating the pupil and allowing more spherical aberration from the paracentral cornea to affect the measurements of refraction and visual acuity. One study by Holladay and colleagues attempted to control accommodation with cycloplegia and control spherical aberration by refracting through an aperture the same diameter as the resting pupil, presently the best method of examination. The accurate measurement of refraction after refractive keratotomy remains somewhat elusive because of the increased asphericity of the cornea.

Demonstration of possible refractive outcomes. For the particularly inquisitive patient, it is helpful to demonstrate clinically the different possible outcomes of the surgery. This is done easily with a phoropter or trial lens without cycloplegia. Allow the patient to read the chart without correction to appreciate the patient's preoperative uncorrected visual acuity. Then add minus power gradually with an explanation. For example, a patient who has a refraction of −5.00 D is shown a "50% correction" with a −2.50 D lens, a "75% correction" with a −3.75 D lens, and a "100% correction" with a −5.00 D lens. A variation of this approach is to show the patient the range within which the most probable outcome will lie—that is, the range within which the surgeon would expect 90% of the eyes to fall using his technique. For example, using the PERK technique on a 35-year-old patient with −5.00 D of myopia, the surgeon would set a −5.00 D lens in place to show the "perfect" correction, then dial in a −7.00 D lens to demonstrate an overcorrection of 2.00 D, and then gradually dial down to a −3.00 D lens to demonstrate a 2.00 D undercorrection. This technique shows the patient the ±2.00 D range within which the outcome is 90% likely to fall.

Refractive astigmatism. Careful measurement of the cylindrical correction with refinement using a crossed cylinder will determine the power and the axis of the cylinder. The measured amount of astigmatism should be compared with the keratometric astigmatism to determine how much astigmatism is induced by the lens. Surgeons still debate on which measure of astigmatism should be the basis for preoperative calculations. Keratometric astigmatism would seem logical, since astigmatic keratotomy modifies corneal shape; refractive astigmatism would seem logical, since that is the amount of astigmatism requiring correction for emmetropia. I prefer refractive astigmatism. The matter is not resolved and is discussed in more detail in Chapter 31, Keratotomy for Astigmatism, and Chapter 32, Atlas of Astigmatic Keratotomy.

Expressing the refractive cylinder in plus cylinder form will identify the steep meridian as the axis of the plus cylinder. However, for astigmatic surgery, the refraction should be expressed in minus cylinder form, which will allow correction of the spherical amount of myopia first and then the residual astigmatic amount of myopia, as explained in Chapter 3, Optics and Topography of Radial Keratotomy.

Age of the patient and stability of refraction

The second most common criterion used to screen patients is age. Generally patients younger than 21 years of age are not offered keratotomy, because their refraction may not be stable and because the patient cannot give independent consent for surgery in most states.

Deitz[10] points out the following four drawbacks of operating on individuals in their late teens or early 20s:

1. Younger individuals do not achieve as much surgical correction with the same amount of surgery as older individuals and therefore require either a smaller clear zone or more incisions.
2. Younger people are more likely to have unrealistic expectations from the keratotomy surgery than are older individuals who have had more life experiences.
3. Younger individuals may not have given contact lenses a sincere and thorough trial.
4. Younger individuals will have to live with their keratotomy for the rest of their lives, and since knowledge of the long-term effects is not completely available yet, they are taking a somewhat greater risk than are older patients.

Simple and intermediate myopias have the greatest rates of progression during the first and second decades of life, generally stabilizing in the early 20s.[7,9] Therefore refractive keratotomy generally should not be performed on teenagers. O'Dell and Wyzinski[29] reported a series of bilateral radial keratotomy in 27 teenagers, reporting results that were roughly comparable to those achieved in adults, 64% of the eyes being within ±1 D of emmetropia an average of 22 months after surgery (range 3 to 54 months). They emphasized the problems of overcorrection, induced astigmatism, and the need for glasses after surgery. They also emphasized the high amount of patient satisfaction after surgery. They used repeated "touch-up" radial keratotomies to deal with increases in myopia that occur at a later age. Smith,[43] in a companion opinion to the O'Dell and Wyzinski study, listed five reasons for not doing radial keratotomy in teenagers: (1) teenagers cannot give adequate informed consent; (2) inadequate consent increases medical-legal questions; (3) teenagers may rationalize the need for surgery on an emotional or inadequately objective basis; (4) wound healing may be different in teenagers than in adults and affect the outcome of the surgery; and (5) natural increases in myopia in teenagers might offset the effect of the surgery.

Technically there is no upper age limit for keratotomy surgery, although practically, few patients older than 50 years of age seek the surgery. The average age of patients in the PERK study[51] was 33.5 years (SD 7.28, range 21 to 58); in the Arrowsmith study[2] the average age was 30 years; in the Deitz study[11] the average age was 32 years (range 18-57); and in the Sawelson study[38] the average age was 33 years (SD 9.6, range 19-75). Since keratotomy produces a greater effect in older people than in younger people—approximately 0.70 D more effect per decade—the surgeon must exercise caution and the patient must know the greater risk of overcorrection when operating on individuals older than 45 years of age. For example, using refractive keratotomy to treat myopia resulting from intraocular lens implantation at cataract surgery will require careful calculation in these older patients.

The effect of patient age on change in refraction is discussed in detail in Chapter 13, Predictability of Refractive Keratotomy.[34,35]

Methods to document a stable refraction include the age of onset of wearing of glasses (an earlier age of onset suggesting a longer time of progression) and

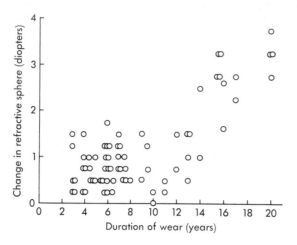

Figure 12-1
Change in refractive sphere correlated with duration of wear of PMMA hard contact lenses in 50 eyes that developed changes in corneal curvature during lens wear. (Levenson DS: CLAO J 1983;9:121-125.)

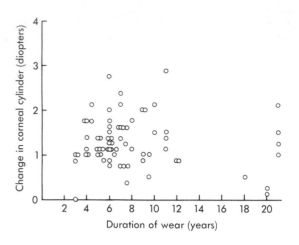

Figure 12-2
Change in keratometric astigmatism correlated with duration of PMMA hard contact lenses in 50 eyes with changes in corneal curvature associated with contact lens wear. (Levenson DS: CLAO J 1983;9:121-125.)

previous refractions from old glasses or previous clinical records (larger refractive errors are more likely to progress for a longer time). A fundus examination should be performed. Eyes with intermediate myopia (a scleral crescent or a tessellated fundus) are more likely to have progressive myopia for a longer time and therefore require more documentation of refractive stability.

Finally, patients should stop wearing contact lenses. Contact lens wear can change corneal curvature. This occurs most commonly with polymethylmethacrylate (PMMA) lenses that have been worn for many years, and the problem is much rarer in patients who wear rigid, gas-permeable and soft, hydrophilic contact lenses. Many patients seeking radial keratotomy had been successful contact lens wearers in the past, but became contact lens intolerant. In the 1980s many of these patients had worn PMMA lenses. Two causes exist for the change in corneal curvature induced by contact lenses (commonly called corneal warpage). The first is quickly reversible (a matter of hours to days) and consists of metabolic alterations in the cornea, such as mild hypoxia that induces slight edema. The second takes longer to reverse and results from a remolding of the cornea, as occurs in orthokeratology. For practical purposes in screening patients for radial keratotomy, leaving the contact lenses of any sort out for approximately 1 week seems to be a reasonable amount of time to allow stabilization of the refraction and to allow detection of any residual corneal warpage.

The problem of warpage caused by contact lens wear can be particularly bothersome. Levenson[19,20] studied 50 patients with changes in refraction induced by PMMA contact lenses; 28 developed 1.00 to 2.00 D of astigmatism, 17 developed 2.00 to 3.00 D of astigmatism, and five developed keratoconus. In this group, 49 of the patients had myopia and in most patients, excluding those that developed keratoconus, flattening of the cornea occurred, with more flattening in the horizontal than the vertical meridian, increasing the with-the-rule astigmatism. All of the patients had worn contact lenses for 3 years or more, and those who wore them for 12 years or more developed the most severe changes in sphere, but not in cylinder (Figs. 12-1 and 12-2). Some of the patients had inadvertently undergone orthokeratology, the flattened corneas being progressively fitted with flatter contact lenses. Many of the patients were refit success-

Table 12-5

Visual Acuity of Patients in the PERK Study, Pupil Undilated (%)*

Snellen visual acuity†	Spectacle corrected baseline (435 eyes)‡		Spectacle corrected 3 years postoperatively (413 eyes)		Uncorrected 3 years postoperatively (414 eyes)§	
20/40			0.2%		6.3%	
20/30			0.2%		7.2%	
20/25			2.2%		12.6%	
20/20	22.4%		13.1%		24.2%	
20/16	53.2%		51.3%		21.5%	
20/12	22.8%	78%	30.0%	84%	4.6%	27%
20/10	1.6%		3.0%		.2%	

*Data not previously published.
†NIH visual acuity charts.
‡Number of eyes, one eye per patient.
§23.4% saw 20/50 or worse.

fully with rigid gas-permeable contact lenses. Corneal warpage has also been reported with soft contact lenses.[26]

The time it takes for a warped cornea to rebound to its original or at least a new stable shape is unknown. Most will do so within 1 week of discontinuing contact lens wear, but some corneas remain warped permanently with high amounts of astigmatism.[4] Whether the keratoconus that occurred and produced steepening of the cornea resulted from contact lens wear is unknown.[17] The potential errors of performing radial keratotomy without discontinuing contact lens wear are obvious. Those patients with flattened corneas may have miscalculation of the surgical plan of 1.00 to 4.00 D for the sphere and of 1.00 to 3.00 D in the cylinder. Those eyes that developed keratoconus should not have radial keratotomy at all, as mentioned under slit-lamp microscopy.

Visual acuity

The best spectacle-corrected visual acuity is an important basis for case selection, since individuals who cannot be corrected better than approximately 20/40 are seldom considered for keratotomy surgery, including individuals with amblyopia from mild strabismus, maculopathy from previous trauma or systemic disease, myopes with previous retinal detachment, and higher myopes with chorioretinal degeneration. Some surgeons argue that performing keratotomy to allow the patient to discard corrective lenses is an advantage, regardless of their visual acuity.

Best visual acuity. The majority of myopic individuals have a spectacle-corrected visual acuity better than 20/20 (Table 12-5). For example, in the PERK study, approximately 80% of the patients could see 20/16 or better with best spectacle correction both before and after surgery, while one fourth to one third could see 20/12 or better. Thus it is important to use visual acuity charts that can measure these finer distinctions, not only for clinical trials, but also for routine refractive surgical practice. For example, a patient who could see 20/12 before surgery best corrected and 20/20 after surgery best corrected has a loss of two Snellen lines, which would be undetected using visual acuity charts that stop at 20/20.

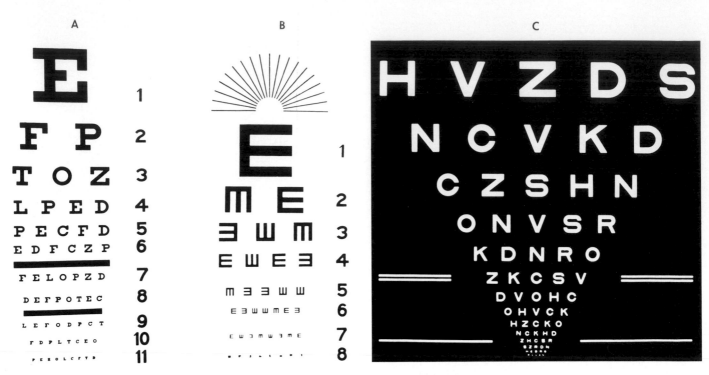

Figure 12-3
A, Standard Snellen eye chart. **B,** Snellen "E" eye chart. **C,** NEI eye chart.

National Eye Institute visual acuity charts. A discussion of visual acuity and optotypes charts is beyond the scope of this book. However, the standard projected Snellen chart has great limitations in the practice of refractive surgery (Fig. 12-3).

These charts have a different number of letters on each line; therefore, one mistake per line has a different meaning at different levels of acuity. Most charts do not have a regular progression of letter size from the easiest to the most difficult lines, so that the visual angle from one line to another varies, making it difficult to interpret a change in visual acuity measured in "the number of lines gained or lost." Snellen letters vary widely in difficulty; for example, the letters "A" and "L" are easier to distinguish than the letter "E." The smallest line on most Snellen charts is 20/20 or 20/15, making it impossible to measure the best possible visual acuity for many myopes.

Therefore we prefer to use the National Eye Institute Visual Acuity Chart, described by Ferris and associates.[13,14] The charts are inexpensive and are available from Lighthouse Low Vision Products, 3602 Northern Blvd., Long Island, NY 11101. The chart (Fig. 12-3, *C*) has the following advantages:

1. Each line has five letters with equal spacing between the lines and a geometric progression in letter height from one line to the next.
2. Each line contains letters of equal difficulty, similar to the difficulty of the Landolt ring. None of the letters spell out words or acronyms.
3. The charts contain 14 lines, with visual acuity measuring from 20/200 to 20/10 (Table 12-6).
4. Three different but comparable charts are available, one to be used for refraction, one for testing the right eye, and one for testing the left eye so that the patient sees the test charts very few times, which minimizes the chance of memorizing the letters.
5. The charts can be mounted in a special box for standardized illumination.

Table 12-6

Equivalent Visual Acuity Measurements

Snellen visual acuities				
4 Meters	**6 Meters**	**20 Feet**	**Decimal fraction**	**LogMAR**
4/40	6/60	20/200	0.10	+1.0
4/32	6/48	20/160	0.125	+0.9
4/25	6/38	20/125	0.16	+0.8
4/20	6/30	20/100	0.20	+0.7
4/16	6/24	20/80	0.25	+0.6
4/12.6	6/20	20/63	0.32	+0.5
4/10	6/15	20/50	0.40	+0.4
4/8	6/12	20/40	0.50	+0.3
4/6.3	6/10	20/32	0.63	+0.2
4/5	6/7.5	20/25	0.80	+0.1
4/4	6/6	20/20	1.00	0.0
4/3.2	6/5	20/16	1.25	−0.1
4/2.5	6/3.75	20/12.5	1.60	−0.2
4/2	6/3	20/10	2.00	−0.3

From Ferris III FL, Kassoff A, Bresnick GH, and Bailey I: Am J Ophthalmol 1982;94:91-96.

Method of visual acuity measurements. The methods by which the visual acuity is measured in a patient can affect the level of the acuity in many ways. For routine clinical practice simply having the patient read as far down on the chart as possible may be adequate, but for clinical trials to obtain the most accurate measurements of acuity, as required in refractive surgery, some attention to detail is necessary. The distance to the acuity chart must be properly measured. In the PERK study we had patients read from 4 meters, as recommended by the National Academy of Sciences–National Research Council on Vision.[42,52] The 4-meter distance has the following advantages:

1. The subtraction of 0.25 D from the spherical component of the refractive correction found at 4 meters solves the problem of obtaining maximal acuity for distances approaching infinity.
2. Conversion of Snellen fractions from 20 feet to their equivalent at 4 meters and vice versa is simple, requiring multiplication by 5. This is easier than the conversion for the 6-meter test, which requires multiplication by 3.333.
3. When space is limited, the 4-meter test is more convenient. The illumination of the chart should be at 75 to 100 footcandles when measured with a photometer held 4 feet from the floor and directed toward the ceiling.

The occluded eye must be well covered to prevent inadvertent peaking. The patient is instructed to begin reading the visual acuity chart at the smallest line in which all of the letters are easily visible. It is helpful if the examiner stands beside the chart and indicates by pointing which line is being read. This obviates the monotonous reading of the entire chart. The examiner encourages the patient to read all letters possible and when a letter is not completely clear, the patient is encouraged to guess at it, committing to a single alternative. The patient must avoid leaning forward to decrease the reading distance or squinting to create a pinhole effect. The patient is encouraged to read all possible letters on the chart, even individual letters on the smaller lines. The examiner records each letter identified correctly, and the raw visual acuity is the total number of letters read on the chart.

Measuring the best uncorrected visual acuity in myopic patients before surgery can be done by having the patient walk slowly toward the chart until the top line can be read, recording the distance from the chart as the numerator of a new Snellen fraction, such as 5/200 (instead of the usual 20/200).

Calculation of visual acuity. Visual acuity can be reported in two ways. The customary method is to identify the smallest line on which three or more letters are read. However, this does not give the patient credit for other letters that can be read below this line. The second method is to count the total number of letters on the chart, dividing by five (each line has five letters) to determine the position on the chart where the patient would have stopped if all letters had been read in sequence with none missed. The smallest line on which three or more letters are "read" is selected as the Snellen notation for the visual acuity. In the PERK study, we compared statistically these two methods of reporting the visual acuity, found no significant difference between them, and used the method of counting the total number of letters as easier for the examiner and probably the most accurate.

Some examiners will simply average the denominator of the Snellen fraction to report the visual acuity in a group of eyes. For example, "the average uncorrected visual acuity in these 57 eyes at 1 year after radial keratotomy was 20/58." Although this may be a mathematically convenient way of representing the information, it is not a very meaningful one. It is better to report the percentage of eyes within a given refractive range such as "the average uncorrected visual acuity in these 57 eyes at 1 year after radial keratotomy was 20/20 or better in 51%, 20/40 in 82%, and 20/100 or better in 98%."

A less familiar method of counting for all letters read is to use the logarithm of the minimal angle of resolution (LogMAR) (Table 12-6). This is calculated by taking the Snellen fraction, converting it to a decimal visual acuity by dividing the numerator by the denominator, and taking the reciprocal of this decimal acuity to approximate the logarithm of the minimal angle of resolution.[51] The convenient thing about the LogMAR score is that it is linear, decreasing by 0.1 unit for each lower line on the NIH Visual Acuity Chart. Since there is a 0.1 Log-MAR unit difference between the lines on these charts and since each line has five letters, a score can be created by assigning 0.02 LogMAR unit for each letter read correctly on this chart. Thus by adding all the scores, a visual acuity score can be created that is a single number and allows changes in visual acuity to be tested statistically over time. For example, if all of the letters down to and including the 20/25 (4/5) line (LogMAR +0.1) are correctly read, and three letters on the 20/20 (4/4) line (LogMAR 0.0) are correctly read, an interpolated Log-Mar score of +0.04 (that is, +0.1 −[3 × 0.02]) can be used to represent the visual acuity. The lower the score, the better the acuity.[13]

The conditions for measuring visual acuity should be reported. "Best corrected visual acuity" usually means best spectacle-corrected visual acuity. A trial contact lens can be used to neutralize irregular corneal astigmatism and improve visual acuity, and therefore a contact lens−corrected visual acuity is often the "best corrected" after refractive surgery. Visual acuity is probably best reported, particularly after refractive keratotomy, with the pupil in its normal constricted state because the dilated pupil might induce more spherical aberration and might allow more glare to interfere with measured acuity.

Slit-lamp microscopy

Establishing that the cornea has a normal anatomy is a prerequisite for keratotomy surgery. A careful slit-lamp microscope examination can reveal the following findings:

1. Early keratoconus with its faint Fleischer's ring and Vogt's lines
2. Preexisting corneal scars that might interfere with the keratotomy incisions
3. Pigment dispersion and iris transillumination defects characteristic of the pigmentary dispersion syndrome with the possible development of future elevations of intraocular pressure
4. Mild lens opacities such as nuclear sclerosis that can increase myopia
5. Subluxation of the lens that might induce astigmatism
6. Syneretic cavities in the vitreous suggesting pathologic myopia or Wagner's vitreoretinal degeneration.

In general, keratotomy surgery is done only on eyes that have a structurally normal anterior segment and are devoid of progressive vitreoretinal disease.

Detailed methods of slit-lamp microscopy are described by Martonyi, Bahn, and Meyer[21] and in the classical textbooks of Berliner,[3] Vogt,[48] and Meyner.[23]

Intraocular pressure

As discussed in Chapter 13, Predictability of Refractive Keratotomy, and Chapter 14, Computerized Predictability Formulas for Refractive Keratotomy, intraocular pressure is the force that changes corneal shape after keratotomy. However, no clinical study of refractive keratotomy, including those using regression analysis, has been able to isolate and quantify the effect of intraocular pressure within the physiologic range. Therefore the major object of measuring intraocular pressure before surgery is to identify individuals who have elevated pressure and exclude them from keratotomy surgery. This screening is particularly important, since myopes are more likely to develop elevated intraocular pressure and glaucoma than emmetropes (see Chapter 1, Myopia: A Brief Overview).

The most accurate type of instrument used to measure intraocular pressure is the applanation tonometer because it is not affected by the decrease in scleral rigidity that occurs in intermediate and higher myopes. The two most commonly used applanation tonometers are the Goldmann instrument and the pneumotonometer. McKay-Marg electronic applanation tonometers are no longer manufactured, and the Maklikov tonometer, the simplest and first practical applanation tonometer invented in 1885, is used in the Soviet Union. Accuracy of indentation tonometry, such as the Schiøtz, decreases with increases in myopia because of the decreased ocular rigidity associated with increases in myopia. The noncontact, air-puff tonometer is used in some offices. More detailed discussions of tonometers and the clinical technique of tonometry are presented by Brubaker[8] and by Shields.[41]

Eyes with intraocular pressure in the normal range of approximately 10 to 20 mm Hg are acceptable for keratotomy. Eyes with pressure lower than this theoretically may have a decreased response to the surgery. Eyes with 21 mm Hg of pressure or more should have further examinations to detect ocular hypertension or glaucoma.

Surgeons should be especially alert for young male myopes with pigment dispersion who, even despite normal intraocular pressures during the examination, are at greater risk of developing glaucoma in the future and should be cautioned about later problems of fluctuating vision if they develop glaucoma after refractive keratotomy.[18,45] Surgeons should search specifically for a Krukenberg spindle on the posterior cornea, patchy radial transillumination of the iris, pigment deposits on the lens surface, and increased pigmentation in the trabecular meshwork.

During funduscopy, inspection of the optic disc is important, not only to detect changes that suggest pathologic myopia, but also to look for changes that suggest glaucoma, which may be difficult to detect if the scleral crescent is large and the disc is slightly tilted.

Surgeons should not perform refractive keratotomy on patients with elevated or fluctuating intraocular pressure without a glaucoma work up and extensive informed consent.

A family history of glaucoma should also signal patients to reconsider keratotomy surgery because of the increased chance that they will develop glaucoma.

Central keratometry

We discuss keratometry in detail in Chapter 3, Optics and Topography of Radial Keratotomy, and its effect on the outcome of surgery in Chapter 13, Predictability of Refractive Keratotomy, and Chapter 14, Computerized Predictability Formulas for Refractive Keratotomy.

Little correlation exists between preoperative central keratometric power and the effect of keratotomy. Some contend that steeper corneas achieve more change in refraction[37]; others find more change in refraction in flatter corneas.[1,31] Still others contend that it is the overall corneal topography that affects the outcome, not just the central keratometric power. Even though many formulas and nomograms include keratometric power, the preoperative keratometric power plays little role in designing the surgical plan.

However, as with intraocular pressure, patients with extreme refractive values outside the normal range of 39.00 to 48.00 D should be regarded with suspicion because they may have an abnormal response to conventional surgery. Steep corneas should spark a search for other signs of keratoconus, particularly examination of the keratometry and keratoscopy mires for irregular astigmatism and a slit-lamp microscopic search for the Fleischer ring. Similarly, irregular keratometry mires in contact lens wearers with somewhat flattened corneas may suggest contact lens warpage. Patients with irregular astigmatism usually should not have keratotomy performed.

Keratometric astigmatism should be approximately the same as refractive astigmatism in the unoperated eye unless there is a contribution by the lens.

The practical, clinical use of keratometers is described by other authors.[12,32,36] The major practical points to consider when using a keratometer are the following:

1. The instrument should be calibrated on a steel test ball that usually measures 45.00 D. If the reading is not 45.00 D, readjust the eyepiece; if an accurate reading cannot be obtained, the instrument must be recalibrated by the manufacturer.

2. A properly adjusted eyepiece is necessary to prevent erroneous readings caused by different focusing distances inducing different magnifications. The eyepiece is adjusted by focusing on the steel ball or the white-backed occluder on the instrument, turning the eyepiece counterclockwise to the plus side, rotating it slowly in the clockwise direction to come from the plus side and avoid stimulating accommodation, and stopping when the mires are in sharp focus. The proper setting for the eyepiece is noted on the calibrated scale around the eyecap and should be used for each examination.

3. Ensure that patients are seated comfortably at the end of the instrument and that they understand how to view the fixation light so that the same area on the cornea is measured each time. If there is no fixation light within the instrument, patients should see the reflection of their eyes in the keratometer tube and fixate on the image of the circular mire in the center of their pupil images. The examiner must align the instrument centrally by ensuring that the cross hairs are near the center of the focusing circle so that the optical axis of the instrument coincides with the patient's line of sight.

4. On normal corneas, standard techniques of alignment of the horizontal (+) and vertical (−) mires can be used. However, I prefer to use the crosses to measure each axis, particularly after keratotomy surgery where some irregular astigmatism may be present or where the principal meridians may not be 90° apart. The crosses allow alignment in two directions and therefore are somewhat more accurate. The focusing mires must be kept in sharp focus throughout the measurement so that a constant distance from the eye can be maintained, ensuring accurate measurement of the image size. The measurements are taken by rotating the drums on the side of the instrument and reading the power off the drum or off the illuminated dial within the instrument. The axis of astigmatism is read from the meridian indicators on the keratometer. The examiner performs many functions simultaneously—focusing the central mire, maintaining central alignment, aligning the crosses by rotating the keratometer, and focusing the crosses for power reading by rotating the drums.

5. The range should be extended for flat corneas. Because radial keratotomy flattens the cornea, often beyond the range of the keratometer, a −1.25 D trial lens may be taped over the front of the keratometer with a convex side out. A nomogram chart is used to convert the drum reading to the true keratometric reading.

Keratography

Keratography is discussed in detail in Chapter 3, Optics and Topography of Radial Keratotomy. Qualitative keratography has a minor role in evaluating radial keratotomy patients for myopia, but qualitative keratography identifies individuals who may have irregular astigmatism associated with keratoconus or warpage caused by contact lens wear. In addition, qualitative keratography plays a major role in planning surgery for astigmatism, particularly surgery following penetrating keratoplasty or ocular trauma, where asymmetric, irregular astigmatism may be present, as discussed in Chapters 30 to 34 on astigmatism surgery.

Quantitative keratoscopy can measure the change in corneal curvature and topography induced by keratotomy surgery, but it currently has a minor role in selecting patients. In the future, measurements of corneal topography will probably play a greater role in patient selection as more is understood about the effect of the shape of the cornea on the outcome of keratotomy surgery.[31]

Measurement of corneal thickness

Corneal pachometry is discussed in detail in Chapter 15, Surgical Instruments Used in Refractive Keratotomy. Since corneal thickness does not seem to affect surgical outcome, the measurement of thickness is not variable in case selection. However, for surgeons who use the preoperative corneal thickness measurement as the guide for selecting the length of the knife blade, accurate and precise optical or ultrasonic measurement is extremely important. I prefer intraoperative ultrasonic corneal pachometry because it measures the thickness of the cornea just before the incision is made.

Fundus examination

Indirect ophthalmoscopy with visualization of the ora serrata is important because of the increased propensity of myopes, particularly intermediate and pathologic myopes, to develop lattice degeneration of the retina, retinal holes, and retinal detachment. Patients with these lesions should have keratotomy surgery performed only if the need for the surgery is clearly indicated and the patient clearly understands future risks. Repair of retinal detachment can be more difficult in eyes that have had keratotomy than in eyes with normal corneas, as discussed in Chapter 23, Complications of Refractive Keratotomy.

Examination of the optic disc with a direct ophthalmoscope or a high-powered indirect ophthalmoscopy lens will help detect any signs of glaucomatous damage and of peripapillary myopic change.

Ocular dominance

Many surgeons prefer to operate on a patient's nondominant eye so that if complications occur, the presumably more valuable dominant eye can be left unoperated.

The dominant eye is not always the same as the dominant hand. Asking patients which eye they use to sight a gun or camera will reveal the dominant eye. It is more appropriate to test directly for ocular dominance by a simple clinical maneuver, such as creating a hole in a piece of paper, having patients hold it at arm's length in front of their face and sight a distant object binocularly through the hole, pull the paper toward them as they maintain fixation on the object, and finding that the hole centers on the dominant eye's line of sight.[24]

Ocular rigidity

Ocular rigidity plays no practical role in patient selection, and its role in determining the outcome of refractive keratotomy remains speculative. The distensibility of the sclera and cornea varies in different parts of the same eye and among different individuals and therefore the identical radial keratotomy technique in two eyes with different ocular distensibilities might be expected to give different results if all other variables were equal. However, no published data have isolated the effect of ocular rigidity. Some surgeons have speculated that eyes with greater ocular rigidity would have a greater effect from keratotomy (see Chapter 13, Predictability of Refractive Keratotomy). It is possible that the increased ocular rigidity that occurs with age might account in part for the increased effect of keratotomy surgery in older individuals. However, none of this information is of practical use to keratotomy surgery as it is currently performed.

Details of the measurement of ocular rigidity are beyond the scope of this chapter. The combined intraocular pressure readings with a Schiøtz and applanation tonometry can be used in Friedenwald's formula and nomogram to determine the coefficient of ocular rigidity.[27]

Corneal diameter

Corneal diameter is not a factor for patient selection and has not been shown to affect the outcome of keratotomy surgery. Accurate measurement of corneal diameter using calipers on the anterior corneal surface is difficult because of scleral overriding superiorly and the lack of clear-cut landmarks at the corneoscleral limbus.

Specular microscopy of the endothelium

Endothelial specular microscopy is discussed in Chapter 23, Complications of Refractive Keratotomy. Endothelial morphology does not play a role in case selection for radial keratotomy. Specular microscopy of the endothelium is limited to studies in which careful preoperative and postoperative examinations are done in the same locations in the central cornea and in the areas of the incisions. It might be of value in eyes with previous cataract or corneal transplant surgery before astigmatic keratotomy.[22]

Axial length of the globe

Axial length measurement of the globe does not play a role in selecting patients for keratotomy surgery. As discussed in Chapter 1, Myopia: A Brief Overview, physiologic myopes have a normal axial length and intermediate myopes a somewhat longer axial length. Eyes with pathologic myopia that manifest a posterior staphyloma and a greatly increased axial length usually have too much myopia to warrant keratotomy surgery, and these eyes can be detected by routine funduscopy without the need for ultrasonic measurement of the axial length.

Corneal sensation

It is not necessary to measure corneal sensation before keratotomy surgery. Although the radial and transverse cuts may sever some corneal nerves, reduced corneal sensation and neurotrophic keratopathy have not been described as clinical complications of the surgery.

Detailed studies of the accommodative convergence/accommodation ratio

Roszka-Duggan and colleagues in the PERK study (unpublished data) evaluated the AC/A ratio in 16 patients before and after radial keratotomy. With the manifest refraction in place, the near measurement of the AC/A ratio was taken and then repeated using the lens gradient method with +3.00 D spherical lenses over the refraction. At 5 years after surgery, all patients had a decrease in their myopia, ranging from 1 to 11 D change. Before surgery the most common AC/A ratio was 2:1. Fifty-six percent of the eyes had a low AC/A ratio of less than 3:1. The remainder had ratios of 3:1 to 5:1. Five years after surgery, the most frequent ratio was 1:1 in 25% of eyes, and the median ratio was 3:1. Thirty-seven percent had a low AC/A ratio of less than 3:1, 56% had a normal AC/A ratio of 3:1 to 5:1, and only one eye had a high AC/A ratio. Thus the change between preoperative and postoperative showed that 37% of the patients demonstrated no change in the AC/A ratio, 25% decreased by one to two prism diopters, and 38% demonstrated an increase of one to three prism diopters. Thus there is no specific directional change that can be identified in terms of the AC/A ratio for myopia patients based on these measurements (Fig. 12-4).

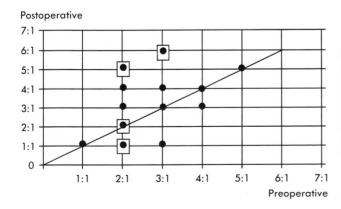

Figure 12-4
Change in accommodative convergence/accommodation (AC/A) ratio in 16 eyes in the PERK study. AC/A ratio is indicated in prism diopters with the preoperative values on the x-axis and the postoperative values on the y-axis. Each symbol indicates one eye. Ratios can increase or decrease after radial keratotomy surgery. (Courtesy of Vicki Roszka-Duggan.)

CONSULTING WITH PATIENTS ABOUT REFRACTIVE KERATOTOMY

One of the most important aspects of talking to patients about radial keratotomy is to determine quickly their preexisting attitudes, premises, and judgments about the surgery. The patient must also determine the underlying attitudes and motives of the surgeon.

Preexisting attitudes of patients

The determined: "I am going to have RK. When can we do it?" These are individuals who have already made up their mind. Nothing the surgeon says will dissuade them. The statement, "You know, there is a chance that you could go stone blind after this operation," often elicits a brief pause, followed by "Yes, when can we schedule the surgery?" The most important thing in dealing with these individuals is to identify whether the basis on which they have decided to have the surgery is realistic. Frequently it is. These individuals often have given considerable thought and inquiry to the subject for months or years, have consulted other surgeons who perform refractive keratotomy, and are well informed. They may say, "I never want to wear glasses or contacts again." Individuals who expect a perfect result from refractive keratotomy have been misled by the good experience of others, enthusiastic endorsements of ophthalmologists, or reports of "miracles" in the popular press. The ophthalmologist should help these optimistic individuals understand the inherent unpredictability of keratotomy and review in detail with them the possibilities of undercorrection, overcorrection, symptomatic presbyopia, and irregular astigmatism. Sometimes these individuals will counter with the contention that a second keratotomy operation can be done to fine-tune the results of the first operation or that "medical progress" will solve any problems that arise. If these patients cling to these unrealistic expectations, it is best not to operate on them.

The surgeon must be particularly careful in recommending surgery to individuals with highly compulsive, demanding personalities, to those with jobs that require extremely good uncorrected acuity, such as surgeons or engineers, and particularly to individuals who have had a good objective outcome in one eye but are subjectively dissatisfied and are seeking a different surgeon for the second eye. Such patients may have an unrealistic understanding of what keratotomy surgery can do for them.

The inquisitive: "What is pinwheel surgery?" These individuals know little about refractive keratotomy and are the easiest to deal with, because they are seeking information with minimal prejudice. A concise presentation of the benefits, risks, predictability, and stability of the surgery is usually all that is necessary to help these individuals decide realistically about the operation.

The data gatherer: "Do you use four or eight incisions?" These cautious, well-informed patients are seeking objective and factual information as they struggle with their own ambivalence about refractive keratotomy. I often provide them with reprints of scientific articles, such as the results of the PERK study,[50] help them interpret information they have already gathered, and invite them to make a return appointment for further discussion.

Preexisting attitudes of surgeons

Ophthalmic surgeons bring their own prejudices to the discussion of refractive surgery with their patients. For the patient to make an autonomous, well-informed decision, the ophthalmologists should disclose their prejudices during the discussion.

The enthusiast: "Refractive keratotomy is my business." This positive attitude is expressed by those who are convinced that refractive keratotomy is safe, effective, and predictable. The attitude especially characterizes the entrepreneurial ophthalmologists who advertise and promote the procedure. It is, of course, possible for these ophthalmologists to provide patients with enough information to allow them to make an independent decision concerning the surgery, but it is more likely that these ophthalmologists will emphasize the positive aspects of keratotomy at the expense of the negative, with a tone more characteristic of a sales person than of a patient advocate. When this orientation prevails on the part of the physician, the patient should assume a "let the buyer beware" attitude. Such enthusiastic physicians might ensure that a more neutral person, such as an independent staff member, counsel individual patients about the strengths and weaknesses of keratotomy.

The opponent: "Refractive keratotomy is unnecessary experimental madness." Many ophthalmologists believe that elective refractive surgery is unnecessary and should be done only under exceptional circumstances—at least at its current stage of development. These strong prejudices result from some physicians' resentment of their entrepreneurial colleagues, from misinformation about scientific and clinical facts, from reticence to operate on a structurally normal eye, and from paternalistic attitudes toward patients. Such attitudes do a disservice to intelligent patients who are genuinely interested in surgically reducing or eliminating their myopia or astigmatism. Ophthalmologists who think refractive keratotomy is madness should admit their prejudices to patients and refer the patients to a respected colleague who does keratotomy.

The selective: "I do refractive keratotomy on selected patients who have a demonstrable need for and reasonable expectations of the operation." This is my attitude. I assume patients have the right to make autonomous decisions about their health care based on adequate information. I do not, however, take the passive role of a mere purveyor of facts. I try to understand individuals' needs, goals, and preconceptions and to help them make decisions most consistent with their autonomous desires. With this attitude, I find that roughly half the patients decide to have keratotomy and the other half decide against it.

Consultation with an individual patient

The major goal of consulting with patients about keratotomy surgery is to give them realistic expectations of the results of surgery. After reviewing the basic facts about keratotomy surgery and alternative methods of treatment—often with video presentations and informative booklets—I emphasize these points, usually in order:

1. Based on my personal experience and published statistics, I tell the patient the odds of achieving 20/40 uncorrected visual acuity (unrestricted driver's license vision in most states), the chance of having a residual refractive error within 1 D of emmetropia, and the chance of being able to go without glasses.
2. Based on the patient's expressed motivation and goals for the surgery, I discuss whether this result is or is not likely to allow them to achieve their goals.
3. I think that the single most important statement to make to a prospective keratotomy candidate is, "I am unable to predict for you the exact outcome of the surgery in your case. Even though I will do everything possible to eliminate your need for glasses or contact lenses, you may end up still nearsighted or actually become farsighted and you must be willing to accept these results before committing yourself to the surgery." For the curious, I demonstrate with lenses the kind of acuity that can be expected with residual undercorrection and overcorrection.

4. I discuss that it will be necessary to wear reading glasses sooner if keratotomy surgery is done than if no surgery is done, realizing how few pre-presbyopic patients care about this. For patients aged 40 years and older I emphasize that after the onset of presbyopia they will have exchanged distance glasses for reading glasses.

5. I emphasize the lack of modifiability and reversibility of the procedure, ("There is no eraser at the end of a diamond knife.") and I contrast this with the easy modifiability of glasses and contact lenses.

6. I point out the most common complications after surgery: fluctuating vision and a starburst pattern of glare. I discuss the nature of daily fluctuation of vision and the possibility of a long-term drift in the direction of continued effect of the surgery. Where appropriate I show pictures of the starburst pattern, but emphasize that disability glare is extremely rare.

7. I emphasize that glasses can restore preoperative visual acuity in almost all cases and can be easily worn after keratotomy if necessary. Fitting contact lenses is more difficult after keratotomy, but can be accomplished. I warn in advance against the use of soft contact lenses after surgery.

8. Finally I discuss the vision-threatening complications of keratitis, endophthalmitis, cataract, and irregular astigmatism, emphasizing the rarity of such occurrences, but stating, "Of course, if these things happen to you, you may go blind." To dwell on a long catalog of the possibly disastrous results that may occur after keratotomy surgery seems inappropriate because the purpose of counseling patients is to present fairly and neutrally the pertinent information and not to terrorize them with grotesque stories of unlikely outcomes.

The box on p. 333 presents a recommended list of eligibility criteria to guide the selection of patients for refractive keratotomy.

SURGERY ON THE SECOND EYE
Timing of surgery on the second eye

There are no published studies of outcomes of radial keratotomy using the interval between surgeries on two eyes in the same patient as the independent variable. Most keratotomy surgeons report waiting 2 to 4 months before operating on a patient's second eye; some wait 1 week or so; a few do simultaneous bilateral surgery.

One year between eyes—the PERK study. When the PERK protocol was designed in 1980, there was little published scientific information about radial keratotomy. Therefore the PERK investigators took an extreme approach to separating surgery on the two eyes, requiring patients to wait 1 year. The purpose for this was to achieve maximum safety for the patient in case unexpected complications arose. Even though 99% of the patients adhered to the design and delayed surgery on the second eye for at least 1 year (five had the second eye done 4 to 10 months after the first), the situation was artificial, peculiar to the PERK study, and is inappropriate and impractical for routine clinical practice.

Months between eyes. The most common practice is to wait approximately 2 to 3 months between surgery on a patient's first and second eye. This is based on the clinical observations of surgeons since the early 1980s and on the PERK study data (Chapter 24, Stability of Refraction after Refractive Keratotomy) that most of the change in refraction after keratotomy occurs by 3 months after the surgery and that sudden large changes in refraction rarely occur after 3 months. Just where between 2 weeks and 3 months this relative stability occurs is unknown. The major advantage of waiting these few months between the first and second eye is to identify the unexpected "over-responders" who have an initial unexpected response and "under-responders" who, despite an initial good re-

Criteria for Patient Selection for Refractive Keratotomy

1. A perceived need to see better without optical correction; selection of surgical correction instead of optical correction of the refractive error.
2. A realistic understanding of the probable results of keratotomy in their case, including an understanding of the less-than-perfect predictability of outcome and of the effects of presbyopia.
3. An understanding of the complications of the surgery, both mild and vision threatening.
4. A clear understanding of the probability that keratotomy surgery will allow the patient to achieve his or her stated personal and professional goals, particularly where employment is concerned.
5. A cycloplegic spherical refractive error within the range of correction achievable by the surgeon with his technique, most commonly between 1.50 and 6.00 D of myopia. An astigmatic refractive error that can be corrected by the surgeon, usually 1.50 to 4.00 D for radial keratotomy, and greater for astigmatic keratotomy.
6. Age of 18 to 21 years or older.
7. Documentation of a stable refraction for at least 1 year, and preferably longer, including removal of contact lenses.
8. Visual acuity correctable at least 20/40 or better, but usually to 20/20 or better, with spectacles.
9. Absence of corneal disease, especially early keratoconus, and of ocular inflammatory disease.
10. Intraocular pressure within the normal range with no signs of a likelihood of developing future glaucoma.
11. Absence of pathologic myopia and specific retinal changes that might lead to retinal detachment.
12. Caution in patients who have systemic diseases likely to affect corneal wound healing after keratotomy, including atopy (eczema, asthma, hay fever), pregnancy, corrective tissue disease, and systemic corticosteroids.
13. Surgeon's experience, skill, and instruments commensurate with the complexity of the case.

sult, show a progressive loss of effect during the first few months. Because these individuals cannot be identified in advance, it is prudent to allow 2 to 3 months between the two eyes in all cases rather than to render a few patients bilaterally +3.00 or −3.00 D. (See Chapter 24, Stability of Refraction after Refractive Keratotomy.)

Having the result of the first eye at 3 months enables the surgeon to plan surgery for the second eye, assuming a symmetric pattern of response. Patients with a result that they consider unsatisfactory in the first eye may wish to delay surgery on the second and consider a repeated operation on the first. For patients with an emmetropic outcome in the first eye, the surgeon may aim to undercorrect the second eye, leaving slight myopia as a hedge against presbyopia. Certainly, patients with a marked overcorrection or undercorrection in the first eye who want the second eye done should have a modification in the surgical plan. In addition, the surgeon may want to do a repeat operation on the first eye before tackling the second. Patients showing marked fluctuation in vision at 3 months should delay surgery in the second eye until a more stable outcome is determined in the first.

The delay period also gives time for the initial positive—sometimes ecstatic—response of patients to subside so that they can address the reality of the refractive outcome and cooperate better with the surgeon in deciding what should be done on the second eye.

Many patients are so thrilled with the improved unaided vision apparent in the first few days after surgery on the first eye that they will press for immediate surgery on the second eye. Those patients who insist—sometimes to the point of threatening to go to another surgeon—will require more time in explaining the possibilities of a delayed loss of effect, the need to determine the outcome in the first eye as a basis for computing the surgical plan on the second, and the necessity for allowing the surgeon's experience and judgment to take precedence over the patient's enthusiasm. The best approach is to explain the required waiting period before the first surgery.

Days between surgery. Some surgeons perform keratotomy on the two eyes a few days apart. This is advantageous for patients who come from a long distance.[15] The delay allows identification of patients with an aberrant initial response so that surgery on the second eye can be modified based on the initial response in the first. However, this approach will fail to identify those individuals with an ideal initial outcome who show marked changes in the first weeks to months after surgery.

Simultaneous bilateral surgery A few surgeons, such as Shepard,[39,40] perform keratotomy on both eyes at once. This has the advantage for the patient of consolidating the unpleasant surgery and postoperative course at one sitting. It also decreases the expense of operating room fees and the amount of time the surgeon must invest to complete surgery on an individual patient. (Two eyes at once can be done much quicker than two eyes at different sittings.) Since the two eyes of each patient are likely to respond similarly and since the surgeon is likely to use an identical technique on these two eyes, there will probably be a symmetrical outcome. If both eyes are undercorrected, a repeat operation can be done later if desired. However, most surgeons consider this approach inappropriate, because of the relatively unpredictable outcome of individual patients and because of the remote danger of bilateral severe complications, such as keratitis or endophthalmitis. Results of bilateral simultaneous surgery have been reported by Villasenor.

Management of the unoperated second eye

The anisometropia created by surgery on the first eye is difficult for some patients to manage, but with a little encouragement and direction from the surgeon and the office staff, most patients adjust easily. Witness the fact that 99% of the 435 PERK patients waited 1 year between surgery on the first and second eyes. In patients with an immediate good outcome in the first eye, the easiest thing to do is to discontinue the wearing of spectacles a week or so after surgery, and allow them to use their operated eye alone. The visual acuity in the uncorrected unoperated eye is usually so blurry that it does not interfere greatly with general daily function. A second approach is to wear a contact lens on the unoperated eye. Even though many patients seek radial keratotomy because of contact lens intolerance, most can adjust to a contact for a few months, if they know that they will not have to wear it indefinitely. Some patients will even purchase a new contact lens for the unoperated eye for use on a temporary basis. Clearly individuals with a good result in the first eye cannot wear a full correction on each eye, because the aniseikonia will create visual confusion and make the patient uncomfortable.

If the first operated eye is overcorrected or undercorrected so it cannot be used for everyday functioning, it is easy to replace the spectacle lens over that eye with a plano lens to leave the operated eye blurry for a while, using the corrected unoperated eye for function. Buying a new spectacle lens for the operated eye in the first few weeks after surgery seems imprudent, because the eye is

Table 12-7

**Surgery on the Second Eye
in the PERK Study**

Number of patients (one eye per patient)	
Total	435
Surgery on second eye	353(81%)
No surgery on second eye	82(19%)
Time (months) between surgery on the first and second eyes (N = 353) (Mean, 16.6 mo; SD, 7; range, 4-61)	
0-12	1%
12-18	77%
18-24	11%
24-36	7%
36-61	4%

Unpublished PERK data courtesy of Michael Lynn, M.S., PERK Biostatistical Coordinating Center.

likely to undergo subsequent refractive changes; this is, however, an option for some fastidious patients, who cannot tolerate the aniseikonia.

In the PERK study, of the 410 patients who waited 1 year between surgery on the first and second eyes, 39% predominantly wore no correction on the unoperated second eye, 29% predominantly wore a spectacle correction, and 32% predominantly wore a contact lens.

Surgery on the second eye in the PERK study

Time between surgery in the two eyes. Because of the anomalous delay of 1 year between surgery on the first and second eyes in the PERK protocol, patients had a long time to think about having surgery on the second eye.

Of the 435 patients in the PERK study, 82 chose not to have surgery on their second eye (Table 12-7). We sought the reasons for this in two ways. First, we conducted a telephone survey of each patient to find out personal and expressed reasons for not having the second surgery. Eighty-one of the 82 patients were contacted and the primary reasons given included the following:

1. Unhappy with the results of the first eye (47%). This included problems such as decreased vision at night, fluctuating vision, undercorrected, double vision, and development of glaucoma in the first eye.
2. Prefer the current situation (26%). This included reasons such as not wanting to wear bifocals, using contact lens on unoperated eye with good results, prefers/likes monovision (good vision at distance with one eye and near vision with the other).
3. Still considering surgery on the second eye (17%). This included reasons such as being too busy to have the second surgery, consulting other ophthalmologists outside the PERK study about surgery in the second eye.
4. Medical contraindications to surgery (5%), including the development of glaucoma in the first eye, advised against surgery by another ophthalmologist, recurrent erosions and base membrane dystrophy in the first eye, and desirous of reoperation on first eye, not surgery on second eye.
5. Other reasons (5%).

Second, we sent a formal questionnaire to the 82 patients. Of these, 56 responded, indicating the following reasons for not having surgery in the second eye (some patients expressed more than one reason):

1. Bad experience with the first eye—38%
2. Glare—34%
3. Fluctuating vision—36%
4. Concerned regarding long-term side effects—32%
5. Pain—10%
6. Inability to wear contact lenses after first surgery—18%

Clearly, it is difficult to get accurate assessments on the basis of such subjective appraisal, but the PERK study concluded that patients had both positive and negative reasons for not having surgery on the second eye.

Most of the patients (88%) who had surgery on their second eye did so within 12 months after the 1-year waiting period.

ECONOMICS OF REFRACTIVE KERATOTOMY

The economic aspects of refractive keratotomy play some role in patient selection. The impact of economics on the motivation of ophthalmologists to do refractive keratotomy is addressed informally in Chapter 8, Development of Refractive Keratotomy in the United States, 1978–1990.

Surgeon's fees

There are many factors that affect the cost of refractive keratotomy surgery for the patient. The most expensive part of refractive keratotomy is the fee charged by the surgeon. This varies greatly from one area of the country to another and from one office to another. In the early 1980s, a fee of approximately $1500 per eye was charged by many surgeons. Since then, fees have fluctuated, dropping below $1000 in some locales, particularly when driven by the market forces of competitive pricing. This cost for the operation perplexes some patients who see the surgery advertised as a "quick and painless 5-minute procedure" and who compute that this amounts to a wage of $18,000 per hour for the surgery (computed at $1500/eye). Surgeons justify these fees by citing the amount of training necessary to learn the procedure, the cost of equipment, the higher malpractice rates they must pay in many areas to do refractive keratotomy, and the personal stress and risk taken in doing surgery on structurally normal eyes. In addition, some simply cite the forces of the marketplace, charging "what the market will bear."

Some reports of fee-splitting between optometrists and ophthalmologists have surfaced, in which the optometrists act as case finders, referring refractive keratotomy patients to an ophthalmologist for surgery and then receiving them back for follow-up care and refraction; the surgeon also pays a fee to the optometrist.

Operating room cost

This cost varies greatly, depending on whether the surgery is done in a hospital operating room, an ambulatory surgical center, or the doctor's office. Patients should certainly be aware that a few hundred dollars will be added to the bill each time, depending on the local rates, the duration of surgery, whether or not anesthesia personnel are involved, and whether or not instrument-use charges are included. Medication costs for postoperative steroids and antibiotics should also be included.

Insurance coverage

Insurance payments for refractive surgery in general and refractive keratotomy in particular vary considerably from one company to another. Some companies simply refuse to pay for what they consider elective (and sometimes incorrectly, cosmetic) surgery, whereas other companies readily include refractive keratotomy in their plan. The amount of reimbursement depends on the conditions of the insurance policy. Patients should check directly with their insurance carrier before surgery to determine the type of coverage available. Some companies can be persuaded to pay for the surgery on the basis of a justifying letter from the surgeon. Some patients have gone so far as to sue their insurance company for payment for the surgery.

Cost of refractive keratotomy versus spectacles and contact lenses

Few patients will decide whether to have refractive keratotomy on the basis of the total cost over a lifetime of refractive correction, but the figures make interesting consideration. The cost of refractive keratotomy surgery for a theoretical patient can be tabulated as follows:

Surgeon's fee for two eyes: $3000
Operating room cost for two surgical sessions: $1000
Preoperative and postoperative clinical visits outside those covered by the surgery: $400
Ancillary charges: variable
Total: $4400

Assuming the surgery is successful and allows the patient not to wear an optical correction, the patient need not spend more money on glasses or contact lenses. Of course if the surgery is unsuccessful, new glasses and new contact lenses may be required, and these may even be increased expense because of frequent changes of the lenses and an extended period required for contact lens fitting.

Cost of spectacles and contact lenses

Assuming that a 70-year-old person with simple physiologic myopia started wearing spectacles at age 9 years and wore them throughout life, changing the glasses once a year between ages 9 and 18 years, and once every 2 years thereafter including the incorporation of a presbyopic correction, and assuming that the patient lives to be 70 years of age, and assuming that a refraction costs $50 and that a new pair of spectacles costs $200, this average myope will have spent $7000.00 dollars for glasses during a lifetime. If a person had radial keratotomy at age 25, an approximate savings of $2500 in new glasses and refractions would be realized between the ages of 25 and 45 (excluding the cost of the surgery and assuming a refraction costs $50 every 2 years and new glasses cost $200 every 2 years).

Similar computations can be done for contact lenses, although it is more difficult to generalize the cost of contact lenses, the frequency of change of the lenses, and the fees charged by fitters. In any case, most contact lens wearers will have spectacles. Currently a pair of single curve, rigid, gas-permeable contact lenses costs approximately $150, and the fee for fitting a new pair of lenses is approximately $75. Contact lenses are replaced approximately every 3 years. Assuming they are worn between ages 15 and 35 years, the total cost for contact lenses would be $1575.

Impact of economics on patient selection

Clearly, the economic factors surrounding the correction of myopia are complex. The most important factor is that patients be well informed about the cost of the surgery to them and realize that if the surgery is unsuccessful, new glasses or contact lenses will be required, and if the surgery is successful, presbyopic correction will be required in the fifth decade.

UNFINISHED BUSINESS

Additional studies on the motivation of patients to have refractive surgery, including refractive keratotomy, are badly needed. Many ophthalmologists still have a prejudicial attitude that patients seeking refractive surgery to avoid use of glasses and contact lenses have frivolous, cosmetic, or ill-informed motivations. The paucity of studies on patients' psychological attitudes towards dependence on glasses and contact lenses simply emphasizes the need for information in this area. Such studies could be carried out as population-based studies, not necessarily involving individuals seeking refractive surgery but involving individuals with myopia or astigmatism, to assess attitudes toward optical correction. Similarly, there is a need to study the attitudes of patients who have had radial keratotomy about the onset of presbyopia. Are myopic patients in their early 40s who are able to read without glasses negatively affected by their accelerated dependence on reading glasses? Similarly, accurate information about the benefits of refractive keratotomy and its safety record must be disseminated to governmental agencies and employers. Too often such agencies make decisions on the basis of prejudicial statements without evaluating the scientific and clinical facts. Organizations such as the International Society of Refractive Keratoplasty and the American Academy of Ophthalmology have published factual summaries about refractive keratotomy that can be used by such agencies (see Appendix B).

Continued research on optimal methods of assessing visual function after refractive keratotomy is necessary. Subtler measures of outcome, such as contrast sensitivity testing, sophisticated glare testing, and quantitative measurements of corneal topography are necessary to measure accurately the effect of such surgery on ocular and patient function. The proper role of conventional clinical measurements such as nondilated manifest refraction, cycloplegic refraction, and visual acuity measurements using high contrast Snellen charts should be better defined. Is a standard projected Snellen acuity chart acceptable for a critical evaluation of the results of refractive keratotomy, or is a more sophisticated chart, such as the NEI chart, necessary? What is the role of cycloplegic refraction in evaluating patients? Methods of measuring the achieved depth of the incision are presently crude, and little research has been devoted to automated methods to more accurately identify the actual depth and contour of the incisions—a most important variable in determining the outcome. Intraocular pressure is generally accepted as the most active force that pushes the cornea into a new shape after refractive keratotomy, and yet no study had demonstrated that variations in intraocular pressure within the normal range (between approximately 12 and 20 mm Hg) can make a predictable difference in the outcome. Why not? Certainly very low pressure and very high pressures can be demonstrated to affect the outcome. Questions surrounding the use of keratometry and keratography as preoperative predictors and postoperative evaluators of refractive keratotomy are discussed in Chapter 3, Optics and Topography of Radial Keratotomy. The most intriguing measurement of all, that of the biomechanical properties of the individual cornea, presents the greatest current challenge. It is likely that until methods evolve to measure the mechanical properties and stress distribution within individual corneas, refractive keratotomy will not be as predictable as desired. A related subject is the measurement of ocular rigidity and its correlation with the importance of age as a preoperative variable. This is a field in which biomechanical engineers and ophthalmologists could collaborate fruitfully.

Further research on the timing of surgery on the second eye is necessary.

Even though most ophthalmologists have a strong bias against operating on both eyes at the same time, perhaps this approach would give the most uniform results in refractive keratotomy. This may be particularly true if techniques are devised that can predictably undercorrect patients and possibly allow for a second stage of the procedure, a "touch-up" operation. Careful prospective studies of alternative methods of timing surgery would do service to the profession.

Finally, there is an important need to convey accurate information to insurance companies about refractive keratotomy. They must understand that this is not cosmetic surgery in most instances and that it may legitimately fall within the purview of payments of some insurance policies. Insurers who do not wish to pay for elective refractive surgery should clearly state this in their policies and not hide behind language such as "experimental" in regard to procedures for which enough information is known to make a rational decision.

REFERENCES

1. Arrowsmith PN and Marks RG: Four year update on predictability of radial keratotomy, J Refrac Surg 1988;4:37-45.
2. Arrowsmith PN, Sanders DR, and Marks RG: Visual, refractive, and keratometric results of radial keratotomy, Arch Ophthalmol 1983;101:873-881.
3. Berliner ML: Biomicroscopy of the eye, New York, 1949, Paul B Hoeber, 1949.
4. Binder PS: Orthokeratology. In Binder et al, editors: Symposium on the cornea. Transactions of the New Orleans Academy of Ophthalmology, St Louis, 1980, The CV Mosby Co, pp 149-166.
5. Bourque LB, Cosand BB, Drews C, et al: Reported satisfaction, fluctuation of vision and glare among patients one year after surgery in PERK, Arch Ophthalmol 1986;104:356-363.
6. Bourque LB, Rubenstein R, Cosand B, Waring GO, and the PERK Study Group: Psychosocial characteristics of candidates for the Prospective Evaluation of Radial Keratotomy (PERK) Study, Arch Ophthalmol 1984;102:1187-1192.
7. Brown EVL: Net average yearly changes in refraction in atropinized eyes from birth to beyond middle life, Arch Ophthalmol 1938;19:719.
8. Brubaker RF: Tonometry. In Duane TD and Jaeger EA, editors: Clinical ophthalmology, vol 3, Philadelphia, 1987, Harper & Row.
9. Curtin BJ: The myopias: basic science and clinical management, Philadelphia, 1985, Harper & Row.
10. Deitz MR: Patient selection and counseling. In Sanders DR, Hofmann RF, and Salz JJ, editors: Refractive corneal surgery, Thorofare, NJ, 1986, Slack, Inc, p 43.
11. Deitz MR, Sanders DR, and Marks RG: Radial keratotomy: an overview of the Kansas City study, Ophthalmology 1984;91:467-478.
12. Duane TD and Jaeger EA: Biomedical foundations of ophthalmology, vol 1, Philadelphia, 1987, Harper & Row.
13. Ferris FL, Kasoff A, Bresnick GH, and Bailey I: New visual acuity charts for clinical research, Am J Ophthalmol 1982;94:91-96.
14. Ferris FL and Sperduto RD: Standardized illumination for visual acuity testing in clinical research, Am J Ophthalmol 1982;94:97-98.
15. Fyodorov SN: Personal communication, January 1988.
16. Fyodorov SN, Veklich OK, and Curasova TP: Radial keratotomy and the rehabilitation of pilots in surgery for anomalies of ocular refraction: a collection of scientific works, Moscow, 1981, Moscow Research Institute for Ocular Surgery, Ministry of Health, USSR, pp 39-42.
17. Gasset AR, Houde WL, and Barcia-Bengochea M: Hard contact lens wear as an environmental risk in keratoconus, Am J Ophthalmol 1978;85:339-341.
18. Goldwyn R, Waltman SR, and Becker B: Primary open-angle glaucoma in adolescents and young adults, Arch Ophthalmol 1970;84:579-582.
19. Levenson DS: Changes in corneal curvature with longterm PMMA contact lens wear, CLAO J 1983;9:121-125.
20. Levenson DS and Barry CV: Findings on follow-up of corneal warpage patients, CLAO J 1983;9:126-129.
21. Martonyi CL, Bahn CF, and Meyer RF: Clinical slit-lamp biomicroscopy and photo slit-lamp biomicrography, J Ophthalmic Photog 1984;7:1-80.
22. Mayer DJ: Clinical wide-field specular microscopy, London, 1984, Bailliere Tindal.
23. Meyner EM: Atlas of slit-lamp photography, Stuttgart, 1976, Ferdinand Enke.
24. Milder B and Rubin ML: The fine art of prescribing glasses without making a spectacle of yourself, Gainesville, Fla, 1978, Triad Scientific Publishers.
25. Mohrman R: The keratometer. In Duane TD and Jaeger EA, editors: Clinical ophthalmology, vol 1, Philadelphia, 1981, Harper & Row.
26. Morgan JF: Induced corneal astigmatism with hydrophilic contact lenses, Can J Ophthalmol 1975;10:207-213.
27. Moses RA: Intraocular pressure. In Moses RA and Hart W Jr, editors: Adler's physiology of the eye: clinical application, ed 8, St Louis, 1987, The CV Mosby Co, pp 223-245.
28. Nakajima A: Effects of antero-posterior incision of cornea on myopia, Japanese J Clin Ophthalmol 1960;14:1943-1945.
29. O'Dell LW and Wyzinski P: Radial keratotomy in teenagers: a practical approach, Refract Corneal Surg 1989;5:315-320.
30. Powers MK, Meyerowitz BE, Arrowsmith PN, and Marks G: Psychosocial findings in radial keratotomy patients two years after surgery, Ophthalmology 1984;91:1193-1198.
31. Rowsey JJ, Balyeat HD, Monlux R, et al: Prospective evaluation of radial keratotomy: photokeratoscope corneal topography, Ophthalmology 1988;95:322-334.
32. Rubin M: Contact lens practice, Baltimore, 1975, Williams & Wilkins, pp 104-130.
33. Salz JJ: Multiple complications following radial keratotomy in an elderly patient, Ophthal Surg 1980;16:579-580.

34. Salz JJ, Reader AL, and Hofmann RF: Radial keratotomy for overcorrected pseudophakia: results of an informal survey, J Refrac Surg 1987;3:137-139.

35. Salz JJ and Salz MS: Results of 4- and 8-incision radial keratotomy for 6 to 11 diopters of myopia, J Refract Surg 1988;4:46-50.

36. Sampson WG, and Soper JW: Keratometry. In Girard LJ, Soper JW, and Sampson WG, editors: Corneal contact lenses, ed 2, St Louis, 1970, The CV Mosby Co, pp 65-92.

37. Sanders DR, Deitz MR, and Gallagher D: Factors affecting predictability of radial keratotomy, Ophthalmology 1985; 92:1237-1243.

38. Sawelson H and Marks RG: Two-year results of radial keratotomy, Arch Ophthalmol 1985;103:505-510.

39. Shepard DD: Radial keratotomy: analysis of efficacy and predictability in 1,058 consecutive cases. Part I. Efficacy, J Cataract Refract Surg 1986;12:632-643.

40. Shepard DD: Radial keratotomy: analysis of efficacy and predictability in 1,058 consecutive cases. Part II. Predictability, J Cataract Refract Surg 1987;13:32-34.

41. Shields MB: Textbook of glaucoma, ed 2, Baltimore, 1987, Williams & Wilkins.

42. Sloan LL: Needs for precise measures of acuity: equipment to meet these needs, Arch Ophthalmol 1980;98:286-290.

43. Smith RS: Radial keratotomy in teenagers: a dubious idea, Refractive Corneal Surg 1989;5:315-320.

44. Sperduto RD, Segal D, Roberts J, et al: Prevalence of myopia in the United States, Arch Ophthalmol 1983;101: 405-407.

45. Sugar HS: Pigmentary glaucoma, Am J Ophthalmol 1966;62:499-507.

46. Tredeici TJ: USAF position on radial keratotomy, Ophthalmic Surg 1983; 14:790.

47. Vetach RM: The patient as partner: a theory of human-experimentation ethics, Indianapolis, 1987, Indiana University Press.

48. Voght A: Textbook and atlas of slit-lamp microscopy of the living eye. Vol 1. Principles and methods of cornea and anterior chamber, Bonn, 1981, Wayneborgh.

49. Volkov VV: Medical indications for radial keratotomy, Oftalmologichesky 1988;8:491-494.

50. Waring GO, Lynn MJ, Culbertson W, et al: Three-year results of PERK study, Ophthalmol 1987;94:1339-1354.

51. Waring GO, Lynn MJ, Gelender H, et al: Results of PERK study one year after surgery, Ophthalmology 1985;92:177-198.

52. Working Group 39, Committee on Vision, Assembly of Behavioral and Social Sciences, National Research Council: Recommended standard procedures for the clinical measurement of specifications of visual acuity, Adv Ophthalmol 1980;41:103-148.

Predictability of Refractive Keratotomy

Michael J. Lynn

George O. Waring III

Michael H. Kutner

THE SEARCH FOR PREDICTABILITY

Every person who has refractive keratotomy harbors one overriding concern: "How well will I see? Will I still have to wear glasses or contact lenses?" The surgeon's concern is similar: "What can I do to tailor the operation to achieve a perfect result for this person?" Patients and surgeons want to know the outcome ahead of time. This desire has led to a perennial debate about the surgery: Is it predictable?

Most published reports have indicated a precision for predicting the refractive outcome of about ±2 D for 80% to 90% of eyes.[1-3,26,40] Therefore some authors contend that refractive keratotomy is predictable because the precision is similar to that of intraocular lens implantation after cataract surgery.[3] Others counter that this is an inappropriate comparison because refractive keratotomy is an elective operation for a non–vision threatening refractive error for which the current standard of care is glasses and contact lenses that can be fit with a refractive outcome of better than ±0.50 D; refractive keratotomy should have a similar predictability. Whether this stringent standard can ever be achieved with refractive surgery is unknown. Currently there are no absolute standards for acceptable predictability in refractive keratotomy; many patients and ophthalmic surgeons are willing to accept the less-than-desirable predictability to eliminate the drawbacks of prosthetic glasses and contact lenses.

BACKGROUND AND ACKNOWLEDGMENTS

The information on which this chapter is based is drawn from the published literature as cited. The majority of information derives from the three major studies of the predictability of radial keratotomy: the Prospective Evaluation of Radial Keratotomy (PERK) study[26]; Sanders, Deitz, Gallagher[40]; and Arrowsmith and Marks.[1,2] Throughout this chapter these three studies are referred to as the PERK study, the Sanders study, and the Arrowsmith study. The chapter was written out of the PERK Statistical Coordinating Center at Emory University and supported by National Institutes of Health grant EY03752. We acknowledge the assistance of our colleagues Azhar Nizam and Brooke Fielding, and the staff of the coordinating center—Portia Griffin, Brenda Henderson, and Phyllis Newman.

Investigators have long sought to identify and control the patient characteristics and elements of surgical technique that determine the refractive outcome. Attempts to examine these factors have included plastic models of the ocular anterior segment,[21] mathematical models of the cornea[42] (see Section VI, Corneal Biomechanics and Computer Modeling of Refractive Keratotomy), experiments on enucleated animal and human eyes,[20,36,37] and statistical analyses of clinical results.[1-3,26,40] We have discussed in previous chapters the prediction factors used by Sato (Chapter 6, Development of Radial Keratotomy in Japan, 1939-1960) and Fyodorov (Chapter 7, Development of Refractive Keratotomy in the Soviet Union, 1960-1990).

This chapter discusses the predictability of refractive keratotomy using primarily the results from three clinical studies.

The nomograms, formulas, and computer software programs designed to improve the predictability of refractive keratotomy are discussed separately in Chapter 14, Computerized Predictability Formulas for Refractive Keratotomy.

DEFINITION AND MEASUREMENT OF PREDICTABILITY

Prediction is determining in advance what an outcome is likely to be. In the case of refractive keratotomy this means specifying before surgery the refractive error a patient can expect at some time after surgery. If the procedure were completely predictable, we could specify the outcome at any time after surgery. Since the predictability of refractive keratotomy is less than perfect, the best we can do is to predict that the result is likely to fall within a particular range of outcomes. For example, we might say to patients with 4.00 D of myopia that their refractive error will probably be between −2.00 and +1.00 D 1 year after surgery. The size or width of this range of refractive error is a measure of the predictability of refractive keratotomy.

Basis for predictability

Predictions about future events are usually based on past experience, unless one happens to have a crystal ball. In medical practice predictions are often clinical impressions based on the overall results of a previous informal series of cases. In this situation the physician may have a general idea of the likely outcome but is probably unable to give any detailed, quantitative evidence for this prediction; acquiring such evidence requires a scientifically valid study. If the results of this more rigorous type study show that the outcome is reasonably reproducible—that is, if the procedure yields similar results when applied to patients with similar characteristics—the range for the predicted outcome in a new patient will be small and the predictability will be considered good. If, on the other hand, similar patients have different results, this will be reflected in a wider range for the predicted outcome and the procedure will be considered unpredictable. Thus the ability to adequately predict future outcomes depends on how reproducible the results have been previously.

Regression analysis and prediction intervals

All studies of refractive keratotomy have reported considerable variability in the refractive change 1 year or more after surgery, even among eyes that had a similar keratotomy operation. For example, in the PERK study[48] among operated eyes with a 3.5-mm clear zone and a standardized technique, the change in refraction varied between 0.75 and 6.63 D. Can this large variation be explained by some difference among the eyes that was measured before surgery? Regression analysis helps answer this question. A regression model or regression equation expresses mathematically the relationship between an outcome factor, for example, change in refraction, and a set of explanatory factors, for example, age, keratometric power, and diameter of clear zone. The challenge is in both finding the important explanatory factors that should be included in the equation and devising the correct form of the equation.

One measure of the adequacy of a regression equation is the R^2 value, which is the percent of the overall variation in the outcome that is explained by the equation: this is the R^2 value.[30] For example, in the PERK study[26] the combination of clear zone diameter, patient age, and depth of incision scar had an R^2 value of 0.44; thus, these three variables explained 44% of the variability in refractive change. However, the R^2 value has little use in evaluating how accurately the equation predicts the outcome for an individual patient. For this a different measure is required—one that can specify the range for the expected outcome in an individual new patient. This range is called the prediction interval. If the range is sufficiently narrow, the predictability is adequate.

The prediction interval is similar to a confidence interval, a term that may be more familiar. Both provide a range of values for predicting an outcome. However, the confidence interval specifies a range for the mean value in a series of new patients and the prediction interval specifies a range for a single new patient. Since there is more uncertainty in predicting for an individual than for a group of individuals, the prediction interval is usually wider than the corresponding confidence interval. If the surgeon wants to know the probable outcome for an individual patient, the prediction interval is the more appropriate measure. These statistical techniques are described fully by Neter and associates.[30] Seigel[43] discusses the use of regression analysis in ophthalmology.

The major thesis of this chapter is that the predictability of refractive keratotomy is not an ethereal property based on opinion ("RK is predictable; No it ain't."), but rather a variable that can be quantified. Predictability formulas can be quantified by using the R^2 value, but this value is not as clinically meaningful as the prediction interval, the derivation and meaning of which are explained in the appendix.

For example, to measure the predictability of radial keratotomy in the PERK[26] study, we determined the 90% prediction interval for the change in refraction for an individual patient. The midpoint of the prediction interval is the predicted change in refraction, which is determined for an individual patient by putting the diameter of the central clear zone, patient age, and the depth of incision scar into the regression equation. For example, using this equation for all clear zone groups combined and putting the mean values for these factors into the equation (clear zone = 3.5 mm, age = 33 years, depth of incision = 75%), the predicted change in refraction was 3.56 D with a 90% prediction interval of 1.85 to 5.27 D (3.56 ± 1.71 D). The width of this prediction interval, 3.42 D, indicates the precision with which the outcome of refractive keratotomy can be predicted for an individual patient (see Table 13-2).

The width of the prediction interval was also determined for each clear zone group. The smaller the diameter of the clear zone, the wider the 90% prediction interval: 4.0 mm, 2.49 D; 3.5 mm, 3.38 D; and 3.0 mm, 4.12 D (see Table 13-2). Thus, predictability was better for patients with lower myopia who received a larger clear zone.

Standard deviation and standard error of the mean

Investigators often summarize data using two quantities: the mean, which is a measure of central tendency, and the standard error of the mean or the standard deviation, both of which measure dispersion. The primary reason for reporting the arithmetic mean, the standard error of the mean, and the standard deviation as summary measures is because they are good estimates if we believe either that our data come from a normal (Gaussian) distribution or that our sample size is relatively large. Here we explain the distinction between the standard deviation and the standard error of the mean.

Two parameters that uniquely identify a normal (Gaussian) distribution are the population mean (denoted μ) and the population standard deviation (denoted σ). Since studies often do not involve the entire population, a sample of the population must be taken. Thus we estimate parameters in a population by measuring the sample mean (denoted $\overline{Y}$) and the sample standard deviation (denoted s.) These two estimated quantities and the sample size allow us to perform tests of statistical significance and to find prediction intervals for these two parameters. The distinction between the standard deviation and the standard error of the mean is that each estimates dispersion but for different random variables. If we are interested in estimating dispersion in a normal population, then the sample standard deviation is the proper estimate to report. As the sample size increases, the sample standard deviation simply better approximates the true population standard deviation. The standard error of the mean is a good measure of dispersion of the sample means. For a relatively large sample size, the distribution of sample means is also approximately normally distributed, so the standard error of the mean is the proper estimate of the dispersion of these means. As the sample size increases, the standard error of the mean gets smaller and smaller, approaching zero as the sample size approaches infinity. This is true because we are estimating the dispersion of sample means, which also depends on the sample size.

Therefore if we wish to make inferences about mean values in the population, then a good estimate is the standard error of the mean. If, on the other hand, our primary interest is in estimating the parameters in an entire population, then a good measure of dispersion is the sample standard deviation.

Predicted versus actual change in refraction

Another way to judge the predictability of a technique of refractive keratotomy clinically is to compare the change in refraction predicted before surgery with the change in refraction actually obtained in the series of eyes. This approach has been taken by Sanders[40] and by Arrowsmith.[2] For example, in the PERK study, using the equation for all clear zone groups combined, the difference between the actual change in refraction and the predicted change was 1.00 D or less for 69% of eyes, 2.00 D or less for 95% of eyes, and 3.00 D or less for 99% of eyes.

IDENTIFICATION OF PREDICTIVE FACTORS

In addition to predicting the refractive outcome, the clinician is also concerned with identifying the determinants of the outcome and using them to create a surgical technique that will achieve the desired result for an individual patient. The most common example in clinical ophthalmology is the calculation of intraocular lens (IOL) power. The use of regression formulas based on clinical experience to calculate intraocular lens power has been found superior to the use of theoretic optical formulas based on the model eye. Regression analysis showed that the two most important patient variables were the central keratometric measurements and the axial length. Also included was the specific "A constant" for each intraocular lens, which allowed the surgeon to customize the calculations for individual lens styles and surgical techniques.

In contrast, identification of factors that predict the outcome of refractive keratotomy has fostered considerable disagreement. Some surgeons use only one or two factors, others use six or eight factors.

Evidence now indicates that one patient factor, age, and three surgical factors, diameter of central clear zone, depth of incisions, and number of incisions, are the most important factors in determining the outcome of refractive keratotomy. This evidence comes from laboratory studies in animal and eyebank eyes, large series of cases analyzed by regression analysis, and individual trials that have studied individual factors.

Regression analysis in laboratory studies

Jester and colleagues[20] used stepwise multiple regression analysis to study the variables affecting outcomes of 14 human cadaver eyes, each of which had a 4 mm diameter central clear zone. They studied the acute change in curvature with a Terry operating keratometer. They identified the average depth of incision, as determined histologically, as the most important factor, deeper incisions giving more effect. The length of incision was negatively correlated with the outcome, especially when extended across to the limbus. Preoperative corneal curvature was next most important with steeper corneas achieving greater effect. Interestingly the effect of varying the diameter of the clear zone and the number of incisions could *not* be studied because they were fixed at 4 mm and 16 incisions, respectively.

Regression analysis in clinical trials

Three clinical studies that have identified predictive factors are the PERK study,[26] the study of Sanders,[40] and the study of Arrowsmith.[1,2] We review here the overall results of the diamond blade cases for these three studies at the longest follow-up.

The PERK study had nearly four times as many eyes as the other two studies (see Table 13-5). Follow-up time was 12 months for PERK, 3 months for Sanders, and 2 years for Arrowsmith, indicating that the Sanders study reported their findings at a time when the results may not have been as stable as the other two studies. The surgical technique and the methods of making postoperative measurements varied markedly among the studies, making the similarities of the results of the three predictability analyses even more remarkable (see Tables 13-1 to 13-5).

In general, the three studies agreed regarding the factors that affect outcome, each concluding that the diameter of the clear zone, the age of the patient, and the depth of the incision scar, including both deepening incisions and microperforations for Arrowsmith, were important (Table 13-1). Both Sanders and Arrowsmith identified the number of incisions as important, but in the PERK study, eight incisions were used in all cases. Sanders reported that the average baseline keratometric power had a small effect; Arrowsmith included average baseline keratometric power in the equations at 2 and 4 years, but not for earlier follow-up points. None of the studies found that patient sex, baseline intraocular pressure, corneal diameter, central corneal thickness, or ocular rigidity significantly affected the outcome. Corneal topography was not studied (Tables 13-2 to 13-4).

The R^2 values were almost identical in the Sanders study (0.78) and the Arrowsmith study (0.73). Both these values were higher than the R^2 value in the PERK study (0.44). A possible explanation for the difference in R^2 is that the PERK study had less total variability in refractive change than the other two studies because there was a single surgical technique and the range of preoperative myopia was smaller. The other two studies may have explained a higher percentage of the total variability, resulting in a higher R^2 value. However, the important consideration for evaluating predictability is the magnitude of the unexplained variability rather than the percentage.

The differences between the predicted and actual changes in refraction were similar in the three studies (Table 13-5), indicating roughly similar degrees of

Table 13-1

Factors Affecting Outcome of Radial Keratotomy in Three Studies*

Factor	PERK[26]	Sanders[40]	Arrowsmith[2]
Clear zone	1	1	7
Age of patient	2	5	6
Depth of incision scar	3†	2†	2‡
Number of incisions	(8 only)	3	1
Average central kera-tometry	No	4	3
Microperforations	No	No	5

Modified from Lynn MJ, Waring GO, Sperduto RD, et al: Arch Ophthalmol 1987;105:42-51.
*Numbers indicate order of entry into regression equation.
†Single-pass incisions.
‡Deepening incisions in some cases.

Table 13-2

Fitted Regression Coefficients for Final Regression Model in the Study of Sanders and Colleagues

	Coefficient	Cumulative R^2
Clear zone diameter	−0.2891	0.52
Mean incision depth	0.0771	0.59
Number of incisions	0.189	0.66
Preoperative average K	0.2347	0.70
Age	0.044	0.72

Modified from Sanders D, Deitz M, and Gallagher D: Ophthalmology 1985;92:1237-1243.

predictability. But there were definite differences. The results obtained by Deitz were better than those in PERK, which in turn were better than those of Arrowsmith. Thus theoretically a surgeon could turn to the Deitz article, identify the surgical techniques that were different from those used in the PERK and Arrowsmith studies, and adopt those to improve these techniques that have produced superior results. Unfortunately, the papers by Deitz and Sanders[10,40] do not specify the surgical technique in enough detail for it to be replicated. The ranges within which the difference between the predicted and achieved values fell for 90% of the eyes were approximately ±1.75 D for the PERK study, ±1.25 D for the Sanders study, and ±2.75 D for the Arrowsmith study.

Although the overall predictability of refractive keratotomy is similar in these three studies, the authors came to different conclusions. Arrowsmith, with the widest interval, stated that refractive keratotomy "seems to be highly predict-

Table 13-3

Regression Coefficients, R^2, and 90% Prediction Interval for Predicted Change in Refraction in the PERK Study at One Year after Surgery

	Three groups combined	Diameter of central clear zone		
		4.0 mm	3.5 mm	3.0 mm
90% Prediction interval (D)	1.85-5.27	1.48-3.97	1.75-5.11	2.39-6.51
Width of interval (D)	3.42	2.49	3.38	4.12
Regression coefficients for:				
Diameter of clear zone	−1.6297	—	—	—
Age	0.0649	0.0506	0.0706	0.0695
Depth of incision scar	0.0203	0.0108	0.0226	0.0287
Intercept (constant term)	5.5987	0.2737	−.5389	−.0368
R^2	.44	.22	.24	.22
Mean square error	1.0766	0.5568	1.0333	1.5368

From Lynn MJ, Waring GO, Sperduto RD, et al: Arch Ophthalmol 1987;105:42-51.

Table 13-4

Factors Significant in 2-Year Predictability of Radial Keratotomy For 1982 Diamond Knife Cases in Arrowsmith and Marks Study

R^2*	Factor	Model Coefficient
—	Intercept	125.80
.520	Number of incisions	†
.094	(Incision depth)^2	0.01434
.034	Number of tertiary incisions	0.14
.034	Average keratometry	−.429
.034	Incision depth	−2.415
.018	Primary incision perforation	1.35
.016	Age × number of incisions	0.006
.027	Incision depth × optical zone	−1.15
.006	Number of perforations in secondary incisions	0.49

From Arrowsmith PN and Marks RG: J Refract Surg 1988;4:37-45.
*R^2 = 78%.
†This was the first factor selected in the stepwise regression, but was removed after Step 7 by the computer program.

Table 13-5

Comparison of Three Studies of the Predictability of Radial Keratotomy

	PERK[26]	Sanders[40]	Arrowsmith[4]
Number of eyes	411	106	90
Follow-up time (months)	12	3	24
R^2	.44	.73	.78
Difference between predicted and actual change in refraction (%)			
Within 1.00 D	69	84	59
Within 1.50 D	86	94	—
Within 2.00 D	95	—	83
Within 3.00 D	99	—	92

Modified from Lynn MJ, Waring GO, Sperduto RD, et al: Arch Ophthalmol 1987;105:42-51.

able."[1] Sanders[40] did not present a specific value judgment, but stated that results provided a "basis for a clinical tool" to aid surgeons in selecting their surgical techniques. The PERK study concluded that a 90% prediction interval approximately 3.50 D wide indicates inadequate predictability because it compared poorly to the estimated interval for fitting glasses or contact lenses, on the order of 0.50 D. We discuss the results of the PERK study in detail in the next section.

Kremer and Steer[22] examined the prediction of refractive correction using age, intraocular pressure, central corneal thickness, number of incisions, number of zones, and size of central optical zone. However, most of their paper discussed the relationship between these factors and "the amount of correction required to achieve emmetropia," which was the *preoperative* refractive error. Since the surgical factors were chosen according to the amount of preoperative myopia, it is not surprising that these factors would correlate well with the preoperative refractive error, and indeed the regression equation had an R^2 value of .99. This exercise in circular reasoning regarding the preoperative refractive error did not justify the statement of Kremer and Steer that their study "indicates a high level of predictability for the correction of myopia."

In one paragraph of their paper, Kremer and Steer mentioned the *postoperative* refractive error and showed the correlation with the following factors: age, 0.11; intraocular pressure, 0.13; central corneal thickness, −0.01; number of incisions, −0.18; number of zones, −0.31; and size of central optical zone, 0.08.

PREDICTABILITY IN THE PERK STUDY

Table 13-6 summarizes the factors evaluated in the PERK study of predictability. Multiple regression analysis was done for the three baseline myopia groups individually and combined (see Table 13-3).

Table 13-6

Characteristics of Patients in the PERK Study*

Factor	Number	Mean	Standard deviation	Minimum	Maximum
Baseline cycloplegic refraction (D)	411	−4.09	1.42	−2.00	−8.00
Age (years)	411	33.5	7.3	21	58
Baseline average central keratometry (D)	411	44.06	1.39	40.25	48.88
Baseline central corneal thickness (mm)	410	0.53	0.04	0.41	0.65
Baseline horizontal corneal diameter (mm)	396	11.9	0.5	11.0	13.5
Baseline intraocular pressure (mm Hg)	410	14.4	3.1	7.0	25.0
Baseline ocular rigidity	410	0.02	0.007	0.002	0.042
Depth of incision scar (%)†	411	72.8	12.5	36.5	87.5
Change in refraction at one year (D)	411	3.60	1.38	0.38	8.63
Diameter of central clear zone (baseline refractive error):					
4.0 mm (−2.00 to −3.12 D)	124 (30%)				
3.5 mm (−3.25 to −4.37 D)	138 (34%)				
3.0 mm (−4.50 to −8.00 D)	149 (36%)				
Sex: Male	215 (52%)				
Female	196 (48%)				

From Lynn MJ, Waring GO, Sperduto RD, et al: Arch Ophthalmol 1987;105:42-51.
*One eye per patient.
†Depth score derived from all eight incisions. Maximum possible value was 87.5%.

Identification of important factors

The analysis for all clear zone groups combined showed that the diameter of the central clear zone was the most important factor. Because the patients in the three clear zone groups had different amounts of preoperative myopia, the clear zone factor in the equation represented the combined effect of both clear zone diameter and baseline refractive error; therefore the effect of the amount of preoperative myopia cannot be analyzed separately. The R^2 value for the diameter of the central clear zone was 0.28, indicating that this factor explained 28% of the variability in the change in refraction. The inclusion of age and the average depth of the incision scar explained an additional 12% and 4% of the variability, respectively. The R^2 value for the equation with these three factors was 0.44. No other factors, including various nonlinear and interaction terms, significantly improved the fit of the model (see Table 13-8).

Results of the analyses of the three individual clear zone groups were similar to those of the groups combined; age was the most important variable, followed by average depth of incision scar. The R^2 values were approximately 0.20 for each clear zone group (see Table 13-3).

Interpretation of regression coefficients in PERK

The regression coefficients (Table 13-3) indicate the effect of each factor on the change in refraction. In the analysis of the three clear zone groups combined, the regression coefficient for the diameter of the central clear zone was -1.63, indicating that a reduction of the clear zone by 1 mm was related to an added average change in refraction of 1.63 D. The coefficient for age was 0.065, so an increase of 10 years in age was related to an average additional change in refraction of 0.65 D. The coefficient for the average depth of the incision scar was 0.02, indicating, for example, that a 25% increase in the average depth of the eight incisions was related to an additional change in refraction of 0.50 D. Of course these are average effects, and because of the variability in patient response, these relationships would not necessarily be accurate for individual patients. Similar coefficients resulted from the analyses of the clear zone groups separately.

INDIVIDUAL PREDICTIVE FACTORS IN REFRACTIVE KERATOTOMY

We now turn our attention to the discussion of specific surgical and patient variables that may affect the outcome of refractive keratotomy, discussing in detail the evidence for and against the effect of each. The surgical variables are discussed in detail in Chapter 17, Atlas of Surgical Techniques of Radial Keratotomy.

Diameter of central clear zone (optical zone)

Sato used a central clear zone diameter of 6 mm, marked with a hair placed in a circular pattern on the cornea (Chapter 6, Development of Radial Keratotomy in Japan, 1939-1960). Fyodorov and Durnev[14] suggested varying the diameter of the clear zone as a method of calibrating the length of the incisions, such that a smaller diameter clear zone and longer incisions would produce a greater decrease in myopia. Since then, varying the diameter of the clear zone to control the outcome has become a veritable canon of keratotomy surgery.*

*References 2, 5, 17, 31, 35, 38, 40, 42.

Table 13-7

Acute Change in Central Keratometric Power Correlated with the Diameter of the Central Clear Zone in an Eyebank Eye Study by Salz and Colleagues

Clear zone (mm)	Change in Terry keratometry (D)*	
	4 incisions	8 incisions
3.0	7.75($\pm$1.19)	9.06($\pm$1.69)
4.0	5.34($\pm$1.65)	6.44($\pm$1.29)†
5.0	3.60($\pm$1.44)	5.23($\pm$1.48)†
6.0	1.23($\pm$0.68)	2.29($\pm$0.70)
F test for difference (P)	27.26($<$.0001)	26.40($<$.0001)
F test for linearity (P)	81.46($<$.0001)	77.45($<$.0001)

From Salz JJ, Rowsey JJ, Caroline P, et al: Arch Ophthalmol 1985;103:590-594.
*Values reported as spherical equivalents in diopters ($\pm$ standard deviations).
†Means do not differ from each other statistically.

Table 13-8

Change in the Spherical Equivalent of the Cycloplegic Refraction 1 Year after Radial Keratotomy by Age and Clear Zone in the PERK Study

Age (years)	Diameter of central clear zone (mm)											
	4.0				3.5				3.0			
	No. of eyes	Mean change (D)	Standard deviation	Difference (D)	No. of eyes	Mean change (D)	Standard deviation	Difference (D)	No. of eyes	Mean change (D)	Standard deviation	Difference (D)
20 to 29	42	2.26	0.63	0.64	51	2.97	1.14	0.57	44	3.98	1.41	0.49
30 to 39	64	2.90	0.85	0.32	67	3.54	1.00	0.58	76	4.47	1.18	0.82
40 to 58	18	3.22	0.75		20	4.12	1.31		29	5.29	1.55	

From Lynn MJ, Waring GO, Sperduto RD, et al: Arch Ophthalmol 1987;105:42-51.

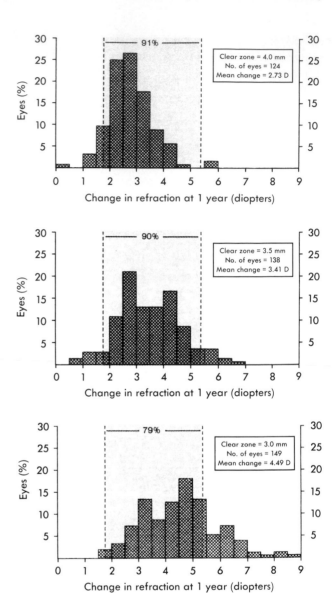

Figure 13-1

Effect of diameter of central clear zone on change in refraction in the PERK study. Each bar graph represents one of the three clear zone groups: 4.0 mm *(top)*, 3.5 mm *(middle)*, 3.0 mm *(bottom)*. The change in spherical equivalent of the cycloplegic refraction 1 year after surgery is indicated across the horizontal axis on each bar graph. The percentage of eyes in each group is indicated on the vertical axis. Graphs demonstrate that the average change in refraction increased for smaller clear zones but that there was considerable variation within each clear zone group and marked overlap among clear zone groups. Percentage of patients with refraction in the range of 1.75 to 5.37 D is given for each group *(shaded area between broken lines)*. (From Lynn MJ, Waring GO, Sperduto RD, et al: Arch Ophthalmol 1987;105:31-51.)

Laboratory study of clear zone diameter. A study of the effect of clear zone size by Salz and colleagues[38] in human cadaver eyes showed a statistically significant effect of decreasing clear zone diameter for both 4 and 8 incisions (Table 13-7). Mathematical models of radial keratotomy have arrived at similar conclusions.[42] (See Chapter 28, A Finite Element Model of Radial Keratotomy Surgery, and Chapter 29, Preliminary Computer Simulation of Radial Keratotomy.)

Clinical studies of clear zone diameter. Clinical studies have also documented an increasing effect of the surgery with decreasing diameter of the clear zone. For example, Sanders[40] noted that reducing the diameter by 0.5 mm resulted in slightly less than 1.00 D of additional refractive change.

Findings in the PERK study[26] were similar (see Fig. 13-1, Tables 13-3 and 13-6 to 13-9). Eyes with smaller clear zones had a greater average decrease in myopia: a 4.0-mm clear zone produced a 2.73 D decrease in myopia; a 3.5-mm, clear zone produced a 3.41 D decrease in myopia; and a 3.0-mm clear zone produced a 4.49 D decrease in myopia. Thus a 0.5 mm reduction in the diameter of clear zone from 4.0 mm to 3.5 mm was related to an increase in the average change in refraction of 0.68 D—a reduction in the diameter of the clear zone from 3.5 mm to 3.0 mm, the increase in change of refraction was 1.08 D.

Interestingly the regression analysis of Arrowsmith and Marks for diamond-knife cases did not include the diameter of the clear zone between 1 and 24 months after surgery, except as an interaction term "incision depth × optical zone size," a factor that had minimal influence (increase in $R^2 = 0.027$). The amount of baseline myopia is also absent from Arrowsmith and Marks's regression equation. One wonders why these two variables, so important in other people's calculations, were absent.

The effect of the diameter of the clear zone is not as clear-cut as generally thought. The histograms from the PERK study in Fig. 13-1 demonstrate the

Table 13-9

Change in R^2 and Width of 90% Prediction Interval as Factors Added to the PERK Regression Equation

Factor	R^2*	Width of 90% prediction interval (D)†
Diameter of clear zone	.28	3.87
Age	.40	3.52
Depth of incision scar	.44	3.42
Baseline refractive error	.45	3.36
Horizontal corneal diameter	.47	3.32
Average central keratometric power	.48	3.29
Intraocular pressure	.49	3.28
Sex	.49	3.28
Central corneal thickness	.49	3.28
Ocular rigidity	.49	3.28

From Lynn MJ, Waring GO, Sperduto RD, et al: Arch Ophthalmol 1987;105:42-51.
*R^2 gives percentage of variation in outcome explained by regression equation.
†Width of prediction interval gives the precision for predicting outcome.

marked variation in the change in refraction within a single clear zone. Furthermore there was a marked overlap in the change in refraction among the three clear-zone groups. To quantify this overlap, we used the range of the refractive change for the middle 90% of eyes in the 3.5-mm clear zone (1.75 to 5.37 D) and determined that 91% of eyes in the 4.0-mm clear zone group and 79% of eyes in the 3.0-mm group were also in this range (areas between broken lines in Fig. 13-1). Although there was a shift toward greater average change in refraction as the clear zone diameter decreased, the majority of eyes in all three clear zones fell in the same range of refractive change.

These results show how the differences in the response among individual patients can overwhelm the relatively smaller effect of changing the diameter of the clear zone by 0.5 mm. Some surgeons vary the clear zone diameter in 0.25 mm steps, but in view of the marked variability, this may be an unnecessary refinement. No studies have compared results of 0.25-mm and 0.50-mm steps.

The optimal diameter of the central clear zone has evolved through clinical experience with help from laboratory studies. Fyodorov[13] initially advocated a clear zone 2.4 mm in diameter but later used a minimum size of 3 mm. The current accepted diameters range from 3.0 to 5.0 mm. Cutting inside the 3-mm zone will increase the effect of the surgery but is associated with increased glare as documented by Smith and Cutro.[44] Diameters greater than 5 mm have much less effect (see Table 13-7); this explains in part the low results achieved by Sato's 6-mm clear zone.

Baseline refractive error and clear zone diameter

The effect of the baseline refractive error in clinical studies cannot be evaluated independently of the diameter of the clear zone because the clear zone is determined by the baseline refractive error. One way to study these factors independently would be to assign a clear zone randomly to patients with the same baseline refraction. This is not now acceptable because all evidence suggests that the clear zone is an important factor for controlling the effect of surgery.[14] In the PERK study the correlation between the baseline refractive error and the change in refraction was approximately -0.20 D in each clear zone group, indicating a slight trend for the amount of correction to increase as the preoperative myopia increased (Fig. 13-2).

Figure 13-2
Effect of baseline refraction on the change of refraction in the PERK study at 1 year. Symbols for each clear zone group and correlations are given in the boxed insert. (From Lynn MJ, Waring GO, Sperduto RD, et al: Arch Ophthalmol 1987;105:42-51.)

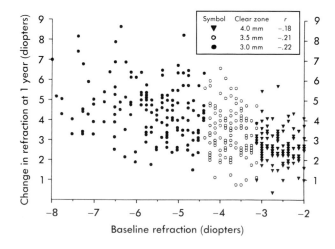

Symbol	Clear zone	r
▼	4.0 mm	−.18
○	3.5 mm	−.21
●	3.0 mm	−.22

Length of incisions

No comparison of short versus long incisions and no careful measurement of actual incision length have been reported in human studies. Currently many surgeons make the incision between the edge of the clear zone mark and the end of the corneal vascular arcade.

Altering the diameter of the clear zone is the most common way to alter the length of the incisions, but since the center of the clear zone is usually located nasal to the geometric center of the cornea, the incisions are not of uniform length, the temporal incisions being longer than the nasal incisions. Both Sato and Fyodorov extended the peripheral part of the incision into the sclera, Fyodorov postulating that this cut the peripheral ligament of the cornea, increasing the effect of the surgery—thus the title of his initial article, "Operation of Dosaged Dissection of Corneal Surgical Ligament in Cases of Myopia of Mild Degree."[14] This practice was abandoned when clinical experience, laboratory testing[20] (Fig. 13-3), and mechanical modeling[21,42] demonstrated no significant difference between incisions confined to the cornea and those extending across the limbus.

Laboratory studies of incision length. In experiments on human cadaver eyes using a 4 mm diameter clear zone, Jester and colleagues[20] demonstrated a negative correlation between the length of the incision extending beyond the corneal limbus and the effect of the surgery (Fig. 13-4). Cutting across the lim-

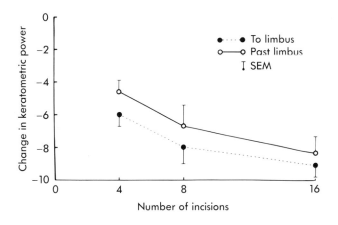

Figure 13-3
Effect of the number of incisions on the change in keratometric power using 4, 8, and 16 incisions in a cadaver eye model. There was no statistical difference between incisions that were confined to the cornea *(closed circles)*. Sixty percent of the total effect was achieved with 4 incisions, 80% with 8 incisions, and 100% with 16 incisions. (From Salz JJ, Lee JS, Jester JV, et al: Ophthalmology 1981;88:742-746.)

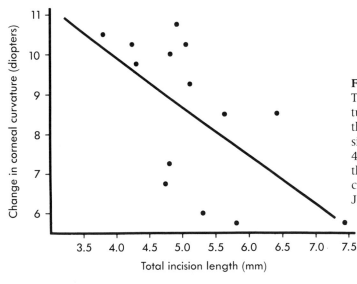

Figure 13-4
The effect of incision length on change in corneal curvature in an eye bank eye model. Longer incisions reduced the amount of corneal flattening, indicating that incisions across the limbus are less effective. Incisions 3.5 to 4.5 mm long (the length used in keratotomy confined to the cornea) did not show this effect. Correlation coefficient = −0.61 ($p < .05$). (From Jester JV, Venet T, Lee J, et al: Am J Ophthalmol 1981;92:172-177.)

Table 13-10

Comparison of Change in Keratometric Power (D) Produced by Diamond-Knife Radial Incisions from Clear Zone to Limbus (Long Incisions) and Paracentrally Outside the Clear Zone (Short Incisions) in the Acute Eyebank Eye Study

	Change in keratometric power (D)	
	Four incisions	**Eight incisions**
To limbus		
Mean length, 4.0 ± 0.2		
Mean*	6.8	9.5
Standard deviation	±1.6	±1.0
Percentage of change†	71	—
Short incisions		
Mean length, 2.6 ± 0.2 mm		
Mean*	3.7	5.8
Standard deviation	±1.5	±1.1
Percentage of change†	63	—
P value‡	t = 3.430	t = 5.986
	p = 0.0064	p < 0.0001

From Salz JJ, Lee T, Jester J, et al: Ophthalmology 1983;90:655-659.
*Values reported as mean difference compared with preoperative readings.
†Percent change as compared with eight incision results.
‡P value obtained by two-sample t-test.

bus was also abandoned because it increased the amount of blood in the wounds. There has been no study of interference with aqueous humor outflow or intraocular pressure from cutting across the limbus.

Based on mathematical modeling, Schachar[42] suggested that most of the effect of the incisions results from the portion in the paracentral cornea adjacent to the clear zone and that the peripheral part contributes less effect. His calculations predicted the following correlations between incision length and decrease in myopia: a 4.5-mm incision into limbus produced a 3.97 D decrease in myopia; a 3.5-mm incision produced a 3.83 D decrease in myopia; and a 2.5-mm incision produced a 3.64 D decrease in myopia. Salz[36] found that 4-mm incisions gave approximately twice the effect of 2.6-mm incisions (Table 13-10).

O'Donnell[32] used six rabbits, a 3-mm diameter clear zone, and eight incisions to compare 2.5-mm incisions in one eye with incisions extending to the limbus, length unspecified, in the second eye. One month after surgery, the short incisions had produced only half the effect of the long incisions, but 12 weeks after surgery the change in keratometric power was similar in the two groups—6.12 D in eyes with short incisions and 6.60 D in eyes with long incisions. The use of the rabbit model and the small number of eyes rendered the study inconclusive.

Clinical studies of incision length. An attempt in the early 1980s to standardize the length of the incision used an 11.0 mm diameter marker that was placed concentric to the clear zone mark. Some incisions were therefore confined completely to the cornea, whereas others extended into the limbus. No data have been published using this technique, which has been abandoned.

Patient age—clinical studies

The role of patient age as a prediction factor was not recognized until the early 1980s. Sato did not mention it. Fyodorov[12] did not include it in his original formula, but did include ocular rigidity as a major variable. Since it is known that ocular rigidity increases with age, there may be a correlation between these two factors. However, the measurement of ocular rigidity has never been shown to affect the outcome, as discussed below. Schachar concluded that age had no effect on outcome.[42] Clinical experience has demonstrated greater effect of the surgery in older patients.[2,26,31,35,40] The predictability analyses from the PERK, Sanders, and Arrowsmith studies all found the age of the patient important, moreso in the PERK study than in the other two studies (see Tables 13-1 to 13-4, 13-7, and 13-8).

In the PERK study there was a trend toward a greater change in refraction as age increased (correlation = 0.4). However, in each clear zone group there was considerable variation in the refractive change for a given age (Fig. 13-5). The average change in refraction increased in each successive 10-year age-group by approximately 0.60 D (Table 13-8). Other studies have documented the effect of

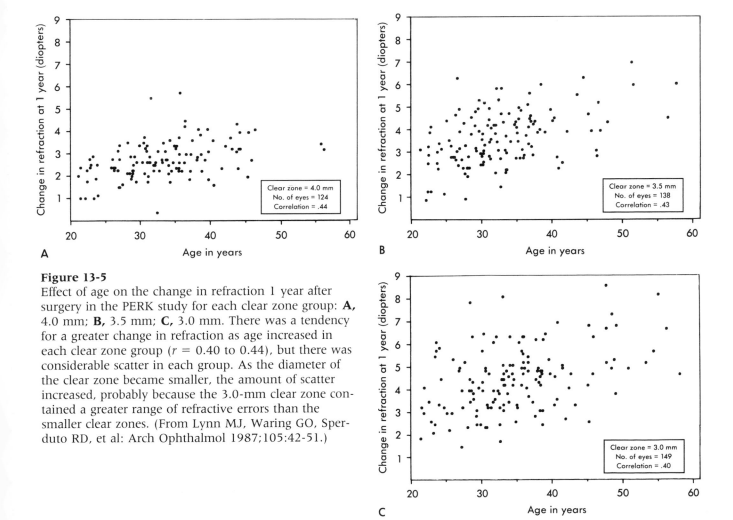

Figure 13-5

Effect of age on the change in refraction 1 year after surgery in the PERK study for each clear zone group: **A,** 4.0 mm; **B,** 3.5 mm; **C,** 3.0 mm. There was a tendency for a greater change in refraction as age increased in each clear zone group (r = 0.40 to 0.44), but there was considerable scatter in each group. As the diameter of the clear zone became smaller, the amount of scatter increased, probably because the 3.0-mm clear zone contained a greater range of refractive errors than the smaller clear zones. (From Lynn MJ, Waring GO, Sperduto RD, et al: Arch Ophthalmol 1987;105:42-51.)

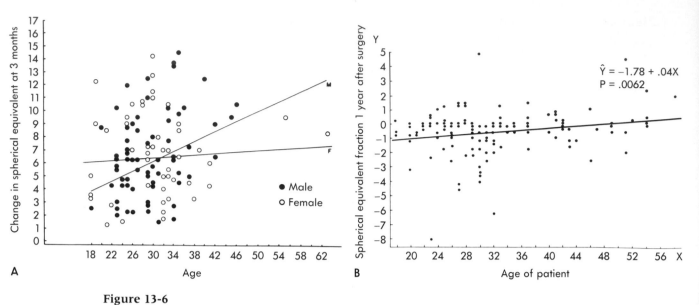

Figure 13-6

Effect of age on change in refraction. **A,** Effect of patient age and sex on change in refraction 3 months after surgery in the study of Arrowsmith and Marks. Although regression lines can be drawn through the data points, no clear relationship between age and change in refraction can be identified for the scatter. The lines show that younger women achieve a greater effect than do younger men, but that this is reversed as age increases. **B,** Scattergram compares age of patient and the spherical equivalent refraction 1 year after surgery in the series of Neumann, involving 147 eyes. (**A** from Arrowsmith PN and Marks RG: Ophthalmology 1985;92:331-338; **B** from Neumann AC, Osher RH, and Fenzl RE: Doc Ophthalmol 1984;56:275-301.)

Figure 13-7

Overall correlation between patient age and change in refraction (D) for three different clear zone groups *(OZ)* and two numbers of incisions (8,16) 3 months after surgery. Increasing age is associated with greater effect of the surgery in the 3.0 and 3.5 mm groups, but not the 4.0 mm group. (From Rowsey JJ, Balyeat HD, Rabinovitch B, et al: Ophthalmology 1983;90:642-654.)

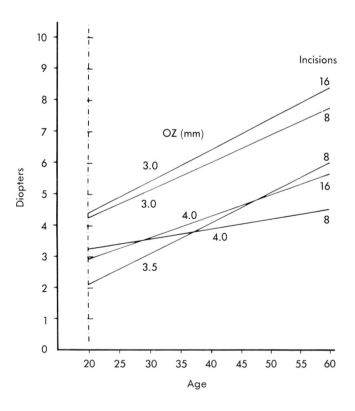

age (Figs. 13-6 and 13-7) and have also emphasized the great scatter of effect at a given age.

Three studies using regression analysis have identified a similar effect of age: PERK,[26] 0.60 D greater effect per decade; Sanders,[40] 0.40 D greater effect per decade; and Arrowsmith,[2] 0.48 D greater effect per decade with eight incisions.

Depth of incision in refractive keratotomy

Early observations. The depth of refractive keratotomy incisions, expressed as a percentage of corneal thickness, has been considered an important variable since the late 1890s, deeper incisions achieving more effect.[4,23] Sato[41] emphasized the need for exquisitely sharp knives to achieve deep incisions and observed that incisions through the posterior surface of the cornea seemed to have more effect than those through the anterior surface. Interestingly Fyodorov and Durnev[15] did not discuss the depth of the incision in their early descriptions.

Measurement of depth of incision. It is difficult to measure the depth of an incision scar accurately and therefore difficult to calculate accurately the effect of incision depth on the change in refraction. The incision depth is usually less than the length of the extended knife blade because of tissue displacement, variability in blade sharpness, variation in surgical technique, and possible variation in the sectility (cutability) of individual corneas. The depth of a single incision is not uniform from one end to another, and the depths of all the incisions in a single eye are not uniform. Therefore any overall calculation of depth of incision for a single case is the result of some type of averaging.

Measuring the depth of the incision scar is difficult. Intraoperative dipsticks are inaccurate because of corneal swelling and the displacement of posterior stroma. Visual inspection with a slit-lamp microscope is inaccurate because different observers will estimate different depths, particularly when trying to distinguish between 75% and 95%. Nevertheless, this is the most commonly used method and was used in the PERK study.[26] The PERK study design used a cross-sectional drawing of each incision scar with an estimate of the depth of the incision at three different locations, which were averaged. The PERK study estimated incision depth in quartiles—0% to 24%, 25% to 50%, 51% to 75%, and 76% to 100%. Although this avoids the misleading accuracy that is sometimes seen in the literature where estimates of "92% or 95%" are given, it fails to distinguish moderately deep incisions (90%) from extremely deep incisions (perforation).

The most accurate reported method of measuring the depth of the incision scar is that of Deitz[9] who used an optical pachometer to measure the full thickness of the cornea over the scar and then the depth of the scar itself, a time-consuming procedure made difficult by the patient's microsaccades.

Optical coherence domain reflectometry has been used to measure the depth of freshly made incisions. This method uses a diode laser light source to achieve high spatial resolution. A spatial resolution of 10 μm can be achieved.[18] The depth of the incision is measured by the time delay of optical signals reflected from the base of the incision using a correlation technique.

Laboratory studies of incision depth. Because of the difficulty of measuring incision depth in living animals, histologic studies provided early documentation that deeper incisions produced a greater effect. The depth of the incision scar can be measured in histologic cross sections of the cornea, assuming the cross sections are made perpendicular to the plane of the scar.

The acute eyebank eye model study of Jester and colleagues,[20] using a metal blade and regression analysis, demonstrated that the depth of the incision was the most important predictor of change in corneal curvature after refractive

Table 13-11

Acute Effect of Peripheral Deepening Incisions Compared with Values after Eight Initial Incisions in the Eyebank Eye Study by Salz and Colleagues

Clear zone (mm)	Terry keratometry*
3	0.06 ($\pm$1.16)
4	0.27 ($\pm$0.39)
5	0.35 ($\pm$1.12)
6	0.19 ($\pm$0.90)

From Salz JJ, Rowsey JJ, Caroline P, et al: Arch Ophthalmol 1985;103:590-594.
*Values reported as diopters (spherical equivalents) ($\pm$ standard deviations).

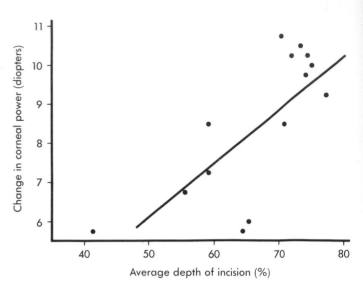

Figure 13-8
Relationship between the depth of incision and change in corneal power in an eye bank eye model. Deeper incisions are associated with the greater change in corneal curvature ($r = 0.76$, $p < .01$). (From Jester JV, Venet T, Lee J, et al: Am J Ophthalmol 1981;92:172-177.)

keratotomy, explaining 56% of the variability of the outcome (Fig. 13-8). In another study by the same group using similar methodology,[36] histologic examination showed great variability in the depth of the incisions, ranging from 38.2% to 84.4% of corneal thickness. However, the depths of the incisions were reasonably uniform from one end to the other: paracentral incisions were 64.8% $\pm$ 2.8% of corneal thickness; middle incisions were 66% $\pm$ 2.7% of corneal thickness; and peripheral incisions were 69% $\pm$ 3.0% of corneal thickness. A report by Ingraham et al.[19] of the depth of radial incisions on a human eye obtained at autopsy used serial histologic sections to demonstrate the reasonable uniformity of depth along and among incisions, although the ends of incisions were shallower than the middle of most.

Salz and colleagues[36] compared the depth of incision achieved with a Feather razor blade and a KOI diamond blade set to 100% of the thinnest of four paracentral ultrasonic pachometry readings in the human eyebank eye model. They found no statistical difference between the depth of the incisions of the two types of blades. The metal blade achieved an average depth of 87% $\pm$ 7% of corneal thickness (range 66% to 97%), and the diamond blade achieved an average depth of 84% $\pm$ 4% of corneal thickness (range 61% to 98%). Of course these results cannot be generalized to other metal or diamond blades.

The role of peripheral deepening incisions is not completely clear. The study by Salz and colleagues[36] of peripheral deepening incisions in the acute eyebank eye model demonstrated no significant increase in the amount of corneal flattening from these incisions (Table 13-11).

Computer and biomechanical models of incision depth. The change in refraction is not directly proportionate to the depth of the incision; that is, incisions of less than 50% of corneal thickness depth produce little effect, whereas incisions of 80% to 90% of corneal thickness produce proportionately much greater effect. It is difficult to make these measurements clinically, but this nonlinear relation-

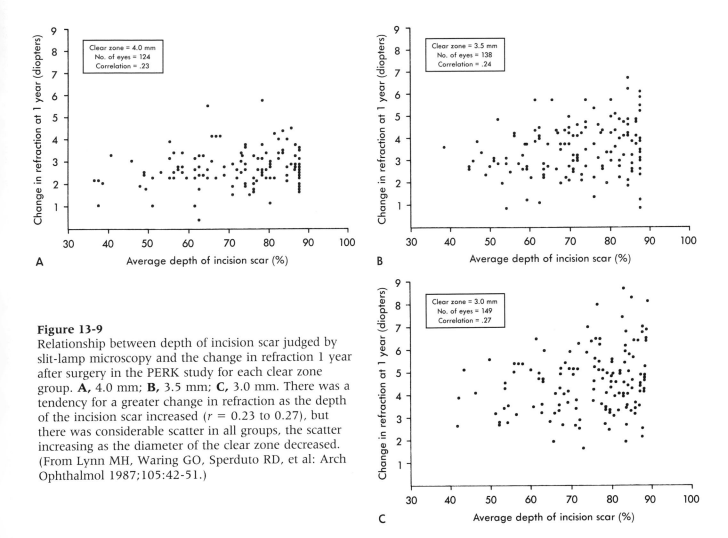

Figure 13-9

Relationship between depth of incision scar judged by slit-lamp microscopy and the change in refraction 1 year after surgery in the PERK study for each clear zone group. **A,** 4.0 mm; **B,** 3.5 mm; **C,** 3.0 mm. There was a tendency for a greater change in refraction as the depth of the incision scar increased ($r = 0.23$ to 0.27), but there was considerable scatter in all groups, the scatter increasing as the diameter of the clear zone decreased. (From Lynn MH, Waring GO, Sperduto RD, et al: Arch Ophthalmol 1987;105:42-51.)

ship can be seen in computer models of acute change after radial incisions (see Chapter 28, A Finite Element Model of Radial Keratotomy Surgery, and Chapter 29, Preliminary Computer Simulation of Radial Keratotomy) where the variables can be isolated in a quantitative way. Excimer lasers hold the promise of making these distinctions more accurately because the depth of a linear laser excision can be calculated with reasonable accuracy by measuring the number of pulses and the pulse energy, which indicate the amount of tissue removed (see Chapter 19, Laser Corneal Surgery). Using a combination of cuts and clinical experience with laser transverse cuts in humans and biomechanical computer modeling, Seiler has demonstrated that the amount of change in refraction increases markedly after the incision depth reaches 80% of corneal thickness (see Chapter 33, Biomechanics of Transverse Incisions of the Cornea).

Clinical studies of incision depth. Most clinicians attempt to achieve a uniformly deep incision on the order of 80% to 90% of corneal thickness in all cases and to adjust the outcome by changing the diameter of the clear zone or the number of incisions. In all three clinical regression analysis studies[2,26,40] the depth of the incision scar was an important variable affecting the outcome (see Table 13-1).

In the PERK study there was a relationship between the depth of the incision scar and the change in refraction (Fig. 13-9). In general, eyes with deeper inci-

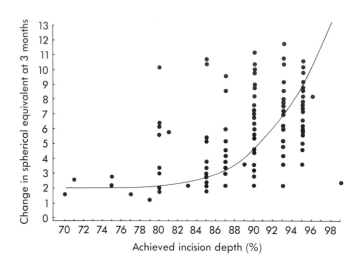

Figure 13-10
Relationship between achieved incision depth as judged by slit-lamp microscopy and the change in refraction at 3 months in the Arrowsmith study. The scattergram shows a tendency for greater change in refraction with deeper incisions, but there is considerable scatter. Scars less than 80% deep have minimal effect, and scars from 80% to 96% deep cover the range from 1.5 to 11 D of change. (From Arrowsmith PN and Marks RG: Ophthalmology 1985;92:331-338.)

sions demonstrated greater flattening of the central cornea (correlation = 0.24). However, even among patients in whom the average depth of incision was near the maximum value (76% to 100%), there was a wide range in the refractive change, as seen in the scattergrams. A similar scatter is seen in Arrowsmith's study (Fig. 13-10).

The regression analyses of Arrowsmith[40] contain a number of terms related to the depth of the incision: incision depth, number of tertiary incisions, primary incision perforation, incision depth × optical zone size, and number of perforations in secondary incisions. Thus the role of the incision depth is emphasized in various ways (see Table 13-4). The authors point out that the role of incision depth takes a quadratic term in the regression equation, indicating that the effect of surgery grows almost exponentially when the incision depth exceeds 90% of corneal thickness. This may be another reason that the corneal perforation terms come into their equation. This prompted their recommendation that the goal of the incision depth be 80% to 90% of corneal thickness, because the very deep incisions and the perforated incisions had a greater and more uncontrolled effect on the outcome, increasing the number of overcorrections.

Deitz and colleagues, using optical pachometry, reported an average incision depth made with a double-edged diamond knife for 611 eyes of 89.3% ± 4.9% of corneal thickness (range 69% to 98%),[10] but did not specifically analyze the effect of incision depth. In the clinical study of Sanders and Deitz[40] second-pass incisions were made in an unspecified manner and were apparently not studied in the regression analysis. The PERK study made no deepening incisions and could not study this aspect.

Leroux Les Jardins and colleagues[24] compared the results in two series of eyes undergoing operation during the same time frame by the same surgeon with the same instruments, all with 3-mm diameter clear zones and eight centrifugal radial incisions. Thirty-two eyes had the incisions made with a single pass at a single depth. Twenty-four eyes had deepening incisions made from 6 mm to the limbus. For eyes with a single pass incision, the average change in manifest spherical equivalent refraction was 3.62 D (range, 1.75 to 6.50 D). For the eyes receiving deepening incisions, the average change in refraction was 4.25 D (range, 2.50 to 6.75 D). The authors concluded that deepening incisions increased the effect of the surgery.

As discussed in Chapter 17, Atlas of Surgical Techniques of Radial Keratotomy, centripetal incisions made from the limbus to the clear zone using the vertical edge of the knife blade generally make deeper, more uniform incisions than

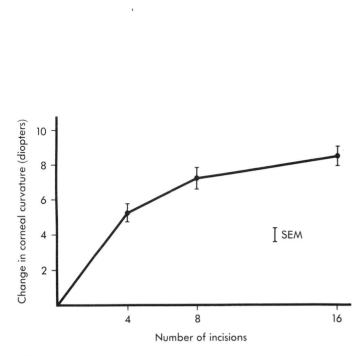

Figure 13-11
Relationship of incisions and change in corneal curvature in human eye bank eye model indicates that 4 incisions achieve 7.25 D of change (85%), and 16 incisions achieve 8.50 D of change (100%). The range of effect is wide for each group, however: 1.50 = 8.75 D; 8 = 3.50 to 10.25 D; 16 = 5.75 to 10.75 D. (From Jester JV, Venet T, Lee J, et al: Am J Ophthalmol 1981;92:172-177.)

Figure 13-12
Effect of 8 and 16 radial incisions in owl monkey eyes followed over 12 weeks. There is no significant difference between 8 or 16 incisions. Much of the initial effect is lost by 6 weeks, indicating that the monkey may be a poor model for radial keratotomy. (From Steel D, Jester JV, Salz JJ, et al: Ophthalmology 1981;88:747-754.)

those made centrifugally from the clear zone to the limbus with an angled knife blade. Thus if all other variables are equal, a greater change in refraction should be achieved from centripetal incisions because of deeper, more uniform incisions.

The overall conclusions are quite clear: deeper incisions, no matter how they are achieved, produce a greater change in refraction, and the portion of the incision from approximately 70% to 99% creates the greatest part of this change.

Number of incisions

The number of incisions used for the correction of both myopia and astigmatism has steadily declined during the past 45 years. Sato made approximately 80 incisions (40 anterior and 40 posterior); Yenaliev made 32 incisions but decreased the number of incisions to 16 and then 12; Fyodorov began with 32 incisions, found that 16 incisions produced an equal effect, and then recommended 8. Keratotomy surgeons generally used 16 incisions in the late 1970s and early 1980s but switched to 8 incisions and in the late 1980s have preferred 4 for lower myopia. These declining numbers reflect the fact that most of the corneal flattening occurs with the first few incisions and that the contribution of additional incisions declines as their number increases.

Laboratory study of number of incisions. In the eyebank eye model Jester and colleagues[20] demonstrated that 4 incisions produced 62% of the change in corneal curvature, 8 incisions produced 85% of the change, and 16 incisions produced 100% of the change in corneal curvature (Fig. 13-11). Additional studies confirmed these findings: 4 incisions produced 70% to 85% of the effect

Table 13-12

Effect of Number of Incisions on Change in Refraction at 6 Months after Radial Keratotomy in the Series of Rowsey and Colleagues

| Diameter of clear zone (mm) | Number of incisions | | | |
| | 8 | | 16 | |
	Change in refraction*	Number of eyes	Change in refraction*	Number of eyes
3.0	5.20 ± 2.28	69	5.47 ± 1.84	36
3.5	3.78 ± 1.15	15	Not reported	
4.0	3.05 ± 1.06	9	3.34 ± 1.06	11

From Rowsey JJ, Balyeat HD, Rabinovitch B, et al: Ophthalmology 1983;90:642-654.
*Spherical equivalent in diopters, mean ± standard deviation.

of 8 incisions (see Tables 13-7 and 13-10).[36,38] Steel and colleagues[46] found no difference in the effect of 8 and 16 incisions in two separate groups of monkey experiments (Fig. 13-12).

Clinical studies of number of incisions. All clinical series have confirmed the findings of the eyebank eye model. One of the difficulties with clinical studies of the effect of the number of incisions is that patients who have many incisions generally have smaller clear zones. Patients with 4 incisions are more likely to have a larger clear zone than patients with 8 or 16 incisions. Thus it is difficult to isolate the effect of the number of incisions because any group of eyes with 8 incisions will have an average clear zone diameter larger than a group of eyes with 16 incisions. One exception to this is the report of Rowsey and colleagues[35] who found no difference in the change produced by 8 or 16 incisions in eyes that had the same diameter clear zone and the same depth of blade (Table 13-12).

Three, six, and 12 incisions have also been used for radial keratotomy, but there is little published information about such cases. The general principle of a greater amount of effect with the earlier incisions would hold for these eyes as well.

The analysis reported by Sanders[40] indicated an approximately 1.50 D greater change in spherical equivalent refraction with 16 incisions than with 8 (Fig. 13-13). The analyses of Arrowsmith and Marks[1,2] found that the number of inci-

Figure 13-13
The effect of patient and surgical variables on the change in spherical equivalent refraction as predicted by regression equations derived from two different series of patients in the Deitz and Sanders study. Mean or median values for the other factors known to affect spherical equivalent in the regression equations were used when each variable was examined individually. All graphs have the same Y scale so that the steepness of the curves reflects the relative effect of each variable on refractive outcome within the physiologic range. The following variables were found to affect outcome. **A,** Optical zone size. Nonlinear representation is due to the use of the area rather than diameter of the central zone in the equation. **B,** Mean incision depth. **C,** Patient age and sex. **D,** Number of incisions. **E,** Preoperative intraocular pressure. **F,** Preoperative average keratometry. (From Sanders DR, Deitz MR, and Gallagher D: Ophthalmology 1985;92:1237-1243.)

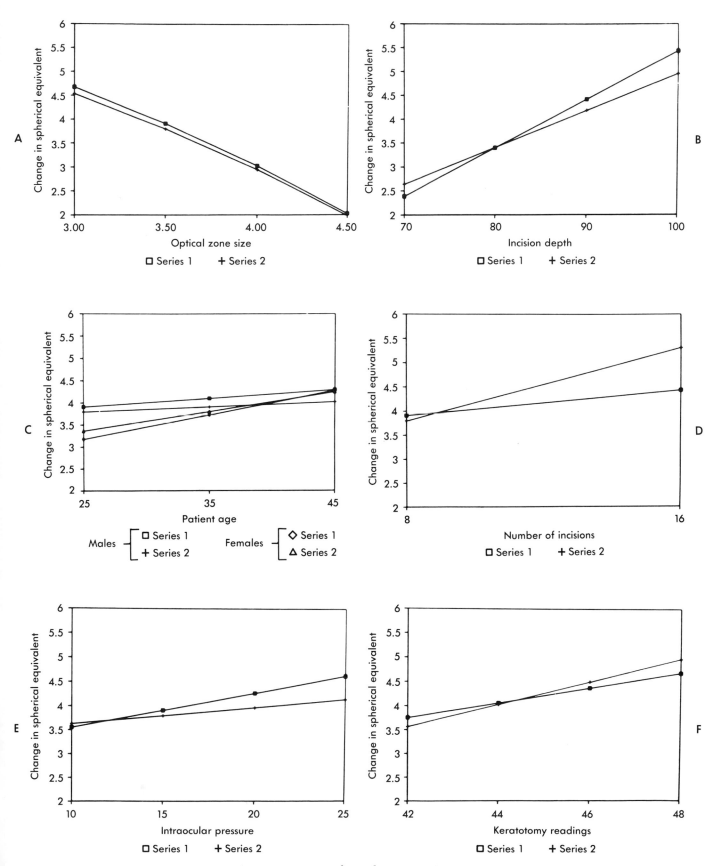

Figure 13-13 For legend see opposite page.

Table 13-13

Comparison of Results of Four and Eight Radial Incisions in Five Different Studies

Amount of preoperative myopia (D)	Outcome variable	Eight incisions: Deitz[21]	Eight incisions: Deitz[42]	Eight incisions: PERK[2]	Four incisions: Salz[38]	Four incisions: University of Minnesota[37]
Low: −2.00 to −3.12	Percent of eyes 20/40 or better uncorrected	97%	95%	92%	86%	93%
	Within 1.00 D of emmetropia	71%	95%	84%	90%	90%
	Overcorrected >1.00 D	29%	0%	11%	4%	9%
Moderate: −3.25 to −4.37	Percent of eyes 20/40 or better uncorrected	87%	90%	81%	68%	0%
	Within 1.00 D of emmetropia	67%	86%	62%	75%	92%
	Overcorrected >1.00 D	24%	7%	7%	0%	0%

From Spigelman AV, Williams PA, Nichols BD, et al: J Cataract Refract Surg 1988;14:125-128.

Table 13-14

Estimated Effect of Four-Incision Radial Keratotomy as a Percent of Eight Incisions in a 30-Year-Old Patient

Number of incisions	Clear zone diameter (mm)	Refractive change as compared to eight incisions(%)*
8	3.0	100
4	3.0	70
4	3.5	50
4	4.0	40
4	4.5	30
4	5.0	20

From Spiegelman AV, Williams PA, Nichols BD, et al: J Cataract Refract Surg 1988;14:125-128.
*Based on cadaver eye studies.

sions affected the outcome in the steel knife cases but not in the diamond knife cases. They stated that the number of incisions was selected by the computer first but was removed after step 7 in the computer program, indicating that the inclusion of other variables replaced the contribution of the number of incisions.

In the PERK study[26] the effect of the number of incisions could not be studied because all eyes had eight incisions. Spigelman and colleagues[45] compared retrospectively five different studies and found equal or better results with four incisions compared with eight (Table 13-13). The authors acknowledge that the eyes with four incisions were operated on more recently and with different techniques, so direct comparison was difficult. Table 13-14 presents the author's estimated comparison of the effect of four incisions as compared with eight incisions based on cadaver eye studies. Surgery with four incisions has been established as clinically useful (see Chapter 21, Published Results of Refractive Keratotomy).

Intraocular pressure

Intraocular pressure causes the cornea to change shape after keratotomy; one would therefore expect the level of intraocular pressure to play a meaningful role in determining the outcome. However, laboratory and clinical data all indicate that intraocular pressure within the physiologic range does not play an identifiable role. This is not true for extremely low or high pressures where a higher pressure increases the amount of central corneal flattening.

Laboratory studies of intraocular pressure. Maloney and colleagues[28] found in the human cadaver eye model that most of the change in refraction was produced at pressures less than 10 mm Hg: 0.5 mm Hg produced 20% of maximum effect; 2 mm Hg produced 77% of the maximum effect; and 10 mm Hg produced 97% of the maximum effect. In the physiologic range of pressure between 10 and 20 mm Hg, little change occurred in the shape of the cornea (Fig. 13-14).

Similarly the study of the effect of intraocular pressure on corneal curvature after radial keratomy in monkey eyes by Busin and colleagues[6] demonstrated that changes in pressure from 10 to 20 mm Hg do not significantly decrease the corneal curvature between 1 week and 6 months after surgery. However, elevated intraocular pressure did flatten the cornea further: 40 mm Hg decreased the keratometric power an average of 0.30 to 0.80 D, and 60 to 80 mm Hg flattened the cornea 0.60 to 1.65 D (Table 13-15).

Similar findings were observed in rabbit experiments.[8] Increases in intraocular pressure between 10 and 20 mm Hg 1 week to 4 months after radial keratotomy produced a decrease of approximately 0.50 D (range 0.00 to 0.75 D) in keratometric power. However, elevations of intraocular pressure from 20 to 80 mm Hg produced an average decrease of central keratometric power by approximately 1.00 to 1.75 D.

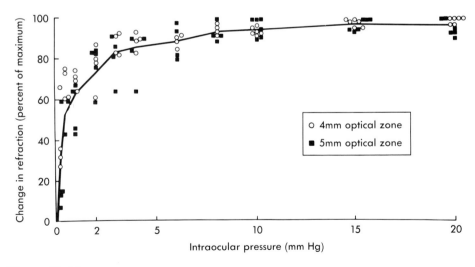

Figure 13-14
The effect of intraocular pressure on the percentage of refractive change after radial keratotomy in human eye bank eyes. The refractive change induced by radial keratotomy increases with increasing intraocular pressure from 0 to 10 mm Hg. However, in the physiologic range from 10 to 20 mm Hg, there is minimal variation in refractive effect as measured by keratometric power. Line represents best fit for scattergram of the data. Two optical zone sizes were used, 4 mm and 5 mm diameter. (From Maloney RK: Ophthalmology 1990;97:927-933.)

Table 13-15

Reduction in Central Corneal Keratometric Power (Mean Reduction in Diopters ± SD) Induced by Increasing Intraocular Pressure at Different Times after Surgery in the Monkey Eye Study of Busin and Colleagues

Time after radial keratotomy	Intraocular pressure interval (mm Hg)			
	10 to 20	10 to 40	10 to 50	10 to 80
1 week	0.23± 0.25	0.55±0.34*	1.05±0.37*	1.62 ± 0.48*
3 months	0.25± 0.32	0.83± 0.55	1.29± 0.42	1.65 ± 0.46*
6 months	0.15±0.21*	0.30±0.54*	0.60±0.39*	0.97 ± 0.30*
Control	0.00	0.00	0.00	0.00

From Busin M, Arffa RC, McDonald MB, et al: CLAO J 1988;14:110-112.

*Five values are averaged, compared with six values in the other groups. Keratometric readings were unobtainable in one eye of each of these groups for technical reasons.

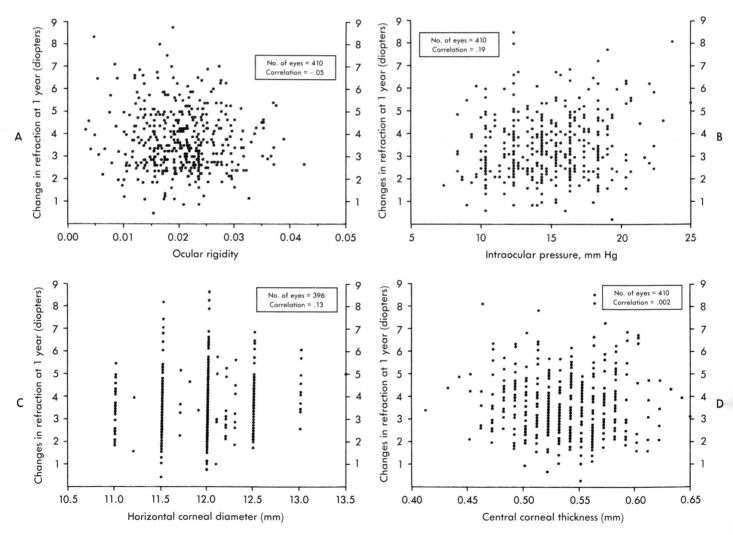

Figure 13-15
Scattergrams demonstrate the effect of ocular rigidity **(A)**, intraocular pressure **(B)**, horizontal corneal diameter **(C)**, and central corneal thickness **(D)** on the change in refraction 1 year after surgery in the PERK study. Number of eyes and correlation coefficients are presented in the boxes. None of these factors had a statistically significant or clinically meaningful effect on the change in refraction. (From Lynn MJ, Waring GO, Sperduto RD, et al: Arch Ophthalmol 1987;105:42-51.)

These experiments indicate that a preoperative intraocular pressure within the normal range has minimal effect on the change in corneal curvature after radial keratotomy and that even the effect of elevated intraocular pressure becomes less as the time after surgery increases. However, elevations in intraocular pressure after radial keratotomy can decrease central corneal curvature.

Clinical studies of the effect of normal intraocular pressure. None of the three series of regression analysis identified intraocular pressure as an important variable in outcome of refractive keratotomy (see Figs. 13-13 and 13-15 and Tables 13-1 to 13-4 and 13-9). Other individual studies have found little or no relationship, including those of Neumann and colleagues.[31] Thus there is no basis for using normal preoperative intraocular pressure as a factor in computing the surgical plan for refractive keratotomy.

Effect of elevated intraocular pressure on refraction after refractive keratotomy. Feldman and colleagues[11] demonstrated that increased intraocular pressure outside the normal range flattened the cornea after refractive keratotomy. They used an ingenious experimental setup in humans, studying the change in intraocular pressure and keratometry readings while the subject was seated and then while the subject was hanging by his feet head down using gravity inversion boots. In patients with normal eyes and no radial keratotomy, the intraocular pressure rose from approximately 14 mm Hg to approximately 25 mm Hg on inversion, but the average keratometric power did not change, remaining stable at 44 D. In the patients who had had radial keratotomy, the pressure rose a similar amount, from 13 mm Hg to 26 mm Hg, and the keratometric power decreased, from 44.3 D to 41.6 D (*SD* = 1.8 D). The decrease in keratometric power was statistically significant. After patients returned to the upright position, the intraocular pressure returned to baseline levels within 1 minute, but it was 5 to 45 minutes before the corneal curvature returned to its preinversion levels.

Numerous other reports have documented that elevations in intraocular pressure after radial keratotomy further flatten the central cornea. Sanders[39] described a nurse who had radial keratotomy, was a steroid responder, and used topical steroids to raise her intraocular pressure, thus improving the effect of her surgery (Fig. 13-16). Busin and colleagues[7] have described elevated intraocular pressure producing an increased effect after radial keratotomy (see the box on p. 368).

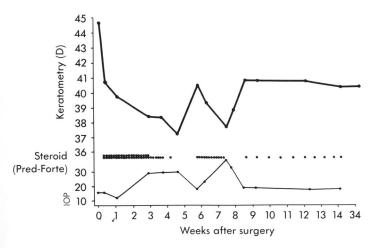

Figure 13-16
Individual case demonstrates the relationship between corneal curvature and increased intraocular pressure induced by topical corticosteroids. Elevations in intraocular pressure (IOP) are associated with a decrease in corneal power. (From Sanders DR and Deitz MR. In Sanders DR, Hofmann RF, and Salz J, editors: Refractive corneal surgery, Thorofare, NJ, 1986, Slack, Inc, pp 79-90.)

Elevated Intraocular Pressure Flattens the Cornea after Radial Keratotomy

A 45-year-old woman had a cycloplegic refraction of −2.50 + 0.50 × 30, keratometric readings of 43.87/45.75 × 90, and an intraocular pressure of 8 mm Hg. She entered the PERK study and received radial keratotomy with eight incisions and a 4-mm diameter clear zone with the diamond-knife blade extended to 100% of the thinnest paracentral pachometry reading. One year after surgery, her refraction was +1.50 + 1.25 × 105, with keratometry readings of 39.75/39.50 × 90 and an intraocular pressure of 11 mm Hg.

Two years after surgery, she noticed sudden worsening of visual acuity. Her cycloplegic refraction was +5.00 D +1.75 × 45 with keratometric readings of 38.25/38.62 × 99 and an intraocular pressure of 26 mm Hg. Timolol maleate 0.5% was administered twice daily, lowering the intraocular pressure to 10 mm Hg and decreasing the hyperopia to +1.25 +1.00 × 135.

Three months later, the patient stopped taking the timolol, and the pressure rose to 20 mm Hg, with a concomitant increase in her hyperopia to +4.00 +2.00 × 40 and steepening of her keratometry readings. This case clearly documents the relationship between elevated intraocular pressure and flattening of the central cornea after radial keratotomy.

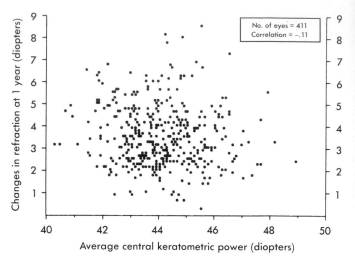

Figure 13-17
Relationship between average central keratometric power and change in the refraction 1 year after surgery in the PERK study shows no significant correlation. (From Lynn MJ, Waring GO, Sperduto RD, et al: Arch Ophthalmol 1987;105;42-51.)

Central corneal curvature

No subject is more confused in the area of predictability of radial keratotomy than the role of corneal curvature. Fyodorov thought that steeper corneas achieved more effect from surgery and included the radius of corneal curvature in his initial formula. Early in the development of radial keratotomy in the United States, bulletins were circulated to warn against surgery on patients with flatter corneas, based on the theory that a steeper cornea had further to flatten than a flatter cornea. Subsequently the published data have led to many different conclusions.

Laboratory studies of corneal curvature. Salz and colleagues,[37] working with a human eyebank model, initially observed that preoperative keratotomy readings were not helpful in predicting the final result, but in a subsequent study, using regression analysis in a separate series of eyes, preoperative corneal curvature was thought to play a role (r = 0.36), steeper corneas getting more effect.

Clinical studies of corneal curvature. The analysis of Arrowsmith[2] 2 years after surgery showed a negative correlation between corneal curvature and long-term effect of radial keratotomy (see Table 13-4). Corneas steeper preoperatively were predicted to have a lesser long-term effect than flatter corneas. For an eye with average preoperative keratotometry of 45.00 D, 1.00 D less effect will be achieved than for an eye with average preoperative keratotomy of 42.00 D. They found a similar effect in the 2-year analysis of the steel knife series. This result contradicts the earlier theory and their own findings at 1 year. It is possible that steeper corneas could obtain more results in the early months after surgery but then regress more over a longer period.

On the other hand, Sanders,[40] analyzing results at 6 months after surgery, found a positive correlation of preoperative average central keratometry and change in refraction, producing approximately 1 diopter increase in refractive change over the keratometric range from 42 to 46 diopters (see Table 13-2 and Fig. 13-13).

The PERK study[26] (see Tables 13-1 and 13-9 and Fig. 13-17), and the study of Neumann, Osher, and Fenzl[31] found no relationship between preoperative keratometric measurements and the change in refraction. Grady[16] concluded that corneas with steeper preoperative keratometry readings had greater postoperative flattening; however, when Rowsey[35] reexamined Grady's data, he found no relationship between the preoperative keratometric power and the change in refractive power.

Thus, with some studies suggesting more keratotomy surgery for patients with steeper corneas and others suggesting less, and with the general opinion that keratometric readings play at best a minor role in predicting the outcome, this variable currently has little value in creating a surgical plan.

Corneal topography

One possible reason for the confusion over using keratometric measurements as a predictive factor is that keratometry samples only the radius of curvature at two points approximately 3 mm apart, assuming that the cornea is a sphere (see Chapter 3, Optics and Topography of Radial Keratotomy). It is likely that the measurement of the entire shape of the cornea by videokeratography might identify patterns of corneal curvature that could correlate with change in refraction. At the time of this writing, little is published on this matter because it is so difficult to quantify the entire corneal surface from keratographs and because the effect of corneal shape on the change in refraction is probably small. Nevertheless, some authors think it is significant.

For example, Rowsey and colleagues[33] in the PERK study used a nine ring photokeratoscope to quantify central and paracentral corneal topography. They estimated corneal shape by comparing the radii of curvature around the second ring and the seventh ring. They found that eyes with a 3-mm diameter clear zone (and therefore longer incisions) showed an influence of corneal topography. The overall effect of this in the one clear zone group was approximately 7%, making topography a minor predictive variable.

Both Lipshitz and Ellis[25] have used topogometry with a Javal keratometer to measure radii of curvature in the central, paracentral, and peripheral cornea. Measurements are taken 2 mm and 4 mm from the center with the patient looking 10 degrees and 20 degrees off center following a fixation light. They think the corneal topography can act as a predictive factor in refractive keratotomy. The important factor they identified is the change in curvature from the center to the periphery, such that corneas with greater asphericity have more effect from refractive keratotomy. For example, two corneas that both have central average keratometric readings of 43 D might have different topographies, such that one might flatten from 43 to 39 D, whereas the other would flatten from 43 to 41 D. The first cornea, with the greater asphericity and the greater change from central to periphery, would change more.

Patient sex

Gender was not found to affect the change in refraction in the regression analyses in the PERK study,[26] or in the studies of Sanders[40] and Arrowsmith[2] (see Tables 13-1, 13-3, 13-4, and 13-9).

In the PERK study the 3.0-mm clear zone group showed an average change in refraction of 0.50 D greater for male than female patients ($p = .02$). Comparison of male and female subjects in the successive 10-year age-groups demonstrated a difference only in the patients older than 40 years of age in 3.5-mm and 3.0-mm clear zone groups. In these groups, on the average, older male pa-

Table 13-16

Change in the Spherical Equivalent of the Cycloplegic Refraction (D) 1 Year after Radial Keratotomy for Males and Females in the PERK Study

	Diameter of central clear zone										
	4.0 mm				3.5 mm				3.0 mm		
Sex	No. of eyes	Mean	Standard deviation	Difference	No. of eyes	Mean	Standard deviation	Difference	No. of eyes	Mean	Standard deviation	Difference
Male	56	2.70	0.83		74	3.56	1.25		85	4.72	1.43	
				0.05				0.32				0.54
Female	68	2.75	0.86		64	3.24	1.03		64	4.18	1.30	

From Lynn MJ, Waring GO, Sperduto RD, et al: Arch Ophthalmol 1987;105:42-51.

tients had a change in refraction approximately 1.50 D greater than did females. In the 3.5-mm clear zone group males had a 4.79 D change in refraction and females had a 3.45 D change in refraction; in the 3.0-mm clear zone group males had a 5.82 D change in refraction and females had a 4.63 D change in refraction (Table 13-16). This overall pattern differs from the findings of Sanders and associates,[40] who found that younger male patients experienced a greater effect than younger female patients and that the difference between male and female subjects disappeared in older patients (see Fig. 13-13).

Clearly, sex is not a major predictor of the outcome of refractive keratotomy.

Corneal thickness and corneal hydration

Corneal thickness. Central corneal thickness has no measurable effect on the outcome of refractive keratotomy based on regression analysis. Of course, corneal thickness is partially compensated for by setting the length of the knife blade as a percentage of the corneal thickness itself. This still would leave different thicknesses of uncut tissue based on the original corneal thickness if every cornea were cut to 90% depth. Theoretically, these different remaining thicknesses might have different effects on the biomechanical properties of the eye. In fact, biomechanical models tend to demonstrate an effect of corneal thickness for this reason: a knife blade set at a fixed percentage of corneal thickness will leave more uncut tissue behind in the thicker cornea than in a thinner cornea, thus changing the biomechanical calculations and demonstrating that thicker corneas achieve less effect than thinner corneas. Nevertheless, no clinical studies have been able to identify corneal thickness as a significant predictive variable. Theoretically, one might wish to leave behind a fixed amount of tissue, for example 50 μm, across the entire depth of an incision for every cornea, but this is not now possible clinically.

Corneal hydration. Measurements of corneal thickness are proportionate to the swelling of the cornea, that is, to corneal hydration. Thus thickness measurements can be used to estimate the percentage of water in the stroma. In the normal cornea there are small variations in thickness that presumably result from hydration. The cornea is thickest in the morning on awakening (presumably because tears do not evaporate as much at night) and therefore is more hypotonic than normal, since osmotically less water is drawn out of the cornea. For example, it is a common finding in Fuch's endothelial corneal dystrophy that corneas are thicker and the vision hazier during the first few hours after awakening, and then this clears gradually.

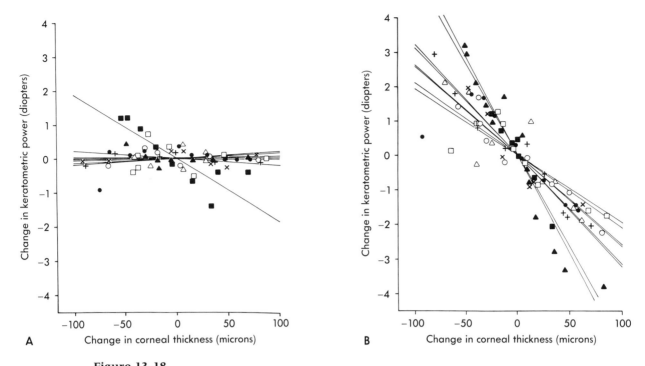

Figure 13-18
Effect of change in corneal thickness on change in keratometric power in normal
cadaver eyes and in cadaver eyes after radial keratotomy. Each line on the graphs
represents one cadaver eye. Changes in corneal thickness and keratometric power
are referenced to their mean values. **A,** In normal eyes there is no significant
change in keratometric power as corneal thickness changes in seven of eight eyes.
B, After radial keratotomy changes in corneal thickness induce marked changes in
keratometric power (average 0.33 D per 10 micron change in corneal thickness).
This evidence suggests that diurnal fluctuations in refractive power are due to diurnal fluctuations corneal hydration. (From Maloney RK: Ophthalmology
1990;97:927-933.)

Maloney[27] demonstrated that changes in corneal thickness in normal eye
bank eyes produce little change in keratometric power (Fig. 13-18, *A*); however,
acutely after radial keratotomy a change in corneal thickness produces a marked
change in keratometric power, thicker corneas inducing a flattening of the cornea and thinner corneas producing a steepening of the cornea (Fig. 13-18, *B*).
Although this is only an acute model, it demonstrates that the cornea after radial
keratotomy is more sensitive to changes in hydration. Although this does not
form a basis for preoperative calculations and predicting the outcome of surgery,
it does form a partial explanation for diurnal fluctuations in refraction, the cornea being thicker and flatter on arising. It also forms some explanation for the
gradual loss of effect in the first few days to weeks after surgery, when the post-
surgical edema is disappearing (See Chapter 3, Optics and Topography of Radial
Keratotomy, and Chapter 24, Stability of Refraction after Refractive Keratotomy).

For example, as Maloney points out, if 4% is taken as a conservative estimate
of the diurnal fluctuation and corneal thickness after radial keratotomy, then the
average morning-to-evening change in corneal thickness would be 4% of 500
mm, which is the normal corneal thickness, or approximately 20 μm of thinning. In his cadaver eye model, the 20 μm decrease in corneal thickness resulted
in approximately 0.66 D increase in corneal power with an increase in myopia.
This correlates roughly with the clinically measured morning-to-evening change
in refraction.

Ocular rigidity

Ocular rigidity was not found to correlate with the outcome in the PERK studies[1,2,26,39] (see Tables 13-1, 13-2, 13-4, and 13-9 and Fig. 13-15). Fyodorov[12] included ocular rigidity in his original formula, so eyes with greater rigidity had more effect from radial keratotomy; Bores and colleagues[5] found this factor "important in the outcome" in a clinical series. Most subsequent studies have supported these conclusions.

It is possible that changes in ocular rigidity underlie the well-documented effect of age on radial keratotomy. The cornea and sclera become stiffer with age, and incising a stiffer structure might be expected to give a greater change than incising a more flexible structure.

Corneal diameter

No studies have documented correlation between corneal diameter and the outcome of refractive keratotomy, despite the early postulates of Fyodorov.[12] It might be logical to expect corneas with a greater diameter to exhibit a greater change after refractive keratotomy because the incisions would be longer, given the fixed diameter of the central clear zone. Possibly, diameter does not play a predictive role because the peripheral portions of the incisions may have a minimal effect on the final outcome, so variations of approximately 0.25 mm do not create a clinically meaningful result.

Intraoperative keratoscopy and keratometry

Theoretically, it might be possible to monitor the changes in corneal curvature and power during surgery, either using currently available operating keratometers and keratoscopes or futuristically using real time corneal topography. Since it is reasonable to assume different corneas with the same curvature might have different stresses within them, graded keratotomies and measurements of change during surgery might allow the surgeon to judge directly the appropriate amount of surgery for each cornea. Thus a standard conservative operation could be done with a larger clear zone and fewer and shallower incisions, and then these variables could be increased according to the surgeon's preference or published nomograms until the desired outcome was reached on the table.

Unfortunately, this approach probably will not work using current methodologies because of the swelling induced in the corneal incisions shortly after they are made (swelling that is aggravated by flooding the surface of the cornea with fluid to get good keratoscopy or keratometry readings). In addition, the vagaries of the ability to make the incisions exactly as desired and of variability in corneal wound healing confound the attempt to "set" the cornea exactly during surgery.

Williams and colleagues[50] performed a retrospective study using intraoperative Terry keratometry and postoperative Bausch and Lomb keratometry and concluded that the correlation between the two was not enough to use intraoperative keratometry solely for surgical planning.

PREDICTABILITY FOR REPEATED OPERATIONS

There are no published studies of calculating the predictability for repeated operations. The published studies of the results of repeated operations indicate more variability than occurs with a primary operation (see Chapter 18, Repeated Surgery for Residual Myopia and Hyperopia after Refractive Corneal Surgery).

CLINICAL APPLICATIONS

Since there is no generally accepted criterion for acceptable predictability of refractive keratotomy, individual surgeons and patients must decide whether the present level of predictability is sufficient to warrant use of current surgical techniques as a treatment for myopia.

When surgeons consult with patients who are considering refractive keratotomy, they should tell patients three things about the expected refractive result. First, they should describe the ideal results, usually slight residual myopia. Second, they should give the average expected result for this patient, based on their previous experiences. Third, surgeons should describe the range of expected refractive outcome, as provided by the prediction interval.

For example, a surgeon might say to a 33-year-old patient with 4.00 D of myopia, "Assuming I make the incisions approximately as I have done in the past and you have an average result, you will probably retain about half a diopter of myopia. However, I cannot tell exactly where you will end up. I am 90% confident that you will be between 2.25 D undercorrected and 1.12 D overcorrected 1 year after surgery. Let me explain this in terms of your vision."

Thus we are left with the problem that for two patients with the same measurable characteristics on whom the same surgical technique of refractive keratotomy is performed, the outcomes can be quite different. Unless we learn to control this variability, refractive keratotomy will not be as predictable as desired, but it can be predictable enough for clinical acceptability.

The only practical hopes for improving the predictability of refractive keratotomy are to improve the accuracy and repeatability of the surgical technique (see Chapter 15, Surgical Instruments Used in Refractive Keratotomy; Chapter 17, Atlas of Surgical Techniques of Radial Keratotomy; and Chapter 19, Laser Corneal Surgery) and the individual variation in corneal wound healing (see Chapter 20, Corneal Wound Healing and Its Pharmacologic Modification after Refractive Keratotomy).

PREDICTION INTERVAL

In this section we present a more detailed explanation of what a prediction interval is and how it can be used to measure predictability. An example is presented using data from the PERK study. This section is intended for illustrative purposes and does not present a full analysis of the PERK data.

Example from the PERK study

In the PERK study, three clear zones were used. For this example we chose eyes having a 3.5-mm clear zone. A 3.5-mm clear zone was used for 138 eyes with a cycloplegic refractive error between −3.25 and −4.37 D. These 138 eyes had similar baseline refractive errors and received surgery according to the same protocol. If the effect of the surgery were highly reproducible, we would expect to see a similar refractive change in these eyes.

Fig. 13-19 is a histogram showing the change in refractive error between baseline and 1 year for the 3.5-mm clear zone group. The mean value was 3.41 D and the standard deviation was 1.16 D. The smallest and largest changes in refractive error were 0.75 and 6.75 D, respectively. For approximately 84% of the patients the change in refractive error was between 2.00 and 5.00 D. There is variability in the refractive change even though the same technique was attempted in all the eyes. Based on these results what can we tell a new patient about the likely outcome of radial keratotomy surgery?

Suppose a patient with 4.00 D of myopia wishes to have radial keratotomy. If the PERK technique is used with a 3.5-mm clear zone, we could use the mean refractive change in the PERK study, 3.41 D, to predict the outcome in the new patient. However, the variability in outcome among the patients in the PERK study makes it unlikely that a patient will obtain exactly 3.41 D of refractive change. Using statistical methods it is possible to calculate a range with 3.41 D at the middle that would have some probability (say 90%) of including the change in refraction that will actually occur. This range is called the 90% prediction interval. The wider this interval is, the less predictable is the outcome.

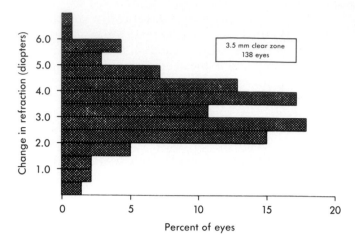

Figure 13-19
Histogram of the change in refraction between baseline and 1 year after surgery in the PERK study. The surgical technique included a 3.5-mm clear zone with eight incisions using a diamond blade knife set at 100% of the thinnest intraoperative paracentral corneal ultrasonic pachometry measurement. (From Lynn MJ and Waring GO: J Refract Surg 1987;3:193-196.)

Calculation of the prediction interval

The approximate formula for the limits of the 90% prediction interval when the sample size is larger than 30 eyes is as follows:

$$\text{Mean refractive change} \pm \text{standard deviation} \times 1.645$$

The value 1.645 is the 95th percentile from the normal distribution. The mean change is 3.41 D and the standard deviation is 1.16. Substituting these values into the formula we obtain 90% prediction limits of 3.41 ± 1.91 D. Thus we have 90% confidence that the refractive change will be between 1.50 and 5.32 D. For a patient with 4.00 D of myopia, we can be 90% certain that the refraction at 1 year will be between −2.50 and +1.32 D.

Effect of age on predictability

The above analysis does not take into account the effect that preoperative patient characteristics such as age might have on the amount of refractive change. These factors might be used to predict the patient outcome more accurately and precisely. How can the effect of age be estimated and then used to predict patient outcome? Will this help reduce the width of the prediction interval?

Fig. 13-20 is a series of scattergrams showing the relationship of age and the change in refractive error between baseline and 1 year after surgery for the 138 eyes with a 3.5-mm clear zone. There is a trend for older patients to have a greater change in refractive error than younger patients, but there is still considerable variation in the change in refraction even among patients of the same age.

Recall that the mean refractive change for all 138 eyes in the PERK study was 3.41 D and that this value was used to predict the outcome in a new patient. Fig. 13-18 suggests that the mean change is probably greater than 3.41 D among older patients and less than 3.41 D among younger patients. To predict the refractive change taking into account the effect of age, we need a method to determine how the mean change in refraction varies with age. Fig. 13-20, *A*, contains a line through the data that appears to follow the mean change in refraction as age varies. The equation of this line could be used to estimate the mean change in refraction for a given age. Using regression analysis, the equation of this line can be determined. The line is called the regression line, and the equation for the data in Fig. 13-20 is as follows:

$$\text{Mean refractive change} = 1.095 \text{ D} + (0.07 \times \text{age})$$

Since the coefficient for age in the equation is 0.07, a 10-year increase in age is related to a 0.70 D increase in the average change in refraction.

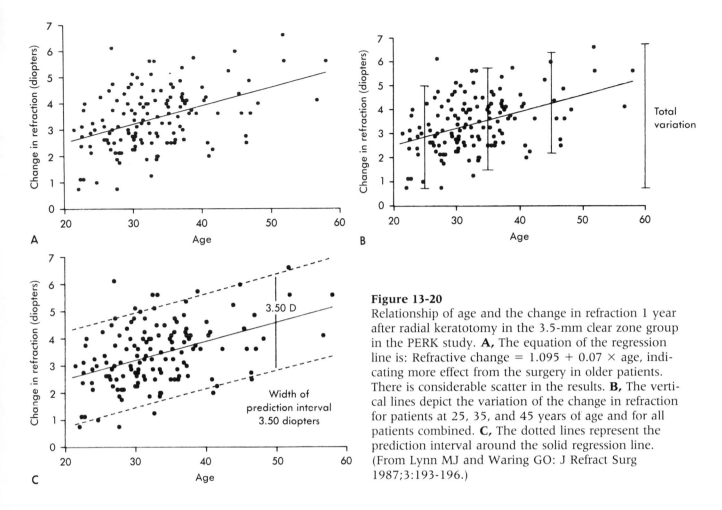

Figure 13-20
Relationship of age and the change in refraction 1 year after radial keratotomy in the 3.5-mm clear zone group in the PERK study. **A,** The equation of the regression line is: Refractive change = 1.095 + 0.07 × age, indicating more effect from the surgery in older patients. There is considerable scatter in the results. **B,** The vertical lines depict the variation of the change in refraction for patients at 25, 35, and 45 years of age and for all patients combined. **C,** The dotted lines represent the prediction interval around the solid regression line. (From Lynn MJ and Waring GO: J Refract Surg 1987;3:193-196.)

Earlier we used the mean change in refraction for the whole group, 3.41 D, to predict the outcome for a new patient. Now we can substitute a patient's age into the regression equation and obtain a predicted value that is an estimate of the mean refractive change for all patients of that age. For example, the predicted value for a 25-year-old patient is 2.85 D (1.095 D + [0.07 × 25] = 2.85 D) and the predicted value for a 45-year-old patient is 4.25 D (1.095 D + [0.07 × 45] = 4.25 D). Since there is a large amount of scatter around the regression line in Fig. 13-20, we would not expect a new 45-year-old patient to obtain exactly 4.25 D of change. Therefore a prediction interval is needed.

Recall that we previously used the standard deviation of the change in refraction for the entire group to calculate the prediction interval. The standard deviation is a measure of the variation around the mean value for the entire group. In Fig. 13-20, *B*, we have represented the variation of the entire group with the vertical line labeled "total variation" that shows the range for the change in refraction. Can consideration of age improve the predictability?

Calculating the prediction interval using the regression equation requires a measure of the variation around the regression line, that is, a measure of the variation of the change in refraction for each age. We demonstrate the variation around the regression line in Fig. 13-20, *B*. For each of the ages, 25, 35, and 45, the variation of the change in refraction is represented by a vertical line. The lines show the range of the refractive change for patients of these three ages. These vertical lines are slightly shorter than the line for the total variation. Thus some of the total variation in the refractive change was due to older patients having a greater average change in refraction than younger patients. However, a considerable amount of variation is still present around the regression line. In other words, patients of the same age differed in the amount by which their refraction changed. The amount of variation around the regression line determines the width of the prediction interval.

We will not burden the reader with the mathematics of the calculation of the variation around the regression line and the determination of the prediction interval. The methods can be found in standard statistical textbooks.[30] For the data in Fig. 13-20, *C,* we determined that the 90% prediction limits are found by adding and subtracting 1.73 D from the predicted refractive change calculated from the regression equation. Therefore the prediction interval is approximately 3.50 D wide. (Prediction intervals tend to be narrower at the mean value for the explanatory factor, age in this example, and wider for values away from the mean. In this example there was little difference in the width of the confidence interval for different values of age.)

Fig. 13-4 shows how the prediction interval for refractive change varies with age. For example, using the regression equation the predicted value for a 25-year-old patient is 2.85 D (1.095 + [0.07 × 25] = 2.85). The 90% prediction interval is 2.85 ± 1.73 D (1.12 to 4.58 D). For a 45-year-old patient the 90% prediction interval is 4.25 ± 1.73 D (2.52 to 5.98 D). How does the prediction interval using the regression equation compare with the previous prediction interval when age was not considered? The prediction interval is now narrower by 0.36 D—a 10% improvement in the width of the prediction interval. Only the diameter of the central clear zone had a greater influence on the change in refraction after surgery.

Clinical use of the statistical analysis

After the statistical analysis has identified the factors that affect the outcome of surgery, the question for the surgeon is how to use the information to refine the surgical technique. It is hoped that the technique can be better tailored to an individual patient by taking into account important patient characteristics and by choosing parameters of the surgical technique that will achieve the desired amount of correction. In this section we will discuss the use and limitations of the results of the analysis for improving the outcome of surgery in future patients.

To illustrate, we will use the previous example from the PERK study and consider the result of modifying the surgical technique to take into account the effect of age. Fig. 13-21, *A,* again shows the relationship of age and the change in refraction 1 year after surgery for patients in the PERK study with a preoperative refraction between −3.12 and −4.37 D who had a 3.5-mm clear zone. The line in the figure is the regression line. The average change in refraction was 3.41 D and the correlation between age and the change in refraction is 0.43.

Fig. 13-21, *B,* shows the relationship of age and the refraction at 1 year after surgery. The average refraction was −0.33 D and 62% of the eyes were within ± 1.00 D of emmetropia. As the graph shows, among younger patients undercorrections were more frequent than overcorrections and among older patients the opposite was true.

Therefore using the effect of age to adjust the surgical technique would be planned to create more correction for younger patients and less correction for older patients. Fig. 13-22, *A,* shows *simulated* data resulting from taking the data in Fig. 13-21, *A,* and adjusting the change in refraction so that it is decreased among older patients and increased among younger patients. The average change in refraction is the same, 3.41 D, but there is no correlation between age and the change in refraction. The regression line is horizontal; that is, the slope is zero. This simulates what we would hope to accomplish by modifying the surgical technique to adjust for the effect of age.

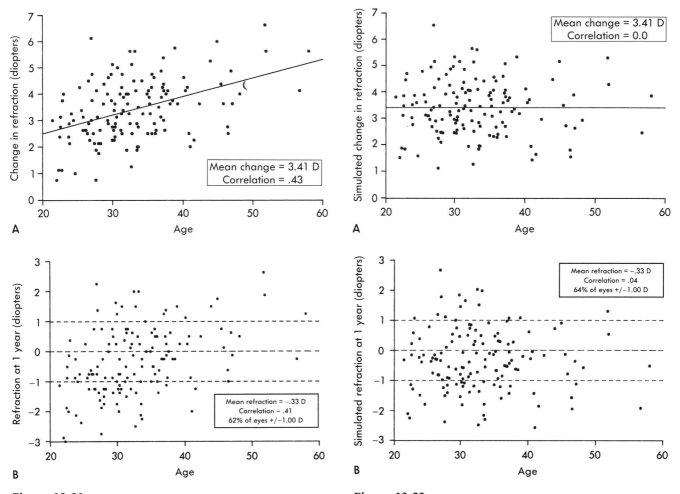

Figure 13-21
A, Relationship of age and the change in refraction at 1 year for the 3.5-mm clear zone group in the PERK study. There is a correlation coefficient of 0.43, indicating a moderate relationship. **B,** Relationship of age and the residual refraction at 1 year. Undercorrections are more prevalent among patients under 40 years of age.

Figure 13-22
Simulated data: **A,** Relationship of age and change in refraction adjusted for age. There is no correlation between age and change in refraction in this simulated example. **B,** Relationship of age and residual refraction adjusted for age. There is a slight increase in the percentage of patients within 1 D of emmetropia with the simulated data compared with the actual data (64% compared with 62%).

What is readily apparent from Fig. 13-22, *A,* is that the scatter around the regression line is the same as in Fig. 13-21, *A.* Adjusting for the effect of age has not increased the precision of the surgical technique. For example, in this *simulation,* patients 20 to 25 years of age have achieved a greater average change in refraction, but there is still considerable variation in the effect of the surgery, even though these patients had the same surgical technique.

Fig. 13-22, *B,* shows the simulated refractive error 1 year after surgery and age. Compared with Fig. 13-21, *B,* there has been a shift toward fewer undercorrections in younger patients and fewer overcorrections in older patients, but the wide scatter persists. We can also evaluate the result on the efficacy of the procedure of the age adjustment by comparing the simulated and actual refractive errors (Table 13-17). The adjustment for age has resulted in a few more patients with a desirable refraction. For example, there are 64% rather than 62% within 1.00 D of emmetropia.

Table 13-17

Refraction Results 1 Year after Surgery in the PERK Study: Comparison of Actual Results with Simulated Adjustment for Age

Refraction range (D)	Percentage of eyes	
	Actual results	Simulated age adjustment
+1.12 to +2.63	12	10
+0.62 to +1.00	9	10
−0.50 to +0.50	33	36
−0.62 to −1.00	20	18
−1.12 to −2.00	20	21
−2.12 to −3.00	6	5
−0.50 to +0.50	33	36
−1.00 to +1.00	62	64

Two published reports[2,40] have applied the results of regression analysis to a new series of patients. These evaluations have focused only on how well the regression equation based on the initial series predicted the refractive change for the new series. However, to evaluate whether there were better results in the new series of patients after applying the information from the initial series, we would have to know the actual refractive or visual acuity outcomes in the new series of patients. This information was not provided in either study.

Two main points result from this example. First, adjusting the surgical technique according to preoperative characteristics can give better results, but will not reduce the inherent variability in the surgical procedure or in the patient response. Stated another way, the only way to reduce the width of the prediction interval is to improve the precision of the surgical technique or to reduce the variation in patient response. The problem remains that two patients with similar characteristics can vary in an interval of about ±1.75 D.

Second there is the problem of how to identify the optimal surgical technique for an individual patient. The best way to acquire the necessary information is to design a clinical trial in which specific combinations of the surgical parameters are tested in a systematic fashion. For example, a study could test different surgical techniques in which the diameter of the clear zone, number of incisions, and depth of the cut are varied and the patients would be stratified according to preoperative characteristics such as age and the amount of myopia. Such a study has not yet been done. The PERK study was limited to a single surgical technique in which the diameter of the clear zone was changed according to the amount of myopia. Other clinical studies have included more varied surgical techniques, but the specification of the technique was not rigorously controlled. Of course ultimately surgeons will have to choose the techniques with which they are most comfortable for their patients.

UNFINISHED BUSINESS

Identification of the factors that determine the outcome of refractive keratotomy is one way to improve predictability (two others being more accurate surgical techniques and control of corneal wound healing). Continued studies of keratotomy surgery are needed to isolate and quantify the effect of additional variables that may influence the outcome. Included in this list are corneal topography (do aspheric corneas respond differently than more spherical corneas?), corneal diameter (do larger corneas allow longer incisions with a greater effect?), intraocular pressure (can an intraocular pressure profile be created that will help to predict the outcome in individual eyes?), and scleral rigidity (what is the relationship between age and ocular rigidity, and can ocular rigidity be measured well enough to serve as a useful predictor?). In addition, new variables should be sought to better predict the outcome of surgery for individual eyes. For example, preoperative measurements of the stress in a given cornea or a given globe might identify corneas that repond more or less than expected given the surgical plan. Can holographic techniques or biomechanical techniques be developed to measure such parameters in the living eye? More accurate intraoperative monitoring of surgical results (sometimes called real time monitoring) should be explored. Can intraoperative keratometry or corneal topography monitor the effect of incisions as they are made and help titrate the operation during its performance to customize the results for individual eyes? The ultimate method of predicting the result of refractive keratotomy will use computational mechanics to create computerized models on which a sequence of simulated operations will be done until the exact desired result is obtained. The surgeon then can perform that specific operative technique on the patient (see Section VI, Corneal Biomechanics and Computer Modeling of Refractive Keratotomy).

REFERENCES

1. Arrowsmith PN and Marks RG: Evaluating the predictability of radial keratotomy, Ophthalmology 1985;92:331-338.
2. Arrowsmith PN and Marks RG: Four-year update on predictability of radial keratotomy, J Refract Surg 1988;4:37-45.
3. Arrowsmith PN and Marks RG: How predictable is radial keratotomy? Cataract 1986;3:7-14.
4. Bates WH: A suggestion of an operation to correct astigmatism, Arch Ophthalmol 1894;23:9-13.
5. Bores LD, Myers W, and Cowden J: Radial keratotomy: an analysis of the American experience, Ann Ophthalmol 1981;13:941-948.
6. Busin M, Arffa RC, McDonald MB, and Kaufman HE: Change in corneal curvature with elevation of intraocular pressure after radial keratotomy in the primate eye, CLAO J 1988;14:110-112.
7. Busin M, Suarez H, Bieber S, et al: Overcorrected visual acuity improved by antiglaucoma medication after radial keratotomy, Am J Ophthalmol 1986;101:374-375.
8. Busin M, Yau CW, Avini I, McDonald M, and Kaufman H: The effect of changes in intraocular pressure on corneal curvature after radial keratotomy in the rabbit eye, Ophthalmol 1986;93:331-334.
9. Deitz M, Sanders DR, and Marks RG: Radial keratotomy: an overview of the Kansas City study, Ophthalmology 1984;91:467-478.
10. Deitz MR, Sanders DR, and Raanan MG: A consecutive series (1982-1985) of radial keratotomies performed with the diamond blade, Am J Ophthalmol 1987;103:417-422.
11. Feldman FT, Frucht-Pery J, Weinrab RN, Chaye TA, Dreher AW, and Brown SI: The effect of increased intraocular pressure on visual acuity and corneal curvature after radial keratotomy, Am J Ophthalmol 1989;108:126-129.
12. Fyodorov SN: Methods of radial keratotomy. In Schachar RA, Levy NS, and Schachar L, editors: Radial keratotomy, Denison, Tex, 1980, LAL Publishing Co, pp 35-66.
13. Fyodorov SN: Surgical correction of myopia and astigmatism. In Schachar AR, Levi S, and Schachar S, editors: Keratorefraction, Dennison, Tex, 1980, LAL Publishing Co, pp 141-172.
14. Fyodorov SN and Durnev VV: Operation of dosaged dissection of corneal circular ligament in cases of myopia of mild degree, Ann Ophthalmol 1979;11:1885-1890.
15. Fyodorov SN, Durnev VV, Ivashina AI, and Gudechkov VB: Calculation of the effect of the surgical correction of myopia (radial keratotomy). In Fyodorov SN, editor: Surgery for anomalies in ocular refraction, Moscow, 1987, Institute for Ocular Microsurgery, p 135.
16. Grady FJ: Experience with radial keratotomy for astigmatism, Ann Ophthalmol 1984;16:942-944.
17. Hoffer K, Darin J, Pettit T, et al: Three years experience with radial keratotomy: the UCLA study, Ophthalmology 1983;90:627-636.

18. Huang D, Lin C, Huang J, Fujaimoto JG, and Puliafito CA: High resolution measurement of anterior and corneal eye structures using optical coherence domain reflectometry, Invest Ophthalmol Vis Sci 1990;31(suppl):245.

19. Ingraham HJ, Guber D, and Green WR: Radial keratotomy: clinicopathologic case report, Arch Ophthalmol 1985;103:683-688.

20. Jester JV, Venet T, Lee J, et al: A statistical analysis of radial keratotomy in human cadaver eyes, Am J Ophthalmol 1981;92:172-177.

21. Knauss W, Rapacz P, Sene K, et al: Curvature changes induced by radial keratotomy in solithane model of eye, Invest Ophthalmol Vis Sci 1982; 20(suppl):69.

22. Kremer FB and Steer RA: Prediction of refractive correction with radial keratotomy, Ann Ophthalmol 1985;17:660-663.

23. Lans LJ: Experimentelle Untersuchungen uber Entstehung von Astigmatismus durch nicht-perforirende Corneawunden: Albrecht von Graefes, Arch Ophthalmol 1889;45:117-152.

24. Les Jardins L et al: Personal communication, November 1989.

25. Lipshitz and Ellis: Personal communication, International Society of Refractive Keratoplasty meeting, Singapore, March 18-24, 1990.

26. Lynn MJ, Waring GO, Sperduto RD, et al: Factors affecting outcome and predictability of radial keratotomy in the PERK study, Arch Ophthalmol 1987;105:42-51.

27. Maloney RK: Effect of corneal hydration and intraocular pressure on keratometric power after experimental radial keratotomy, Ophthalmology 1990;97:927-933.

28. Maloney RK, Stark WJ, and McCally RL: Intraocular pressure causes refractive change after radial keratotomy, Invest Ophthalmol Vis Sci 1987;28(suppl):224.

29. Moiseyenko GS, Durnev VV, and Ivashina AI: About the possibility of maximum lengthening of incisions in anterior keratotomy. In Fyodorov SN: Surgery for anomalies in ocular refraction, Moscow, 1981, Research Institute for Ocular Microsurgery, p 135.

30. Neter J, Wasserman W, and Kutner M: Applied linear statistical models: regression analysis of variance and experimental designs, Homewood, Ill, 1985, Richard D Irwin, Inc.

31. Neumann AC, Osher RH, and Fenzl RE: Radial keratotomy: a comprehensive evaluation, Doc Ophthalmol 1984; 56:275-301.

32. O'Donnell FE: Short incision radial keratotomy: a comparative study in rabbits, J Refract Surg 1987;3:102-108.

33. Rowsey JJ, Monlux R, Balyeat HD, Stevens HX, Gelender H, Holladay J, and the PERK study group: Accuracy and the reproducibility of KeraScanner analysis in the PERK corneal topography, Curr Eye Res 1989;8:661-674.

34. Rowsey JJ, Balyeat HD, Monlux R, et al: Prospective evaluation of radial keratotomy: photokeratoscope corneal topography, Ophthalmology 1988;95: 322-334.

35. Rowsey JJ, Balyeat HD, Rabinovitch B, et al: Predicting the results of radial keratotomy, Ophthalmology 1983; 90:642-654.

36. Salz JJ, Lee T, Jester JV, et al: Analysis of incision depth following experimental radial keratotomy, Ophthalmology 1983;90:655-659.

37. Salz JJ, Lee J, Jester JV, et al: Radial keratotomy in fresh human cadaver eyes, Ophthalmology 1981;88:742-746.

38. Salz JJ, Rowsey JJ, Caroline P, et al: A study of optical zone size and incision redeepening in experimental radial keratotomy, Arch Ophthalmol 1985;103:590-594.

39. Sanders DR and Deitz MR: Factors affecting predictability of radial keratotomy. In Sanders DR, Hofmann RF, and Salz J, editors: Refractive corneal surgery, Thorofare, NJ, 1986, Slack, Inc, pp 79-90.

40. Sanders D, Dietz M, and Gallagher D: Factors affecting predictability of radial keratotomy, Ophthalmology 1985; 92:1237-1243.

41. Sato T, Akiyama K, and Shibata H: A new surgical approach to myopia, Am J Ophthalmol 1953;36:823-829.

42. Schachar R, Black T, and Huang T: Understanding radial keratotomy, Denison, Tex, 1981, LAL Publishing Co, pp 12-37.

43. Seigel D: Regression (editorial), Arch Ophthalmol 1987;105:185-186.

44. Smith RS and Cutro J: Computer analysis of radial keratotomy, CLAO J 1984;10:241-248.

45. Spigelman AV, Williams PA, Nichols BD, et al: Four incision radial keratotomy, J Cataract Refract Surg 1988; 14:125-128.

46. Steel D, Jester JV, Salz JJ, et al: Modification of corneal curvature following radial keratotomy in primates, Ophthalmology 1981;88:747-754.

47. Waring GO, Lynn MJ, Culbertson W, et al: Three-year results of the prospective evaluation of radial keratotomy (PERK) study, Ophthalmology 1987;94:1339-1354.

48. Waring GO, Lynn MJ, Gelender H, et al: Results of the prospective evaluation of radial keratotomy (PERK) study one year after surgery, Ophthalmology 1985;92:177-198.

49. Waring GO, Moffitt SD, Gelender H, et al: Rationale for and design of the National Eye Institute prospective evaluation of radial keratotomy (PERK) study, Ophthalmology 1983;90:40-58.

50. Williams PA, Chin V, Choi KY, Skelnik DL, and Lindstrom RL: The intraoperative and postoperative changes in K readings following four incision radial keratotomy, Invest Ophthalmol Vis Sci 1990;31(suppl):30.

Computerized Predictability Formulas for Refractive Keratotomy

Donald R. Sanders

Ophthalmologists attempting refractive keratotomy for the first time may realize that no standard and universally accepted approach exists for determining the parameters of surgery for an individual patient. In an effort to systematize refractive keratotomy and improve postoperative results, many surgeons have developed formulas (prediction formulas, software, nomograms, computer programs, or guides) that serve as guides to the surgery (Figs. 14-1 to 14-6). These formulas relate patient variables—such as amount of myopia and patient age—to surgical variables—such as the diameter of the central clear zone (optical zone), the number of incisions, and the depths of the incisions. The number of factors in a formula and the complexity of their relationship varies greatly. In all instances the formulas are based on the experience of a single surgeon and tacitly include the artistic and technical nuances used by that surgeon. Therefore if a given formula is used with the technique most similar to that of the surgeon who derived it, results may be better than if the formula were adapted to different surgical techniques.

BACKGROUND AND ACKNOWLEDGMENTS

This chapter is modified from previous publications that compare and review six predictability formulas based on information developed and analyzed by Drs. Donald Sanders and James Salz.[9,10,16] Other published sources of information are cited in the references. Programs that are trademarked are indicated in their initial citation in the chapter, but for reasons of simplicity we omit the trademark symbol thereafter.

The nomograms included at the end of the chapter were taken from previously published sources. In comparing predictability formulas, we do not endorse or favor any nomogram or commercially available software. We leave those judgments to the surgeon.

Analysis of data was performed at the Center for Clinical Research in Anterior Segment Surgery at the University of Illinois Medical School in Chicago, which is funded by the American Society of Cataract and Refractive Surgery, the International Society of Refractive Keratoplasty, and private donations.

ASSESSMENT OF REFRACTIVE KERATOTOMY FORMULAS

Formulas are available as printed nomograms and computer software packages. Selected nomograms are presented in Figs. 14-16 to 14-21. The available computerized software programs are summarized in Table 14-1. There are no published formulas to guide the surgeon for repeated keratotomy. This subject is discussed in detail in Chapter 18, Repeated Surgery for Residual Myopia and Hyperopia after Refractive Corneal Surgery.

The individual variables that affect the outcome of surgery are discussed in detail in Chapter 13, Predictability of Refractive Keratotomy. In this chapter, the discussion is confined to the overall formulas contained in computer programs and nomograms, comparing their use with predicted effect of specific patient and surgical variables.

Useful questions to ask about refractive keratotomy formulas, in addition to the technical information presented in Table 14-1, include the following:

1. What is the basis on which the formula was developed: number of eyes and type of analysis? For example, a formula may be derived from thousands of eyes, an unspecified percentage of which are analyzed retrospectively to give the general recommendations. A better approach is to study a few hundred consecutive eyes using regression analysis to identify the effect of specific variables.

2. What evidence is presented to justify the inclusion of each variable in the formula? For example, is it well demonstrated that the age of the patient makes a difference in planning the surgery or that the use of peripheral deepening incisions achieves a greater effect?

3. Does the formula also include an adjustable surgeon's factor, also known as a practical coefficient of correction, a depth factor, or a fudge factor? How important is this factor in the overall formula?

4. Is the entire formula disclosed so that surgeons know what they are doing when making the surgical plan? A nondisclosed, proprietary formula commits the surgeon to planning an operation without knowing exactly how the plan is derived.

5. Has the specific formula been tested on one or more series of patients and have the results been published? Such testing provides a yardstick against which other surgeons can measure the effectiveness of their use of the particular formula.

6. Has the formula been tested in comparison with other formulas on similar groups of patients by the same surgeon or different surgeons? Two published papers, both retrospective studies, compare clinical results of refractive keratotomy formulas: Sanders and colleagues[22] compare the DRS[TM] and AMark[TM] formulas and Lavery[13] compares the Sawelson, Thornton, and Ellis nomograms.

COMPONENTS OF REFRACTIVE KERATOTOMY FORMULAS

Refractive keratotomy formulas comprise three components—two specified and one unspecified.

The first component is patient variables, which may include some or all of the following:

1. Refraction (spherical equivalent or sphere and cylinder for astigmatism)
2. Age
3. Central average keratometric corneal power
4. Sex
5. Topographic or shape factors

6. Preoperative intraocular pressure
7. Corneal thickness (central, paracentral, peripheral, or all three)
8. Corneal diameter (usually horizontal)
9. Ocular rigidity

Of course, the way in which each of these variables is used may differ among formulas. For example, the refraction may be given using cycloplegic, manifest, or spherical equivalent units of measure or divided into spherical and cylindric components. The patient's age may be entered as years or deciles. The corneal thickness may be measured by optical or ultrasonic pachometry at a single point (for example, central) or at multiple points, either preoperatively or intraoperatively. Whether these subtleties make a difference in the outcome is unknown.

The second component is the surgical variables, including the following:

1. Diameter of central clear zone (optical zone) (This determines the length of the incisions.)
2. Number of incisions
3. Knife-blade length (This affects the depth of the incisions.)
4. Direction of incisions
5. Number, type, and depth of deepening incisions

Most formulas were derived on the basis of eight or 16 incisions; formulas using data from eyes that had four incisions are being developed. All published formulas assume centrifugal incisions; those formulas will have to be recomputed if centripetal incisions are used. The pattern of deepening incisions varies greatly from one formula to another.

The third component, which is unspecified in the formulas, is the surgical technique, including the instruments used (especially which knife), the methods of controlling intraoperative intraocular pressure used, the specific manual techniques of executing the incisions used, and postoperative medications used, including corticosteroids. Some formulas attempt to encompass these variations in technique by including an adjustable factor specific for the surgeon—the surgeon factor, practical coefficient of correction, or depth factor—which is probably necessary when individual formulas are adapted from one surgeon to another.

Depending on how a formula uses the three preceding components, it can vary in the type of result it gives a surgeon for an individual case. Some formulas present a single recommended set of surgical variables; others present a number of alternatives so that the surgeon can mix and match the different variables to achieve a similar outcome. For example, a larger clear zone with a deeper knife setting or a smaller clear zone with a shallower knife setting could give the same results.

DESCRIPTIONS OF INDIVIDUAL FORMULAS
DRS formulas

The Deitz-Retzlaff-Sanders (DRS) series of formulas[23] provides a method for surgeons to estimate the amount of surgery required for individual patients and to modify this estimation based on their own surgical experience and technique. All three formulas of the DRS program are based on regression analysis of data collected by Deitz on cases between 1979 and 1983 using metal and diamond knife blades and are modified by clinical judgment in areas where data were sparse. The effects of different variables used in the formula were defined by Sanders and colleagues and based on their regression analysis,[21] but the exact relationships used in the DRS formula are not published.

These RK Eprom software packages guide the user through calculations with

Table 14-1

Consumers' Guide to Refractive Keratotomy Predictive Software

Program	Deitz, Retzlaff, Sanders (DRS)	Thornton Guide (TG)	R.K. Data Master (RKD)	R.K. Predictor (RKP)	AMark	Kremer (KR)	RK—STAT*
Authors	Michael Deitz, MD; Donald Sanders, MD; John Retzlaff, MD	Spencer Thornton, MD	Leo Bores, MD; Svyatoslav Fyodorov, MD	Frank Grady, MD	Peter Arrowsmith, MD; Ronald Marks, PhD	Frederic Kremer, MD	George Simon, MD
Formula based on	Multiple regression analysis and clinical experience	Clinical experience	Multiple regression analysis and clinical experience	Clinical experience	Multiple regression analysis and clinical experience	Multiple regression analysis	Regression analysis and clinical experience
Patients in data base (No.)	450	Hundreds	10,000	4000	1000	Not indicated	Over 5000
Patient variables	Refraction, K, IOP, sex, age	Refraction, K, IOP, sex, age, corneal thickness	Refraction, K, sex, age, IOP, corneal rigidity	Refraction, K, IOP, sex, age, corneal thickness	Refraction, age, sex, IOP requested (but not used)	Refraction, age, sex, IOP, central corneal thickness	Refraction, age, sex, K, IOP, thickness, diameter
Surgical variables							
Incisions (No.)	8, 16, 4†	8, 16	6-20	8, 12	3-16	8, 12, 16	8-16
Clear zone diameter	2.75-5.5 0.10 mm steps rounded to nearest 0.25 by surgeon	3.0-4.75 0.25 mm steps	2.75-5.00 0.25 mm steps	2.8-4.50 0.25 mm steps	3.0-4.0 0.25 steps 4.0 to 6.0 0.50 steps	3.00 0.25 mm steps	3.0-? 0.25 mm steps
Blade setting based on	Operative paracentral thickness	Preoperative paracentral thickness	Operative % of paracentral thickness + "penetration factor"	Preoperative paracentral thickness	Operative paracentral thickness	Operative paracentral thickness	Not indicated

Modified from Sanders DR: Computerized RK predictability programs. In Sanders DR, Hofmann RF, and Salz JJ, editors: Refractive corneal surgery, Thorofare, NJ, 1985, Slack, Inc, pp 91-108 and Salz JJ: J Refract Surg 1985; 1:60-69.

*Data on RK-STAT from Refractive Surgery Institute advertisement.

†Accuracy not established for 4 incisions.

‡Surgeon's personal depth factor can be adjusted to allow for deepening incision.

§Cost in US dollars in 1988.

Table 14-1

Consumers' Guide to Refractive Keratotomy Predictive Software—cont'd

Program	Deitz, Retzlaff, Sanders (DRS)	Thornton Guide (TG)	R.K. Data Master (RKD)	R.K. Predictor (RKP)	AMark	Kremer (KR)	RK—STAT*
Deepening incisions	No‡	2 zones	3 zones	3 zones	3 zones	3 zones	2 zones
Astigmatism program	No	T cuts for up to 2 D	Yes	Yes	Yes	No	Yes, flag incisions
Computer hardware	Texas Instruments compact CC40 IBM	Texas Instruments compact CC40 IBM	Apple, IBM	Apple, IBM	Apple, IBM, Radio Shack, Digital	Texas Instruments compact, Computer 40, IBM	Not indicated
Special features	Personalized depth factor—"Quick Calc" allows for predicted myopia decrease for a given patient; IOL program also available for CC40	Suggest location of T cuts for up to 2 D of astigmatism	Provides several combinations of number of incisions, and incision depth for a given patient	Draws graphics and suggested incision patterns for astigmatism	Multiple combinations of number of incisions, and CZ, and incision depths integrated with data base program, graphic printout		Graphic printout of surgery
Cost§	$1100-1300 includes computer and DRS; IBM 5950	$1100-1300 includes computer and TG; IBM 5950	Apple $500 IBM $625	$2800 Apple or IBM $175 for individual case analysis (applies to purchase price)	$3995 includes data base program	$4000 Includes TI CC 40 computer	$995 + $100 for annual update
Vendor	Slack Inc, 6900 Grove Road, Thorofare, NJ 08086; Cilco; Storz; KOI; DGH Pilling; Jedmed	Slack Inc, 6900 Grove Road, Thorofare, NJ 08086; Cilco; Storz; KOI; DGH Pilling; Jedmed	Leo Bores, MD, 7350 E. Stetson #203, Scottsdale, AZ 85251	Brazosport Eye Facility, Inc, 103 Parking Way, Lake Jackson, TX 77566	Ophthalmic Prediction Software, Inc, PO Box 14627, Gainesville, FL 32604	Accutome, 490 Lancaster Ave, Frazer, PA 19355	RK-STAT, Refractive Surgery Institute, 2299 Bacon St, Concord, CA 94520

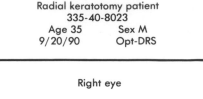

Radial keratotomy patient
335-40-8023
Age 35   Sex M
9/20/90   Opt-DRS

Right eye

−3.50   +0.00 × 0
43.00/ 43.25 K
IOP 15

Depth factor 85

8 incisions

Optic zone	Myopia decrease
3.50	3.94
3.77	3.50
4.00	3.09

Figure 14-1
Sample printout of DRS (Deitz, Retzlaff, and Sanders) formula. (From Sanders DR: J Refract Surg 1985;1:110.)

a series of menus that create a customized procedure. When the computer with a chip in place is turned on, it moves slowly through a flashing display of a numbered series of the following choices:

1. DRS formulas
2. Quick calculations
3. DRS personalized depth factor
4. Thornton guide

Press *1*, and the program asks you to choose which of the three DRS formulas you wish to use. After you choose one of them (or if you had chosen *2, 3,* or *4* from the first menu), you are prompted to insert patient and surgical information, including patient name, age, sex, which eye, intraocular pressure, keratometry, and refraction. The program is extensively "error trapped" in that it will not allow the surgeon or technician to enter nonphysiologic data. For example, the program will not allow input of preoperative keratometry measurements less than 35.00 D or more than 50.00 D. This feature is extremely important, and any refractive keratotomy predictability software package being considered should be tested to see that it rejects inappropriate data.

The first DRS formula, "Calculate optic zone size," asks for patient age, sex, preoperative intraocular pressure, and preoperative keratometry, the amount of myopia the surgeon wishes to correct, and an incision depth factor, which is the average percent incision depth that the surgeons believe they routinely attain. The DRS program calculates the clear zone size predicted by the formula to produce the desired myopia correction for the particular patient (Fig. 14-1). This DRS formula is the one compared with the other predictability software programs discussed in this chapter.

Radial keratotomy patient
335-40-8023
Age 35   Sex M
9/20/90   Opt-DRS

Right eye

−3.50   +0.00 × 0
43.00/43.25 K
IOP 15

8 incisions

98% deep at optic zone

Optic zone 3.50

Figure 14-2
Sample printout of Thornton guide formula. (From
Sanders DR: J Refract Surg 1985;1:110.)

The second DRS formula, "Calculate myopia decrease," asks for the clear
zone size the surgeon plans to use, the patient information previously described,
and the surgeon's incision depth factor. The program will calculate the amount
of myopia correction expected for that patient with that surgical technique.

The third DRS formula is used to "Calculate incision depth factor" and to obtain the "Personalized depth factor." The first part calculates the incision depth
needed to correct a specific amount of myopia with a given clear zone size. The
second part, "Personalized depth factor," enables surgeons to tailor a predictability formula to their own surgery. This formula asks for the amount of myopia
actually corrected, the clear zone size, the number of incisions used, and the patient information. The program then calculates an individual incision depth factor for the case. This formula was devised to deal with differences in refractive
outcome reported by different surgeons using similar techniques even when patient age, sex, keratometry, and preoperative intraocular pressure are taken into
account.

To overcome these differences, whatever their cause, the DRS "Personalized
depth factor" enables the surgeon to tailor a predictability formula for refractive
keratotomy in a manner similar to the successful tailoring achieved by the
Sanders-Retzlaff-Kraff (SRK) formula for intraocular lens power calculation in
which the surgeon can personalize the "A" constant. In effect, surgeons compare
their results with those of Deitz. If the results are similar, the depth factor will be
about 90%, which is what Deitz usually achieves. If the surgeon consistently
achieves less effect than Deitz on similar cases, the depth factor must be increased to greater than 90%; if the surgeon achieves a greater effect than Deitz,
the depth factor should be decreased to less than 90%.

The DRS formula does not contain programs for the correction of astigmatism.

Thornton guide

The Thornton guide is derived from Thornton's analysis[24] of his own clinical
experience (Fig. 14-2). The guide requires refraction in minus cylinder form and
for eyes with astigmatism over 0.75 D; the spherical portion of the refraction is

Figure 14-3
Sample printout of the Bores and Fyodorov RK Data Master formula. (From Sanders DR: J Refract Surg 1985;1:110.)

R.K. Patient—Male	Age 25	Right Eye Date—9/25/85

MOST MYOPIA [MM] . . . . − 3.00 diopters
LEAST MYOPIA [ML] . . . . − 3.00 diopters
CORNEAL DIAMETER [CD] . . . . 11.7 mm.
STEEPEST K (IN DPTRS OR MM/S) [RS] . . . . 43.00 diopters
FLATTEST K (IN DPTRS OR MM/S) [RF] . . . . 43.00 diopters
CORNEAL RIGIDITY [CR] 0.95

OPTICAL ZONE/ID COEFFICIENT COMBINATIONS (OPTIMUM ZONES IN BRACKETS)

Incision Depth:	INCISIONS:			
	6	8	12	16
1.3	2.60	>3.10<	>3.63<	>4.22<
1.6	>3.00<	>3.55<	>4.10<	>4.74<
2.0	>3.19<	>3.76<	>4.34<	>4.98<
2.5	>3.54<	>4.14<	>4.74<	5.40

used to calculate the radial incisions and the cylindric portion of the refraction to calculate the placement of transverse incisions between the radial incisions. The depth is constant at 98% of the corneal thickness as measured at the margin of the clear zone. For deepening incisions, the depth is indicated as "redeepening to Descemet's membrane." This nomogram has been incorporated as a series of computer programs in the same hardware/software system as the DRS formula. A printout from this is shown in Fig. 14-2. Patient age, sex, preoperative refraction, average central keratometry, and preoperative intraocular pressure are used in the calculation. The program indicates the diameter of central clear zone, the number of incisions, and the pattern of deepening incisions. The program calculates surgery up to eight incisions with a 3-mm clear zone, and if the patient's myopia and other parameters require more surgery than this, peripheral deepening incisions are added, followed by a change from eight to 16 incisions.

RK Data Master formula

The RK Data Master formula was derived by Bores and Fyodorov. The basis for the formula is unclear, and the formula has not been published. It is derived from a data base of "approximately 10,000 patients." The only publications that might be related to this formula are those of Bores in 1981.[4,6] The method was based on the use of metal-bladed knives and includes freehand deepening to Descemet's membrane, which are techniques that are now largely abandoned. Calculation of the corneal rigidity factor requires the use of Maklikov tonometry, which is not readily available in the United States. Patient age and sex, the amount of myopia to be corrected, corneal diameter, central keratometry measurements, and corneal rigidity factor are entered into the program, which produces a table providing several combinations of surgical techniques and options for various numbers of incisions.

A typical printout is shown in Fig. 14-3. The numbers at the top correspond to the number of incisions that could be used for the desired result. The numbers in the left column (1.3, 1.6, 2.0, and 2.5) refer to Fyodorov's four surgical factors. Factor 1.3 indicates single-pass incisions with blade length set at the paracentral optical pachometry thickness minus 0.08 mm, which is approximately equal to 80% observed incision scar depth. Factor 1.6 indicates single-pass incisions with blade length set at paracentral optical pachometry thickness minus 0.05 mm, which is approximately 90% of the observed incision scar depth. Factor 2.0 indicates initial single-pass initial incisions as in Factor 1.6, with the addition of peripheral deepening of all incisions at a blade setting of the midperipheral optical pachometry thickness minus 0.05 mm. Factor 2.5 indicates initial single-pass incisions and peripheral deepening as in Factor 2.0, with the addition of freehand deepening to Descemet's membrane in four to eight incisions, depending on the amount of myopia.

The numbers in the body of Fig. 14-3 refer to recommended clear zone diameters. For example, for an eight-incision case attempting approximately 90% depth (surgical factor 1.6), RK Data Master suggests a clear zone diameter of 3.55 mm.

AMark formula

The AMark software is based on the analysis of refractive keratotomy surgeries performed by Arrowsmith. The formula was developed through the use of multiple regression analysis. The original formula developed in 1981 was based on Arrowsmith's first 156 operations using a steel blade.[3] This formula was tested prospectively on more than 200 cases until a new model was developed at the end of 1982, based on Arrowsmith's first 142 operations performed using a diamond knife. This formula was tested in more than 1000 cases in 1983 and 1984. The type of regression analysis on which the formula is based was published with analysis of the clinical data,[1,2] but the formula incorporated in the AMark program has not been published.

The major patient variables used in the formula are refractive error, age, sex, and central keratometry. Keratometry is used to determine the limit of the effect that can be achieved. A clinical adjustment for intraocular pressure is suggested if the intraocular pressure is low or high, but this factor is not an integral part of the calculation on each case. The program allows the user to review the predicted results for 152 different combinations of number of incisions, clear zone, incision depth, and deepening incisions. Predicted results can be obtained for keratotomies using the following variables:

1. Three, four, six, and eight primary incisions
2. Deepening using eight, 12, and 16 incisions
3. Clear zones from 3 to 6 mm in diameter
4. Achieved incision depths of 80% to 95% of corneal thickness

The formula also contains recommendations for transverse incisions to correct astigmatism. Given these options, surgeons must select the surgical plan that they consider most appropriate, based on personal techniques.

The AMark software includes a graphic sketch of the eye with the location of the incisions, including their length and depth. This sketch can be printed. The program also contains data base management software that will store preoperative information, surgical data, and postoperative data.

A typical printout from the AMark refractive keratotomy prediction formula is shown in Fig. 14-4. Patient age is the only requested factor that appears to affect the values produced in the figure; thus Fig. 14-4 applies to all 25-year-old patients regardless of sex, refraction, keratometry, or intraocular pressure. Note that the AMark formula predicts the same or 0.01 D less effect by increasing the depth of incision from 80% to 85%. The maximum myopia correction obtained for a 25-year-old patient by cutting at 85% corneal depth is 2.32 D with a 3-mm clear zone and no deepening. The maximum correction that one could obtain by cutting 90% corneal depth is 2.98 D.

Peripheral deepening is a part of the AMark technique. The formula predicts that by adding eight secondary incisions and four tertiary incisions (changing from eight incursions to 20 incursions into the cornea), a surgeon can obtain 0.44 D of additional effect. By adding four more tertiary incisions (a total of 24 incursions), an additional 0.44 D can be obtained.

Sixteen primary incisions are performed only with 16 secondary and at least

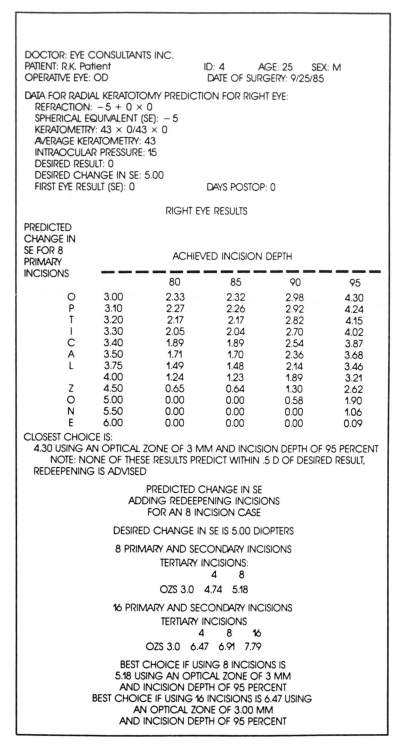

DOCTOR: EYE CONSULTANTS INC.
PATIENT: R.K. Patient   ID: 4   AGE: 25   SEX: M
OPERATIVE EYE: OD   DATE OF SURGERY: 9/25/85

DATA FOR RADIAL KERATOTOMY PREDICTION FOR RIGHT EYE:
  REFRACTION: $-5 + 0 \times 0$
  SPHERICAL EQUIVALENT (SE): -5
  KERATOMETRY: $43 \times 0/43 \times 0$
  AVERAGE KERATOMETRY: 43
  INTRAOCULAR PRESSURE: 15
  DESIRED RESULT: 0
  DESIRED CHANGE IN SE: 5.00
  FIRST EYE RESULT (SE): 0   DAYS POSTOP: 0

RIGHT EYE RESULTS

PREDICTED
CHANGE IN
SE FOR 8 PRIMARY INCISIONS

ACHIEVED INCISION DEPTH

		80	85	90	95
O	3.00	2.33	2.32	2.98	4.30
P	3.10	2.27	2.26	2.92	4.24
T	3.20	2.17	2.17	2.82	4.15
I	3.30	2.05	2.04	2.70	4.02
C	3.40	1.89	1.89	2.54	3.87
A	3.50	1.71	1.70	2.36	3.68
L	3.75	1.49	1.48	2.14	3.46
	4.00	1.24	1.23	1.89	3.21
Z	4.50	0.65	0.64	1.30	2.62
O	5.00	0.00	0.00	0.58	1.90
N	5.50	0.00	0.00	0.00	1.06
E	6.00	0.00	0.00	0.00	0.09

CLOSEST CHOICE IS:
  4.30 USING AN OPTICAL ZONE OF 3 MM AND INCISION DEPTH OF 95 PERCENT
     NOTE: NONE OF THESE RESULTS PREDICT WITHIN .5 D OF DESIRED RESULT,
REDEEPENING IS ADVISED

PREDICTED CHANGE IN SE
ADDING REDEEPENING INCISIONS
FOR AN 8 INCISION CASE

DESIRED CHANGE IN SE IS 5.00 DIOPTERS

8 PRIMARY AND SECONDARY INCISIONS
TERTIARY INCISIONS:
        4   8
OZS 3.0 4.74 5.18

16 PRIMARY AND SECONDARY INCISIONS
TERTIARY INCISIONS
        4   8   16
OZS 3.0 6.47 6.91 7.79

BEST CHOICE IF USING 8 INCISIONS IS
5.18 USING AN OPTICAL ZONE OF 3 MM
AND INCISION DEPTH OF 95 PERCENT
BEST CHOICE IF USING 16 INCISIONS IS 6.47 USING
AN OPTICAL ZONE OF 3.00 MM
AND INCISION DEPTH OF 95 PERCENT

Figure 14-4
Sample printout of AMark formula. (From Sanders DR: J Refract Surg 1985;1:111.)

Date	09-25-1985
Patient's Name	R.K. Patient
Eye	OD
Desired Change-Spher. Equiv.	4
Patient's Age	25
Intraocular Pressure	15
Central Corneal Thickness	.55
Sex	Male
Predict Change-Spher. Equiv.	4.24
Central Optical Zone Size	3.00
Number of Incisions	8
Number of Zones	1.5

Figure 14-5
Sample printout of Kremer-Accutome RK spherical myopia program. (From Sanders DR: J Refract Surg 1985;1:112.)

four tertiary incisions. Thus the surgeon must be prepared for at least 36 incursions into the cornea if "16-incision" cases are to be performed. The AMark formula predicts 1.73 D more effect with 16 incisions than with the corresponding eight incisions.

Kremer formula

The Kremer formula was developed on the basis of multiple regression analysis of a series of cases.[12] A critical review of the methods used in this regression analysis reveals circular calculations, in which the desired correction is used as the basis to determine the achieved correction, obtaining R^2 values of 0.99 (see Chapter 13, Predictability of Refractive Keratotomy). The Kremer formula was evaluated by Sanders,[18] but Kremer chose not to respond to the questionnaire submitted by Salz.[16]

A sample printout from the Kremer Accutome RK Spherical Myopia program is shown in Fig. 14-5. Information requested includes desired change in spherical equivalent, patient age, sex, refraction, intraocular pressure, and central corneal thickness. Then the clear zone size, number of incisions, and amount and type of deepening (number of zones) required to produce a specific change in the refraction are calculated and printed.

The logic used by the Kremer formula is to begin by using eight incisions without deepening incisions, then progressively reducing the clear zone diameter to 3 mm to get increasingly more effect. Once a 3-mm clear zone is reached, the formula uses the concept of multiple "zones" to attain further effect. The term "one-and-one-half zones" refers to eight primary incisions at the 3-mm clear zone (one complete zone) and one half that number of incisions (four) in the 5-mm, or secondary, incision zone. "Two zones" refers to the same number of incisions at the 3-mm and 5-mm zones, regardless of whether this is eight, 12, or 16 incisions. "Two-and-one-half zones" refers to 16 incisions at the 3-mm and 5-mm zones and one half that number (eight incisions) at the 7-mm, or tertiary, incision zone. "Three zones" refers to 16 incisions at the 3-mm, 5-mm, and 7-mm zones.

Once eight incisions at the 3-mm clear zone are predicted to undercorrect the myopia, four peripheral deepening incisions are added at the 5-mm zone (1.5 zones) for an additional 0.56 D of effect. If still more effect is needed, an additional four deepening incisions are placed at the 5-mm zone (2.0 zones), which the Kremer formula predicts will add an additional 0.55 D of effect. The next step is to add four additional primary and deepening incisions at the 5-mm zone (for example, 12 primary and secondary incisions, or two complete zones),

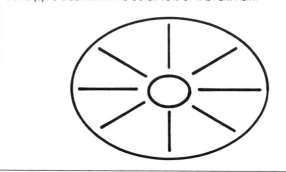

THIS PROGRAM IS INTENDED TO AID THE SURGEON PERFORMING A RADIAL KERATOTOMY. IN NO WAY SHOULD THESE CALCULATIONS AND PREDICTIONS BE SUBSTITUTED FOR SOUND SURGICAL JUDGEMENT.

PATIENT: JOHN JONES   AGE: 48   SEX: MALE   EYE: R
HORIZONTAL K READING 46.25   DIOPTERS
VERTICAL K READING: 46.25   DIOPTERS
INTRAOCULAR PRESSURE: 22   MM HG
REFRACTIVE SPHERE: −7.5   DIOPTERS
REFRACTIVE CYLINDER: 0   DIOPTERS
CYLINDER AXIS: 0   DEGREES
PACHOMETRY OF CORNEA: .57   MM

THE OPTICAL ZONE IS LESS THAN 3.0 MM AND NON-STANDARD. USE A 2.8MM STORZ WITH THE FOLLOWING INSTRUCTIONS FOR INCISIONS
EIGHT (8) RADIAL INCISIONS AT AN INITIAL DEPTH OF .54 MM. DEEPEN ALL INCISIONS (8) TO 0.62 MM IN THE OUTER 90% OF THE PERIPHERY.

Figure 14-6
Sample printout of the Grady RK predictor formula. (From Salz JJ: J Refract Surg 1985;1:64.)

which is predicted to add 0.58 D of effect. Kremer then recommends 16 primary and 16 secondary incisions (predicted to add another 0.58 D of effect). If more effect is needed, eight additional tertiary incisions (2.5 zones) are made at the 7-mm zone added for an additional 0.75 D of effect and finally another eight tertiary incisions (3 zones) are made for an additional 0.75 D of effect.

Thus for a hypothetical 25-year-old male with an intraocular pressure of 15 mm Hg and central corneal thickness of 0.55 mm, maximal surgery consisting of 16 primary incisions at a 3-mm clear zone, 16 secondary incisions at a 5-mm zone, and 16 tertiary incisions at a 7-mm zone should result in a predicted change in spherical equivalent of 7.45 D.

The Kremer formula is the only one that uses central corneal thickness as a variable in calculating the predicted outcome. Corneal thickness appears to have a greater effect on the outcome than the other factors, with the exception of preoperative myopia. When we specifically analyzed Deitz's data, we found no effect of corneal thickness.[21] Arrowsmith and Marks[1,2] also have not found central corneal thickness to be an important predictive factor.

RK predictor formula

The RK predictor was developed by Grady based on clinical analysis of approximately 4000 patients. Statistical methods used and the formula itself have not been published, although Grady[9] did publish a series of early cases.

The patient variables entered are refractive error, age, sex, intraocular pressure, central keratometry, and corneal thickness. The surgical technique varies from 8 to 12 incisions with clear zones varying from 2.8 to 4.5 mm in diameter. Deepening of incisions is recommended for up to three different peripheral zones. The blade length settings are based on a single preoperative paracentral pachometry reading.

A schematic graphic depiction of the location of the incisions, including astigmatic incisions, can be seen on the screen and printed separately (Fig. 14-6).

Grady will provide recommendations on specific cases for a consultation fee.

The program suggests a specific combination of clear zone diameter and incision number, pattern, and depth but does not allow the surgeon to enter independently a proposed clear zone and number of incisions to determine the amount of predicted myopia reduction.

RK Stat program

The RK Stat program was developed by Simon based on regression analysis of more than 5000 radial keratotomy operations during 3 years. No published information is available concerning this formula.

COMPARISON OF VARIABLES
IN FIVE SOFTWARE FORMULAS

To compare the predictions of the five major refractive keratotomy software predictability programs, we studied a hypothetical case: a 25-year-old male with 3.00 D of myopia, average central keratometry of 43.00 D, and an intraocular pressure of 15 mm Hg.

To separate the effect of each predictor variable in turn, only the variable being studied was changed; all other variables were kept constant. We chose 93.00 D of myopia correction for the hypothetical test case because all the formulas predicted clear zones of 3 mm or less without resorting to peripheral deepening or more than eight incisions. For the AMark formula, we assumed a relative incision depth of 95%. For the RK Data Master (Bores/Fyodorov) formula, we used a Fyodorov surgical factor of 1.6, which corresponds to an approximate incision depth of 90%. These depth factors were chosen because they were the deepest incisions recommended. The DRS formula was used with an assumed incision depth of 90%. The only predictions shown in the graphs are those clear zones predicted for eight incision cases without peripheral deepening.

Figs. 14-8 to 14-12 compare the effect of different variables in five formulas.

Incision depth

Only two formulas (AMark and DRS) allow the surgeon to vary the incision depth to change the amount of effect of keratotomy. The predicted relationship between change in spherical equivalent, refraction, and depth of incision with the AMark and DRS formulas is shown in Fig. 14-7. The other three assume a constant depth of incision in all cases. This is an important point because it is difficult for a surgeon to attain a uniform depth of incision throughout a single cut and to attain a uniform depth of incision for all of the cuts in a particular eye. Uniformity of cuts is even more difficult when two or three deepening incisions are made in a given location. Thus although depth of incision is emphasized either as a variable in two of the formulas or as a constant factor in three formulas, the ability of a surgeon to achieve an accurate and constant incision depth is questionable; furthermore the ability to measure the depth of an incision scar accurately has never been adequately demonstrated, except possibly with Deitz's data.[7,11,14,17]

With the exception of the DRS formula, all of the software programs suggest the use of peripheral deepening incisions. The DRS formula is based largely on single-pass, single-blade-setting radial keratotomy using a diamond knife without deepening; this technique is similar to the one used in the PERK study.[25-27]

Diameter of clear zone (optical zone)

Fig. 14-8 shows the effect of clear zone diameter for different amounts of preoperative myopia. With 2.00 D or less of myopia, the predictions of the Bores, Kremer, DRS, and AMark formulas seemed to cluster together, but the Thornton

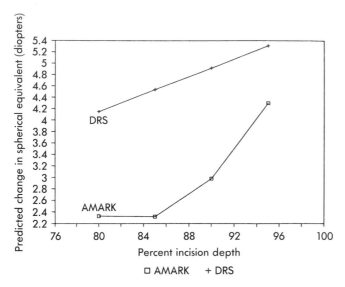

Figure 14-7
Predicted relationship between change in spherical equivalent refraction and depth of incision with the AMark and Deitz, Retzlaff, and Sanders *(DRS)* formulas. Results are for a hypothetical 25-year-old man with average keratometry measurements of 43 D and an intraocular pressure of 15 mm Hg. (From Sanders DR: J Refract Surg 1985;1:112.)

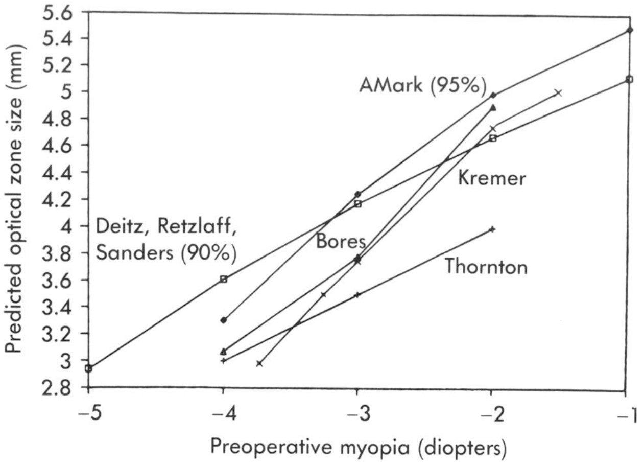

Figure 14-8
Comparison of five prediction programs in calculating the effect of preoperative myopia on predicted clear zone diameter. (From Sanders DR: J Refract Surg 1985;1:110.)

guide predicted the need for a smaller clear zone. With 3.00 to 4.00 D of myopia, the Thornton, Kremer, and Bores formulas clustered together, but the AMark and DRS formulas required somewhat larger clear zone diameter.

Age and sex

Fig. 14-9 shows the effect of age on clear zone size for men. For males younger than age 30, AMark and DRS formulas were similar and the Kremer formula and Thornton guide were similar, with the prediction of the Bores formula falling between these two. With increasing patient age, the AMark formula predicted the largest clear zone, the DRS and Kremer formulas intermediate, and the Thornton guide and Bores formula the smallest.

There was a greater scatter among the recommendations for formulas for females of varying ages (Fig. 14-10) with clear zone diameters ranging from 3.5 to 4.5 mm for a 35-year-old female.

Corneal curvature. The effect of preoperative keratometry on selection of clear zone diameter is shown in Fig. 14-11. Neither the AMark nor the Kremer formulas use preoperative keratometry in the clear zone diameter prediction; therefore they both describe horizontal lines. With the DRS, Thornton, and to a lesser extent the Bores formulas, patients with flatter corneas require smaller clear zone diameters to get the predicted correction.

Intraocular pressure. The effect of preoperative intraocular pressure on selection of clear zone diameter is shown in Fig. 14-12. Only the Kremer formula shows a significant effect of intraocular pressure, suggesting a 3.5 mm diameter clear zone at 10 mm Hg and a 4.2 mm diameter at 24 mm Hg. The other formulas do not indicate a significant role of intraocular pressure, except for the Thornton guide, which increases the diameter 0.25 mm for pressures greater than 20 mm Hg. There is considerable spread in the diameter of the clear zone requested at any given intraocular pressure among the five formulas, ranging from 3.5 to 4.3 mm.

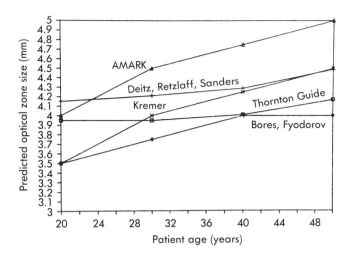

Figure 14-9

Comparison of five prediction programs in calculating the effect of age (in men) on clear zone diameter. (From Sanders DR: J Refract Surg 1985;1:116.)

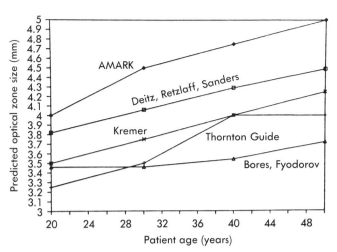

Figure 14-10

Comparison of five prediction programs in calculating the effect of age (in women) on clear zone diameter. (From Sanders DR: J Refract Surg 1985;1:116.)

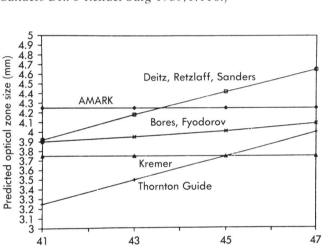

Figure 14-11

Comparison of five prediction programs in calculating the effect of preoperative keratometric measurements on predicted clear zone diameter. (From Sanders DR: J Refract Surg 1985;1:116.)

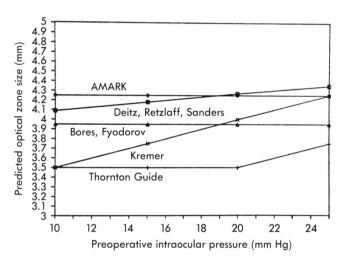

Figure 14-12

Comparison of various prediction programs in calculating the effect of preoperative intraocular pressure on predicted clear zone diameter. (From Sanders DR: J Refract Surg 1985;1:116.)

EVALUATION OF TWO DIRECTLY COMPARABLE PROGRAMS: DRS AND AMARK

The DRS and AMark programs can be compared retrospectively using an independent clinical series of radial keratotomy procedures without astigmatic correction. We have computed the decreases in myopia that each of the formulas would have predicted given the patient parameters and clear zones used in two series of radial keratotomy cases: Lindstrom's data—67 eyes with eight incisions—and Salz's data—96 eyes with eight incisions and 100 eyes with four incisions. Details have been published elsewhere.[22]

For purposes of comparison, we optimized the prediction of each formula. To optimize the DRS formula predictions, we computed the personalized depth fac-

Table 14-2

Depth Factors Used for Comparison of DRS and AMark Formulas

	DRS average depth factor (%)	AMark optimized depth factor (%)
Lindstrom	78	90
Salz 4 incision	74	90
Salz 8 incision	86	95

tor for each case and averaged these values (Table 14-2). Then we substituted the averaged value to determine the predicted decrease in myopia. To optimize the AMark data, we used the AMark software to compute predicted corrections for incisions with depths of 80%, 85%, 90%, and 95% and chose the best prediction based on percentage of cases whose actual corrections were within 0.50 D, 1.00 D, 1.50 D, and 2.00 D of predicted values.

Next we compared results for each of the series by using the percentage of cases whose actual corrections were within 0.50 D, 1.00 D, 1.50 D, and 2.00 D of predicted values (Table 14-3). We then computed the standard errors of the predictions and compared between the two formulas for each series. In this way we could evaluate the spread around the predictions. These evaluations were the basis of comparison for the DRS and AMark formulas. The average depth factors used to compute the optimized DRS predictions are presented in Table 14-2 along with the AMark optimized depth factors chosen as described.

Results of comparisons between the DRS and AMark formulas are presented in Tables 14-2 and 14-3 and in Figs. 14-13 to 14-15 for each of the case series.

Table 14-3

Prediction Accuracy of DRS and AMark Formulas in Three Series of Cases

Case series	Predicted interval of refractive correction (ID)	Percentage of cases within predicted interval	
		DRS formula	AMark formula (%)
Lindstrom	0.50	52	40
	1.00	85	77
	1.50	92	90
	2.00	97	94
Salz 4 incision	0.50	49	47
	1.00	80	76
	1.50	92	94
	2.00	96	96
Salz 8 incision	0.50	28	24
	1.00	57	55
	1.50	76	78
	2.00	85	92

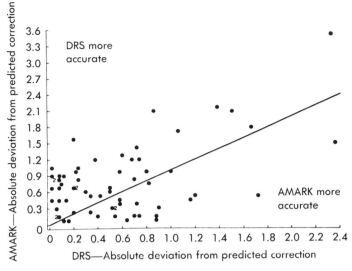

Figure 14-13
Comparison of the accuracy of the DRS (Deitz, Retzlaff, Sanders) and AMark formulas in predicting the outcome of a series of 67 radial keratotomy cases using eight incisions by Dr. Lindstrom. The oblique line represents the equivalence line. Circles indicate individual cases. Points with multiple cases are indicated by numbers. (Similar notations are used in Figs. 14-14 and 14-15.) The scattergram indicates the DRS formula was more accurate in this series of cases. (From Sanders DR, Deitz MR, Lindstrom RL, and Salz JJ: J Refract Surg 1986;2:120.)

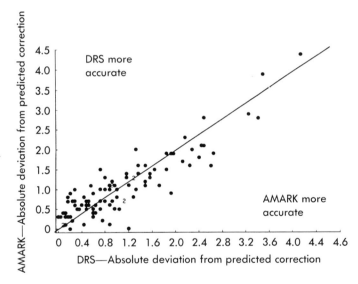

Figure 14-14
Scatterplot comparing the absolute deviation of actual correction predicted by the DRS and AMark formulas for a series of 98 radial keratotomy cases using eight incisions by Dr. Salz. Scattergram indicates a similar prediction by both formulas. (From Sanders DR, Deitz MR, Lindstrom RL, and Salz JJ: J Refract Surg 1986;2:121.)

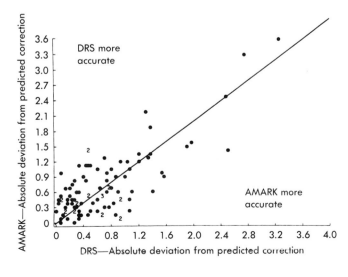

Figure 14-15
Scatterplot comparing the absolute deviation of actual correction as predicted by the DRS and AMark formulas in a series of 100 radial keratotomy cases using four incisions by Dr. Salz. The scattergram suggests a similar accuracy of prediction for both formulas. (From Sanders DR, Deitz MR, Lindstrom RL, and Salz JJ: J Refract Surg 1986;2:121.)

In Lindstrom's series, the DRS predictions were found to be consistently more accurate than the optimized AMark predictions (Fig. 14-13). Clinical corrections within 0.50 D and 1.00 D of the DRS predictions were found in 52% of the cases. The AMark predictions were 40% for 0.50 D and 77% for 1.00 D. Comparison of the standard errors of the two predictions [F test] showed that this difference in accuracy was significant [$p = <0.025$]).

With regard to Salz's series, the DRS and AMark formulas performed similarly with respect to accuracy of the predictions (Figs. 14-14 and 14-15 and Table 14-3). A slightly higher proportion of cases in the four- and eight-incision series had corrections within 0.50 D and 1.00 D of the DRS predictions than within 0.50 D and 1.00 D of the AMark predictions. However, the two predictions were not significantly different statistically with respect to accuracy or consistency.

In a separate evaluation of only the DRS formula,[21] we compared two series of Deitz's patients, one performed before the development of the DRS formula and the other performed using the DRS formula. The two series were compared using clinical refractive results. The use of the DRS formula resulted in a small increase in patients within 1.00 D of emmetropia (4%). However, use of the DRS formula decreased the proportion of cases deviating from emmetropia by more than 2.00 D by 75% (8% versus 2%) (Table 14-4).

Observations on comparison of formulas

Comparison of the five programs shows that there are more similarities than differences in the predicted outcomes. Where formulas differ, there is no way of knowing which method is most accurate because no method has been tested by many surgeons in many of the cases. The only published comparison of the use of different refractive keratotomy formulas by a single surgeon in similar groups of patients is that of Lavery,[13] who compared the nomograms of Sawelson, Thornton, and Ellis, as previously discussed.

One problem in testing or comparing the various formulas, with the exception of the AMark and DRS programs, is that there is no means of determining how accurate a method would have been if a surgeon did not follow exactly the surgical parameters recommended by the predictability program. Another problem is that surgeons sometimes use their clinical experience and intuition to modify the recommendations of the predictability formulas—even those surgeons who have developed their own formulas. Thus it is difficult to quantify the effect of the formula. Nevertheless, well-informed ophthalmologists can use comparisons of predictive accuracy among formulas, such as those described here, to help in the selection process.

Table 14-4

Postoperative Refractive Outcome in Series with and without Use of DRS Formula

Postoperative deviation from emmetropia	Deitz series 1 without DRS (12 months) (%)	Deitz series 2 with DRS (3 months) (%)
Within 1.00 D	76	80
>2.00 D	8	2
>3.00 D	2	1

Although none of the currently available predictability formulas can guarantee an accurate outcome, they can provide approximate figures on which surgeons can build and modify, based on their own experience.

NONCOMPUTERIZED REFRACTIVE KERATOTOMY NOMOGRAMS

Numerous nomograms have been published to guide surgeons in refractive keratotomy surgery. These have varied from the simple PERK nomogram in which the only patient variable used was the spherical equivalent of the cycloplegic refraction (Table 14-5) to highly complex nomograms that require multiple zones of deepening incisions. With the exception of the comparison of three nomograms by Lavery,[13] no critical comparison of the use of these nomograms in practice has been published.

The nomograms follow the same principles as the computerized formulas previously discussed. Indeed, the Thornton nomogram is a good example of how a simple table with a set of modifiers can be programmed into a computer.

Figs. 14-16 to 14-21 show a series of published nomograms without evaluative or comparative comment.

Preoperative Keratometry	Degree of Preoperative Myopia (Modified)								
	−1.50	−1.75	−2.00	−2.25	−2.62 to −3.00	−3.12 to −3.50	−3.62 to −4.00	−4.12 to −5.00	−5.12 to −6.00
41.00-43.00	4.50/4*	4.25/4	4.00/4	3.75/4	3.50/6	3.25/6	3.25/8	3.00/8	3.00/12
43.00-45.00	4.75/4	4.50/4	4.25/4	4.00/4	4.00/6	3.75/6	3.50/8	3.25/8	3.25/12
45.12-47.00	5.00/4	4.75/4	4.50/4	4.25/4	4.25/6	4.00/6	3.75/8	3.50/8	3.50/12

Modifiers:			
Age/Sex	M	20's	−0.75**
	F	20's	−1.00**
	(M/F)	30's	−0.50**
	(M/F)	>35	+0.00**
	(M/F) Early	40's	+0.50**
	(M/F) Late	40's	+1.00**
	(M/F)	50's	+1.50**
IOP	+0.20D/mmHg>17**		
	−0.20D/mmHg<14**		
Corneal Diameter	−0.50D if <11.5mm(H)**		
Corneal Thickness	+0.25D/10μ>.56**		
	−0.25D/10μ<.52**		

Assume:

1) Assume thinnest paracentral (100%) Add 10μ per 0.25mm O.Z. greater than 3.0mm O.Z.
2) Double-edged diamond blade
3) Thornton Ring Fixation
4) Expect −0.50D at 6 months postoperatively

---

* Number in front of slash represents proposed optical zone size
Number after slash represents number of incisions
** Add indicated value (+ or −) to preoperative myopia

Figure 14-16
The nomogram developed by Dr. Robert Hofmann for radial keratotomy. (From Hofmann RF and Lindstrom RL: In Sanders DR, editor: Radial keratotomy surgical techniques, Thorofare, NJ, 1986, Slack, Inc, p 40.)

Table 14-5

Assignment of Central Clear Zone Diameter Based on Preoperative Refraction in PERK Study*

Group	Spherical equivalent of the cycloplegic refraction (D)	Diameter of the central clear zone (mm)	No. of eyes (%)
Lower	−2.00 to −3.12	4.0	121 (30)
Middle	−3.25 to −4.37	3.5	135 (34)
Higher	−4.50 to −8.00	3.0	145 (36)
TOTAL			401

From Waring GO et al: Ophthalmology 1987;94:1339.
*All eyes had eight incisions. Patient age was not included in the calculations.

Keratometry	Myopia 1.50-2.11	2.12-2.61	2.62-3.11	3.12-3.73	3.74-4.36	4.37-5.11	5.12-6.11	6.12-8.00	>8.00
38.00-42.00	4.00(8) or 3.50(4)	3.75(8) or 3.50(6)	3.50(8) or 3.25(4)	3.25(8)	3.00(8)	3.00(8) redeepen peripheral 1/3	3.00(8) redeepen peripheral 1/2	3.00 16 cuts redeepen peripheral 1/2	3.00 16 cuts differential redeepen
42.12-44.00	4.25(8) or 3.50(4)	4.00(8) or 3.50(6)	3.75(8) or 3.50(6)	3.50(8)	3.25(8)	3.00(8)	3.00(8) redeepen peripheral 1/3	3.00 16 cuts	3.00 16 cuts differential redeepen 1/2
44.12-46.25	4.50(8) or 3.75(4)	4.25(8) or 3.75(6)	4.00(8) or 3.50(6)	3.75(8)	3.50(8)	3.25(8)	3.00(8)	3.00(8) redeepen peripheral 1/2	3.00 16 cuts redeepen peripheral 1/2 of 8 cuts
46.37-50.00	4.75(8) or 4.00(4)	4.50(8) or 3.75(4)	4.25(8) or 3.75(6)	4.00(8)	3.75(8)	3.50(8)	3.25(8)	3.00(8)	3.00 16 cuts redeepen peripheral 1/3 of 8 cuts

Note: Redeepening for higher powers should be carried to 95% of corneal thickness as measured by pachymetry in the mid-periphery and periphery (ie, essentially to Descemet's membrane).

Peripheral 1/3 = Begin cuts 2.5mm from the 3mm optical zone margin and carry to the limbus; that is, use an 8mm optical zone for the deepening cuts.

Peripheral 1/2 = Begin cuts 1.5mm from the 3mm optical zone margin and carry to the limbus; that is, use a 6mm optical zone for the deepening cuts.

Copyright 1981, 1982, 1984, 1986, Spencer P. Thornton, MD, FACS.

Figure 14-17
Thornton guide for optical zone size with four, six, eight, and sixteen incisions. For every year above age 30, subtract 2% from the myopic error to age 50 then 1% per year thereafter. For women patients, subtract 3 years from the age before calculating the myopic error. For every millimeter below 11, add 2% to the myopic refractive error. For every millimeter above 18, subtract 2% from the myopic refractive error. (From Hofmann RF and Lindstrom RL: In Sanders DR, editor: Radial keratotomy surgical techniques, Thorofare, NJ, 1986, Slack, Inc, p 42.)

Neumann Guide
Approximate Optical Zone (mm)*
Myopic Refractive Error
(Diopters: Use Minus Cylinder)

Keratometry (D)	1.50-2.00	2.25-3.00	3.25-4.00	4.25-5.00	5.25-6.00	6.00
41.00-42.00	4.00	3.50	3.00	2.75	**	***
42.25-44.00	4.25	3.75	3.25	3.00	**	***
44.25-46.00	4.50	4.00	3.50	3.25	3.00	***
46.25-48.00	5.00	4.50	4.00	3.50	3.00	***

Convert refraction to minus cylinder form and ignore cylinder component for optical zone determination.
* This guide assumes 8 incisions of 95% paracentral corneal thickness (front-cutting blade: 100% central specular microscopic pachymetry value)
** May require Fyodorov multiple depth incision or, rarely, a second set of 4 or 8 radial incisions.
*** 8 or 16 incisions and/or multiple depth required.

Schachar IOP Guide +

Preop	Add to Refraction	Preop	Add to Refraction
10	−3.00	15	−1.25
11	−2.75	16	−0.75
12	−2.25	17	−0.50
13	−2.00	18	−0.00
14	−1.50	21	+0.50
		22	+0.75

+ Add to the preoperative sphere values listed in the Neumann Guide before choosing the optical zone size.

Figure 14-18
Neumann and Schachar guides for radial keratotomy. (From Neumann AC and McCarty GC: In Sanders DR, editor: Radial keratotomy surgical techniques, Thorofare, NJ, 1986, Slack, Inc, p 75.)

Modifiers: To The Myopic Refractive Error in Minus Diopters, Add:

IOP		AGE			FOUR CUT GUIDE	
IOP	Modifier	Years	Male	Female	Original Modified Refractive Error	New Modified Refractive Error
12	-1.50	45 & over	+1.50	+1.25	-1.0	-1.67
14	-1.00	40	+1.00	+0.75	-1.5	-2.5
16	-0.50	35	+0.50	+0.25	-2.0	-3.37
18	-0.00	30	-0.00	-0.25	-2.5	-4.12
20	+0.25	25	-0.50	-0.75	-3.0	-5.00
22	+0.50	20	-1.00	-1.25	-3.5	-5.57

OPTIC ZONE SIZE IN MM					
Modified Refractive Error / K-Readings	1.5 / 2.0	2.12 / 3.0	3.12 / 4.0	4.12 / 5.0	5.12 / 6.0
41.00-42.00	4.00	3.50	3.00	** 3.00	*** 3.00
42.12-44.00	4.25	3.75	3.25	* 3.00	*** 3.00
44.12-46.00	4.5	4.00	3.50	* 3.25	** 3.00
46.12-48.00	5.00	4.50	4.00	3.50	** 3.00

REDEEPEN
One Step
* 4 Cuts
** 8 Cuts
Two Steps
*** 8 Cuts

Interpolation of values near borders of range is recommended.
After Neumann[5] and Thornton[11].

Figure 14-19
Tate nomogram for radial keratotomy. (From Tate GW: In Sanders DR, editor: Radial keratotomy surgical techniques, Thorofare, NJ, 1986, Slack, Inc, p 95.)

Radial Keratotomy Technique

Assumptions: 90% achieved depth, centrifugal incision, noncycloplegic refraction
Factors considered: Refractive error, age, gender, intraocular pressure, corneal thickness
Factors not considered: Corneal diameter, keratometry

Refractive error (working sphere)	Number of incisions	Optical zone		
−0.50	3	5.00		
−0.75	3	4.50		
−1.00	6	4.50		
−1.25	6	4.25		
−1.50	6	4.00		
−2.00	8	4.00		
−2.50	8	3.75		
−3.00	8	3.50		
−3.50	8	3.25		
−4.00	8	3.00		
−4.50	8	3.00	5.00	
−5.00	8	3.00	5.00	7.00
−5.50	8	3.00	5.00	7.00
−6.00	16	3.00	5.00	
−6.50	16	3.00	5.00	7.00
−7.00	16	3.00	5.00	7.00
−7.50	16	3.00	5.00	7.00

Age factor

Age	18-23	24-27	28-31	32-34	35-37	38-41	42-45	46-48	49-53	54-57	58 and above
0− −2.00	−.75	−.50	0	+.25	+.50	+.75	+1.00	+1.25	+1.50	+1.50	+1.75
−2.25− −4.75	−1.0	−.50	0	+.25	+.50	+.75	+1.00	+1.25	+1.50	+1.50	+1.75
−5.00 + more	−1.5	−.75	−.25	0	+.50	+.50	+1.00	+1.25	+1.50	+1.50	+1.75

Corneal thickness factor

If central corneal thickness is less than 0.49 mm, add −0.50 D to refractive error if original refractive error is −2.00 D or greater. If central thickness is greater than 0.57 mm, add +0.50 to refractive error.

Intraocular pressure factor

Add −0.25 D for every 2 mm Hg less than 15 mm Hg. If intraocular pressure is greater than 22 mm Hg, control it as appropriate and consider undercorrection.

Gender factor

Females: Age 24 to 34 add −0.50 D to refractive error.

Figure 14-20
Nordan nomogram of radial keratotomy. (Courtesy Lee Nordan, M.D., October 1985.)

Parameter Selection Table for Standard Radial Keratotomy Procedure

Myopia (D)	Age (yr)	Optical zone(mm)	Number of incisions	Peripheral redeepening
1	18 to 25	4.50	4	No
1	26 to 35	4.75	4	No
1	36 to 40	5.00	4	No
1	Over 40	5.00	4	No
1.5	18 to 25	4.25	4	No
1.5	26 to 35	4.50	4	No
1.5	36 to 40	4.75	4	No
1.5	Over 40	4.75	4	No
2	18 to 25	4.00	4	No
2	26 to 35	4.25	4	No
2	36 to 40	4.50	4	No
2	Over 40	4.75	4	No
2.5	18 to 25	3.75	4	No
2.5	26 to 35	4.00	4	No
2.5	36 to 40	4.25	4	No
2.5	Over 40	4.50	4	No
3	18 to 25	3.50	4	No
3	26 to 35	3.50	4	No
3	36 to 40	3.75	4	No
3	Over 40	4.00	4	No
3.5	18 to 25	3.25	6	No
3.5	26 to 35	3.50	6	No
3.5	36 to 40	3.75	6	No
3.5	Over 40	3.75	6	No
4	18 to 25	3.25	8	No
4	26 to 35	3.25	8	No
4	36 to 40	3.75	8	No
4	Over 40	3.75	8	No
4.5	18 to 25	3.25	8	No
4.5	26 to 35	3.25	8	No
4.5	36 to 40	3.75	8	No
4.5	Over 40	3.75	8	No
5	18 to 25	3.25	8	No
5	26 to 35	3.25	8	No
5	36 to 40	3.25	8	No
5	Over 40	3.50	8	No
5.5	18 to 25	3.00	8	No
5.5	26 to 35	3.25	8	No
5.5	36 to 40	3.25	8	No
5.5	Over 40	3.25	8	No
6	18 to 25	3.00	8	No
6	26 to 35	3.00	8	No
6	36 to 40	3.00	8	No
6	Over 40	3.00	8	No
6.5	18 to 25	3.00	8	Yes
6.5	26 to 35	3.00	8	Yes
6.5	36 to 40	3.00	8	Yes
6.5	Over 40	3.00	8	No
7	18 to 25	3.00	8	Yes
7	26 to 35	3.00	8	Yes
7	36 to 40	3.00	8	Yes
7	Over 40	3.00	8	Yes
7.5	18 to 25	3.00	8	Yes
7.5	26 to 35	3.00	8	Yes
7.5	36 to 40	3.00	8	Yes
7.5	Over 40	3.00	8	Yes

Figure 14-21
Ellis parameter selection table for determining optical zone size at an incisional depth of 90% to 95% of corneal thickness. (From Ellis W: Radial keratotomy and astigmatism surgery, Irvine, Calif, 1986, Medical Aesthetics, Inc, Keith Terry & Assoc, p 39.)

Peripheral redeepening is started from an optical zone of 6 mm and extended to the limbus. All cuts 90% to 95% depth at optical zone border. Never do more than eight initial cuts. If more are required, do them 3 months later.

UNFINISHED BUSINESS

The most daunting practical challenge for the surgeon seeking a preoperative planning nomogram or formula is to know which variables should be used in the formula. This chapter amply demonstrates differences of opinion, some formulas even calling for information that apparently is not used. Although most surgeons agree that preoperative myopia and patient age are indispensable variables for planning, the role of central keratometry, patient sex, intraocular pressure, corneal thickness, and other variables have not been well established, as discussed in Chapter 13, Predictability of Refractive Keratotomy. How can the surgeon decide what variables to use for preoperative planning? The information presented in this chapter represents a useful theoretical comparison of the different radial keratotomy nomograms, formulas, and computer programs. There are no clinical studies in which an individual surgeon has used the same instruments to compare two different programs or nomograms. There are few clinical studies in which specific variables are used in one series of eyes and not in another series to see if they make a difference. Thus potential users of nomograms should be highly critical of the information in them and require a reasonable demonstration of its usefulness.

Until there is more standardization of instruments so that surgeons can be assured of making the exact length and depth of incisions, computerized programs and nomograms will remain only useful starting points that individual surgeons will modify based on their own experience. The "universal" formula has yet to be devised.

REFERENCES

1. Arrowsmith PN and Marks RG: Evaluating the predictability of radial keratometry, Ophthalmology 1985;92:331-338.
2. Arrowsmith PN and Marks RG: Four-year update on predictability of radial keratometry, J Refract Surg 1988;4:37-45.
3. Arrowsmith PN, Sanders DR, and Marks RG: Visual, refractive, and keratometric results of radial keratometry, Arch Ophthalmol 1983;101:873-881.
4. Bores LD, Myers WD, and Cowden J: Radial keratotomy: an analysis of the American experience, Ann Ophthalmol 1981;13:941-948.
5. Cowden JW: Radial keratotomy: a retrospective study of cases observed at the Kresge Eye Institute for six months, Arch Ophthalmol 1982;100:578-580.
6. Cowden J and Bores L: A clinical investigation of the surgical correction of myopia by the method of Fyodorov, Ophthalmology 1981;88:737-741.
7. Deitz M, Sanders DR, and Marks R: Radial keratotomy: an overview of the Kansas City study, Ophthalmology 1984;91(5):467-477.
8. Fyodorov S: Surgical correction of myopia and astigmatism. In Schachar RA, Levy NS, and Schachar L, eds: Keratorefraction, 1980, Denison, Tex, LAL Publishing, pp 141-170.
9. Grady FJ: Experience with radial keratotomy, Ophthalmic Surg 1982;13:395-399.

10. Hoffer KJ, Darin JJ, Pettit TH, et al: UCLA clinical trial of radial keratotomy, Ophthalmology 1981;88:729-736.
11. Kogan L: Advantages of shallow radial keratotomy incisions cited, IOL & Ocular Surgery News 1984;2(7):1.
12. Kremer FB and Steer RA: Prediction of refractive correction with radial keratotomy, Ann Ophthalmol 1985;17:660-663.
13. Lavery FL: Comparative results of 200 consecutive radial keratometry cases using three different nomograms, J Refract Surg 1987;3:88-91.
14. Nirankari VS, Katzen LE, Richards RD, et al: Prospective clinical study of radial keratotomy, Ophthalmology 1982;89:677-683.
15. Rowsey JJ and Balyeat HD: Preliminary results and complications of radial keratotomy, Am J Ophthalmol 1982;93:437-455.
16. Salz JJ: A consumer's guide to radial keratotomy predictive software, J Refract Surg 1985;1:60-69.
17. Salz J: Thirty-two many, IOL Ocular Surgery News 1984; 2(11):4 (editorial).
18. Sanders DR: Computerized RK predictability programs. In Sanders DR, Hofmann RF, and Salz JJ, editors: Refractive corneal surgery, Thorofare, NJ, 1985, Slack, Inc, pp 91-107.
19. Sanders DR: Computerized radial keratometry predictability programs, J Refract Surg 1985;1:109-117.

20. Sanders DR, editor: Radial keratotomy: ARK study group, Thorofare, NJ, 1984, Slack, Inc.
21. Sanders DR, Deitz MR, and Gallagher D: Factors affecting predictability of radial keratotomy, Ophthalmology 1985; 92:1237-1243.
22. Sanders DR, Deitz MR, Lindstrom RL, and Salz JJ: Computer-aided radial keratotomy predictability programs: comparison of DRS and AMark formulas, J Refract Surg 1986;2:119-123.
23. Sanders DR, Retzlaff J, and Deitz MR: Deitz-Retzlaff-Sanders (DRS) formulas: determination of radial keratometry surgical parameters, J Refract Surg 1985;1:75-79.
24. Thornton SP: Thornton guide for radial keratotomy incision in optical zone size, J. Refract Surg 1985;1:28-51.
25. Waring GO, Lynn MJ, Gelender H, et al: Results of the Prospective Evaluation of Radial Keratotomy (PERK) study one year after surgery, Ophthalmology 1985;92:177-198.
26. Waring GO, Lynn MS, Culbertson N, et al: Three-year results of the Prospective Evaluation of Radial Keratotomy (PERK) study, Ophthalmology 1987; 94:1339-1354.
27. Waring GO, Moffitt SD, Gelender H, et al: Rationale for and design of the National Eye Institute Prospective Evaluation of Radial Keratotomy (PERK) study, Ophthalmology 1983;90:40-58.

Surgery

Surgical Instruments Used in Refractive Keratotomy

Spencer P. Thornton
Susanne K. Gardner
George O. Waring III

We discuss here the surgical instruments used for refractive keratotomy. In this chapter we also discuss the fundamental principles of the instruments to help surgeons choose intelligently among new designs and alternatives. However, we have not done side-by-side clinical testing, as one might find in *Consumer Reports.* The box on p. 408 provides a checklist for the types of instruments needed for keratotomy.

Because there are no industrial standards for the manufacture of refractive keratotomy instruments, there is an expected lack of uniformity. Therefore we emphasize continuously that each set of surgical instruments has its own per-

BACKGROUND AND ACKNOWLEDGMENTS
We have drawn on numerous sources for the information in this chapter. Many individuals in the instrument manufacturing industry have contributed information. Where a specific instrument or manufacturer is discussed or illustrated, the source of the information and instrument is cited. In addition, numerous individuals have contributed details and background information on instruments that would not be readily available otherwise. These include Magnum Diamond, Inc., Mr. William Knepshield, Jr., of KMI, Inc., Mr. Bill Ballard of LAB Instruments, Mr. Keith Yeisley of Metico Instruments, and Mr. Earl Henderson of DGH, Inc.

Whenever evaluation of commercially available instruments is undertaken, there is always the danger of favoritism, loss of objectivity, inaccurate information, and out-of-date information. We have sought to avoid these pitfalls as rigorously as possible. We have tried to fairly represent different styles of instruments and different manufacturers, without being mindlessly exhaustive. We have double-checked information as carefully as possible, although in many cases we have had to simply take the word of manufacturers for technical parameters. We have tried to present the information in a way that does not endorse or denigrate any specific product, but objectively evaluates design and performance. We are aware that by the time this information is published, some of it will be out-of-date. It is thus up to the reader to critically evaluate what we present on instruments used for refractive keratotomy and draw personal conclusions.

Dr. Thornton has presented descriptions of diamond knives and pachometers in previous publications, and these are extensively updated here. Of course, we have drawn as extensively as possible on published scientific literature concerning instruments.

Instruments and Supplies Used for Refractive Keratotomy Performed Under Topical Anesthesia

Surgical instruments

Operating microscope
Ultrasonic pachometer and calibration device
Wire eyelid speculum
Centering device
Blunt intraocular lens (IOL) hook (center marker)
Circular zone markers
Incision pattern markers
Astigmatism axis protractor and markers
Micrometer crystal-bladed knife
Knife gauge block or calibration microscope
Fixation forceps or ring
Instrument tray

Instruments available for suturing perforation

Needle holder
0.12-mm toothed forceps
Tying forceps
10-0 nylon suture

Supplies

Written surgical plan
Preoperative sedative (as needed)
Oxygen mask, tubing, and source
Sterile preparation, drapes, gowns, and gloves
Topical anesthetic (for example, 0.5% proparacaine)
Fine-tipped methylene blue marking pen (if used)
Surgical microsponges
Hydrogen peroxide and distilled water (to clean diamond)
Balanced salt solution
Small syringe
Cannulas, 19 and 30 gauge
Topical antibiotic solution
Eye pads (optional) and shield
Oral analgesics and sedatives after surgery

sonality. Even in the hands of the same surgeon under the same operating conditions, different brands and styles of pachometers, knives, and fixation devices will create different types of incisions with different clinical results. For example, the surgeon who uses a pachometer that gives relatively thick measurements, a zone marker whose diameters are slightly larger than stated, a knife that cuts relatively shallowly, and a fixation device that minimally elevates the intraocular pressure during surgery is likely to get less correction than a surgeon who uses a group of instruments with biases in the opposite direction.

Thus surgeons must know not only the effect of their surgical plan and manual techniques, but also the individual characteristics of their instruments.[11] Indeed instruments with identical designs should be numbered separately, by either the manufacturer or the surgeon so that some adjustment can be made for individual performance.

MEASUREMENT OF CORNEAL THICKNESS

Instruments designed to measure corneal thickness enhance our understanding and management of disorders of the corneal endothelium, such as Fuchs' endothelial dystrophy, trauma from cataract surgery, contact lens wear, and penetrating keratoplasty. However, corneal pachometry became a more integral part of clinical practice when radial keratotomy and other types of refractive surgery made accurate measurement of corneal thickness a necessity (Fig. 15-1).

Terminology

Etymologically, pachometer comes from the Greek terms *pachy* (thick) and *metron* (to measure). Pachometer can also be spelled *pachymeter,* and both spellings are acknowledged by the *Oxford English Dictionary.* The spelling, *pachometer,* was introduced into ophthalmology by David Maurice[16,19] on the advice of Sir Stuart Duke-Elder, who was a classical scholar. Sir Stuart preferred to derive the term from the Greek noun for thickness, πάοσ, rather than the Greek adjective for thick, παχθσ. The adjective form is used most commonly, as in pachyderm, because the adjective "thick" describes the suffix noun "skin." In considering the term "pachometer," it is not the meter that is thick but rather the meter that measures the thickness; therefore the noun form pachometer seems preferable, as pointed out by Maurice.

Corneal thickness measurements can be expressed in millimeters (for example, 0.52 mm) or in microns (for example, 520 μm). Optical pachometry values have conventionally been expressed in millimeters because they are accurate to .01 mm, but with the increased precision of ultrasonic pachometry and the accuracy sought in refractive surgery, expressing values in microns is preferable as long as one remembers that the variability in measurements in microns is on the order of 10 μm, not 1 μm.

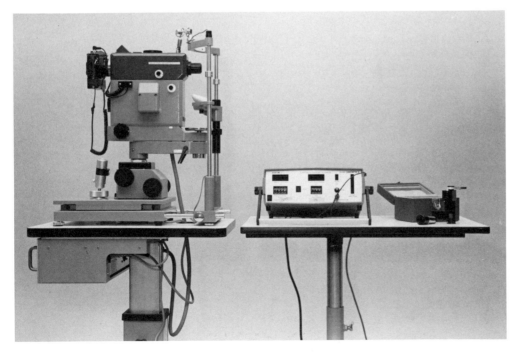

Figure 15-1
Three types of instruments used to measure corneal thickness. Left to right: specular microscope, ultrasonic pachometer, optical pachometer.

Methods of measuring corneal thickness

There are three contemporary methods of measuring corneal thickness: specular microscopy, optical pachometry, and ultrasonic pachometry (Fig. 15-1). An ideal pachometer includes accurate reading of the corneal thickness; reproducible measurements by all trained operators; ease of operation that avoids adjustments, alignments, or manual recording of the readings; portability for use in the office or operating room; ability to be used by one unassisted person; and durability with adequate warranty and repair service.

The oldest method of measuring corneal thickness is specular microscopy, which focuses the instrument on the anterior and posterior surfaces of the cornea and measures the distance traversed. This method may be complicated by changes in the refractive index of the cornea. The technique is described by Mishima and Hedbys.[18] Modern specular microscopes are fitted with a digital readout that records the corneal thickness. This can be used in radial keratotomy by measuring the corneal thickness before surgery, but it is difficult to know exactly where the reading was taken. Specular microscopes are impractical for use in the operating room. We do not discuss specular microscope pachometry further.

Optical pachometers have been used clinically since 1949, using principles recognized by Helmholz. Repeated precise measurements of the corneal thickness require great attention to detail, including standardizing the conditions of use of the pachometer and using auxiliary alignment lights. Even with these precautions, errors among observers can be up to 0.02 mm (Table 15-1). Optical pachometry is discussed later.

The ultrasonic pachometer, developed by Henderson, Gillian, Detweiler, and Kremer in 1980,[12,13] is currently the preferred method of measuring corneal thickness for keratotomy because of its ease of use, precision, portability, and ability to measure corneal thickness eccentrically. Therefore this is the method discussed in detail here.

Normal corneal thickness

Optical pachometry served as the standard for measuring normal corneal thickness, and the reported values in the literature are remarkably consistent (Table 15-2). Five different studies using five different optical pachometers all

Table 15-1

Comparison of Three Instruments Used for the Clinical Measurement of Corneal Thickness

	Ultrasonic	Optical	Specular microscope
Accuracy by one observer	Good	Good	Good
Repeatability of measurements by multiple observers	Good	Fair	Fair
Endpoint measurement	Electronic	Visual	Visual
Difficulty of use	Least	Most	Middle
Location of reliable measurements	Entire cornea	Central	Central
Portability	Good	Poor (slit-lamp microscope required)	Poor (specular microscope required)
Cost	Middle	Least	Most

showed mean central corneal thickness values of 0.51 to 0.52 mm (standard deviation, .02 to .04 mm). Kremer's original calibration for the ultrasonic pachometer settled on a speed of sound in the cornea of 1640 m/sec, which corresponded to central average thickness readings of 0.512 ± 0.035 mm in 175 eyes.[13] Subsequent studies of corneal thickness measurements by ultrasonic pachometry show more variation as indicated by the comparison of nine different pachometers by Reader and Salz[25] (Tables 15-2 and 15-3); the most frequently obtained central thickness readings are between 0.52 and 0.54 mm.

Novak and colleagues[21] compared optical (Haag-Streit 900 with Mishima-Hedbys attachment), specular microscopic (PRO-Koester), and ultrasonic (Accutome, 1630 ± 10 m/sec) pachometry in 93 consecutive patients in the PERK study, using the mean value of three central corneal thickness measurement readings for each instrument on each eye. Mean values were: optical, 0.554 ±0.028 mm; specular microscopy, 0.551 ±0.037 mm; and ultrasound 0.542 ±0.035 mm. Analysis of variance showed no significant difference between the optical and specular readings ($p > 0.05$) but significant differences between the ultrasonic pachometer and the optical and specular microscopic instruments ($p < 0.0001$). To make the ultrasonic readings consistent with the two specular readings, the velocity of sound in the cornea would have to be increased from the standard 1640 m/sec to approximately 1670 m/sec. The consequence of an ultrasonic corneal reading 10 μm thinner than presumed normal might be an increased incidence of corneal perforation during keratotomy surgery. The accuracy and precision of ultrasonic pachometers has been evaluated by Salz and Thornton.[28,34]

Ultrasonic pachometry

Principles of ultrasonic pachometer function. An ultrasonic pachometer uses the principles of A-scan ultrasonography.[2] The basic component is an electronic pulser that provides short voltage pulses. A piezoelectric crystal changes its shape with each electronic pulse and generates an ultrasonic pulse that is propagated through the cornea, reflected off Descemet's membrane, and received back by the piezoelectric crystal. The impact of the ultrasonic waves on the crystal deform it once again, generating an electronic pulse that is sent to a receiver, where it is detected, amplified, and then displayed on an oscilloscope screen or registered on a digital display. The frequency of the excitation voltages deter-

---

Table 15-2

Human Central Corneal Thicknesses Reported in the Literature

Author	Year	Corneal thickness (mm), x ± SD	Eyes measured	Pachometer used
Von Bahr	1948	0.565 ±0.035	224	Von Bahr
Maurice and Giardini	1951	0.507 ±0.028	44	Maurice and Giardini
Lavernge and Kelcom	1962	0.51 ±0.04	198	Goldmann
Donaldson	1965	0.518 ±0.041	268	Donaldson
Mishima and Hedbys	1968	0.518 ±0.02	40	Haag-Streit
Kremer et al	1983	0.512 ±0.035	175	Kremer ultrasonic

From Kremer FB, Walton P, and Genshimer G: Ann Ophthalmol 1985;17:506-507.
SD, Standard deviation.

mines the frequency with which the transducer surface vibrates back and forth. Using high frequencies near 10 MHz and small wavelengths near 150 μm gives better resolution.

The instrument functions by measuring the amount of time (transit time) needed for the ultrasound pulse to pass from the end of the transducer to Descemet's membrane and back to the transducer. This creates the following basic relationship: transit time in seconds = 2 × the thickness of the cornea in meters divided by the ultrasonic propagation velocity in the cornea in meters per second:

$$T \ (\text{sec}) = \frac{2 \times \text{thickness (m)}}{C \ (\text{m/sec})}$$

The ultrasound waves travel through the cornea at a speed *(C)* that is determined by the density and the compressibility of the cornea—the velocity of propagation. Since the cornea is 78% water, it exhibits a relatively slow propagation velocity of approximately 1600 m/sec. The propagation velocity of water is 1524 m/sec. In contrast, the propagation velocity in a dense, noncompressible substance, such as steel, is approximately 6000 m/sec.

Thus it is important that the propagation velocity of the cornea be known accurately because this variable can be set on many ultrasonic pachometers, and different settings will change the apparent thickness of the cornea:

$$\text{Corneal thickness} = \frac{\text{Transit time} \times \text{propagation velocity}}{2}$$

Thus setting the "speed of sound in the cornea" at 1000 m/sec on the pachometer will give a reading half as thick as a setting of 2000 m/sec. That is, the faster the speed of sound is thought to travel in the cornea, the thicker the cornea will appear.

Speed of sound in the cornea. One of the difficult problems in standardizing ultrasonic pachometry is deciding the propagation velocity (speed) of sound in the cornea. The current standard is 1640 m/sec. Numerous velocities of sound ranging from 1550 to 1639 m/sec have been reported for the cornea in cows, pigs, and humans as summarized by Coleman.[2] The best measurements in humans show a value of 1639 m/sec.[36,38] Kremer[13] selected 1640 m/sec because that measurement gave corneal thickness readings of 0.512 ±0.035 in 175 eyes, which agrees with that reported with optical pachometry. The laboratory research of Dybbs and colleagues[1,10] documented a propagation velocity of 1636 m/sec (see the box on p. 413). A value of 1640 m/sec was used in the instruments in the PERK study.

The speed of sound in the cornea is higher than the 1550 m/sec value used for the whole eye in intraocular lens calculations. The lower value for the whole eye stems in large part from the slower propagation velocity of sound in the vitreous.

Practical clinical interpretation of ultrasonic corneal pachometry measurements. The variability in corneal thickness measurements by different ultrasonic pachometers leads to several conclusions. The measurement of optical pachometry should be still considered the standard reference value, 510 to 520 μm. The speed of sound in the cornea should be considered 1636 to 1640 m/sec. Although it would be ideal for surgeons to know whether their pachometers tend to read thinner or thicker than these normal values, that is difficult information to determine. Manufacturers do not provide it; there are no industry standards for ultrasonic pachometers to which the surgeon can refer. Most surgeons have

Determination of the Speed of Sound in the Cornea

A-mode ultrasonography provides a convenient means of measuring corneal thickness. To determine the central corneal thickness, the ultrasonic beam is aligned precisely perpendicular to the central corneal surface. Ultrasonic echoes are obtained from the anterior and posterior surface of the cornea. The time interval between the corneal echoes can be used to determine the corneal thickness if the ultrasonic speed of propagation in the cornea is known. The corneal thickness is the speed of sound in the cornea multiplied by the time interval between corneal echoes divided by 2. The factor of 2 arises, since T represents the round-trip transit time. The accuracy of the thickness determination is predominantly limited by the accuracy of the assumed speed of sound in the cornea. Currently it is not possible to measure the acoustic velocity in the cornea in vivo, so investigators have employed in vitro techniques on excised corneas.

Human eye bank corneas and rabbit corneas were removed as corneoscleral shells and placed in moisture chambers using balanced salt solution as the medium at a temperature of 34° C. Twenty-eight data points were obtained from four human corneas and 52 data points were obtained from 15 rabbit corneas. Each individual cornea was used for several data points, so the speed of sound was determined over a relatively wide range of hydration. The hydration of the cornea was determined by the tonicity of the bathing medium, but the hydration was not measured directly. The time of arrival difference for ultrasonic pulses traveling from the anterior to the posterior surface of the cornea was chosen as the independent variable for the velocity measurements. Once the speed of sound in the cornea was determined for a particular time of arrival difference measurement, the corneal thickness was calculated from the foregoing equation.

Table 15-3

Relationship Between Time of Arrival Difference (TOAD), Thickness, Hydration, and Speed of Sound in the Human Cornea

TOAD (ns)	Thickness (mm)	Hydration (mg water/mg dry wt)	Speed of sound (m/sec)
550	0.456	2.58	1656
600	0.493	2.84	1644
650	0.531	3.11	1633
700	0.568	3.37	1624
750	0.606	3.64	1616

Modified from Lazzara SC, Dybbs A, Hazony D, and Greber I: The ultrasonic measurement of corneal thickness, Detroit, 1983, Case Western Reserve University.

When the corneal thickness was plotted against the time of arrival difference for the human cornea, a regression analysis yielded $t = 0.000752 \, T_1 + 0.042$, in which t represents the corneal thickness and T_1 time of arrival difference. The correlation coefficient for the points fitted to this line is 0.999, indicating an extraordinarily good correlation. Thus the speed of sound in the human cornea varied from 1616 to 1656 m/sec for the range of hydration that occurs in vivo.

The average speed of sound in the human cornea is 1636 m/sec. Errors incurred by changes of hydration in the normal range are insignificant, and only for very dehydrated or edematous corneas does the error amount to more than 1% of the total thickness. The assumption of a constant speed of sound of 1636 m/sec can result in a maximum error of 1.8%. If variations with hydration are accounted for, the human corneal thickness can be determined to within $\pm 0.4\%$.

The authors concluded that A-mode ultrasound should provide a more accurate and reproducible means of clinically measuring corneal thickness than was previously possible with optical methods.

Modified from Lazzara SC, Dybbs A, Hazony D, and Greber I: The ultrasonic measurement of corneal thickness: the effects of hydration on the speed of sound in the cornea, unpublished thesis, Detroit, 1983, Department of Mechanical and Aerospace Engineering, Case Western Reserve University.

neither the time nor the willingness to calibrate their ultrasonic pachometers against an optical pachometer or a specular microscope. Therefore most surgeons follow the manufacturer's instructions for calibrating the instrument and interpreting their own clinical experience, employing the following fudge factors:

1. Changing the setting for the speed of sound in the cornea on the instrument; for example, if microperforations occur too frequently during keratotomy surgery, the speed of sound on the instrument could be decreased from 1640 to 1630 m/sec, which would give an apparent thinner measurement and result in setting the knife blade shorter.
2. Employing a bias factor in setting the length of the knife blade; for example, if corneal perforation is occurring too frequently with the knife blade set at 110% of the paracentral corneal thickness reading, the knife blade would be set at 105% or 100% of the reading.

(Of course, there are other reasons for frequent corneal perforation.) Unfortunately, this type of trial-and-error calibration of instruments in refractive surgery ("microsurgery") reflects the lack of industry standards and the variation in surgical technique among surgeons.

Is accuracy in measuring the corneal thickness more important than accuracy in executing the incisions with a diamond knife? Using modern techniques, the manual execution of the incisions is more important. Ultrasonic pachometers can repeatedly measure the thickness of the cornea in the same area with a precision of approximately ± 2 μm. Therefore once surgeons have decided on the proper settings for their pachometers and the proper settings for their knife blades, they can be reasonably assured of repeatability (precision) in the measurements. This potential error of 4 μm is approximately 0.4% of the average central corneal thickness of 0.52 mm. This is far less a variation than achieved in the depth of keratotomy incisions. Therefore as Hofmann and Lindstrom[11] emphasize it is the variability in manual technique and the knife blade that is more important than the variation in the ultrasonic pachometry readings.

Components of ultrasonic pachometers. Ultrasonic pachometers generally consist of three major components: the probe handle with its transducer and tip; the housing of the instrument; and accessories and convenience features. The surgeon should not confuse the highly advertised accessories and convenience features with the most important aspects—the handle and the fundamental components in the housing.

Pachometer probe handle. The ultrasound mechanism is contained in the pachometer probe handle and has the piezoelectric crystal that emits an ultrasonic beam of approximately 20 MHz (less in some instances). All probes are hand held; smaller and lighter probes are easier to use clinically. Visualization of the tip of a straight probe is sometimes difficult under the operating microscope; angled probe handles allow viewing down the tip of the probe with the handle out of the way to help ensure perpendicular application to the corneal surface. Some handles contain a digital readout so that the surgeon can see the results without searching for the console (Fig. 15-2).

Transducer. The transducer sends the beam of ultrasound waves through the probe tip into the cornea and receives them on return. The width of the transducer beam is related to the size of the emitting crystal and the width and configuration of the probe through which it passes. A wide probe tip and a wide transducer beam reduce the accuracy of the corneal thickness reading at a single point.

The transducer is not usually fragile but has a limited lifetime of approximately 150 to 200 cases, after which it loses some of its accuracy and precision,

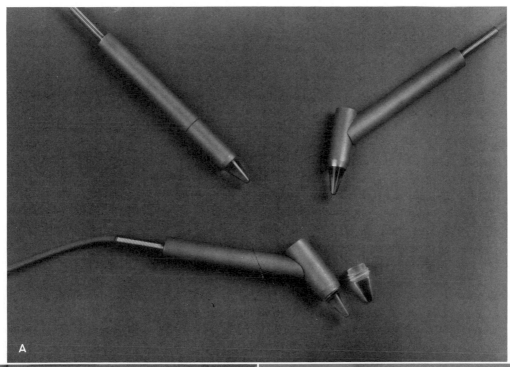

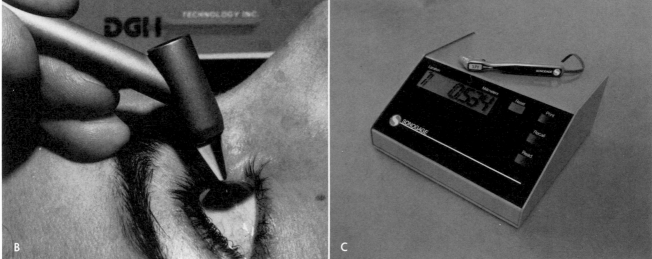

Figure 15-2
Probe handles and tips. **A,** DGH ultrasonic pachometer. Upper left: Straight probe. Upper right: Angled probe. Below: Tip removed to show need for periodic refilling of gel coupling. Company has since introduced completely solid-tip probe without gel coupling. **B,** Angled probe handle is easily held and improves the tip on the cornea under the operating microscope. **C,** Sonogage II handle has digital readout.

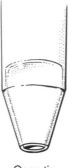
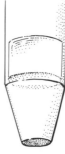
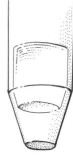

Open tip
water replaceable

Solid tip
gel replaceable

Solid probe
couplant permanent

Figure 15-3
Three types of ultrasonic pachometry probe tips.

Figure 15-4
Open tip Accutome probe shows air bubble *(arrow)* in chamber and small-gauge cannula used to refill the tip.

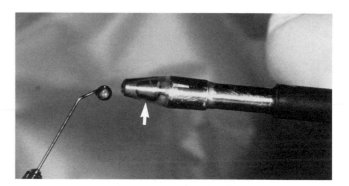

especially in the thicker peripheral cornea. When readings become increasingly variable on the calibration block, the probe should be changed.

Probe tip. The probe tip is the interface between the cornea and the transducer. The ultrasonic beam has a limited spread that is affected by the geometry of the probe tip. The transducer focuses the beam at a point beyond the probe tip. The internal steepness of the walls, the probe diameter, and its configuration all contribute to the internal reflections of the beam and its ultimate focusing point. Therefore the material in the probe tip should not attenuate the ultrasound beam, and the geometric design of the probe tip should facilitate its optimal transmission.

The diameter of the tip should be 2 mm or less to diminish the area over which the ultrasound beam is spread and to allow the observer to see exactly where the tip is placed on the cornea. The surface of the tip should be smooth so that the corneal epithelium is not damaged.

Three basic probe designs in current use (Fig. 15-3) are the open, water-filled type that requires frequent refilling; the solid tip containing an internal fluid reservoir that is refilled periodically; and the all-solid probe with no internal reservoir and no refilling. Each can provide accurate and precise measurements, but convenience and practicality vary.

The open, water-filled tips were used in earlier designs because they provided an accurate echo response with a good standoff and coupling. They are inconvenient to use, however, because as fluid is pulled out of the tip by surface tension and capillary action, air bubbles enter and give erroneous readings (Fig. 15-4). Even though the tips are easily refilled using a blunt 30-gauge cannula on a small syringe, they have almost disappeared from use, being replaced by solid-tip probes.

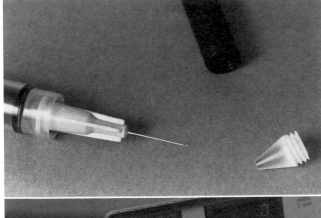

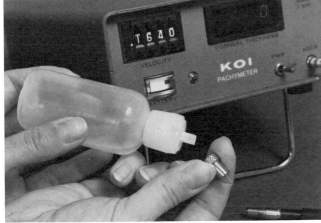

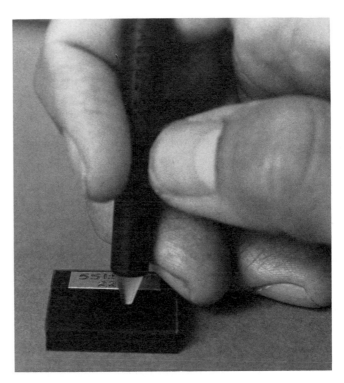

Figure 15-5
A, Probe handle from Humphrey shows the applanation tip removed and the syringe loaded with coupling gel, which would be injected into the end of the handle, free of bubbles, before the applanation tip is screwed back into place. **B,** Solid-tipped KOI pachometer probe being filled with coupling fluid.

Figure 15-6
Humphrey straight ultrasonic solid-tipped pachometer probe being applied to test block to verify accuracy of reading.

The solid-tipped probes contain a replaceable couplant (gel or oil) and are more convenient (Fig. 15-5). The frequency of refilling varies from once a week to once a year, depending on the design. The Teknar Ophthasonic pachometer has an oil interface that needs to be checked only about once a year. The CooperVision KOI 3000X has a water interface that requires periodic maintenance. The DGH unit with its gel interface can easily be changed by the user; the need to add more gel is indicated automatically by the unit.

The all-solid tip probes eliminate replaceable couplants. These tips, made of a polystyrene, are more convenient to handle and require less maintenance (Fig. 15-6). Instruments with an all-solid tip probe include the Accutome Corneometer, Pach-Pen, Sonogage, and Humphrey pachometers.

Cleanliness of probe tips. Solid-tipped probes require cleaning following the same precepts as those for tonometers. The probe should be wiped with alcohol or peroxide at the end of each use. Prophylaxis against the inadvertent spreading of human immunodeficiency virus through the tears must be kept in mind; standards in the profession for management of instruments that contact the eye are evolving.

Type of pachometer and accuracy of measurement. All pachometers average a series of thickness measurements to give the single, final readout display of corneal thickness. Instruments average from approximately 30 to 500 measurements in a fraction of a second. The important factor is the range of readings that is accepted by the instrument. There are two methods by which instruments create an average reading. The first is the pulse-locked method, in which the unit will record all readings that are within 5 to 10 degrees of perpendicularity or within 5 to 10 μm of each other, rejecting those outside that range. When the required number of acceptable readings has accumulated, the thickness is computed. The second is the averaging method, in which a fixed number of consecutive measurements must be within 5 to 10 degrees of perpendicularity (or 5 to 10 μm of each other) before these are averaged. If the probe is not perpendicular or the readings are too disparate, the series is rejected and must be begun again.

The resolution of the instrument is the smallest unit measurable by the machine, which is 1 μm. The time-based accuracy of ultrasound transmission measurement within the cornea is claimed by manufacturers to be 0.001% to 0.002%. Although most instruments claim clinical accuracy of $\pm$5 to 10 μm, no independent verification of these claims has been published. Such accuracy is beyond that needed for doing radial keratotomy because current manual techniques are much more variable. When the tissue displacement produced by knives of varying configuration and sharpness is also considered, measuring corneal thickness to an accuracy greater than 10 μm loses clinical meaning.

Ultrasonic corneal pachometers can measure thicknesses ranging from approximately 200 to 2000 μm; the range varies among units. For radial keratotomy, a range of 400 to 800 μm is adequate, since normal corneal thicknesses do not exceed these limits.

Alignment signal. Several units give a tone signal when the probe is off perpendicular. Other units simply refuse the reading and will give an indication that the reading should be repeated.

The DGH instrument is interesting in that a short tone sounds when there are enough measurements in an acceptable range with the probe perpendicular, but a long tone sounds if the alignment is off or if the readings are not within an acceptable range; therefore the operator knows without looking at the screen when the readings are not proper.

Calibration. Most pachometers have a selected speed of sound in the cornea of approximately 1640 m/sec. Some units allow adjustment of the speed of sound, so operators can select faster or slower velocities as part of the adjustment of their techniques. Selection of a faster velocity will produce a thicker corneal reading.

Many instruments have an internal calibration to determine that the speed of sound is properly set. If it is set at 1640 m/sec, for example, this setting can be verified by an internal calibration mechanism that is adjusted for the specific probe length and transducer. There is no means for the user to verify the accuracy of this setting or mechanism; it is a function of the unit's technology.

Other units offer a separate test block for the user to verify accurate readings (see Fig. 15-6). The probe is placed on the test block of known thickness. If the pachometer reading is different from that on the block, the user must adjust the speed of sound setting or the gain until the proper reading is obtained. Changes in temperature and humidity can affect the actual thickness of the block, but the extent of these changes has not been measured.

Test block readings indicate consistency of the transducer sensitivity, not the actual thickness of the test block, because the transducer and probe are calibrated for corneal tissue, not the test block material. In our laboratory, measurements of a given test block thickness varied depending on the ultrasonic probe used, but the readings were generally consistent with each probe.

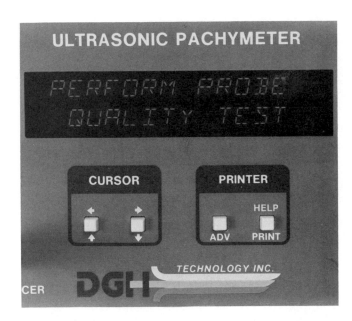

Figure 15-7
DGH pachometer automatically performs a probe quality test that confirms an acceptable interface with the gel in the probe tip. The instrument will not take readings without performing this function.

Quality check pachometer functions. Automatic functions that illustrate how instrument design can help ensure accurate readings (Fig. 15-7) are contained in the DGH 2000 pachometer. Many other brands of ultrasonic pachometers have similar safeguards. When the instrument is turned on, the instrument goes through a self-test of the internal electronics and then gives a short beep when this is complete. Without the beep, the instrument will not function and indicates an internal failure. The operator then presses a probe quality-test button on the front panel, and the instrument tests how well the probe cavity has been filled with the ultrasonic gel by sending and receiving an echo and comparing the magnitude of the signal with the magnitude of the echo signal when the unit was originally calibrated at the factory. Depending on the results of this comparison, a "percentage quality" of the probe fill is displayed on the front panel. A reading of 85% or more is necessary for the probe to be used, otherwise the instrument will not accept readings. In that case, the instrument will indicate a number of alternatives, such as "check probe fill," "plug in probe," and "self-test fail," the last indicating a hardware failure requiring a factory repair. During use, a short beep indicates that the probe is perpendicular and readings are accepted and displayed. A long beep indicates the probe is not properly positioned and readings are not accepted.

Pachometer console functions and displays. The design of ultrasonic pachometers ranges from simple to complex; some units give only a readout of the individual measured thickness, and other units have many options, including function as a small computer (Fig. 15-8).

Thickness display. The corneal thickness is displayed on a digital readout on the front of the housing or on the handle of the probe. The display should appear promptly on the screen to prevent delays between readings and should be easily seen from a distance so that the surgeon can read it comfortably in the operating room. The Storz unit offers a voice synthesizer that allows the surgeon to hear the progress of the measurements and the results of the readings with a mean and standard deviation. This convenience allows the surgeon not to look up from the eye but is slower than glancing at an LED display. Sometimes the voice requires an explanation for the patient.

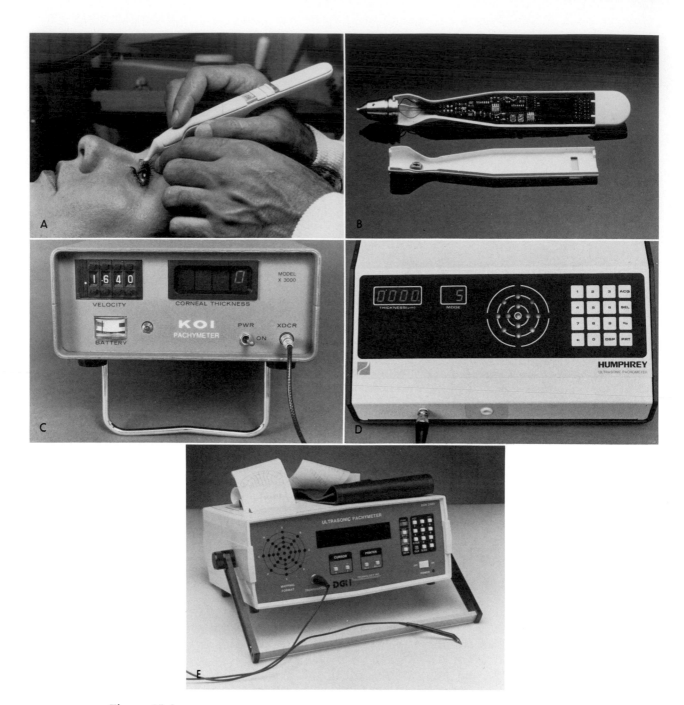

Figure 15-8

Four types of ultrasonic pachometers. **A,** Pach-Pen is a single self-contained unit held in the hand. Note the readout on the top. **B,** Inside of Pach-Pen. It has a transducer in the tip and a microprocessor in the handle. **C,** KOI console is uncomplicated, with speed of sound setting, battery charge indicator, and corneal thickness readout. There is no printer. **D,** Humphrey console has thickness readout, pattern selection mode, pattern indicator, and programmable buttons to set speed of sound and other variables. **E,** DGH console has a complex format: pattern indicator, message and thickness readout panel, cursor for identifying location of thickness measurement, printer operation, series of function selection buttons including one for setting the speed of sound, numerical buttons for programming variables, off-on switch, and power indicator.

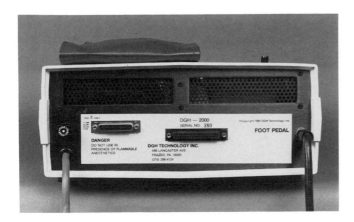

Figure 15-9
External connections on DGH 2000 ultrasonic pachometer show fuse box, power cord, two connectors for external computer interfaces, and foot pedal cord.

Memory storage. Some units will store multiple measurements for later printout. This is useful when multiple areas of the cornea are being measured.

Thickness bias. A useful feature is the ability to set a unit to compute a percentage of thickness, known as the surgeon's bias (Fig. 15-8, *C* and *D*). Many surgeons set the length of the knife blade shorter or longer than the actual corneal thickness reading; it is convenient to have this percentage computed as the readings are displayed. The percent bias must be programmed into the instrument before taking the readings.

Mapping corneal thickness. Surgeons who wish to measure the corneal thickness at different zones and in different meridians may prefer a unit that offers a mapping format. The examiner can program the sequence of readings into the console. A map of the cornea with LEDs at specific locations (central, paracentral, or peripheral, with four to eight lights around each zone) will guide the sequence of measurements. The measurement for a particular location can then be recalled from the memory by selecting the appropriate buttons or the entire map can be printed out. Some instruments print out the thickness across a single meridian, giving a cross-sectional profile of the cornea (Fig. 15-8, *C* and *D*; see Fig. 15-11).

Predictability formulas. Many units contain software programs that contain predictability formulas based on nomograms or multiple regression analysis, such as the DRS formula, the Thornton Guide, or the Bores-Fyodorov formula. Some units come with these programs already loaded, and others allow the surgeon to select a particular program. To use these programs, the operator enters preoperative patient information, such as age, sex, and keratometry readings. Some programs are flexible and can be modified according to the surgeon's experience by the use of a practical surgeon's coefficient or "depth factor." The use of such programs is discussed in Chapter 14, Computerized Predictability Formulas for Refractive Keratotomy.

External computer port. Many consoles have an RS232 output port that allows the information measured by the pachometer to be transferred to a computer system or a printer (an advantage when measurements are being fed into a centralized data base) (Fig. 15-9) and allows coupling of a computerized predictability program to the pachometer.

Ancillary features of pachometers

Foot pedal design. Most foot pedals have a simple, flat, off-on design. The pedal is depressed and released to obtain a reading. When the pedal is depressed and released again, the instrument is reset to allow for the next reading. Some

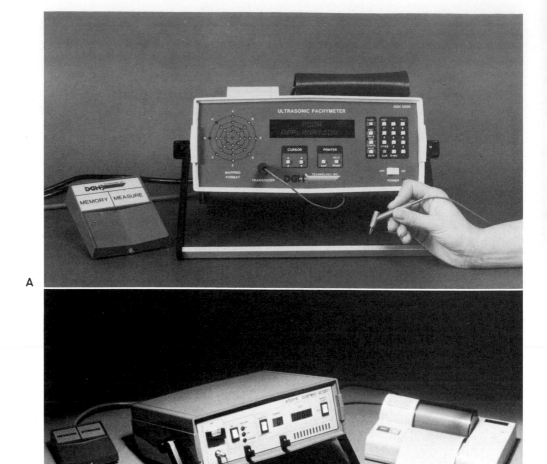

Figure 15-10
Examples of printers. **A,** DGH 2000 has built-in printer at top left of console. Foot pedal has both measurement and memory functions. **B,** Storz Corneoscan 1000 has separate printer unit and foot pedal that both displays and stores information.

pedals have two sides: one to obtain the thickness reading and the other to enter the reading into the memory (Fig. 15-10).

Printers. If only the illuminated LED thickness display is present, an observer must manually record the readings as they are obtained. A printer, either as part of the console or as an ancillary device, makes this task easier. Patient identification information can be entered and printed out, along with the thickness readings and computation of the thinner or thicker bias. Many printouts also present a map of thickness readings in different locations (Fig. 15-11). These printouts are not only convenient but also an accurate method of collecting data, preventing transcription errors, and providing good documentation.

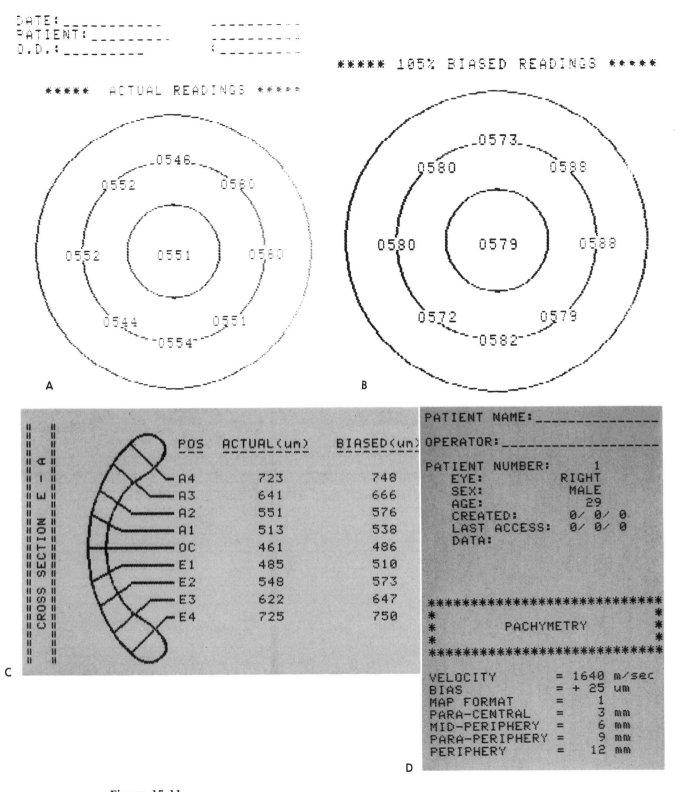

Figure 15-11
Examples of printouts from ultrasonic pachometers. **A,** Humphrey model 850 shows patient identification information, a map of the actual thickness readings, and **B,** a map of the readings calculated with a 105% bias. **C,** DGH 2000 printout shows a cross section of the cornea with both actual and bias computed (+25 μm) thickness readings. **D,** Average measurements around a given circumference.

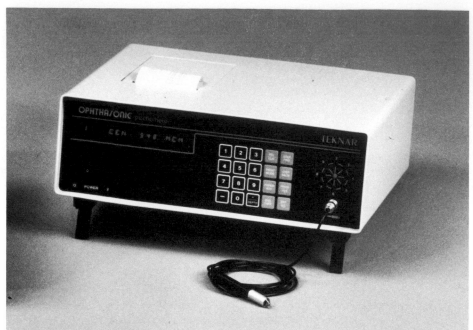

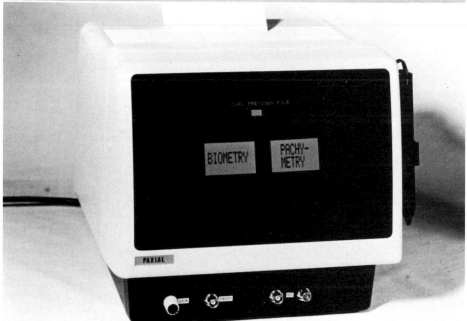

Figure 15-12
Combined ultrasonic corneal pachometer and axial length measurement. **A,**
JedMed Axipac II shows printer on top, LED readout on left, buttons for selection
of type and pattern of measurement on right, and two different probes, one for cor-
neal pachometry (right probe) and one for axial length measurements (left probe).
B, Biophysic Medical Paxial Unit with interactive computer screen.

Combination units. Ultrasound consoles that measure corneal thickness and axial length are available, offering convenience and some cost savings over the purchase of two separate units (Fig. 15-12). Their larger size reduces portability.

Power. All instruments use a standard 110-volt line current in the United States and a 220- to 250-volt line current in most other countries. Many offer a battery option for portability. Batteries last for 7 or 8 hours and most can be recharged in 16 to 20 hours. A battery strength indicator is important because batteries with a lower charge can cause inaccurate measurements and may fail during use. The battery unit should be rechargeable while the pachometer is in use on electrical power; a replaceable back-up battery pack is an added safety feature. The Underwriters Laboratories (UL) certify the electrical safety of some of these units, but certification has nothing to do with ultrasonic accuracy.

Size and weight. It is convenient to have a separate pachometer in each location where it is used, such as the office and the operating room. However, it may be necessary to transport the pachometer from one location to another, and the ease of portability is determined by the size and weight of the unit. This varies greatly among available pachometers, from the small hand-held size of the Pach-Pen (see Fig. 15-8, *A*) to the larger consoles, such as the Humphrey and Biophysic units. Generally, more features increase bulk, although microprocessor technology is rapidly offering greater capability in units of smaller size and weight.

Price and warranty. Purchasing an ultrasonic pachometer is similar to purchasing any other piece of equipment. Purchase price is important but so are service and warranty. Some manufacturers provide separate warranties for the probe and the console. If computerized functions are included, the purchaser should inquire about provision for updates and improvements in the software. Service contracts are also available.

The ophthalmologist should use caution when buying new units or new designs; be sure that the unit will have longevity and that the company will remain in business and provide support.

Comparison of ultrasonic pachometers

Quantitative comparison. Two studies by Reader, Salz, and colleagues[25,28] have compared the relative corneal thickness measurements with different ultrasonic pachometers. One study[25] compared nine different ultrasonic pachometers (1640 msec) on six different patients. Triplicate measurements were taken at central, paracentral, and peripheral zones at different times of the day. Table 15-4 and Fig. 15-13 present the results. Central and paracentral readings were much more consistent than peripheral ones.

Thickness readings among instruments varied significantly. Values had a range of 49 μm centrally and 59 μm paracentrally among the instruments. For example, a cornea actually 535 μm thick could be measured as thin as 521 μm or as thick as 578 μm by different instruments. The authors offered some explanations for the variability in readings. The Cilco unit with a 4.2-mm diameter probe tip gave among the thickest readings, possibly because of displacement of the cornea by the large tip and possibly because of the method in which the ultrasonic waves exited the large tip. The company has replaced the probe tip with a 2-mm diameter tip, but it is still internally calibrated to match the readings in the larger tip. Both the DGH and Storz CS II are solid-tipped probes with a replaceable gel interface in the transducer tip. Both gave consistently higher readings, possibly because of the additional impedance of the coupling gel, although the exact reason is unknown. The Humphrey unit gave consistently thinner readings, and this is the only unit that has a solid probe with no replaceable coupling medium and the only one that uses a 12 MHz transducer instead of the standard 20 MHz. These variations may account for the lower readings.

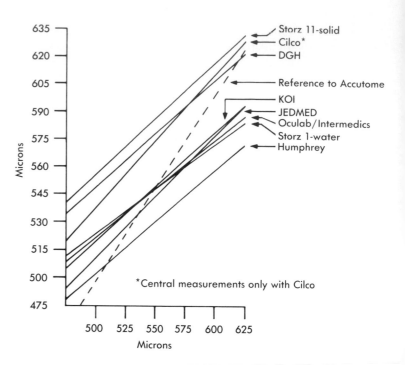

Figure 15-13
Comparison of nine different pachometers. Horizontal x-axis shows the paracentral measurements. Vertical y-axis shows the central measurements. Variability ranges up to 50 to 75 μm among instruments. (From Reader AL and Salz JJ: J Refract Surg 1987;3:7-11.)

Table 15-4

Mean Corneal Thickness at Each of Nine Positions Measured with Nine Ultrasonic Pachometers (Average ± Standard Deviation in Micrometers)*

	Accutome ±8.8†	Cilco ±3†	DGH ±4.6†	Humphrey ±10.8†	Oculab/ Intermedics ±8.6†	Jedmed ±9.6†	KOI ±4.6†	Storz CS1000 ±7†	Storz CS II ±12.4†
Central	535 ±6	560 ±3	556 ±5	520 ±6	520 ±5	521 ±5	536 ±2	535 ±3	569 ±4
Paracentral superior	609 ±10	—	627 ±10	590 ±12	593 ±11	591 ±11	585 ±4	586 ±9	620 ±13
Paracentral nasal	621 ±8	—	619 ±9	582 ±9	581 ±8	572 ±10	583 ±6	580 ±9	631 ±22
Paracentral inferior	599 ±11	—	599 ±10	579 ±14	571 ±8	572 ±11	577 ±7	578 ±7	626 ±15
Paracentral temporal	601 ±9	—	607 ±12	587 ±13	575 ±11	579 ±11	588 ±4	576 ±7	612 ±8
Peripheral superior	736	—	706	691	706	707	711	710	751
Peripheral nasal	756	—	747	759	716	774	760	733	804
Peripheral inferior	777	—	741	760	718	757	780	736	830
Peripheral temporal	769	—	771	861	715	764	778	746	796

From Reader AL and Salz JJ: J Refract Surg 1987;3:7-11.
*Speed of sound in cornea.
†Overall average of standard deviations of the central and four paracentral readings.

Five of the instruments were used to obtain central readings in eight eyes of four subjects, adjusting the speed of sound on each instrument until the thickness readings were the same. The box on p. 427 shows that the adjusted velocities ranged from 1475 to 1640 m/sec.

These disturbing findings emphasize two practical conclusions. First, variation in the performance among pachometers is one of the factors that produces variations in surgical technique and outcome among surgeons. Second, there is a need for industry standards—a need which should be addressed by cooperative work among companies that make ultrasonic pachometers. As instrument designs and technology improve, further comparative testing will be needed.

> ### Adjusted Speed of Sound in Five Ultrasonic Pachometers on Six Human Corneas Required to Obtain Identical Corneal Thickness Readings (m/sec)
>
> | | |
> |---|---|
> | Cilco | 1475 |
> | DGH | 1530 |
> | Humphrey | 1640 |
> | Storz CS 1000 (Water) | 1575 |
> | Storz CS II (Solid) | 1495 |
>
> From Reader AL and Salz JJ: J Refract Surg 1987;3:7-11.

Qualitative comparison of features among pachometers. Thornton compared features of pachometers and performed a qualitative comparison of different pachometers in office practice in 1986 (Tables 15-5 and 15-6). The goal was to compare the ability of an office technician to obtain consistent measurements of corneal thickness. Ratings from 1 to 10 were established, with 10 as the best. The final ratings took into account the technician's experience, the surgeon's experience, and other physicians using similar units in 1987.

The performance evaluation (Table 15-6) included the following. Readings taken in one location judged reproducibility. Ease of operation was judged by the technician's ability to learn to use the instrument and obtain reasonably consistent readings. Surgical and postoperative verifications were the estimate of how well the instrument provided the correct thickness measurement for accuracy in surgery with a minimal number of perforations and apparent proper depth setting on the micrometer knife as determined by postoperative slit-lamp microscope examination. The maintenance record was judged by the number of failures and the response of the company to remedy these failures. Portability was judged by the ease of carrying the instrument from one location to another.

The Myocure and Sonogage units were not available for office use, and the ratings are based on limited experience. The speed of sound in the cornea of 1640 m/sec was used for all instruments.

The features of the designs listed in Table 15-5 may have changed since 1986. As modifications and improvements in each unit are made, the performance evaluation (Table 15-6) will be less valid; here we present a few observations to amplify our experience.

Several units operated on a rechargeable battery, and, although we had no problems with battery tests, some surgeons reported batteries losing charge during a series of measurements. Manufacturers are now supplying extra rechargeable battery packs with all battery-operated units so that the packs can be interchanged as needed.

Most units could be managed by one operator who would place the probe on the cornea, elicit a thickness reading, and then see the reading on the screen. An assistant would have to record the findings unless a memory function in the foot pedal or a memory function integrated into the console allowed storage of information. The Cilco unit was rated the lowest because it gave continuous readings, which required monitoring by a second person to identify the readings that appeared most frequently and to select the final reading. The Myocure and KOI units were slightly more awkward to use. The Storz unit with a synthesized voice was convenient but much slower because of the need to wait for the voice

Table 15-5

Features of Pachometers in Office Practice

Instrument	Price (1987 U.S. dollars)	Weight (pounds)	Probe tip size (mm)	Probe tip type	Measurement method	Alignment signal	Transducer (MHz)	Battery compatible	Printer	Mapping format	Instrument accuracy (microns)
Allergan-Humphrey Pachometer	6500	15.0	1.5	Solid	Pulse locked	Tone	12	No	Yes	Yes	±5
Kremer II Corneometer	6500	10.0	1.8	Solid	Pulse locked	Tone and visual	20	No	Yes	No	±5
Alcon 55 Villasenor	6000	4.0	4.2 2.0 (optional)	Solid	Averaged	None	20	Yes	No	Yes	±10
BioRad Pach-Pen	3100	0.0125	1.5	Solid	Averaged	Tone and visual	20	Yes	Optional	Yes	±5
Teknar Pachysonic II	5200	8.0	2.1	Solid (oil interface)	Averaged	Tone	20	No	Yes	Yes	±5
Storz CS 1000 Omega	5000 (4350 without printer)	10.0	1.6	Water	Averaged	Audio	20	No	Optional	Yes	±5
DGH 2000	6500	8.0	1.5	Solid (gel interface)	Averaged	Tone	20	No	Yes	Yes	±5
Myocure Pachometer*	4600	3.4	1.5	Solid	Averaged	Visual	20	Yes	No	No	±10
Alcon Biophysique KOI 3000X	4000	5.0	1.5	Solid (water interface)	Averaged	None	20	Yes	No	No	±10
Sonogage Corneogage II	6200	3.0	1.5	Solid	Averaged	Tone	20	Yes	Optional	No	±5

From Thornton SP: J Cataract Refract Surg 1986;12:416-419.
*Instrument not available as of 1991.

Table 15-6

Performance Evaluation of Pachometers

Instrument	One operator	Reproducibility	Ease of operation	Surgical and postoperative verification	Maintenance record	Portability
Allergan-Humphrey Pachometer	9*	10	7	8	8	3
Kremer Corneometer	9	10	6	8	7	4
Alcon 55 Villasenor	5	2	7	6 (with smaller 20 mm probe tip)	7	8
BioRad Pach Pen	10	10	9	8	9	10
Teknar Pachysonic II†	9	10	7	6	NR	6
Storz CS 1000 Omega	9	9	7	8	7	3
DGH 2000	10	10	8	8	8	6
Myocure Pachometer‡	8	NR	7	NR	NR	8
KOI 3000X	8	9	7	8	6	8
Sonogage Corneogage II†	10	10	7	NR	NR	8

From Thornton SP: J Cataract Refract Surg 1986;12:416-419.
*Scale 1-10 with *1*, poor; *5*, average; *10*, excellent; *NR*, not rated (too little experience).
†Manufacturer allowed only limited testing in the office.
‡Instrument not available as of 1991.

to pronounce each individual reading. Storz now offers an instrument without a voice readout but with the standard digital display. The KOI pachometer did not have an audible signal to indicate when a properly aligned measurement had been achieved, requiring the operator to glance frequently at the digital readout.

We estimated but did not quantify the reproducibility of the units and found them generally reliable in taking sequential measurements in a single area by one observer. An exception was the Cilco unit, which gave more variable readings, partly because it presented readings continuously. We tested the instruments primarily for central readings and agree with Reader and Salz[25] that the reproducibility of central readings for an individual instrument is quite good. They found that the standard deviation for central readings with eight different instruments ranged from 2 to 6 μm. There was more variability in paracentral readings; Reader's standard deviations ranged from 4 to 22 μm and the variability in peripheral readings was so large that Reader did not report them.

No instrument received a 10 rating for ease of operation because Thornton found some areas in which he thought each instrument could be improved. Most disruptive was refilling and managing of the probe tips. The fluid-filled tips of the Storz instrument required continued refilling, and the tip has since been updated with a solid tip. The KOI instrument had a solid tip but a water-coupling medium, so the tip had to be taken apart and dried each day; there were enough pieces in this probe tip to make losing one likely, since it was disassembled so frequently. This tip has also been replaced with an all-solid tip. The JedMed Pachysonic unit read slow (one reading per second), prolonging the measurement process and requiring drying of the tip between each reading.

Programmable mapping of a pattern of readings with a printer was offered by the Humphrey, JedMed, and DGH units. The JedMed and Humphrey units had a limited number of readings; for example, the JedMed was limited to nine points on the cornea, so the entire cycle had to be run again to obtain more readings. The DGH 2000 was the most versatile unit; it had the ability to program and print out any number of readings in any pattern desired.

The maintenance record was not perfect. Some instruments functioned incorrectly, and the response by the companies for repairs varied; none experienced major breakdown. JedMed, Myocure, and Sonogage instruments were not left in the office long enough to estimate maintenance problems.

The Intermedics Pach-Pen rated highest in portability because it is the smallest (weighing 2 oz) of the full-function ultrasonic pachometers, fitting easily into the hand (see Fig. 15-8, *A*). Its accuracy and precision were comparable with the larger consoles. Both the Cilco and Myocure units were lightweight and portable but were ranked lower on other functions. DGH has made a smaller lightweight console unit, the Pachette, with modular features that can be added as needed. The large console units (Humphrey, DGH, Accutome, Storz) are portable but cumbersome.

Optical pachometry

The original method of measuring corneal thickness was optical pachometry, as summarized by Duke-Elder.[4] The major problem in the practical, clinical use of an optical pachometer has been repeatability of measurements, particularly among observers. This variability stems from the following four major sources[20]:

1. Lack of a small fixation target for the patient, which is located in a fixed position relative to the instrument
2. Lack of a known alignment of the pachometer with the cornea in a reproducible position so that the slit beam intersects the cornea at the same angle for consistent thickness readings
3. Lack of a consistent endpoint for the overlap of the split image of the slit beam by the observer, which is done on the basis of subjective visual inspection
4. Lack of an identified reproducible slit beam for consistency and the lack of compensation for the beam width in the measurement process

Optical pachometry has advantages. It does not touch the corneal surface and therefore does not damage the epithelium, which can sometimes happen with the contact methods of ultrasonic pachometry and specular microscopy. The location on the cornea that is being measured can be identified visually, although it is not easy to return to that specific point without auxiliary fixation devices; the ultrasonic pachometer probe tip, which is about 3 mm in diameter, can be located fairly accurately, but the large tip of the specular microscope is difficult to relocate in the same position. The optical pachometer can measure different layers of the cornea, which might be desired in lamellar refractive surgical procedures, such as intracorneal lenses, as can the specular microscope. Optical pachometry measures all the layers of the cornea down to the first reflective layer. Measurement of eccentric areas on the cornea is more difficult with the optical pachometer, as it is with the specular microscope. This process is easier with the ultrasonic pachometer because the probe tip can be placed perpendicular to the surface of the cornea in any location, particularly when it is used in the operating room. The errors in accuracy and precision inherent in the optical pachometer are minimized when the instrument is used by a single observer and the errors are less than 10 μm, an acceptable error for practical, clinical refractive keratotomy. However, the error increases to 20 μm or more with multiple users, and this is unacceptable.[22,23]

As Mondell and colleagues[20] emphasize, the problems in optical pachometry can be minimized with the use of alignment lights that serve for patient fixation, particularly when the alignment lights are located centrally between the slit beam and the microscope observation path.

The method chosen by the examiner to overlap the split image of the slit-beam mires varies. There are two criteria that are generally used. The first is the "just touch" criterion, in which the alignment is made such that an imaginary line extends from the endothelial border of the upper image to the epithelial border of the lower image. The second criterion is the "overlap" method, in which the imaginary extension of the bright portion of the endothelial image is overlapped with the bright portion of the epithelial image because the bright portions are actually produced by the finite width of the slit-lamp beam as it passes through each surface of the cornea. In practice there is considerable individual difference in the appearance of the bright portion and in the methods of alignment used by observers. The "just touch" method is easier to align for most observers.

Currently used models of optical pachometers are a bit cumbersome because the scale reading must be read by the observer or by a second person and recorded separately. It would not be difficult to modify the scale so that when it is moved manually the thickness reading is recorded electronically, displayed on a screen, and recorded automatically, as done in ultrasonic pachometers, but such a technologic improvement is not commercially available.

One major drawback of optical pachometry is that any system of alignment and fixation lights makes reading locations in the paracentral and peripheral cornea difficult. Since corneal thickness in these areas is important in setting the length of the knife blade, this is an important drawback. A system with an array of fixation lights would be required to control patient fixation.

Because optical pachometers require slit lamps, they are not easily portable and are not usable in the operating room.

Thus, although optical pachometry can be used by single observers under controlled conditions accurately in both the laboratory and the clinic, it is used much less commonly than ultrasonic pachometry for refractive keratotomy.

KNIFE BLADES AND HANDLES USED FOR REFRACTIVE KERATOTOMY

During the 15 years that Sato worked to refine keratotomy, he repeatedly emphasized the importance of high-quality, exquisitely sharp blades. Modern keratotomy has further heightened this demand with emergence of high-quality, guarded, diamond micrometer knives that allow the surgeon to make exquisite incisions into the cornea with minimal disruption of adjacent tissues (Fig. 15-14).

Knife blades

Of the knife blades available, diamonds are by far the most frequently used, followed by ruby, sapphire, and then stainless steel (Table 15-7).

Terminology. Diamond, ruby, and sapphire blades are collectively referred to as gem or crystal blades. We prefer the term "crystal" because the sapphire and ruby blades are often synthetic and therefore are not gems.

Designation of blades as front-cutting or back-cutting is often confusing (Fig. 15-15). The best convention is to adopt that used for ordinary cutlery and pocket knives: the curved, sharp cutting surface is the front of the blade and the straight, dull, noncutting surface is the back. Therefore front-cutting usually refers to cutting with the oblique edge of the blade whereas back-cutting usually refers to the use of the vertical edge of the blade; in this case it is sharp!

The "Russian" technique of radial keratotomy uses a centripetal cut made

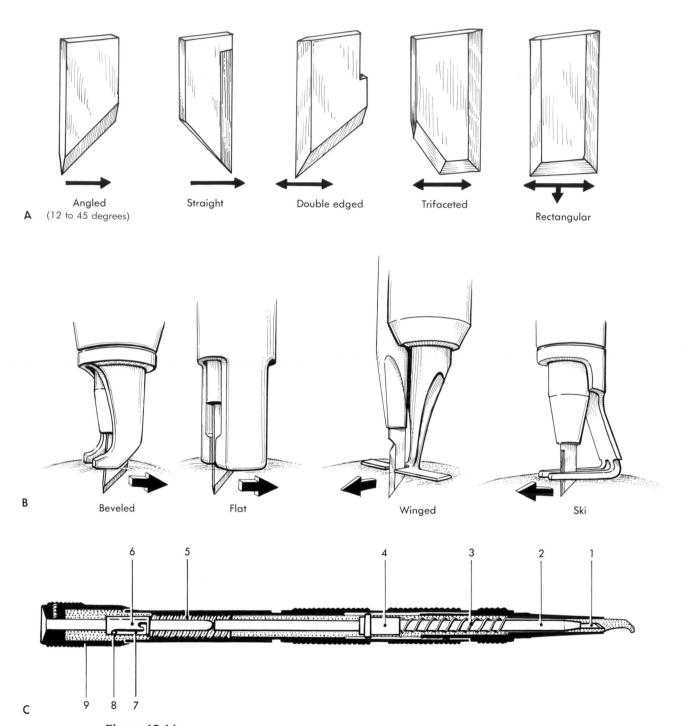

Figure 15-14
Configuration of components in guarded, crystal-bladed micrometer knives for keratotomy. There are three basic components: the blade, the footplate, and the micrometer handle. **A,** Crystalline blades of five alternative configurations. **B,** Footplates of four alternative designs. **C,** Micrometer handle. The basic components are *(1)* the crystalline blade, *(2)* the central shaft that carries the blade, *(3)* the spring that keeps the blade and micrometer taut, *(4)* the pin-guide that keeps the shaft and blade from rotating, *(5)* micrometer screw threads, *(6)* the bayonet locking slot and pin, *(7)* the rotating plunger attached to the micrometer handle, *(8)* the pin that allows extension or retraction of the blade, *(9)* micrometer handle and the housing within which the shaft and blade can retract.

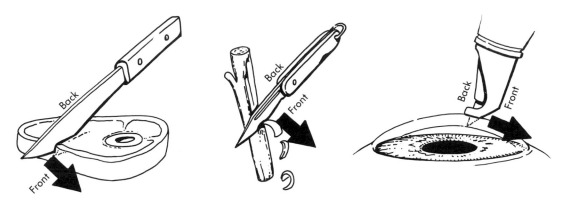

Figure 15-15
Convention designates the front of a knife blade as the curved part of the blade.
Thus the term "front cutting" refers to cutting with the angled edge of the crystal
blade, and "back cutting" refers to cutting with the vertical edge.

Table 15-7

Knife Blades Used for Keratotomy

Characteristic	Diamond	Ruby/Sapphire	Metal
Material	Carbon	Al_2O_3 (corundum)	Stainless or mild carbon steel (iron)
Hardness*	5.18	1.00	0.50
Durability	Excellent	Poor (sapphire greater than ruby)	Disposable
Edge quality	Excellent	Excellent (new)	Very good to poor
Approximate number of cases	100s	10 (sapphire greater than ruby)	1
Cost of raw material	$75 to $250	$0.50	$0.01
Difficulty of manufacture	Extreme	Moderate	Slight
Repairability	Fair	None	None
Cost value per case	Excellent	Poor	Fair

*Knoop-Ridgeway scale.

"uphill" from the limbus to the clear zone with the vertical knife edge (back-cutting), whereas the "American" technique involves a centrifugal cut made "downhill" from the clear zone to the limbus with the oblique knife edge (front-cutting). Transverse incisions are usually made with the vertical edge (back-cutting).

Confusion arises because some surgeons use this terminology to refer to the direction in which the hand is moving, so that pushing the knife forward toward the front of the hand (usually cutting with the vertical edge) is called "front-cutting" and pulling the knife toward the back of the hand is called "back-cutting." This confusing custom should be abandoned.

Diamond knife blade. A diamond is simply carbon in crystalline form; however, when its properties are compared with other materials, the diamond is usually described in superlatives. It is by several multiples the hardest of all materials and therefore among the most durable. Relative hardness is usually rated on the Knoop-Ridgeway indentation scale[26]: diamond, 5.180; ruby and sapphire, 1.000; topaz, 0.766; fluorite, 0.100. A less accurate comparison of hardness is Mohs' exponential scale: diamond, 10; ruby and sapphire, 9; topaz, 8; stainless steel, 6; fluorspar, 4; fingernail, 2.5. Diamond is also the most inert solid material, making it resistant to chemical damage. It is virtually incompressible, and thereby retains its shape. It is the best heat conductor, having a very low coefficient of expansion, which allows cleaning by autoclaving. The crystal can be polished into a near perfect mirror, which plays beautifully with the light, reflecting approximately 90% of the light because its refractive index is the highest known. The luster from a polished gem diamond, whether used for jewelry or for surgical blades, is so deep and beautiful that it has been given its own name: *adamantine,* derived from the Greek, "I tame, I subdue." The root is also the origin of the word "adamant," a derivation that captures the struggle necessary to convert this extremely hard stone into a useful surgical blade.

Mining and selling diamonds. Diamond is formed when carbon (graphite) is subjected to extreme temperatures on the order of 3300° C (5970° F) and pressure on the order of 115 kilobars (1700 pounds per square inch). Geologically, diamonds are found in relatively young kimberlites. Australia is currently the top producer of diamonds, followed by South Africa. Mining diamonds is a technical (and political) challenge; it takes approximately 1 billion tons of diamondiferous ore to yield approximately 1 ton of gem-quality diamonds. Diamonds are mined from river beds or from large rock columns and are separated from the crushed ore by taking advantage of their hydrophobic quality. The ore is passed over a sluice covered with axle grease, and the hydrophobic diamonds stick to the grease while the other materials wash through. There are many other ways to separate diamonds, including x-ray fluorescence and hand sorting.

Synthetic diamonds are currently being made using hydrogen (approximately 90%) and methane (approximately 10%), which are bombarded by microwaves, producing a continuous deposition process.

The raw diamonds are sent to the Diamond Producers' Association in Johannesburg or to the Diamond Corporation offices in London where they are divided into gem-quality and industrial-quality stones, which are distributed through a separate organization.

The process by which diamonds are selected is fascinating. Gem rough sorters are highly trained workers who can instantly identify subtle differences in the crystals and who work at tables covered with fresh white paper. They first divide the rough diamonds into different sizes by hand or by sieving and then subdivide them on the basis of the shape of the crystals—the regular unbroken ones being more valuable than the irregularly shaped, fragmented crystals. In descending order of value the crystals are designated stones, shapes, cleavages, macles, or flats.

Using a magnifying loop, the sorters identify inclusions and blemishes within the stone that were caused by fissures during natural growth or by the inclusion of small pieces of other minerals (graphite-type carbon, iron, and garnet) or of nitrogen. They look for solid inclusions, transparent bubbles, clouds, cleavage cracks, graining, jagged growth lines, and radial fringe cracks, grading the stones on a scale of 1 to 10, 1 to 5 generally being gem quality and 6 to 10 industrial quality. Sorting for color involves removing the less desirable brown stones, separating the useful uniform yellow, blue, or pink ones, and then grading the remaining tints of white on a 1 to 10 scale, 1 through 6 generally being classified as gem-quality stones. (Some manufacturers use brown stones for surgical blades.)

Gem-quality diamonds are sold 10 times a year to approximately 220 dealers, who distribute them to the wholesale trade through an ancient market organization in the form of the Diamond Club for rough stones and The Diamond Bourse for polished stones, both located in the main diamond cities of Antwerp, New York, Tel Aviv, London, and Amsterdam. The industrial purchaser must buy diamonds 10 times a year at specified sites. Each purchaser must accept a sealed box of diamonds for a set price. From this the purchaser must select the stones that are suitable for making diamond-bladed surgical knives; the buyer must sell the remainder of the stones elsewhere or devise other uses. This creates a temptation to use the residual, poorer quality stones for surgical knives. Most manufacturers of diamond blades purchase their diamonds from a site buyer, specifying color, shape, size, and the presence or absence of flaws.

The manufacturers and dealers of diamond surgical knives fall into the following three general groups: (1) firms that purchase and cut their own diamonds and therefore can control quality firsthand, (2) firms that buy ready-made knife blades and assemble their own knives, and (3) firms that buy ready-made knives and put their brand name on them. Clearly the probability of maintaining high quality of the diamond blade diminishes along this spectrum. Unfortunately, until industry-wide standards are established through cooperation among different companies, the ophthalmologist and the patient remain at the mercy of manufacturers and dealers.

Manufacturing diamond blades for surgical knives. Diamonds used for making surgical blades should be gem quality. Although there are industry-wide standards that define "gem quality" for diamonds used as jewels, there are no such standards for the diamonds used as surgical blades.

The basic quality of a diamond is determined by the four "C's:" carat weight, color, clarity, and cut. In manufacturing a diamond knife blade, the carat weight is not important, but the length of the diamond oriented along selected crystalline structures determines the length of the finished blade. Diamonds weighing 1 to 3 carats yield blades 5 to 7 mm long. Color plays a role, because white and yellow stones have a more regular crystalline structure, whereas brown stones tend toward the irregular graphitic state of carbon. The clarity is extremely important, not for appearances, but because flaws within the diamond blade affect its strength and longevity. The artistic cut of a diamond blade is not as important as it is for jewelry, but the ability to cut a fine edge is obviously important for surgery.

The most conscientious manufacturer who selects high-quality stones for blades may end up with rubbish because cutting and polishing diamonds depends on a thorough understanding of the internal structure of the diamond, as deduced from the unique macrostructure of each stone. The chemical structure of all diamonds is similar. Every carbon atom is bonded to four neighboring atoms by its four valences; each atom extends equidistantly to form a tight tetrahedral lattice. This structure builds into a crystalline form, the most common of which is the octahedron, a solid that has eight identical triangular sides and is shaped like two pyramids stacked together on their square base. The shape and crystalline structure of diamonds are as different as snowflakes.

These raw diamonds, known as glassies, are shaped to the final dimensional specifications for each style of knife (for example, tri-facet, 45 degree, and sphere) by skilled diamond cutters who are able to identify the natural crystal and cleavage planes within the stone, much like a woodcutter finds the grain in wood or a marble-carver finds planes in marble. In the past, cutters used mallets and wedge-shaped tools to cleave the stone into slabs and plates that looked like pieces of broken glass, but the process is now done with fine saws or lasers. The

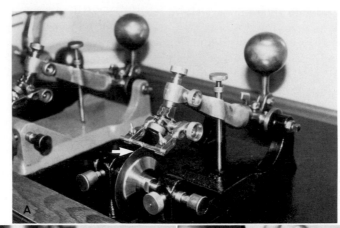

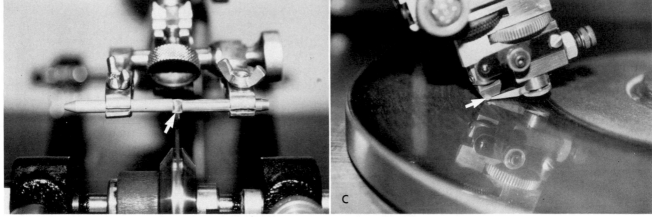

Figure 15-16

Steps in the manufacture of diamond knives. **A,** Cleavage of the raw stone is accomplished with a diamond-edged saw *(arrow)*. **B,** The rough diamond *(arrow)* is held between the end of two metal pincers and the saw is used to cut the stone into several slabs along the natural crystalline cleavage planes. **C,** Sharp knife blade edge is created by honing and polishing (not grinding) with the diamond held on the end of the metal shank *(arrow)* where it is placed on the surface of a large, flat rotating wheel that uses diamond grit for the polishing. (Courtesy Magnum Diamond.)

shape of the stone is refined by cutting it with a diamond-charged, phosphur-bronzed saw blade or a laser into properly oriented stones. The orientation must be performed within ±3 degrees of the crystalline planes of the stone, or the slabs are useless for knife production. Trying to get too many slabs from one stone will decrease the quality of the final knife blade (Fig. 15-16).

The diamond edge is the hardest cutting surface known. The unique crystalline structure of diamonds allows the creation of extremely sharp edges by splitting, without honing. This same crystalline structure, however, imposes limitations on blade design and configuration because diamonds cannot be manipulated into smooth curves or made extremely thin, processes that are possible with steel and synthetic crystalline blades.

To create the knife blade, the diamond must be sharpened by honing and polishing—not by grinding—the most exacting part of the entire process (Fig. 15-16). The sawed plate is welded to a metal shank by a skilled worker, a faceter, who hones and polishes the edge on large, flat, rotating wheels that use diamond grit for polishing and vegetable oil for cooling. The skill of the faceter determines the quality of the blade edge because the stone glued onto its "dop"

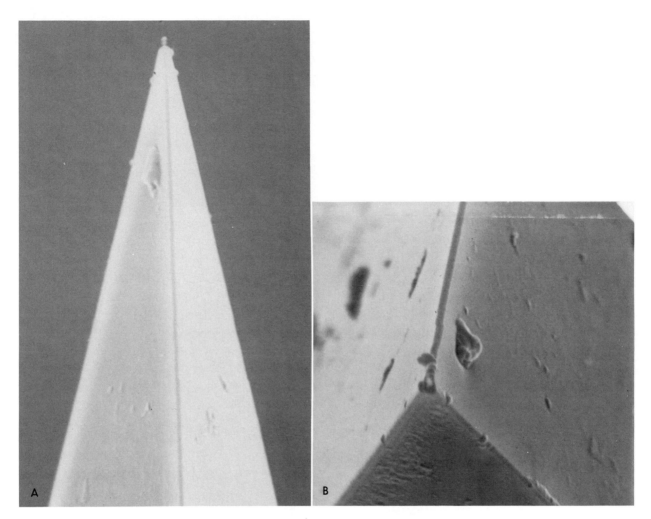

Figure 15-17
Scanning electron micrographs demonstrates sharp tip **(A)** and smooth cutting edge
at rear of blade **(B)** of a high-quality diamond knife polished by honing. The average
radius of curvature of the blade edge is 0.13 to 0.15 μm (**A,** ×10,500; **B,** ×21,000).
(Courtesy William Knepshield, Jr., KMI, Inc.)

must have its surfaces oriented precisely to the platen wheels, which are aligned
with micron accuracy; these processes are sometimes guided by x-ray diffraction. The more edges required on a blade, the more skill required by the faceter.

Diamond polishing is analogous to sanding wood; the final surface is
smoother when it is sanded with the grain and not across it. The size of the diamond dust particles varies during polishing; it is initially larger to remove more
material and subsequently finer to obtain the smoothest surface. Since only 1%
to 2% of the diamond dust on the platen wheel will be aligned properly to actually cut and polish the surface of the crystal, the work is slow and tedious.
Since the hardness of diamonds varies by a factor of 10 to 100 in different directions, the faceter must work the diamonds in different directions. Polishing creates a smooth, hard surface that decreases tissue drag and damage.

Manufacturers work under 500 magnification to produce diamond blades,
examining each edge up to 40 times during the manufacturing process and using
cross-polarization to check for internal stress that may cause fracturing.

The ideal diamond blade has a perfectly sharp tip and an edge devoid of even
the smallest nicks (Figs. 15-17 to 15-19). It is devoid of internal flaws in the

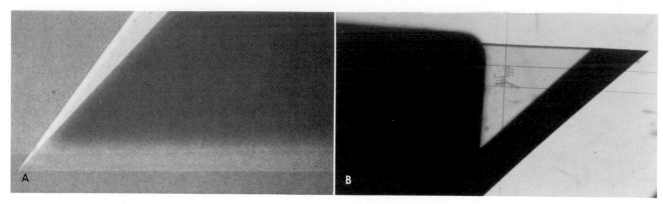

Figure 15-18
Side views of high-quality diamond knife blade. **A,** Scanning electron micrograph shows sharp tip and smooth edge (×1000). **B,** View of sharp tip and edge and clean blade through a light microscope (×100). (**A** courtesy Myocure, Inc; **B** courtesy Magnum Diamond.)

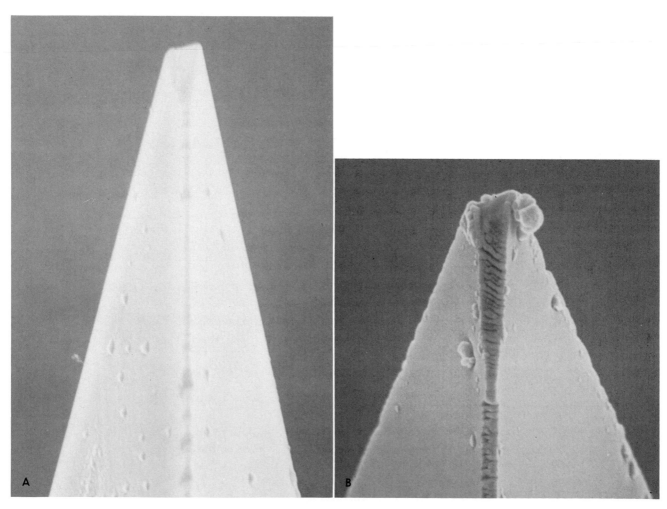

Figure 15-19
Scanning electron micrographs of poorly manufactured diamond knives show chipped tips **(A)** and nicked, dull edges **(B).** (×10,500.) (Courtesy William Knepshield, Jr., KMI, Inc.)

crystalline structure (Figs. 15-20 and 15-21). The surface is polished smooth and optically flat, without lapp marks (Fig. 15-22). Companies skilled in this technical cut include Antoine-Meyer in Switzerland, Moria in France, and LAB in Nevada.

Unfortunately, no industry standards exist for the manufacture of diamond knife blades, as there are for diamonds used in jewelry. Because most ophthalmologists are incapable of judging the quality of a diamond blade before they purchase it (even magnification of 100× to 200× will reveal only gross damage, not subtle internal edges or flaws), the ophthalmologist must rely on the successive judgments of several individuals: the gem sorter, the diamond purchaser, the diamond blade manufacturer, the distributor, and the sales person. Fortunately, standards for diamond selection in the ophthalmic industry are improving. In the mid 1980s, when there was a rush to purchase diamond knives for keratotomy, quality standards fell as manufacturers sought to fill the orders of surgeons less aware of the need for high-quality diamonds in producing these

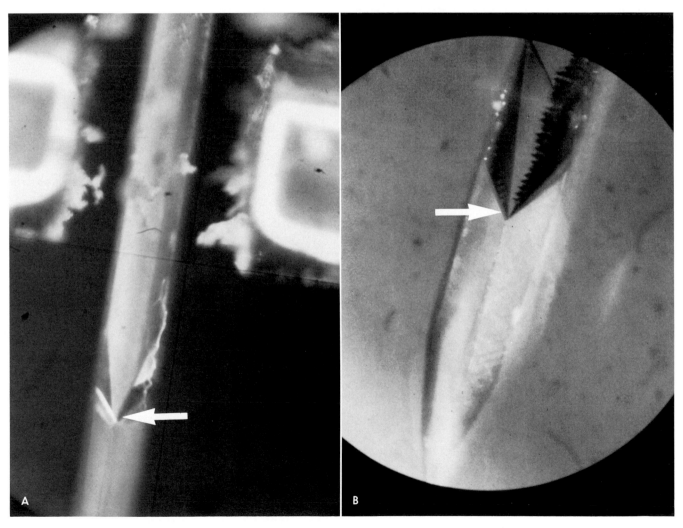

Figure 15-20
Two microscopic views of diamond knife blades show the internal crystalline structure of the knife, appearing as a sharp facet within the blade. This may predispose to fracture of the blade (×100). (Courtesy Magnum Diamond.)

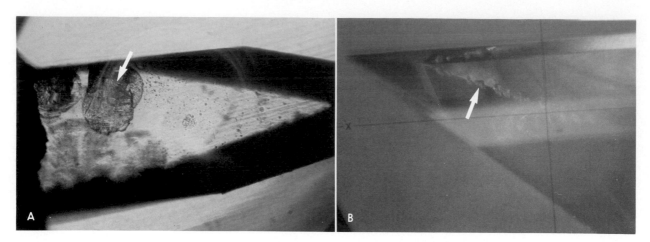

Figure 15-21
Diamond knife blade seen with light microscope demonstrates flaws in the crystalline structure. **A,** Rounded inclusions *(arrow.)* **B,** Linear sheets *(arrow).* (**A,** × 200; **B,** ×100). (Courtesy Magnum Diamond.)

Figure 15-22
Poorly manufactured diamond knife blade seen with light microscope demonstrates chipped tip *(circle)* and coarse lapp marks parallel to the edge from poor honing *(arrows)* (×100). (Courtesy Magnum Diamond.)

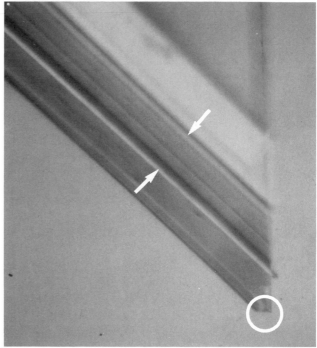

blades. Now, both manufacturers and ophthalmologists are more critical in their evaluation of these crystalline blades.

The hardness of a diamond is a great advantage when used for jewelry because of its extraordinary durability, but in surgery it is an advantage and disadvantage, because the hardness makes the finely honed tip and edge of a diamond knife brittle and at great risk of fracture (Fig. 15-23).

Probably the most common source of fracture is improper cleaning and handling of the knife blade, as discussed later. Internal flaws in the knife blade are a second source of fracture, and this depends on the quality of the gem itself.

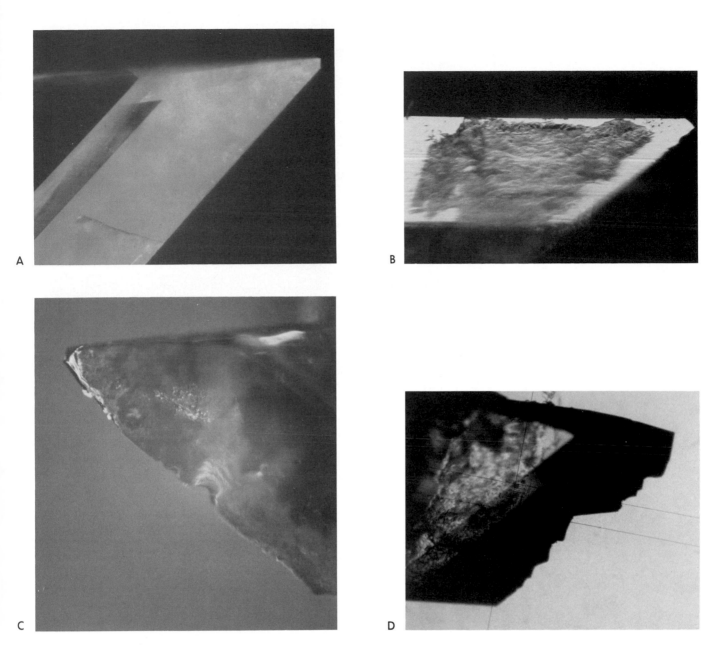

Figure 15-23
Used diamond knife blades showing various amounts of chipping and edge fracture.
A, Mild, broken tip. **B,** Moderate. **C,** Ruby blade, severe. **D,** Extreme (×100).
(Courtesy of Magnum Diamond.)

Fortunately, a coated or chipped diamond blade can be repaired or replaced by the manufacturer. When a surgeon thinks the diamond blade is cutting poorly or finds it damaged, chipped, or coated, the blade should be returned promptly. The manufacturer will do one of three things: replace the blade with a new one; replace the blade from inventory with one that has already been resharpened; or resharpen the blade. Replacing the blade out of inventory is much quicker than resharpening the blade, which can take weeks. A diamond blade can be repaired and resharpened only two or three times because some of the crystalline structure is removed and the entire diamond becomes shorter.

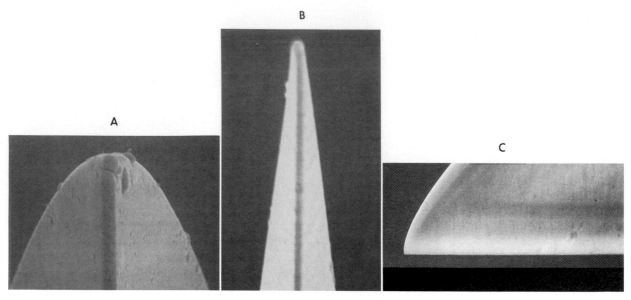

Figure 15-24
Comparison of tips of two crystalline knife blades for radial keratotomy as seen by scanning electron microscopy. **A,** Sapphire with average radius of curvature of 1.1 μm. **B,** Diamond blade with average radius of curvature of 0.15 μm (×10,500). **C,** Unused sapphire knife blade shows relatively blunted tip (SEM, ×1000). (**A** and **B** courtesy William Knepshield, Jr., KMI, Inc.; **C** courtesy Myocure, Inc.)

The ophthalmologist must deal with a knowledgeable, reputable manufacturer. One doctor tells the story of receiving his blade back from repair, only to find that the dull vertical back edge of the blade had been sharpened, leaving the oblique, original cutting edge damaged.

Ruby and sapphire knife blades. Ruby and sapphire blades are made from synthetic crystals of aluminum oxide (Al_2O_3, corundum). The two crystals are essentially the same; the ruby contains a few parts per million more chromium that gives it its red color.

Two different crystalline forms are grown synthetically: a single crystal and a matrix crystal. Although both the ruby and sapphire are rated with a hardness of 1.00 on the Knoop-Ridgeway scale, they are not equally durable. The sapphire is much more resistant to damage than the ruby. Ruby and sapphire edges are ground directly, in the same way as metal blades, since no internal crystalline structure limits the process. However, the ruby and sapphire blades are so much softer than a diamond (at least 140 times softer) that a very fine edge can chip easily, so honing to a very sharp edge and tip is unrealistic (Fig. 15-24). In general, a sapphire blade can be used for 10 to 20 cases, whereas a ruby blade can be used for only a few. After the first or second cut, the ruby blade becomes noticeably duller in the same way that a metal blade does.

A sapphire blade can be cleaned similar to a diamond blade, but the ruby blade must not be stabbed into or wiped on any cleaning material because the blade will be damaged. Of course, the durability of a blade is influenced by how well it is cleaned and how carefully it is used, so a slovenly or clumsy surgeon may find the diamond blade less durable than the sapphire blade used by a fastidious, compulsive colleague.

Sapphire and ruby blades cannot be repaired; they are simply replaced. In fact, many manufacturers sell replaceable blades that can be exchanged by the surgeon.

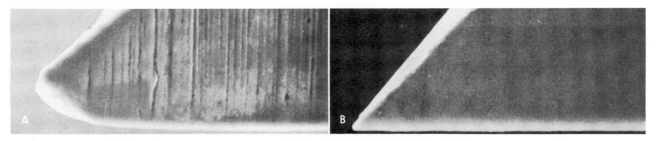

Figure 15-25
Metal knife blades. **A,** Stainless steel blade shows rounded tip, coarse honing marks, and somewhat dull edge. **B,** High—carbon steel blade shows sharp edge and tip with smooth side devoid of honing marks. (Courtesy Myocure, Inc.)

Cost of crystal-bladed knives. The cost of crystal-bladed knives varies greatly. It is clear, however, that the cost of the raw diamonds and the manufacture of a high-quality diamond blade is much greater than the cost of the materials and manufacture for ruby and sapphire blades (see Table 15-7). Yet the differential cost among these knives in the marketplace is not very great; the manufacturers of the ruby and sapphire blades identify overall manufacturing expense and marketing costs as the reason.

Metal blades. The stainless steel surgical blade had been the standard scalpel for ophthalmic surgeons until diamond blades were introduced in 1966.[5] Compared with the smooth edge that can be produced on a diamond, the edge on a stainless steel blade is like the silhouette of the Grand Teton Mountains. Early in the development of radial keratotomy, surgeons used stainless steel blades, for example, blades made by the Beaver Company, Vxtra PS, Wilkinson, Gillette, Schick, and others (Fig. 15-25). However, the tough cornea presented considerable resistance, and the rough blades caused drag and made faltering incisions with jagged edges, which was a particular problem with centripetal incisions that were difficult to stop at the margin of the central clear zone. Surgeons then began using high—carbon steel razor blades, for example, blades made by Feather, Gillette, and Clay-Adams, because they made better incisions. But breaking the blades and inserting them into the blade holder or chuck and adjusting their length manually was tedious and variable. The coating used on commercial razor blades to lubricate the blade and prevent rusting increased tissue drag. Therefore uncoated high—carbon steel blades with highly polished edges, such as Vxtra, Myocule, and Sputnik, were designed for surgical use (see Fig. 15-25).

Metal blades are approximately 0.10 mm thick and have an included cutting angle of 12° to 15°.[32] These excellent design characteristics are offset by the softness of the blade, which cannot be ground as sharp as a diamond and which dulls rapidly with use.

The surgeon using a metal blade to incise the cornea feels resistance and drag in contrast to the feel of a sharp diamond blade, which seems to float through the tissue. The drag with the metal knives produces a kinesthetic sense that the surgeon can use to control the blade, whereas with a sharp crystal blade, control is almost completely visual.

Microscopic study of the quality of the incision made by stainless steel and diamond blades has demonstrated a rougher epithelial surface and stromal margin with the steel blade, presumably because the steel blade displaces tissue before it cuts, whereas the diamond cuts quicker (Fig. 15-26).[8] On the other hand, the histologic features and the depth of the incisions made with carbon steel blades and diamond blades appear similar in cadaver eye models.[29]

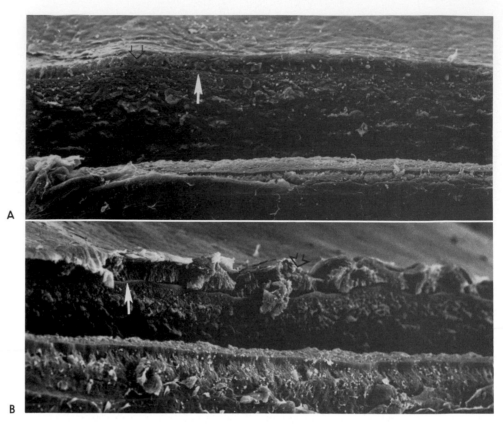

Figure 15-26
Comparison of incision in the cornea made by diamond blade **(A)** and razor blade fragment **(B)** shows greater disruption of the epithelium *(open arrow)* and Bowman's layer *(white arrow)* caused by the razor blade (SEM, ×150). (From Goldberg EJ: Ophthalmic Surg 1984; 15:203-204.)

Configuration of crystal knife blades. Given an exquisitely sharp, clean crystal blade, its design and configuration determine its cutting characteristics during surgery, as discussed by Eisner.[6] Diamond blade characteristics are described in the box on p. 445 and in Fig. 15-27.

Width of the blade. When viewed from the side, blades have a width from back to front that varies from approximately 1 to 2 mm at the base and tapers down to a few microns at the tip. Wider blades are more stable during cutting than a narrow blade because they track a straight line better.

Thickness of the blade. Blades have a side-to-side thickness at the base of approximately 0.08 to 0.3 mm (80 to 300 μm), tapering down to a few microns at the tip. The base thickness is not an important characteristic because the thick part of the blade usually does not enter the tissue. However, the thickness of the back of the blade affects stability during cutting—wider backs creating a more stable wedge but more drag.

Included angle. The angle formed by the two sides of the blade as they taper toward the cutting edge is called the included (or alpha) angle. It varies from approximately 30° to 45° and determines the functional "thickness" of the blade that separates the tissue. A larger included angle creates more wedge effect and tissue drag as the blade is plunged into or pulled through the tissue. This increased resistance makes the knife feel "duller" to the surgeon, even though the edge is exquisitely sharp.

Characteristics of Diamond Knife Blades

Desirable qualities

Hardness	5.18 on Knoop-Ridgeway scale
	10 on Mohs' scale
Gem quality	Clarity 1 to 5
	Color scale 1 to 6
Weight	1.5 to 2.5 carats
Blemishes (clarity)	No inclusions, cracks, bubbles
Surface	Smooth without lapp or polishing lines

Blade configuration

Width (back to front)	1 to 2 mm
Thickness (side-to-side)	
Regular	.2 to .3 mm
Thin	120 to 150 μm
Very thin	80 to 100 μm
Included cutting angle (approximate alpha angle)	25°, 30°, 45°
Cutting edge thickness	5 μm
Cutting edge radius of curvature	.15 to .5 μm
Number of cutting edges	1—oblique or vertical
	2—oblique, vertical, or both
	3—square, trifaceted
	Many—curved
Angle of cutting edges	12°, 30°, 45°, 90°
Quality of tip and edge	Sharp and regular at 100× to 1000× magnification

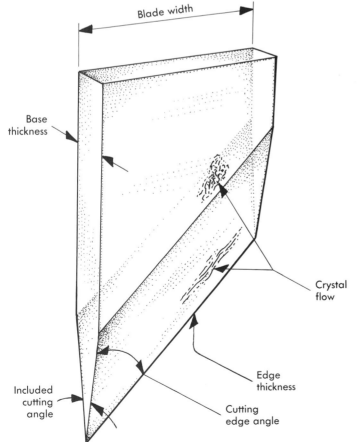

Figure 15-27
Characteristics of diamond knife blade. The configuration of each diamond knife blade may be different and will determine the feel and function of the blade during surgery.

Included angle and width of blade. The thickness of the blade and the included angle are the two variables that determine the maximal incision depth that can be reached before the full thickness of the blade is reached (Fig. 15-28). For a blade of a given width, a smaller included angle allows a deeper incision to be made before the full width of the blade is reached. Conversely, for a given included angle, a wider blade allows a deeper incision to be made before the full width of the blade is reached. The feel of the blade to the surgeon as it is cutting through the cornea varies with the blade configuration. A thicker blade with smaller included angles cuts only with the beveled part of the blade, which decreases tissue drag; however, a thinner blade that is cutting with the full width of the blade in the tissue may have less tissue drag because of the thinness of the blade, assuming that all the knives are equally sharp. Thus as with many hand instruments in ophthalmic surgery the surgeon's own sensibilities determine the preferable configuration.

Thickness of cutting edge. Knives cut tissue by concentrating the mechanical force applied to the handle at the edge of the blade. The thinner the edge, the more force concentrated on it and the sharper the knife. A blade edge ground to a point has an infinite amount of force applied to it. Because of its crystalline structure and hardness, a diamond can be honed to a thin cutting edge, approximately 5 μm (30 carbon atoms) thick. When examined by scanning electron microscopy, the edge is sometimes measured in micrometer radius of curvature because a gold coating is necessary for observation. The coating actually obscures the real cutting edge. The finer the edge, the more brittle it is, with a greater chance of fracturing because of internal flaws or mechanical damage. Examination of the edge under high magnification (approximately 250 to 400×) can help the surgeon identify irregularities.

Angle of the cutting edge. The cutting edge is most commonly angled at 45 degrees or is vertical at 90 degrees; blades are sometimes cut at 30 degrees or with multiple angles in those multifaceted edges. As discussed in Chapter 17, Atlas of Surgical Techniques of Radial Keratotomy, an obliquely angled blade cuts the layers of the cornea sequentially from anterior to posterior, exerting vector forces both forward and downward with resultant posterior displacement of tissue; the vertically edged blade cuts the anterior and posterior layers simultaneously, exerting a vector force forward and displacing less tissue posteriorly. A dull or chipped vertical edge will cut the tissue more poorly because it must be pushed frontally against the tissue, whereas a dull or chipped angled edge will cut relatively better because of the combined vector forces.

Number and orientation of edges. Configurations of knife edges include one cutting edge angled either obliquely (front-cutting) or vertically (back-cutting); two cutting edges that are both oblique and vertical; three cutting edges that may be on three sides of a rectangularly shaped blade or along the curved edge of a trifaceted blade; and many edges in a multifaceted blade. In general, blades with more edges are higher quality diamonds because the splitting and honing are more difficult.

Each surgeon determines how he or she will use a given knife-blade configuration. In general, an angled blade is used for centrifugal radial incisions from the clear zone to the limbus; a vertical blade is used for centripetal radial incisions from the limbus to the clear zone and for transverse incisions; a double- or triple-edged blade has the potential for use in any of these directions. In general, diamond-bladed micrometer knives designed for radial keratotomy are not useful for freehand dissection in other types of anterior segment surgery because the footplates obscure the view of the cutting edge and the blade does not extend far enough beyond the footplates.

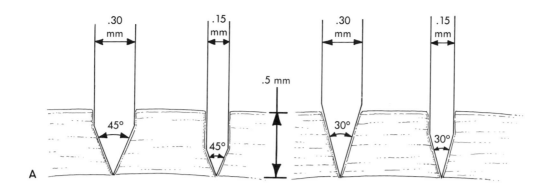

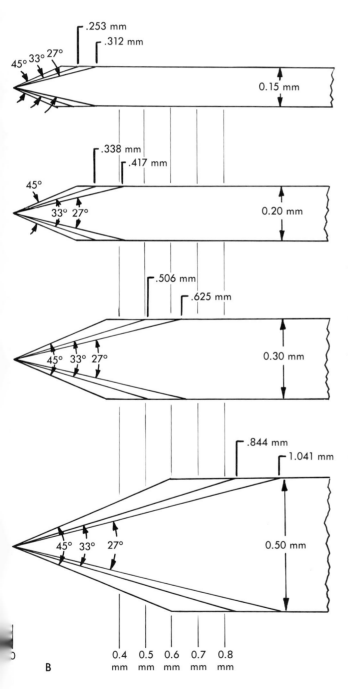

Maximum Incision Spread

Incision depth	0.15 Thick			0.20 Thick			0.30 Thick			0.50 Thick
	27°	33°	45°	27°	33°	45°	27°	33°	45°	45°
0.40 mm	.15	.15	.15	.192	.20	.20	.192	.237	.30	.33
0.50 mm	.15	.15	.15	.20	.20	.20	.240	.296	.30	.42
0.60 mm	.15	.15	.15	.20	.20	.20	.288	.30	.30	.50
0.70 mm	.15	.15	.15	.20	.20	.20	.30	.30	.30	.50
0.80 mm	.15	.15	.15	.20	.20	.20	.30	.30	.30	.50

Figure 15-28
The relationship of the thickness of the knife blade and the included angle. **A,** For blades of a given thickness, those with a smaller included angle will cut deeper before the full width of the blade is reached. Conversely, for blades with a given included angle, those that are thicker will cut deeper before the full thickness of the blade is reached. In general, tissue drag increases once the full thickness of the blade enters the tissue. **B,** Drawing shows the relationship between the following variables concerning knife blade: thickness of the blade, included angle of the blade, depth of the incision, depth of the incision before the maximal thickness of the blade is reached, and maximal spread of the incision. The table of maximal incision spread relates the three variables of blade thickness, included angle, and incision depth. It demonstrates that thinner blades (0.15 and 0.20 mm) use their full thickness in cutting no matter what the included angle or depth. On the other hand, thicker blades (0.3 and 0.5 mm) cut only with the beveled part of the blade when the included angle is smaller (27°, 33°) or when the depth of the incision is shallower (0.4 to 0.5 mm). These factors give a different feel of sharpness and tissue resistance for different knife blade configurations. (Courtesy William Knepshield, Jr., KMI, Inc.)

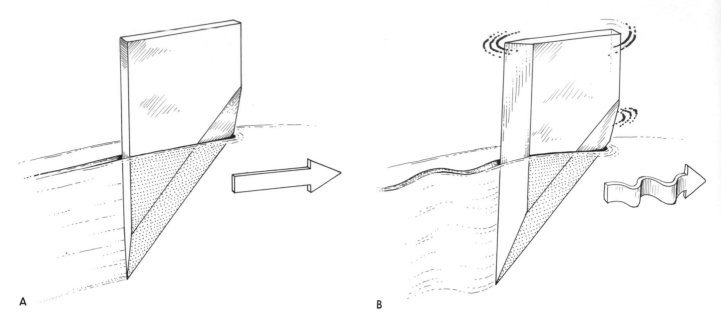

Figure 15-29
The amount of contact between the surface of the knife blade and the tissue is determined by the configuration of the blade and the number of edges. Single-edged blades **(A)** have more contact than double-edged blades **(B).** Greater contact creates more tissue drag.

Cutting characteristics of different blade configurations. The combination of all of the variables listed in the box on p. 445 and illustrated in Figs. 15-27 and 15-28 creates the personality of a knife blade, which must be added to the personality of the footplate and handle. The sharpness of the blade is the most important characteristic. Second is the amount of tissue drag created by the blade configuration. The more blade area that contacts the tissue during cutting and the rougher the blade surface, the greater the drag. For example, using a single-edged, oblique blade creates more tissue contact than the same design with a double edge because the tapered sharp back vertical edge does not contact the tissue as much (Fig. 15-29). Early designs of diamond knife blades used for radial keratotomy had a wide included angle with a wide, flat back edge that sometimes split the tissue at the paracentral end of the incision, forming a T-patterned incision. Improved designs have made the crystal blades thinner, the included angles smaller, and the number of cutting edges greater, so the amount of contact between the blade and the tissue is reduced.

Knives with different configurations cut differently (Fig. 15-30). A thicker blade with a greater included angle and a single cutting edge tends to track better in a straight line through the tissue because the back edge acts as a rudder, whereas a thinner blade with a smaller included angle and double edge tends to wobble through the tissue because there is less directional stability. Similarly a double-edged blade can easily cut in both directions, so a surgeon who allows the blade to drift toward the clear zone after inserting it paracentrally will find the incision extended in the wrong direction, something that would not happen with the single-edged blade.

Surgeons must know the personality of their knife blades and the types of incisions they make to predict the outcome of the surgery more accurately.

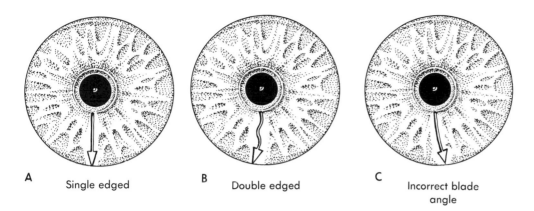

A	B	C
Single edged	Double edged	Incorrect blade angle

Figure 15-30
Knife blades of different configurations will have different cutting characteristics. **A,** A single-edged, wide blade with a thick trailing surface tends to track straighter in tissue and make a straighter cut. **B,** A thinner, double-edged blade will track less well and tend to wobble in the tissue, making a more irregular cut. **C,** A blade that is set at a wrong angle on the end of the shaft or that has asymmetrical grinding or roughness may tend to veer in one direction.

Assessment of knife blades

Quality control of the manufacture of diamond blades. Neumann and co-workers[20a] using a microscope examined seven knives purchased directly from the manufacturer. Their findings may not apply to all blades manufactured by a company. Their descriptions were as follows: two Micra blades had broken tips; Metico blade had a flawless edge and a smooth surface; one KOI blade had good quality; one Bausch & Lomb blade had no obvious flaws in the diamond but an extremely rough surface; of two Storz blades, one had on internal flaw and both were misaligned between the footplate.

Comparison of cutting characteristics. Huebscher and colleagues[11a] compared the power necessary to incise a pig cornea with different knife blades and discovered the following: a new diamond required the least power; resharpened diamonds required somewhat more power; blades made individually from razor blade fragments were the next most effective; ruby knives varied in their sharpness; and knives manufactured in bulk from razor blade fragments as well as conventional steel bladed knives were relatively dull. Examples are presented in the box on p. 450.

Attachment of crystal blade to knife handle

A crystal blade is shaped as a long rectangle, the butt of which is sunk into the end of a rod that acts as the support and transport mechanism within the knife handle (see Fig. 15-14). The blade is secured to the rod with epoxy or other cement, and the quality of this mounting is important, not only to maintain the alignment of the blade between the footplates and to hold the blade absolutely secure during cutting and cleaning, but also to resist chemical erosion from tissues and cleaning fluids and acoustic damage from ultrasonic cleaners.

Comparison of Power Required for Different Knife Blades to Make a Linear Incision to a Depth of 0.5 mm in Porcine Corneas

Instrument type and example	Power range mN (milliNewton)
Knives with diamond blades	
Diamond knife (new)—Geuder	44
Diamond knife (resharpened)—Meyko	74
Instruments made individually from razor blades	100-120
Nelson Safety Razor Blades—Eisfeld	
Sputnik—Soviet Union	
Knives with ruby blades	
Ruby knife (lancett)—Grieshaber	96-200
Instruments manufactured from razor blades with a manufactured handle	
Microsurgical knife—Weck	140-190
Instruments manufactured from razor blades	
Razor blade pieces—Klein	176-280
Special blades with a handle	186-530
Micro-sharp blade—Beaver	
Microsurgical knife—Sharpoint	
Conventional scalpels and steel knives	
Discission knife—MLW	430-510

Modified from Huebscher HJ, Goder GJ, and Lommatzsch PK: Ophthalmic Surg 1989;20:120-123.

This factor is most important with diamond-bladed knives, where hundreds of uses are expected out of a single blade. Attachment of ruby and sapphire blades that come on disposable chucks need not meet as exacting standards.

Maintenance and cleaning of crystal knife blades

Cleaning diamond blades. A clean diamond blade reduces tissue drag during cutting (Fig. 15-31). A properly cleaned, properly handled diamond blade will remain useful for hundreds of keratotomy cases, assuming good initial quality of stone. Because of its extreme hardness and surface resistance, the surface of the diamond is not damaged by the accumulation of tissue residues or salts from surgical solutions. Fastidious and compulsive maintenance is required by the surgeon, who will be more likely to preserve the use of a diamond knife if he follows two rules: the surgeon should be the only person to handle the knife when the diamond blade is extended, and the surgeon should clean the blade immediately after making the last incision, before the blade is retracted. It is difficult to decide exactly what method to use for cleaning a diamond blade because there is considerable variation among manufacturers' recommendations and among the opinions of individuals who claim to be knowledgeable about diamonds. We review the different recommendations here step-by-step.

Cleaning fluids. What fluids should be used for immediate cleaning? Mineral-containing water, such as saline and balanced salt solution, should be avoided because salts crystallize and coat the surface of the blade and the steel parts of the knife. Distilled water is preferred, but since the diamond is hydrophobic, simply squirting or wiping water over the surface will not provide good cleaning.

A   B   C

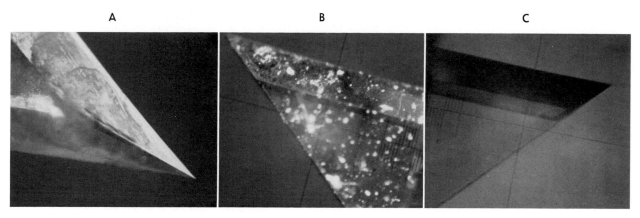

Figure 15-31
Clean and dirty diamond knife blades. **A,** A double-edged diamond knife blade with smooth edges and a sharp tip, but with debris coating the surface. **B,** Single-edged diamond knife blade with chipped tip and surface festooned with plaques and particles of debris. **C,** A clean diamond knife blade with smooth edges and a sharp tip. (Courtesy Magnum Diamond.)

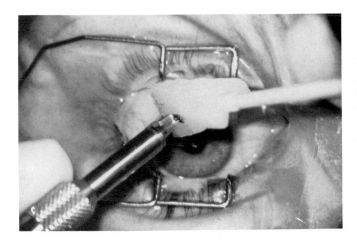

Figure 15-32
Intraoperative cleaning of diamond knife blade is done immediately after the last incision. The knife blade is extended fully and pulled through a microsponge soaked in hydrogen peroxide and then through another microsponge soaked in distilled water. The blade is retracted and the footplates cleaned with peroxide and water. Only the surgeon should handle the knife when the blade is extended.

Cleaners such as acetone are dangerous on the surgical field if they contact tissues; they can damage the epoxy-based mounting adhesives of the blade. Industrial diamond-cleaning liquids are not generally available. Cleaning solutions designed especially for diamond knives used in ophthalmology are commercially available, for example, Neutrad CRC from Magnum Diamond, Inc. Undiluted 3% hydrogen peroxide is an inexpensive, effective cleaning solution for these knives (Fig. 15-32). The hydrogen peroxide can be placed in a properly labeled medicine cup on the back instrument table and used only at the moment of cleaning, removing it from the surgical field immediately to prevent inadvertent instillation into the eye. The peroxide oxidizes tissue particles and fluid precipitates that are on the blade. The peroxide and debris are rinsed off with distilled water.

To remove debris that is caked onto the blade, a soapy cleaner can be used. Another way to remove residues is to use a soft–contact lens enzyme cleaner, soaking the knife for approximately 6 to 12 hours in a pan of water containing two enzyme tablets. Enzyme cleaning is ineffective if the residues have been baked on by autoclaving or if the knives are soaked for only short periods.

All cleaning liquids can be picked up into the mechanism of the micrometer handle, possibly damaging the mechanism and possibly damaging the eye of the next patient. Therefore the knife must be thoroughly rinsed and dried after cleaning.

Manual cleaning. Mechanical cleaning of the knife blade is necessary immediately at the conclusion of surgery to completely remove tissue fluids and debris (see Fig. 15-31). Simple irrigation is inadequate. A microsponge of cellulose, Merocel, cotton, or styrofoam will do the job. Never use dry material; always have it completely wet with peroxide or distilled water. The diamond is much harder than any of these substances and will not be damaged by them. After extending the blade fully, the surgeon should gently plunge the knife into the material and cut it with the knife. This gently wipes the surface of the blade against the material. The surgeon should not twist the knife blade within the material, which will tend to fracture the diamond edge and loosen the blade mounting, and should not strike the blade on the plastic, wooden, or metal holder (see Fig. 15-32).

We prefer to soak one microsponge in hydrogen peroxide for the initial cleaning and a second sponge in distilled water for the final cleaning. Then the knife blade is retracted into the handle, and the footplates can be cleaned by wiping them on the microsponges.

Cleaning machines. Manufacturers and experts disagree about ultrasonic cleaning of diamonds. There is no question that ultrasonic cleaning machines can remove caked-on debris, blood, and tissue fluids. However, since ultrasonic cleaning machines use different amounts of power to generate different frequencies of ultrasound, a diamond may sustain some damage to the edge. Diamonds with intrinsic flaws can suffer acoustic damage as the sound waves and the imploding air bubbles in the fluid strike the crystal, causing vibrations that may crack the stone—failure by harmonic restitution. The ultrasound can also damage the metal finishes and mounting cements of the knife. If ultrasonic cleaning is used, the knife must be held securely in a cradle with the blade retracted so that it does not contact the metal tray.

On the other hand, a properly controlled ultrasonic cleaning of diamond blades can be done safely with a small, jewelry-type cleaner using hydrogen peroxide as the fluid. The blade and the footplates are immersed in the fluid, but the rest of the handle is left out in air. The time for ultrasonic cleaning is approximately 15 seconds, after which the knife is rinsed in distilled water. It is not necessary to immerse the handle completely.

Meticulous cleaning of the blade and footplates immediately after the last incision of every procedure may obviate the need for ultrasonic cleaning.

A water-pic instrument designed for cleaning teeth can be used to squirt distilled water against the diamond blade, adding some power to help remove surface debris.

Cleaning sapphire blades. Because sapphires are softer than diamonds, they must be cleaned more gently. Ultrasound should never be used. The blade is hard enough to cut surgical microsponges, which allows cleaning with peroxide and distilled water as described in the diamond blade cleaning section.

Cleaning ruby blades. As the softest of the crystal blades, ruby blades must be cleaned most gently, irrigating with hydrogen peroxide or distilled water. Forcefully squirting the fluid onto the blade through a syringe and needle may provide some mechanical force to remove debris without damaging the blade. Ruby blades must not be cleaned by cutting through any material, and ultrasound should not be used. Ruby blades are used for only a few cases, then discarded.

Sterilization of knives. Manual and mechanical cleaning does not sterilize the knife or its blade. Steam autoclaving is a standard and safe procedure, but the operating room staff must avoid producing sudden changes in temperature for the knife, such as placing the recently autoclaved hot knife in a cold water bath, which can produce thermal shock because of the different expansion coefficients of the diamond and its housing, loosening the diamond blade. Fortunately modern epoxy glues are made to expand, so they are not as adversely affected by these temperature changes. Gas sterilization is also effective.

Knife footplates

Function of footplates. The footplates at the end of the knife handle straddle either side of the knife blade and serve numerous functions. They determine the extension of the knife blade and therefore the depth of the incision. In this sense the knives are called guarded knives because the footplates guard the knife blade from extending too far and cutting too deeply. The footplates stabilize the tissue on either side of the knife blade as it cuts, displacing the tissue posteriorly and flattening it to increase the cutability (sectility) of the cornea.[6] The footplates stabilize the knife handle and help the surgeon make the incision of the exact desired configuration. The blades allow the knife to glide smoothly over the surface of the cornea without damaging the epithelium.

Of course each of these functions requires specific design features. If the footplates on either side of the blade are aligned unevenly or are curved, it is difficult to measure the extension of the blade accurately. Narrow footplates provide less stability for the knife, and they may slide into the incision during a second pass. Narrow footplates increase the visibility of the knife blade. Broad footplates may depress the cornea too much as the incision is made and obscure the view of the blade, although they may stabilize the knife better. Rough footplates abrade the corneal epithelium.

Design of footplates. Footplates can be divided into three common designs (Figs. 15-14 and 15-33). The first is the beveled or angled footplate (PERK-style, American-style) (Fig. 15-33, *A* to *D*) that has a relatively small surface touching the cornea. The leading edge of the footplate is beveled away from the cornea so that the cutting edge of the blade encounters the tissue directly without the footplates wrinkling up or pushing the tissue away from the edge of the blade. This design also allows the knife to be tilted forward or backward on the cornea without changing the depth to which the blade cuts.[27] The dimensions of this footplate are approximately 2 mm by 1.5 mm. Most knives of this style have a semicircular opening cut out of the back of the footplate to improve visualization of the blade during cutting, but this is generally ineffective; the cutting edge of the blade is obscured in most positions.

The second style of footplate (Fig. 15-33, *E* and *F*) is a simpler, flat design that has a half cylinder or two struts extending down on either side of the knife blade, with the entire blade encased between the footplates. This configuration is usually used with an angled cutting edge or a double-cutting edge and allows minimal visualization of the blade during cutting.

The third type of footplate is the ski-shape or "sewing machine" shape (as in the Fyodorov-Neumann knife) (Fig. 15-33, *H* to *K*). It consists of two supports that extend down from the end of the handle, curve backward, and extend on either side of the blade, protruding beyond the cutting edge. This configuration is used with either a vertical or oblique cutting edge. The cutting edge may face either the open end or closed end of the footplates. Because the side of the footplate is open, it allows good visualization of the knife blade while cutting both from the side and from the front.

Two other footplate designs require further clinical use before their role can be assessed. The first is the single loop that extends down on one side of a

Text continued on p. 458.

Figure 15-33
Comparison of 12 commercially available diamond blade and footplate designs. Each is viewed from the side (left), from the cutting edge of the blade (middle), and obliquely (right). Each knife was supplied in late 1987 by the manufacturer at the request of the authors. Some of the knives were used for commercial demonstration and were not intended for clinical use. The photographs were taken by Mr. Steve Carlton at the Emory Eye Center.

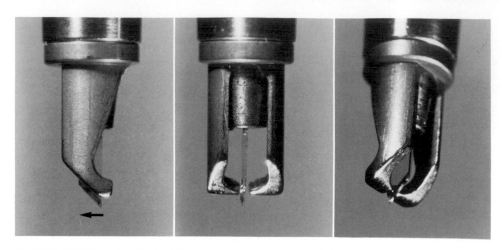

A, KOI, PERK-style. Blade: Diamond, single edge, angled. Footplate: Marked bevel with blade edge exposed.

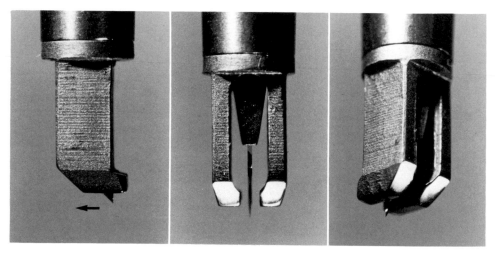

B, Pilling. Blade: Diamond, single edge, angled. Footplate: Flat with slight bevel, blade edge not exposed.

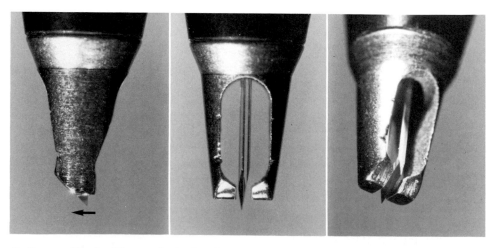

C, Beaver. Blade: Diamond, single edge, angled. Footplate: Moderate bevel, blade edge sometimes exposed.

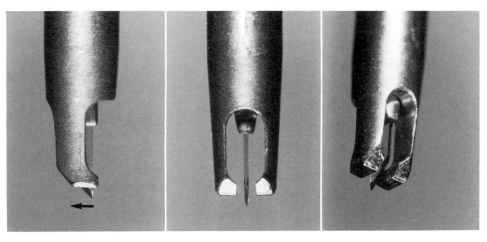

D, Storz. Blade: Diamond, single edge, angled. Footplate: Flat with slight bevel, blade edge sometimes exposed.

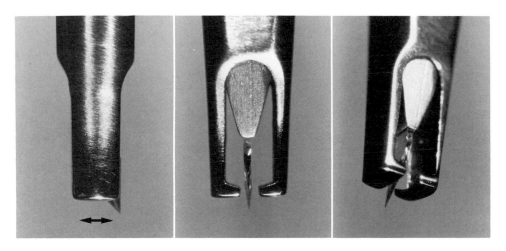

E, Metico. Blade: Diamond, double edge, angled and straight. Footplate: Square and flat, straight blade edge exposed, angled blade edge not exposed.

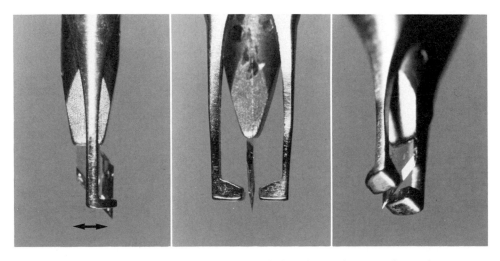

F, Metico. Blade: Diamond, double edge, angled and straight. Footplate: Flat L-shape, blade edges not exposed. *Continued.*

Figure 15-33, cont'd
Comparison of 12 commercially available diamond blade and footplate designs. Each is viewed from the side (left), from the cutting edge of the blade (middle), and obliquely (right). Each knife was supplied in late 1987 by the manufacturer at the request of the authors. Some of the knives were used for commercial demonstration and were not intended for clinical use. The photographs were taken by Mr. Steve Carlton at the Emory Eye Center.

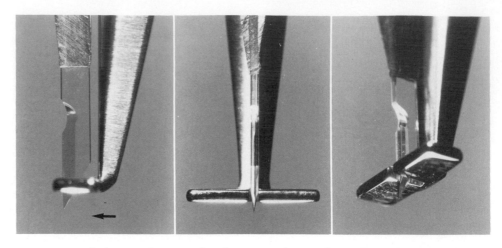

G, Katena. Blade: Sapphire, single edge, vertical. Footplate: Flat with wings, blade edge not exposed.

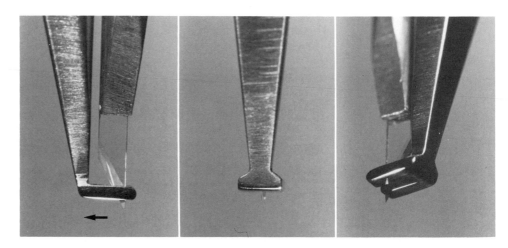

H, Katena. Blade: Sapphire, single edge, angled. Footplate: Flat L-shaped, blade edge not exposed.

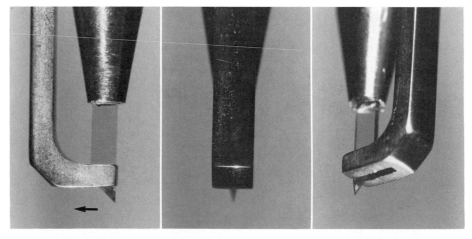

I, Bausch & Lomb. Blade: Diamond, single edge, angled. Footplate: Flat, L-shaped, slight bevel, blade edge not exposed.

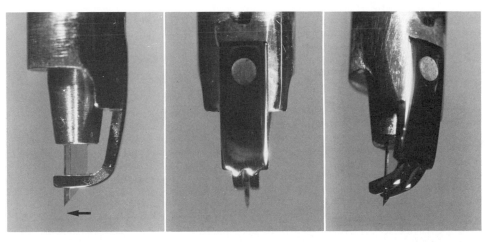

J, KMI. Blade: Diamond, single edge, vertical. Footplate: Flat, **L**-shaped with slight bevel, blade edge not exposed.

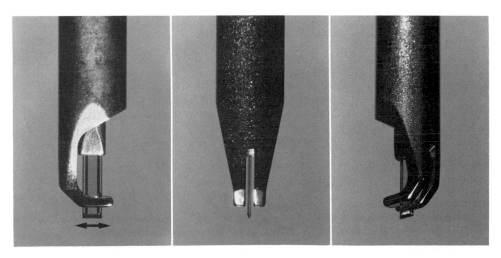

K, Keeler. Blade: Diamond, rectangle, three edges. Footplate: Flat, **L**-shaped, slight bevel.

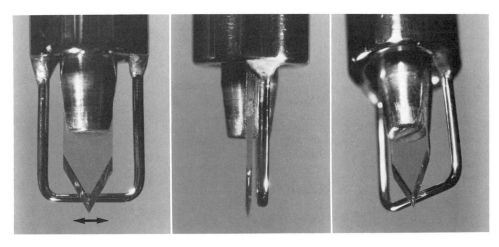

L, KOI. Blade: Diamond, double edge, angled. Footplate: One side, flat wire, blade edge exposed.

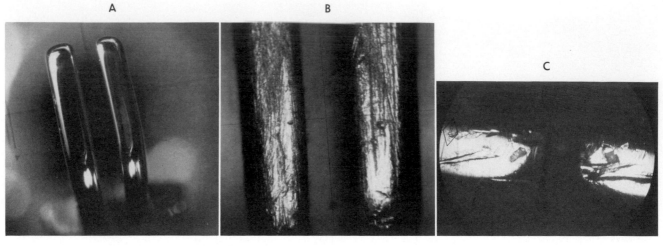

Figure 15-34
Surface of footplates. **A,** Smooth footplate after polishing and gold plating. **B,** Moderate scratching of footplate surfaces by edge of gauge block. **C,** Severely gouged footplate surfaces will abrade epithelium (×100 to 200). (Courtesy Magnum Diamond.)

double-angled blade (Stulting) and is designed for cutting arcuate incisions and wedge resections. The second configuration has two broad wings that stick out to the side (Fig. 15-33, *G*) and are designed to help keep the blade perpendicular and stabilized during the incision.

Footplates vary in width from 0.4 to 1.0 mm and in length from 0.8 to 3.0 mm in most knives.

The considerable variation in design translates into variations in surgical technique and variations in the depth and contour of the incisions, emphasizing that surgeons must know the performance characteristics of each knife they use.

Visibility of blade. The visibility of the knife blade during cutting varies with the design of the footplate and the orientation of the incision. Visibility is better with the straight vertical "back-cutting" blades in the sewing-machine footplates than with the angled oblique "front-cutting" blades in the cylindric or beveled footplates. Visualization of the blade for centrifugal incisions is not as important as it is for centripetal incisions, where the knife must be stopped exactly at the margin of the clear zone. Similarly blade visibility is important in transverse incisions because transverse incisions must not intersect the radial incisions. If transverse incisions are made first, it is an important advantage to see the edge of the blade while the radial incisions are being made to prevent intersecting previously made transverse incisions.

Surface of footplates. Footplates must have smooth bottom surfaces to reduce tissue drag and epithelial trauma (Fig. 15-34). Polishing of the surfaces to a mirror finish is often completed by hand. This smooth surface must be maintained by proper handling. A damaged surface is usually caused by scraping the footplate along the edge of a gauge block; to prevent this, the footplate should be applied perpendicularly to the side of the gauge block over the setting desired, without sliding it along the side of the block.

The footplates can be coated with gold or Teflon to make the surface even smoother and to increase the ease of sliding. After repeated autoclaving, the Teflon or gold coating can flake off, leaving sharp edges that can abrade the epithelial surface. When properly applied, however, gold plating can present an exquisite surface for contact with the cornea. Replating the stainless steel footplates with gold or Teflon after it has peeled off requires stripping, etching, and replat-

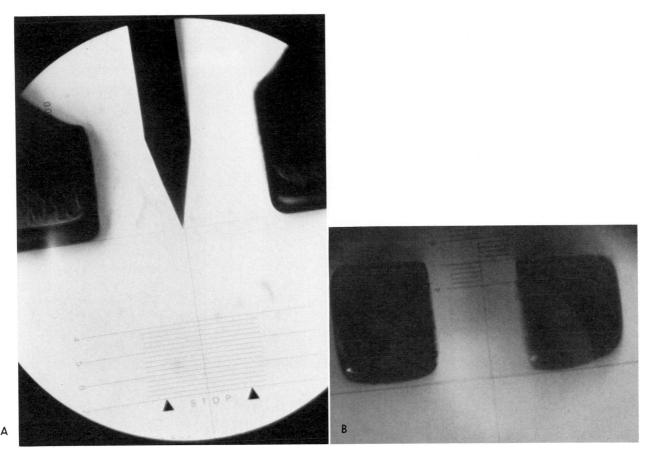

Figure 15-35
Alignment of footplates. **A,** Footplates are aligned equally and are flat. **B,** Footplates are unequal and are not flat, predisposing to inaccurate setting of the blade length and variability in cutting depth (×100). (Courtesy Magnum Diamond.)

ing. It is best to have the footplates properly honed and polished by the manufacturer and kept in pristine condition by the surgeon.

Alignment of the footplates. Both footplates should be equal in length and exactly parallel to each other (Fig. 15-35). If one footplate is longer than the other, the length of the knife blade setting will be different, depending on which of the footplates abuts the gauge block (a longer knife-blade setting for the shorter footplate).

The bottom surface of the footplate should be flat because if it is rocker-shaped, a knife blade setting may also be less accurate (Fig. 15-36). Each footplate should be equidistant from the knife blade and must not be so misaligned that the advancing blade strikes the footplate (Figs. 15-35 and 15-37). The surgeon should inspect the alignment of the extended blade and the footplates frequently, using 100× to 200× magnification, and should have misalignments corrected by the manufacturer. Most footplates are attached to the end of the knife handle as a separate piece, and this attachment sometimes works loose.

Cleaning and maintenance of footplates. The footplate is cleaned after the blade has been retracted by the methods described. The knife should be stored in its own cradle or foam-lined compartment so that the footplates are not abraded by other metal surfaces.

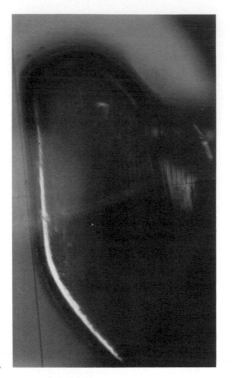

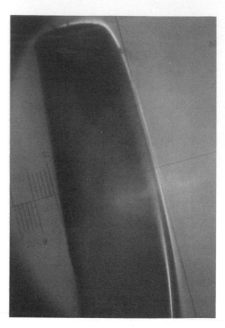

Figure 15-36
Flatness of footplates. **A,** Footplate is flat from one end to the other and smooth.
B, Footplate is curved (rocker-shaped), creating less accurate knife blade settings
(×100). (Courtesy Magnum Diamond.)

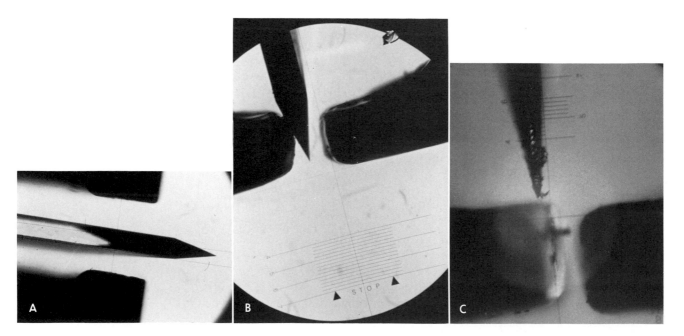

Figure 15-37
Misalignment of footplates can cause damage to the blade. **A,** Slightly off-center
blade. **B,** Blade striking inside edge of footplate. **C,** Blade striking surface of footplate
(×100). (Courtesy Magnum Diamond.)

Knife handle

Configuration of handle. The knife handle serves as the carrier and protective scabbard for the blade and the delicate micrometer.

Knife handles are made of high-quality surgical stainless steel (such as type 303 chromium-nickel) that is nonmagnetic, corrosion resistant, easily machined, and smoothly functioning. Metico and Micra use titanium for a lighter, nonmagnetic handle. Some manufacturers use a plastic, disposable handle.

Most knife handles are approximately 100 mm long, ranging from 70 to 140 mm, with an average diameter of approximately 8 mm. The instruments vary in shape and balance to satisfy individual preferences of surgeons (Fig. 15-38).

Most knives designed for keratotomy have a straight handle, making it difficult to see the footplates and blade of the knife during the paracentral part of the incision, when the knife should be held perpendicular to the surface of the cornea (see Chapter 17, Atlas of Surgical Techniques of Radial Keratotomy). To solve this problem, Metico has marketed the Hofmann/Osher knife in which the carrier for the footplate and the blade is angled approximately 30 degrees from the knife handle itself, allowing the knife to be held similar to a pencil and allowing better visualization of the tip (Fig. 15-39).

Disposable knives with carbon steel blades of preset length were manufactured by Myocure. The blade extensions range from 435 to 685 μm in 10-μm steps, obviating need for a micrometer or gauge block. Drawbacks of this approach include the need for a large inventory, the use of two or three knives per case if incisions of different depth are made, and the requirement of exquisite quality control on the part of the manufacturer.

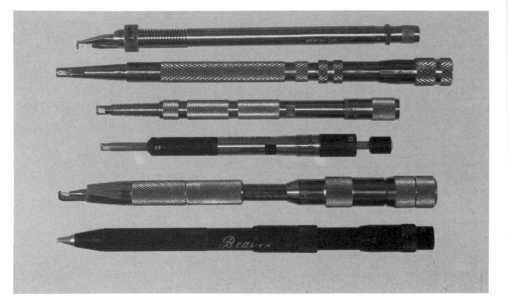

Figure 15-38
Keratotomy micrometer knife handles show considerable variation in design and size. From above to below: Katena with replaceable sapphire blade, Metico straight handle, KOI PERK knife, Storz, Bausch & Lomb, Beaver with external bayonet retracting mechanism.

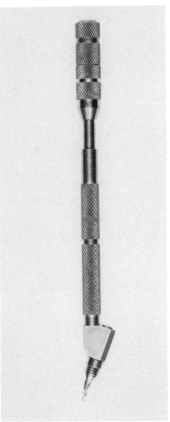

Figure 15-39
Angled knife handle by Metico, Hofmann/Osher design.

Retraction mechanism. To protect the crystal blade when not in use, most knives provide a mechanism for retracting the blade into the barrel of the handle (Fig. 15-40). This mechanism has three designs.

The bayonet design for retraction (Fig. 15-41) uses a spring-mounted mechanism to allow the blade carrier to retract into the barrel when not in use. In this design a pin extending from the outer barrel slides along a groove on the inner carrier. At either end of the groove is an **L**-shaped notch. To advance or retract

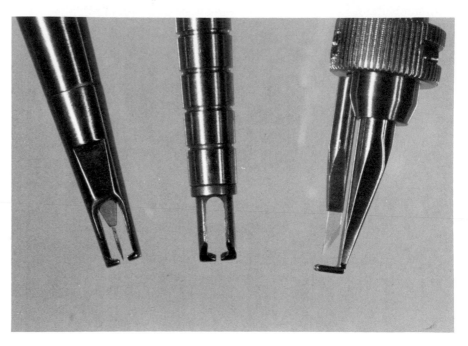

Figure 15-40
Types of blade-retraction mechanisms. Left: Metico knife with blade near zero setting between footplates; a retraction mechanism is present for blade protection. Middle: KOI PERK knife with blade retracted into handle. Right: Katena sapphire blade has no retraction mechanism; the blade can be protected by a soft cover.

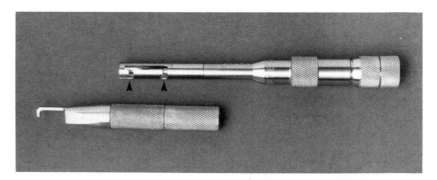

Figure 15-41
Disassembled Bausch & Lomb handle shows internal bayonet retracting mechanism. The grooves at the end of the inner tube *(arrows)* engage a pin that allows the blade to be locked in the retracted or extended position. If the surfaces of the bayonet become worn in the extended position, the zero setting of the knife may be inaccurate.

the blade, the micrometer is rotated to disengage the securing pin from the notch, advanced or retracted by the spring, and then rotated again to engage the pin in the notch at the other end. When the blade is extended, the spring is compressed and the blade is held out by the pin that fits in a small notch. If this notch becomes worn or the spring does not seat the pin properly, the zero setting of the knife may be inaccurate. The mechanism may be located on the inside or the outside of the barrel. This is the most common design used in keratotomy knife handles. In the Katena and some Magnum Diamond styles, the blade remains unprotected outside the barrel (see Fig. 15-40).

In the second design for retraction (Micra, IOLAB), the entire footplate and blade mechanism retract into the sleeve. The retracting bayonet mechanism does not play a role in the extension of the knife blade and therefore cannot get out of calibration. The micrometer is dialed directly with one full turn of the micrometer handle being 50-μm advancement of the knife blade. This is less extension per rotation than knives with other retraction designs.

The third design for retraction uses a micrometer with more threads on it, so the blade is advanced and retracted by many rotations of the handle; there is no spring mechanism. Although it takes slightly longer to expose and retract the blade, this mechanism obviates the potential inaccuracies of a worn bayonet mechanism. Metico and Magnum Diamond make this style.

Micrometer screw mechanism. The heart of most micrometers is the spring-mounted, threaded screw mechanism at the distal end of the knife handle (see Fig. 15-14). The handle advances a rod inside of the knife that pushes the knife blade forward against tension of a spring. A 360-degree turn of the micrometer handle advances the micrometer either 100 or 500 μm, depending on the number of threads and the pitch of the threads.

The micrometer handle should advance the blade with no lateral motion or wobble. In some poorly manufactured knives, the lateral motion is enough to allow the blade to strike the side of the footplate and to cause an incision to veer from the intended straight path (see Fig. 15-37). Many of the new diamond micrometer knives examined by Neumann and colleagues showed wobble during the advancement of the blade.[7,20a]

Use of the micrometer. The calibration scales on micrometers differ (Fig. 15-42). Most have a scale calibrated in steps of 500 μm (0.5 mm) with subdivisions of 100 μm (.10 mm). Those that do not have these fine calibrations allow the

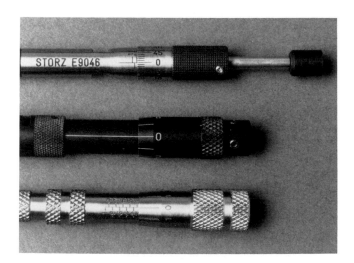

Figure 15-42
Three types of micrometer scales. Above: With Storz handle, a single rotation advances the blade 500 μm. Calibration on outer barrel is in 10-μm steps. Calibration on inner barrel is in 500-μm steps. The extension at top of handle controls the bayonet retracting mechanism. Middle: With Beaver handle, one revolution advances the blade 500 μm. The outer barrel is calibrated in 500-μm steps. The inner barrel is not calibrated. Bottom: With Metico handle, one rotation advances the blade 100 μm. The outer and inner barrels are calibrated in 100-μm steps.

surgeon to lose track of how far the blade has been extended, so when this happens the surgeon may have to retract the blade to the zero point and begin again.

Operating the micrometer is simple. The zero mark on the outer barrel is aligned with the zero mark on the inner barrel so that the tip of the knife blade is flush with the surface of the footplates. The outer barrel is turned clockwise to the desired setting. For example, on a knife in which a single rotation advances the blade 500 μm, the scale on the outer barrel is calibrated into five large units, each representing a distance of 100 μm with 10 small divisions in between, each representing 10 μm. To set the knife blade to a length of 580 μm, the surgeon sets the micrometer to zero, turns the outer barrel clockwise one complete revolution (500 μm), and then continues to turn it clockwise eight more small divisions for a total of 580 μm.

It is a good idea always to set the blade length while advancing the micrometer forward (clockwise) against the spring. If there is some play in the micrometer mechanism, setting the blade in the counterclockwise direction may give a different extension than setting it in the clockwise direction. In other words, surgeons should always set the blade length while advancing the blade. The Katena sapphire knife has no internal spring.

Accuracy of micrometers. The micrometer is simply a calibrated screw designed to fine tolerance. A high-quality micrometer will control the blade length with an accuracy of ± 10 μm (0.01 mm), a tolerance acceptable for human keratotomy. Some companies claim an accuracy of ± 5 μm. To achieve an accuracy greater than ± 5 microns, one consultant from industry (Doug Mastel, Magnum Diamond) listed the following conditions:

1. Because metal expands and contracts with temperature changes, the operating room temperature must be at 68° F with no temperature variation and the knife must contain a thermal transducer to verify the temperature.
2. A minimum of 1 or 2 hours for temperature stabilization of the knives and gauge blocks must be allowed.
3. There must be a method of detecting a broken blade tip using high magnification. Any chip of the tip would reduce the length of the knife blade.
4. Even if the blade could be set to ± 5 μm accuracy, a method of measuring the corneal thickness with similar accuracy and allowing for swelling or dehydration of the cornea during the procedure to achieve the required depth of the incision would require some type of real time servomechanism feedback that could adjust the length of the blade constantly during the incision.

Clearly these conditions are too exacting for current technology.

Because no industry standards for ophthalmic micrometer knives exist, the quality of manufacturing varies considerably. The surgeon can take two steps to ensure accuracy of the knife. The first is to require a warranty from the manufacturer or distributor stating the accuracy of the micrometer. The second is to check the accuracy of the micrometer on an instrument such as a shadowgraph or MicronScope. A high-quality micrometer should not get out of adjustment unless the threads wear down, which would take many years of constant use, or unless the blade guard becomes loose in its mount. However, a poorly manufactured instrument with too much play in the threads can be inaccurate. In addition, a mishandled instrument that sustains mechanical damage or fouling of the threads by the buildup of salts and debris during use may get out of adjustment.

An accurate, properly functioning micrometer and a knife blade with a sharp tip would obviate the need for a gauge block.

Care of the micrometer. Micrometers on keratotomy knives will last indefinitely if properly maintained. They should not be forced at either end. They

A   B   C

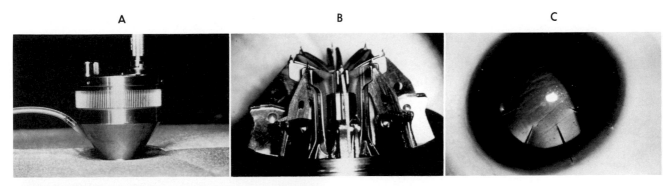

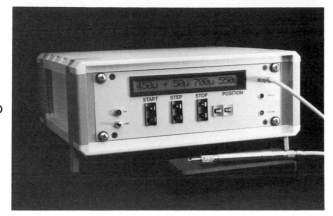

D

Figure 15-43

Mechanical keratotomy knives: Hanna radial microkeratome. **A,** The instrument is shaped as a truncated cone. The outer suction cone attaches it to the surface of the globe and raises the intraocular pressure. **B,** Eight diamond blades are present in grooves. The blades are retracted upward and then released by spring action to make eight simultaneous centrifugal incisions. **C,** Human eye showing eight simultaneous incisions. **D,** Krumeich electronic diamond knife consists of a motorized console with digital display of the blade extension. The starting extension, the extension at each graduated step, the full extension of the blade that is allowed, and the current extension of the blade during the procedure are all indicated on the console. Each value can be set independently. The extension of the blade is controlled electronically by a motor incorporated into the handle, which is controlled by a foot pedal. Each step of the pedal advances the knife by the amount preset in the console. (**A-C** courtesy Khalil Hanna; **D** courtesy Jorg Krumeich.)

should not be soaked in saline, and tissue fluids should not enter the barrel of the knife because they will clog the threads. The bayonet-locking mechanism should be treated gently to prevent disrupting the zero point.

Mechanized knife systems

Radial microkeratome. To increase the accuracy and precision of the incisions, Hanna[24] designed a radial microkeratome shaped like a truncated cone, similar to a Goldmann gonioscopy lens (Fig. 15-43). It consists of an outer suction cone that uses a syringe or machine suction to secure the apparatus to the limbal conjunctiva and raises intraocular pressure slightly to press the cornea against a reference surface. An inner mechanism has eight diamond blades spaced equidistantly around its circumference, each blade associated with a guarded slit. The length of each can be set individually. A lever cocks the blades up into the instrument. When the surgeon pushes the release lever, the eight spring-loaded blades descend simultaneously, cutting from the clear zone to the limbus. The depth of the cut is 150 μm deeper in the periphery than in the paracentral area because the blades descend in an arc of increasing radius. The length of the incision also can be adjusted. Because all four or eight incisions are made simultaneously, the blades are confronted with an identical resistance, helping create identical incisions.

Initial experiments on human eye bank eyes and limited clinical experience document the feasibility of this instrument. A smaller overall size and a better method to verify the length of the blade setting are needed. The instrument is not commercially available as of 1991.

Electronic radial keratotomy knife. An electromechanical knife that can change the length of the knife blade during surgery while the blade is within the corneal tissue has been designed by Krumeich. The knife is designed so that the surgeon can advance or retract the blade during an incision, thus achieving finer control of incision depth. For example, in cutting from the clear zone to the limbus, the blade might be extended because the cornea becomes thicker towards the periphery. Similarly, in cutting from the limbus toward the center the blade could be retracted during the incision. The console is simply programmed to advance and retract the blade a set number of microns each time the surgeon presses on the foot pedal. The console displays four numbers: the initial length of the blade at the beginning of the incision, the length that the blade is extended or retracted with each press on the foot pedal, the maximum length to which the blade can be extended by the instrument, and the present length of the blade. Each of these values can be set independently. To use the knife, the surgeon takes a series of ultrasonic pachometry readings and calculates the four numbers indicated above, programming each one into the instrument. The initial length of the blade is set (for example, 700 μm); the blade is plunged into the tissue and advanced as far as the surgeon wishes for cutting at that depth (for example, 1 mm); the surgeon pushes on the foot pedal to advance (or retract) the knife blade the set amount; the incision is made longer and the length of the blade adjusted again repetitively until the total length of the incision is completed. As a safety factor, the maximum extension of the blade can be set so that the surgeon does not inadvertently allow the blade to become too long. The knife is available from Eye Tech (Bochum, Germany).

Computer-controlled knives. Most keratotomy surgeons dream of a knife equipped with a feedback mechanism that could measure the thickness of the uncut posterior stroma and change the length of the blade in real time during the incision so that the depth of the incision would be a uniform percentage of corneal thickness throughout. Prototypes have been built, but none has been marketed. For example, the Metico "microcomputer knife for radial keratotomy" provided electronic verification of the blade depth on a digital readout.

GAUGE BLOCKS
Purpose and development

Gauge blocks verify the length of the extension of the knife blade beyond the footplate in attempt to calibrate the depth of the incisions. In the late 1970s and early 1980s when metal blade fragments were held in blade holders, a time-consuming part of the operation was the seating of the blade at the proper length using a ruler-style gauge block with a calibrated line or notches along the edge. Resetting the blade during surgery to replace a dull one or to extend it for deepening incisions was tedious.

Micrometer knife handles that could dial the blade to a desired extension theoretically obviated gauge blocks. However, experience with inaccurate micrometers perpetuated the need for gauges and led to a second generation of systems in which the knife was mounted in a cradle on a platform and the blade extended over an elevated ridge of calibrated width. Recognition of the problems of parallax led to the development of microscopes fitted with calibrated reticles and micrometer stages, as well as the development of more accurate micrometer knife handles.

Accuracy of gauges

Two problems undermine the surgeon's confidence that a gauge block will guarantee an accurate extension of the blade. The first problem is the assumption that the gauge block is accurate. Most are. Many manufacturers guarantee accuracy; one described independent verification to an accuracy of 0.00000254 mm—good enough. For example, the accuracy of the coin gauge blocks used in the PERK study was verified by an independent testing facility. When the nine blade gauges were tested at four different reference values, 100% were within 11 μm, 97% were within 10 μm, and 64% were within 5 μm of the stated value. However, in testing commercial gauge blocks, Neumann and colleagues[20a] found numerous inconsistencies. Some gauge blocks were accurate, but others measured 16 μm or more too thick, and some had different errors on either side of the gauge block. In general, the errors show an actual reading higher than the stated reading, that is, the knife would be set longer than desired, increasing the chance of corneal perforation. Without industry standards, surgeons are left to verify the accuracy of their own gauge blocks with an independent tester.

The second, more significant problem with ensuring accuracy of gauge blocks is the surgeon's inability to align the tip of the blade exactly along the edge of the gauge mark. The surgeon must be sure that the same side of the footplate is applied to the edge of the gauge block each time because the two footplates are

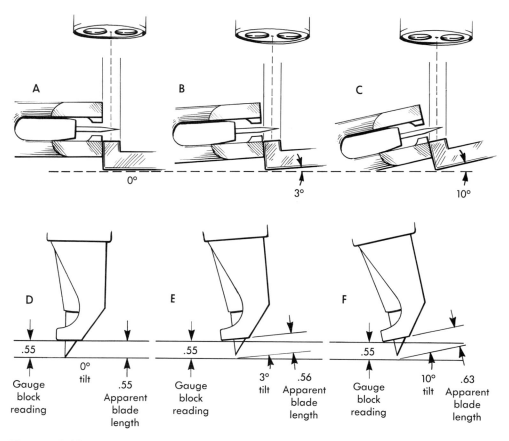

Figure 15-44
Tilting the knife or gauge can induce parallax error by not having the footplate applied perpendicularly to the edge of the gauge. **A,** Perfect alignment with proper reading. **B,** Three-degree tilt requires extension of blade and induces a 0.08-mm error. **C,** Ten-degree tilt requires extension of blade and induces a 0.29-mm error. **D, E,** and **F,** Tilt of knife at edge of gauge block induces longer than desired knife blade lengths. (Redrawn from Hofmann RF and Lindstrom RL: J Refract Surg 1987;3:215-223.)

Figure 15-45
Holding a coin gauge block beneath the operating microscope demonstrates the difficulty of keeping the platform horizontal and the danger of inducing parallax.

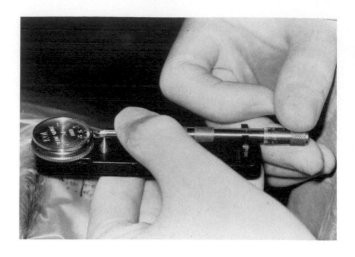

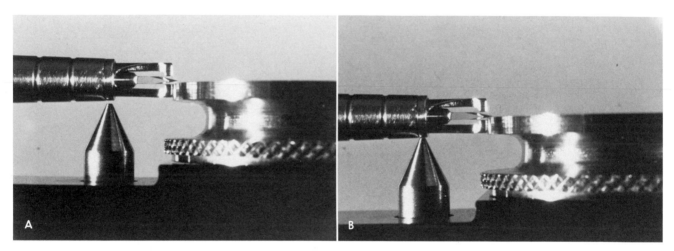

Figure 15-46
The further the blade from the ridge, the greater the parallax. **A,** End of handle is not pressed on conical rest so that blade is elevated above ridge. **B,** End of handle is pressed on conical rest so that blade is close to, but not touching, the ridge.

not always parallel. This can be done by orienting one of the markings on the knife handle up each time. Holding the handle and footplates steadily against the edge of the gauge is facilitated by using a built-in cradle, but even under ideal circumstances, tilting the knife or gauge creates parallax, as discussed in detail in Chapter 17, Atlas of Surgical Techniques of Radial Keratotomy.

The farther the knife blade is from the surface of the gauge block and the more the gauge block is tilted from an exact orthogonal orientation to the microscope, the more parallax is induced (Figs. 15-44 to 15-46). Of course surgeons do not want their crystal blades to be damaged by touching the gauge block, so there is always distance between the blade and the block. It is impractical to place the gauge block on a fixed flat surface, such as a table, exactly parallel to the surface of the microscope. Therefore the surgeon has the task of tilting the gauge block back and forth and sighting the tip of the knife exactly down the edge of the gauge to minimize parallax. It is easy to highlight the problem of parallax: simply ask three surgeons to set the extension of a single knife to 0.5

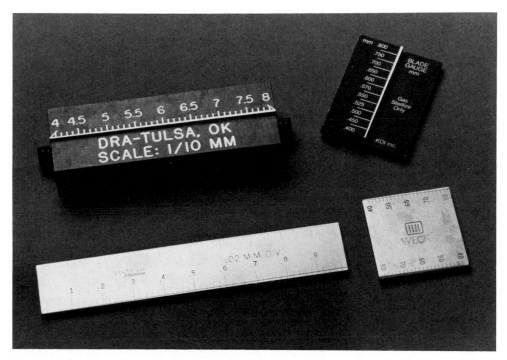

Figure 15-47
Ruler-style gauge blocks. Above: Two styles of gauge blocks with central elevated ridge. Below: Two styles of gauge blocks with etched line along edge. The scales vary: upper left, 0.01 mm; upper right, variable; lower left and right, 0.02 mm.

mm using a micrometer and gauge block, and then verify the real length of the blade under 150× with a calibration microscope. Readings often vary from one surgeon to another—part of the "art" of radial keratotomy.

These problems of parallax and inaccurate micrometers can be obviated by using a micrometer mounted on a compound microscope or a shadowgraph with magnification of 100× to 200× and a calibrated reticle; with this the surgeon can measure the extension of the blade, check the alignment of the blade and the footplates, and check for any damage to the blade. For example, at the conclusion of a course in radial keratotomy, six surgeons used a drum (ridge) gauge system to set the blade extension of a knife at 0.60 mm. The actual settings as determined by the MicronScope were 0.68, 0.82, 0.70, 0.83, 0.70, and 0.72 mm. Au and colleagues[1a] found different measurement errrors: KOI micrometer knife handle, 3%; KOI coin blade gauge block, 0.07%; Magnum optical micrometer, 0.04%. The authors preferred the optical micrometer.

Types of gauge blocks

There are three types of gauge blocks currently available for measuring radial keratotomy blade extension: the ruler-style gauge block, the ridge-style gauge block, usually coupled to a cradle, and magnifying instruments that contain a reticle.

Ruler gauge blocks. Ruler gauge blocks have a flat plate of steel or glass with a groove, etched line, or step along one edge (Fig. 15-47). The distance between the line and the edge increases from one end to the other. Most, but not all, blocks are calibrated in 0.01-mm divisions.

Most companies that manufacture radial keratotomy instruments make a

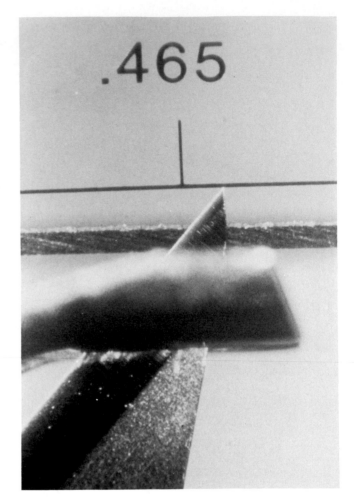

Figure 15-48
Aligning tip of blade along side of ruler-style block requires selection of outer, middle, or inner part of the line.

stainless steel gauge block that carries an eponym such as Kremer, Bores, Neumann, or Shepard. Myocure manufactured a gauge block out of glass using photolithography and vacuum deposition of the reference lines (Fig. 15-48).

The problems with the ruler-type gauge block include the danger of damaging the knife blade on the block; the difficulty of maintaining the footplate perpendicular to the side of the block during reading; the uncertainty of whether to align the blade tip with the outer edge, the center, or the inner edge of the groove; the inaccuracies of parallax; and the necessity of putting down the block to adjust the micrometer (Fig. 15-49).

Cradle and ridge gauge blocks. It is probably easier and more accurate to align the tip of the knife blade with the edge of a ridge than with the width of a groove, so manufacturers have designed gauge blocks in which the reference surface is a gradually widening ridge calibrated in 10-μm steps. A cradle with Y-shaped forks that slide into grooves in the knife handle holds the knife in a stable, fixed position (Fig. 15-50). This design allows placement of the calibrated ridge beneath the blade without danger of touching the blade and allows the surgeon to hold the knife and gauge block in one hand while the other hand is free to adjust the micrometer. The surgeon must tilt the cradle and gauge back and forth until the ridge is in a perfectly vertical position and the tip of the blade

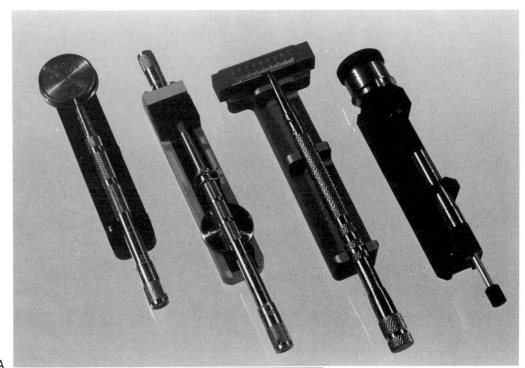

A

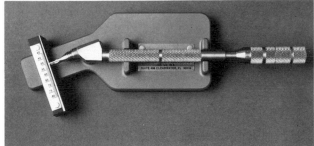

B

Figure 15-49
Gauge blocks with a knife cradle and a ridge-style calibration block. **A,** From left to right: KOI coin, Pilling double micrometer, Metico slide, Storz barrel. **B,** Metico angled cradle with slide gauge for angled knife.

is aligned with the edge of the ridge (see Figs. 15-44 and 15-45). Use of these blocks during surgery is described in Chapter 17, Atlas of Surgical Techniques of Radial Keratotomy.

Gauges with micrometer stage and magnified reticle. Two instruments have been designed for inspection and calibration of the knife blades before surgery: the Magnum Diamond MicronScope is a compound microscope (150×) fitted with a micromanipulator stage (Fig. 15-51), and the Xtal-800 Shadowgraph (200×) that is similar to that used for examining contact lenses (Fig. 15-52). Both instruments require that the knife be mounted on a carrier stage that is moved into position under the microscope. The surgeon views the knife against a reticle calibrated in 10-μm steps. The handle and platform of these instruments can be sterilized. The knife is examined and calibrated before or during surgery.

To set the blade, the surgeon mounts the knife handle on the stage, moves the stage to bring the knife into view, aligns one footplate along the zero baseline of the reticle, and uses the knife micrometer to extend the blade to the desired length on the reticle. The discrepancy between the micrometer handle reading and the reticle reading is recorded, and this is used as an adjustment factor when the blade is set during surgery.

Using these instruments requires care. The knife must be aligned and seated

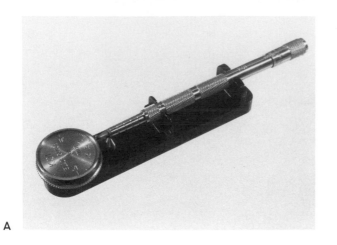

A

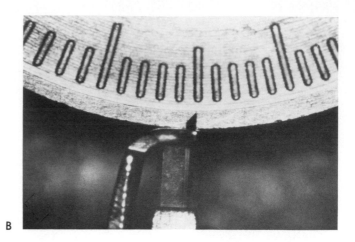

B

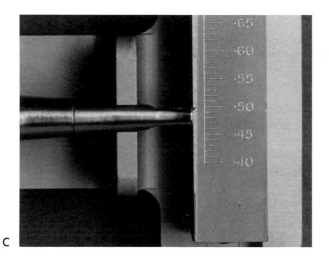

C

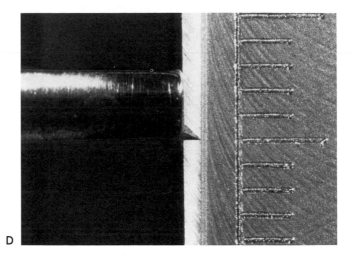

D

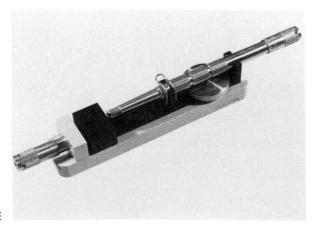

E

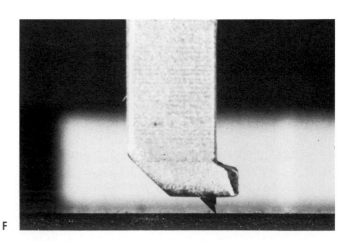

F

Figure 15-50
Figure legend see opposite page.

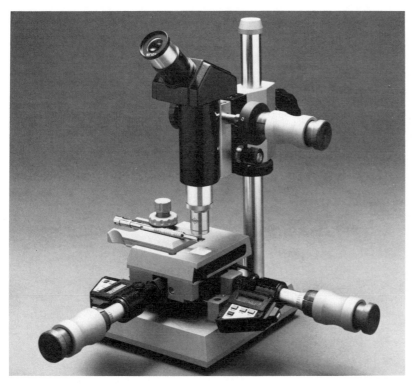

Figure 15-51
Magnum Diamond MicronScope consists of compound microscope, retroillumina-tion around the objective lens, a movable micrometer stage that clamps the knife onto its surface, and a digital micrometer readout. (See Figs. 15-35 to 15-37 for views through MicronScope.) (Courtesy Magnum Diamond.)

Figure 15-50
Varieties of alignment between knife blade and gauge block ridge. **A,** KOI coin gauge: knife handle lies in the cradle with the footplate abutting the edge of the coin gauge. **B,** KOI coin gauge: coin is turned until blade is opposite desired setting and micrometer on knife is turned until the tip of blade is aligned with the inner edge of the ridge. **C,** Metico slide gauge: knife is held in cradle with blade tip over calibrated slide. **D,** Metico slide gauge: the slide is moved until the blade is opposite the de-sired setting and then the micrometer handle is turned until the blade is aligned with the inner edge of ridge. The tip of the blade is separated by some distance from the calibration marks. **E,** Pilling double micrometer: the knife is snapped into the cradle. The micrometer on the gauge block is set to zero and the knife footplate abutted on the block. The micrometer on the gauge block retracts the reference surface the de-sired extension of the blade. **F,** Then the micrometer on the knife handle advances the blade until it overlaps the edge of the reference surface. (Photographs by Steven Carlton.)

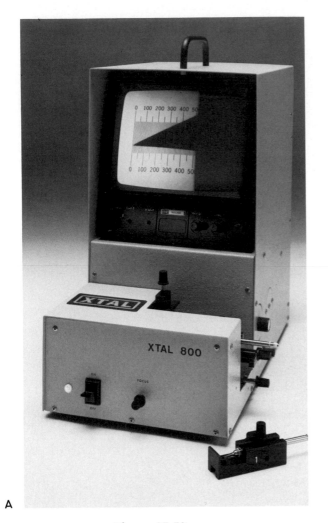

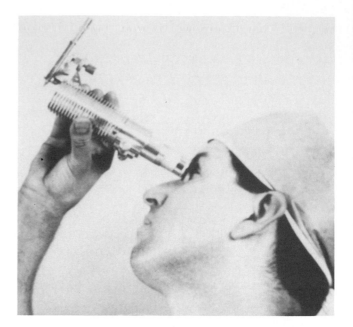

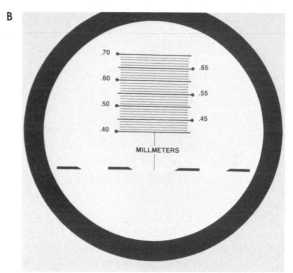

Figure 15-52

A, Xtal shadowgraph comparator consists of knife carrier (lower right) that is inserted into side of console so that profile of blade is projected onto screen. Footplate is aligned at reading of desired blade extension and micrometer of knife extends blade to zero point. **B,** (top and bottom), A gauge system that combines magnification with a reticle but without micrometer control is manufactured by Precision Corneal Instruments. The knife is mounted at the end of the cone that contains the magnifier. The surgeon views the end of the knife through the magnifier against a background light, so the length of the blade can be adjusted with the micrometer handle and calibrated on the reticle. (**A** courtesy Gil Weatherly; **B** courtesy Richard Villasenor.)

properly in the carrier. The MicronScope will hold all styles of handles. The Xtal-800 Shadowgraph uses a different carrier for each style handle. Readings are taken with the blade extended, exposing the blade to damage. The knife must be oriented so that the footplates and the blade are parallel to the surface of the reticle without tilt. Alignment of the footplates along the reticle marks is difficult if the footplates are curved because it is not possible to focus on an exact sharp edge of the footplate, so the microscope must be focused up and down until the point of farthest extension of the footplate is identified. At magnifications of 500×, considerable wobble can be seen as the knife blade is extended and retracted with the micrometer. The blade should be read with the micrometer moving in the advancing direction and the blade centered between the footplates. Blades with a chipped tip can be compensated for by setting the blade longer, although the tip will not cut as well.

A gauge system that combines magnification with the reticle, but without micrometer control, is manufactured by Precision Corneal Instruments. The knife is mounted at the end of a cone containing a magnifier. The surgeon views the end of the knife through the magnifier against a background light, so the length of the blade can be adjusted with the micrometer handle and calibrated on the reticle at the end of the magnifier (Fig. 15-52, *B*).

Care of gauge blocks

Short of major mechanical damage, little disrupts the accuracy of the gauge block, so ordinary cleaning and maintenance are adequate. The MicronScope and Xtal-800 Shadowgraph require appropriate gentle handling and care. Batteries must be replaced.

ZONE AND INCISION MARKERS
Purpose and design of markers

Zone and incision markers guide the proper placement of the incisions by making indentations or ink marks in the corneal epithelium during surgery.

The two types of markers are the circular zone markers that determine the length of the incisions and the radial and transverse markers that determine the placement and spacing of the incisions (Fig. 15-53).

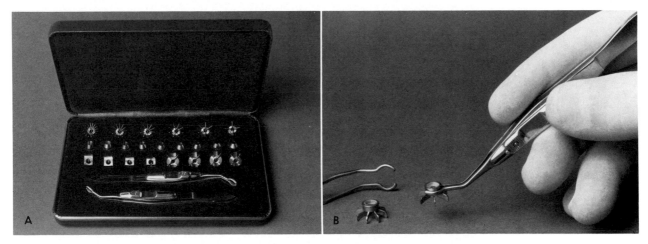

Figure 15-53
Set of Fyodorov markers. **A,** Top row: Radial markers. Middle row: Zone markers. Bottom row: Astigmatism markers (transverse and trapezoidal). Holding forceps below. **B,** A pair of forceps grasps the markers by their shank. (**A** courtesy Bausch & Lomb.)

Blades on markers

All markers, whether circular or linear, have tapering metal blades that form a dull, smoothly polished edge. If the edges are sharp or rough, they may lacerate the epithelium and even Bowman's layer.

The markers are pressed onto the surface of the cornea where they indent the epithelium; the indentation marks last for 15 to 30 minutes. It is not necessary to twist or slide the markers because this might cut into Bowman's layer. Balanced salt solution on the epithelium obscures the marks, but they are quickly revealed when the fluid over the marks is dried with a microsponge.

Centering of markers

A blunt intraocular lens hook is an ideal instrument to mark the center of the surgical procedure because it is readily available and angled, allowing the surgeon to sight along the tip, and because it has a small tip, making a minimal dimple in the epithelium. Using a needle may be dangerous because it may lacerate Bowman's layer and create a scar in the center of the visual axis, although this technique was used on over 500 eyes in the PERK study without creating any scar.

Circular zone markers

Terminology. Many surgeons refer to any circular mark on the cornea as an "optical zone" mark, as in, "I deepened the incisions from the 7-mm optical zone to the limbus." Of course, there is no such thing as a 7-mm optical zone; the optical zone of the cornea is limited to the central 3 to 4 mm. Therefore we refer only to "zone markers," whether they are marking the true optical zone, the uncut clear zone inside the incisions, or a circular zone delimited by a specific diameter.

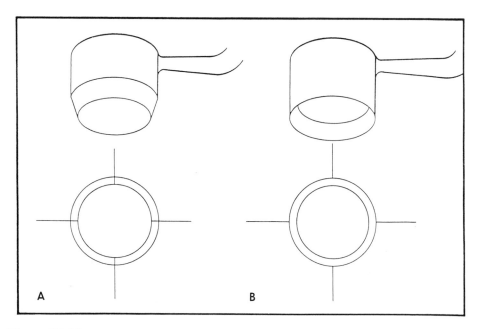

Figure 15-54
The diameter of the circular zone marker is measured from the vertical edge. **A,** A bevel on the outside places the vertical edge on the inside, so the incision should extend to the inner part of the mark. **B,** A bevel on the inside makes the vertical edge outside and the incision should extend to the outer edge of the epithelial mark. (Courtesy Mr. John Guckes, Storz, Inc.)

Configuration of zone markers. To create the fine, blunt edge on a zone marker, manufacturers begin with a stainless steel cylinder and taper the end. This tapering or beveling may occur on the inside or the outside of the cylinder (Fig. 15-54 and Table 15-8). Manufacturers designate the diameter of the marker from the vertical edge, so the surgeon must know whether the vertical edge of the marker is on the inside, as it is in most styles, or on the outside. If the vertical edge is on the inside of the marker, the incision should be carried across the width of the mark in the epithelium to the inside edge. If the vertical edge is on the outside of the marker, the incision should be carried only to the

Table 15-8

Configuration of Circular Zone Markers

Company	Product number	Description	Vertical edge inside	Vertical edge outside
Storz	E9011 Series	Hoffer	X	
	E9023 Series	Neumann-Shepard	X	
	E9030 Series	Thornton		X
I-Tech	RK—105-109	Shepard	X	
	RK—115-119	Hoffer		X
	RK—145-153	Neumann-Shepard	X	
	RK—180-188	Thornton	X	
Katena	K3—8129-50	Bores	X	
	K3—8170-76	Berkeley	X	
	K3—8330-434	Hoffer	X	
	K3—8300-12	Thornton	X	
Weck	7113 Series	Weck	X	
	1560 Series	Weck	X	
V. Mueller	OP8909 Series	Round Markers	X	
Pilling	42—7480-88 Series	Neumann-Shepard		X
	42—7490-94 Series	Shepard		X
	42—8350-90 Series	Hoffer		X

Courtesy John Guckes, Storz Instrument Co, St Louis, MO.

Table 15-9

Indicated and Actual Diameter of Central Clear Zone Markers

Indicated diameter (mm)	Actual diameter (mm)*							
	Cilco (ID)	Storz (ID)	I-Tech (OD)	Pilling (ID)	Katena (OD)	Katena (ID)	Stephens (ID)	Harper (OD)
3.00	2.93	2.93	3.19	3.05	2.89	2.98	3.17	2.66
3.25	3.21	3.11			3.19	3.23	3.39	2.96
3.50	3.48	3.49	3.73	3.49	3.45	3.51	3.63	3.17
3.75	3.70	3.64			3.68	3.74	3.84	3.45
4.00	3.99	3.96	4.29	4.03	3.96	4.02	4.13	3.73
4.25	4.24	4.21			4.20	4.28	4.39	3.91
4.50	4.45	4.41	4.71	4.55	4.41	4.5	4.60	4.20
4.75	4.76	4.66			4.67	4.75	4.88	4.47
5.00	4.95		5.23	5.05		5.02	5.14	4.70
6.00							6.25	
7.00							7.03	

Zone markers were sent by practicing surgeons to Magnum Diamond for verification. Readings were taken on the MicronScope. The location of the vertical side of the bevel is indicated by *ID* (inside diameter) and *OD* (outside diameter).

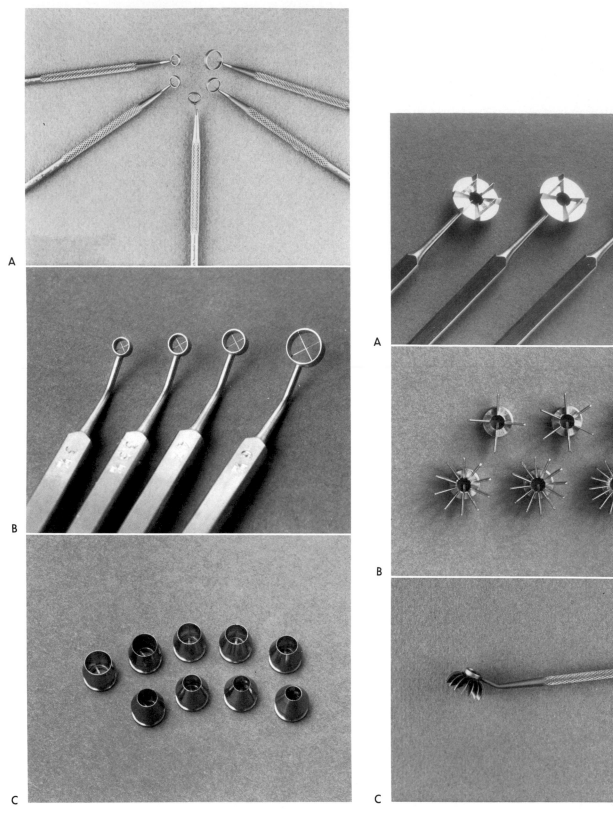

Figure 15-55
Sighting mechanisms on circular zone markers. **A,** Single pin with low profile Thornton marker. **B,** Cross hairs with low profile Hoffer marker. **C,** Fyodorov circular zone markers with sighting hairs far from marking tip. (**A** and **B** courtesy Katena, Inc.; **C** courtesy Bausch & Lomb.)

Figure 15-56
Radial and transverse incision markers. **A,** Blades beneath plate. Left to right: Eight radial and two transverse blades, four radial and two transverse blades, eight radial blades. **B,** Radial markers with four to sixteen blades. **C,** Buttress-style, 16-blade radial marker. (**A** courtesy Katena, Inc.; **B** courtesy Bausch & Lomb.)

outside edge of the mark in the epithelium. The width of the mark is approximately 0.1 mm, which can make a measurable difference in the outcome of surgery.

Some companies provide sets of markers with an inconsistent location of the bevel. For example, one surgeon using a set of eight Katena markers found that the bevel was on the inside in four markers and on the outside in four markers.

Accuracy of zone markers.   In the absence of industry standards to ensure accurate diameters of zone markers, the surgeon must verify the real diameter of the markers. Although some markers are accurate, others vary 0.10 to 0.20 mm from the stated value (Table 15-9). Considerable error in the length of the incisions can be induced by the combination of not cutting from the vertical edge of the marker and having a marker that is inaccurate; if the mark is 0.1 mm wide and the diameter is misrepresented by 0.2 mm, each incision can be 0.2 mm too long or too short—a total of 0.4-mm error along one meridian.

Centering the zone markers.   To facilitate centering many markers are fitted with an alignment sight, such as cross hairs that intersect in the middle, cross hairs with an opening in the middle, or a single shaft that extends to the middle (Fig. 15-55). The center point in the marker is placed over the centering mark in the corneal epithelium.

If the centering sight is far from the surface of the cornea, more parallax occurs when the cylinder is tilted and it is more difficult to center the marker. Therefore a short cylinder approximately 1.2 mm high with the alignment sight mounted near the beveled end of the marker will make alignment easier. To decrease parallax, the surgeon should tilt the cylinder back and forth and view down the inside of the cylinder for 360 degrees just before the marker is pressed into the epithelium. Surgeons should be aware whether they are sighting binocularly or monocularly, as discussed in Chapter 16, Centering Corneal Surgical Procedures.

Size and shape of zone markers.   Most zone markers are circular and vary in diameter from 3 to 5 mm in 0.25-mm steps. Diameters of 6 to 9 mm are also available for locating the deepening or transverse incisions. Markers mounted with concentric rings to delineate concentric zones for deepening incisions are also available, for example, in 3-, 5-, and 7-mm diameters (Fig. 15-56). Historically, oval zone markers were used to allow placing longer incisions in the steeper meridian, but these were found ineffective.

Most markers are made of stainless steel.

Radial incision markers

Radial markers help guide the surgeon in placing the incisions equidistant from each other. The greater the number of incisions, the more useful are the markers. Most surgeons can place four incisions at 3, 6, 9, and 12 o'clock with reasonable accuracy by visual inspection, but if the incisions must be rotated off axis to accommodate transverse incisions, it is necessary to have the marks indented in the epithelium. Aligning the incisions without radial markers is easier when cutting centrifugally than when cutting centripetally. This is because the incision is begun around the smaller clear zone mark when cutting from the inside out, so it is easy to identify the 3, 6, 9, and 12 o'clock locations and then use the width of the footplates to bisect those locations in placing the oblique incisions. However, when cutting from the outside in, the diameter of the limbus is approximately 12 mm, and it is more difficult to align the incisions accurately around this larger circumference, making the use of radial markers more advantageous.

Radial markers come in the following three basic designs (see Fig. 15-56):
1. Flat plate with radial blades mounted beneath the plate and grooves on the top of the plate indicating their location

2. Radial blades arching out from a central circular mount like buttresses on a Gothic cathedral, allowing the surgeon to see the blades as they indent the cornea
3. Radial blades mounted around a clear zone marker so that the circular mark and the radial marks are made at the same time

Some of the radial markers also have a centering alignment sight, making it easier to align them around the central and circular zone marks. When using the incision markers, the surgeon should press them into the cornea in four directions to ensure that all of the radial and transverse edges indent the corneal well. However, excess rocking may make multiple marks that confuse placement of incisions.

The number of blades on radial markers varies from three to 16 but most commonly four and eight are used.

Astigmatism markers

There are four types of astigmatism markers. The first type is a circular protractor that indicates the direction of meridians on the surface of the cornea (Fig. 15-57). This is used to identify the steep corneal meridian. The protractor either has a smooth bottom surface or may contain teeth. Care must be taken during surgery that teeth do not scratch the corneal epithelium. The protractor may consist of a single, flat ring or a rotating ring that allows the fixation plate to remain stable on the cornea while the calibrated ring is rotated on the surface to identify the location of the correct meridian. The steep meridian is marked in the epithelium either using a separate linear marker or using blades mounted on the back of the protractor (see Chapter 32, Atlas of Astigmatic Keratotomy).

The second type of astigmatism marker is a transverse marker that indicates the length and location of the transverse incisions in the steep meridian. The markers have two parallel blades, usually 4 to 7 mm apart, along with a centering cross hair. These may be either mounted separately (Fig. 15-58) or integrated into the radial markers (see Fig. 15-56).

The third type of astigmatism marker is for the trapezoidal pattern (Ruiz) and consists of semiradial and transverse blades. The fourth type of astigmatism marker is a corneal ruler that marks the length of the transverse incision. The ruler has small, parallel blades, each 1 mm long, separated by 0.5 mm, to measure up to 5 mm across the steep meridian (see Fig. 15-58).[31] Straight (Thornton) and arcuate (Lindstrom) rulers are available.

To use the separate transverse markers, the surgeon places the transverse blades between or straddling the radial marks. Using multiple independent markers is difficult because of problems aligning the center mark, the clear zone mark, the radial marks, and the transverse marks around the same point. Some eccentricity is bound to creep in; therefore it is more convenient to have markers that outline all of the incisions used for a given operation, including the clear zone, in one instrument. Most instrument makers do not make sets with such diversity, which would require four to eight different clear zones with two to three different radial patterns and six different transverse patterns—a total of some 50 different instruments.

FIXATION INSTRUMENTS

Fixation instruments help the surgeon control the position and movement of the globe during surgery, a goal best achieved with instruments that provide multiple points of fixation. They also elevate the intraocular pressure during surgery to provide more uniform corneal resistance for each incision. The intraocular pressure during radial keratotomy has been studied under controlled laboratory conditions by Mendelsohn and colleagues[17] (see Chapter 17, Atlas of Sur-

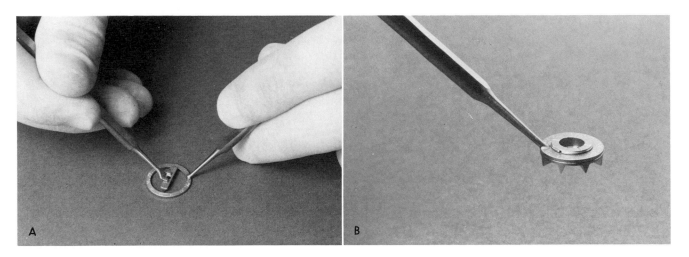

Figure 15-57
Limbal protractor for marking steep astigmatism meridian. **A,** Circular protractor (Mendez) is marked in 10-degree intervals (0 to 180 degrees) and comes with or without teeth on posterior surface that stabilize the ring at the conjunctival limbus. Meridian marker (Bores) is aligned with steep refractive axis. **B,** Rotating eight radial marker with protractor (Grandon) allows alignment of radial marks to accommodate exact meridian of astigmatism. (**B** courtesy Katena, Inc.)

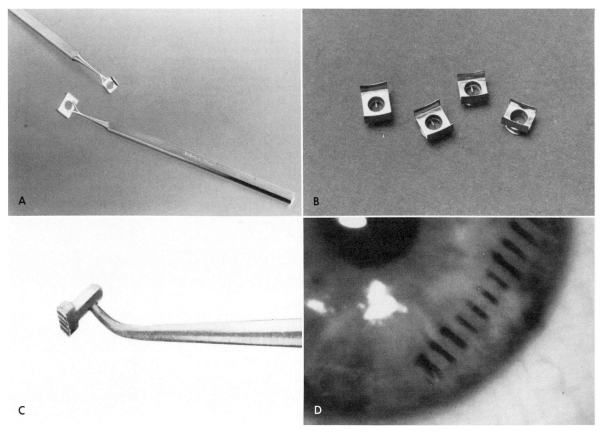

Figure 15-58
Markers for transverse incisions. **A,** Two markers (Bores) for placement of T-incisions at 5- and 7-mm zones. **B,** Astigmatism markers (Fyodorov) with blades 4 to 7 mm apart and sighting pin. **C** and **D,** Astigmatism ruler marker (Thornton). (**A** courtesy Katena, Inc.; **B** courtesy Bausch & Lomb.)

gical Techniques of Radial Keratotomy), who demonstrated that forceps, compression rings, and suction rings all elevate the intraocular pressure during surgery, with forceps being the most erratic and suction rings being the least.

The four types of fixation devices are the single-pronged forceps, the double-pronged forceps, compression rings, and suction rings (Fig. 15-59). Most commonly used are double-pronged forceps and compression rings.

Single-pronged forceps

Early in the development of modern radial keratotomy, a conventional fine-toothed, single-pronged forceps was used to fixate the limbus opposite the incisions or to grasp the inside of the wound opposite the subsequent incisions. The single point of fixation had the disadvantage that the globe could torque around the tip. Therefore forceps with coarser ends, such as the Bracken-Farkus forceps, were designed with a stabilizing tip on the end. Few surgeons use these today because of their instability.

Double-pronged fixation forceps

To gain more stability, U-shaped, double-pronged, toothed forceps were developed to fixate the limbus, with the tips separated by a distance of 3 mm (Bores), 5 mm (Suarez),[30] 7 mm (Hofmann), or 13 mm (Kremer). Most of these are manufactured with straight and angled handles. The first three types are usually positioned opposite each incision. The Kremer 13-mm forceps spans the cornea and has a lock on the handle that allows it to adhere to the limbal conjunctiva in a single location during the procedure (Fig. 15-60).

Compression rings

The compression ring designed by Thornton is a 14- to 16-mm diameter ring studded with a dozen dull teeth (Fig. 15-61). The ring is applied to the surface of the anesthetized conjunctiva and pressed onto the globe, providing torsion-free fixation and movement in all directions. The ring retropulses the globe into the orbit, and the surgeon must compensate for this by a downward focus of the microscope. The displacement of the globe can be reduced by using peribulbar anesthetic, which pushes the globe forward.

The compression ring has disadvantages. It must be repositioned every time the knife changes hands. It can slip on the surface if downward pressure is released. If the teeth are too sharp, they may lacerate the conjunctiva and hurt the patient. The surgeon can rotate the eye by pressing the ring onto the surface but may have difficulty moving the eye nasally if the patient has a large nose that obstructs the movement of the handle.

Suction fixation rings

The logic of borrowing the Barraquer suction ring from lamellar refractive surgical procedures and applying it to keratotomy procedures was based on its ability to fixate the globe and to elevate the intraocular pressure uniformly. Barraquer and Ruiz routinely used this ring for radial keratotomy in the early 1980s, raising the intraocular pressure to 60 mm Hg, which could be tolerated because the patients were under general anesthesia. Both of these surgeons have abandoned the use of the ring and now prefer a compression ring or fixation forceps.

Gelender and Parel[9] have described a limbal conjunctival suction fixation ring that uses a suction pump and raises the intraocular pressure to 40 mm Hg (Fig. 15-62). Cowden and colleagues[3] used this suction ring in a series of reoperations, observing that they got more effect with the suction ring than with fixation forceps alone. They attribute the greater effect to the elevated intraocular

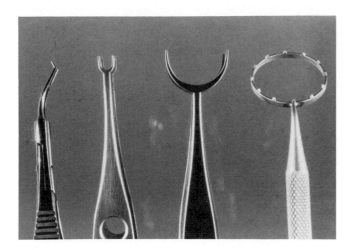

Figure 15-59
Fixation instruments for keratotomy. Left to right:
Single-pronged Colibri forceps, double-pronged forceps
with 3-mm spread (Bores), double-pronged spanning
forceps with 13-mm spread (Kremer), and compression
ring (Thornton).

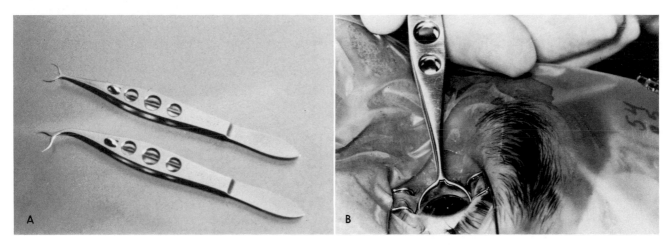

Figure 15-60
Spanning-style fixation forceps (Kremer). **A,** Straight and angled handles **B,** The
13-mm spanning forceps fixate the limbal conjunctiva during surgery. (**A** courtesy
Katena, Inc.)

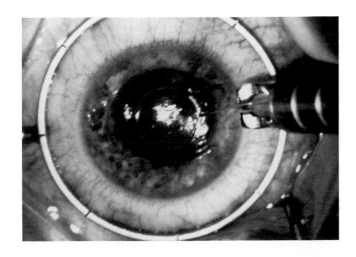

Figure 15-61
Compression fixation ring (Thornton). Ring compresses
the perilimbal conjunctiva and retropulses the globe
during surgery.

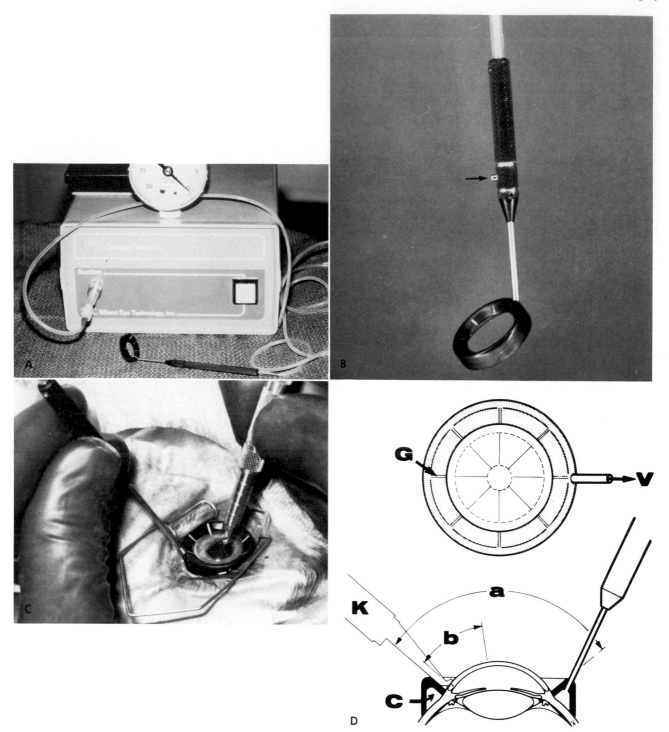

Figure 15-62

Suction fixation ring (Gelender). **A,** Suction console is connected to suction ring by tubing. Suction pressure applied is indicated by the gauge on the top. **B,** Fixation ring has eight radial markings and escape valve that allows instant release of suction pressure *(arrow).* **C,** Intraoperative photograph of ring fixating the globe during radial incision. **D,** Schematic of vacuum fixation ring as viewed from above and in cross section. Vacuum line *(V)* is connected to vacuum system and evacuates the hollow ring *(C).* As the sclera is pulled outward, the intraocular pressure is elevated and the cornea made rigid. Guided by the ring grooves *(G),* the radial keratotomy knife *(K)* cuts the cornea across the incision angle *(b).* The knife freedom angle *(a)* is limited by the slanted wall of the vacuum fixation ring, which protects the knife blade from inadvertent damage. (**A** courtesy John Cowden; **B, C,** and **D** from Gelender H and Parel J-M: Ophthalmic Surg 1984;15:126-127.)

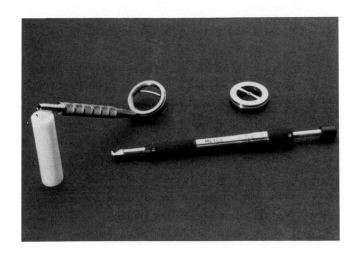

Figure 15-63
Krumeich radial keratotomy suction bridge consists of a suction ring handle with an eccentric arch over it (upper left). The diamond knife (below) is braced against the arch during the incision to create a straighter cut and to give support to the knife for a more uniform depth. A centering ring (upper right) can be inserted into the suction bridge. (Courtesy Jorg Krumeich, M.D.)

pressure and the more rigid cornea. Disadvantages include patient discomfort and conjunctival hemorrhages and chemosis.

Radial keratotomy bridge. Krumeich[14] designed a suction ring with a slightly eccentric arching bridge to guide the knife handle (Fig. 15-63). The suction ring is approximately 14 mm in diameter and is powered by a suction pump, applying 800 millibars of pressure to secure the ring firmly to the globe, raising the intraocular pressure to only approximately 20 mm Hg. A centering plate with a round gunsight in the middle is used to center the ring over the centering mark. The plate is removed, and the bridge, which can be rotated into four or eight different positions, is locked in place for the first incision. The knife blade is extended to the desired length and is then plunged into the cornea so that the flattened side of the end of the knife is applied to the side of the arching bridge. The incision is made by guiding the knife along the side of the bridge, which helps maintain the knife handle perpendicular to the surface of the cornea and create a more uniform depth of incision. The side of the footplates must be modified to have a flat rectangular shape, which is different from the round shape of most knife handles. Since the distance between the blade and the side of the knife is different for different knives, the location of the bridge must be properly aligned for each type of knife by applying the suction ring in the exact desired position on the globe.

OTHER INSTRUMENTS USED FOR RADIAL KERATOTOMY

Other instruments not peculiar to radial keratotomy are used during the operation.

Eyelid speculums

We prefer a Barraquer-style, wire eyelid speculum that exerts minimal pressure on the lids. Ptosis has been described after radial keratotomy using topical anesthetic and a rigid lid speculum that locks in the open position and may damage the levator aponeurosis.[15]

Depth gauges

Dipsticks and devices that estimate the depth of the incision have no practical role in radial keratotomy. Dipsticks are inaccurate because the incisions are made with a tolerance in excess of that estimated by dipsticks, the cornea swells shortly after it is cut, and the deep uncut stroma and Descemet's membrane are easily displaced. Incision spreaders are a convenient way to examine the inside of a wound but tend to tear the base of the wound and split the collagen lamellae if spread too wide.

Wound openers

A blunt, angled intraocular lens hook (Sinsky, Clayman) is useful for opening keratotomy wounds that are going to be recut because of undercorrection. When the intraocular lens hook is pressed into the wound, it pops through the residual epithelial plug easily and passes to the depth of the scar. It can be pushed and pulled along the length of the wound, spreading open the weak scar with almost no danger of perforating the cornea.

Irrigating cannulas

A 19-gauge cannula is useful to spread some topical anesthetic in the conjunctival cul-de-sac and to drop balanced saline solution on the surface of the cornea. A blunt angled 27- or 30-gauge cannula is useful for irrigating epithelium and debris out of the wounds at the end of the procedure.

ACCURACY IN MANUFACTURE AND USE OF INSTRUMENTS FOR KERATOTOMY

The absence of industry standards for the manufacture of instruments used in keratotomy is a concern. Perhaps such standards are not necessary, since radial keratotomy is a surgical art form and a few microns difference in instrument accuracy one way or the other will not make any practical, clinical difference. This reasoning is erroneous, not only because small variations in the depth of the incision (particularly around 90% depth) can make a big difference in the surgical outcome, but also because small inaccuracies may have a cumulative effect in a single direction during one operation.

Pachometers

We discussed in the section on pachometers the variability of different instruments measuring the same corneas with the same assumed speed of sound (1640 msec). Under the most ideal circumstances, a properly calibrated pachometer can measure with an error of ± 10 μm ($+1.8\%$), or a range of 3.6%. The comparison of nine different pachometers by Reader and Salz[25] found a range of approximately 10% difference among the pachometers.

Knife blades

Quality control in the manufacture of crystal knife blades is difficult to quantify, particularly since the blades can be damaged during use. Clearly, a blade with a sharp tip and edge will cut deeper, displacing less tissue, than a blade with a chipped tip and dull edge. The design of the knife blade—including its thickness, number of edges, and included angle—also affects its cutting characteristics in a way that cannot be easily quantified.

Micrometer handles

The micrometer in the knife handle must have an accurate zero setting as determined by the bayonet mount and the micrometer screw and an accurate advancement of the blade based on the accuracy of and play among the threads and the wobble in the advancement mechanism. Inaccuracies on the order of 100 μm have been reported.

Knife footplates

If the footplates are misaligned, gauge block readings or micrometer readings may be inaccurate by the difference between the alignment of the two footplates. Footplates with curved rocker shapes and those that are not equidistant from the blade may allow the blade to enter the cornea at other than the desired perpendicular orientation.

Gauge blocks

While most gauge blocks are manufactured to a high tolerance of ± 10 μm, some coin-gauge and ruler-style blocks can be off 10% or more. Probably a greater source of variability in the use of these blocks, however, is the surgeon's alignment of the knife, which is rendered inaccurate both by parallax and by not knowing exactly where to align the tip of the blade (for example, outer edge, center, or inner edge of the line on a ruler-gauge). As Hofmann and Lindstrom[11] have pointed out, tilting of the knife on the gauge block by only 3 degrees can induce a 2% to 15% error in the measurement of the length of the blade.

Clear zone markers

Variation in the accuracy of the stated diameter of central clear zone markers ranges from none to 0.3 mm. An error of 0.2 mm is common. In addition, many surgeons do not know whether their markers are beveled on the inside or the outside, so they may be cutting from the wrong portion of the clear zone mark, inducing an error of approximately 0.2 mm.

Centering mark

As demonstrated by Uozato and Guyton,[37] use of commercially available centering devices viewed monocularly can induce a decentration of 0.2 mm. This has only a small effect on the accuracy of the procedure, since the decreased length of the incisions in the direction of decentration will be compensated for by the increased length of the incisions in the opposite direction.

UNFINISHED BUSINESS

The technical goal of the surgeon performing refractive keratotomy is to make each incision in the cornea accurately (a specifically defined location, depth, and length) and to maintain this accuracy for each incision. Currently, using manual techniques and diamond bladed micrometer knives, surgeons can approximate but not achieve this goal because there is variability in the configuration and depth of incisions—even in those made in an individual cornea during the same surgical session. Thus the major item of unfinished business in the development of instruments used in refractive keratotomy is to design instruments that can improve the accuracy and precision of the incisions. Developments such as improved configuration of diamond knife blades, guides such as the Krumeich bridge, mechanical devices such as knives that allow intraoperative adjustment of the length of the blade, and ultimately a knife that can automatically adjust the blade length to leave a consistent and known amount of posterior stromal tissue along the entire length of that incision will all potentially help the surgeon achieve the technical goals of refractive surgery. Active collaboration between engineers and ophthalmologists will foster the development of such instruments.

When excimer lasers were first introduced into ophthalmic surgery, the hope that the laser would be able to make a uniformly contoured incision with great predictability was short-lived, when it was found that the instrument actually created a 100-μm micron wide trough in the cornea and that the width of the trough itself was not accurately controllable. Nevertheless, other types of lasers may fulfill the promise of using lasers to make radial cuts in the cornea, whether through Bowman's membrane or intrastromally.

Completely missing from the field of instruments for refractive keratotomy are industry standards in instrument manufacture. Although manufacturers may compete with each other in the business world, they should cooperate with each other in the scientific world so that conventional standards can be applied to make more accurate ultrasonic pachometers, micrometer handles, corneal markers, and the like. Industry would do well to cooperate with committees of ophthalmic organizations, such as the International Society of Refractive Keratoplasty and the American Society of Cataract and Refractive Surgery, in defining and establishing such standards. If industries such as those that manufacture spectacle lenses can conform to national standards, then industries that manufacture precision surgical instruments should be able to as well.

REFERENCES

1. Abramson J, Dybbs A, Breber I, and Hazony D: Echo enhancement techniques in corneal ultrasonography, Invest Ophthalmol Vis Sci 1981;20 (suppl):156.

1a. Au YK, Reynolds MD, and Chadalavada RC: A study of the optical micrometer, the coin gauge, and the diamond knife micrometer in diamond knife calibration, Refract Corneal Surg (in press).

2. Coleman DJ, Lizzi FL, and Jack RL: Ultrasonography of the eye and orbit, Philadelphia, 1977, Lea & Febiger, pp 112-114.

3. Cowden JW, Lynn MJ, Waring GO, et al: Repeated radial keratotomy in the Prospective Evaluation of Radial Keratotomy (PERK) study, Am J Ophthalmol 1987;103:423-431.

4. Duke-Elder S and Smith RJH: The foundations of ophthalmology, vol III. In Duke-Elder S: System of ophthalmology, St Louis, 1962, The CV Mosby Co, pp 263-266.

5. Durham DG and Luntz MN: Diamond knife in cataract surgery, Br J Ophthalmol 1968;52:206-209.

6. Eisner G: Eye surgery: an introduction to operative techniques, Berlin, 1980, Springer-Verlag.

7. Fenzl R, Neumann A, Shepard D, Simon G, and Thornton S: Gauges, knives, gem blades: care and feeding, Oc Surg News 1986;4:68-71.

8. Galbaby EJ: Use of diamond knives in ocular surgery, Ophthalmic Surg 1984;15:203-205.

9. Gelender H and Parel J-M: Vacuum fixation ring for radial keratotomy, Ophthalmic Surg 1984;15:126-127.

10. Hazony D, Lazzara S, Greber I, and Dybbs A: The speed of sound in the human and rabbit cornea, Invest Ophthalmol Vis Sci 1983;24(suppl):128.

11. Hofmann RF and Lindstrom RL: Sources of error in keratotomy knife incision, J Refract Surg 1987;3:215-223.

11a. Huebscher JH, Goder GJ, and Lommatzsch PK: The sharpness of incision instruments in corneal tissue, Ophthalmic Surg 1989;20:120-123.

12. Kremer FB: A new instrument for clinical pachymetry. In Schachar RA et al, editors: Radial keratotomy, Dennison, Tex, 1980, LAL Publishers, pp 201-212.

13. Kremer FB, Walton P, and Genshimer G: Determination of corneal thickness using ultrasonic pachometry, Ann Ophthalmol 1985;17:506-507.

14. Krumeich JH: The RK bridge, J Refract Surg 1986;2:265-266.

15. Linberg JV, McDonald MB, Safir A, and Googe JM: Ptosis following radial keratotomy, Ophthalmology 1986;93:1509-1512.

16. Maurice DM: Letter to the editor, Ophthalmology 1986;93:422.

17. Mendelsohn AD, Parel J-M, Dennis JJ, et al: Intraocular pressure during radial keratotomy, J Refract Surg 1987;3:79-87.

18. Mishima S and Hedbys BO: Measurement of corneal thickness with the Haig-Streit pachymeter, Arch Ophthalmol 1981;80:710-713.

19. Mishima S and Maurice DM: The oily layer of the tear film and evaporation from the corneal surface, Exp Eye Res 1961;1:39-45.

20. Mondell RB, Polse KA, and Bonanno J: Reassessment of optical pachometry. In Cavanagh HD, editor: The cornea: transactions of world congress on the cornea III, New York, 1988, Raven Press, pp 201-205.

20a. Neumann AC, McCarty GR, Copello B, and Mastel D: Enhanced accuracy is necessary for refractive surgery instrumentation, J Cataract Refract Surg 1989;15:220-226.

21. Novak AE, Lindstrom RL, Williams RA, and Everson M: Corneal pachymetry prior to radial keratotomy: a comparison of techniques, J Refract Surg 1985;1:151-153.

22. Olson T, Neilson CB, and Ehlers N: On the optical measurement of corneal thickness. I. Optical principle and sources of error, Acta Ophthalmologica 1980;58:760-766.

23. Olson T, Neilson CB, and Ehlers N: On the optical measurement of corneal thickness. III. The measuring conditions and sources of error, Acta Ophthalmologica 1980;58:975-984.

24. Pouliquen Y, Hanna K, and Saragoussi J: The Hanna radial microkeratome: presentation and first experiment, Dev Ophthalmol 1987;14:132-136.

25. Reader AL and Salz JJ: Differences among ultrasonic pachymeters in measuring corneal thickness, J Refract Surg 1987;3:7-11.

26. Ridgeway RR, Balland AH, and Bailey BL: Hardness values for electrochemical products, The Electrochemical Society 1933;63:15.

27. Rowsey JJ, Balyeat HD, and Yeisley KP: Diamond knife, Ophthalmic Surg 1982;13:279-282.

28. Salz JJ, Azen SP, Berstein J, et al: Evaluation and comparison of sources of variability in the measurement of corneal thickness with ultrasonic and optical pachymeters, Ophthalmic Surg 1983;14:750-754.

29. Salz JJ, Lee T, Jester JV, Villasenor RA, et al: Analysis of incision depth following experimental radial keratotomy, Ophthalmology 1983;90:655-659.

30. Suarez E, Arffa RC, McDonald MB, and Kaufman HE: Suarez double fixation forceps for radial keratotomy, J Refract Surg 1985;1:236.

31. Thornton SP: Corneal press-on ruler for astigmatic keratotomy, J Cataract Refract Surg 1989;15:96-100.

32. Thornton SP: Cutting instruments. In Sanders DR, Hofmann RF, and Salz JJ, editors: Refractive corneal surgery, Thorofare NJ, 1986, Slack, Inc, pp 145-162.

33. Thornton SP: A guide to pachymeters, Ophthalmic Surg 1984;15:993-995.

34. Thornton SP: A guide to ultrasonic pachymeters, J Cat Ref Surg 1986;12:416-419.

35. Thornton SP: Surgical armamentarium. In Sanders DR, Hofmann RF, and Salz JJ, editors: Refractive corneal surgery, Thorofare NJ, 1986, Slack, Inc, pp 129-145.

36. Tschewnenko AA: Velocity of ultrasound in ocular tissues, Wiss Z Humboldt Univ Berlin (Math Naturwiss) 1965;14:67-69. (International symposium on diagnostic ultrasound in ophthalmology, Berlin, 1964.)

37. Uozato H and Guyton DL: Centering corneal surgical problems, Am J Ophthalmol 1987;103:264-275.

38. Vanysek J, Preisova J, and Obraz J: Measurement of the distances in the eye. In Ultrasonography in ophthalmology, London, 1969, Butterworth's, pp 203-209.

Centering Corneal Surgical Procedures

Hiroshi Uozato

David L. Guyton

George O. Waring III

Most corneal surgical procedures require proper centration on the cornea. Eccentric placement of corneal grafts may produce asymmetric wound healing, irregular astigmatism, vascularization, and graft failure. Many corneal refractive surgical procedures cause unavoidable paracentral distortion and scarring, leaving only a small, central, regular optical zone. If this optical zone is too small or is not centered properly, irregular astigmatism and glare can interfere seriously with visual function.

Where should the optical zone of corneal surgical procedures be centered? Although many authorities suggest that the procedure should be centered on the visual axis, either they do not define the visual axis or they define it improperly. We believe that the center of the entrance pupil, not the visual axis, should be used for centering corneal surgical procedures.[11]

ENTRANCE PUPIL AND LINE OF SIGHT

When we look at an eye, we do not actually see the real pupil and iris; we see a virtual image of the pupil and iris formed by the cornea. The virtual image of the pupil is called the entrance pupil of the eye. From the dimensions of Gullstrand's schematic eye, the entrance pupil is approximately 0.5 mm closer to us and about 14% larger than the real pupil (Fig. 16-1).[1] Because the entrance pupil is conjugate to the real pupil, light rays directed toward the entrance pupil will be refracted by the cornea and will pass through the real pupil.

BACKGROUND AND ACKNOWLEDGMENTS

In 1983, Steinberg and Waring described the technique of marking the visual axis on the cornea during radial keratotomy, which was used in the PERK study, comparing this to the Osher alignment system.[7] In a letter to the editor, Walsh and Guyton[11] criticized the clinical attempt to mark the intersection of the visual axis with the cornea, asserting that it was the center of the entrance pupil around which corneal surgical procedures should be centered. This fostered a reexamination of the PERK techniques and the thorough analysis published by Uozato and Guyton.[9] This chapter is a revision and expansion of their important article. Ophthalmologists and companies who contributed material and illustrations of instruments are acknowledged in the text.

Light rays from a point fixated by the patient fall on the entire eye, but only that bundle of rays bounded by the entrance pupil will enter the eye. Consequently the only portion of the cornea used to see the fixation point is the portion that overlies the entrance pupil and is centered on the line connecting the fixation point with the center of the entrance pupil; this line is called the "line of sight." In theory this area of the cornea is simple to locate by starting from the fovea. Rays of light emanating from a theoretic point source of light at the fovea will exit the pupil and describe an almost circular area on the cornea (Fig. 16-2, *A*). If the patient has 1.00 D of myopia, an image of the point source will be formed 1 m in front of the cornea. Because ray paths are reversible, an object (point source) placed 1 m in front of the eye will produce an image point on the fovea, passing through the same area of the cornea—the area that overlays the pupil (Fig. 16-2, *B*).*

The line of sight corresponds in geometric optics terms to the chief ray of the bundle of rays passing through the pupil and reaching the fovea.[5] For best optical performance therefore it is the intersection of the line of sight with the cornea that marks the desired center for the optical zone of corneal surgical procedures, including refractive keratotomy.

This principle can be illustrated using a patient with correctopia, or an eccentric pupil (Figs. 16-2, *C,* and 16-2, *D*). The patient is asked to fixate on the target while the surgeon observes from immediately behind the target and marks an optical zone concentric with the pupil. The properly located optical zone of the cornea will be significantly decentered, even though the corneal light reflex is in the same location as in a normal eye.

Any corneal irregularity or scarring that overlays the entrance pupil will cause irregular refraction and glare. Conversely, any irregularity or scarring periph-

*The relationship between corneal topography and the entrance pupil after refractive keratotomy is discussed in Chapter 3, Optics and Topography of Radial Keratotomy.

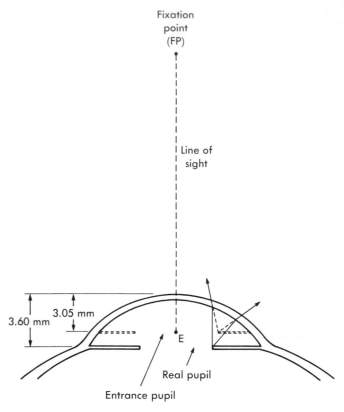

Figure 16-1
The entrance pupil of the eye is the virtual image of the real pupil formed by refraction of light at the cornea. The line of sight connects the fixation point *(FP)* with the center of the entrance pupil *(E)*. (From Uozato H and Guyton DL: Am J Ophthalmol 1987;103:264-275.)

eral to the portion of the cornea that overlays the entrance pupil cannot affect the light reaching the fovea.

If the only optically important part of the cornea is that overlying the entrance pupil, why is the cornea as large as it is? Light from peripheral points in the visual field must pass through peripheral portions of the cornea to fill the entrance pupil (Fig. 16-3). Irregularity

Figure 16-2
Rationale for using the center of the entrance pupil as the center point for keratotomy. **A,** To visualize the area of the cornea that forms the foveal image, place an imaginary point source of light at the fovea. Note that the light emerging from the eye is formed into a circular cone by the pupil and traverses only the area of the cornea overlying the pupil, the optical zone of the cornea. For a 1.00-diopter myope, the image of the theoretical foveal light source will be one meter in front of the eye. **B,** Now turn the situation around, since light ray paths are reversible, and place the object point source of light one meter from the eye. Only the light that strikes the optical zone of the cornea passes through the pupil to the fovea, centered around the line of sight. **C,** In an eye with an eccentric pupil, the optical zone of the cornea is the portion that overlies the pupil, far from the geometric center of the cornea and far from the corneal light reflection. (Courtesy Jack Holladay, M.D.)

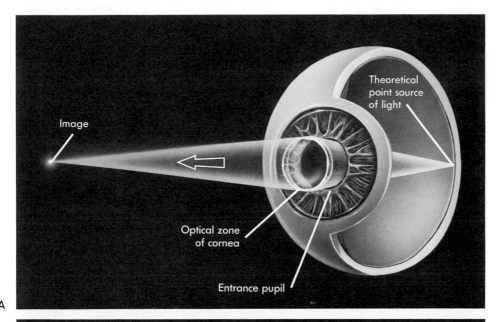

A

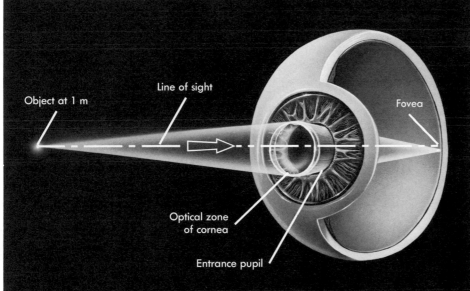

B

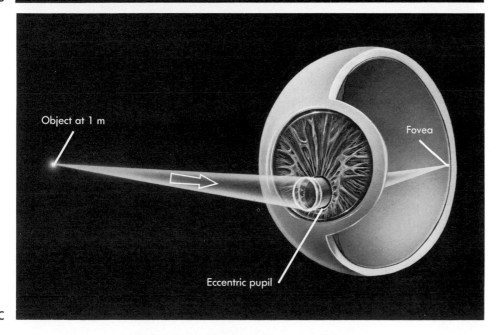

C

Figure 16-2 For legend see opposite page.

Continued.

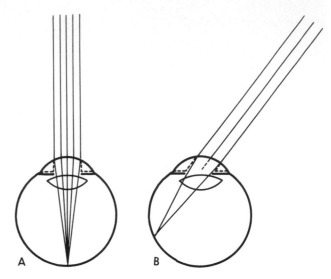

Figure 16-3

A different portion of the cornea is involved in the formation of each image point. **A,** Foveal rays pass through the central portion of the cornea directly overlying the entrance pupil. **B,** Peripheral rays pass through eccentric portions of the cornea to reach the entrance pupil. Peripheral corneal irregularity or scarring can thus affect peripheral image quality. (From Uozato H and Guyton DL: Am J Ophthalmol 1987;103:264-275.)

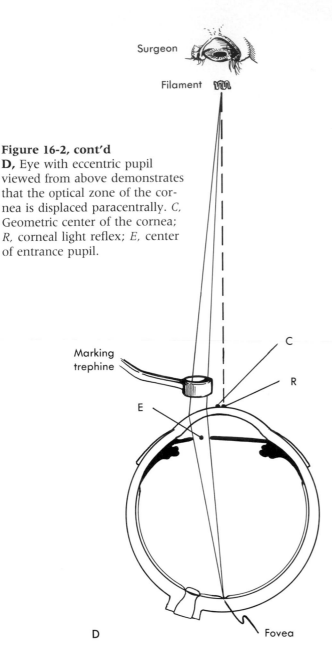

Figure 16-2, cont'd
D, Eye with eccentric pupil viewed from above demonstrates that the optical zone of the cornea is displaced paracentrally. *C,* Geometric center of the cornea; *R,* corneal light reflex; *E,* center of entrance pupil.

and scarring in the periphery of the cornea therefore cause irregular blur and glare in peripheral vision. For a patient to have a zone of glare-free vision centered on the point of fixation, the optical zone of the cornea must be larger than the entrance pupil. The larger the optical zone, the larger the field of glare-free vision (Table 16-1). No matter how large the optical zone of the cornea, it must still be centered on the line of sight if the zone of glare-free vision is to be centered on the fixation point.

Another reason for centering on the entrance pupil is the Stiles-Crawford effect: because the photoreceptors are aimed toward the center of the normal pupil, light passing through the center of the pupil is more effective in stimulating the photoreceptors than light passing through the peripheral pupil. With eccentric pupils, Enoch and Laties[4] and Bonds and MacLeod[2] have demonstrated that photoreceptors actively orient themselves toward the center of the eccentric pupil. The pupil therefore remains the proper optical reference for centering corneal surgical procedures.

The natural pupil is optimally used for centering corneal surgical procedures because medications used for dilating or constricting the pupil can sometimes shift its center. However, we could not find published data on whether the pupil constricts or dilates eccentrically.

There are of course mechanical and biologic reasons for using the geometric center of the cornea instead of the entrance pupil to center corneal surgical procedures, especially penetrating keratoplasty. However, if the geometric center is used and the pupil is markedly eccentric, glare will result from the scars that overlie the pupil. An iridoplasty can recenter the pupil in some eyes. If the glare is primarily in the peripheral visual field, it may be tolerable. Fortunately most pupils are close enough to the geometric center of the cornea that centering the corneal surgical procedure on the line of sight causes no problem with glare from corneal wounds.

Table 16-1

Diameter of Clear Optical Zone for Glare-Free Distance Vision*

| | Entrance pupil diameter (mm) | | | | | |
	2.00	3.00	4.00	5.00	6.00	7.00
Visual field radius in degrees (angular subtense)	Necessary diameter of clear optical zone (mm)					
0 (fixation point only)	2.00	3.00	4.00	5.00	6.00	7.00
5	2.52	3.50	4.48	5.45	6.41	7.37
15	3.53	4.46	5.38	6.28	7.17	8.04
30	5.04	5.86	6.66	7.43	8.18	8.91
45	6.62	7.29	7.93	8.55	9.14	9.71
60	8.36	8.83	9.27	9.70	10.12	10.51

From Bennett AG and Francis JL: The eye as an optical system. In Davson H, editor: The eye, vol 4, New York, 1962, Academic Press.
*Calculated for visual fields of various radii using the dimensions of Gullstrand's schematic eye.

CORNEAL LIGHT REFLEX

The corneal light reflex is often used for centering purposes, but its actual location is not widely understood. Many surgeons believe it is on the cornea, in the anterior chamber, or in the plane of the entrance pupil. On the basis of calculations from Gullstrand's schematic eye, it is actually about 0.85 mm posterior to the plane of the entrance pupil (Fig. 16-4). The corneal light reflex is formed by reflection of light from the anterior surface of the cornea. It is a virtual image of the light source and is more properly known as the first Purkinje-Sanson image. If the light source is at infinity, the corneal light reflex is located exactly at the focal point of the convex corneal surface. Because the focal point is halfway back to the center of curvature with the center of curvature 7.80 mm behind the front corneal surface, the corneal light reflex is 3.90 mm behind the front surface of the cornea. In clinical practice the light source is often held 33 cm from the eye or even closer. This simply moves the corneal light reflex a few hundredths of a millimeter closer to the cornea. For practical purposes, we will consider the corneal light reflex to be located 4 mm behind the front corneal surface, or simply 4 mm.

Where exactly is the entrance pupil? The entrance pupil is also a virtual image that is formed by light from the real pupil refracted by the cornea (see Fig. 16-1). It is located approximately 3 mm posterior to the front surface of the cornea. When the eye is fixating on a light source, the corneal light reflex, which is 4 mm posterior to the front surface of the cornea, is therefore about 1 mm posterior to the entrance pupil (see Fig. 16-4). The location of the corneal light reflex, however, is not constant. Instead, it depends on the direction of gaze of the eye with respect to the position of the light source. It is most convenient to consider the corneal light reflex to be 4 mm behind the front

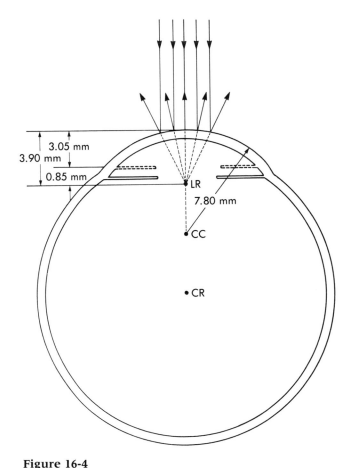

Figure 16-4
The corneal light reflex *(LR)* of a distant light source is a virtual image formed at the focal point of the convex mirror formed by the anterior corneal surface. It lies approximately 4 mm behind the front surface of the cornea and behind the entrance pupil (dotted line), on a line connecting the fixation point with the center of curvature *(CC)* of the cornea. The center of rotation of the eye *(CR)* is farther back and is not involved with the formation of the corneal light reflex. (From Uozato H and Guyton DL: Am J Ophthalmol 1987;103:264-275.)

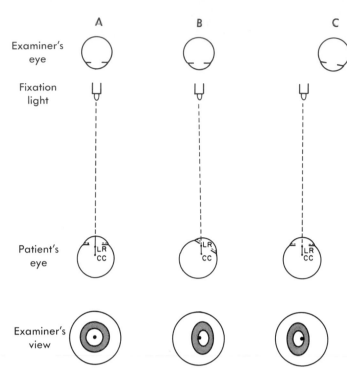

Figure 16-5
The corneal light reflex *(LR)*. **A,** In its proper position with the patient's eye fixing the light. **B,** Displaced by deviation of the patient's eye. **C,** Displaced by misalignment of the examiner's eye from its proper position behind the fixation light. *CC,* Center of curvature of the cornea. (From Uozato H and Guyton DL: Am J Ophthalmol 1987;103:264-275.)

surface of the cornea on an imaginary string connecting the light source with the center of curvature of the cornea (not the center of rotation of the eye, which is farther behind the front surface of the cornea) (Fig. 16-5). An examiner behind the light source sees the corneal light reflex move laterally as the eye's direction of gaze changes. In addition, because of the parallax between the entrance pupil and the corneal light reflex, the exact projection of the corneal light reflex onto the patient's entrance pupil depends on the position of the examiner's eye behind the light source. The examiner's eye is usually held directly behind the light source to prevent this parallax effect when viewing the corneal light reflex. To understand the relationship of the customarily viewed corneal light reflex to the various methods used for centering corneal surgical procedures, one must also be familiar with the various axes of the eye.

AXES OF THE EYE

Many axes of the eye have been described in the history of physiologic optics, occasionally with confus-

ing and conflicting definitions. These include such axes as the optical axis, visual axis, pupillary axis, line of sight, and fixation line.[6] The definitions and significance of some of these axes will be reviewed briefly as they relate to centering corneal surgery.

A true optical axis for the eye cannot be defined because the eye is not a centered optical system. For the eye's optical system to be centered, the optical axis of the crystalline lens would have to pass through both the center of curvature of the cornea and the fovea. Because the axis generally passes through neither center, an overall optical axis cannot be defined. The line that most closely connects the fixation light with the four Purkinje-Sanson images is our best approximation of an optical axis.

The visual axis is usually defined as the broken line that connects the fixation point with the fovea and passes through the nodal points.[6] This definition has nothing to do with the pupil, corneal light reflex, entrance pupil, or line of sight. If the eye was a centered optical system, with the fovea on the optical axis, the visual axis would coincide with the optical axis. Because of the noncentered optics of the eye, however, it is difficult, if not impossible, to locate the true visual axis experimentally.[10] The visual axis is thus of no practical use, and the term should not be used clinically.

The pupillary axis is easily defined and easily located. It is the line perpendicular to the cornea that passes through the center of the entrance pupil. It also passes through the center of curvature of the anterior corneal surface. Given the previous description of the corneal light reflex, it should be obvious that the pupillary axis can be located by an examiner's centering the corneal light reflex in a patient's pupil while being careful to sight from directly behind the light source.

The pupillary axis generally does *not* coincide with the line of sight. Although both pass through the center of the entrance pupil, the line of sight passes through the fixation point, whereas the pupillary axis usually passes through the cornea temporal to the line of sight. The angle between the pupillary axis and the line of sight is known as the angle lambda (Fig. 16-6). Lambda can be measured precisely and is used here instead of the angle kappa, which is defined as the angle between the pupillary axis and the nondeterminable visual axis. In Figs. 16-5, 16-6, and 16-7, the eye is fixating on the light source. The corneal light reflex usually lies nasal to the line of sight and the pupillary axis. If the examiner's eye is directly behind the fixation light, the corneal light reflex appears decentered nasally in the patient's pupil. The projection of the corneal light reflex onto the anterior corneal surface is therefore nasal to the intersection of the line of

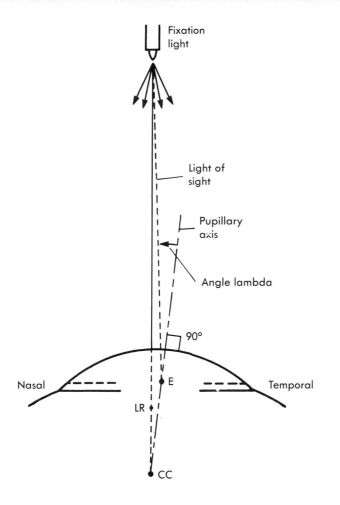

Figure 16-6
The pupillary axis and line of sight both pass through the center of the entrance pupil *(E)*. The angle between the two, the angle lambda, is normally 3 to 6 degrees, with the pupillary axis passing more temporally through the cornea. The corneal light reflex *(LR)* is nasal to both the pupillary axis and the line of sight when the eye is fixating on the light. *CC,* Center of curvature of cornea. (From Uozato H and Guyton DL: Am J Ophthalmol 1987;103:264-275.)

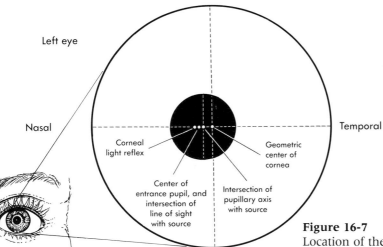

Figure 16-7
Location of the intersection of various axes with the cornea, assuming that the patient is looking at the fixation light, the examiner is sighting in line with the fixation light, and there is a small, positive angle lambda. As drawn, the entrance pupil is usually slightly nasal to the geometric center of the cornea. The pupillary axis passes through the center of the entrance pupil and is perpendicular to the surface of the cornea, intersecting the cornea just nasal to the geometric center. The line of sight connects the fixation point with the center of the entrance pupil, intersecting the cornea just nasal to the intersection by the pupillary axis. The corneal light reflex is located still further nasal to the line of sight.

sight with the cornea and thus nasal to the desired centration point for corneal surgical procedures.

For further discussion of axes of the eye, see Duke-Elder.[3]

CURRENT METHODS OF CENTERING CORNEAL SURGERY

Various methods have been described for centering corneal surgical procedures with the operating microscope.

PERK technique

Steinberg and Waring[7] described the technique used in the PERK study. Patients fixated on the coiled microscope light filament that emerged from the microscope toward 6 o'clock from the viewing tubes (Fig. 16-8). This displaced reflection of the microscope light filament from the cornea toward 12 o'clock (Fig. 16-8). The corneal light reflex was also displaced to the right when viewed monocularly through the right

ocular. Therefore a compensation was made. Viewing through the right microscope ocular, the surgeon marked the corneal epithelium at the left end of the rectangular filament reflection and one half to one width of the filament inferiorly (toward 6 o'clock) with the tip of a hypodermic needle (Fig. 16-8). This generally resulted in a centering mark slightly nasal to the center of the entrance pupil. They concluded incorrectly that, "because the visual axis is not aligned with the pupillary axis, the center of the pupil cannot be used as a reference point."[7]

They compared this method with the Osher centering device, showing that both methods identified approximately the same spot on the corneal surface in a series of 34 eyes,[7] a spot 0.2 mm to 0.5 mm nasal to the center of the entrance pupil, as shown. This method can produce errors resulting from the patient not fixing the center of the light source, from the offset estimation required of the surgeon, and from the use of the corneal light reflex in the first place.

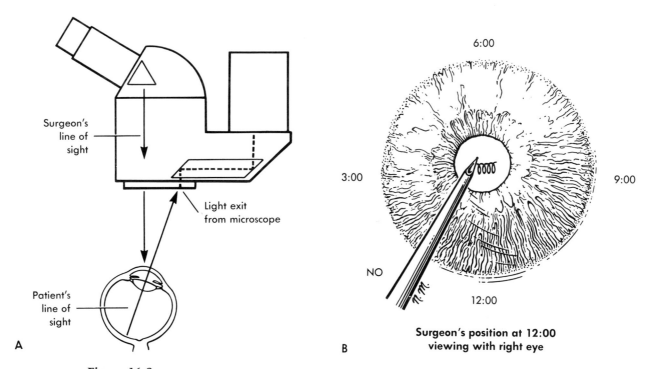

Figure 16-8
Obsolete PERK method of using microscope light reflection to mark the center of the optical zone. **A,** Because the microscope light does not exit the microscope coaxial to the surgeon's line of sight, the patient will look eccentrically, approximately 7 degrees inferiorly to see it, displacing the apparent position of corneal light reflection on the surface of the cornea. **B,** To compensate for the displaced corneal light reflection and the parallax induced by monocular viewing with the right eye, the surgeon placed the mark on the cornea at the left and beneath the light reflection. This resulted in a centering mark that was displaced nasal to the desired location at the center of the patient's entrance pupil. This technique should be abandoned in favor of marking the center of the entrance pupil. (From Steinberg EB and Waring GO: Am J Ophthalmol 1983;96:605.)

Several arrangements have been described to decrease the potential error from such noncoaxial sighting by the examiner. Each is prone to error either from the use of the corneal light reflex or from reliance on binocular sighting in surgeons who may not be able to do so. An analysis of the error involved with each of these methods follows.

Osher's optical centering device

Osher's optical center device (JEDMED, St. Louis), covers the operation microscope's objective lenses, occluding the light source and one of the viewing tubes. It channels some of the light through a fiberoptic bundle to emerge from a spot in the exact center of the open viewing tube[7] (Fig. 16-9). The patient fixates the

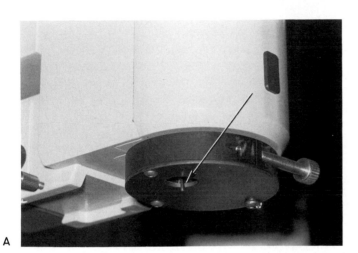

A

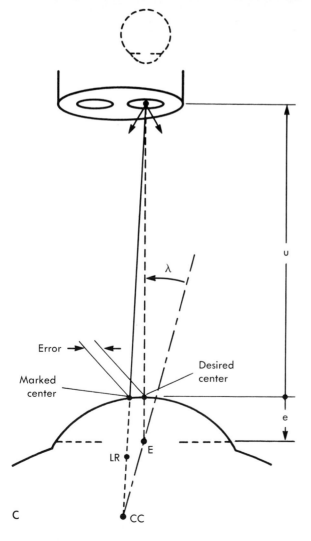

C

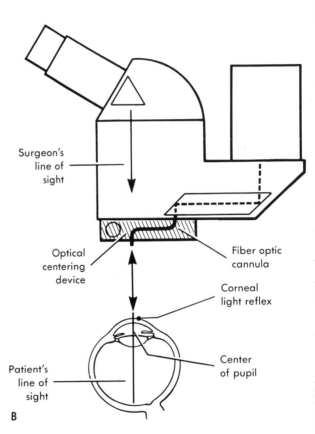

B

Figure 16-9
Osher optical centering device. **A,** The device is attached over the objective lens of the operating microscope. Arrow points to fiberoptic fixation light. **B,** Drawing demonstrates that the fiberoptic light spot is placed in the center of the one objective lens of the microscope, but the light reflection on the cornea is not centered over the patient's line of sight in the center of the entrance pupil. **C,** Schematic illustration of the error in corneal centering produced by Osher's optical centering device. The fixation light is centered in one viewing tube of the operating microscope. The other viewing tube is covered. If the center of the entrance pupil *(E)* were used for sighting, rather than the corneal light reflex *(LR)*, the desired center would be located. (**A** and **B** from Steinberg EB and Waring GO: Am J Ophthalmol 1983;96:605; **C** from Uozato H and Guyton DL: Am J Ophthalmol 1987;103:264-265.)

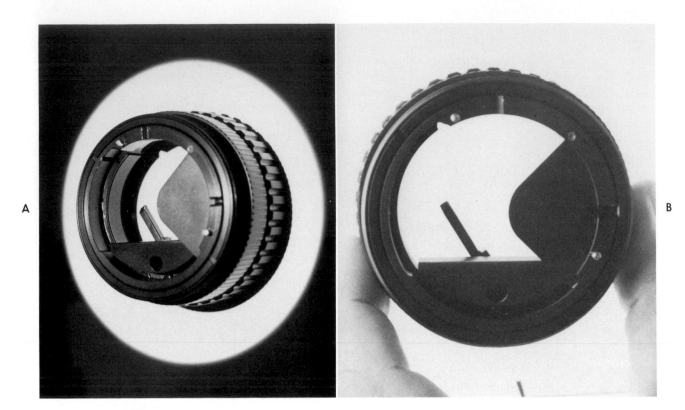

Figure 16-10

Microscope centering device. **A,** The attachment screws on over the objective lens of the microscope. The triangular guard blocks out one viewing tube. **B,** The thin rectangular rod houses a small light on its tip, which is centered beneath the other viewing tube. The patient fixates the light and the surgeon sights down the viewing tube, marking the center of the entrance pupil.

spot of light, the examiner views monocularly through the viewing tube, and the "visual axis" is marked as coinciding with the apparent position of the corneal light reflex. With this optical arrangement, the surgeon views the corneal light reflex coaxially with the fixation light (see Fig. 16-10). Error in corneal centering occurs whenever lambda is not zero. Table 16-2 lists the error calculated[11] for values of lambda between 3 and 6 degrees, using the dimensions of Gullstrand's schematic eye. The error is greater when lambda is larger, approaching 0.5 mm when lambda equals 6 degrees.

There are two other drawbacks to Osher's optical centering device: attaching it to and removing it from the microscope take time. If the screw-clamp is not fastened securely, the device can fall on the patient's eye, although a guard chain is provided to prevent this. The light emitted by the fiberoptic tip is dim, making it difficult to see its reflection in the cornea and impossible to see the pupil.

Table 16-2

Centering Error with Osher's Centering Device*

	Angle lambda (in degrees)			
	3	4	5	6
Working distance (mm)	Centering error (mm)			
150	0.237	0.316	0.395	0.475
175	0.238	0.318	0.398	0.478
200	0.240	0.320	0.401	0.481

*Calculated for customary working distances of the operating microscope and for various normal values of the angle lambda.

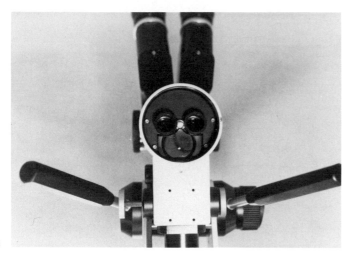

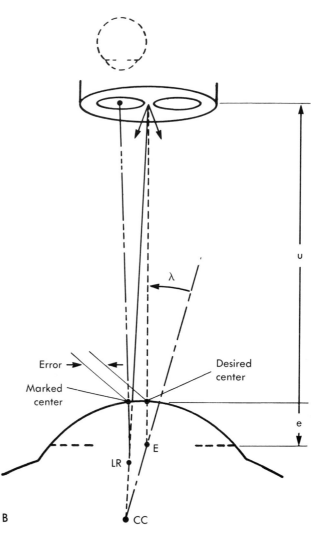

Figure 16-11
A, Centering device mounted on a Weck microscope places a small, red fixation light between the two viewing tubes. The light is turned on for centering and is turned off when not in use. **B,** Schematic illustration of the maximal error in corneal centering caused by monocular sighting of the corneal light reflex as the patient fixates the Zeiss or Weck fixation device. (**A** courtesy Weck Instruments). (From Uozato H and Guyton DL: Am J Ophthalmol 1987;103:264-275.)

A similar fixation/centering device is being designed for the Wild microscope by E. Leitz, Inc. in Rockleigh, N.J. (Fig. 16-10). This device not only aligns the lines of sight of the patient and the surgeon, but also allows the surgeon to see the entrance pupil and mark its center.

Fixation target between microscope viewing tubes

Two methods of centering use a fixation target centered between the microscope viewing tubes: a fixation light in the Zeiss and Weck centering devices and a nonluminous fixation spot in Thornton's methods.

Weck and Zeiss light reflex target

Attachments to the Weck and Zeiss microscopes (Weck Surgical Systems, Research Triangle Park, N.C.; Carl Zeiss, Inc., Thornwood, N.Y.) place a fixation light exactly between the two viewing tubes. The patient fixates on the light and the examiner sights the corneal light reflex of the fixation light binocularly, marking its apparent position as the "visual axis." Centering error results not only from the angle lambda in sighting the corneal light reflex, but also from the surgeon sighting monocularly because the fixation light is not coaxial with either viewing tube (Fig. 16-11). The errors from these two sources tend to balance one another when the surgeon marks one eye of the patient, but the errors combine when both patient eyes are marked. From trigonometric analysis we can calculate the worse-case error. Table 16-3 lists the maximum error calculated for values of lambda between 3 and 6 degrees, using microscope working distances of 150, 175, and 200 mm. The two viewing tubes are separated by 25 mm between centers. The error is greater when lambda is large and the working distance is short. The error approaches 0.8 mm when lambda equals 6 degrees and the working distance equals 150 mm. If surgeons use only their right eye to sight the patient's right eye, and only their left eye to sight the patient's left eye, the centering error will be much less (0.0 to 0.2 mm) (Table 16-3).

Table 16-3

Centering Error with the Zeiss or Weck Fixation Device*

Working distance (mm)	Centering error (mm)	Angle lambda (in degrees)		
		3	4	5	6

Working distance (mm)	Centering error (mm) 3	4	5	6
150	0.553	0.631	0.710	0.789
	(−0.008)	(−0.001)	(−0.078)	(0.157)
175	0.518	0.597	0.677	0.756
	(−0.042)	(0.038)	(0.117)	(0.196)
200	0.478	0.558	0.638	0.717
	(0.001)	(0.080)	(0.160)	(0.240)

*The worst-case error when sighting the corneal light reflex is calculated for customary working distances of the operating microscope and for various normal values of lambda. If surgeons use only their right eye for sighting the patient's right eye, and only their left eye for sighting the patient's left eye, the centering error is much less, as given by the values in parentheses.

Thornton's fixation target

Thornton's fixation target is a round, brightly colored, nonluminous adhesive spot placed between the two viewing tubes of the microscope on the objective lens.[8] The microscope light is turned off, and the room lights are left on, decreasing the patient's light sensi-

tivity and removing the corneal light reflection. The contralateral eye is covered, and the patient is told to fixate the dot in the center of the microscope lens. The surgeon views monocularly and marks the center of the entrance pupil (Fig. 16-12). A centering error results only when the surgeon does not sight binocu-

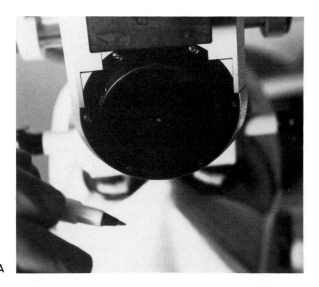

A

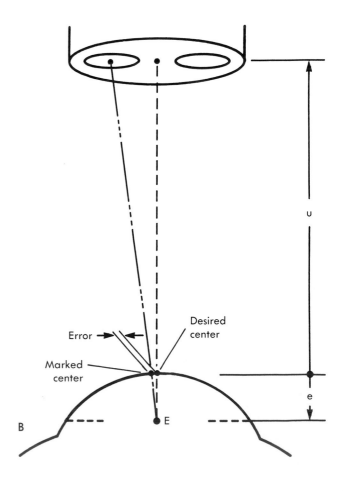

B

Figure 16-12
A, Thornton's nonluminous adhesive spot is placed between the two viewing tubes and is fixated by the patient's eye with the microscope light off. The surgeon uses a pen to mark the center of the pupil. **B,** Schematic illustration of the error in corneal centering caused by monocular sighting of the center of the pupil as the patient fixates Thornton's fixation target. (**A** from Thornton SP: In Sanders DR, Hofmann RF, and Salz JJ, editors: Refractive corneal surgery, Thorofare, NJ, 1986, Slack, Inc, p 134; **B** from Uozato H and Guyton DL: Am J Ophthalmol 1987;103:264-275.)

Table 16-4

Centering Error When Sighting Monocularly with Thornton's Fixation Target

Working distance (mm)	Centering error (mm)
150	0.249
175	0.214
200	0.188

larly. In the case of monocular sighting, the error can be derived.[9] The error is approximately 0.2 mm in all cases, assuming the viewing tubes are separated by 25 mm between centers (Table 16-4).

BINOCULAR SIGHTING

Centering methods using binocular sighting have been based on the assumption that binocular sighting is valid. When a point on the surface of the cornea is marked as being in line with the corneal light reflex, 4 mm posterior to the surface of the cornea, or in line with the center of the entrance pupil, 3 mm posterior to the surface of the cornea, should the sighting be performed stereoscopically or primarily with one eye? Because of our suspicion that monocular sighting is often used, we investigated this question more thoroughly.

The Zeiss Keratolux Fixation Device was mounted on a Zeiss 6-SFC operating microscope, providing a small, bright, white light source exactly between the viewing tubes behind the objective lens of the microscope. A sewing needle was mounted in the vertical meridian of a chrome-plated keratometer calibration sphere so that the tip of the needle could be moved precisely across the surface of the sphere in the horizontal meridian. We asked 27 ophthalmic surgeons to focus the microscope on the tip of the needle and to move the needle transversely to center the tip on the light reflex. Three different magnifications were used, and the alignment was performed under three viewing conditions: with only the right eye fixing, with only the left eye fixing, and with both eyes open. By comparing the binocular setting with the two monocular settings, we determined the frequency and accuracy of binocular sighting under each magnification for the 27 surgeons.[9]

The results of this experiment showed that approximately one sixth of the surgeons sighted monocularly, approximately one half sighted binocularly, and the remaining third somewhere in between. Only half of the five surgeons who sighted monocularly were aware that they customarily did so. Monocular sighting leads to centering errors in sighting techniques that rely on binocular sighting.

The frequency of binocular sighting increased with increasing magnification. The tiny corneal light reflex of the fixation light was seen double (physiologic diplopia) by most observers under the higher magnifications, and the needle was simply centered between the double images. The surgeons who sighted monocularly saw only a single image. A solution to the problem of monocular sighting was noted during the experiment. By looking first with one eye and then with the other, most monocular sighters could learn to balance the position of the needle between the two positions of the corneal light reflex.

OPTIMAL CENTERING FOR REFRACTIVE KERATOTOMY

Our main conclusions are that the corneal light reflex is not the appropriate reference mark for centering refractive keratotomy and other corneal surgical procedures; the center of the entrance pupil is the optimal optical center for the corneal surgeon. Fortunately our theoretic analysis of currently used methods for corneal centering indicates errors that are clinically insignificant in most situations, 0.2 to 0.4 mm. For example, even though the centering mark in the PERK study was decentered nasally from the entrance pupil by approximately 0.2 to 0.4 mm, problems from glare were minimal (see Fig. 16-8).[12]

On the other hand, centering errors of 0.5 to 0.8 mm can be significant, especially with central clear zones that have a diameter of only 3.0 mm. Because refractive surgery is "microsurgery," every adjustment toward the most desirable procedure should be made. Because it is easy and practical to mark the center of the entrance pupil during surgery, that is the advised procedure. This will be appreciated by patients who are particularly sensitive to glare, patients who may have large pupils, and surgeons who are fastidious about detail.

Optimal corneal centering requires the patient to have a natural undilated pupil and to fixate on a light or target that is coaxial with the examiner's sighting eye. Practically speaking this means the patient must fixate on a target and the observer must view the patient's eye from the position of the target before marking a zone concentric with the pupil. The position of the corneal light reflex is irrelevant and often misleading.

None of the commercial fixation devices available in 1989 fulfilled these criteria. A simple approach can be used: the operating microscope can be used with a small fixation spot placed in the exact center of one of

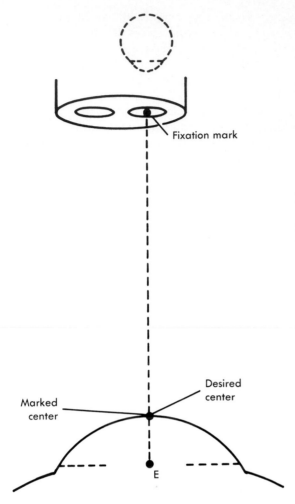

Fixation mark

Desired
center

Marked
center

E

Figure 16-13
Optimal corneal centering. The patient sights a fixation mark placed in the center of one of the viewing tubes of the microscope, and the surgeon views monocularly through that tube and marks the patient's cornea in line with the center of the entrance pupil *(E)*. (From Uozato H and Guyton DL: Am J Ophthalmol 1987;103:264-275.)

the viewing tubes (Fig. 16-13). A 1- or 2-mm mark will not interfere significantly with the optics. The surgeon should sight monocularly through the tube with the fixation spot and mark the cornea at the center of the patient's entrance pupil.

Alternatively, the marking procedure can be performed at the slit-lamp microscope with a similar fixation spot centered in one objective of the slit-lamp microscope.

The direct ophthalmoscope can also be used to locate the center of a patient's pupil. The patient should look exactly at the light of the ophthalmoscope, and the surgeon should sight monocularly through the ophthalmoscope to mark the center of the pupil. By

dialing in plus sphere to provide a "reading add" to focus the pupil clearly, examiners can obtain a magnified view of the patient's pupil if they move in close enough. The patient's line of sight and examiner's line of sight are not exactly coaxial because of the slight displacement of the illuminating light from the peephole in the ophthalmoscope, but the two axes are very close. The closer one moves, to the patient's eye, however, the less coaxial these axes become.

The procedure can also be performed without magnification, albeit with more chance for error, provided the patient fixates the surgeon's sighting eye while the surgeon marks the cornea at the center of the patient's entrance pupil.

UNFINISHED BUSINESS

Further study of the role of the entrance pupil of the eye in corneal surgery is needed, especially in terms of the aspheric optics that are created by refractive corneal procedures. For example, the surgeon doing penetrating keratoplasty faces a dilemma in cases of eccentric pupils. It is advantageous to center the keratoplasty geometrically to keep the donor tissue as far away from the limbus as possible to prevent its detection by the immune system, but it is also advantageous to center the graft over the pupil for optical purposes, since the center of the graft has the best optical function. There is a need for further studies of the role of the cornea over the pupil after refractive keratotomy with better definition of the optimal diameter of the central optical zone and of the role of asphericity and corneal scars in the production of multifocal images, decreased contrast sensitivity, and glare. Development of simple instruments is needed to help ensure proper centering of refractive surgical procedures.

REFERENCES

1. Bennett AG and Francis JL: The eye as an optical system. In Davson H, editor: The eye, vol 4, New York, 1962, Academic Press, p 101.
2. Bonds AB and MacLeod DIA: A displaced Stiles-Crawford effect associated with an eccentric pupil, Invest Ophthalmol Vis Sci 1978;17:754.
3. Duke-Elder S and Abrams D: Ophthalmic optics and refraction, Vol V. In Duke-Elder S, editor: System of ophthalmology, St Louis, 1970, The CV Mosby Co, pp 134-138.
4. Enoch JM and Laties AM: An analysis of retinal receptor orientation. II. Prediction for psychophysical tests, Invest Ophthalmol 1971;10:959.
5. Fry GA: Geometrical optics, Philadelphia, 1969, Chilton Book Co, p 110.
6. Lancaster WB: Terminology in ocular motility and allied subjects, Am J Ophthalmol 1943;26:122.
7. Steinberg EB and Waring GO: Comparison of two methods of marking the visual axis on the cornea during radial keratotomy, Am J Ophthalmol 1983; 96:605.
8. Thornton SP: Surgical armamentarium. In Sanders DR, Hofmann RF, and Salz JJ, editors: Refractive corneal surgery, Thorofare, NJ, 1986, Slack, Inc, p 134.
9. Uozato H and Guyton DL: Centering corneal surgical procedures, Am J Ophthalmol 1987;103:264.
10. Uozato H, Makino H, Saishin M, and Nakao S: Measurement of visual axis using a laser beam. In Breinin GM and Siegel IM, editors: Advances in diagnostic visual optics, Berlin, 1983, Springer-Verlag, p 22.
11. Walsh PM and Guyton DL: Comparison of two methods of marking the visual axis on the cornea during radial keratotomy (correspondence), Am J Ophthalmol 1984;97:660.
12. Waring GO, Lynn MJ, Gelender H, Laibson PR, Lindstrom RL, Myers WD, Obstbaum SA, Rowsey JJ, McDonald MB, Schanzlin DJ, Sperduto RD, Bourque LB, and the PERK Study Group: Results of the prospective evaluation of radial keratotomy (PERK) study one year after surgery, Ophthalmology 1985;92:177-198.

Atlas of Surgical Techniques of Radial Keratotomy

George O. Waring III

There are many ways to describe the surgical technique of radial keratotomy. One is to detail the steps in the surgery. This has been done in most publications on radial keratotomy; I cover the basic steps in Plate 17-1. This provides a useful outline but details neither alternative techniques nor the specific artistic and manual nuances necessary for successful surgery.

A second approach is to tell "how I do it," giving my specific idiosyncratic details of planning and executing the operation. Such detailed personal descriptions are available and useful for the surgeon who seeks to emulate a colleague, although they provide no perspective on alternative approaches and variations.

A third approach is simply to list all of the alternative techniques that have been described by surgeons doing radial keratotomy. This approach presents a useful inventory but provides a poor guide for the surgeon seeking to perform the operation.

BACKGROUND AND ACKNOWLEDGMENTS

In a sense, this entire textbook provides the background and acknowledgments for this atlas because the atlas tries to distill the surgical techniques that have developed over the past 100 years. I gratefully and humbly acknowledge the contributions of the many surgeons, who contributed to this development, particularly those cited in Section II, Development of Refractive Keratotomy.

Numerous descriptions of the techniques of radial keratotomy have been previously published, some providing a historical record of the development of the surgery and others practical advice about current performance. These contributions include Ronald Schachar,[9] *Understanding Radial Keratotomy* (1981); Donald Sanders and the ARK study group[7], *Radial Keratotomy* (1984); Andrew Lewicky's chapter, "Surgical Techniques and Related Complications," in Sanders, Hofmann, and Salz's[4] *Refractive Corneal Surgery* (1986); William Ellis,[1] *A Textbook of Radial Keratotomy and Astigmatism Surgery* (1986); the contributions of Hofmann, Lindstrom, Neumann, Salz, Tate, and Thornton[8] in *Radial Keratotomy—Surgical Techniques* (1986); and the PERK technique by Waring and the PERK study group, "Design and Rationale of the Prospective Evaluation of Radial Keratotomy (PERK) Study."[10] I have drawn from these publications, personal communication with keratotomy surgeons, and my own experience for this atlas.

Because the techniques of keratotomy have gradually evolved through trial-and-error refinement and through informal communication, it is difficult to attribute a particular technique to its true originator. I have therefore avoided trying to acknowledge the innovator of each, a task left to the published documentation in the literature.

A fourth approach—the one adopted here—includes aspects of all three. By breaking down the operation into individual steps, I try to detail the sequence through which the surgeon will proceed during the operation. By presenting alternative techniques in each step, I try to describe strengths and weaknesses and present a fair opinion about which are preferable. By detailing fine points of technique, in both the text and drawings, I have tried to depict surgical reality. No single "standardized" method is presented.

"But wait a minute," you may object, "I'm reading this book to learn how to do radial keratotomy. What is the correct preferred technique?" As this chapter adequately demonstrates, there is currently no correct "preferred technique" of radial keratotomy. My effort here is to describe in detail the steps and subtleties in keratotomy surgery and to point out the strengths and weaknesses of different approaches. It is impossible for me to distill from the information available a technique that clearly emerges as superior. Therefore in addition to digesting the techniques in this atlas, you must take a course, train with someone who has developed artistic and surgical skills in radial keratotomy, and refine your own personal techniques.

The goal of keratotomy surgery—and that of any refractive surgical procedure—is to achieve an accurate outcome that is at least as predictable as the result of fitting glasses and contact lenses. We have not yet realized that goal. In its present stage of development, radial keratotomy is a combination of science and art: science, because there are numerous objective, verifiable, replicable aspects to the procedure, and art, because there is so much individual variability among surgeons that all must create their own techniques by combining information gleaned from others, personalized modifications, and subtle nuances.

Many factors are subject to individual variation that will affect the outcome of the procedure. These include the following:

1. Cooperation of the patient during surgery
2. Use of topical versus peribulbar anesthesia
3. Method of determining the center of the clear zone
4. Surgical plan—the relationship between the amount of myopia, patient age, clear zone diameter, and the number and depth of the incisions
5. Selection of the area to measure the corneal thickness that is used as the reference value for setting the knife blade
6. Pachometer used to measure corneal thickness and the method of calibration

7. Design and configuration of the knife blade (width, blade angle, sharpness) and the footplate
8. Percent bias that the length of the knife blade is set and the method by which it is verified
9. Hydration of the cornea during the procedure
10. Method of fixation of the eye and the level of the intraocular pressure during the incisions
11. Method of spacing the incisions
12. Sequence in which the incisions are made
13. Direction in which the incisions are cut: centrifugal versus centripetal
14. Manual kinesthetic techniques of executing the incision, including the perpendicularity of the knife blade and the pressure exerted on the knife during the incision
15. Speed at which the incisions are made
16. Length of the incisions, as determined by their termination near the limbus and the clear zone
17. Achieved depth of the incisions, including deepening incisions
18. Frequency and size of corneal perforations
19. Amount of manipulation and irrigation of the incisions
20. Types of postoperative medications used; for example, corticosteroids

Each of these variables affects the outcome to a different degree (see Chapter 26, Summary of Factors That Affect the Outcome of Refractive Keratotomy). For illustrative purposes, assume that the 20 factors increase the effect by 1% each for one surgeon and decrease the effect by 1% each for another surgeon. This would make a 40% difference in outcome for the two surgeons—2.00 D difference for a −5.00 D myopic patient. Therefore, keratotomy requires individual surgeons to develop their own personal technique. Only by careful, unbiased studies of the scientific and artistic aspects of radial keratotomy can we wrest it from the individual idiosyncrasies of art and ground it in the objective generalities of science.

The surgical instruments used in refractive keratotomy are described in detail in Chapter 15, so only their practical use during surgery is included in this atlas. Although I discuss some aspects of astigmatic keratotomy here, the details are left for Chapter 32, Atlas of Astigmatic Keratotomy. The steps in preoperative planning and the nomograms used to quantify the variables during surgery are covered in Chapter 13, Predictability of Refractive Keratotomy, and in Chapter 14, Computerized Predictability Formulas for Refractive Keratotomy.

PLATE 17-1:   Steps in Keratotomy Surgery (Figs. 17-1 to 17-14)

To provide an overall orientation to radial keratotomy surgery, Plate 17-1 presents the basic steps in the operation as a series of paired photographs, one taken through the operating microscope to depict the surgeon's view and the other taken from the side to depict the orientation of the eye and the surgeon's hands. Details of each step are presented in the remainder of the atlas in Plates 17-2 through 17-22 (See insert for color versions of Figs. 17-1 to 17-13.)

FIGURE 17-1   TOPICAL ANESTHESIA

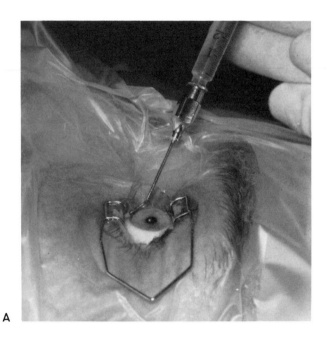
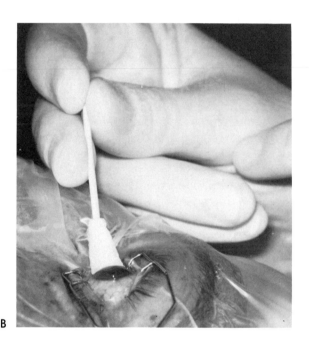

A   B

Topical anesthesia. In addition to application of topical drops, flushing of fornices with anesthetic through a blunt cannula **(A)** and application of anesthetic on a sponge at the limbus **(B)** enhance topical anesthesia.

FIGURE 17-2   MARKING THE CENTER OF THE PUPIL

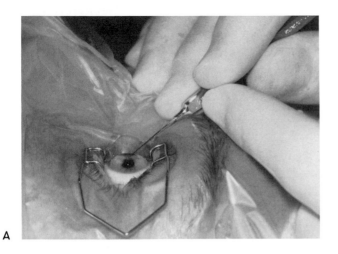

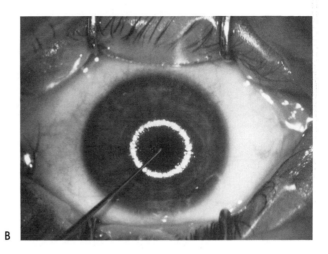

A

B

Marking the center of the pupil. A, A blunt instrument, such as an IOL hook, marks the cornea by indenting it over the center of the pupil. **B,** Circular light reflection from indentation of the cornea.

FIGURE 17-3   MARKING THE CENTRAL CLEAR ZONE

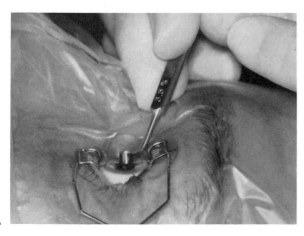

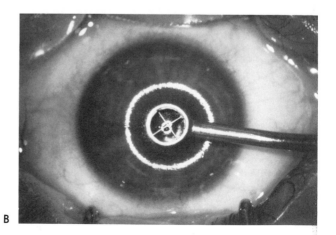

A

B

Marking the central clear zone. A, A clear zone marker of appropriate diameter indents the cornea. **B,** Centering mark with cross hairs seen with circular light reflection from indentation of the cornea.

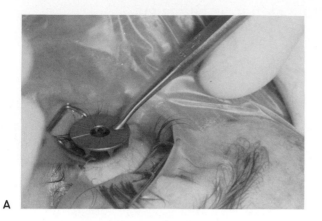

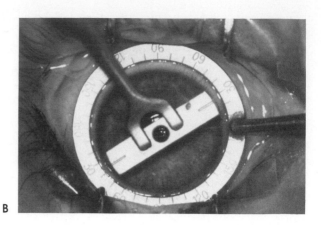

Marking the location of incisions. A, A marker with ridges imprints the location of the incisions in the epithelium as it is depressed on the cornea. **B,** The meridian for astigmatism surgery may be marked using a circular protractor and linear marker.

FIGURE 17-5   MEASURING CORNEAL THICKNESS WITH AN ULTRASONIC PACHOMETER

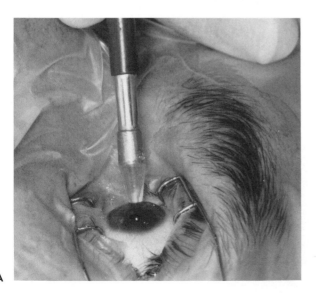

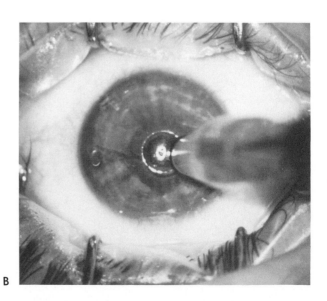

Measuring corneal thickness with an ultrasonic pachometer. A, The fluid-filled probe tip is held perpendicular to the corneal surface. **B,** The instrument obtains paracentral measurements just outside the circular clear zone mark.

FIGURE 17-6   MEASURING PERIPHERAL CORNEAL THICKNESS   513

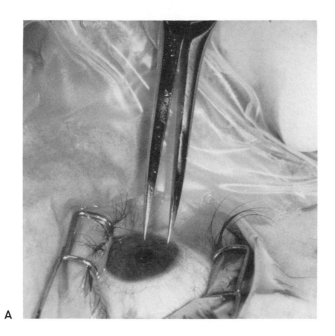
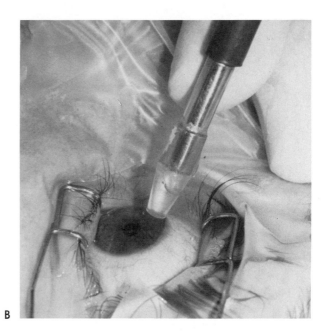

A

B

Measuring peripheral corneal thickness. A, The location of transverse or deepening incisions is marked with a caliper or incision marker. **B,** The ultrasonic pachometer probe is applied perpendicularly to the peripheral cornea.

FIGURE 17-7   SETTING THE LENGTH OF THE KNIFE BLADE WITH A MICROMETER

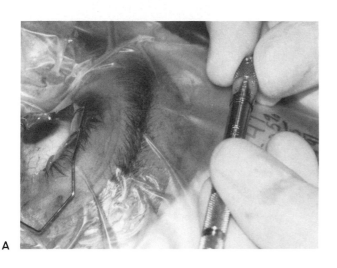
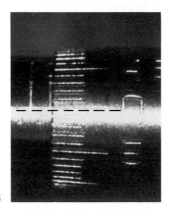
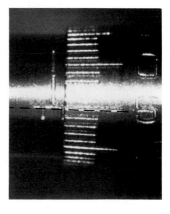

A

B

C

Setting the length of the knife blade with a micrometer. A, Micrometer setting is done away from the surface of the patient's eye. **B,** Initial setting is on zero. **C,** The micrometer is turned forward until the desired setting is achieved (500 μm).

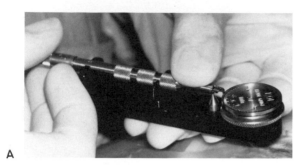

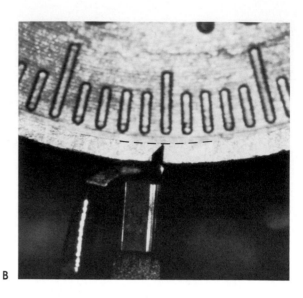

A   B

Verifying the length of the knife blade. A, The micrometer handle is placed in a gauge block cradle. **B,** Under high magnification, the tip of the blade is aligned with the edge of the gauge block at an appropriate setting, avoiding parallax.

FIGURE 17-9   CALIBRATING THE LENGTH OF THE KNIFE BLADE

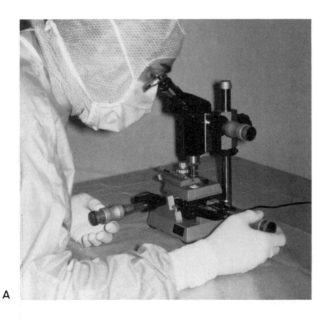

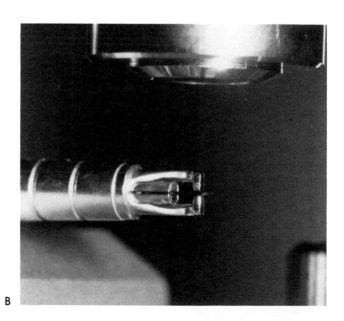

A   B

Calibrating the length of the knife blade. A, Compound microscope with micrometer stage is used to inspect the knife blade and measure the accuracy of its extension. **B,** The microscope objective lens allows inspection and calibration under magnification of approximately 150×.

FIGURE 17-10   REMOVING EXCESS SURFACE FLUID 515

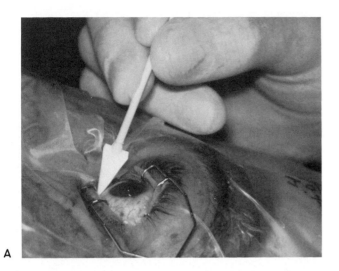
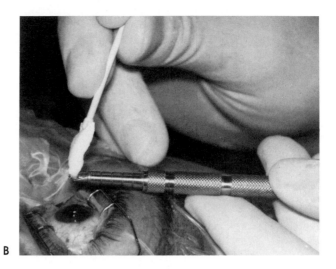

Removing excess surface fluid. A, The ocular surface, fornices, and, **B,** the tip of the knife are dried to prevent misinterpretation of surface fluid as aqueous from corneal perforation.

FIGURE 17-11   CENTRIFUGAL INCISION WITH AN OBLIQUE KNIFE BLADE

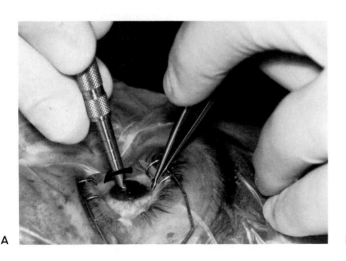
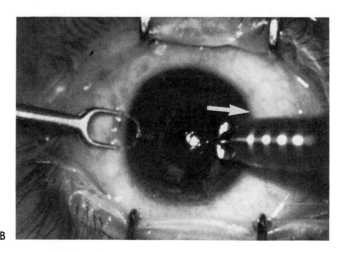

Centrifugal incision with an oblique knife blade. A and **B,** Double-pronged forceps fixate the globe at the limbus, and the knife is held perpendicular to the corneal surface at the edge of the clear zone, commencing a centrifugal incision (arrow).

FIGURE 17-12   CENTRIPETAL INCISION WITH A VERTICAL KNIFE BLADE

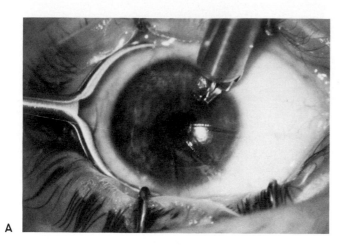
A

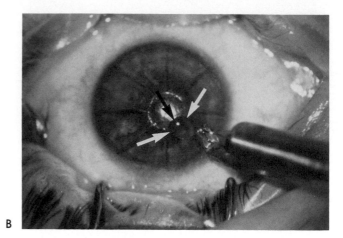
B

Centripetal incision with a vertical knife blade. A, The globe is fixated at the limbus with a spanning forceps, and the knife blade is inserted into the cornea adjacent to the limbus. **B,** Perforation of the cornea results in a bead of aqueous on the dry corneal surface (arrows).

FIGURE 17-13   TRANSVERSE INCISION WITH A VERTICAL KNIFE BLADE

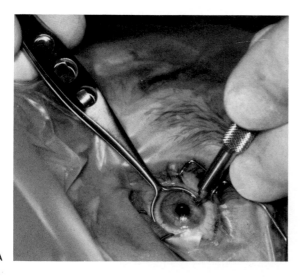
A

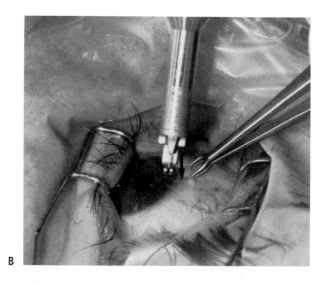
B

Transverse incision with a vertical knife blade. A, A knife with a vertical blade cuts a transverse incision for astigmatism. **B,** A double-pronged forceps fixates the globe adjacent to a transverse incision (arrow).

FIGURE 17-14   CLEANING THE DIAMOND KNIFE AND IRRIGATING THE WOUNDS

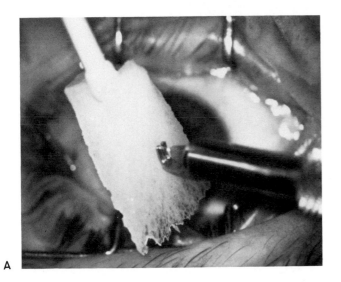

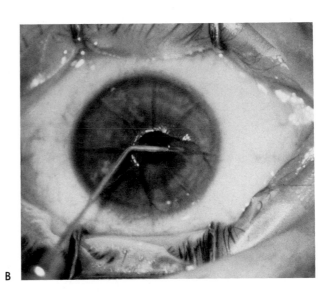

Cleaning the diamond knife and irrigating the wounds. A, Final cleansing of the knife is done with hydrogen peroxide and distilled water, using a fully extended knife blade to cut through the cellulose sponge. **B,** Blood and foreign material are irrigated from the wounds using a fine blunt cannula and irrigating parallel to the corneal surface.

PLATE 17-2: Orientation of Drawings (Fig. 17-15)

All drawings in this chapter depict surgery on the right eye and are represented from the view of the surgeon, seated at the head of the table. The brow and the 12-o'clock limbus are oriented toward the bottom of the page, the nose on the left of the page. The pupil is displaced slightly nasally.

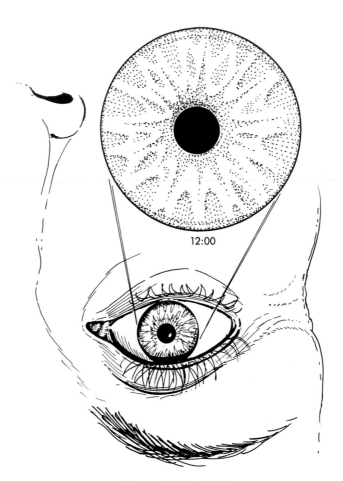

12:00

Surgeon's view of right eye

Goals:

1. Inform the patient about what to expect during the surgical procedure, making it as positive an experience as possible
2. Reduce the patient's fear and anxiety
3. Administer appropriate topical drops and sedative/hypnotic drugs as needed
4. Plan the exact surgical procedure
5. Select the surgical instruments in advance

FIGURE 17-16   PREOPERATIVE EXPLANATION, REASSURANCE, AND PREPARATION

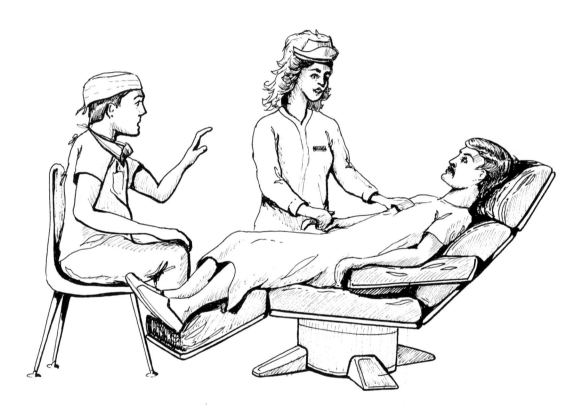

Preoperative explanation, reassurance, and preparation. The surgeon and operating room staff should use nontechnical language and a comforting tone to explain the procedure step-by-step to the patient. Fewer surprises result in a more cooperative patient.

A fool proof system of identifying the eye for surgery should be part of any ocular surgical procedure. This may include marking the patient's forehead, examining the patient's chart immediately before administration of a topical anesthetic, and prominently identifying the eye for surgery on the preoperative planning sheet.

The location of surgery and the amount of preoperative patient preparation vary widely among surgeons. Some surgeons tilt back a chair in an examining room, swing in a portable microscope, and commence the surgery. Others go through the same steps as for intraocular surgery. Each surgeon must follow the precepts of the highest quality patient care with the lowest risk of complications. Proper sterilization of the instruments is imperative. Cold sterilization by soaking can lead to multiple infections from contaminated solutions.

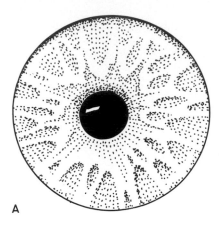

A

Natural pupil

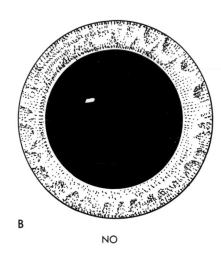

B

NO

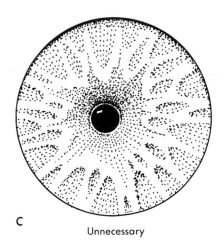

C

Unnecessary

Management of the pupil and preoperative medication. A, The pupil's natural diameter need not be altered. The bright light of the microscope usually constricts the pupil enough to make marking the center easy and reduces the patient's light sensitivity. The intraoperative pupillary diameter in 363 eyes in the PERK study was 2.7 ± 0.5 mm. **B,** A dilated pupil makes the patient more sensitive to light during the procedure (decreasing cooperation), makes marking the center of the pupil more difficult, exposes the lens more directly to laceration if the knife enters the anterior chamber, and can predispose to phototoxic maculopathy. **C,** Topical pilocarpine further constricts the pupil but is unnecessary and sometimes produces a brow ache.

Preoperative topical antibiotics, such as tobramycin, gentamicin, or a broader spectrum combination such as neomycin, bacitracin, and polymyxin B (Neosporin), given 15 minutes apart for four applications immediately before surgery can decrease the normal conjunctival bacterial flora, but there is no evidence that they decrease the rate of infection after keratotomy. There is no role for prophylactic intramuscular or oral antibiotics.

Systemic sedation is seldom necessary because the patient's cooperation can be elicited by a thorough preoperative explanation, supportive reassurance, and practical hypnotic suggestion. Anxious patients may need a mild relaxant such as diazepam (Valium) 5 to 10 mg orally or intramuscularly or midazolam (Versed) 1 to 3 mg intramuscularly approximately 30 minutes before surgery.

An intravenous line, blood pressure monitor, and electrocardiogram are usually unnecessary. In fact, the beeping noise that sometimes accompanies such monitors and the periodic inflation of the blood pressure cuff around the arm may agitate the patient during the procedure.

FIGURE 17-18   POSTING OF THE SURGICAL PLAN

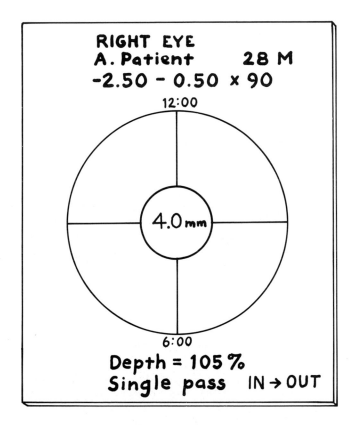

Posting of the surgical plan. A drawing of the exact surgical procedure to be performed for each patient is placed within easy view of the surgeon. Identifying information includes the patient's name and age, the eye to be operated on, and the refraction written in minus cylinder form. The chart should indicate the diameter of the central clear zone, the number and location of the incisions, the planned length of the knife blade, the direction of the incisions, and the number of passes or deepening incisions at each location. Some surgeons prefer to position the drawing so that it is seen from the surgeon's view, with 12:00 at the bottom.

PLATE 17-4:   **Preparation in the Operating Room** (Figs. 17-19 to 17-21)

Goals:

1. Ensure a calm, relaxed attitude and behavior on the part of the patient
2. Ensure patient comfort
3. Inspect all surgical equipment and verify proper function

FIGURE 17-19   DEPICTION OF PATIENT'S FEARS WHEN RECLINING ON THE OPERATING ROOM TABLE

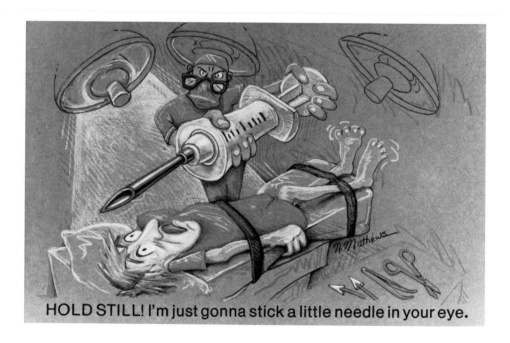

HOLD STILL! I'm just gonna stick a little needle in your eye.

FIGURE 17-20   PRACTICAL HYPNOTIC SUGGESTION

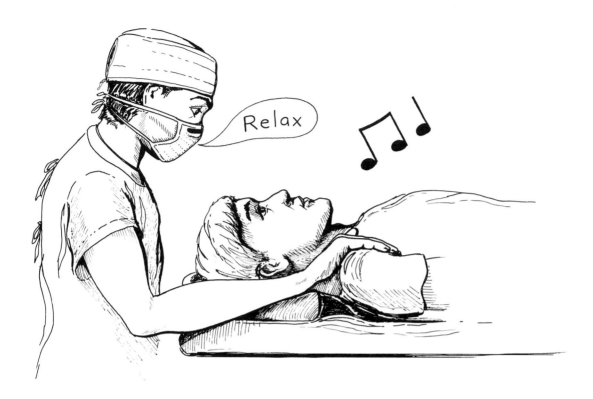

Practical hypnotic suggestion. Refractive keratotomy may be easily performed without systemic sedation, especially if the surgeon uses practical hypnotic suggestion to encourage the patient to relax and cooperate during the procedure. A quiet operating theater and a slow, reassuring tone provide a good atmosphere in which to ask the patient to take a series of deep breaths with slow exhalation and to let each body part relax and go limp, from face to toes. The surgeon calms the patient: "You will feel me working, but nothing I do will bother you." These techniques are similar to those used in natural childbirth and hypnosis.

With a calm, relaxed attitude the surgeon also should personally verify that the microscope is properly positioned and working, the ultrasonic pachometer is calibrated, the surgical instruments are properly selected, and the micrometer knife works properly. An experienced, competent technical assistant or nurse makes the operation easier.

FIGURE 17-21   COMFORT FOR THE PATIENT

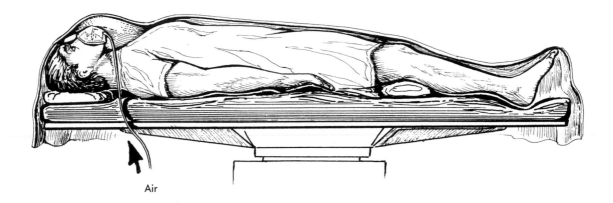

Air

Comfort for the patient. Comfort on the operating room table with good ventilation helps ensure patient cooperation. A padded table, a pillow beneath the patient's knees, and a soft headrest increase comfort. The patient should uncross his or her legs and let the arms relax comfortably on the side of the table, tucked in if needed. Many patients experience a sense of claustrophobic panic once the drapes are put over their face. Reassurance from the surgeon, elevation of drapes over a support, and a good flow of air and oxygen through a face mask or nasal cannula make it easier for the patient to breathe and relax. The surgeon tells the patient to ask for more air if needed. Full draping is unnecessary for keratotomy surgery.

Topical anesthetic and an eye shield for the unoperated eye help the patient keep both eyes open during surgery. Alternatively, the unoperated eye may be taped shut.

PLATE 17-5: Anesthetizing the Eye (Figs. 17-22 to 17-26)

Goals:

1. Maintain anesthesia of the cornea, limbus, and conjunctiva
2. Control the eyelids and globe throughout the operation

FIGURE 17-22   TOPICAL ANESTHESIA

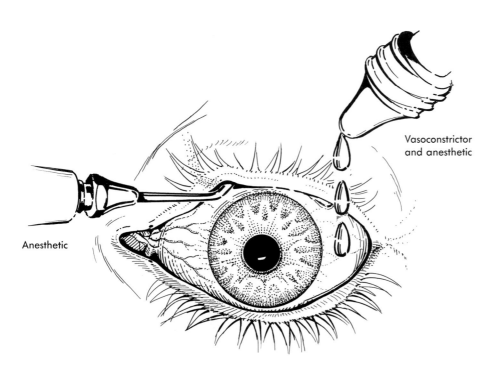

Vasoconstrictor
and anesthetic

Anesthetic

Topical anesthesia. Topical anesthesia is sufficient for refractive keratotomy. It is inexpensive, is quickly administered, and prevents the discomfort and potential complications of seventh nerve blocks and intraorbital injections. Most patients remember the pain of the anesthetic injections far more than the transient apprehension of the procedure performed under topical anesthesia.

A few drops of topical anesthetic easily anesthetize the cornea itself, which remains anesthetized throughout the operation. The conjunctiva is more difficult to anesthetize, particularly at the limbus. Therefore irrigation of an anesthetic into the conjunctival cul-de-sac through a blunt cannula increases patient comfort. In addition, dabbing topical anesthetic along the limbus with a microsponge ensures that the patient will not feel the fixation forceps during the procedure and prevents excess anesthetic on the corneal epithelium, which damages the superficial squamous cells and increases the chance of epithelial abrasion.

The most commonly used topical anesthetic for refractive keratotomy is tetracaine because it is packaged in sterile unit dose vials. Tetracaine causes stinging for 30 seconds or so after application. Proparacaine 0.5% (Ophthetic, Alcaine, Ak-Taine, Ocu-Caine) stings less but contains preservatives. It does not come in a sterile, unit dose vial, but it can be decanted into a sterile medicine glass on the instrument tray or dropped on the eye by an assistant. Some surgeons use topical 4% lidocaine (Xylocaine), which seems to be the least toxic to the epithelium. Topical cocaine should be avoided because it damages and softens the epithelium.

A topical vasoconstrictor such as naphthazoline (Vasocon, Albalon, Naphcon, Akcon) decreases the chance of conjunctival hemorrhage during fixation of the globe at the limbus.

FIGURE 17-23   COMPARISON OF PROPARACAINE AND COCAINE

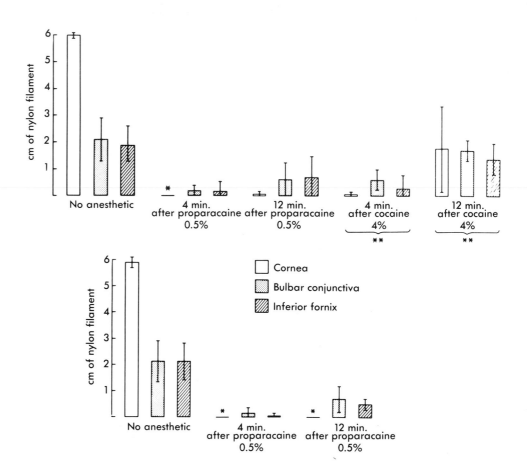

Comparison of proparacaine and cocaine. Jordan and Baum[3] instilled three drops each of 0.5% proparacaine and 4% cocaine in 22 eyes (** = 18 eyes) of subjects 25 to 45 years of age *(above)* and 12 eyes of subjects 57 to 71 years of age *(below)*. They used the Cochet-Bonnet esthesiometer to measure anesthesia of the ocular surface before and 4 and 12 minutes after instillation. Proparacaine achieved better anesthesia than cocaine. The cornea remained completely anesthetized with proparacaine for 12 minutes, long enough to complete keratotomy surgery. (From Jordan A and Baum J: Basic tear flow. Does it exist? Ophthalmology 1980;87:920-930.)

FIGURE 17-24   SEVENTH NERVE BLOCK

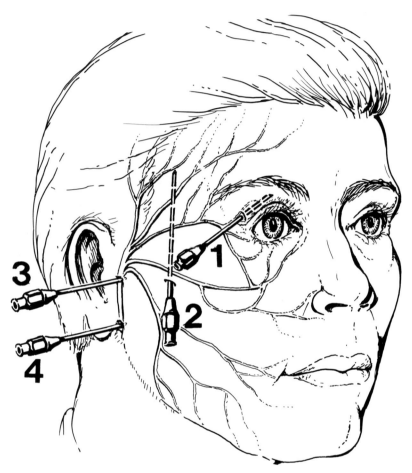

Seventh nerve block. A seventh nerve block is seldom necessary for refractive keratotomy and should be reserved for those few anxious patients who continuously force their eyelids shut. The surgeon should use his or her most reliable technique: *1,* VanLint; *2,* Atkinson; *3,* O'Brien; or *4,* Nadbath.

FIGURE 17-25 PERIBULBAR AND GENERAL ANESTHESIA

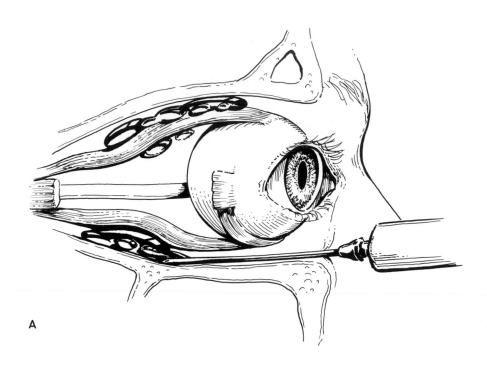

A

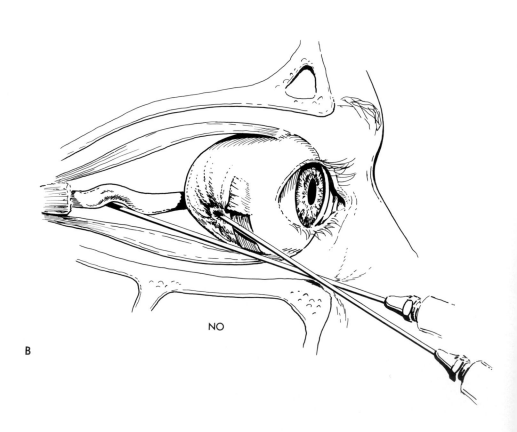

NO

B

Peribulbar and general anesthesia. A, A peribulbar anesthetic is probably safer than a retrobulbar anesthetic because it can produce acceptable akinesia and anesthesia of the globe without, **B,** the danger of damaging the optic nerve or perforating the sclera, a particular danger in individuals with elongated globes associated with their myopia. Both complications have occurred during refractive keratotomy.

In contrast to retrobulbar anesthesia, peribulbar anesthesia attempts to place the tip of the needle outside the muscle cone and uses a larger volume of anesthetic. It also may require injections in the superior and inferior orbit. A superior orbital injection involves introducing the needle just below the orbital rim at approximately a 45-degree angle to the orbital plane, in the superior lateral part of the orbit and directing the tip toward the top of the head until the superior orbit is encountered (approximately 1 cm, approximately 15 mm to get past the equator of the globe) when the needle is then redirected toward the occiput and slowly advanced until the posterior wall of the orbit is encountered. The inferior approach is similar, the needle being inserted in the inferior lateral orbit and directed inferiorly past the equator and then posteriorly to the apex of the orbit. Directing the needle away from the globe decreases the chance of injuring the globe, and keeping the needle outside the muscle cone eliminates the chance of damaging the optic nerve. The bevel of the needle is always directed toward the globe to decrease the chance of the tip of the needle catching the sclera. Anesthetic (4 to 6 ml) is injected in each location, which will fill the orbit and press the globe anteriorly. If some anesthetic is injected during withdrawal of the needle, some seventh nerve block will also result. The surgeon must be careful not to inject close to the globe so that the anesthetic does not balloon up the conjunctiva, making fixation of the globe more difficult. Gentle manual compression of the globe into the orbit for a minute or two will redistribute the anesthetic in the orbit, but prolonged ocular compression is avoided before refractive keratotomy so that the intraocular pressure will remain normal or slightly elevated during the incisions.

The anesthetic agents used vary from surgeon to surgeon; most prefer 0.75% bupivacaine (Marcaine) for its long action, and some combine this with 2% lidocaine (Xylocaine) for more rapid onset of effect. Hyaluronidase and epinephrine are used as needed.

General anesthesia is indicated in the rare circumstance of complete patient uncooperation under topical or regional anesthesia or when the indications for refractive keratotomy warrant the increased risk of a general anesthetic.

FIGURE 17-26   INTRAORBITAL ANESTHESIA

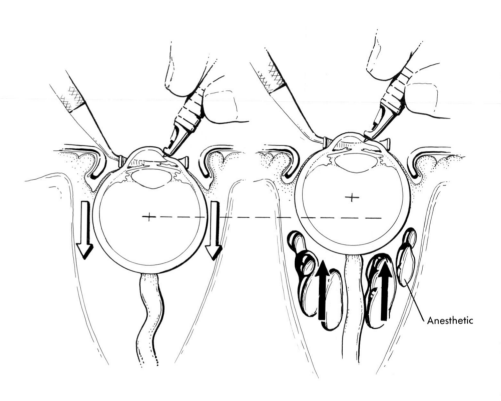

Anesthetic

Intraorbital anesthesia. An intraorbital anesthetic is indicated under two circumstances. The first circumstance is determined by the surgical technique. For example, the surgeon may wish to increase the orbital volume for purposes of increasing the intraocular pressure and decreasing the retropulsion of the globe during surgery, (arrows), especially if a compression fixation ring is used to stabilize the globe. The anesthetic decreases the pain associated with the teeth of the fixation ring. The second circumstance is to produce ocular akinesia and anesthesia in an anxious, uncooperative patient.

VIDEOKERATOGRAPHY

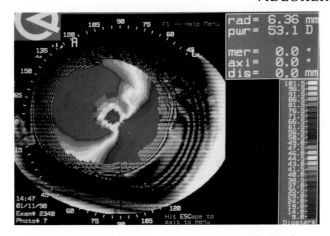

Eccentric corneal vertex *(purple area)* after myopic epikeratoplasty with patient looking directly ahead. (See Figure 2 on p. 52.)

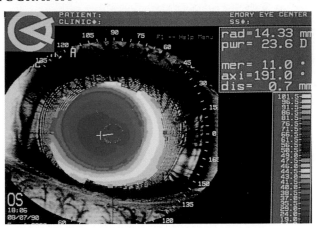

When patient looks eccentrically the vertex area becomes more uniform *(dark blue central zone)*. (See Figure 4 on p. 53.)

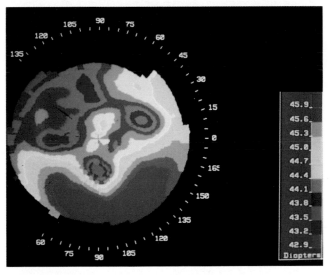

Videokeratograph demonstrating irregular pattern with irregular shape after radial keratotomy. (See Fig. 3-55, *G.*)

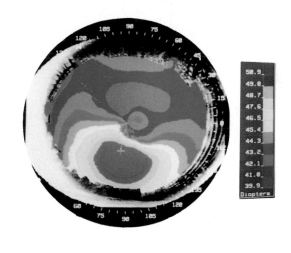

Videokeratograph of eye with keratoconus shows steep inferior cornea. (See Fig. 3-29, *A.*)

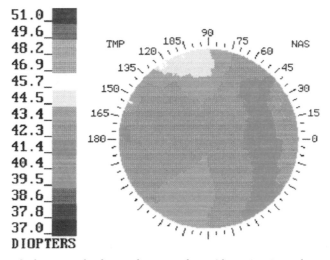

Videokeratograph of normal cornea taken with EyeSys Corneal Analysis System. (See Fig. 3-52, *A.*)

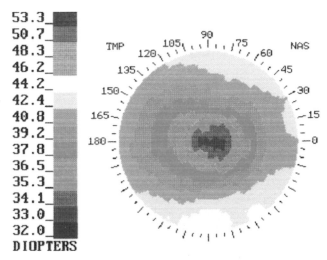

Videokeratograph of eye after radial keratotomy taken with EyeSys System. Note flatter central cornea. (See Fig. 3-52, *B.*)

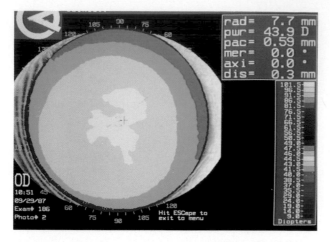

Videokeratograph of normal cornea taken with Corneal Modeling System (CMS) using absolute scale. (See Fig. 3-51, *E.*)

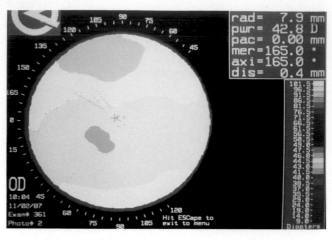

Videokeratograph of cornea after radial keratotomy (note central flattening) taken with CMS using absolute scale. (See Fig. 3-51, *F.*)

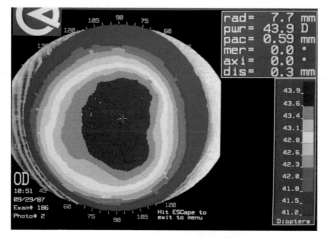

Videokeratograph of normal cornea taken with CMS using normalized scale; central cornea is steeper. (See Fig. 3-51, *G.*)

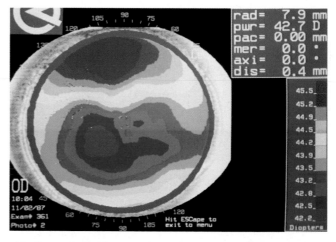

Videokeratograph of cornea after radial keratotomy with CMS; central cornea is flatter with polygonal pattern. (See Fig. 3-51, *H.*)

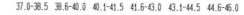

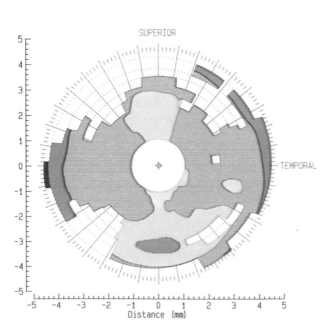

Manually digitized Nidek photokeratograph of normal cornea. Note absent central data. (See Fig. 3-50, *C.*)

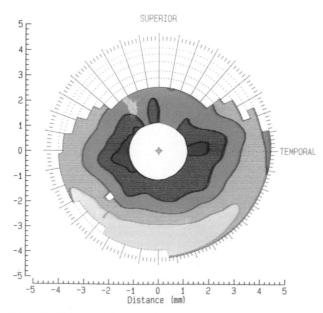

Manually digitized Nidek photokeratograph of cornea after radial keratotomy. Note central flattening. (See Fig. 3-50, *F.*)

Five Videokeratographic Patterns of Normal Corneal Topography
Using the Normal Eye Scale *(bottom right)*

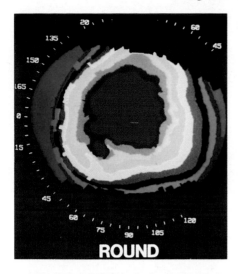

ROUND

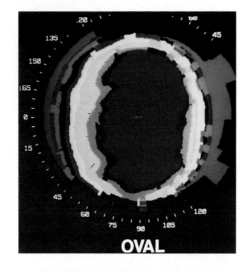

OVAL

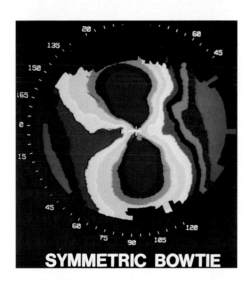

SYMMETRIC BOWTIE

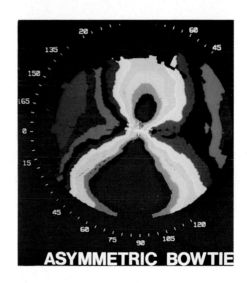

ASYMMETRIC BOWTIE

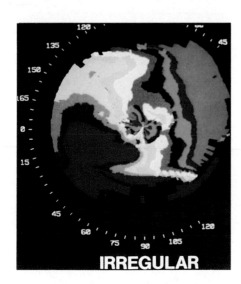

IRREGULAR

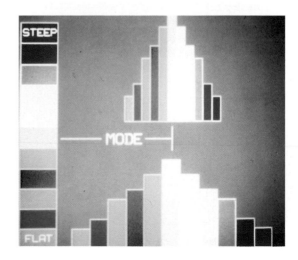

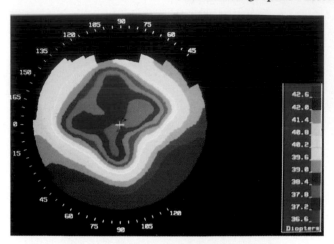

Polygonal pattern, oblate shape, flatter centrally and steeper peripherally. (See Fig. 3-55, *A.*)

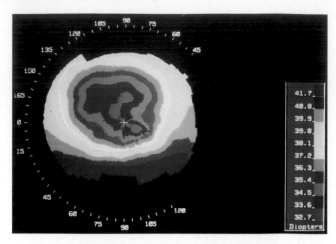

Round pattern, oblate shape, flatter centrally and steeper peripherally. (See Fig. 3-55, *B.*)

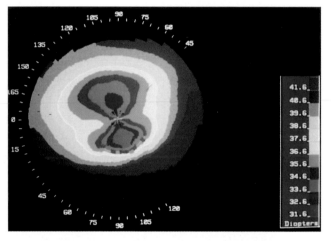

Symmetric bowtie pattern, oblate shape, flatter centrally and steeper peripherally. (See Fig. 3-55, *C.*)

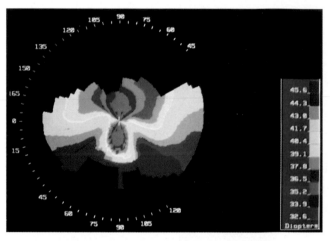

Asymmetric bowtie pattern, oblate shape, flatter centrally and steeper peripherally. (See Fig. 3-55, *D.*)

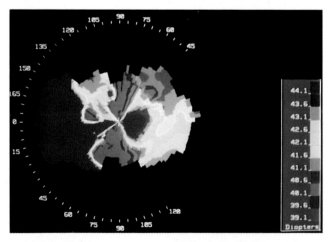

Bowtie pattern, mixed prolate/oblate shape, flatter vertically and steeper horizontally. (See Fig. 3-55, *E.*)

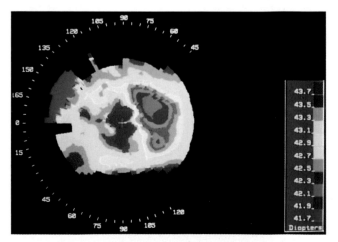

Polygonal pattern, oblate shape with a focal central steep nipple. (See Fig. 3-55, *F.*)

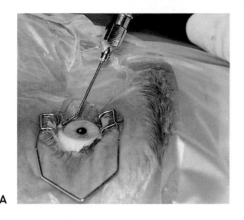

A

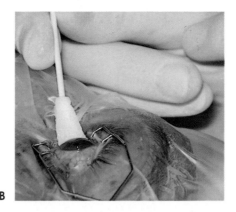

B

Topical anesthesia. In addition to application of topical drops, flushing of fornices with anesthetic through a blunt cannula (**A**) and application of anesthetic on a sponge at the limbus (**B**) enhance topical anesthesia. (See Fig. 17-1.)

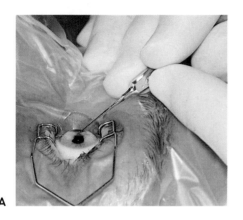

A

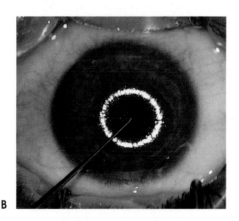

B

Marking the center of the pupil. **A,** A blunt instrument, such as an IOL hook, marks the cornea by indenting it over the center of the pupil. **B,** Circular light reflection from indentation of the cornea. (See Fig. 17-2.)

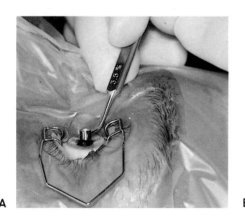

A

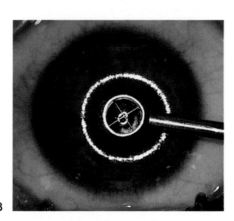

B

Marking the central clear zone. **A,** A clear zone marker of appropriate diameter indents the cornea. **B,** Centering mark with cross hairs seen with circular light reflection from indentation of the cornea. (See. Fig. 17-3.)

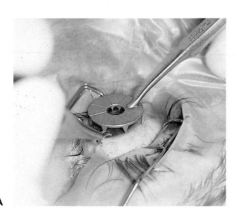

A

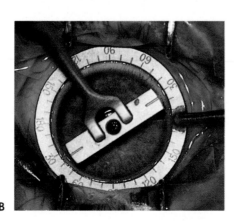

B

Marking the location of incisions. **A,** A marker with ridges imprints the location of the incisions in the epithelium as it is depressed on the cornea. **B,** The meridian for astigmatism surgery may be marked using a circular protractor and linear marker. (See Fig. 17-4.)

Measuring corneal thickness with an ultrasonic pachometer. **A,** The fluid filled probe tip is held perpendicular to the corneal surface. **B,** The instrument obtains paracentral measurements just outside the circular clear zone mark. (See Fig. 17-5.)

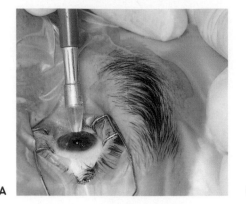

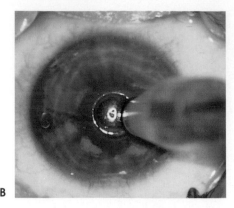

Measuring peripheral corneal thickness. **A,** The location of transverse or deepening incisions is marked with a caliper or incision marker. **B,** The ultrasonic pachometer probe is applied perpendicularly to the peripheral cornea. (See Fig. 17-6.)

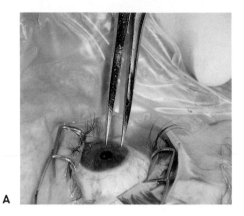

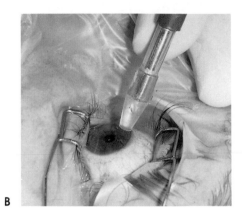

Setting the length of the knife blade with a micrometer. **A,** Micrometer setting is done away from the surface of the patient's eye. **B,** Initial setting is on zero. **C,** The micrometer is turned forward until the desired setting is achieved (500 μm). (See Fig. 17-7.)

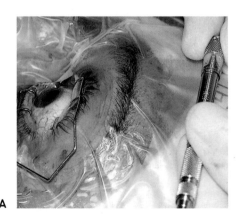

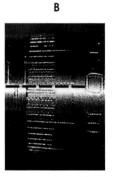

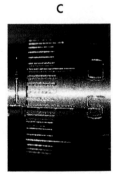

Verifying the length of the knife blade. **A,** The micrometer handle is placed in a gauge block cradle. **B,** Under high magnification, the tip of the blade is aligned with the edge of the gauge block at an appropriate setting, avoiding parallax. (See Fig. 17-8.)

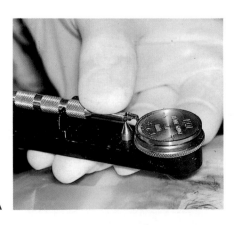

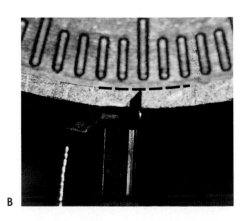

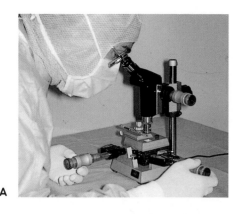

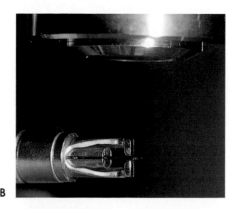

Calibrating the length of the knife blade. **A,** Compound microscope with micrometer stage is used to inspect the knife blade and measure the accuracy of its extension. **B,** The microscope objective lens allows inspection and calibration under magnification of approximately 150×. (See Fig. 17-9.)

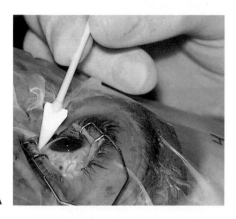

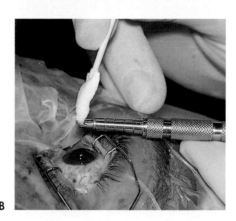

Removing excess surface fluid. **A,** The ocular surface, fornices, and, **B,** the tip of the knife are dried to prevent misinterpretation of surface fluid as aqueous from corneal perforation. (See Fig. 17-10.)

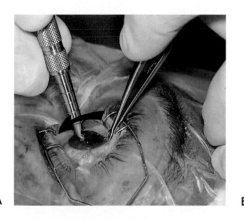

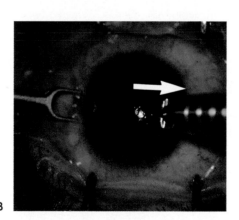

Centrifugal incision with an oblique knife blade. **A** and **B,** Double-pronged forceps fixate the globe at the limbus, and the knife is held perpendicular to the corneal surface at the edge of the clear zone, commencing a centrifugal incision *(arrows).* (See Fig. 17-11.)

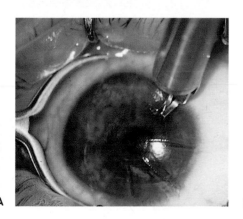

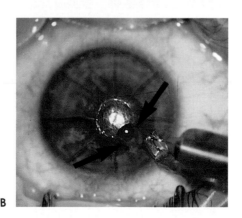

Centripetal incision with a vertical knife blade. **A,** The globe is fixated at the limbus with a spanning forceps, and the knife blade is inserted into the cornea adjacent to the limbus. **B,** Perforation of the cornea results in a bead of aqueous on the dry corneal surface *(arrows).* (See Fig. 17-12).

Transverse incision with a vertical knife blade. **A,** A knife with a vertical blade cuts a transverse incision for astigmatism. **B,** A double-pronged forceps fixates the globe adjacent to a transverse incision *(arrow).* (See Fig. 17-13.)

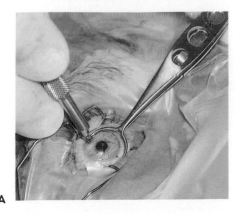

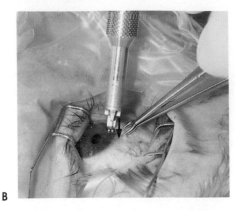

A

B

COMPUTER SIMULATION OF REFRACTIVE KERATOTOMY

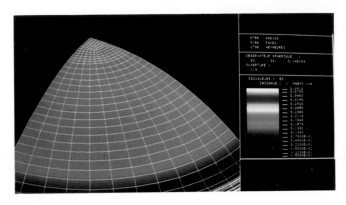

Group stress in normal cornea is distributed uniformly. (See Fig. 34-2, *A.*)

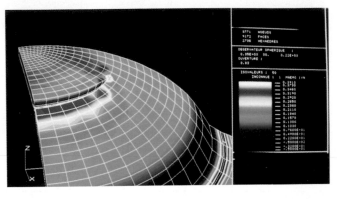

Arcuate keratotomy creates increased hoop stress on either side of incision. (See Fig. 34-2, *B.*)

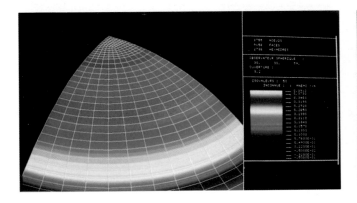

Meridional stress is greater near limbus in normal cornea. (See Fig. 34-2, *C.*)

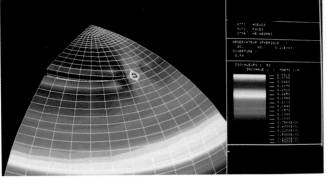

Arcuate keratotomy creates increased meridional stress at end of incision. (See. Fig. 34-2, *D.*)

Shear stress is increased at the ends of the arcuate transverse incision. (See Fig. 34-2, *E.*)

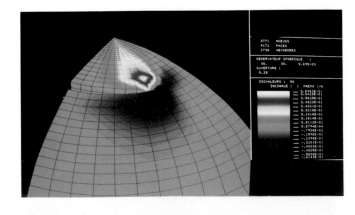

Goals:

1. Achieve a sterile operative field
2. Achieve good exposure of the cornea without causing postoperative ptosis

FIGURE 17-27   PREPARATION OF THE SKIN AND INSERTION OF EYELID SPECULUM

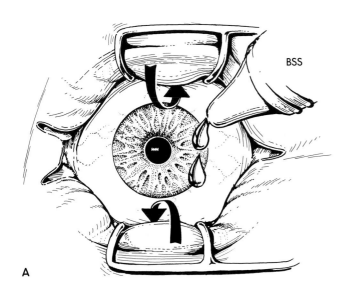

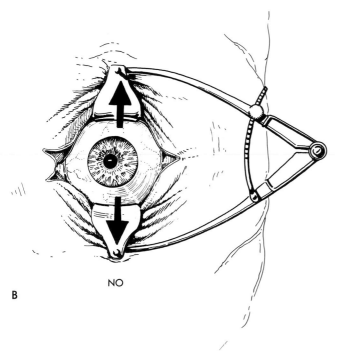

Preparation of the skin and insertion of eyelid speculum. The eyelids should be cleansed and prepared in the same manner as for intraocular surgery. Povidone-iodine (Betadine) solution (not soap) is a good antimicrobial agent that does not require scrubbing—just prolonged contact, particularly when dry, with the skin. The skin of the lids, nose, and face is swabbed with this solution. A cotton swab soaked in this solution is used to cleanse the eyelashes and eyelid margins. Some surgeons intentionally place the solution on the ocular surface and in the cul-de-sac (it does not damage the surface epithelial cells) and then irrigate it to help remove the mucus thread and sterilize the conjunctival surface.

A, Sterile drapes are applied; the amount of draping varies among surgeons. A fenestrated plastic drape is commonly used. A nonfenestrated, adhesive plastic drape can be wrapped around the eyelid margin. The upper and lower lids are pulled open with the blunt end of an instrument or cotton applicator, everting the lashes and allowing the adhesive drape to hold the lashes against the eyelid skin. An **H**-shaped incision is made in the drape with blunt scissors, along the palpebral fissure, with small vertical incisions to allow the surgeon to wrap the drape around the margin of the eyelid (arrows). This seals off the lashes, meibomian glands, and lid margin from the surgical field to enhance sterility. The cornea is kept moist with topical balanced salt solution *(BSS)* to prevent drying and thinning.

A light wire eyelid speculum, such as a Barraquer speculum, holds the drape in place and retracts the lid without excessive pressure. An open-bladed speculum without a crosswire allows room for the knife handle when making the 6-o'clock and 12-o'clock incisions. **B,** Application of excess force with a heavy eyelid speculum to gain better exposure of the cornea may damage the levator palpebrae aponeurosis and produce postoperative ptosis.

FIGURE 17-28   FINAL PREOPERATIVE CHECK

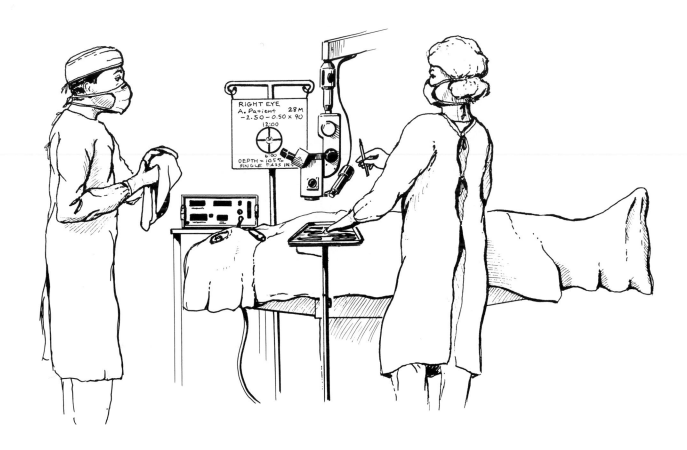

Final preoperative check. At the commencement of surgery, the surgeon verifies that the patient is calm and comfortable, all equipment is available, and the surgical plan is correct and readily visible. Not all surgeons use the full operating room gown and drape illustrated here.

PLATE 17-7: Manipulation of the Microscope (Figs. 17-29 to 17-31)

Goals:
1. Maintain adequate focus of the microscope throughout the procedure
2. Keep light intensity low so that the patient is comfortable

FIGURE 17-29   POSITIONING THE MICROSCOPE

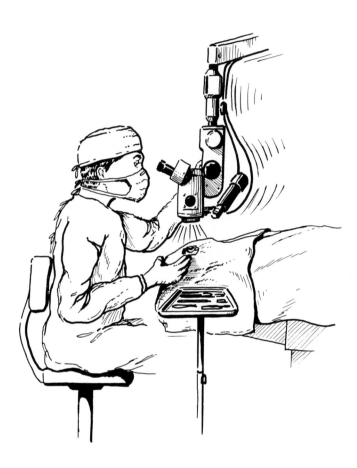

Positioning the microscope. As the microscope is swung into position over the patient's eye, the surgeon must have good verbal and emotional contact with the patient to prevent scaring the patient and inducing photophobia and blepharospasm.

FIGURE 17-30   CONTROL OF MICROSCOPE LIGHT INTENSITY

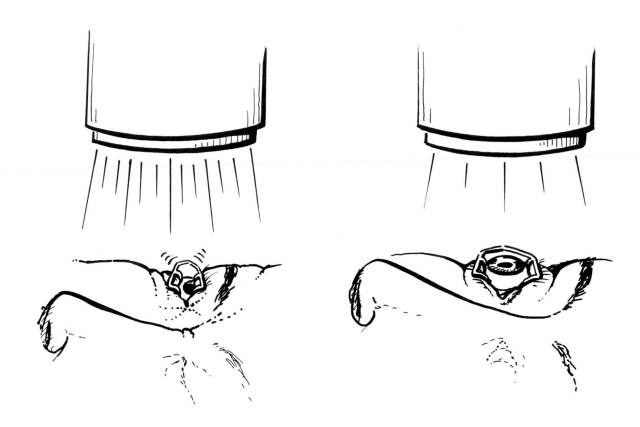

Control of microscope light intensity. The microscope light is dimmed to the minimum brightness necessary to perform the operation by turning down the rheostat and, if necessary, inserting a neutral density or other filter in place of the cobalt blue filter. The surgeon must warn the patient of the bright light: "I'm going to shine a bright light in your eye. It will be like going outside on a bright, sunny day. You will get used to it, and it won't bother you." Invariably the patient will try to close his or her eye, inducing a transient Bell's reflex. After a moment, the surgeon asks the patient to look at the coiled filament of the bright microscope light, and the globe recenters between the eyelids.

FIGURE 17-31   FOCUS OF THE MICROSCOPE DURING MARKING OF THE CENTER

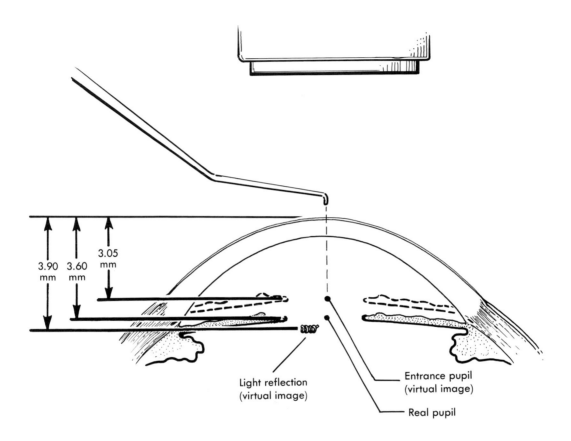

3.90 mm   3.60 mm   3.05 mm

Light reflection (virtual image)

Entrance pupil (virtual image)

Real pupil

Focus of the microscope during marking of the center. Marking the center of the optical clear zone on the corneal surface is complicated by the fact that the images of the pupil and the light reflection are 3 to 4 mm behind the cornea. Thus when they are in focus the corneal surface is out of focus. First, the surgeon focuses the microscope on the epithelial surface, views binocularly for stereopsis, and lowers the marking instrument close to the corneal surface. Then, the microscope is focused down to the plane of the pupil, which is viewed monocularly. The surgeon places the marking instrument on the surface and indents the cornea.

PLATE 17-8:   Marking the Center of the Optical Clear Zone
(Figs. 17-32 to 17-34)

Goal:

Mark the center of the uncut clear optical zone to minimize glare and irregular astigmatism over the entrance pupil. (This topic is discussed in detail in Chapter 16, Centering Corneal Surgical Procedures.)

FIGURE 17-32   MARKING THE OPTICAL CLEAR ZONE OVER THE PUPIL

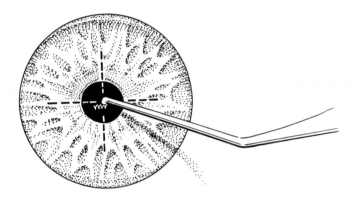

Marking the optical clear zone over the pupil. The corneal surface is dried with a microsponge. It is preferable to place the center of the clear zone over the center of the pupil, not over the corneal light reflection, which is displaced somewhat nasally. A fine, blunt instrument, such as a 0.2 mm–tipped intraocular lens hook, will not lacerate Bowman's layer as might a sharp instrument, such as a hypodermic needle. It indents the epithelium, leaving a mark that lasts throughout the operation.

If the centering mark is placed in the wrong position, the surgeon should mark the cornea again and maintain a careful visual image of the location of the correct mark, while the circular clear zone marker is brought into the field for proper positioning. Multiple marks can be confusing, especially since they cannot be erased. A dot made with a methylene blue surgical marking pen can identify the correct mark.

**FIGURE 17-33   ALIGNMENT OF THE SURGEON'S AND PATIENT'S LINES
OF SIGHT**

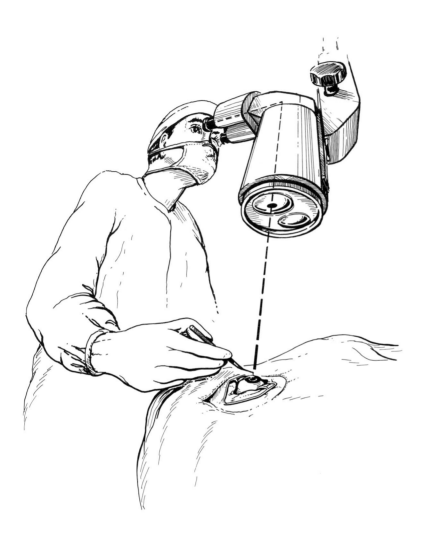

Alignment of the surgeon's and patient's lines of sight. Optimal centering of
the clear zone requires the patient to fixate a target that is coaxial with the examiner's sighting eye. Osher's fixation device satisfies this requirement, as long as the surgeon marks the center of the entrance pupil and not the corneal light reflex. Alternatively, a 1- to 2-mm fixation spot can be placed over the center of one of the viewing tubes of the microscope, where it will not interfere significantly with the optics.
The patient fixates the spot and the surgeon sights monocularly through that tube,
marking the cornea at the center of the patient's entrance pupil.

FIGURE 17-34 OTHER TECHNIQUES OF MARKING THE CENTER OF THE CLEAR ZONE

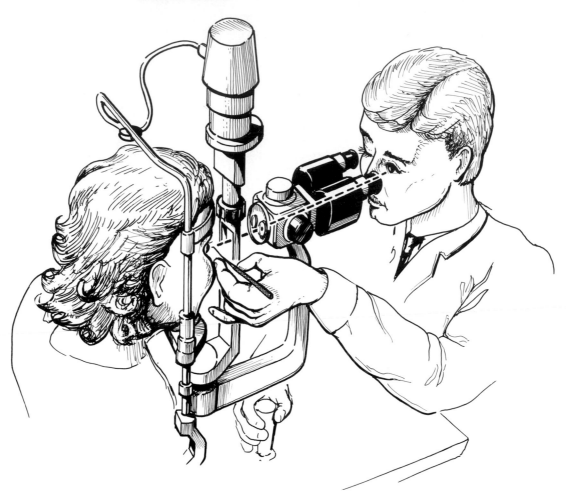

Other techniques of marking the center of the clear zone. The center can be marked before surgery with the slit-lamp microscope. A fixation spot is placed over one of the objective lenses. The surgeon sights with one eye, and the patient fixates the spot, allowing the surgeon to mark the center of the entrance pupil. There is little advantage to this when proper centering can be accomplished in the operating room.

There are many other methods of marking the center of the optical clear zone, most of which involve placing a mark within fractions of a millimeter of the center of the pupil. Because of this similarity, there may be little practical, clinical difference among the methods. No clinical studies have been conducted to compare methods of centering. Some methods are described as follows: (1) placing the centering mark at the opposite end of and just inferior to the corneal light reflection with the patient's gaze fixated on the microscope light filament and the surgeon fixated with one eye (the PERK technique); (2) using a fixation mark or light placed between the two microscope oculars and marking the corneal light reflection; (3) viewing the pupil through a direct ophthalmoscope with the patient looking at the light, and marking the light reflection on the surface of the cornea; (4) using a "centered" keratograph to measure the distance from the center of the smallest ring to the nasal and temporal limbus and then using the fraction obtained by the ratio of these two measurements to multiply the patient's horizontal corneal diameter, which is measured with calipers during surgery; and (5) using an opaque contact lens with a small central opening and rotating it until the patient can see the microscope light through the opening, which serves as a guide to making the center mark.

PLATE 17-9:   Marking the Central Clear Zone and Location of Incisions on the Epithelial Surface (Figs. 17-35 to 17-39)

Goals:

1. Outline the central circular clear zone ("optical zone")
2. Mark the correct location of the radial incisions
3. Retain the marks in the epithelium throughout the procedure
4. Avoid cutting Bowman's layer

Marking for astigmatism surgery is discussed in Chapter 32, Atlas of Astigmatic Keratotomy.

FIGURE 17-35   MULTIPLE CLEAR ZONE MARKS

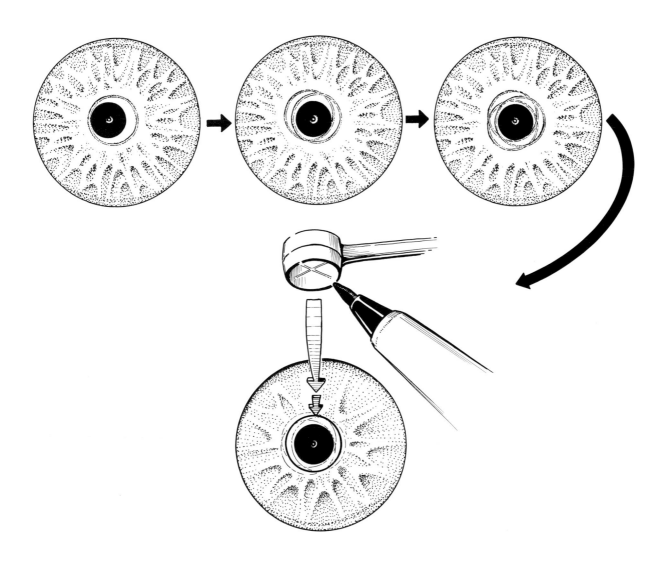

Multiple clear zone marks. Placing the clear zone mark in the proper position on the first try is important because multiple eccentric marks will create confusion when the central clear zone mark is finally made. Coating the edge of the marker with a methylene blue marking pen allows highlighting of the correct mark.

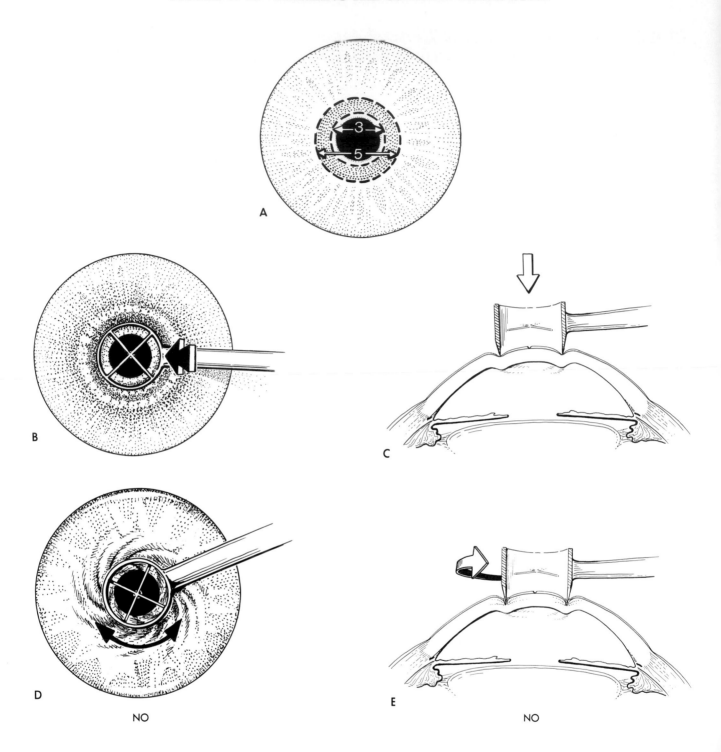

Marking the central clear zone. After marking the center the surgeon quickly refocuses the microscope on the surface of the cornea without moistening the surface. **A,** The diameter of the central clear zone ranges from 3 to 5 mm and is marked in 0.25- or 0.50-mm increments. **B,** A dull circular trephine with thin, smooth edges (the thicker the edge the less distinct the circular mark in the epithelium) is aligned over the center mark with the cross hairs, or pointer, inside the cylinder. **C,** The farther these alignment sights are from the corneal surface, the more parallax occurs, requiring the surgeon to view the sides of the cylinder to be sure it is oriented vertically. The surgeon presses down on the trephine, slightly indents the cornea, and holds it for 2 or 3 seconds to mark the epithelium. As the cornea is indented, a circular light reflection appears on the corneal surface. **D** and **E,** Rotating the trephine is unnecessary and can cut into Bowman's layer if the trephine is sharp or rough.

FIGURE 17-37 MARKING CONCENTRIC ZONES   541

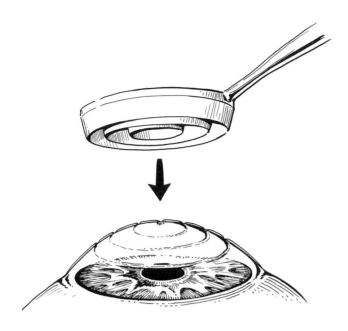

Marking concentric zones. If the surgical plan calls for a longer blade setting in the more peripheral cornea, concentric zones are marked, usually with a 3.0-mm central clear zone diameter, a 5- to 6-mm diameter middle mark, and a 7- to 9-mm diameter outer mark. This can sometimes serve to mark the zone for transverse incisions for astigmatism.

FIGURE 17-38 MARKING THE LOCATION OF RADIAL INCISIONS

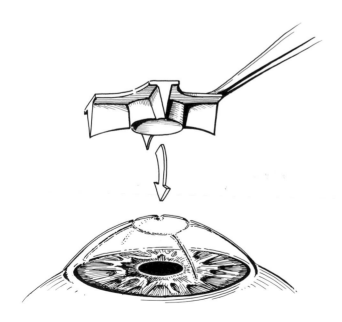

Marking the location of radial incisions. Some surgeons prefer to mark the location of the radial incisions in the epithelium as a guide during surgery. Such marks can help locate the beginning of each incision. However, following these marks with a PERK-style knife cutting from the clear zone to the limbus is difficult because the footplates and blade cover the mark and the cutting edges of the blade cannot be visualized directly. Therefore many surgeons do not use these radial markers for centrifugal incisions and simply locate the position of the incisions by visual inspection. Such markers are more useful when cutting from the limbus toward the clear zone because it is more difficult to locate the proper clock hour for each incision around the larger circle of the limbus than it is around the smaller circle of the clear zone mark and because the vertical cutting edge of the knife blade can be visualized directly and guided along the radial mark.

The markers come with three to eight dull radial ribs that indent the corneal epithelium upon gentle pressure. Some markers combine the circular clear zone mark and the radial ribs. It is unnecessary to coat the edge of the radial markers with a dye such as fluorescein or methylene blue because the indentation in the corneal epithelium remains clearly visible throughout the operation. However, if multiple sets of marks have been made, it is prudent to use a dye to highlight the correct marks. The orientation of the incisions is shown in Plate 17-15 and in Chapter 32, Atlas of Astigmatic Keratotomy.

FIGURE 17-39   MARKING THE LOCATION OF RADIAL INCISIONS

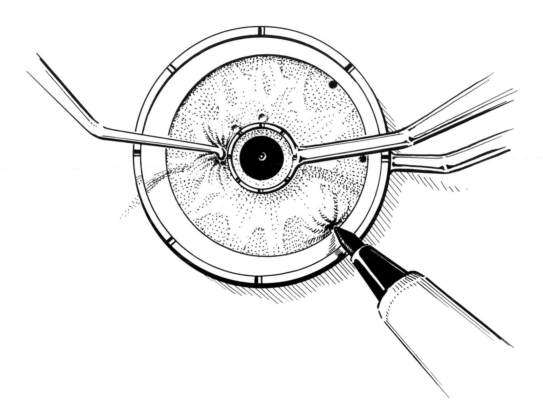

Marking the location of radial incisions. Some clear zone markers and fixation rings have notches in the surface to locate the orientation of the incisions. These allow the surgeon to mark the epithelium with a blunt hook or marking pen, helping to space the incisions equidistantly without trying to follow the lines made by radial markers.

After all marks in the epithelium have been made, a few drops of balanced salt solution moisten the corneal surface to prevent dehydration and thinning.

PLATE 17-10:   Measurement of Corneal Thickness (Figs. 17-40 to 17-47)

Goals:

1. Ensure proper calibration and function of the ultrasonic pachometer
2. Accurately measure corneal thickness
3. Select a consistent location for the measurement of corneal thickness that will serve as a reliable guide for setting of the length of the knife blade

FIGURE 17-40   FILLING THE ULTRASONIC PACHOMETRY PROBE TIP

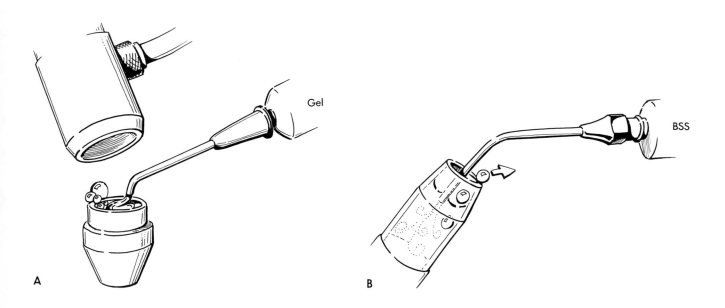

Filling the ultrasonic pachometry probe tip. A, Solid-tipped probes are more convenient to use, but the surgeon must ensure that the reservoir at the base of the probe tip is properly filled with the fluid recommended by the manufacturer without the introduction of air bubbles. **B,** A fluid-filled probe tip must be filled with balanced salt solution *(BSS)* through a small-gauge, blunt irrigating cannula (a sharp-tipped hypodermic needle may scratch the inside surface of the transducer) without introducing air bubbles. It must be refilled anytime air bubbles enter the chamber. Abnormal or inconsistent readings are a reminder to stop and refill the probe tip.

FIGURE 17-41   CALIBRATION AND SETTING OF THE ULTRASONIC PACHOMETER

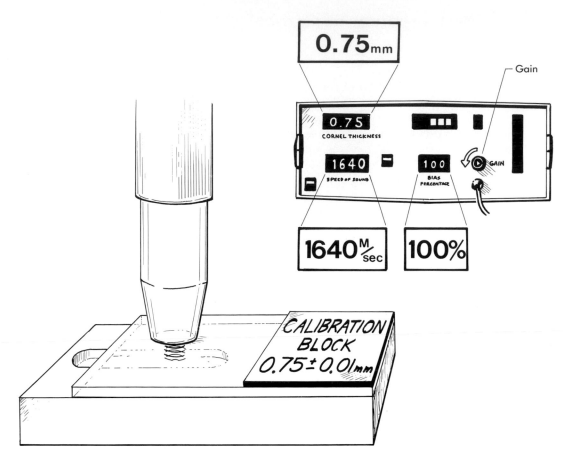

Calibration and setting of the ultrasonic pachometer. The ultrasonic pachometer should be calibrated and its accuracy verified before preparing the patient. If the instrument is broken, this gives time to repair the instrument, substitute a backup ultrasound probe, use an optical pachometer, or cancel the case. Verifying function of the instrument in advance avoids confusion during the surgical procedure.

The accuracy of the pachometer should be checked according to the manufacturer's instructions, using a test block, an internal calibration mechanism, or other methods. Individual features on pachometers, such as the setting of the percent thickness bias, the selection of the pattern of readings, and the use of internal storage or printing devices, should be properly set before surgery.

FIGURE 17-42   LOCATION OF CORNEAL THICKNESS MEASUREMENTS

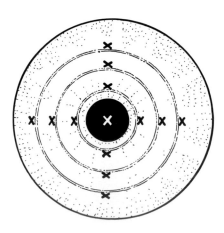

Location of corneal thickness measurements. The location of the corneal thickness measurement that determines the knife blade setting varies from one surgeon to another. Some use the central reading alone as the reference value. Some take readings around the edge of the clear zone, using the thinnest reading or an average reading as the reference value. Those who perform zone cutting often take readings at the edge of each zone.

FIGURE 17-43   SPEED OF SOUND IN THE CORNEA

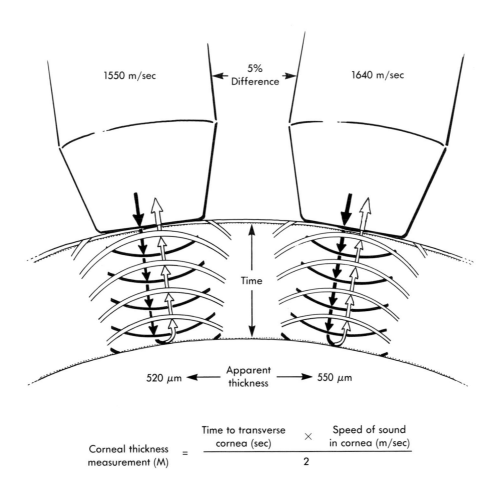

$$\text{Corneal thickness measurement (M)} = \frac{\text{Time to transverse cornea (sec)} \times \text{Speed of sound in cornea (m/sec)}}{2}$$

Speed of sound in the cornea. The corneal thickness measurement is determined by the amount of time it takes the ultrasonic pulse to pass from the transducer to Descemet's membrane and back to the transducer. The speed of sound in the cornea is its propagation velocity, which is an inherent property of the tissue. Many ultrasonic pachometers have the ability to select different propagation velocities. This feature allows adjustment of the pachometer to read the test blocks accurately and to adjust for differences in the thickness readings between different pachometers.

The relationship

$$\text{Time (sec)} = \frac{2 \times \text{Thickness (m)}}{\text{Propagation velocity (m/sec)}}$$

can be written as

$$\text{Thickness (m)} = \frac{\text{Time (sec)} \times \text{Propagation velocity (m/sec)}}{2}$$

This relationship demonstrates that corneal thickness is proportionate to the speed of sound in the cornea that is set on the instrument. The higher the speed is, the thicker the cornea will appear. A speed of 1640 m/sec is usually used.

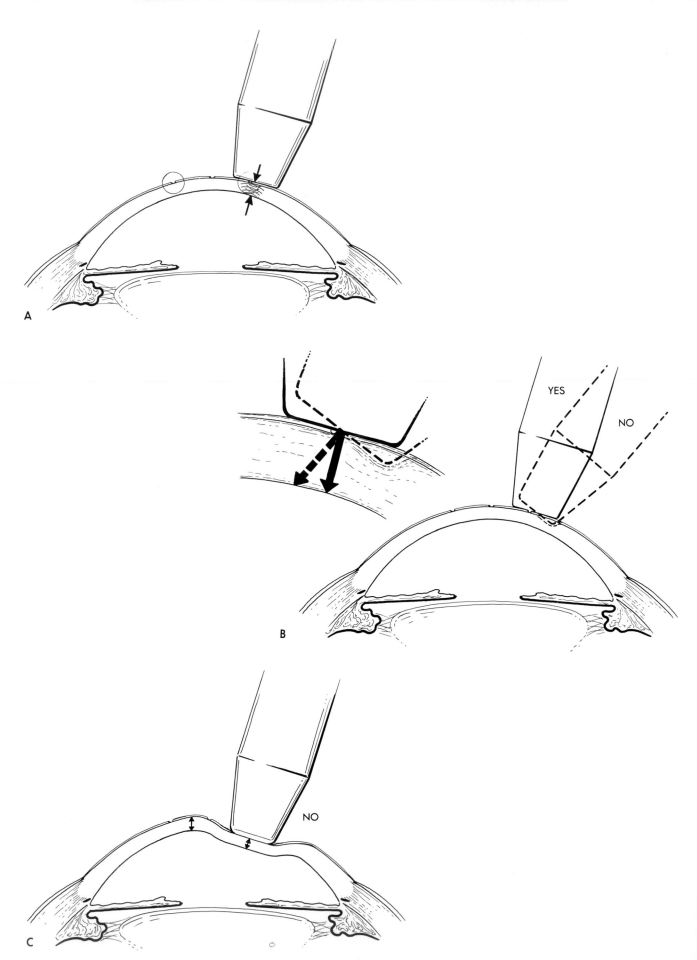

Intraoperative ultrasonic pachometry. The surgeon focuses the operating micro-scope on the corneal surface, dries the clear zone mark to make it visible, and brings the ultrasound probe tip into the surgical field. Fixation of the globe is unnecessary. The probe tip covers an area 3 or 4 mm in diameter, so the surgeon must estimate where the center of the probe is, since that is where the ultrasonic thickness mea-surement is taken.

A, Paracentral readings should be taken with the center of the probe just outside the clear zone mark because that is the thinnest part of the cornea to be incised. The probe is applied perpendicularly to the cornea, so it may be difficult to see exactly where the tip is in some positions. **B,** Most instruments will not give a reading un-less the tip is perpendicular to the corneal surface and a series of readings can be averaged. Therefore obtaining a reading often involves subtle tilting of the probe back and forth. The farther from the central cornea the reading is, the more the probe must be tilted toward the limbus to remain perpendicular to the surface. **C,** The surgeon should apply the tip gently to the surface because indenting the cornea with the tip may give an erroneous thickness measurement.

It is prudent to take two or three readings at each location to ensure a consis-tency of $+0.01$ mm (10 μm). Abnormally thin (less than 0.50 mm) or thick (greater than 0.60 mm) central readings call for caution, refilling of the probe tip, and com-parison with preoperative values, if available. The surgeon must know the thickness readings as they are being obtained to judge the consistency and relative value of the readings. This is done most efficiently by the assistant (or the synthesized voice on the instrument) calling out the values. It is inefficient and distracting for the surgeon to look up from the microscope to see the values.

Some pachometers read to three decimal places, but most micrometer knives can be set only to two decimal places. Therefore, the surgeon should round the pachom-eter readings to two decimal places before setting the knife blade.

FIGURE 17-45   REGIONAL DIFFERENCES IN CORNEAL THICKNESS

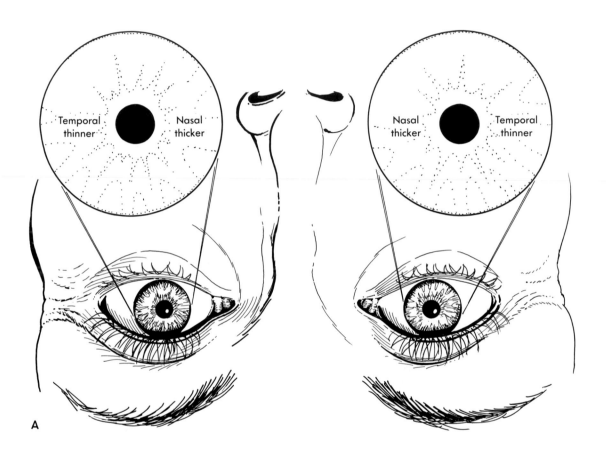

Regional differences in corneal thickness. A, In general, the temporal cornea is thinner than the nasal cornea, a fact that alerts the surgeon to the greater chance of corneal perforation temporally and may influence the selection of the sequence of incisions. A corny but useful crutch to remember comes from combining the two terms: *temp*oral th*inn*er = tempinn; *nas*al th*ick*er = nasick.

FIGURE 17-45, CONT'D

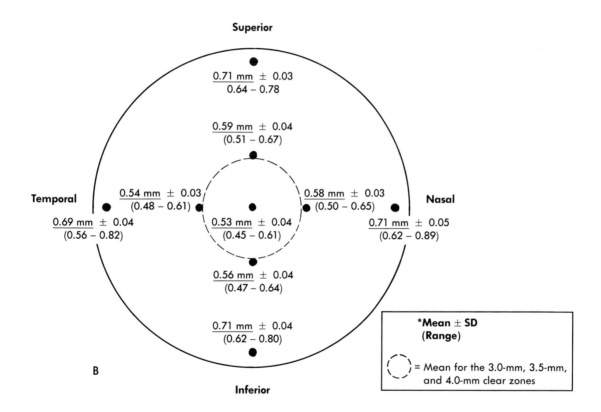

B, Measurements based on a series of 48 consecutive eyes (PERK study, unpublished data) using intraoperative ultrasonic pachometry (1640 m/sec). The values are pooled for the right and left eye. Central values are taken over the centering mark as made in the PERK study. Paracentral values are pooled for all three clear zones (3.0, 3.5, and 4.0 mm), so they do not represent an exact anatomic regional thickness of the cornea, but rather the thickness as obtained just outside the clear zone mark. Peripheral readings were taken at the corneal limbus through clear cornea. The range of readings at each location spanned 0.15 to 0.20 mm. In general, the paracentral cornea became thinner when proceeding from superior to nasal to inferior to temporal locations. There was little difference in average limbal measurements.

FIGURE 17-46   RECORDING CORNEAL THICKNESS AND CALCULATING BLADE LENGTH

CORNEAL THICKNESS RECORD

Eye: right

Name: A. Myope   **Instrument:** Thickometer

Speed of sound: 1640 m/sec

Center: 536

Location:	12:00	3:00	6:00	9:00
Zone:				
3 mm	592	587	561	543
6 mm				
9 mm				

Recording corneal thickness and calculating blade length. Corneal thickness readings should be recorded manually by an assistant in the operating room or printed out by the instrument. The surgeon should be sure the format for recording is easily interpretable, and therefore a properly labeled table is preferable because labels on the drawing of an eye can easily be misinterpreted if the drawing is oriented incorrectly.

To use the corneal thickness measurements as a guide for setting the length of the knife blade, the surgeon must calculate the percentage of the reference value that represents the length of the knife blade, commonly called the "bias."

Calculations can be done by programs in some pachometers (which display both the measured values and the bias values), by a computer program, by calculator, or by hand. If done before surgery, the calculations should be available on the chart in the operating room where they can be verified. If the calculations are done during surgery, an assistant will be required to use a computer or calculator. Alternatively the surgeon can do the calculations by hand, using a sterile marking pen and writing on the drapes. It is always prudent to have the calculations double-checked by a second person to detect errors.

**FIGURE 17-47   OUTPATIENT MEASUREMENT OF CENTRAL
CORNEAL THICKNESS**

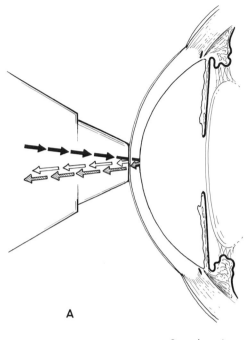

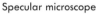

A

Specular microscope

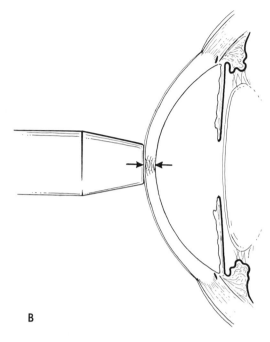

B

Ultrasonic pachometer

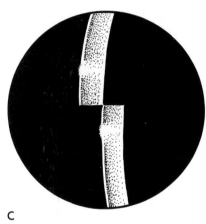

C

Optical pachometer

Outpatient measurement of central corneal thickness. Some surgeons use an ultrasonic pachometer **(A),** specular microscope **(B),** or an optical pachometer **(C)** to measure corneal thickness in the outpatient clinic before surgery. In an outpatient setting, it is difficult to take reliable paracentral thickness measurements with these instruments because there is no clear zone mark to act as a reference point. The advantage of preoperative measurement of corneal thickness is that the operation goes faster and is less complicated, since the pachometry does not have to be done with the patient prepared and draped and since the knife blade can be preset if desired.

Goals:

1. Set the knife blade accurately to the required length
2. Prevent damage to the knife blade
3. Prevent thinning of the patient's cornea during the setting of the knife blade

FIGURE 17-48   POSITION OF THE MICROSCOPE

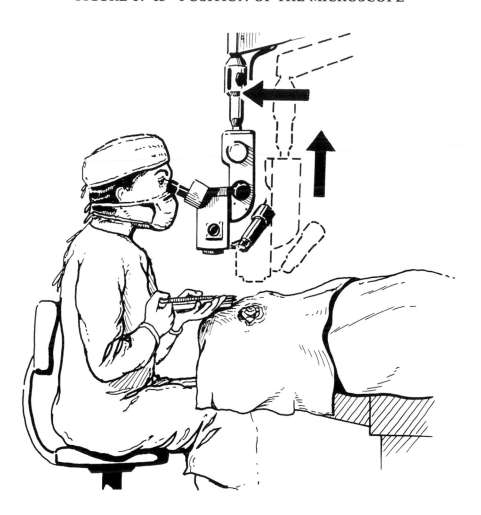

Position of the microscope. The setting and verification of the length of the knife blade are achieved under the microscope. The surgeon swings the microscope over the patient's forehead, a position that has the following advantages: (1) the patient's forehead provides a platform for the gauge block and steadies the surgeon's hands; (2) this decreases the amount of time the cornea is exposed to the heat of the microscope light; and (3) there is no chance of inadvertent contact between the eye and the gauge block.

During the setting of the knife blade, the surgeon must prevent drying of the cornea. Spreading a layer of balanced salt solution over the surface is usually adequate. A moist microsponge also can be placed on the cornea. Some surgeons remove the eyelid speculum and allow the patient to close the lid, but this seems unduly time consuming and complex, particularly when it is manipulation of the eyelid margins, which are not anesthetized, that creates the most discomfort for the patient.

FIGURE 17-49   SETTING THE LENGTH OF THE KNIFE BLADE WITH THE MICROMETER

One full revolution plus six additional marks

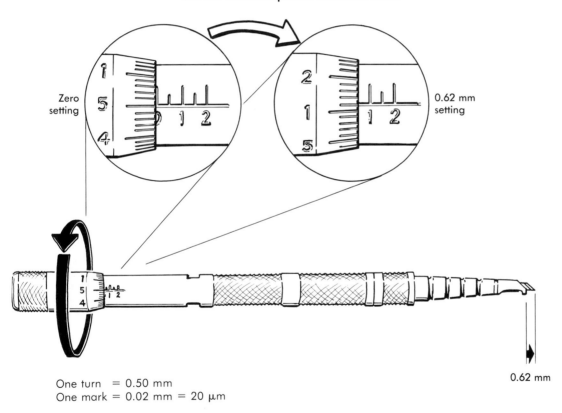

One turn = 0.50 mm
One mark = 0.02 mm = 20 μm

Setting the length of the knife blade with the micrometer. With the microscope on low power, the surgeon turns the micrometer handle until the zero point on the micrometer scale is aligned with the zero line on the barrel. The blade is inspected to be sure the tip is approximately flush with the ends of the footplates. The micrometer handle is then turned clockwise, each scale line advancing the blade 0.02 mm (20 μm) and one complete rotation advancing it 0.50 mm (500 μm), until the desired setting is reached. The micrometer should be turned only in the direction of advancing the blade, stopped as soon as the desired length is reached, and not turned in the reverse direction for setting. If the desired length is exceeded, the blade should be retracted past the desired length and then turned forward again, stopping at the exact point. This technique minimizes the inaccuracy caused by play in the micrometer mechanism.

FIGURE 17-50   ADVANCEMENT OR REMOVAL OF BLADE FROM
                THE PROTECTIVE SLEEVE

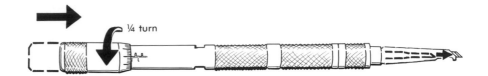

FIGURE 17-51   SETTING THE LENGTH OF AN EXCHANGEABLE
                KNIFE BLADE

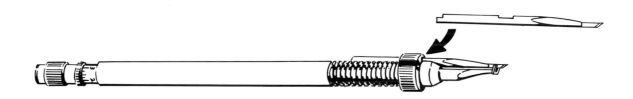

FIGURE 17-52   FIXED BLADES OF PRESET LENGTH

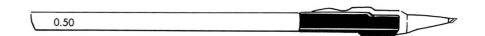

Advancement or removal of blade from the protective sleeve. The best way to ensure that a diamond or other crystal knife blade is not nicked or damaged is for only the surgeon to handle the knife when the blade is extended. Therefore the surgeon should receive the knife from the scrub nurse and return it with the blade retracted in its protective sleeve.

To advance the blade out of the sleeve, the micrometer is set in the middle of its excursion and the inner blade housing is pushed forward with the micrometer handle, rotated one quarter to one half turn, and locked in the extended position.

The surgeon inspects the tip, edge, and alignment of the blade under highest magnification. If the blade is damaged, a backup knife is used or the case is postponed.

Setting the length of an exchangeable knife blade. Knives with exchangeable blades must be handled with even more care because there is greater chance of damaging the blade while it is being attached to the handle. This is especially true for blades that require insertion into the end of the knife through a circular housing or between the tips of the footplate. The blade is locked in position.

Fixed blades of preset length. Disposable knives with fixed blades of preset length are convenient to use but require a large inventory. The blades can be damaged when removed from the factory packaging. Verification of the knife blade length on a gauge block may help detect errors caused by poor quality control. If the blade length seems incorrect, another knife with a correct length should be used.

PLATE 17-12:   Verifying the Length of the Knife Blade (Figs. 17-53 to 17-56)

Goals:

1. Ensure the knife blade is set accurately at the desired length
2. Reduce parallax
3. Prevent damage to the knife blade
4. Identify damage to the blade (chipped tip or cutting edge, dirty surface, flaws within the diamond), wobble on advancement, inaccurate setting, and so forth.

FIGURE 17-53   INSPECTION AND CALIBRATION WITH COMPOUND MICROSCOPE

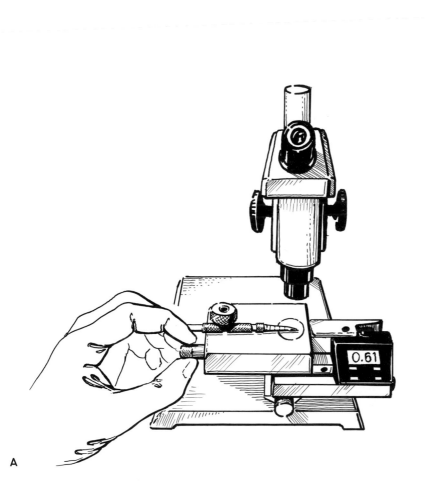

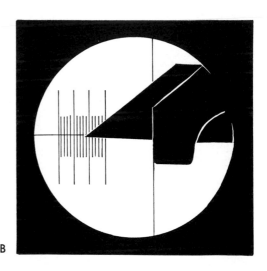

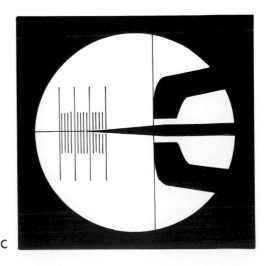

Inspection and calibration with compound microscope. A, A compound microscope fitted with a movable micrometer stage has a number of advantages. **B,** It allows magnification up to 150 times, so the surgeon can inspect the tip and edge of the blade as well as the quality of the footplates. The much lower magnification achievable with the operating microscope does not allow detection of fine defects in the blade or footplates. **C,** The alignment of the footplates and the blade also can be checked to detect whether one footplate is longer than the other, whether the blade is centered between the footplates, and whether the blade moves irregularly when advanced with the micrometer handle. Because the blade is secured on the surface of the micrometer and viewed through the microscope in a perpendicular manner, parallax plays little role, so the blade can be set with great accuracy. One major drawback, however, is finding the exact zero point for the blade, since the footplates are often curved, and it is hard to align the tip of the blade exactly with the edge of the footplate.

There are two basic approaches to using this type of microscope gauge. The first is to use the knife micrometer handle to set the length of the knife blade to a known length, for example 500 microns. The knife is then carefully mounted on the microscope micrometer stage and brought into focus under the microscope. One of the footplates is aligned on the zero line at the cross hairs of the reticule. The micrometer readout is set to zero, and the micrometer stage moved until the tip of the knife blade is on the reticule line. The length of the blade is measured as the distance the micrometer stage moves and is read on the micrometer digital readout as the true extension of the blade. For example, if this reading were 530 microns, then the blade extends 30 microns longer than indicated by the knife micrometer handle, and 30 microns would be subtracted from the knife handle reading when setting the length of the blade. The second approach is to mount the knife on the microscope stage and set both the blade and the footplate on the zero reticule mark. The micrometer stage is advanced a known amount (for example, 500 microns). The blade can then be extended by the knife micrometer until the tip reaches the reticule mark. The knife is then removed and the reading on the knife handle is compared with that on the microscope, the difference being noted as an adjustment factor of the knife handle setting. This approach is less accurate.

FIGURE 17-54   GAUGE BLOCK WITH PLATFORM AND ELEVATED RIDGE

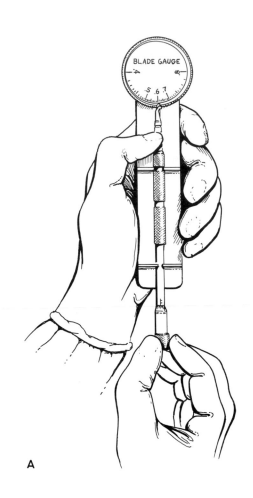

A

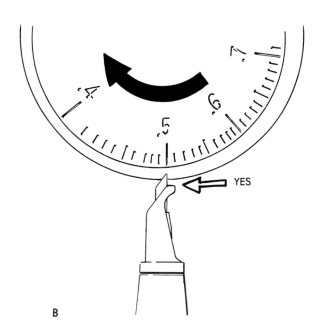

B

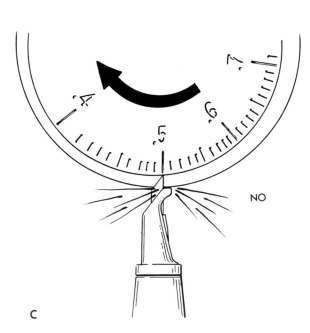

C

Gauge block with platform and elevated ridge. Gauge blocks can be mounted on the end of a platform with fork-shaped cradles that hold the knife handle in a fixed position, usually so that the blade cannot readily contact the gauge block, a valuable safety feature. Many styles are available. The principle is the same: the elevated ridge becomes increasingly wide, as indicated on the accompanying scale, so when the footplate is abutted on one side of the ridge, the length of the knife blade can be measured by aligning the tip of the blade with the other side of the ridge.

A, The surgeon looks away from the microscope to insert the knife into the cradle. Most of these platforms are designed for use with a specific style of knife handle. The notches on the handle are inserted into the cradle. **B,** Because the two footplates on a knife may not be aligned exactly parallel, the handle should be oriented with the same footplate against the gauge block on each occasion for consistency of measurement. This is done by consistently having one of the markings on the knife handle facing up.

The surgeon returns to the microscope (set on low power) and rests the platform and his or her hands on the patient's forehead for stability. The scale on the gauge, usually calibrated in 0.1-mm (10-μm) increments, is moved until the desired value is aligned with the tip of the knife blade. **C,** The gauge block is positioned beneath the knife blade, taking care not to turn or slide the block along the surface of the footplate, to prevent abrading and roughening the surface.

The microscope is then zoomed to highest power, the platform tilted to avoid parallax, and the tip of the blade adjusted with the micrometer so that it is aligned exactly with the edge of the ridge. The microscope is zoomed back to lower power and the knife removed from the cradle without hitting the blade on the gauge. The microscope is recentered over the patient's eye.

The surgeon should observe the actual setting of the micrometer and make note of the difference between the original micrometer setting and the verified setting. This not only indicates the consistency and accuracy of the micrometer, but also can provide the factor needed to adjust the micrometer to an accurate setting for a series of cases, if the gauge block is not used for each case. For example, if the desired knife setting is 0.55 mm and the verified setting is 0.57 mm, the surgeon can add 0.02 mm to the micrometer reading on each of successive cases done with the same knife and avoid the repeated time-consuming verification of the blade length. Of course, this carries the assumption that the micrometer is working exactly the same from one case to another after autoclaving.

The same process applies if a nonsterilizable calibration apparatus is used, such as a compound microscope with micrometer, a shadowgraph, or a helium neon laser. The surgeon determines the difference between the micrometer reading and the actual length setting, sterilizes the knife, and then uses the micrometer with the "fudge factor" to set the length of the blade under the operating microscope.

FIGURE 17-55 CONTROL OF PARALLAX

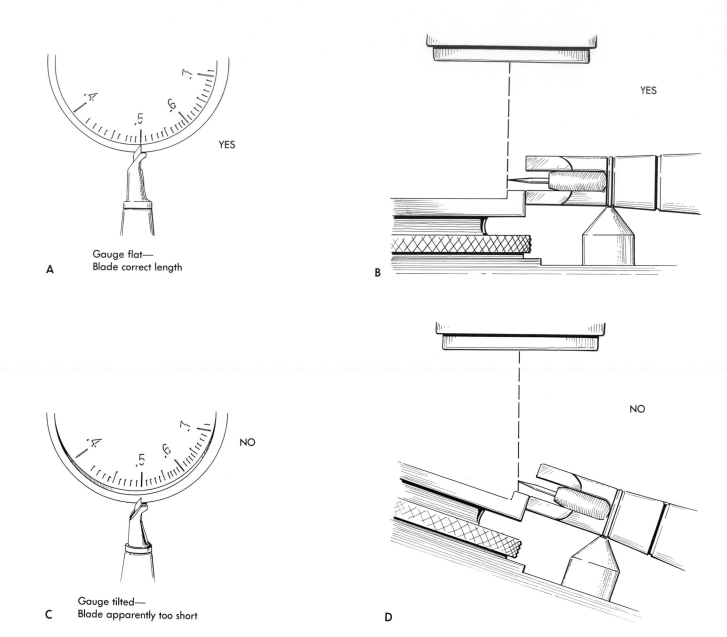

A
Gauge flat—
Blade correct length

B

YES

C
Gauge tilted—
Blade apparently too short

D

NO

Control of parallax. Because the knife blade is not applied directly to the surface of the gauge, the alignment of the tip of the blade over the edge of the ridge varies when the platform is tilted. This is parallax. The greater the distance between the blade and the gauge, the greater the parallax. **A** and **B,** Therefore the surgeon must sight directly down the edge of the ridge (that is, perpendicular to the surface of the gauge) to avoid parallax. Theoretically the problem of parallax can be prevented by placing the gauge platform on a surface parallel to the objective lens, but such a surface is not conveniently available in the operating room. The gauge can be stabilized on the patient's forehead and tilted up and down until it is flat. **C** and **D,** If the platform and gauge are tilted backward so that the surgeon can see inside the ridge, the blade will appear too short. If they are tilted forward so that the inside of the ridge is not visible, the blade will appear too long. The technique for proper alignment is to tilt the gauge so that the inside of the ridge can be seen, and then gradually flatten the gauge until the inside of the ridge just disappears. At this point, parallax is minimized and the blade setting will be the most accurate; sighting is binocular to increase stereopsis. The platform is held in one hand and tilted under the microscope while the other hand steadies the knife and turns the micrometer handle to align the tip of the blade with the edge of the ridge by advancing or retracting it.

FIGURE 17-56   GAUGE BLOCK WITH GROOVES

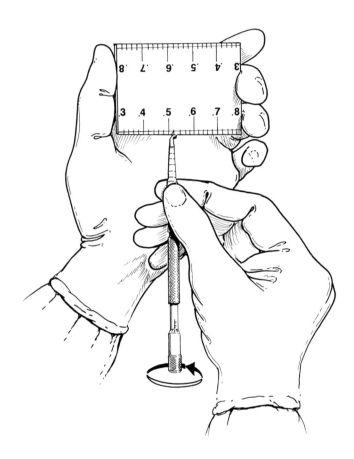

Gauge block with grooves. Another style of gauge is a flat block with grooves etched along the edge. The surgeon holds the gauge block in one hand supported on the patient's forehead and holds the knife in the other. The knife blade is aligned over the desired scale reading and gradually lowered to the surface of the block. The surgeon is careful not to touch the tip or cutting edge of the blade to the block and not to slide the footplate along the edge of the block. The surgeon must be consistent in aligning the tip of the blade with a given point on the groove: the outside edge, the middle, or the inside edge; parallax may play a role. If the blade length is incorrect, the knife must be removed from the gauge block, the micrometer adjusted the presumed amount for a proper setting, and the length of the blade again measured. The process can be accelerated a bit by placing the gauge block on a flat surface or flat on the patient's forehead, and then holding the knife with two hands so that the micrometer can be adjusted while the knife is applied to the gauge.

PLATE 17-13: Moistening the Ocular Surface (Figs. 17-57 to 17-60)

Goals:

1. Ensure good anesthesia of the limbus and cornea
2. Maintain a slightly moist corneal surface for smooth gliding of the knife footplates
3. Prevent a thinning or thickening of the cornea
4. Prevent epithelial abrasions
5. Avoid confusion between surface fluid and aqueous humor

FIGURE 17-57   FINAL TOPICAL ANESTHESIA

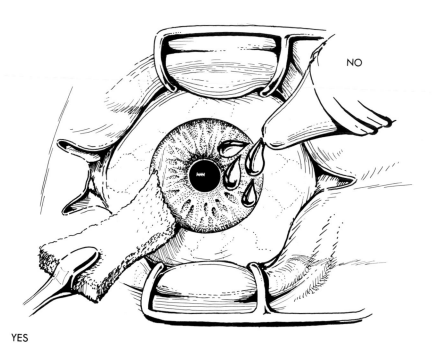

NO

YES

Final topical anesthesia. A microsponge soaked in anesthetic is applied to the limbus to ensure that the patient will not feel the fixation forceps. It is unnecessary to apply additional anesthesia to the cornea. Another way to anesthetize the limbus without excess anesthesia of the cornea is to use a cellulose sponge ring. The ring is placed dry over the limbus and impregnated with anesthetic for 15 to 30 seconds.

FIGURE 17-58   MOISTENING THE OCULAR SURFACE

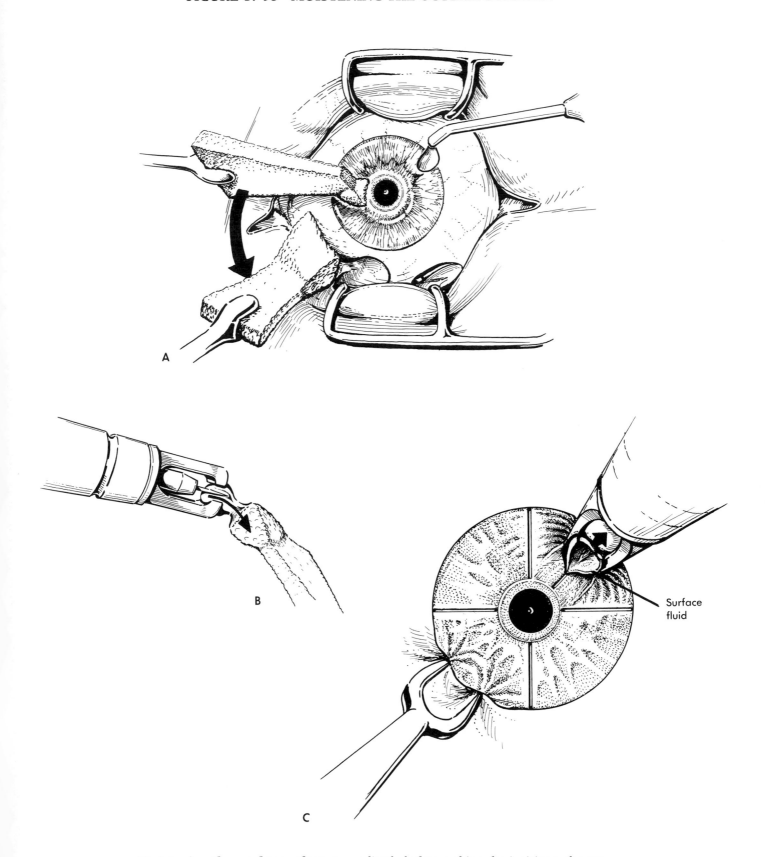

Surface
fluid

Moistening the ocular surface. Immediately before making the incisions, the surgeon moistens the corneal surface with balanced salt solution and then removes fluid from the surface of the conjunctiva and the tear meniscus **(A),** as well as from the knife, footplates, and blade **(B). C,** This prevents surface fluid from appearing around the knife, giving the false appearance of aqueous humor flowing from a corneal perforation.

FIGURE 17-59   MOISTENING THE CORNEAL SURFACE

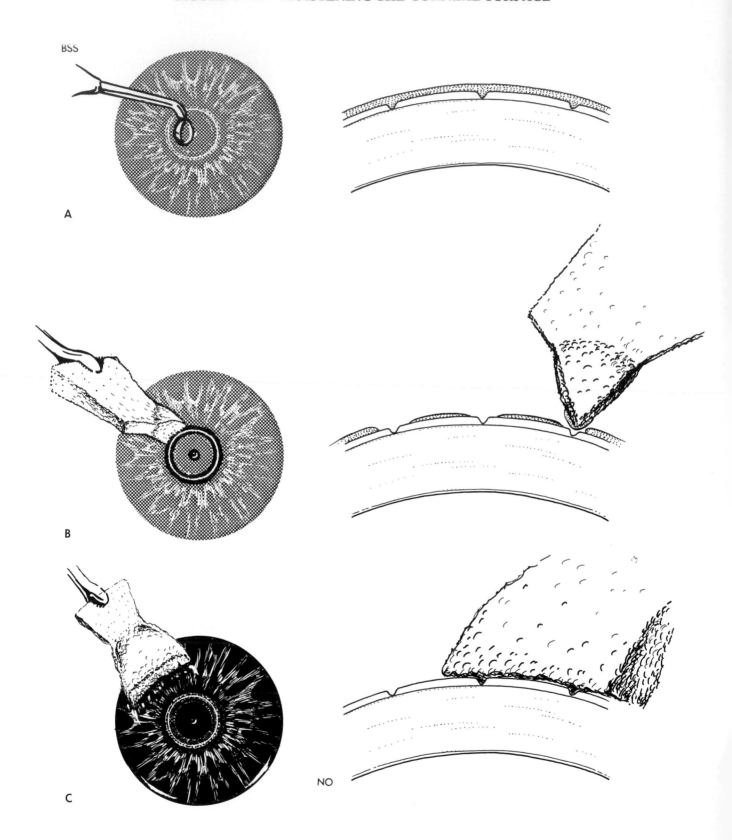

Moistening the corneal surface. A, A meniscus of balanced salt solution *(BSS)* remains over the entire cornea. **B,** The surgeon dries the cornea over the epithelial marks. **C,** A completely dry surface is undesirable because it speeds corneal evaporation and thinning and decreases the smoothness with which footplates slide over the surface. Do not rub the surface because this produces small abrasions of the epithelium and probably increases postoperative pain.

FIGURE 17-60   SURFACE HYDRATION DURING INCISIONS

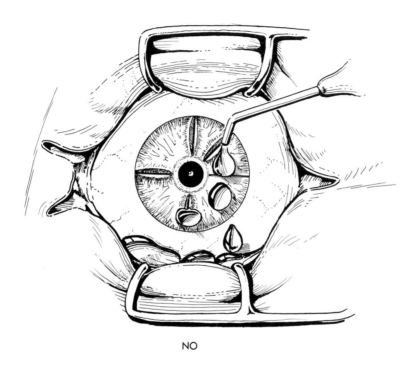

NO

Surface hydration during incisions. The surgeon should try to make all of the incisions without remoistening the corneal surface. Extra balanced salt solution applied to the surface after the incisions are made is soaked up by the stroma; this may produce corneal swelling and make any recutting of the incisions less accurate. However, if the epithelium becomes dry enough to prevent smooth gliding of the footplates or if epithelial abrasions occur, balanced salt solution on a wet microsponge should be spread over the corneal surface in the areas not yet incised.

PLATE 17-14:   Fixation of the Globe (Figs. 17-61 to 17-67)

Goals:

1. Stabilize the globe and control its position so that all incisions are perpendicular and straight
2. Consistently raise the intraocular pressure, providing a firmer cornea on which to cut in an attempt to increase the depth and uniformity of the incisions

FIGURE 17-61   DOUBLE POINT FIXATION OPPOSITE THE INCISION

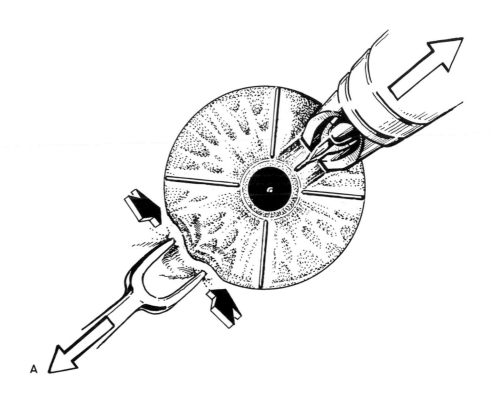

A

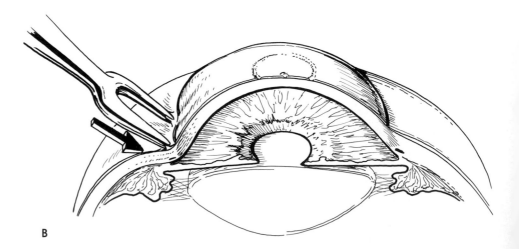

B

FIGURE 17-62 SINGLE POINT FIXATION

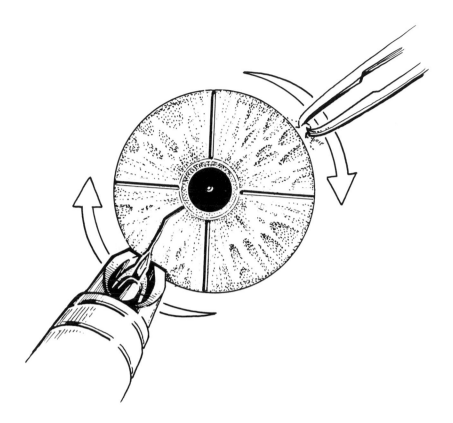

Single point fixation. Fixation with a heavy, single-pronged forceps in the semi-meridian opposite each incision can provide effective fixation as long as the knife and forceps pull in opposite directions. If either pulls off axis, the globe may torque around the single point fixation, producing a crooked incision. Some surgeons use a single-point forceps to grasp the edge of a previously made incision, but this may tear the edge of the incision and still provides only single point fixation.

FIGURE 17-61

Double point fixation opposite the incision. A, Fixation forceps with two prongs 3 to 5 mm apart are placed in the same meridian as the incision, 180 degrees away. The forceps are usually repositioned opposite each incision. They grasp limbal conjunctiva and Tenon's capsule firmly. Too shallow a bite will tear the conjunctiva. Too large a bite may hurt the patient. Preoperative vasoconstriction helps reduce the small hemorrhages that sometimes result from crushing the limbal vessels. **B,** The forceps compress the globe.

The surgeon accomplishes the following with these forceps: (1) the forceps are held steady to stabilize the globe and prevent torquing; (2) the forceps are pulled gently in the direction opposite the knife's movement to provide countertraction (*open arrows*) that facilitates cutting of the blade through the tissue and to move the eye beneath the knife if necessary; and (3) the forceps compress the globe (*black arrows*) to elevate the intraocular pressure, which increases the force on the cornea that opposes the cutting of the knife blade in an attempt to increase the depth and uniformity of the incision.

FIGURE 17-63   DOUBLE POINT FIXATION WITH SPANNING FORCEPS

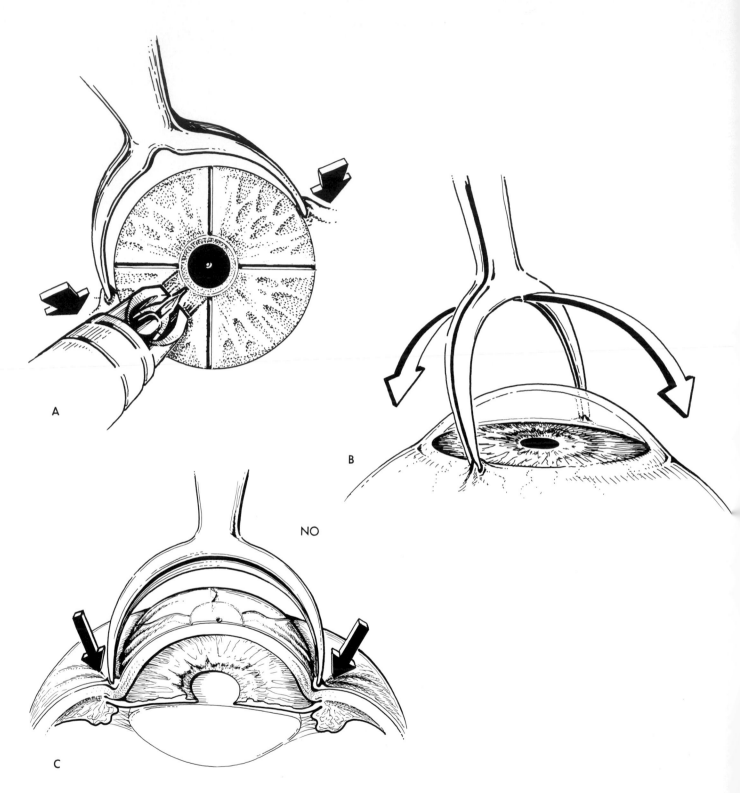

NO

Double point fixation with spanning forceps. A, Double-pronged forceps with tips 13 mm apart span the cornea and fixate the limbal conjunctiva. These forceps have a lock on the handle and are placed in a single position for all of the incisions. The teeth are positioned to lie between two incisions, usually in an oblique direction, so that the forceps do not obstruct the movement of the knife handle. During an incision, a gentle downward force is applied to the globe (*arrows*) to increase the intraocular pressure. **B,** After the first few incisions are made, the forceps are flipped over (*arrows*) and held in the opposite hand, making room for the remaining incisions. **C,** If the forceps clamp too much of the episclera at the limbus or if pressed into the globe with too much force (*arrows*), they will distort the cornea.

FIGURE 17-64 SUCTION FIXATION RING 569

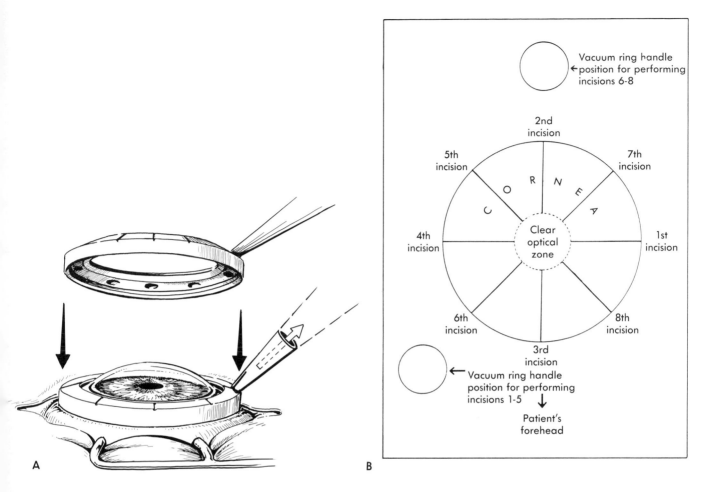

Suction fixation ring. A, Although infrequently used, a suction ring similar to that used for keratomileusis can provide good fixation for the globe. Using suction from a large syringe, a suction console, or wall suction in the operating room, the ring is applied to the anterior bulbar conjunctiva, which occludes the suction ports, allowing adhesion to the surface of the globe.

The suction ring is pressed onto the surface of the conjunctiva and the suction turned on with the foot pedal. With some instruments the surgeon's first finger occludes a vent valve at the base of the handle. The intraocular pressure rises and the pupil dilates. In some instruments the intraocular pressure rises minimally. The handle is oriented in the inferotemporal quadrant. After the surgeon makes the 6 o'clock, 12 o'clock, and nasal incisions, he or she releases the suction ring, changes hands, orients the handle of the ring inferonasally, and completes the temporal incisions. **B,** The position of the handle of the ring is different if the PERK sequence of incisions is used.

If the ring is left on too long for the initial incisions, conjunctival swelling occurs, and it is difficult to apply the ring for the second set of incisions. During the incisions the surgeon holds the ring steady or pulls up slightly on it; it is not necessary to compress the globe with the ring, since the intraocular pressure increases with the suction.

The suction ring is not used for deepening incisions because of the increased danger of corneal perforation. Corneal perforation produces a small squirt of aqueous, but the surgeon can release the finger from the vent hole to break suction quickly. (**B** from Mendelsohn AD, Parel J, Dennis JJ, et al: J Refract Surg 1987;3:79-87.)

FIGURE 17-65   COMPRESSION FIXATION RING

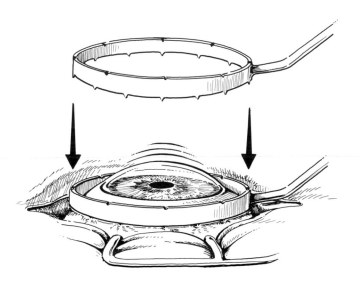

Compression fixation ring. The compression ring holds the globe stable with small, dull teeth that press into the conjunctiva and Tenon's capsule, requiring increased amounts of topical anesthesia. The sharpness and length of the teeth vary among manufacturers. The surgeon must press the ring firmly onto the globe, which pushes it into the orbit. To counteract this, about 6 ml of peribulbar anesthetic can be injected to increase the volume of the orbit, decrease the excursion of the globe, and increase the intraocular pressure. If the downward pressure on the ring is released slightly during the procedure, the ring may slide on the surface of the globe, loosing fixation. The handle of the ring is oriented in the 45-degree or 135-degree meridian to avoid hitting the nose. If necessary, the ring can rotate the globe. After a number of incisions are made, the ring is removed from the globe, the instruments are exchanged to appropriate hands, the ring is reapplied, and another set of incisions is made. Eight notches along the upper surface of the ring help the surgeon sight the direction of the incisions.

FIGURE 17-66   INTRAOCULAR PRESSURE DURING RADIAL KERATOTOMY

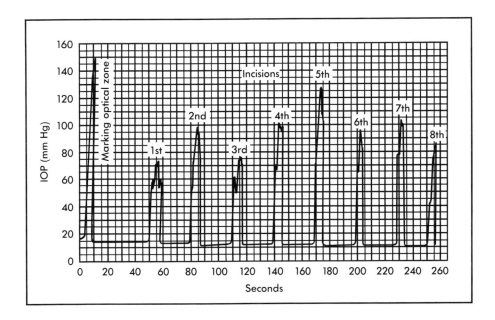

Intraocular pressure during radial keratotomy. Intraocular pressure was measured in human eye bank eyes by direct cannulation of the globe. The globe was fixated with a two-pronged forceps. The continuous reading shows that the pressure was elevated to between 70 mm Hg and 150 mm Hg during the surgery. The number of each incision is indicated on the graph. (From Mendelsohn AD, Parel JM, Dennis JJ, Gelender HH, Forster RK, and Ullman S: J Refract Surg 1987;3:79-86.)

FIGURE 17-67   RESULTS OF LABORATORY EXPERIMENTS MEASURING INTRAOCULAR PRESSURE IN HUMAN EYE BANK EYES WITH THREE DIFFERENT METHODS OF FIXATION DURING RADIAL KERATOTOMY

Results of laboratory experiments measuring intraocular pressure. Graphs **A** to **C** show intraocular pressure during each of eight incisions. **D,** The changes in intraocular pressure during the surgery. There is no published evidence that a higher intraocular pressure or a more stable pressure during surgery produces deeper or more regular incisions. However, the tabular material in **D** indicates systematic differences in corneal flattening in eye bank eyes as measured with keratometry among the three methods of fixation.

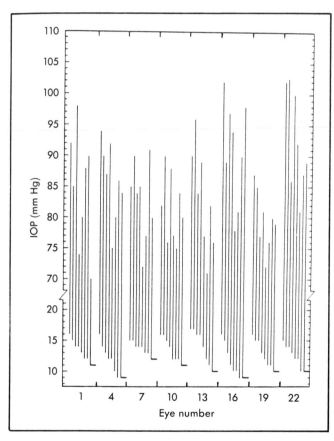

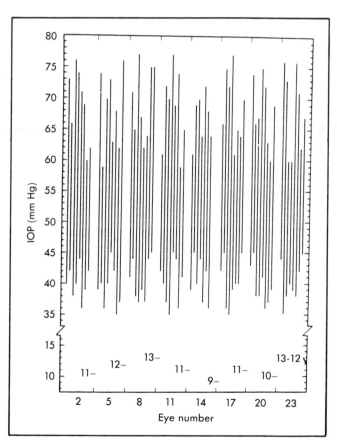

A, Fixation with double-pronged forceps produced the highest intraocular pressure during the incision (100 mm Hg), the lowest intraocular pressure between the incisions (10 mm Hg), and the greatest variability in pressure from one incision to another.

B, Fixation of the eye with a compression ring produced a level of intraocular pressure between that of the double-pronged forceps and the suction ring. There was a reasonably consistent minimum intraocular pressure between incisions (35 to 40 mm Hg), and a moderate variation in intraocular pressure during the surgery.

FIGURE 17-67, CONT'D

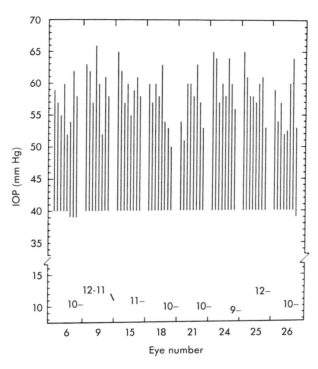

C, The suction fixation ring produced the lowest maximum intraocular pressure during incisions (60 mm Hg) of the three methods and the most consistent minimum intraocular pressure (40 mm Hg), with the least variability in pressure during the operation. (From Mendelsohn AD, Parel JM, Dennis JJ, Gelender H, Forster RK, and Ullman S: J Refract Surg 1987;3:79-86.)

Figure 17-67, D

Intraocular Pressure During Radial Keratotomy Using Three Methods of Fixation

Intraocular pressure	Average values (mm Hg) for operative method (mean ± SD)		
	Two prong	Compression ring	Vacuum ring
Mean peak	85.2 ± 4.6	68.3 ± 1.1	58.3 ± 1.7
Mean trough	13.0 ± 0.9	40.1 ± 0.4	39.9 ± 0.1
Overall range (difference between peak and trough)	72.3 ± 5.2	28.2 ± 1.1	18.4 ± 1.6
Decrease in IOP from surgery	6.8 ± 1.0	5.9 ± 1.2	6.5 ± 0.9
Change in corneal power (D)*	3.5 ± 1.1	4.56 ± 0.6	4.67 ± 0.7

From Mendelsohn AD, Parel JM, Dennis JJ, Gelender H, Forster RK, and Ullman S: J Refract Surg 1987;3:79-87.
*Unpublished data.

PLATE 17-15:   Number and Orientation of Incisions
(Figs. 17-68 to 17-72)

Goals:

1. Use the least number of incisions with the designated clear zone to achieve the desired correction
2. Space the incisions equidistant around the cornea for correction of myopia
3. Orient the incisions around the steep meridian if astigmatism surgery is planned
4. Minimize induced astigmatism

FIGURE 17-68   NUMBER OF INCISIONS

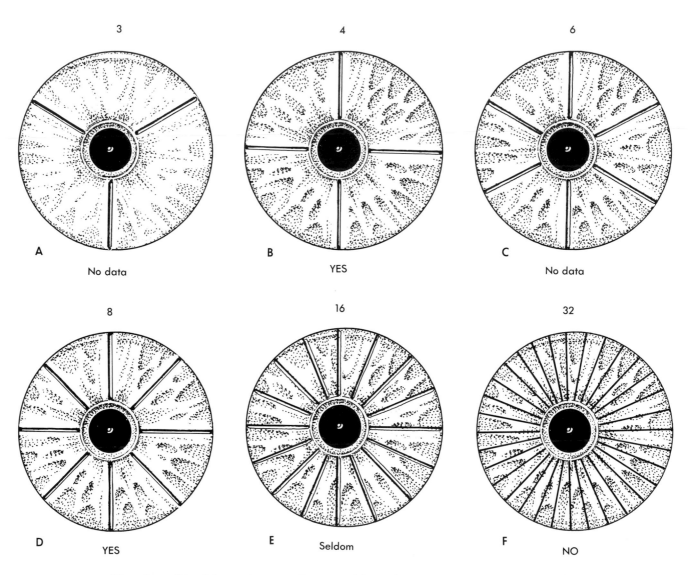

Number of incisions. Surgeons have used from three to 32 primary radial incisions **(A-F).** The number of incisions is determined by the surgeon's individual experience and technique and by the nomogram used to calculate the surgical plan. Most commonly, four incisions are used for lower amounts of myopia and eight for moderate amounts of myopia. There are no published data on cases with three, six, or twelve incisions. Sixteen incisions sometimes are used to correct higher amounts of myopia but produce increased scarring, increase the chance of irregular astigmatism, and have a minimal increased effect over eight incisions. No published evidence supports the use of more than 16 primary radial incisions.

FIGURE 17-69   ORIENTATION OF INCISIONS FOR SPHERICAL MYOPIA

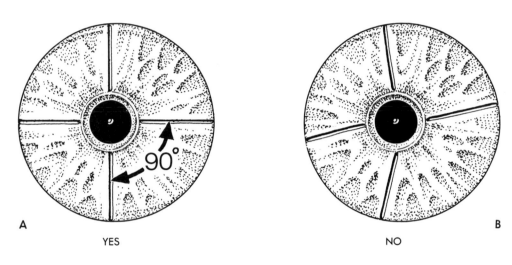

A   YES   NO   B

Orientation of incisions for spherical myopia. To decrease the chance of inducing astigmatism, the radial incisions are spaced equidistantly around the cornea. **A,** Four or eight incisions are placed orthogonally to each other so that the two incisions present in each meridian are oriented perpendicular to those 90 degrees away. Thus four incisions are 90 degrees apart, and eight incisions are 45 degrees apart. The incisions are placed either directly opposite each other, perpendicular to each other, or bisecting the space between the previous ones. Placement is easier with four and eight incisions because of the orthogonal relationship; it is more difficult with three, six, or twelve incisions. **B,** Unevenly spaced incisions are more likely to increase astigmatism.

FIGURE 17-70   ALIGNMENT AND SPACING OF INCISIONS

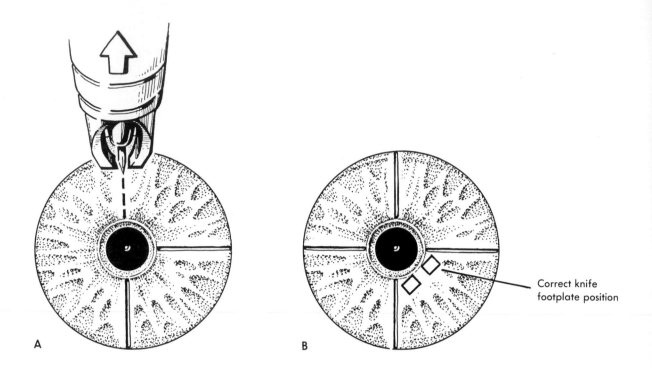

Correct knife
footplate position

Alignment and spacing of incisions. There are many techniques for ensuring proper alignment and spacing of the incisions. **A,** Visually inspecting the initial incisions involves identifying the widest part of the circular clear zone mark and aligning it with the center mark. The surgeon can make a false pass with the knife over the center mark out to the widest part of the circle (like a golfer taking a practice swing) to get a sense of the proper direction and to test hand position (*arrow*). When the surgeon makes a second incision on the opposite side of a single meridian, the first incision, the center mark, and the wide parts of the clear zone circle all serve to assist alignment. **B,** Bisecting the space between previous incisions helps ensure proper alignment. This is easiest when the incisions are made centrifugally because the footplates of the knife can be visually spaced between two previous incisions at the edge of the clear zone mark. It is more difficult when making centripetal incisions beginning at the limbus because of the larger arc between the limbal ends of the incisions.

FIGURE 17-70, CONT'D

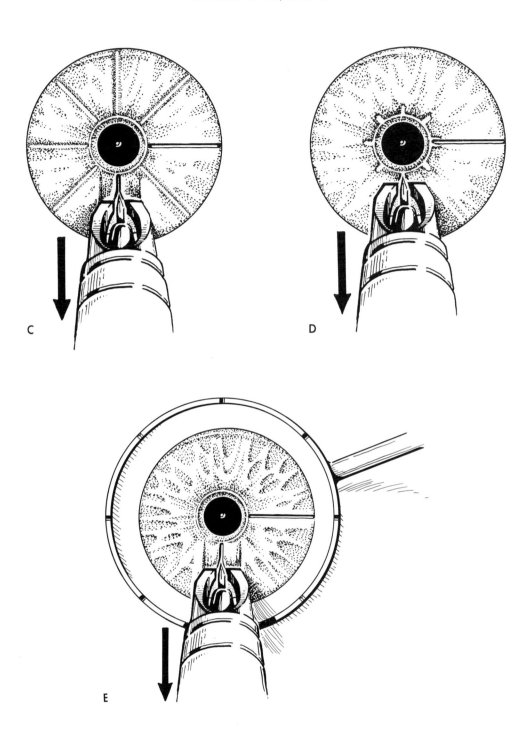

C, Using radial markers can help guide incisions, as discussed in Fig. 17-38. **D,** Some clear zone markers have studs that indicate the orientation of the radial incisions. **E,** Compression fixation rings have notches to help orient the incisions. This is a particular help with centripetal incisions.

FIGURE 17-71   MISPLACED INCISIONS

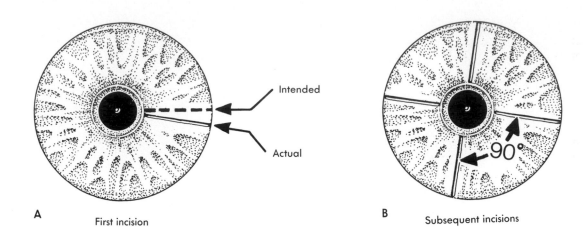

A First incision

B Subsequent incisions

Intended

Actual

90°

Misplaced incisions. If the first incision **(A)** is placed slightly off the intended semimeridian, the subsequent incisions **(B)** should be placed orthogonal to it, using it as a reference point. Unless astigmatism surgery is contemplated, the actual orientation of the incisions is not important as long as the incisions are equally spaced around the cornea.

FIGURE 17-72   ORIENTATION OF RADIAL INCISIONS FOR ASTIGMATISM SURGERY

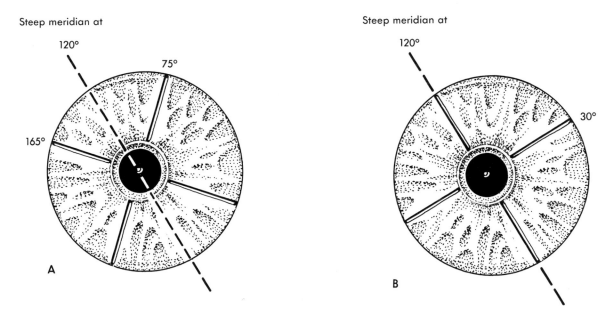

Steep meridian at

120°

75°

165°

A

Steep meridian at

120°

30°

B

Orientation of radial incisions for astigmatism surgery. If 1 D or more of astigmatism is present, the radial incisions should be placed to plan for possible future transverse incisions in the steep meridian. **A,** If the surgeon's technique involves placing transverse incisions between two radial incisions, the radial incisions should straddle the steep meridian. **B,** If the surgeon's technique involves placing transverse incisions on either side of a radial incision ("jump-T," "flag" incisions), one set of radial incisions should be placed in the steep meridian.

PLATE 17-16: **Sequence of Incisions** (Figs. 17-73 to 17-76)

Goals:

1. Prevent corneal perforations
2. Place the incisions with the hand most comfortable for the surgeon in each location
3. Minimize residual astigmatism if the operation is stopped before its completion

Note: The drawings for this plate contain notations for each incision that indicate the number of the incision in the sequence and the hand of the surgeon for an eight-incision case. For example, *1R* indicates the first incision made with the right hand.

FIGURE 17-73 PLACEMENT OF FIRST INCISION

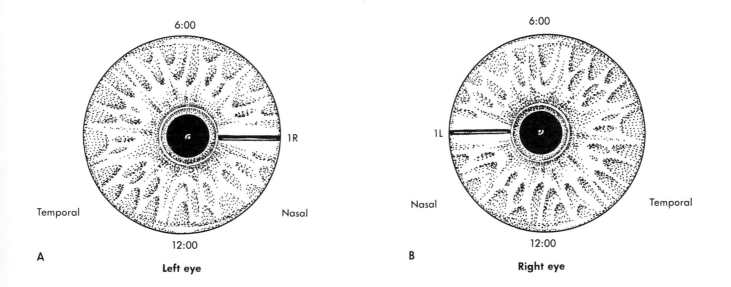

A Left eye

B Right eye

Placement of first incision. Surgeons have different criteria for selecting the location of the first incision.

1. It may be placed nasally because the nasal cornea is usually thickest and therefore there is less chance of perforation producing a soft eye for the remainder of the case.
2. It may be placed in the horizontal meridian because that is mechanically the easiest incision to make; it is good to begin a case with an easy maneuver.
3. It may be placed with the dominant hand because it is easier to start a case in the most secure manner.
4. It may be placed in the vertical meridian, where it always can be made with the dominant hand, even though the 12 o'clock incision is more difficult because it is awkward to hold the knife perpendicular and view directly down the knife handle.
5. It may be placed temporally in the thinnest area of the cornea with the reasoning that the cornea will become thinner under the microscope light during the procedure, and therefore cutting the thickest cornea last will decrease the chance of perforation—a premise that is probably not true if the surface is kept moist with balanced salt solution.

I begin in the thicker nasal cornea in the horizontal semimeridian. **A,** For a left eye I first incise the 9 o'clock semimeridian with my right hand. **B,** For a right eye I first incise the 3 o'clock semimeridian with my left hand.

FIGURE 17-74   ALL NASAL INCISIONS FIRST

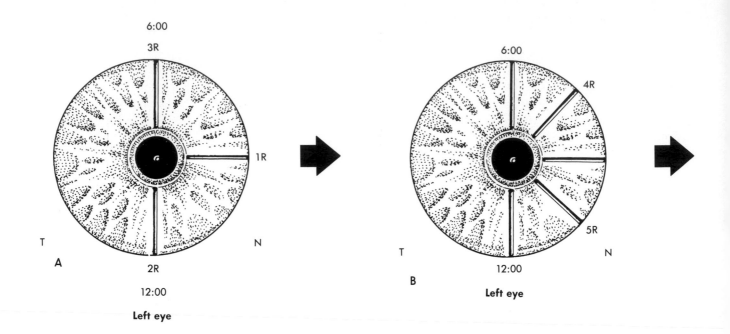

FIGURE 17-75   PERK SEQUENCE

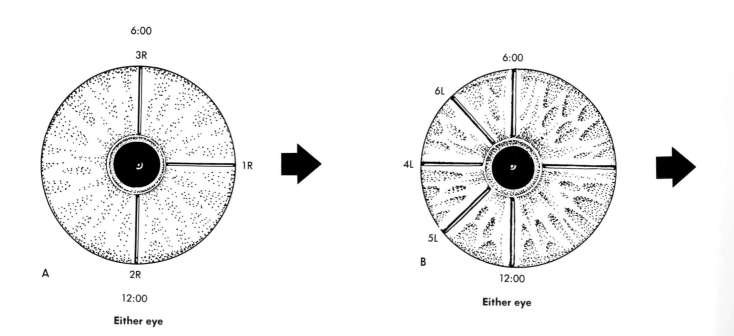

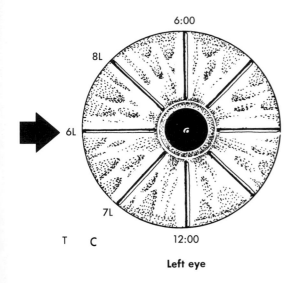

Left eye

FIGURE 17-74

All nasal incisions first. Placing the incisions in the nasal (thickest) cornea first reduces the chance of corneal perforation. **A,** For a left eye the 9 o'clock incision is made first, followed by the 12 o'clock and 6 o'clock. **B,** The two nasal oblique ones are then made—all with the right hand. **C,** Then the knife changes hands (only once) and the temporal incisions are placed, the horizontal one followed by the obliques. The last incision should be placed in the inferotemporal quadrant where the cornea is generally the thinnest. With this approach, a corneal perforation is most likely to occur near the end of the procedure, leaving fewer incisions for the surgeon to complete with a soft eye. This is currently my preferred technique.

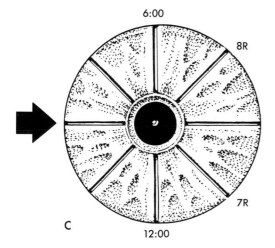

Either eye

FIGURE 17-75

PERK sequence. The technique devised in the PERK protocol **(A-C)** had the following goals: (1) begin with the right hand; (2) make the 3, 6, 9, and 12 o'clock incisions first so the second four incisions could be placed easier by bisecting the space between the first four (no marker was used); and (3) use a sequence such that termination of the case before the eight incisions would have less chance of inducing astigmatism, especially if no other incisions were placed later. The technique has the disadvantage in right eyes of beginning in the temporal (thinnest) cornea. It also requires that the knife change hands twice.

FIGURE 17-76   AROUND-THE-CLOCK SEQUENCE

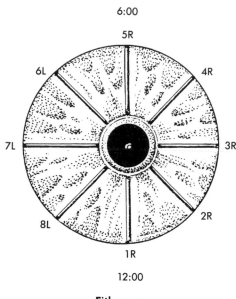

Either eye

Around-the-clock sequence. Starting the incisions at 12 o'clock and simply proceeding with each subsequent incision adjacent to the previous one has the disadvantages of cutting the temporal (thinner) cornea first in right eyes and of not having the orthogonal, horizontal, and vertical incisions in place to help guide the equidistant placement of the oblique incisions. Of course, the use of corneal markers can help placement.

PLATE 17-17:   Direction and Depth of Incisions (Figs. 17-77 to 17-81)

Goals:

1. Cut in a direction that produces a controlled incision
2. Achieve an incision of uniform configuration and depth

FIGURE 17-77   DIRECTION OF INCISIONS

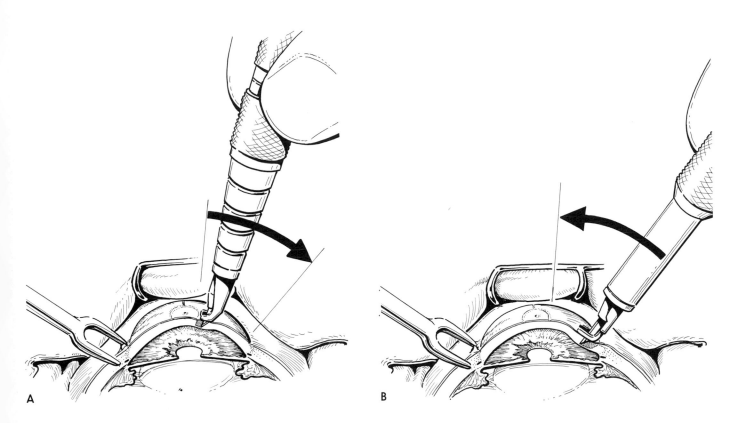

Direction of incisions. There are differences between centrifugal incisions (**A**) made with an angled knife blade and centripetal incisions (**B**) made with a vertical knife blade when both blades are set at the same length and the surgeon uses the same manual technique. The differences listed in **C** are realized by the average surgeon under similar conditions and can certainly become irrelevant when surgeons employ various artistic adjustments and fudge factors: different blade lengths, footplate configurations, rates of cutting, methods of plunging the knife into the cornea, amounts of pressure on the fixation device, and the like.

Luc Haverbeke, MD, of Wilrijk, the Netherlands, performed an informal prospective study of 23 patients, operating on one eye with centrifugal incisions using an angled diamond knife blade (American technique) and on the other eye with centripetal incisions using a straight vertical diamond knife blade (Russian technique). Comparison of the two series and the results are listed in **D**.

Haverbeke[2] concluded that, although more difficult to perform, the centripetal technique with a vertical knife blade achieves a greater effect, allowing the use of fewer incisions with a larger optical clear zone.

FIGURE 17-77, CONT'D

Figure 17-77, C

Comparison of Centrifugal and Centripetal Incisions

	Angled knife blade cutting from clear zone to limbus	Vertical knife blade cutting from limbus to clear zone
Direction of incision	Centrifugal (L., *centrum*, center + *fugio*, to flee)	Centripetal (L., *centrum*, center + *peto*, to seek)
Colloquial designations	American Downhill In and out	Russian Uphill Out and in
Configuration of knife blade	Angled cutting edge ("front" cutting)	Vertical cutting edge ("back" cutting)
Angle of cutting edge in cornea	Oblique	Perpendicular
Blade length setting for specific corneal thickness	Longer	Shorter
Depth of incision acheived for specific blade length	Shallower	Deeper
Visibility of cutting edge	Fair	Good
Configuration of paracentral incision	More curved	More square
Ease of straight incision	Easier	More difficult
Danger of cutting into clear zone	Lesser	Greater

Figure 17-77, D

Comparison of Centripetal and Centrifugal Incisions with Diamond Blades in 23 Patients

	Centrifugal incisions	Centripetal incisions
Population	Eye one of 23 patients	Eye two of 23 patients
Diamond micrometer knife	KOI (USA) oblique	Miklew (USSR) straight
Direction	Centrifugal	Centripetal
Number of incisions	Eight	Eight
Blade length	Same	Same
Pass per incision	Single	Single
Preoperative refraction	Mean −4.6 D (3.0 to 7.5)	Mean −5.5 D (3.5 to 8.0)
Postoperative refraction ±1.00 D	78%	96%
Average difference in effect	1.50 D	

Haverbeke L: Unpublished data, personal written communication, September 1987.

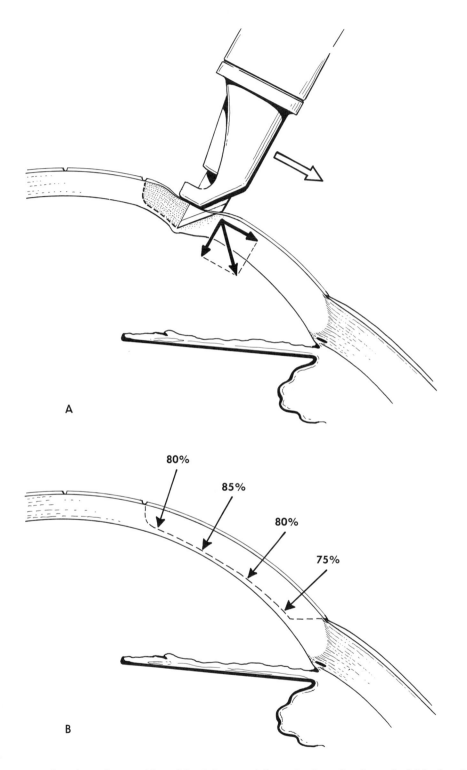

Mechanics of centrifugal incisions with a single-edged angled blade. A, Incisions from the clear zone to the limbus are made with a knife blade with a cutting
edge angled at approximately 45 degrees. The angle exerts vector forces in both the
lateral and posterior directions, which displace some tissue posteriorly without cutting it. Because centrifugal incisions begin near the margin of the clear zone, the
blade has little momentum in the area adjacent to the clear zone, which further
tends to displace rather than cut the tissue. However, as the blade begins to move,
more of the deeper layers are cut because of the lateral force of the blade (cutting
force on the blade = mass of knife × acceleration of hand). **B,** For this reason, centrifugal incisions are somewhat curved and are more shallow adjacent to the clear
zone. The depth is greatest near the middle of the incision.

**FIGURE 17-79 MECHANICS OF CENTRIPETAL INCISIONS WITH A
SINGLE-EDGED VERTICAL BLADE**

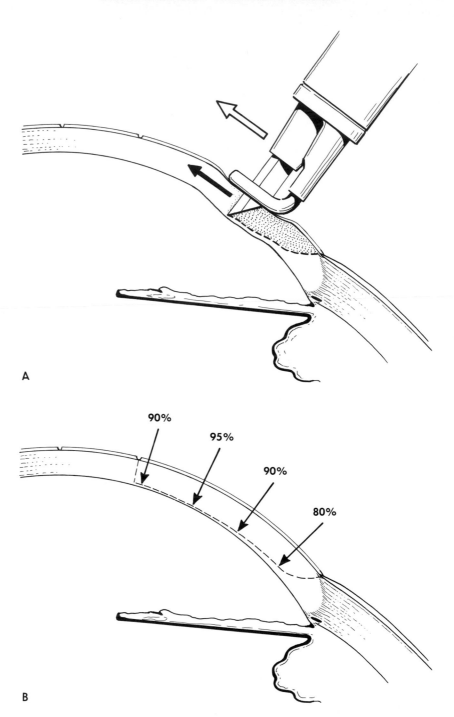

Mechanics of centripetal incisions with a single-edged vertical blade.
A, Centripetal incisions are usually made with a knife blade with a vertical cutting
edge that creates a smaller vector force posteriorly and therefore displaces less tissue.
The incisions begin peripherally, and since the blade has momentum as it travels
centrally up to the clear zone, it is more likely to cut than displace tissue. **B,** For
these reasons, centripetal incisions usually have a squarer configuration adjacent to
the clear zone and are deeper.

FIGURE 17-80   MECHANICS OF CENTRIFUGAL INCISIONS WITH A DOUBLE-EDGED ANGLED BLADE

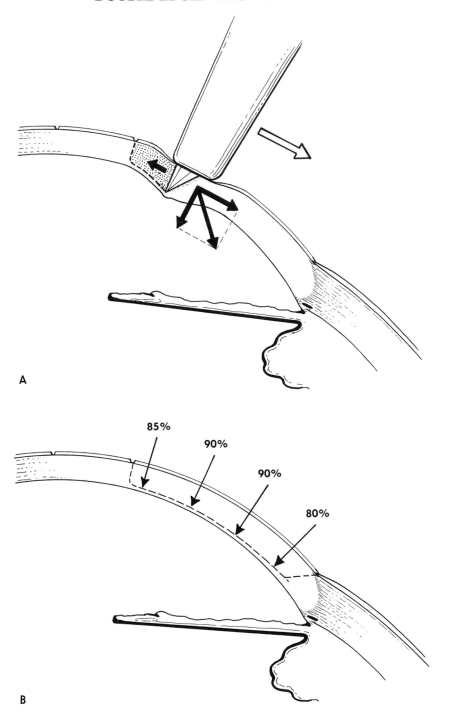

Mechanics of centrifugal incisions with a double-edged angled blade.
A, Incisions can be made from the clear zone to the limbus with a knife blade that has an angled cutting edge in the front and a vertical cutting edge in the back. There is a cutting force in both directions as the knife penetrates the stroma, which allows a somewhat deeper cut adjacent to the clear zone. As the blade moves, deeper layers of the cornea are also cut. **B,** For this reason, centrifugal incisions with a double-edged knife blade are more squared adjacent to the clear zone and have a depth approximately between the single-edged angled blade used centrifugally and the single-edged vertical blade used centripetally. The danger of a double-edged blade is that the surgeon may inadvertently slip the blade centrally, entering the clear zone. Some surgeons intentionally push the vertical edge back toward the center to square up the paracentral end of the incision.

FIGURE 17-81   COMPARISON OF CENTRIPETAL AND CENTRIFUGAL INCISIONS

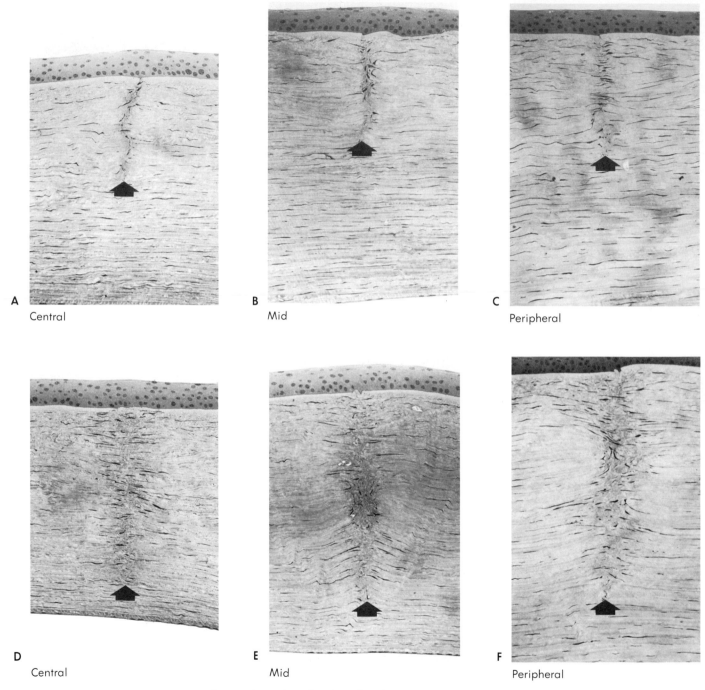

Comparison of centripetal and centrifugal incisions. In a series of monkey eyes, Melles and Binder demonstrated histologically that centripetal incisions were deeper and more uniform than centrifugal incisions. **A** to **C**, Light microscopy sections of one centrifugal incision made from the clear zone to the limbus. **A**, Central portion of the incision. **B**, Midportion of the incision. **C**, Peripheral portion of the incision (toluidine blue O; original magnification ×250). **D** to **F**, Light microscopy sections of one centripetal incision made from the limbus to the clear zone. **D**, Central portion of the incision. **E**, Midportion of the incision. **F**, Peripheral portion of the incision. Arrowheads indicate bottom of incisions. (toluidine blue O; original magnification ×250; bar = 100 μm).   *Continued.*

FIGURE 17-81, CONT'D

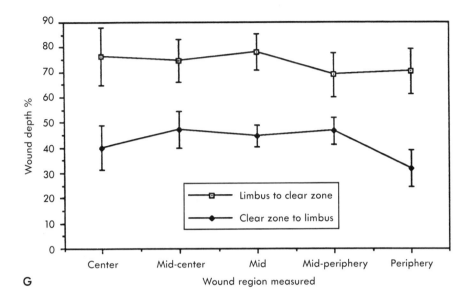

G

G, Graphic representation of average incision depth comparing the centripetal incisions *(upper line, open squares)* with centrifugal incisions *(lower line, closed diamonds).* The bars represent the standard deviation of each measurement.

Gritz and colleagues compared the depth of incisions using four diamond knives. Radial incisions were performed on a series of cadaver eyes, alternating the use of a centripetal limbus-to-clear zone (Russian) cutting technique with a vertical diamond knife blade (200 μ thick with a 45-degree cutting angle and 45-degree tip angle) and a centrifugal clear zone-to-limbus (American) cutting technique with a beveled diamond knife blade (200 μ thick with a 35-degree cutting tip and a 45-degree tip angle), and two ultrathin diamond blades (one 100 μ thick with a 35-degree cutting tip and 35-degree tip angle and another 100 μ thick with a 35-degree cutting tip and 45-degree tip angle). Incisions were examined on serial histological sections to determine the actual depth of the incision along its length, comparing this measurement to the original depth setting of the knife. The vertical cutting blade using the centripetal technique yielded significantly deeper incisions 2.0 mm from the central end of the incision (93% of blade length) than the other three blades using the centrifugal technique (80%, 83%, and 78%). The standard knife yielded significantly shallower incisions at the central end of the incisions compared with the vertical cutting blade and the ultrathin blade with a 35-degree cutting tip and 35-degree tip angle. All of the blades tested produced deeper incisions at the central aspect of the incisions compared with the peripheral aspect of the incisions. (From Gritz DC, Lee M, McDonnell PJ, Salz JJ: Refract Corneal Surg 1991, in press.)

Goals:

1. Orient the knife perpendicularly to the surface of the cornea
2. View along the knife handle with the microscope to see the tip of the blade
3. Hold the handle in a position that accomplishes the above two goals

FIGURE 17-82   FOCUS OF THE MICROSCOPE DURING THE INCISION

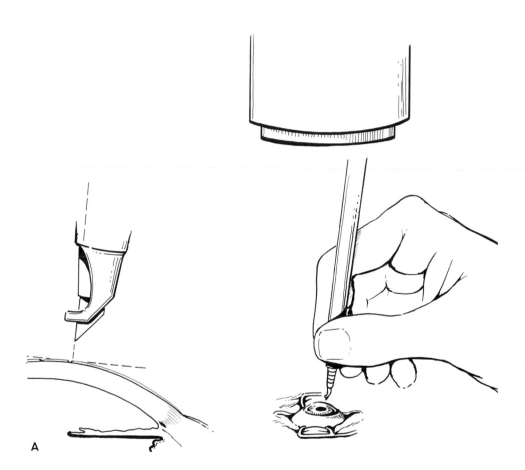

A

Focus of the microscope during the incision. A, Instinctively, most surgeons focus the microscope on the surface of the cornea at the commencement of the incisions. However, the knife displaces the cornea posteriorly when the incision is being made, putting it out of focus.

FIGURE 17-82, CONT'D

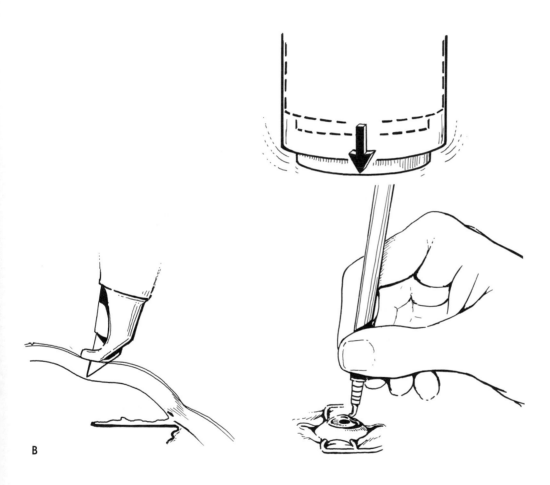

B

B, Therefore the microscope should be focused posterior to the surface of the cornea 2 or 3 mm into the anterior chamber (*arrow*) so that the corneal surface and the knife are in focus *during* the incision.

FIGURE 17-83   ANGLE OF KNIFE DURING INCISION

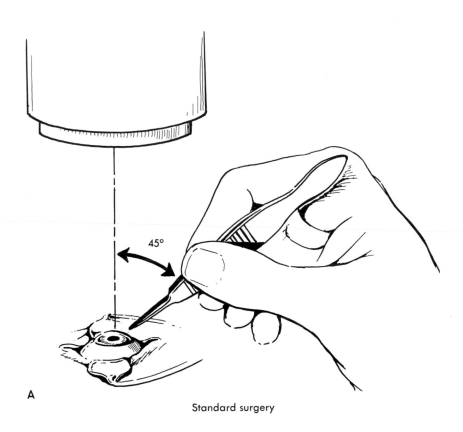

45°

A

Standard surgery

Angle of knife during incision. A, Most surgical instruments are held at approximately a 45-degree angle to the globe during use.

FIGURE 17-83, CONT'D

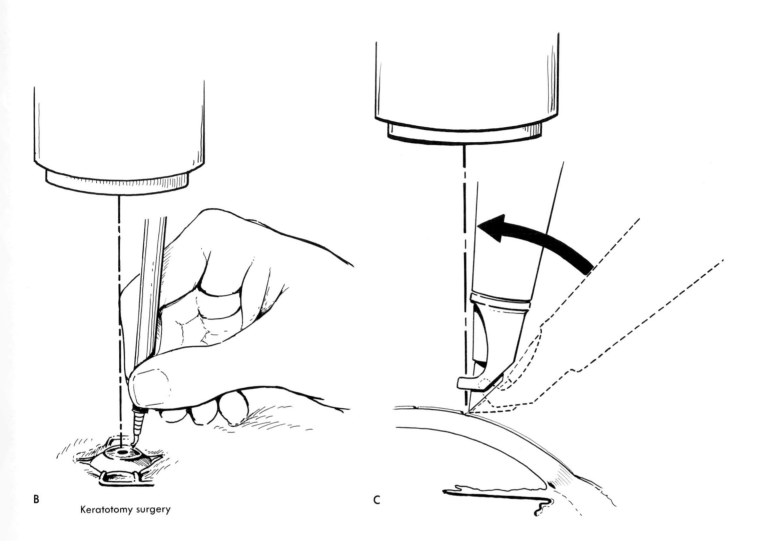

B

Keratotomy surgery

C

B, A radial keratotomy knife is different because it must be maintained perpendicular to the surface of the cornea. **C,** To achieve this, the surgeon brings the knife blade, tilted at an acute angle, into the field of view of the microscope. The tip of the blade is oriented at the edge of the clear zone and then the knife handle is tilted centrally (*arrow*) until it is perpendicular to the surface of the cornea and the surgeon is viewing along the side of the knife handle to the knife blade.

FIGURE 17-84   ENTRY OF THE KNIFE BLADE INTO THE CORNEA

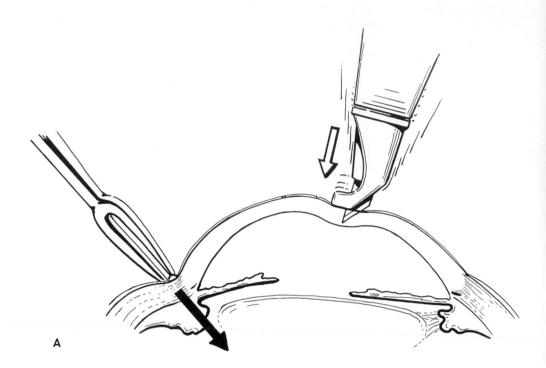

A

Entry of the knife blade into the cornea. A, The surgeon compresses the globe with the fixation forceps to elevate the intraocular pressure (*black arrow*) places the tip of the knife blade near the epithelium adjacent to the center clear zone mark, and plunges the knife into the stroma with a vigorous, short stab (*open arrow*) slightly indenting the cornea. This is no time to be timid. The surgeon must have confidence enough in the corneal thickness reading and the knife blade setting to know that the blade will not perforate the cornea at the beginning of each incision. A hesitant insertion of the knife blade at the edge of the clear zone will create a shallower incision. **B,** To implant the tip of the blade deeper, the surgeon bounces the knife slightly (*arrows*). **C,** The knife is held in a vertical position and bounce gently for approximately 3 seconds (one-a-thousand, two-a-thousand, three-a-thousand) to allow the tip of the knife to cut some of the deep displaced stroma. During this momentary pause, the surgeon can get a feel for the position of his or her hand and fingers and sense whether he or she is able to make a smooth radial incision by pulling the knife handle or whether the globe will have to be rotated beneath the footplates.

FIGURE 17-84, CONT'D

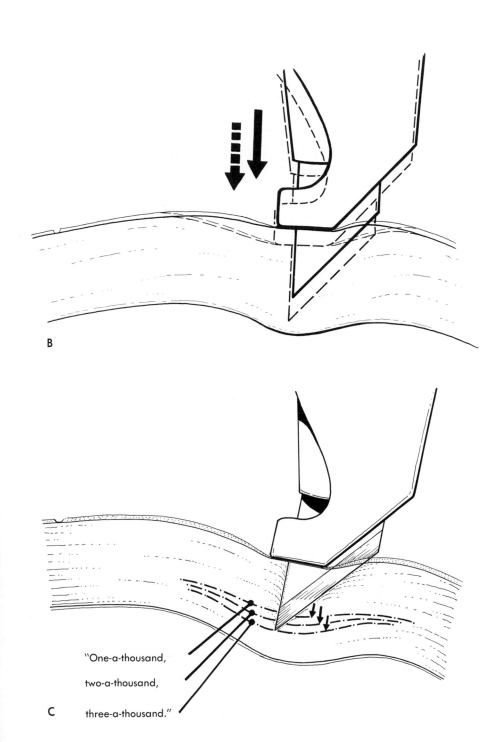

B

"One-a-thousand,

two-a-thousand,

C   three-a-thousand."

FIGURE 17-85　HOLDING THE KNIFE

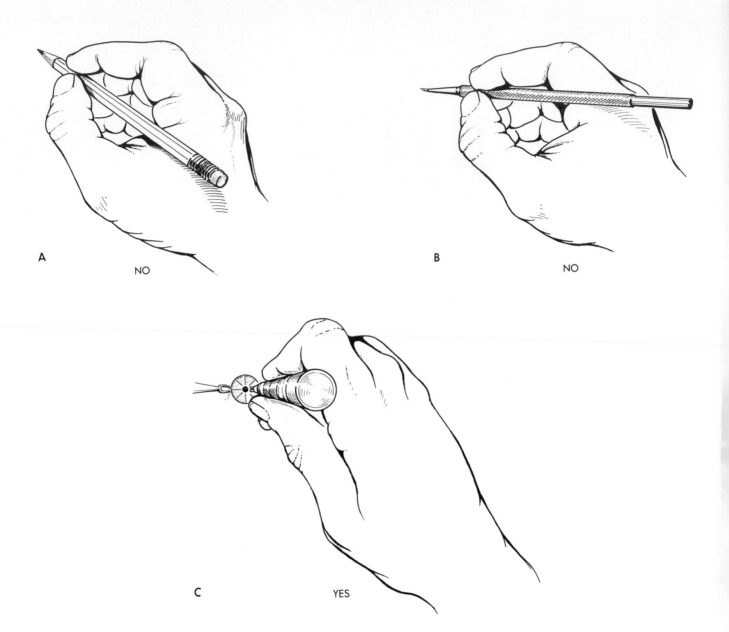

Holding the knife. A, No surgical instrument is held like a pencil, resting in the crotch between the thumb and first finger. **B,** In conventional eye surgery, long instruments the size of a radial keratotomy knife are usually held resting against the first metacarpophalangeal joint, with the thumb and first two fingers encircling the handle. **C,** In contrast, the radial keratotomy knife is held like a dart, with the handle resting along the side of the first metacarpal, supported on either side by the thumb and second finger. A space is left between the end of the thumb and the first finger to allow visualization of the blade along the side of the perpendicularly oriented knife handle. If the thumb and first finger touch, there is a tendency to tilt the knife backwards to visualize the blade, and subsequently the knife is not perpendicular to the corneal surface. The grip on the knife is gentle but firm.

As with other surgical instruments, stability is achieved by resting the side of the fifth finger on the periorbital facial structures.

PLATE 17-19: Execution of the Incisions (Figs. 17-86 to 17-89)

Goals: To make radial incisions that are

1. Perpendicular to the surface
2. Straight
3. Accurate, that is, the desired depth throughout their length
4. Precise, that is, the same configuration and depth for all incisions

FIGURE 17-86 MANUAL TECHNIQUE OF MAKING THE INCISION

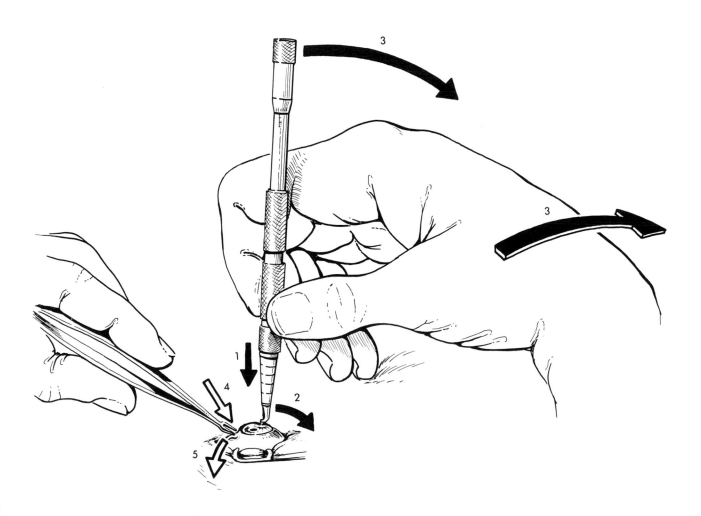

Manual technique of making the incision. Making a straight, perpendicular, uniformly deep radial incision requires five simultaneous, manual motions. The surgeon *(1)* presses to indent the cornea slightly, *(2)* pulls the knife at a uniform speed across the cornea, and *(3)* supinates his or her wrist to tilt the knife and keep it perpendicular to the cornea. With the fixation instrument the surgeon *(4)* compresses the globe and *(5)* pulls in the direction opposite the force of the knife to provide countertraction.

FIGURE 17-87   LATERAL PERPENDICULARITY OF THE KNIFE BLADE

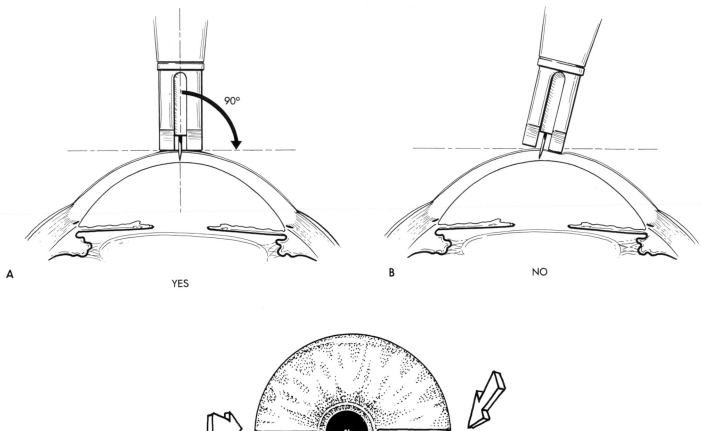

90°

A   YES

B   NO

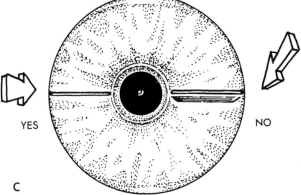

YES   NO

C

Lateral perpendicularity of the knife blade. A, The surgeon maintains the blade perpendicular to the surface of the cornea not only along the axis of incision but also laterally. **B,** If the blade is tilted to one side or another, the incision is undercut, creating a wider incision scar when viewed from the front of the cornea, with possible increased glare **(C).** A radial keratotomy bridge can help support the knife and keep it perpendicular.

FIGURE 17-88   KEEPING THE KNIFE PERPENDICULAR TO THE CORNEA

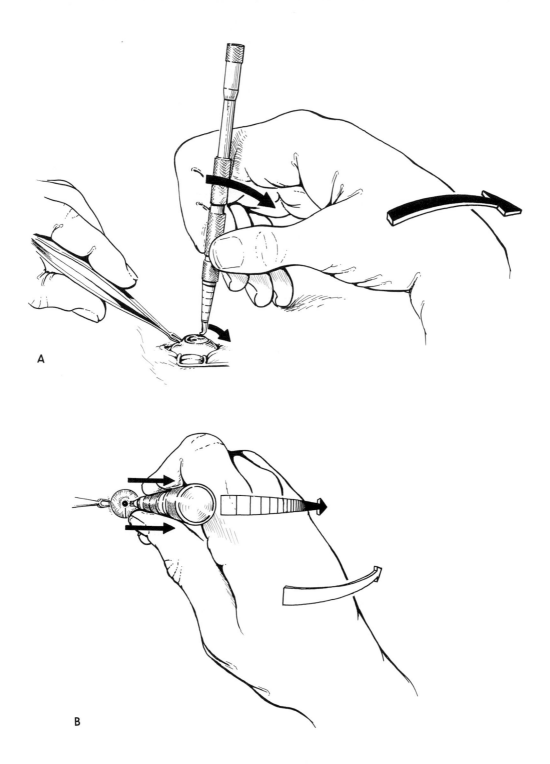

Keeping the knife perpendicular to the cornea. A perpendicular incision requires that the knife follow the curvature of the cornea, a goal accomplished by gradually supinating the hand, wrist, and forearm when cutting from the clear zone to the limbus (**A** and **B**) or gradually pronating the hand, wrist, and forearm when cutting from the limbus to the clear zone. This motion differs from that used with other surgical instruments, where the predominant movement is often rotation of the instrument between the fingers. During the radial incision, there is no rotational movement of the knife between the fingers. A long footplate will flatten the cornea under the blade and more easily produce a perpendicular incision. Because the incisions are relatively short, 3 to 4 mm, the surgeon can also pull (or push) the knife somewhat by moving the first three fingers only, keeping the fourth and fifth fingers stationary on the rim of the orbit and avoiding the coarser movement of sliding the whole hand.   *Continued.*

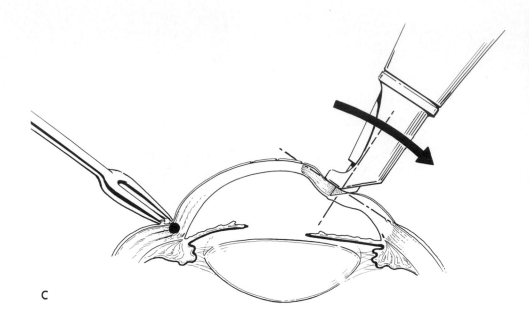

C

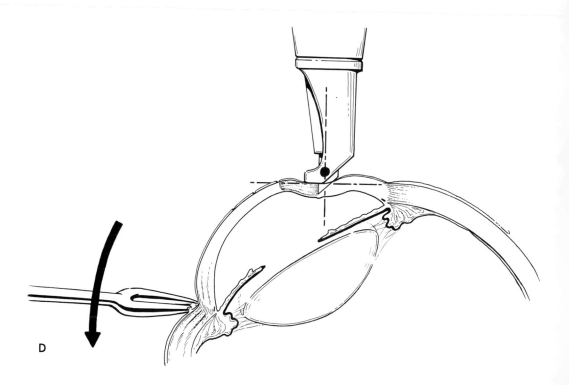

D

C, Generally the globe is held still (*dot*) and the knife is pulled laterally (*arrow*). **D,** Alternatively the knife can be held in a fixed vertical position (*dot*) and the globe can be pulled or pushed beneath the footplates by the fixation instrument (*arrow*). This is a particularly helpful maneuver if the excursion of the knife is limited by the lid speculum, the drape, or an awkward position of the hand.

FIGURE 17-88, CONT'D

601

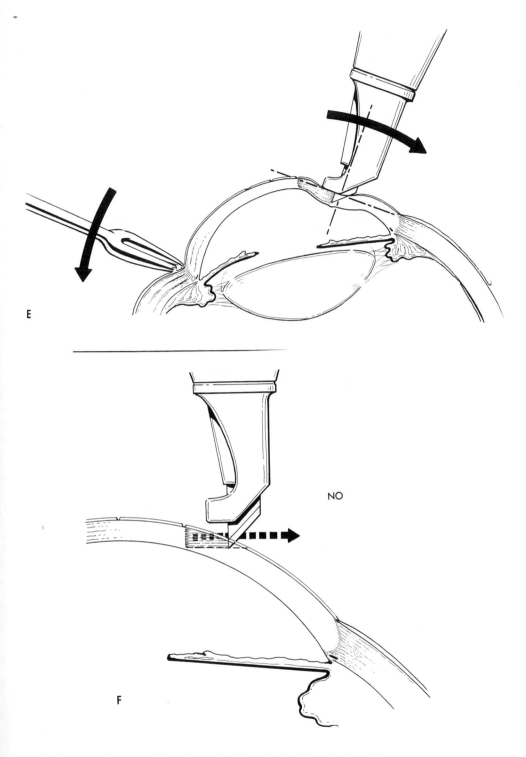

E, Commonly a combination of pulling the knife and the globe in opposite directions is used (*arrows*), since providing some countertraction on the globe is an integral part of making the incision.

Most surgeons find it easier to make a straight incision by moving the knife across the corneal surface because it is a familiar motion and similar to drawing a straight line with a pencil. It is more difficult to move the globe in a straight line with the fixation instrument because the globe is large and there is a greater tendency for it to veer from one side to the other, creating a curved or oblique incision. Moving the globe is made difficult because the patient senses the motion and may fight against it in an attempt to continue to look at the microscope light or may move the eye erratically to respond to the motion of the globe.

F, If the knife does not follow the curve of the cornea and is merely pulled straight laterally, it will cut shallower than desired.

FIGURE 17-89   RATE OF MAKING THE INCISION

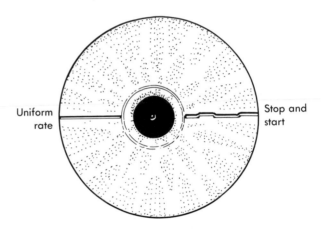

Uniform rate

Stop and start

Rate of making the incision. The pulling or pushing of the knife across the corneal surface is done in a single, smooth motion at a slow, deliberate, uniform rate—taking 3 to 4 seconds per incision. Hesitation or stopping during the incision can create a jagged, misaligned wound. Moving the knife too slowly will decrease the force of the blade against the tissue and, even with a diamond blade, will substitute tissue displacement for tissue cutting. Too fast an excursion decreases the surgeon's control, increasing the chance that a small perforation will become a large laceration, and making it more difficult to control the termination of the incision.

In general, it takes 8 to 10 seconds to make a radial keratotomy incision, including fixating the globe, aligning the blade, plunging the blade into the tissue, waiting for the blade to penetrate the deeper stroma, executing the incision, and removing the blade from the cornea.

Goals:

Make a uniformly deep incision

FIGURE 17-90   PRESSURE ON THE KNIFE

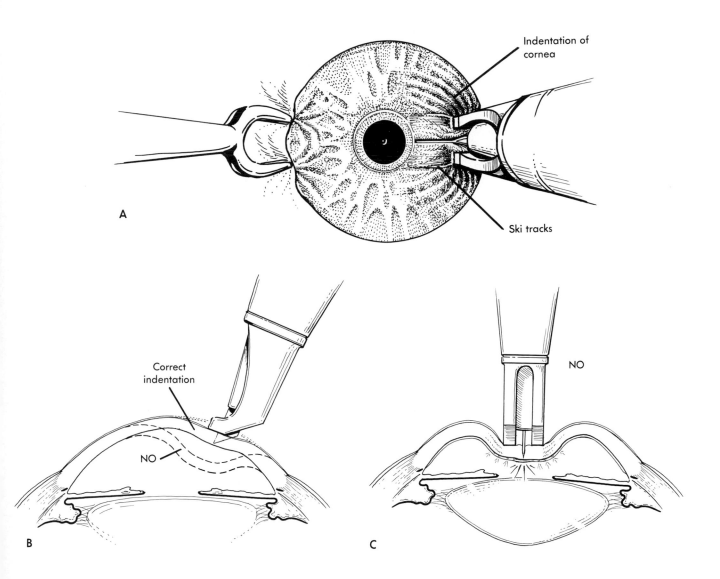

Pressure on the knife. A, During the incision the surgeon must keep gentle, downward pressure on the knife to ensure that the blade remains deeply seated in the tissue. There are two indicators of the proper amount of pressure: a slight indentation of the cornea, which can be seen as a distortion of the surface, and the creation of a pair of parallel tracks (ski tracks) by the footplates in the epithelium. **B,** Increased pressure on the knife does not produce a proportionately deeper cut: the cornea is 78% water and not readily compressible, so it is displaced by the increased pressure. **C,** Excess pressure on the knife may indent the cornea enough to disrupt the endothelium and rub on the lens and iris. A large perforation of the cornea is more likely to occur when excess pressure decreases the surgeon's fine manual control.

FIGURE 17-91   INTRAOCULAR PRESSURE DURING THE INCISIONS

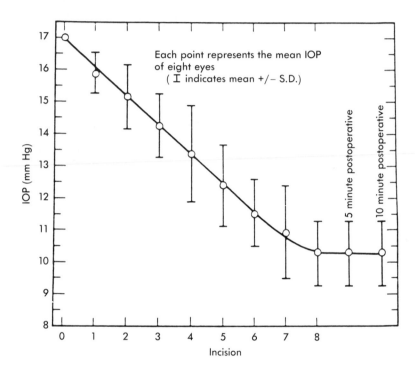

Intraocular pressure during the incisions. As the sequence of incisions is completed, the intraocular pressure gradually falls because the compression of the globe by the fixation instrument and knife forces out intraocular fluid (as in tonography) and because the cornea becomes more flaccid and distensible. The graph indicates the decrease of intraocular pressure in human eye bank eyes in which eight incisions were made, the intraocular pressure being measured by a cannula attached to a pressure transducer. Therefore there must be an increase in force on the fixating instrument and the knife as the operation progresses, since a lower intraocular pressure allows deformation of the posterior cornea, possibly resulting in a shallower incision. (From Mendelsohn AD, Parel JM, Dennis JJ, Gelender H, Forster RK, and Ullman S: J Refract Surg 1987;3:79-86.)

FIGURE 17-92   DEPTH OF INCISION

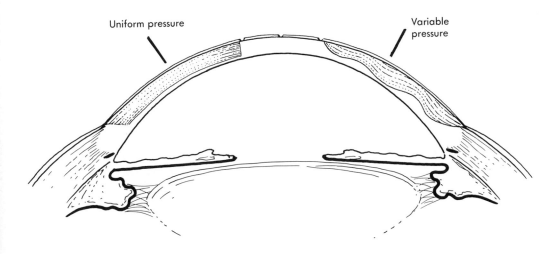

Depth of incision. A uniformly deep incision requires uniform pressure on the knife during cutting, a uniform rate of cutting, and as uniform an intraocular pressure as possible throughout the incisions. Merlin[6a] demonstrated histopathologically that the following factors are associated with a deeper incision: vertical cutting edge, triple-edged knife blade, sharper (newer) knife blade, and a single footplate. Factors associated with a more irregular incision depth included high cutting velocity and low intraocular pressure. Factors that did not affect incision depth included direction of incision, American or Russian techniques, and sequence of incisions.

PLATE 17-21: **Length and Termination of Incisions** (Figs. 17-93 to 17-96)

Goals:

1. Extend the incisions from the edge of the clear zone to the tip of the limbal vascular arcade
2. Create smooth, uniform, vertical ends of the incisions without stopping the incision shorter or longer than its intended position

FIGURE 17-93   LENGTH OF THE INCISIONS

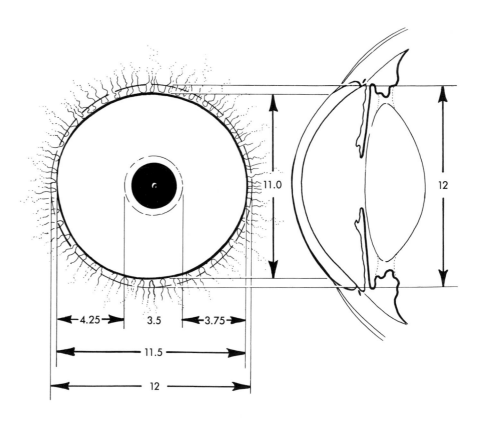

Length of the incisions. Radial keratotomy incisions are 3 to 4 mm long. The length of individual incisions varies, depending on the decentration of the pupil, the diameter of the clear zone, and the diameter of the cornea. The nasal incisions are usually shorter than the temporal ones.

One anatomic fact seldom considered in radial keratotomy is that the posterior limbal ring at the termination of Descemet's membrane is circular, approximately 12 mm in diameter, but the anterior limbal ring at the termination of Bowman's layer is oval, being approximately 1 mm shorter in the vertical than in the horizontal meridian because of physiologic anterior overriding of the sclera. The amount of anterior scleral overriding varies considerably from one individual to another. If it is the anatomic cornea that should be cut and that controls the final outcome, logic dictates that all incisions should extend equidistant from the circular posterior limbal ring and therefore pass into the limbal vascular arcade superiorly and inferiorly.

One technique to achieve this is to use an 11- or 11.5-mm circular marker placed concentric to the clear zone mark to make the length of all the incisions the same. There seems to be anatomic justification for this approach, which was used by some surgeons in the early 1980s but is seldom used now.

Because the paracentral part of the incision seems to have the greatest effect, this variation in the peripheral part may be less important. But, does it contribute to the variability of outcome?

FIGURE 17-94   LOCATION OF ENDS OF INCISIONS

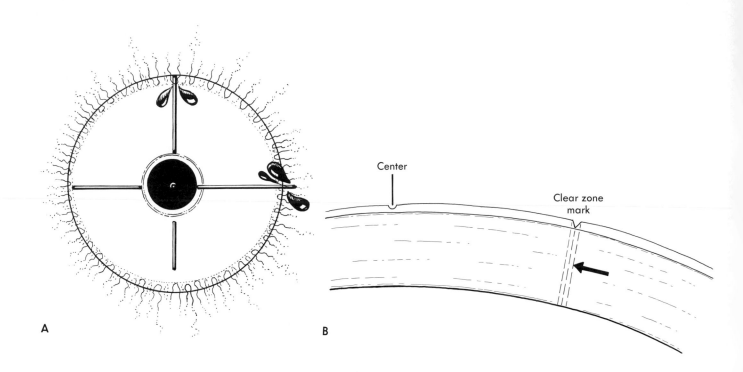

A   B

Location of ends of incisions. A, Incisions that are too short (for example, the 6 o'clock incision), beginning outside the clear zone and stopping more than 1 mm short of the limbal arcade, will not have as much effect as intended. Incisions that are too long (for example, the 12 o'clock and 3 o'clock incisions), extending inside the clear zone or across the vascular arcade, will have more effect. In the late 1970s surgeons extended incisions into the scleral limbus, but this approach causes considerable bleeding and does not enhance the effect of the operation. The correct length (for example, 9 o'clock incision) extends from the edge of the clear zone mark to the tip of the limbal vascular arcade. **B,** However, each surgeon has his or her own concept of the location of these two landmarks. The paracentral end of the incision can terminate just inside, exactly on, or just outside the clear zone mark, depending on the bevel of the marker and the technique of the surgeon. The limbal vascular arcade extends a variable distance onto the cornea. Such subtleties probably affect the outcome.

FIGURE 17-95   TERMINATING THE CENTRIFUGAL INCISIONS   **609**

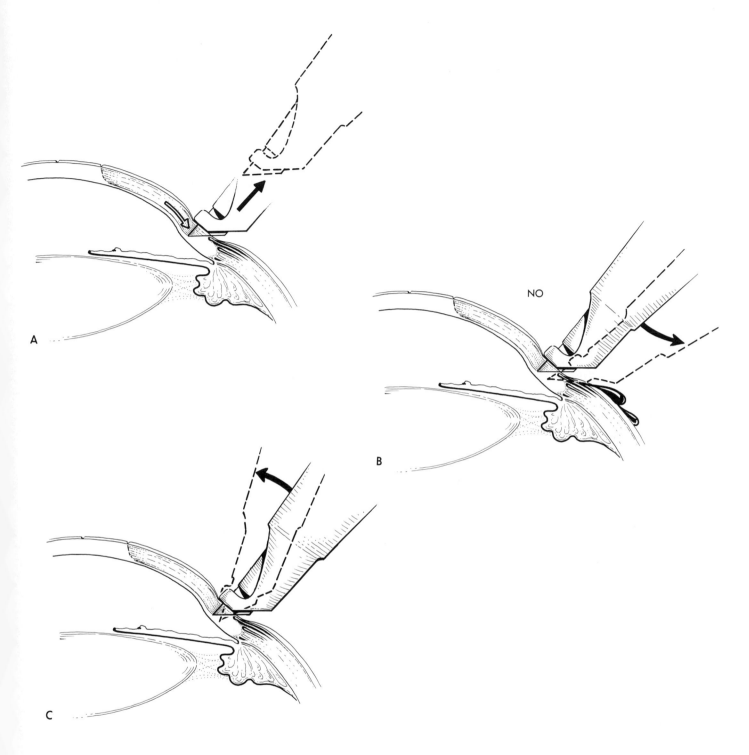

Terminating the centrifugal incisions. A, As the knife approaches the limbus, the surgeon should see the cutting edge of the blade directly or visualize its position mentally. The knife is stopped just short of the limbal vessels (or 0.25 mm into the arcade at 6 o'clock and 12 o'clock), and the knife is lifted out of the wound perpendicular to the surface (*black arrow*). **B,** There is a tendency to let the momentum of the knife carry the incision into the limbus, but dragging the knife across the end of the wound and across the superficial limbus creates excess bleeding and does not enhance the effect of the surgery. **C,** Some surgeons intentionally tilt the knife handle toward the center of the cornea (*arrow*), trying to sweep the tip of the angled blade deeply into the peripheral cornea to create a more vertical, deeper end of the incision—a technique of unproven usefulness.

FIGURE 17-96   TERMINATING THE CENTRIPETAL INCISIONS

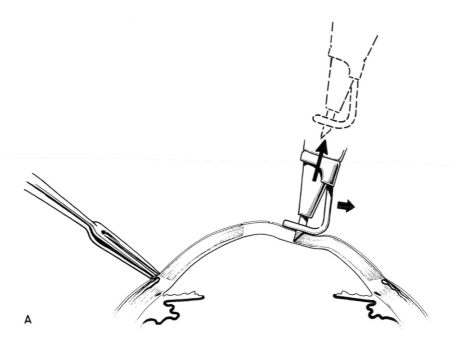

A

Terminating the centripetal incisions. A, As the surgeon pushes the knife toward the edge of the clear zone, the natural deceleration that occurs to avoid cutting into the clear zone must not produce a staggering of the paracentral part of the wound. Rather, the knife blade should cut at a uniform rate up to the edge of the clear zone and then be pulled out perpendicular to the corneal surface and away from the central cornea (*arrows*) to prevent pushing into the clear zone. Above all, the surgeon must avoid continuing the entire incision directly into the clear zone, an error easily prevented by a light touch on the diamond knife, a slow to moderate cutting speed, and a gentle pull of the knife back away from the end of the incision when removing it.

FIGURE 17-96, CONT'D

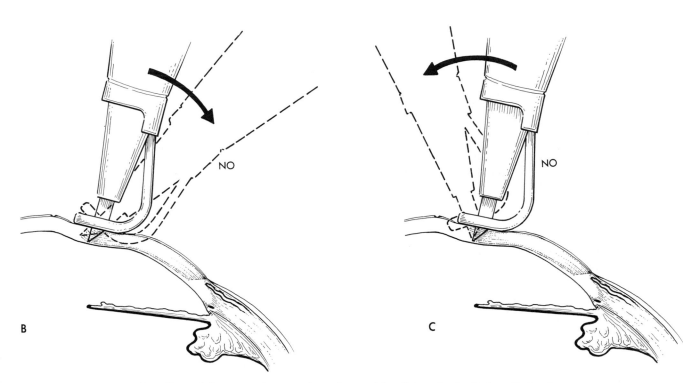

B, The effect of the operation can be enhanced by tilting the knife handle back toward the limbus (*arrow*) and sweeping the tip of the blade in under the edge of the clear zone, rendering the clear zone smaller and making the recorded size of the clear zone and the actual size of the clear zone different. **C**, The surgeon should avoid tilting the knife blade toward the center of the cornea (*arrow*) and dragging it across the edge of the clear zone mark, a maneuver that extends the superficial part of the wound only, enhances the operation minimally, and may increase light scattering over the pupil.

PLATE 17-22: Deepening of Incisions (Figs. 17-97 to 17-101)

Because the cornea becomes thicker from the center to the periphery and because the theoretically ideal radial keratotomy incision is of uniform depth (either the same percentage of corneal thickness throughout or leaving a uniformly thick layer of posterior stroma), surgeons have attempted to make the peripheral part of the incision as deep as the paracentral parts. Because it is difficult to do this with the blade set at a fixed length, surgeons have devised methods of making the incisions in concentric zones, with the knife blade longer when cutting the outer zones. Convincing evidence that zone cutting increases the effect of radial keratotomy has not been published.

There are many variables involved in making deepening incisions in different zones. Goals in making incisions include the following:

1. Obtain incisions of uniform depth from one end to the other
2. Use multiple passes of the knife, multiple blade length settings, or multiple zones to achieve uniformly deep incisions
3. Maintain straight, regular incisions

The surgeon must select among the following on the basis of artistic sense, intuition, experience, previous results, and surgical plan:

1. *Number of zones.* Use two zones or three zones.
2. *Diameter of zones.* Because most zone cutting is performed in patients with a high amount of myopia, the central clear zone usually has a diameter of 3 mm. The diameter of the next zone is usually 6 mm but is sometimes 5 mm. The diameter of the outer zone is usually 9 mm but is sometimes 7 or 8 mm. Markers with three concentric rings—for example, 3, 6, and 9 mm in diameter—allow rapid delimitation of the zones. Some of these markers also contain radial markers to help guide the location of the incisions in each zone.
3. *Number of incisions in each zone.* In general, the same number of incisions is made in each zone, but some surgeons will make eight incisions across all zones and add only four incisions across others.
4. *Direction of incisions.* The direction may be different for different zones. For example, the first and second incisions may be made centripetally to cover all three zones, but the final deepening in the outer zone may be made centrifugally. Different knife blades may be used, depending on the direction of the incisions.
5. *Sequence of cutting zones.* Some surgeons cut across all zones with the first incision, two zones with the second, and one zone with the third. Others prefer to cut each zone separately so that two passes are never made through the same zone.
6. *Selection of knife blade length.* Different techniques for selecting knife blade length for each zone include measuring central corneal thickness and the addition of a fixed length measure (for example, 0.05 mm) or a fixed percent (for example, 10%) for each zone and measuring corneal thickness around each zone mark, typically in the 3, 6, 9, and 12 o'clock meridians, and then either average these readings or select the thinnest of the readings and reset the blade length in each zone based on the readings at that zone. Readings should be recorded in a table.
7. *Method of changing the length of the blade.* Cutting in zones is more time consuming than making single-pass incisions. If too much time is consumed, the cornea thins, possibly requiring irrigation of the surface with a balanced salt solution, which will soak into the wounds and produce thickening. Such changes in corneal thickness will interfere with the attempts at accurate deepening incisions. To prevent this, some surgeons use three separate preset knives, one for each zone, so that the incisions can be

made without any adjustment. Others will simply dial the micrometer and extend the blade (for example, 0.05 mm) for each subsequent zone, without verifying the new blade length. Still other surgeons will reset the blade on the basis of the pachometry readings specifically in each zone and verify the length on a gauge block. (Colloquial jargon has christened these "redeepening" incisions. This is a redundancy. The second and third passes simply "deepen" the incision; they do not *re*-deepen them.)

FIGURE 17-97 TWO PASSES WITH BLADE AT SAME LENGTH

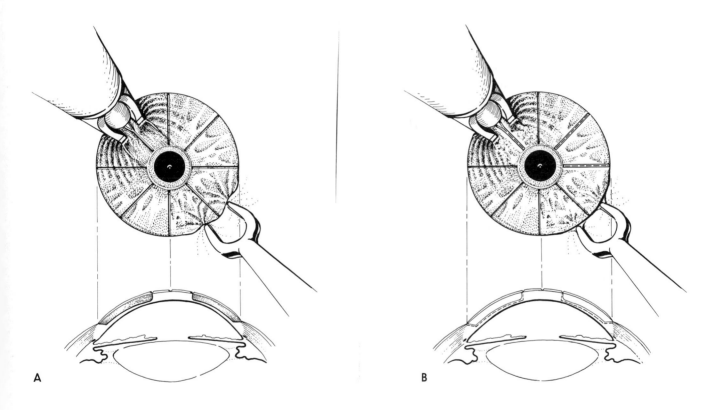

A, B,

Two passes with blade at same length. When the surgeon makes centrifugal incisions with a knife blade that has an angled cutting edge, some of the deep stromal tissue is displaced posteriorly without being cut. Therefore a second pass of the knife through the same incision with the knife blade at the same length will cut some of this deep stromal tissue.

A, The surgeon makes the full number of incisions. **B,** With the knife blade at the same setting and without rewetting the corneal surface or irrigating the incisions, the knife is reinserted in each incision and pulled toward the periphery *(dotted lines)*. On inserting the knife, the blade can be wiggled back and forth slightly to help the tip seat itself in the apex of the previous incision. The downward force on the knife and the pressure on the fixation forceps during the second pass are less than that during the first to avoid perforation; the footplates skate *lightly* along the surface of the epithelium without indenting the cornea. Generally the nasal incisions in the thicker part of the cornea are made first.

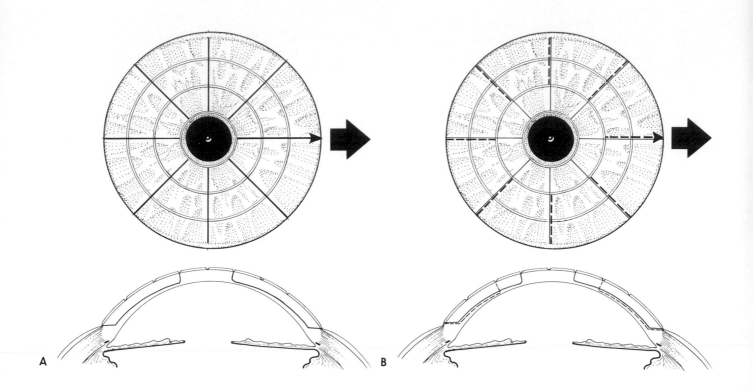

FIGURE 17-98   INCISIONS IN ZONES WITH INCREASING BLADE LENGTH AND FULL EXCURSION

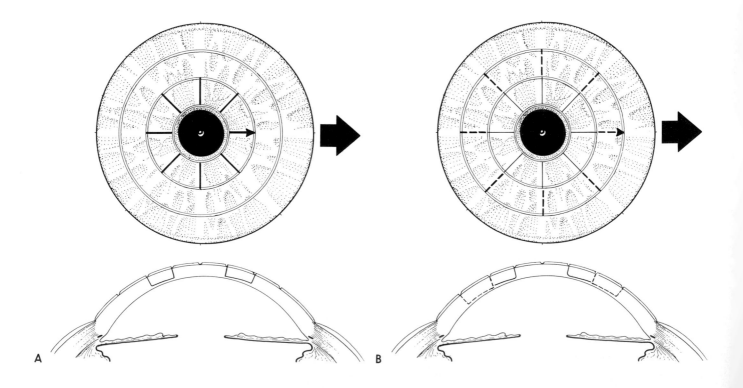

FIGURE 17-99   INCISIONS IN ZONES WITH INCREASING BLADE LENGTH AND PARTIAL EXCURSION IN THE CENTRIFUGAL DIRECTION

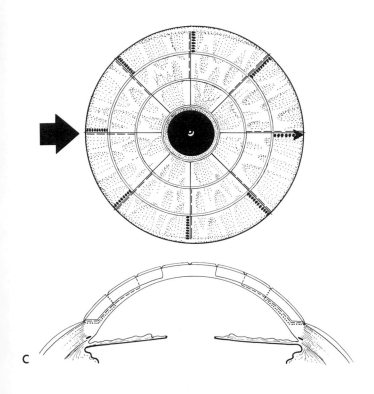

FIGURE 17-98

Incisions in zones with increasing blade length and full excursion. A, The first set of incisions is made from the clear zone to the limbus, as in the standard single pass technique. **B,** The second set of incisions is made from the middle zone mark to the limbus by extending the length of the knife blade and inserting the blade into the previously made wound at the edge of the middle zone mark. The blade usually drops easily into this incision, and very little pressure is applied to the corneal surface as the knife is pulled centrifugally, the surgeon allowing the blade to follow the path of the previous incision. **C,** Cutting the outer zone, which is narrow because it extends from 9 to 11 mm, may be difficult with the angled knife blade because the angle takes up much of the excursion of the short incision. Therefore the outer zone may be cut from the limbus into the 9-mm mark or a vertical cutting blade can be used. The advantage of this approach is that the knife can be lowered into the previous incision easily and the final incision is usually straight.

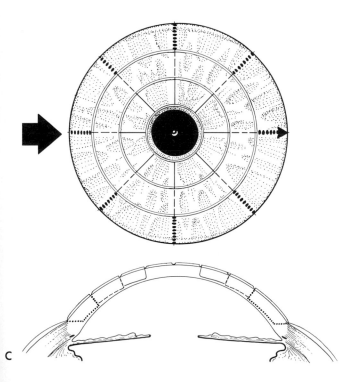

FIGURE 17-99

Incisions in zones with increasing blade length and partial excursion in the centrifugal direction. The premise of this technique is that the paracentral part of the incision is the most important and therefore should be made with the most uniformity. Because the intraocular pressure decreases as more incisions are made, it is difficult to obtain a uniformly deep incision later in the operation. **A,** Therefore the first eight incisions are made in the inner zone only. **B,** These are followed by the second eight incisions in the middle zone. **C,** Then the third eight incisions are made in the outer zone.

The first set of incisions is made as in the standard radial keratotomy technique. The second and third sets are made by dropping the knife into the previous incision and bringing it to the end of that incision, which is then extended to the next zone mark. Cutting the outer zone centrifugally may be difficult, and the surgeon may elect to cut it centripetally or to use a vertical knife blade. The challenge in this technique is to avoid making jagged or S-shaped wounds from misalignment of the three different incisions on the same axis and to avoid leaving tissue bridges between the ends of the three short incisions. This requires inspecting the wound at the end of the procedure and recutting any tissue bridges that may be present.

FIGURE 17-100   INCISIONS IN ZONES WITH INCREASING BLADE LENGTH AND PARTIAL EXCURSION IN THE CENTRIPETAL DIRECTION

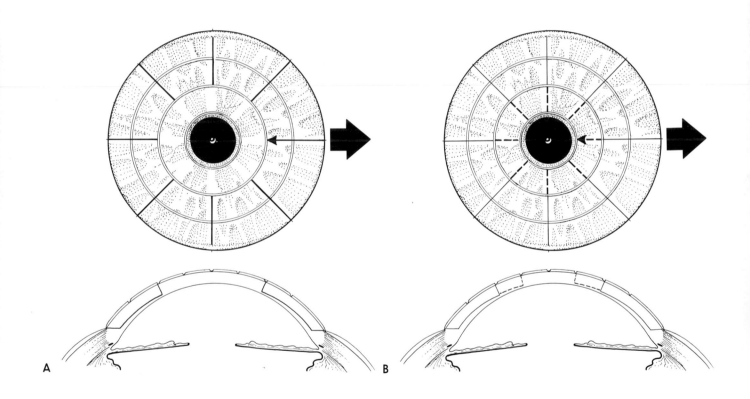

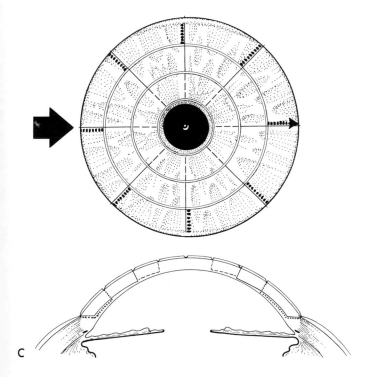

C

FIGURE 17-100

Incisions in zones with increasing blade length and partial excursion in the centripetal direction. **A,** The first set of incisions is made from the limbus to the middle zone mark, covering the outer two zones. **B,** The second set of incisions is made across the inner zone. **C,** If required, the third set of deepening incisions is made in the outer zone.

Using this approach, it is not practical to incise the inner zone first because the surgeon would then be required to make a cut from the limbus to the end of the previous incision in the inner zone, joining the two incisions, which is extremely difficult.

FIGURE 17-101   ERRORS IN DEEPENING INCISIONS

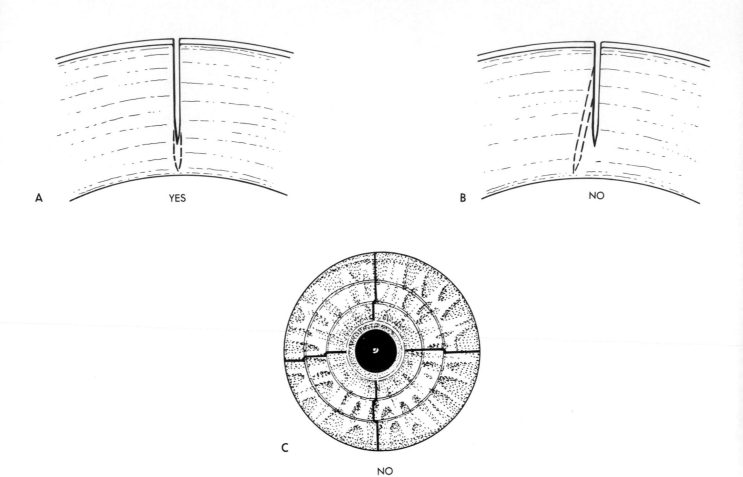

Errors in deepening incisions. A and **B,** When the blade is extended through the same incision area twice, the tip of the blade may not find its way to the deep apex of the incision and will create a second cut in the form of an inverted Y. Whether this has any practical effect on the outcome is unknown. **C,** When joining incisions in different zones, the surgeon must be careful to align the incisions and avoid jagged or S-shaped wounds.

FIGURE 17-101, CONT'D

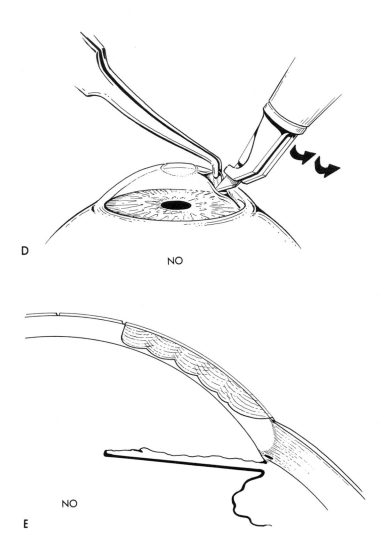

D

NO

NO

E

D and **E,** Surgeons in the early 1980s advocated freehand dissection of the wounds down to Descemet's membrane, an extremely difficult technique that should be avoided because it increases greatly the chance of corneal perforation and usually leaves a nonuniform base.

PLATE 17-23:   Corneal Perforations (Figs. 17-102 to 17-104)

Goals:

1. Minimize the number and length of corneal perforations
2. Complete the operation if a self-sealing small corneal perforation occurs
3. Terminate the operation if a large corneal perforation occurs, suturing the perforation, if needed, and preventing secondary complications

FIGURE 17-102   SMALL CORNEAL PERFORATION (MICROPERFORATION)

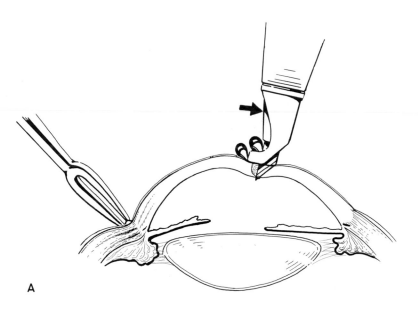

A

Small corneal perforation (microperforation). Perforations commonly occur in three locations:

1. In the *thinner paracentral cornea* just after the incision has begun. Usually the perforation does not occur when the knife blade is plunged into the tissue because tissue is displaced at that moment; rather, perforation occurs after the blade excursion has begun, and some of the acceleration creates a deeper incision and then the perforation.
2. In the *thinner temporal and inferotemporal parts of the cornea.* This is the most common location.
3. *During deepening incisions.* This is most common when a previous incision has been made and the knife is passed through the same area a second time, either with the blade at the same length or extended and especially if it is pressed down too much.

A, The surgeon detects a microperforation by attending carefully to the corneal surface around the knife blade during the incision. The surface must be reasonably dry, without any fluid present between the knife blade footplates or on the surface of the eye at the limbus, both of which can either simulate or mask the appearance of aqueous humor. The first sign of a perforation is the welling up of a drop of aqueous around the knife blade between the footplates. At this moment, the surgeon should stop the excursion of the knife, withdraw it slowly and deliberately from the wound, and simultaneously release the fixation instrument. There should be no "burned finger" reflex, that is, jerking the knife out of the wound and creating an irregular incision.

FIGURE 17-102, CONT'D

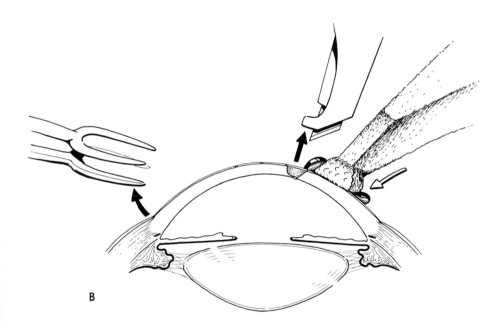

B

B, A very deep nonperforating incision can produce a leak of aqueous, presumably because the fluid percolates through Descemet's membrane. The surface of the wound in the area of the perforation is dried with a microsponge and gentle pressure is applied to estimate the size of the laceration in Descemet's membrane by the amount of aqueous that comes out. Of course, every attempt is made to lose as little aqueous as possible. Most of these small perforations are self-sealing because the stroma swells shut and they do not show a continued leak of aqueous when gently pressed with a microsponge. Therefore suturing is unnecessary, and the operation usually can proceed to conclusion if only one or two small perforations are present and the anterior chamber remains deep. Shortening the length of the knife blade is seldom necessary, assuming an initial accurate setting. Indeed, the surgeon must avoid overreacting and making the rest of the incisions too shallow.   *Continued.*

FIGURE 17-102, CONT'D

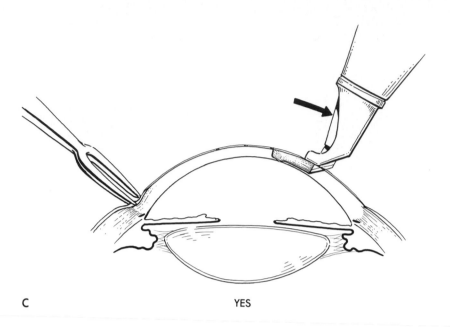

C   YES

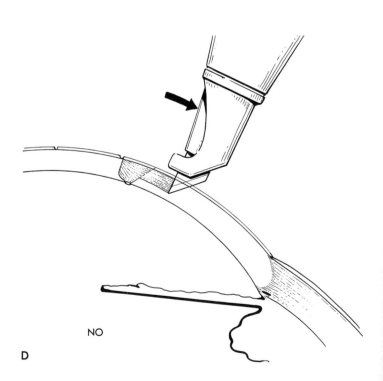

                                NO

                    D

C and **D,** The corneal surface is dried and the knife reinserted into the previously made portion of the incision with slightly less downward pressure. Sometimes reopening the wound with the knife blade causes aqueous to reappear around the tip of the blade through the previous perforation, and the surgeon must make a judgment about whether the knife is causing another perforation or the fluid is coming from the previous one—a difficult judgment indeed. Because the cornea is slightly swollen, the eye is softer, and the surgeon is cutting toward thicker cornea with a centrifugal incision, there is less likelihood that the perforation will be extended. Another strategy is to perform the remaining new incisions and then return to complete the perforated one at the end of the operation. The fixation instrument is reapplied with less pressure on the globe than previously to prevent forcing aqueous humor out of the perforation. However, enough pressure must be applied to make the globe reasonably firm to help make the remaining incisions at the original desired depth. If perforations occur on each of two successive incisions, the blade is clearly set too long and should be shortened 0.01 mm. Alternatively the blade can be checked on the blade gauge if the surgeon thinks the calibration is far off.

FIGURE 17-103   LARGE CORNEAL PERFORATION (MACROPERFORATION)

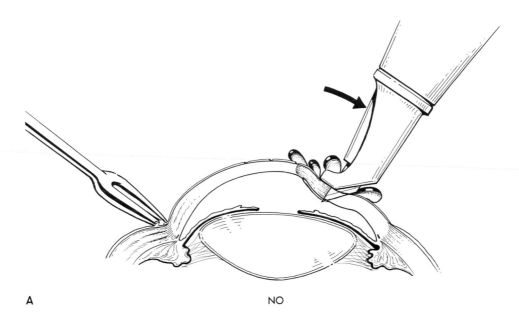

A   NO

Large corneal perforation (macroperforation). A, A large corneal perforation appears when the surgeon continues the incision after puncturing Descemet's membrane. This may occur because of a hurried and careless technique, inattention and failure to recognize the appearance of aqueous humor between the footplates, or mistaken identification of aqueous humor as only surface fluid. Immediately upon recognizing the perforation, the surgeon should stop the incision, remove the knife, and release the fixation instrument. The extent of the perforation is estimated by pressing gently adjacent to the wound with a microsponge.

Continuation of the incision in the face of shallowing of the anterior chamber can lacerate the iris and lens, causing secondary cataract.

FIGURE 17-103, CONT'D

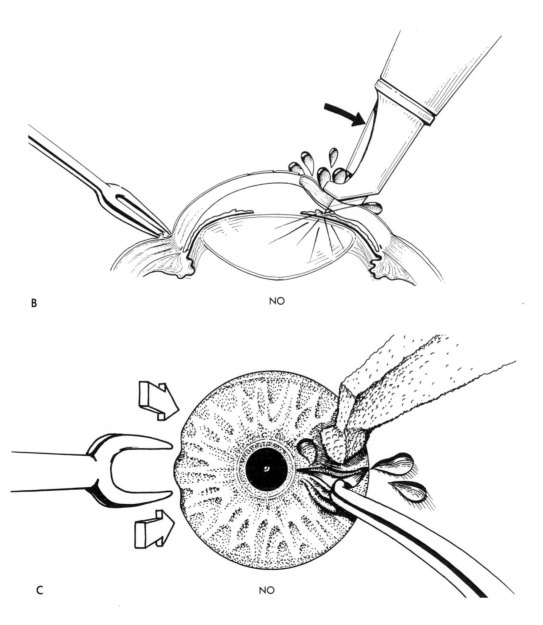

B   NO

C   NO

B, If the laceration is large enough, the anterior chamber becomes shallow. **C,** Wound manipulation should be minimized to prevent shallowing of the anterior chamber.

FIGURE 17-104   MANAGEMENT OF LARGE PERFORATION

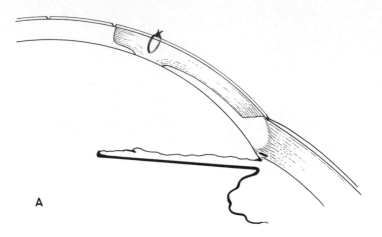

A

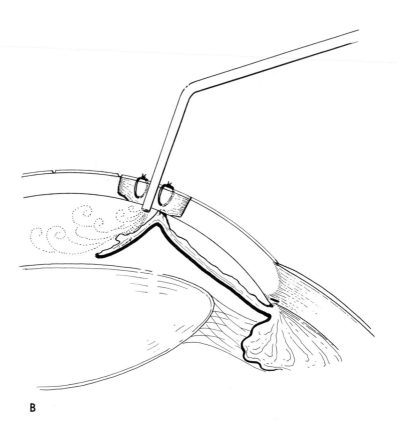

B

FIGURE 17-104, CONT'D

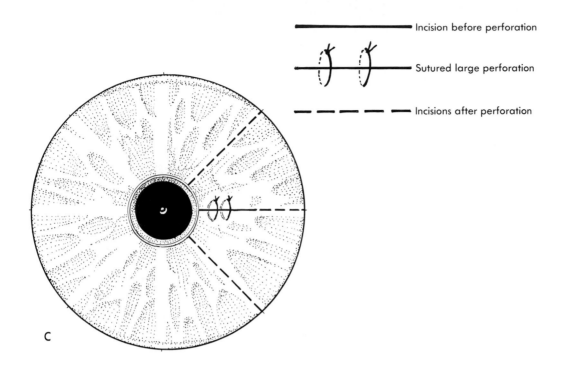

Management of large perforation. A, If a large corneal perforation has a contin-ued spontaneous leak of aqueous with shallowing of the anterior chamber or shows a brisk flow of aqueous from gentle pressure with a microsponge, the wound should be sutured as part of the operative procedure. This is preferable to trying to patch the eye or apply a soft contact lens in the hope that the wound will self-seal, only to be faced with a few days of continued leakage and a later secondary repair, as well as the twin dangers of endophthalmitis and epithelial ingrowth. Placement of two or three 10-0 nylon sutures on a compound curved needle with a straight needle holder accomplishes this. The sutures gently approximate the edges of the wound and need not be placed especially deep or tied especially tightly. **B,** If iris is adherent to the perforation or the anterior chamber is shallow, balanced salt solution can be injected. Injecting fluid in the anterior chamber is not, however, a routine part of managing corneal perforations. **C,** If the anterior chamber remains formed and the pressure in the eye is reasonably firm, it is possible to complete the operation by making the remaining incisions (*dotted lines*). However, if the anterior chamber is shallow and the eye is soft, the surgeon can deepen the chamber with balanced salt solution and complete the operation or can terminate the procedure after suturing and complete the operation a few weeks later. The sutures remain in place for 2 to 3 weeks, at which time they should be removed to minimize scarring.

PLATE 17-24: Verification of Incision Length and Contour
(Figs. 17-105 to 17-107)

Goals:

1. Manipulate the wounds minimally
2. Determine that all incisions are appropriate length
3. Identify suspected irregularities in the bed of the incision

FIGURE 17-105   CHECKING INCISION LENGTH

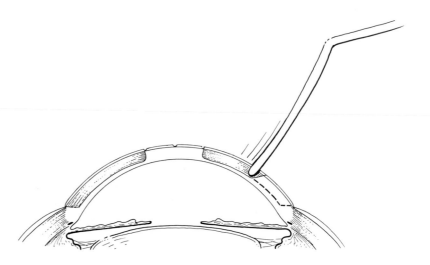

Checking incision length. Each incision should be made full length and depth. If the incisions have been made in a smooth, uncomplicated, routine manner without hesitation or complication, there is no need for inspection or manipulation of the wound. However, if there has been a known lifting of the blade or if joining the incisions in different zones has been irregular, the surgeon can inspect the wound and extend or revise it. Manipulation of the wound produces more stromal swelling and damage to the tissue.

A blunt instrument gently dipped into the incision and swept toward each end can verify the length. If the incision is too short, the knife can be reinserted and the wound lengthened on either end.

FIGURE 17-106   INSPECTION OF INCISION BED

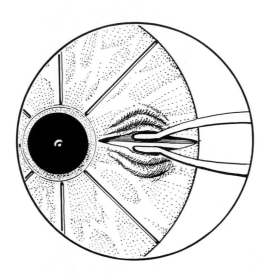

Inspection of incision bed. A wound spreader separates the edges of the incision and allows inspection by zooming the microscope to high power and focusing into the incision bed to identify stromal bridges or shallow areas that may need recutting. This maneuver is seldom used.

FIGURE 17-107   CHECKING INCISION DEPTH

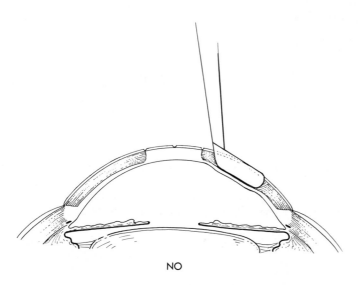

NO

Checking incision depth. There is no reliable way to measure the depth of a radial keratotomy incision intraoperatively. Dipsticks and calibrated gauges are inaccurate because they displace the posterior stromal tissue, do not account for stromal swelling, and are not calibrated in units fine enough to detect subtle variations in the depth of the wound. Therefore they are not useful in this surgery.

PLATE 17-25: Care of the Diamond Knife (Figs. 17-108 to 17-110)

Goals:

1. Prevent any damage to the knife blade during surgery
2. Clean the knife blade meticulously at the end of the operation before storing it

FIGURE 17-108   PROTECTING THE KNIFE BLADE

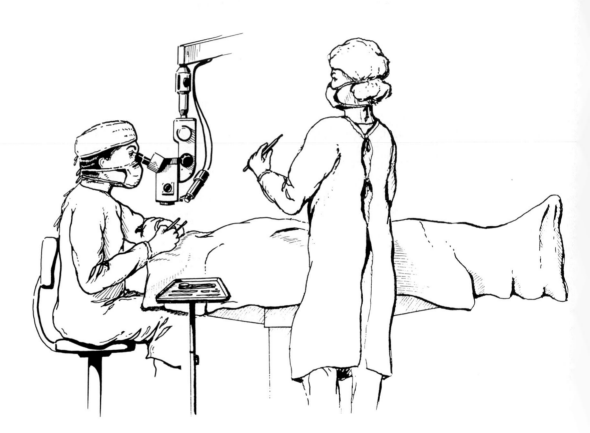

Protecting the knife blade. After the incisions are made, the surgeon may wish to readjust the knife blade or inspect the incisions. The nurse or assistant should hold the knife in the air paying full attention to the blade without doing anything else. A knife with an extended crystal blade should not be laid on the instrument tray.

FIGURE 17-109   CLEANING THE KNIFE BLADE   **631**

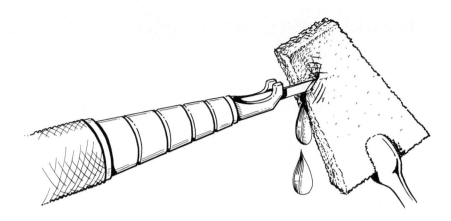

Cleaning the knife blade. Once all incisions have been completed and before irrigating the incisions, the surgeon cleans the knife blade. The blade is fully extended, and a microsponge soaked to saturation in hydrogen peroxide is used to clean the blade and footplates by wiping them and by stabbing the blade into the sponge and cutting the sponge, being careful not to hit the handle. A second sponge saturated with distilled water (balanced salt solution may cause precipitation of salt deposits on or in the knife) is used to wipe the blade and footplates. The blade is inspected under highest magnification. This should be done as quickly as possible after completing the last incision so that debris and fluid do not dry and adhere to the surface of the knife. Using this method can cause the blade to break at its base and the tip of a thin blade to fracture, so it must be performed cautiously. Alternatively, ultrasonic cleaning can be used, as discussed in Chapter 15, Surgical Instruments Used in Refractive Keratotomy.

FIGURE 17-110   RETRACTING THE KNIFE BLADE

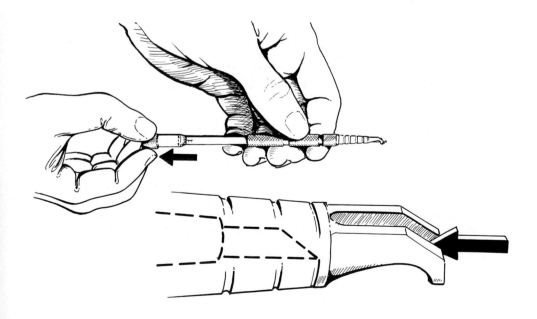

Retracting the knife blade. The surgeon should retract the knife blade into its protective barrel before passing the knife off the surgical field. Damage to the blade is more likely if the cleaning of the knife blade or its retraction is delegated to an assistant.

PLATE 17-26: Cleaning the Incisions (Figs. 17-111 to 17-113)

Goals:

1. Minimize the amount of blood that seeps into the wounds
2. Remove blood, epithelial cells, and foreign bodies from the wounds
3. Minimize corneal edema

FIGURE 17-111 CONTROL OF BLEEDING AT THE LIMBUS

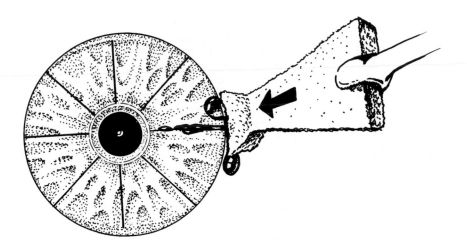

Control of bleeding at the limbus. If the limbal blood vessels are incised, blood will ooze into the incisions and be drawn centrally by capillary action. The surgeon should not stop the surgery to attend to this bleeding because it is more important to complete the sequence of incisions without corneal thinning or swelling. Deepening incisions can be made with blood in the wound.

Usually, by the time the remaining incisions are completed, the bleeding at the limbus has stopped spontaneously. If active bleeding persists, simple compression of the limbal vessels with the end of a microsponge or surgical instrument will stop the bleeding in a minute or so. Vasoconstrictors (naphthazoline or phenylephrine) are unnecessary.

In rare cases where the incision has been carried across the sclera, bleeding may persist. Topical vasoconstrictors may help slow this bleeding. Cautery should not be used in proximity to the cornea, but it could be used to stop conjunctival bleeding. All limbal bleeding must be stopped before irrigation of the wounds.

FIGURE 17-112   REPAIR OF EPITHELIAL ABRASION

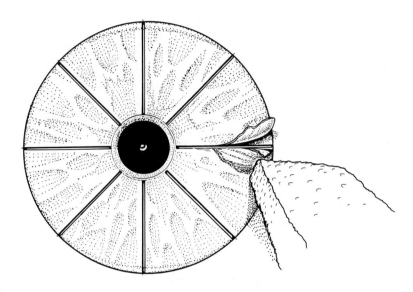

Repair of epithelial abrasion. If an epithelial abrasion occurs and a flap of epithelium is present adjacent to the wound, a moist microsponge can push it back down and recover the defect. If the epithelium has been ripped off completely, it should be left alone.

FIGURE 17-113   IRRIGATION OF INCISIONS

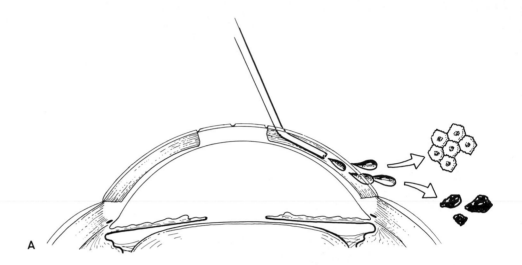

A

Irrigation of incisions. Irrigation of the incisions produces two effects: the desirable removal of foreign material and the undesirable increase in stromal edema, which may increase the amount of correction for a few days after surgery. Some surgeons think irrigation of the wounds increases the patient's pain after surgery. Therefore these effects must be balanced, using the minimal amount of fluid necessary to cleanse the wound, minimizing stromal edema. It is not possible to see fine debris or epithelial cells in the wound during surgery, but they certainly can show up after surgery as foreign bodies or epithelial cysts or pearls.

A, The surgeon irrigates with balanced salt solution using a small syringe or a squeeze bottle with a blunt 26- to 30-gauge cannula. The cannula tip is inserted parallel to the surface of the cornea, rather than perpendicular to the surface, to avoid forcing fluid into the stroma and in front of Descemet's membrane. **B** and **C,** Irrigation is directed from central to peripheral to avoid forcing fluid into the stroma of the clear zone and to wash any material away from the center.

FIGURE 17-113, CONT'D

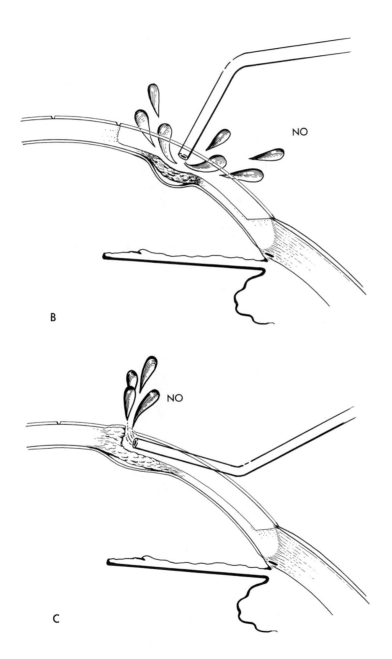

PLATE 17-27:   Concluding the Operation (Figs. 17-114 to 17-116)

Goals:

1. Administer antibiotic prophylaxis
2. Reassure the patient about the technical success of the procedure
3. Minimize pain after surgery

FIGURE 17-114   TOPICAL MEDICATION

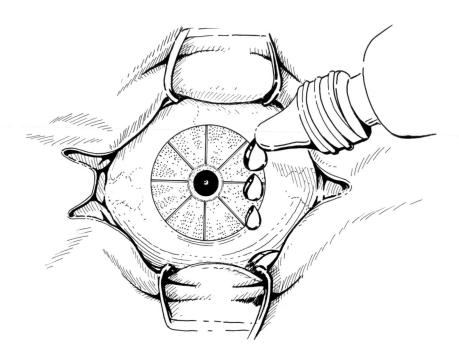

Topical medication. A reasonably broad-spectrum antibiotic should be flooded over the eye at the end of the operation, using a drug such as gentamicin, tobramycin, or neomycin-polymyxin-bacitracin.

If a corneal perforation has occurred, a loading dose of antibiotic to give a rapid high concentration in the corneal stromal and anterior chamber can be administered by flooding the surface of the eye continuously for 2 or 3 minutes while the lid speculum is still in place. This will produce antibiotic levels as high as or higher than those achieved by subconjunctival injection, although they may not last quite as long. Subconjunctival injection of gentamicin (20 mg), cefazolin (100 mg), or both is painful and the most unpleasant and memorable part of the operation for most patients. They are unnecessary.

The use of topical corticosteroids varies among surgeons, and there are no clear-cut guidelines. Steroids used acutely decrease stromal inflammation and slow early stromal wound healing.

FIGURE 17-115   UNNECESSARY ANCILLARY TREATMENTS

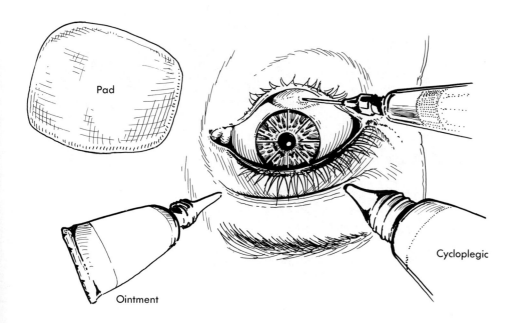

Unnecessary ancillary treatments. The routine use of subconjunctival antibiotics, mydriatic-cycloplegics, topical ointments, and eye pads is unnecessary after radial keratotomy. Mydriatics increase postoperative photophobia, and the cycloplegic effect is usually unnecessary because significant iridocyclitis is rare. Topical ointment may find its way into the incisions as fine, permanent droplets. A pressure patch often increases postoperative pain in an uncomplicated case and is applied only if a corneal perforation has occurred to aid in the sealing of the wound. The patient should be warned before the adhesive drapes are removed so that the pulling on the skin is neither startling nor unpleasant. A shield will provide protection and remind the patient to be careful of the eye.

FIGURE 17-116   REASSURANCE OF THE PATIENT AND RELIEF OF PAIN

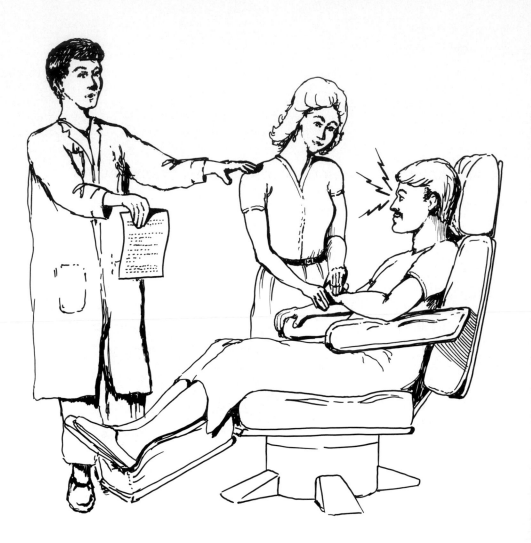

Reassurance of the patient and relief of pain. Communication with the patient during surgery varies widely among surgeons; some chatter throughout the case with banter and reassurance, whereas others remain virtually silent. Whichever approach is used, the surgeon should instill confidence in patients during the operation and reassure them about the technical success of the procedure at its conclusion. If complications have occurred, it is prudent to tell the patient about them at the end of the procedure because a well-informed patient will be more tolerant of postoperative difficulties than one who is kept guessing. Speaking with the patient's family and friends after surgery will also reduce anxiety.

A set of clearly written postoperative instructions, including a description of what to expect after surgery, medication, time and location of follow-up appointments, and emergency procedures should be given to the patient and reviewed verbally by the surgeon, nurse, or assistant.

Prophylactic topical antibiotics such as neomycin-bacitracin-polymyxin, or gentamicin should be used two to four times daily, commencing the day of surgery, for 5 to 7 days (unless the eye is patched). Some surgeons recommend topical hypertonic drops, such as 5% sodium chloride, to decrease edema and transient overcorrection.

Pain after radial keratotomy can be severe for 24 to 48 hours and should be the subject of careful discussion and planning between the surgeon and the patient. The patient should expect severe pain during the night after surgery. The surgeon should provide adequate oral analgesics every 4 hours, using schedule 2 narcotic drugs such as hydromorphone (Dilaudid) 2 mg or meperidine (Demerol) 50 mg or the less effective combination of oxycodone and aspirin (Percodan) one or two tablets. Because it is not possible to know which patients will have severe pain, using the narcotic agents routinely is preferable. There is no reason for the surgeon to withhold these narcotic agents for a short period of time, even though extra effort is required to dispense them. All these drugs may produce gastrointestinal upset. In general, acetaminophen (Tylenol) is inadequate to control pain after radial keratotomy, except in stoic patients. A sedative such as flurazepam (Dalmane) 30 mg will help the patient sleep better the first night or two after surgery. Patients can decrease photophobia by wearing a dark pair of sunglasses. Many patients quickly forget the severity of the pain and blithely tell their friends they had little discomfort.

REFERENCES

1. Ellis W: A textbook of radial keratotomy and astigmatism surgery, Irvine, Calif, 1986, Terry & Associates.
2. Haverbeke L: Personal written communication, September 1987.
3. Jordan A and Baum J: Basic tear flow, Ophthalmology 1980;87:923.
4. Lewicky AO: Surgical technique and related complication. In Sanders DR, Hofmann RF, and Salz JJ, editors: Refractive corneal surgery, Thorofare, NJ, 1986, Slack, Inc, pp 163-196.
5. Mendelsohn AD: Personal written communication, August 1987.
6. Mendelsohn AD, Parel JM, Dennis JJ, Gelender H, Forster RK, and Ullman S: Intraocular pressure during radial keratotomy, J Refract Surg 1987;3:79-86.
6a. Merlin V, Bordin P, Rimondi AP, and Schirollo R: Factors that affect keratotomy depth, Refract Corneal Surg (in press).
7. Sanders DR and Hofmann RF, editors: Refractive surgery: a text of radial keratotomy, Thorofare, NJ, 1985, Slack, Inc.
8. Sanders DR, editor: Radial keratotomy—surgical techniques, Thorofare, NJ, 1986, Slack, Inc.
9. Schachar RA, Black TD, and Wang T: Understanding radial keratotomy, Denison, Tex, 1981, LAL Publishing, pp 52-66.
10. Waring GO, Moffitt SD, Gelender H, et al: Rationale for and design of the National Eye Institute Prospective Evaluation of Radial Keratotomy (PERK) study, Ophthalmology 1983;90:40-58.

Repeated Surgery for Residual Myopia and Hyperopia after Refractive Corneal Surgery

George O. Waring III

Unfortunately the outcome of primary refractive keratotomy does not always meet the goals of the patient or the surgeon; a considerable number of individuals remain unacceptably myopic, become hyperopic, have increased regular astigmatism, or develop irregular astigmatism. The same may happen to patients who have had lamellar refractive surgery such as keratomileusis and epikeratoplasty. These individuals are candidates for further corneal surgery. In contrast to the enormous literature on primary radial and astigmatic keratotomy, a dearth of laboratory and clinical data about repeated keratotomy and other types of secondary corneal surgery has left numerous questions unanswered. Should refractive keratotomy be done as an intentionally staged series of procedures? Should surgery for residual myopia have the incisions placed between or within the original ones? What surgical techniques are available for managing overcorrections? How reliable are lamellar or penetrating surgical techniques for man-

BACKGROUND AND ACKNOWLEDGMENTS

The information on repeated keratotomy and other corneal operations after primary refractive keratotomy comes largely from the published literature. Edward R. Rashid, MD, compiled the information on penetrating keratoplasty, epikeratoplasty, and myopic keratomileusis. Information from the PERK study was provided by the PERK clinical and statistical coordinating centers at Emory University.[6] Kevin H. Charlton, MD, provided unpublished data on the technique of spreading and recutting incisions. Marguerite McDonald, MD, provided information on an unpublished series of epikeratoplasty procedures after radial keratotomy. Richard ·Damiano, MD, and Lance Forstot, MD, provided unpublished information on purse-string sutures for overcorrected radial keratotomy.

agement of residual ametropia or irregular astigmatism? I draw on the few published studies and the personal experience of a number of surgeons to address these and other questions.

CLASSIFICATION AND TERMINOLOGY

There are four types of secondary operations that are done after an initial refractive keratotomy. The first is another keratotomy in an undercorrected eye to further decrease the myopia. I use the term "repeated keratotomy"—and its synonyms, "repeat operation," "reoperation," "second operation"—to mean the placement of additional corneal incisions to decrease residual myopia or astigmatism. (Surgery for residual astigmatism is discussed in Chapter 31, Keratotomy for Astigmatism.) The second type of secondary operation is opening and suturing the wounds ("wound revision") to reduce an overcorrection. The third type is a lamellar refractive keratoplasty (keratomileusis, epikeratoplasty) or penetrating keratoplasty to correct residual ametropia, irregular astigmatism, or both. The fourth type is an operation to repair a structural defect, such as suturing a large perforation (see Chapter 23, Complications of Refractive Keratotomy). I discuss the first three types in this chapter.

ROLE OF REPEATED KERATOTOMY IN CLINICAL SERIES

Reports of clinical studies of keratotomy should indicate clearly the number of eyes that required repeated surgery to achieve the results reported. A series with good results and no repeated operations is quite different than a series in which 30% of the eyes required repeated surgery. For example, in the PERK study the major reported results at 1, 3, and 4 years excluded eyes that had repeated keratotomy because of the desire to identify clearly the result of a single, uniform surgical procedure.[33,34] The results of eyes that had repeated keratotomy were reported separately.[6] The number of repeated operations in other reported series varies greatly, as discussed in Chapter 21, Published Results of Refractive Keratotomy.

STAGING KERATOTOMY SURGERY

There are three ways in which repeated operations for residual myopia come about after an initial keratotomy: (1) the surgeon intends for the first operation to correct the refractive error completely and therefore does "maximum" appropriate surgery, but a resulting undercorrection leads to a second operation[6,8,10,29]; (2) the surgeon purposefully uses less than the maximum appropriate amount of surgery to correct the entire refractive error, leaving some room for further surgery, such as in the use of four initial incisions fol-

lowed by a second set of four incisions in between the previous ones[24]; and (3) the surgeon intends to perform a sequence of operations (staged procedure), as might occur with the use of only radial incisions to correct compound myopic astigmatism, followed later by the use of transverse incisions for the residual astigmatism. There are no published studies of intentionally staged keratotomy.

Staged procedures deserve consideration because the outcome of radial keratotomy is fairly unpredictable (see Chapter 13, Predictability of Refractive Keratotomy), making it desirable to plan for a sequence of operations to fine-tune the final result. Thus an eye with a refraction of $-4.50 -1.75 \times 180°$ might have three operations, the first consisting of four incisions to decrease the myopia and to see what happens to the astigmatism, the second placing transverse incisions to reduce the residual astigmatism, and the third making more radial incisions if myopia persists. The disadvantages are obvious: multiple operations with their inherent chance of complications, increased corneal scarring, prolonged time to achieve the final outcome, increased inconvenience and morbidity for the patient, increased time and work for the surgeon, and increased expense for the patient who may have to pay multiple operating room charges. However, if progressively adjustable surgery can achieve an ideal result, these disadvantages become more acceptable.

Salz and colleagues[24] extolled the virtues of staging surgery in low-to-moderate myopes, performing an initial four incisions, then observing the eyes for a response, adding an additional four incisions or transverse incisions as necessary. They noted, "This staging concept allowed us to increase the percentage of eyes 20/40 or better from 64% to 90% and to improve the percentage of eyes within one diopter of ametropia from 71% to 93% without increasing our rate of overcorrection."

PATIENT SELECTION

Selection of patients for repeated keratotomy is a more subjective and idiosyncratic process than selection of patients for an initial refractive keratotomy (see Chapter 12, Examination and Selection of Patients for Refractive Keratotomy), since the patient's subjective satisfaction with the results of the first surgery is more important than are the objective criteria of refraction or visual acuity in electing additional surgery. For example, a residual refractive error of -2.00 D with an uncorrected visual acuity of 20/50 might be perfectly acceptable to someone who wanted radial keratotomy for the convenience of recreation and athletics but might be intolerable to an individual who was seeking a job that required 20/40. Surgeons differ greatly in their threshold for doing repeated operations, some thinking that a single keratotomy per eye is enough, others reoperating two or three times in an attempt to fine-tune the surgery and achieve a more perfect result.

It is difficult to enunciate specific guidelines for repeated keratotomy, but some principles are clear. Patients must have an especially thorough understanding of the hazards of repeated surgery: increased corneal scarring, glare and fluctuating vision, and overcorrection with early symptomatic presbyopia. Special caution should be exercised in patients with undercorrections of -1.00 to -2.00 D because repeated surgery is more likely to make them hyperopic. Patients with 16 incisions should not have additional incisions. Repeated radial keratotomy can be offered to dissatisfied patients who have an undercorrection of approximately -2 D or more and no specific contraindication because they have a reasonably good chance of improved visual acuity. Patients with a 3-mm diameter clear zone should not have their incisions extended centrally. Patients who already have persistent glare, fluctuating vision, or significant irregular astigmatism should not have further keratotomy. Patients who are fully corrected in one eye and are undercorrected in the other might forego repeated keratotomy in the undercorrected eye, saving it for reading without correction after the onset of presbyopia. Patients with overcorrection who insist on achieving a good result through keratotomy have little alternative but to have some type of suturing of the wounds.

Lamellar refractive keratoplasty and penetrating keratoplasty should be reserved for individuals who experience functional disability from the results of the keratotomy surgery.

I think the cost of repeated keratotomy should be covered by the initial surgeon's fee, to be fair to the patient and to decrease the surgeon's financial incentive to keep operating.

TIMING OF ADDITIONAL SURGERY

There are no studies on which to base opinions about the timing of reoperations, and the matter resolves into two philosophies. The first is to consider an eye that is undercorrected a few weeks after surgery as a surgical failure that needs repair. For example, if the preoperative refraction was -4.00 D and 2 to 4 weeks after surgery the refraction is -2.00 D, it is unlikely that more of the residual myopia will spontaneously disappear. If the surgeon can identify an aspect of the procedure that explains the undercorrection, such as too large a clear zone or too shallow incisions, the decision to reoperate then by spreading the wounds and incising them more deeply or extending them into a smaller clear zone makes good sense. It is easier to

open the wounds in the early preoperative period because they are still full of the epithelial plug. Alternatively, an additional set of incisions could be made.

The second approach is to wait 3 months until most of the postoperative changes from early wound healing have passed and the final result is more reasonably approximated. At this point, patients have had a chance to live with their undercorrection for a while, to see what the functional acuity is, and to experience more stable vision. This approach makes sense if the incisions seem to be the proper length and depth.

Timing of repeated keratotomy for residual myopia or astigmatism

Villasenor and Cox[29] reported a tendency to greater effect from the reoperation when it was done 9 months or more after the original surgery than when it was done before that time. The protocol for the PERK study required that at least 6 months elapse after the initial operation.[6] Of 59 patients meeting this criterion, the time between the initial operation and the repeated operation was 6 to 9 months for 63%, 10 to 19 months for 30%, and 25 to 29 months for 7%.

Timing of wound revision for induced hyperopia

Surgery for hyperopia probably should be performed as soon as it is apparent a marked overcorrection has occurred. Conceptually the surgery aims to revise the wounds, and this is most easily done before they are in an advanced stage of healing. Yet, enough time must be allowed to judge the amount of the overcorrection, so the surgery is optimally done 1 to 3 months after the initial surgery, although it can be performed at any time thereafter.

Timing of lamellar and penetrating keratoplasty

Since these operations require cutting through the initial incisions, the more healed the incisions are the less likely they are to splay apart and the more likely is the result from the new surgery to be stable. Furthermore, many months must pass before the patient can exhibit enough disability to warrant such major surgical intervention. Usually, a year or more passes before keratoplasty is performed.

SURGICAL PLAN FOR REPEATED OPERATIONS

Ideally the surgeon should be able to examine the cornea of an undercorrected patient and determine the reason for the undercorrection. If the incisions were too shallow, they can be deepened; if the clear zone was too large, it can be made smaller by extending the original incisions; if the depth of the incisions and the clear zone size were ideal, additional incisions can be added between the original ones. The logic of this approach is fine, its implementation difficult. Some patients appear to have had a technically adequate radial keratotomy, yet they remain undercorrected, presumably because of some inherent property of their corneas. It is not possible to differentiate clearly the relative effects of the clear zone diameter, the depth of incision, and the number of incisions, so the surgeon must arbitrarily choose which of these variables to adjust in the repeated operation. Finally, the surgeons' own preferences hold sway in the surgical plan, depending on whether they favor reworking the initial incisions or making additional ones.

Predicting the outcome of repeated radial keratotomy is more difficult than predicting the outcome of a primary procedure because the biomechanics of the cornea have been changed by the initial incisions, because there is a paucity of thorough studies to provide guidance, because most surgeons have less experience with reoperations than with initial operations, and because the effect of patient variables such as age or intraocular pressure is not as clear in repeated operations. Therefore it is not possible to create a ratio between the effect of the initial operation and the effect of the repeated operation; that is, the surgeon cannot state that "eight more incisions will give 20% more effect" or "deepening the paracentral part of the incision adds one diopter of effect." There is too much scatter and unpredictability of results for these generalities to be reliable.[6]

There is a detailed discussion of the factors that affect the outcome in Chapter 13, Predictability of Refractive Keratotomy, and Chapter 14, Computerized Predictability Formulas for Refractive Keratotomy.

Diameter of clear zone

Because undercorrection is most common in individuals with larger amounts of myopia (those who have had a 3.0-mm diameter clear zone), making the clear zone smaller is not usually an option, since this will increase the danger of glare and irregular astigmatism. For example, of 59 eyes in the PERK study that had a repeated radial keratotomy, the initial clear zone diameter was 3.0 mm in 66%, 3.5 mm in 29%, and 4.0 mm in 5%. In cases in which the initial clear zone was larger than 3 mm, the initial incisions can be extended centrally or the repeated incisions can be extended to the edge of a new 3-mm clear zone,[1,18,25] to enhance the effect.

Number of incisions

The cumulative effect of increasing the number of incisions drops dramatically after eight.[30,31] In a cor-

nea that has had four initial incisions, four more incisions may enhance the effect measurably[24,26]; a cornea with eight incisions will usually show less response to eight additional ones than to the eight initial ones. I never make more than 16 radial incisions.

Depth and profile of initial incisions

Deeper incisions cause more central corneal flattening.[30,31] Theoretically, repeated operations in eyes with initially shallow incisions should have a greater effect than in eyes with initially deep incisions, presumably because the repeated deeper incisions will cut collagen fibrils that had remained intact, further weakening the cornea. This generality is difficult to implement in practice, because it is difficult to measure the depth of the incisions and their profile accurately. Subjective estimation by visual inspection is an unreliable method because one surgeon's 80% depth is another surgeon's 95% depth. Nevertheless, there are incisions that are obviously shallow along their entire length or that are tapered rather than squared off adjacent to the clear zone, and it seems reasonable to revise these incisions or to add incisions between them.

Depth of incisions. Published studies of the effect of the depth of the initial incisions on the outcome of repeated keratotomy have given conflicting results. Cowden and Weber[7] published a study of repeated radial keratotomy in monkeys, adding eight incisions

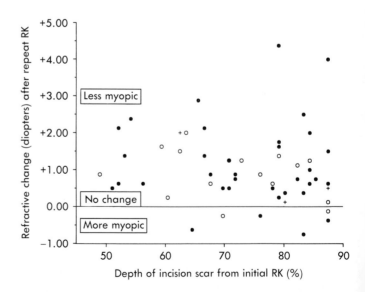

Figure 18-1
Scattergram demonstrates no relationship between the depth of the incision scar resulting from the initial radial keratotomy *(RK)* and the change in refraction after the repeated radial keratotomy (8 + 8 incisions) in the PERK study. Symbols indicate the clear zone groups (plus, 4.0 mm; open circle, 3.5 mm; solid circle, 3.0 mm). (From Cowden JW, Lynn MJ, Waring GO, et al: Am J Ophthalmol 1987;103:423-431.)

between the eight initial ones, and observed that the greatest effect was achieved in eyes with shallower incisions in the initial operation. Villasenor and Cox[29] observed that adding four or eight incisions to six eyes with shallow initial incisions of less than 70% depth produced a mean additional reduction in myopia of 2.16 D (range, 0.50 to 3.75 D), whereas the same procedures in 30 eyes with initially deep incisions produced a mean change of only 0.78 D (range, −1.50 to 3.00 D). Hofmann[10] thought the effect of repeated keratotomy was less in eyes that had good initial depth and length of the incisions.

In contrast, analysis of repeated operations in 62 eyes in the PERK study that received eight additional incisions between the initial eight incisions showed no relationship between the depth of the initial incisions and the change after the repeated operation[6] (Fig. 18-1). The PERK study measured the depth of the incisions by visual inspection with the slit-lamp microscope and graded them in quartiles of corneal thickness (0% to 25%, 26% to 50%, 51% to 75%, and 76% to 100%). Thus an incision that appeared 78% deep was graded in the same category as one that perforated. This method of measurement probably obscured some of the effect of depth of the incisions; this may account for the discrepancy between the findings of the PERK study and the others cited.

Configuration of incisions. Most surgeons think the depth and configuration of the paracentral part of the incision is the most important. The configuration of the incisions in that area differs with different styles of knife blades and surgical techniques: single-edged angled blades passed centrifugally tend to cut a sloping end; double-edged vertical blades passed centripetally tend to cut a square end[8] (see Chapter 17, Atlas of Surgical Techniques of Radial Keratotomy). Wounds that are sloping and shallow paracentrally can be squared off and made deeper with a second operation.

Direction of incision

Deciding whether to cut centrifugally or centripetally during the repeated operation is done on the same basis as for the initial operation (see Chapter 17, Atlas of Surgical Techniques of Radial Keratotomy) and is based on the surgeon's preference, knife style, and surgical technique. For knives with the same blade length, a vertical blade passed centripetally cuts deeper than an angled blade passed centrifugally.

Overall guidelines for repeated keratotomy for residual myopia or astigmatism

Because the techniques used for repeated operations are more idiosyncratic than those for initial keratotomy, generalities are difficult. Achieving a greater

depth and better configuration of the original incisions is a matter of surgical artistry[15] but may be the most effective way of further decreasing myopia because it severs collagen fibrils deeper in the original wound and because it does not add more scar to the cornea. Increasing the number of incisions, particularly if the initial number is four, has been demonstrated to improve the results, although the outcome is not predictable in an individual case. Reducing the diameter of the clear zone to the minimum 3 mm should also enhance the effect if the previous clear zone is larger than that. The patient's age has a less clear-cut relationship to repeated operations than to initial operations, but older patients presumably get more effect. Eyes that already have a 3-mm diameter of clear zone, 16 incisions, and a uniform incision depth greater than 80% probably should not have a repeated keratotomy.

TECHNIQUES OF REPEATED KERATOTOMY FOR RESIDUAL MYOPIA

In this and the succeeding sections, I describe the surgical techniques for repeated corneal surgery (Fig. 18-2) and the published results for each type of technique. The preoperative management, preparation, and draping of the patient is similar to that for an initial operation (Fig. 18-3) (see Chapter 17, Atlas of Surgical Techniques of Radial Keratotomy).

Hofmann[10] reported on repeated operations in 38 patients, which was approximately 4.5% of a series of 820 radial keratotomy operations. The most common technique was to use additional radial incisions between the initial ones or to add transverse incisions.

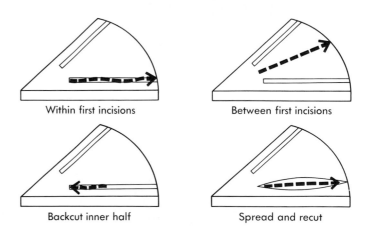

Within first incisions   Between first incisions

Backcut inner half   Spread and recut

Figure 18-2
Four techniques of repeated radial keratotomy. Upper left: recutting initial incisions (not currently in use). Upper right: additional incisions between initial incisions. Lower left: centripetal recutting of the inner portion of the incision. Lower right: spreading of the incision followed by recutting.

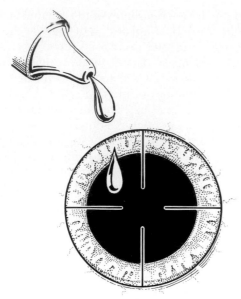

Figure 18-3
Dilation of the pupil increases the visibility of the initial incisions against the red fundus reflection, but also increases the patient's light sensitivity during surgery and exposes the lens to direct damage in the event of a perforation.

Attempts to deepen the original incisions or to decrease the diameter of the clear zone were also carried out. Purse-string sutures were performed in a series of overcorrected eyes. Hofmann emphasized the unpredictability of repeated keratotomy, observing that three eyes in his series actually had an *increase* in myopia. He preferred the techniques of deepening the incisions. Case reports that illustrate the spectrum of results from repeated keratotomy are presented in the box on pp. 650 and 651.

Repeated incisions between initial incisions

This technique simply involves performing a second radial keratotomy. The most difficult part is alignment of the incisions, including recentering the clear zone marker and placing the incisions equidistantly between the initial ones (Figs. 18-4 to 18-7). The technique for making the incisions may be the same one used for the initial operation or may involve efforts to achieve deeper, squared-off incisions (centripetal direction, deepening incisions). I do not make more than 16 total incisions (Fig. 18-8).

Repeated radial keratotomy in PERK study. The most extensive results of repeated operations using a

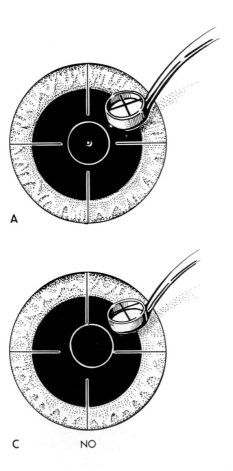

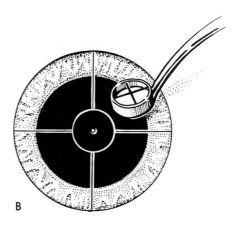

Figure 18-4
Placing the clear zone mark. **A,** The centering mark and clear zone mark are centered over the entrance pupil, as in the initial procedure. If the initial incisions are not properly centered around the entrance pupil, the new clear zone mark should be properly centered. The diameter of the new clear zone depends on the surgical plan, but it can be smaller than the initial one to increase the effect of the repeated operation **(A)** or the same size **(B).** It should not be decentered **(C)** unless the previous incisions are quite eccentric.

second set of incisions placed between the first were reported by Cowden and colleagues[6] in 59 eyes from the PERK study. The surgical technique for the repeated operation was the same as that for the initial operation: eight centrifugal incisions, the same diameter of the central clear zone, and the setting of the blade at 100% of the thinnest of four intraoperative ultrasonic pachometry readings taken adjacent to the clear zone mark. The authors studied one eye of each patient who received a reoperation 6 to 29 months after the initial one. The patients were followed an average of 26 months.

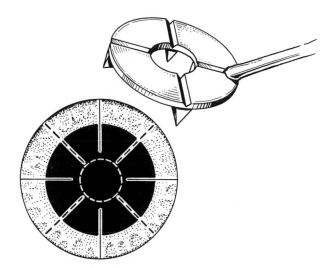

Figure 18-5
A radial marker is often necessary to guide the placement of the new incisions equidistant between the faintly visible initial ones. Alternatively the knife can be visually aligned to bisect the previous incisions. This is easier when beginning the incision adjacent to the clear zone because the size of the footplates can be spaced just adjacent to the ends of the initial incision. It is more difficult to make this alignment when starting at the limbus.

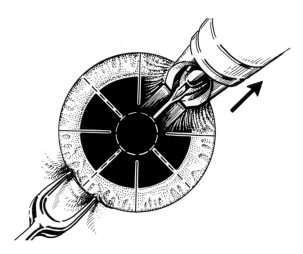

Figure 18-6
The technique for making the additional incisions is identical to that for the initial ones, whether made centrifugally (as illustrated here) or centripetally.

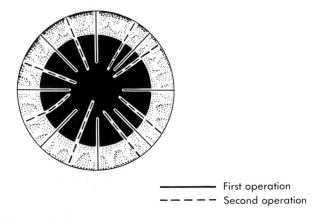

First operation
Second operation

Figure 18-7
Irregular placement of the second set of incisions is more likely to create irregular astigmatism and glare, particularly oblique placement and extension into the clear zone.

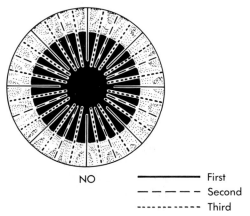

NO   First
Second
Third

Figure 18-8
A third operation is seldom indicated. Avoid more than 16 total incisions.

Most eyes became less myopic after the reoperation (Fig. 18-9). The average change in refraction was a reduction in myopia of 1.09 D (SD, 1.05) (Table 18-1). Twenty percent of the eyes changed by less than half a diopter—interpreted as no effect, a much higher number than expected. Two of the eyes actually became more myopic. In general, patients' eyes were still undercorrected after the repeated operation (Table 18-2); 46% of the eyes had a refractive error of between +0.12 and −1.00 D. Overcorrections were infrequent; only two eyes (3%) were overcorrected by more than one D.

For the majority of the eyes, there was less change in refraction after the reoperation than after the initial operation (Fig. 18-10), but there was no consistent correlation between the two (R, 0.04). Therefore the authors could not predict the result of a reoperation as a fixed percentage of the change in refraction achieved

Table 18-1

Change in the Spherical Equivalent of the Cycloplegic Refraction after Repeated Radial Keratotomy: Eight Initial and Eight Additional Incisions in the PERK Study

Change in refraction (D)	No. of eyes	Percentage
Decrease in myopia		
0.50 to 0.87	18	31
1.00 to 1.87	15	26
2.00 to 2.87	9	15
3.00 to 4.37	3	5
Change <0.50	12	20
Increase in myopia		
0.50 to 0.75	2	3
Total	59	100

From Cowden JW, Lynn MJ, Waring GO, and the PERK Study Group: Am J Ophthalmol 1987;103:423-431.

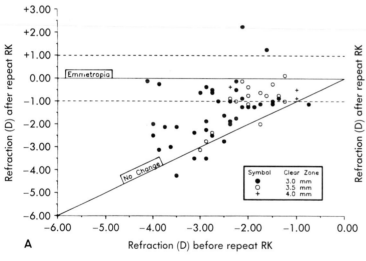

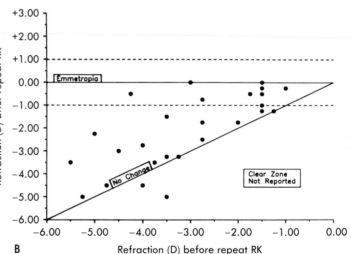

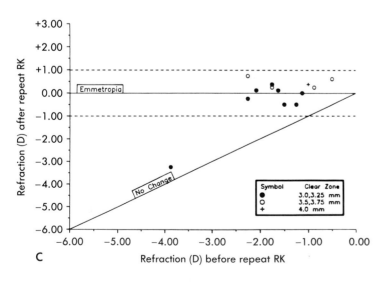

Figure 18-9

Outcome of repeated radial keratotomy in three studies. The desired outcome was emmetropia. **A,** In the PERK study 46% of 59 eyes had a residual refractive error of +0.12 to −1.00 after eight-incision repeated radial keratotomy. Two eyes were overcorrected more than 1 D. Twenty percent had essentially no change after the second set of eight incisions. There was considerable scatter in the results. **B,** Villasenor[28] reported that 50% of 26 eyes got less than 1.00 D of effect from the reoperation (eight-incision radial keratotomy) and 30% fell within ±1.00 D. **C,** Salz and colleagues[24] reported that 12 of 13 eyes fell within ±1.00 D after repeated four-incision radial keratotomy. (**A** from Cowden JW, Lynn MJ, Waring GO, et al: Am J Ophthalmol 1987;103:423-431.)

Table 18-2

Spherical Equivalent of the Cycloplegic Refraction after Repeated Radial Keratotomy: Eight Initial and Eight Additional Incisions in the PERK Study

Refractive error (D)	No. of eyes	Percentage
+1.25 and +2.25	2	3
−0.50 to +0.125	12	21
−0.62 to −1.00	15	25
−1.12 to −2.00	15	25
−2.12 to −3.00	10	17
−3.12 to −4.25	5	9
Total	59	100

From Cowden JE, Lynn MJ, Waring GO, and the PERK Study Group: Am J Ophthalmol 1987;103:423-431.

Table 18-3

Change in Uncorrected Visual Acuity after Repeated Radial Keratotomy: Eight Initial and Eight Additional Incisions in the PERK Study

Change in visual acuity (Snellen lines)	No. of eyes	Percentage
Increase		
2 to 3 lines	16	27
4 to 5 lines	12	20
6 to 7 lines	9	15
8 to 9 lines	8	14
Change ≤ 1 line	13	22
Decrease 3 lines	1	2
Total	59	100

From Cowden JW, Lynn MJ, Waring GO, and the PERK Study Group: Am J Ophthalmol 1987;103:423-431.

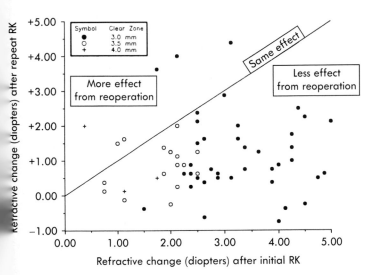

Figure 18-10

Comparison of the change induced by the initial eight incisions and the repeated eight incisions in the PERK study. The vast majority of eyes got less effect from the second set of eight incisions, but no fixed percentage of the initial results could be determined. (From Cowden JW, Lynn MJ, Waring GO, et al: Am J Ophthalmol 1987;103:423-431.)

Table 18-4

Uncorrected Visual Acuity after Repeated Radial Keratotomy: Eight Initial and Eight Additional Incisions in the PERK Study

Uncorrected visual acuity (Snellen lines)	No. of eyes	Percentage
Increase		
20/10 to 20/20	15	25
20/25 to 20/40	23	39
20/50 to 20/160	20	34
20/200 or worse	1	2
Total	59	100

From Cowden JW, Lynn MJ, Waring GO, and the PERK Study Group: Am J Ophthalmol 1987;103:423-431.

by the initial operation. The finding of less effect from the reoperation has been reported by others and is consistent with the observation that most of the effect of a radial keratotomy is achieved with the first few incisions.

The uncorrected visual acuity improved for most patients after the reoperation (Tables 18-3 and 18-4); 70% of the patients gained from two to nine Snellen lines, 64% of them seeing 20/40 or better without cor-

rection after the reoperation, in contrast to only 5% before the reoperation.

The PERK study also found a general lack of correlation between the change in refraction after reoperation and other variables: depth of initial incision scars (R = −0.08) (see Fig. 18-4), depth of repeated incision scars (R = 0.15), diameter of clear zone (p = 0.5), patient age (R = −0.01), central keratometry (R = 0.002), baseline intraocular pressure (R =

Case Reports of Repeated Radial Keratotomies

Case 1: Two repeated keratotomies with a "perfect" result

A 38-year-old woman wore contact lenses for many years to manage her myopia, but keratoconjunctivitis sicca developed and her eyes became intolerant of contact lenses despite vigorous artificial tear therapy and punctal occlusion. Details of her ophthalmic history and her radial keratotomy surgery from her first physician are not complete, but her refraction in the left eye was approximately $-5.00 +1.00 \times 90°$, giving a visual acuity of 20/20. She had an initial radial keratotomy on September 19, 1988, with eight centrifugal incisions using a 3.5-mm clear zone, which left her undercorrected. To manage this, 9 days later later the surgeon opened and deepened the wounds, making centrifugal incisions and extending the clear zone from 3.5 to 3.0 mm.

When the patient was seen at the Emory Eye Center in consultation on November 10, 1988, the refraction in the left eye was $-4.00 +1.50 \times 80°$ and slit-lamp microscopy showed the depth of the incisions to range from 10% to 75%, an average of approximately 50%. Therefore, 2 months after the initial operation, a second repeated radial keratotomy was performed, opening all eight wounds with a blunt intraocular lens hook, cleaning out the epithelial plug, and using a vertically bladed back-cutting knife with the blade set at 95% of the thinnest paracentral corneal thickness reading to make centripetal deepening incisions within the bed of the previous incisions up to a clear zone mark of 3 mm. There were no complications, and 6 months after this operation, her manifest refraction was $-0.25 +0.50 \times 65°$.

Comment: This case emphasizes three points: (1) the importance of the depth of incision in achieving the desired outcome, (2) the difficulty of using an oblique front-cutting knife passed centrifugally to achieve good deepening of previously made incisions, and (3) that this technique can be repeated more than once—sometimes with ideal results.

Case 2: Repeated radial keratotomy with induction of hyperopic astigmatism

A 35-year-old man enrolled in the PERK study in 1981. His visual acuity was 20/16 in each eye, with his cycloplegic refraction of $-4.25 +1.25 \times 29°$ and $-5.25 +1.25 \times 130°$. Keratometry readings were $42.75 \times 135°/43.62 \times 131°$, right eye and $42.87 \times 30°/44.12 \times 115°$, left eye. Surgery was done on the left eye. According to PERK protocol, eight centrifugal radial incisions were made with a 3.0-mm clear zone and the blade set at 100% of paracental corneal thickness. There were no complications.

One year postoperatively, the uncorrected visual acuity of the left eye was 20/100. The visual acuity was 20/12 with the patient's cycloplegic refraction of $-3.25 +1.25 \times 135°$. In 1985, 3 years postoperatively, the refraction was unchanged. At that time a reoperation was performed. Eight centrifugal incisions were placed between the initial incisions, using the angled front-cutting PERK knife and a 3.0-mm diameter clear zone. The incision depth was 100% of the thinnest paracentral pachometry reading. In 1988, 2½ years after the reoperation, the patient's uncorrected visual acuity was 20/30. His visual acuity was 20/20 with the cycloplegic refraction $+0.75 +2.50 \times 145°$. The keratometry readings were $36.50 \times 142°/38.37 \times 25°$.

Comment: The repeated operation decreased the spherical component of the refraction by 4.00 D, but increased the cylinder by 1.25 D. The +2.00 D spherical equivalent overcorrection was compatible with 20/30 acuity for this 42-year-old man, and he wore no distance optical correction, but required reading glasses.

Case Reports of Repeated Radial Keratotomies

Case 3: Residual myopia after two repeated keratotomies

A 21-year-old college student, intolerant of contact lenses, had a cycloplegic refraction in the right eye of −6.50 sphere, 20/20, and in the left eye of −6.75 sphere, 20/20. His keratometry readings were 42.75 × 165°/42.87 × 75° in the right eye and 42.37 × 95°/42.50 × 02° in the left. A radial keratotomy was performed on the left eye in August 1987 using eight centripetal incisions, a 3-mm clear zone, and a blade extension of 95% of the thinnest paracentral corneal thickness reading.

Two weeks postoperatively, his uncorrected visual acuity was 20/20, with a manifest refraction of −1.00 sphere. Keratometry readings were 40.25/40.25 D. Three months after surgery, the manifest refraction was −2.50 +0.50 × 115° (keratometry readings, 40.25 × 05°/40.75 × 95°) and, because the incisions were 75% to 80% deep, all incisions were opened and their depth was increased using centripetal cuts with the knife blade at 100% of paracentral thickness.

Approximately 2 weeks postoperatively, the acuity of the left eye was 20/30, with a refraction of −1.25 +1.75 × 94°. Three months after the repeated operation, the uncorrected visual acuity was 20/80 and the refractive error was −2.75 +0.75 × 138°. Keratometry readings were 39.75 × 60°/40.12 × 150°. In June 1988, 6 months after the repeated deepening keratotomies, eight additional centripetal radial incisions were placed between the previous eight using a 3-mm clear zone and a knife blade extension of the thinnest paracentral pachometry. One day postoperatively, the uncorrected visual acuity was 20/20. His refraction was −1.25 +0.75 × 130°, which yielded a visual acuity of 20/20. One week later, on June 21, 1988, the patient's uncorrected visual acuity was 20/30. His visual acuity was 20/20 with −1.25 +1.75 × 150°. Keratometry readings were 37.82 × 54°/38.75 × 143°. The patient has moved out of state and has been followed by another ophthalmologist. No further postoperative data are available.

Comment: This case illustrates the less-than-satisfactory results that have been sometimes attributed to the patient's cornea through the euphemism "underresponder." In spite of two repeated radial keratotomies, obtaining good incision depth based on slit-lamp examination, the patient remains myopic. Why some corneas respond more readily than others to what is apparently adequate surgery is unknown.

Case 4: Increased myopia after repeated radial keratotomy

A 40-year-old Army major enrolled in the PERK study in 1983 with a cycloplegic refraction of −5.75 +1.25 × 95° in the right eye and −5.50 +1.00 × 90° in the left. His visual acuity was 20/16 bilaterally. Keratometry readings were 43.25 × 20°/44.50 × 98° in the right eye and 43.12 × 15°/44.12 × 85° in the left. Surgery was performed on the left eye using the PERK protocol and a 3.0-mm diameter clear zone.

One year after surgery, the uncorrected visual acuity in the left eye was 20/60 and with a cycloplegic refraction of −2.75 +0.75 × 105°, visual acuity was 20/20. Keratometry readings were 41.50 × 05°/42.62 × 90°. Average incision depth was 75% to 100% of corneal thickness.

Eighteen months after the initial surgery, a repeated operation was performed on the left eye. Eight centrifugal radial incisions were placed between the original incisions with a 3.0-mm clear zone. Four years after the second operation, the uncorrected visual acuity of the left eye was 20/200. The visual acuity was 20/20, with a cycloplegic refraction of −4.50 +1.00 × 90°. Keratometry readings were 41.37 × 15°/42.25 × 95°. The patient wore spectacles for distance correction.

Comment: Paradoxically, the repeated radial keratotomy increased the myopia by 1.50 D—an unusual response.

Table 18-5

Cylinder Power of the Cycloplegic Refraction in the PERK Study

Cylinder power (D)	Baseline		After initial radial keratotomy		After repeated radial keratotomy	
	No. of eyes	Percentage	No. of eyes	Percentage	No. of eyes	Percentage
0.00 to 0.50	33	56	25	42	14	24
0.75 to 1.00	17	29	15	26	24	41
1.25 to 1.50	9	15	15	26	12	20
1.75 to 2.00	0	0	2	3	6	10
2.25 to 2.50	0	0	2	3	3	5
Total	59	100	59	100	59	100

From Cowden MW, Lynn, MJ, Waring GO, and the PERK Study Group: Am J Ophthalmol 1987;103:423-431.

Table 18-6

Effect of Original Incision Depth on Addition of Four or Eight Radial Incisions

No. of eyes	Estimated incision depth	Mean change in refraction (D)	Range (D)	Standard deviation (D)
6	Shallow	2.16	0.50 to 3.75	1.068
30	Deep	0.78	−1.50 to 3.00	0.671

From Villasenor RA and Cox KC: J Refract Surg 1985;1:34-37.

0.074), patient sex ($p = 0.58$), and all other variables tested. Thus the outcome of repeated radial keratotomy is less predictable than that of initial keratotomy.

No patient lost more than one line of spectacle-corrected Snellen visual acuity after the reoperation, but five patients had a spectacle-corrected visual acuity of 20/25, instead of their baseline 20/20 or better. Refractive astigmatism increased by more than 0.50 D in 19% of the eyes. There was a cumulative increase in astigmatism after both the initial and the repeated radial keratotomies (Table 18-5).

Other complications included a small perforation that occurred in one eye and ulcerative keratitis developed along one of the reoperation scars 2 years postoperatively in one patient who was wearing a contact lens.[19]

The general conclusion about repeated radial keratotomy in the PERK Study was that a clinically meaningful improvement in refractive error and uncorrected visual acuity occurred in the majority of eyes.

Published results from other studies. Villasenor and Cox[29] found that adding eight more incisions to eight previous incisions gave a mean decrease of myopia of 1.00 D (range, 1.50 to +3.75 D) (see Fig. 18-9).

When four incisions were added to four or eight previous incisions, a mean decrease in myopia of approximately 0.70 D occurred (range, 0.00 to 1.25 D). In this series, 50% of the eyes achieved less than 1.00 D of effect after the surgery. They emphasized that eyes with shallower initial incisions received more effect from additional incisions than those with deeper incisions (Table 18-6).

Salz et al.,[24] in a study of four-incision radial keratotomy, reported the results of reoperations in 13 eyes. For seven of the 13 eyes the effects of the initial operation and the reoperation were similar (0.50 D or less difference); four of the remaining six eyes obtained more effect from the initial operation and two of them obtained less effect. Adding four incisions to the initial four in 13 eyes produced an average of 1.6 D of additional myopic correction (range, 0.62 to 3.00 D). For the group with low preoperative myopia (−1.12 to −3.12 D), this improved the percentage of eyes with a final refraction of ±1 D from 92% to 95% and with 20/40 or better visual acuity from 86% to 91%. In the moderate refraction group (−3.25 to −4.37 D), the improvement for refraction within ±1 D was from 75% to 93%, and for eyes with 20/40 or better visual

Table 18-7

Results of Repeated Radial Keratotomy with Eight Additional Incisions between Original Incisions in 27 Eyes* Reported by Menezo

		First RK (8 or 16 incisions)		Second RK (8 incisions)	
	Baseline refraction (D)†	Change in refraction (D)†	Refraction 3 wk to 12 mo after first RK (D)	Change in refraction (D)†	Refraction 6 mo or more after second RK (D)
Mean	−6.92	2.72	−4.21	+2.00	−2.21
Range	−4.25 to −11.00	1.24 to 5.00	−1.25 to −6.72	+0.50 to +3.50	0 to −4.50 D

Adapted from Menezo JL, Cisneros AL, and Harto MA: J Refract Surg 1988;4:60-62.
*20 patients, ages 23 to 46 years, clear zone 3.0 mm in 26 eyes, single-pass incisions.
†Spherical equivalent.

acuity was from 68% to 90%.

Spigelman and colleagues[26] emphasized the empirical nature of selecting a surgical plan for repeating operations and illustrated the results that could be obtained with a second set of four incisions by reporting a 61-year-old patient with a preoperative spherical equivalent refraction of −8.37 D. After an initial radial keratotomy with four incisions (presumably because of the patient's age), the residual refractive error was −6.2 D at 3 months. Then, surprisingly, an additional four incisions produced a refraction of +1.00 D 1 year after the repeated surgery.

Menezo et al.[21] reported a series of repeated operations in 27 undercorrected eyes, in which eight additional incisions were made between eight or 16 previous incisions. The results are presented in Table 18-7. All the patients were still emmetropic or undercorrected after the second operation. Menezo observed

that the time of the reoperation after the initial operation did not make any difference in the results: 1 to 3 months (8 eyes) mean change 1.93 D; 3 to 8 months (8 eyes) mean change 2.02 D; 9 months (11 eyes) mean change 1.96 D.

Recutting initial incisions

The first technique described for repeated operations was simply to attempt to recut the first set of incisions.

Surgical technique. It is difficult to place a second incision in the exact location of the healed scar of the first incision because there is nothing to guide the knife blade except the manual skill of the surgeon and the previous faint scar. Invariably, the second incision will be parallel to or stray in and out of the path of the first (Fig. 18-11). The result is often a pattern of interlacing scars; the more scars, the greater the amount of

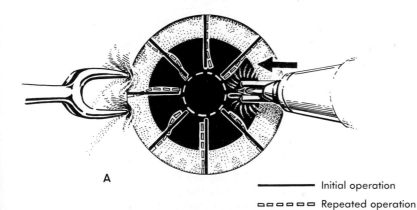
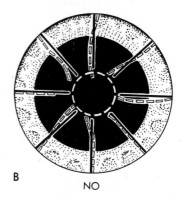

A   ————— Initial operation

    ▫ ▫ ▫ ▫ ▫ ▫ Repeated operation

B   NO

Figure 18-11
Recutting the initial incision scar. **A,** It is difficult to keep the second set of incisions exactly in the first set, simply because it's difficult to control the direction of the diamond blade fine enough to trace the original line. **B,** Invariably the second incision will stray in and out of the path of the first, so surgeons should avoid this technique of repeated radial keratotomy.

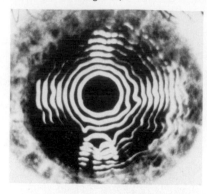

Right eye

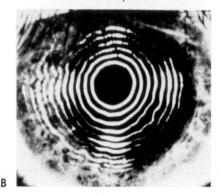

Left eye

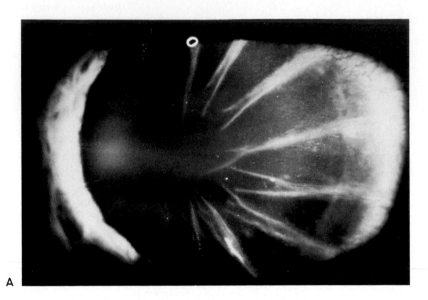

A

B

Figure 18-12

Repeated radial keratotomy by recutting initial incisions. **A,** Cornea of patient who received an initial radial keratotomy in 1981 followed by a repeated radial keratotomy a few months later for undercorrection, producing a double set of scars in the area of each incision, which splay apart paracentrally. **B,** Keratographs from both eyes taken in 1985 show the extensive irregular astigmatism induced by the multiple incisions; presumably this astigmatism is permanent. The patient could not wear contact lenses and functioned with a best spectacle-corrected visual acuity of 20/50 in the right eye and 20/80 in the left. (See case history, "High Expectations" in Chapter 25, The Patient Speaks: Testimonials after Refractive Surgery.)

irregular astigmatism, a problem encountered frequently in the early 1980s when surgeons would make as many as three separate sets of incisions in the same area (two repeated operations) in 16-incision cases for a total of 48 incisions.

Recutting the full length of old incisions is easier with a vertical "back-cutting" blade pushed centripetally from the limbus toward the clear zone because the edge of the blade can be seen and guided along the incision scar. Even with this technique, however, the new incisions do not remain within the original scars. This technique is no longer used.

Results of recutting initial scars. Fyodorov and colleagues[9] observed that there was a reduction in myopia after this approach and that the eyes with finer scars had a greater decrease in central keratometric power (mean, 1.53 D; range, 0.5 to 3.75 D),

whereas eyes with coarser scars and inclusions had a smaller mean decrease in keratometric power of 0.69 D (range, 0 to 2.37 D).

Chen and associates[5] performed a second set of eight incisions over the first set of eight incisions with a metal blade in 20 eyes followed for 3 months and observed an average decrease in refractive error of 1.89 D, but still had a general undercorrection in their patients, with an average residual myopia of 2.08 D.

A case of recutting the original incision scars is captioned "High Expectations, Poor Result, and a Lawsuit" in Chapter 25, The Patient Speaks: Testimonials after Refractive Keratotomy (Fig. 18-12).

Recutting the paracentral part of incision

On the theory that the paracentral part of the incision adjacent to the clear zone creates the most flat-

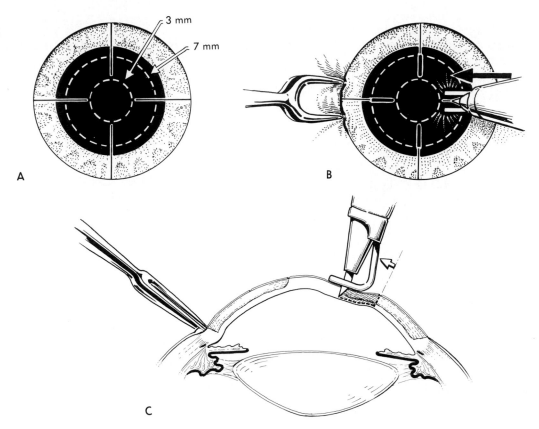

Figure 18-13

Technique for recutting ("back-cutting") the paracentral incision. **A,** The surgeon marks two zones: a new clear zone either at the edge of the previous clear zone or within it (but not smaller than 3 mm) and an outer zone approximately 4 mm larger in diameter so that the paracentral 2 mm of each incision is identified. The wound may be opened (see Fig. 18-14). **B,** The vertical blade, back-cutting knife is plunged into the incision at the outer zone mark and pushed toward the center, stopping either at the end of the previous incision or at the margin of the newly marked clear zone. **C,** The knife blade is carried deeply into the cornea and pushed forward to square off the paracentral edge of the incision.

tening effect and that surgeons who use single-edged, angled, "front-cutting" blades for centrifugal incisions (American technique) often do not achieve a perpendicular, completely deep wound adjacent to the clear zone, Franks[8] developed the technique of re-incising the central 2 mm of each wound using a vertical "back-cutting" blade and cutting centripetally toward the clear zone (Fig. 18-13).

The diameter of the clear zone is left the same or made smaller than that in the original operation. The vertical blade is inserted into the incision scar 2 mm from the clear zone mark and pushed to the edge of the previous clear zone in an attempt to create a squared-off, deep, perpendicular wound.

A similar technique has been used by K. Buzzard, MD,* who uses a vertical blade to make 1-mm incisions at the slit-lamp microscope, which he calls "touch-ups and tickles," to "square up" the paracentral part of the original wounds.

Results of paracentral back-cutting. Franks[8] presented the results at an unspecified follow-up time in 85 eyes with an initial myopia of less than 6 D and a residual refractive error after the first operation of −0.50 to −4.00 D; 71 eyes (84%) achieved a refraction of zero to −1.00 D. Of 43 eyes with an initial myopia greater than 6 D and a residual refraction of −1.00 to −8.00 D, 19 (42%) achieved a refraction of zero to −1.00 D, 14 (32%) having a residual myopia of more than 2 D (Table 18-8).

The author claimed a number of advantages: none of the patients was overcorrected; none had an increase in myopia; there was minimal increase in scarring without an increase in glare; if the "back-cutting"

*Buzzard K: Personal verbal communication, September 1987.

Table 18-8

Results of Paracentral Centripetal (Back-Cutting) Repeated Incisions in 128 Eyes Undercorrected after Initial Radial Keratotomy

Residual spherical equivalent myopia (D) before back-cutting (no. of eyes)	Spherical equivalent refraction (D) after back-cutting						
	±0.50	−0.5 to −1	−1 to −2	−2 to −3	−3 to −4	−4 to −5	−5 to −6
−0.50 to −1.00 (20)	15	3	2				
−1.00 to −2.00 (57)	32	14	8	3			
−2.00 to −3.00 (28)	10	9	5	4			
−3.00 to −4.00 (15)	4	2	6	3			
−4.00 to −5.00 (2)					1		1
−5.00 to −6.00 (2)						1	1
−6.00 to −7.00 (2)					2		
−7.00 to −8.00 (2)		2					
Total eyes	61	30	21	10	3	1	2

From Franks S: J Refract Surg 1986;2:171-173.

of the initial incisions was ineffective, an additional set of incisions could still be added between the initial ones.

Because there is only one published report of the use of this paracentral back-cutting technique, further experience and verification are necessary to confirm its usefulness.

Opening and recutting the wounds

Because of the difficulty in recutting the previous incision scars and because of the undesirability of adding additional scars to the cornea, Kevin Charlton, MD,* has used the technique of reopening the original wounds and cutting the entire length of the wound to make it deeper and to square it off at the central end.

Surgical technique. After the usual anesthesia, preparation and draping, marking of the center, marking of the new clear zone (which may be the same as or smaller than the previous clear zone), and measurement of paracentral corneal thickness with intraoperative ultrasonic pachometry, the surgeon fixates the globe at the limbus and presses a blunt angled intraocular lens hook into the peripheral portion of each incision. It breaks through the residual epithelial plug

*Charlton K: Personal written communication, January 1988.

and is gently pulled back and forth within the incision, breaking the scar tissue and opening the incision to its previous full depth. A vertical-bladed diamond knife is set with the blade extended to a length that depends on the cutting "personality" of the knife. The blade is passed toward the center to deepen the wound and extend, deepen, and square up the paracentral part of the wound. Zone cutting may be used to deepen the peripheral half of the incision. The wounds are irrigated (Figs. 18-13 and 18-14).

It is not difficult to drop the knife blade into the previously opened wound, but the tip of the knife blade may not always find the deep recess of the wound, and a small inverted Y may result (Fig. 18-15). However, this is not usually visible on slit-lamp microscopy. The density of the recut scars is similar to or only slightly greater than the density of the original scars, and any difference is not clinically meaningful.

Results of opening and recutting the wounds. There are no published results on this technique. Charlton has provided the results from his personal experience (Table 18-9). He reported the results on 27 eyes of 20 patients, with a mean follow-up of 8.21 months (range, 1 week to 21 months). The average age was 37.5 years (range, 21 to 54 years). There were 15 men. All eyes had the deepening of eight incisions,

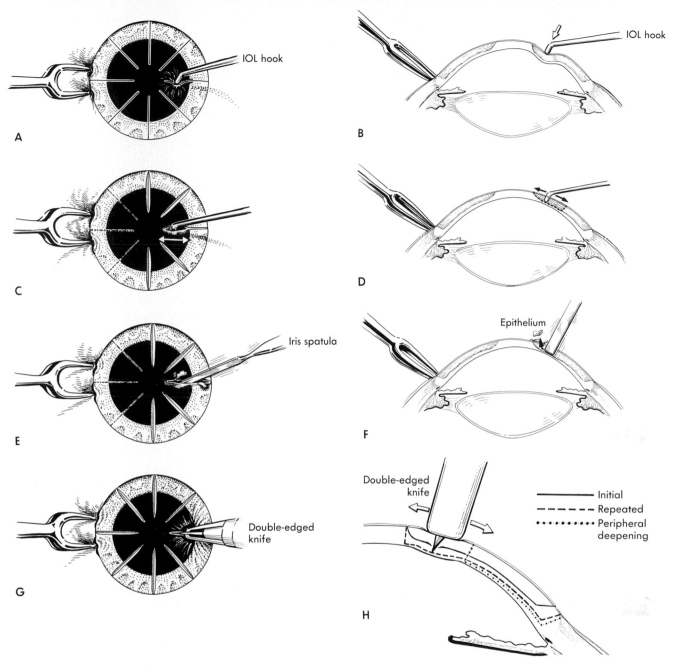

Figure 18-14

Technique of opening and recutting the previous wound. This technique prevents the duplication of scarring and the placement of additional incisions in clear cornea and provides a track for the second incision. **A** and **B,** Fixation is achieved with a double-pronged forceps. **C** and **D,** Using a blunt instrument, such as an intraocular lens *(IOL)* hook or a cyclodialysis spatula, the surgeon reopens the wound by inserting the instrument into the previous scar. **E** and **F,** Because most scars harbor a superficial epithelial plug, there is a tract into which the instrument can be pressed until it pops into the scar. Because the corneal stroma is only partially healed, the incision can be forced open easily. Using a blunt instrument prevents accidental cutting into the adjacent clear cornea and perforation. **G** and **H,** A double-edged knife is set at the calculated length, dropped into the open wound perpendicularly, and passed in a gentle skating motion across the surface of the wound. The vertical edge is pushed centrally to deepen and square up the wound and to extend it to a smaller clear zone diameter if indicated. Then the angled edge is pulled centrifugally, deepening the wound. The maneuver is similar to performing a second pass incision with the knife blade at the same setting during a primary radial keratotomy. Alternatively a vertical, back-cutting knife may be used to recut and extend the opened incisions. The knife blade can be extended to make a second peripheral deepening incision, if indicated by the surgical plan. The wounds are irrigated at the end of the procedure.

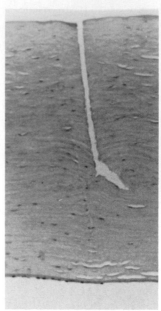

Figure 18-15
Histopathologic section of eye bank cornea after recutting a previously shallow wound shows the potential angled incision that can occur if the knife blade is not dropped perpendicularly into the original wound (H & E ×30).

Table 18-9

Results of Two Techniques of Repeated Radial Keratotomy (Mean, SD, Range, or Percentage of Eyes)

Variable	Open, deepen, and lengthen original eight incisions*	Eight additional incisions between original ones
Number of eyes	27	23
Time of surgery	1985-1987	1985-1987
Patient age (yr)	37.5 ±8(21 to 54)	35 ±7.5 (21 to 53)
Original refraction (D)†	−3.34 ±.86 (−1.63 to −4.75)	−5.95 ±1.00 (−3.75 to −7.63)
Time after original refractive keratotomy (wk)	8.6 ±5.3 (2 to 24)	12.5 ±13 (2 to 52)
Refraction after original refractive keratotomy (D)† (range)	−1.69 ±0.73 (−0.75 to −3.88)	−2.52 ±0.84 (−1.00 to −4.25)
Uncorrected visual acuity after first refractive keratotomy (% ≥ 20/40)	11%	4%
Peripheral deepening incisions	33%	13%
Reduction in clear zone diameter (mm)	0.56 ±0.30 (0.25 to 1.50)	None
Follow-up (mo)	9 ±6 (0.1 to 21)	11 ±8 (1 to 30)
Change in refraction (D)†	+1.51 ±0.74 (+0.38 to +3.00)	+1.54 ±1.33 (−0.88 to +5.38)
Refraction after repeated surgery (D)†	−0.18 ±0.57 (+1.50 to −1.13)	−2.52 ±0.84 (−1.00 to −4.25)
Eyes with refraction ±1.00 D†	93%	44%
Uncorrected visual acuity after repeated surgery (% ≥ 20/40)	96%	65%
Eyes losing two or more Snellen lines of spectacle-corrected visual acuity	0	0

Unpublished data, courtesy Kevin Charlton, MD.
*One eye had four incisions.
†Spherical equivalent.

except one that had the deepening of four. The central clear zone was reduced in diameter by 0.25 to 1.00 mm, depending on the surgical plan, with the minimum of 3.0 mm. Results are presented in Table 18-9. Two eyes experienced microperforation. The average astigmatism did not increase: preoperative = 0.58 D, postoperative = 0.56 D.

An uncorrected visual acuity of 20/20 was achieved by 59% of the eyes and of 20/40 or better by 96% of the eyes. Only one saw worse than 20/40, and this acuity was 20/50 uncorrected. No eyes lost best spectacle-corrected visual acuity.

These excellent results—particularly with regard to visual acuity—probably reflect the initial careful selection of patients, none of whom had more than −4.75 D of myopia before the first operation, as well as the success in the repeated operation. As demonstrated in Table 18-9, the outcome of the opening and recutting of wounds was better than that achieved when using eight additional incisions in between the initial eight incisions, although the two groups were not operated on concomitantly and the initial amount of myopia was greater in the eyes with eight plus eight incisions. Thus opening and recutting the wounds is a useful technique from repeated operations, but published data and independent verification are necessary to evaluate it further.

CORRECTION OF HYPEROPIA AFTER RADIAL KERATOTOMY

The frequency and consequences of overcorrection are discussed in detail in Chapter 23, Complications of Refractive Keratotomy. Since the mechanism by which radial keratotomy flattens the central cornea is gaping and increased volume of the radial incisions, the method by which this can be reversed is closure of the incisions with sutures.

Purse-string suture

The technique of a continuous purse-string suture was described by Starling and Hofmann.[27] Using the eyes of human cadavers, they demonstrated that the placement of a continuous running purse-string suture into each newly opened radial wound and across the tissue bridge between each wound resulted in a circumferential suture that could be gradually tightened with a single knot, using an operating keratometer to monitor the amount of central corneal steepening. They preferred placement of the suture at a 7-mm zone because a 6-mm zone produced excessive irregular central astigmatism and using an 8-mm zone did not give as much effect. They demonstrated a steepening of 5 to 10 D, depending on how tightly the purse-string suture was pulled.

Hofmann[10] reported the results of seven eyes with a purse-string suture. These cases had a mean preoperative spherical equivalent refraction of +3.00 D (range, +1.75 to +4.00 D). One year after surgery with the purse-string suture still in place, the mean spherical equivalent refractive error was +1.4 D (range, +0.50 to +3.75 D). A reduction in hyperopia of 1.00 D or more occurred in five of the seven eyes (70%). None of the eyes became myopic. Two eyes developed a suture-related keratitis.

Damiano and Forstot have presented the most detailed information on using purse-string sutures for reducing hyperopia after radial keratotomy. They used topical anesthesia and marked the visual axis with a hypodermic needle. They marked two zones, 5 mm and 7 mm, with dull zone markers. The preexisting radial incisions were opened with a blunt intraocular lens hook to half depth, cutting from the limbus into the 5-mm zone. The wounds are not opened to full length or full depth. A 10-0 polyester (Mersilene) suture on a 140-degree needle is placed into the wound at half depth, passed along the tissue between the two wounds, and brought out in the adjacent wound. Two purse-string sutures are placed, one along the 7-mm mark and another, starting 90 degrees away from the start of the first, along the 5-mm zone mark. A paracentesis is done to deflate the anterior chamber to half depth. The 7-mm suture is tightened first, giving dramatic steepening of the cornea, followed by tying the 5-mm suture somewhat more gently so as not to loosen the effect of the 7-mm suture. Both sutures are tied and the ends cut within one of the incisions. Postoperatively, topical corticosteroids and antibiotics are used.

The authors have presented their results, which are summarized in Table 18-10. The mean reduction in hyperopia was 3.5 D, reducing the mean refraction from +3.47 D to −1.68 D for the 19 eyes. Even with this very useful reduction, the range in outcome was still wide: +2.50 to −4.25 D.

No information has been published on the stability of refraction after purse-string sutures. If a nylon suture is used, its elasticity would be likely to produce less overall effect but also cause less cheese-wiring of the suture through the stroma. If Mersilene suture is used, its virtual lack of elasticity would be likely to cause some cheese-wiring through the stroma over time. It is possible that the reinforcing technique of two concentric purse-string sutures, as described by Damiano and Forstot, might diminish the overall cheese-wiring effect and increase stability over time, a premise that would need documentation.

Interrupted sutures

Lindquist and colleagues[13,14] have advocated the use of nonbiodegradable polyester (Mersilene) inter-

Table 18-10

Results of Purse-String Suture for Hyperopia after Refractive Keratotomy

Variables	Data
Population	18 patients, 19 eyes 11 men, 7 women
Diagnoses after original refractive keratotomy	9 progressive hyperopia 5 original overcorrection 5 overcorrection
Management before purse-string suture	19 eyes treated with intraocular pressure–lowering medicines 9 eyes treated with molding contact lens
Time from refractive keratotomy to purse-string suture	25 months (range, 8 to 51)
Follow-up	5 patients, 6 months to 1 year 14 patients, ≥1 year (range, 6 to 35 months; mean, 18 months)
Uncorrected visual acuity before purse-string suture	11 eyes 20/100 or worse (58%) 8 eyes 20/50 to 20/100 (42%) (no eye was 20/40 or better uncorrected)
Uncorrected visual acuity after purse-string suture	13 eyes 20/40 or better (69%) 4 eyes 20/50 to 20/80 (21%) 2 eyes 20/100 or worse (10%)
Refraction before purse-string suture	Average: +3.47 D (range, +1.25 to +5.75 D)
Refraction after purse-string suture	Average: −1.68 D (range, +2.50 to −4.25 D)
Change in refraction after purse-string suture	Average: −3.50 D (range, −1.00 to −8.25 D)
Change in keratometry after purse-string suture	Average 4.30 D (range, 1.00 to 9.00 D)
Change in spectacle-corrected visual acuity	15 eyes were the same as before operation or one line better 2 eyes gained two lines or more 2 eyes lost one or two lines

From Damiano RE, Forstot SL, and Dukes DK: Presented at the International Society of Refractive Keratoplasty, New Orleans, October 28, 1989; Personal written communication, November 17, 1989.

rupted sutures across radial or transverse incisions to decrease overcorrection after keratotomy.

The surgical technique involves opening the wounds to full depth and length with an intraocular lens hook or other blunt instrument, cleaning out the epithelial plug by gentle scraping, and placing one or two interrupted sutures across the wound. For radial keratotomy, the sutures are placed at or adjacent to the 7-mm diameter zone. For astigmatic keratotomy, the sutures are placed across the transverse incision. Intraoperative keratometry helps judge the tightness of the suture, which can be adjusted using a slip knot. Tightening the suture to achieve a slight overcorrection will allow for subsequent resolution of surgically induced corneal edema, cheese-wiring of the sutures, and later selective suture removal to modulate the central corneal curvature (Fig. 18-16).

No systematic studies of suturing human radial keratotomy wounds have been published. A study of eyes of cadavers[13] demonstrated that the tension on the slip knots in the sutures could induce considerable steepening of the central cornea from 7.5 to 12.0 D in eyes with four incisions, and from 9 to 15 D in eyes with eight incisions. After astigmatic keratotomy, Lindquist and colleagues[13] have reported a series of six eyes showing a change in central keratometry readings from 0.50 to 12.00 D, representing a reversal of the overcorrection by 41% to 100% (average, 70%). They recommended the sutures be left in place at least 6 to 8 weeks before selective removal, and leaving them indefinitely if an acceptable result is achieved.

PENETRATING AND LAMELLAR KERATOPLASTY AFTER RADIAL KERATOTOMY

Severe irregular astigmatism, glare, and contact lens intolerance develop in some patients after radial keratotomy. These complications are more frequent when large numbers of incisions and multiple repeated operations were used in the early 1980s. These complications are distinctively rare now that only four to eight incisions are used with more refined techniques for repeated surgery. The symptoms may be reduced by creating a new corneal surface, using penetrating keratoplasty, epikeratoplasty, or homoplastic keratomileusis, which can also attempt to correct residual ametropia (see Chapter 4, Development and Classification of Refractive Surgical Procedures). In each of these techniques, a common complicating factor is the dehiscence and opening of the wounds during surgery.

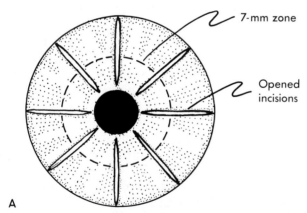

A

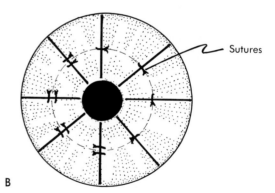

B

Figure 18-16
Interrupted sutures in radial incisions to reduce overcorrection. **A,** A 7-mm zone is marked with a zone marker in the epithelium. The wounds are opened with a blunt instrument, such as an IOL hook. **B,** Interrupted sutures can be placed singly or in pairs across the wounds in approximately 3 months after suturing of radial incisions shows some sutures intact and others that have been removed because of loosening. **C,** Photograph is from case report on p. 662.

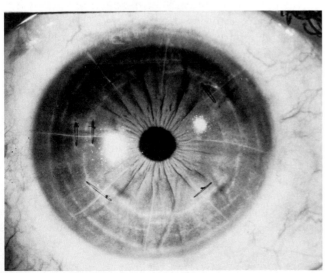

C

Case Report: Early Suturing of Wounds for Marked Overcorrection

A 46-year-old man had a refraction in his right eye of $-4.50 +1.50 \times 80°$ with a corrected visual acuity of 20/20. Central keratometry readings were $42.75 \times 178°$ and $43.50 \times 88°$. He underwent radial keratotomy with a 4-mm diameter clear zone, eight centripetal incisions with the knife blade set at 95% of the thinnest paracentral intraoperative ultrasonic pachometry reading. On the first postoperative day, the incisions were observed to be generally greater than 90% depth and the manifest refraction was $+4.00 +1.00 \times 80°$ postoperatively, with a wound leak in the three o'clock-position incision from a perforation. Central keratometry readings were approximately 36.00 D in all meridians. The wound leak was closed by two interrupted 10-0 nylon sutures. To treat the marked overcorrection, the four incisions in the oblique meridians were irrigated and closed with a single 10-0 nylon suture each, using mild tension without slip knots. All knots were buried in the tissue (Fig 18-18). Over the next 6 months, some of the sutures loosened spontaneously and were removed. One year after surgery, with all sutures removed, the uncorrected visual acuity was 20/30; the manifest refraction was $-0.50 +1.50 \times 90°$, 20/20; central keratometry readings were $37.40 \times 180°$ and $40.20 \times 90°$.

Comment: In this case, it was not possible to distinguish between the effect of the suture closure of the radial keratotomy incisions and the natural disappearance of immediate postoperative edema in terms of reduction of the overcorrection. Under most circumstances, the surgeon would observe the patient for 2 to 4 weeks, allowing the postoperative edema to subside before opening and suturing the wounds.

Penetrating keratoplasty

Beatty and colleagues[2] have discussed in detail the techniques and complications of penetrating keratoplasty after radial keratotomy. They emphasize that the forces created by trephination tend to pull the radial wounds open (Fig. 18-17) and recommended placing sutures across the radial wounds before trephination to hold them closed. Otherwise, aqueous leaks tended to occur at the junction of the separated radial incisions and the circular keratoplasty wound, requiring multiple sutures to obtain a watertight wound.

One case has been reported that required 29 interrupted 10-0 nylon sutures to achieve wound closure.[23] Beatty and colleagues[2] used an eye bank eye model to describe numerous techniques for stabilization of the radial wounds during trephination and for closure of the keratoplasty wound. Their recommendations included: (1) placing two transverse sutures across each radial wound approximately 1.5 mm outside the intended trephine incision before trephination; (2) placing the keratoplasty sutures between the radial keratotomy incision scars; and (3) meticulously closing the junction between the radial keratotomy scars and the trephination wound with a combination of apposition and overlying compression sutures. Overall the authors found double-crossed interrupted and double-running, antitorque suturing techniques to be the most effective.

I have used an intrastromal purse-string suture placed approximately 1.5 mm outside the intended trephination site to hold the wounds closed. This is especially useful when a large number of incisions is present, making placement of individual sutures across each wound impractical. The surgeon does not open the wounds, but simply places the suture bites between each of the previous wounds, inserting each successive bite at the approximate point of exit of the previous one, for a continuous placement. The suture is pulled slightly before the knot is tied, but not enough to distort the cornea during trephination (Figs. 18-17 and 18-18).

No large series of cases of penetrating keratoplasty after radial keratotomy has been published. However, anecdotal reports and our personal experience have demonstrated that preoperative myopia tends to persist after the penetrating keratoplasty because the radius of curvature of the donor corneas either is within the normal range or is steeper. Theoretically, one might use a donor cornea that is the same size or 0.25 to 0.50 mm smaller in diameter than the host opening to try to achieve a flatter postoperative configuration—a technique that has been suggested for keratoconus.

The postoperative course of penetrating keratoplasty after radial keratotomy is similar to that seen in other avascular corneal disorders such as keratoconus

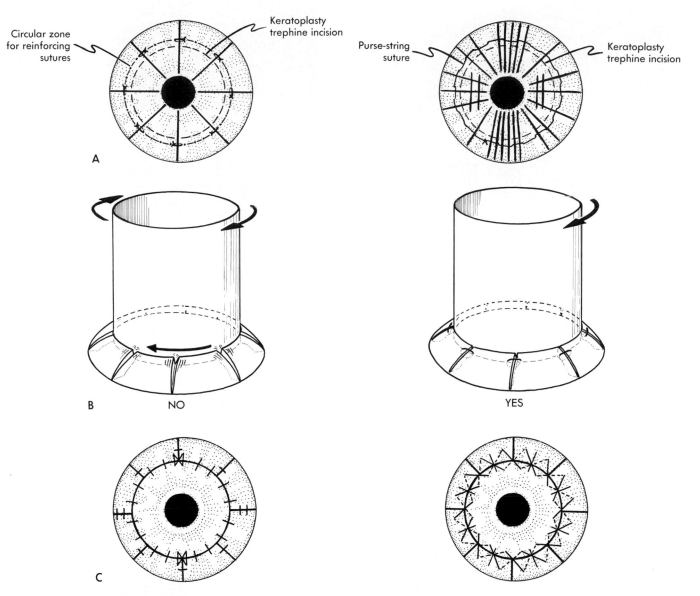

Figure 18-17

Control of radial keratotomy wounds during penetrating keratoplasty. The major challenge is to prevent the wounds from opening during or after surgery. **A,** Before surgery the keratotomy incisions should be sutured shut with either interrupted sutures across each incision *(left)* or a purse-string suture *(right).* The purse-string suture is particularly useful when multiple irregular incisions have been placed close to each other. **B,** During trephination, unsutured wounds may pull open *(left),* but sutured wounds will remain closed *(right).* **C,** Suturing the donor cornea in place involves not only securing the donor to the host, but also securely closing the junction of the end of the keratotomy incision with the keratoplasty wound, either by interrupted and **x**-shaped sutures *(left)* or by interrupted and double running sutures *(right).* (Modified from Beatty RF, Robin JB, and Schanzlin DJ: J Refract Surg 1986;2:207-214.)

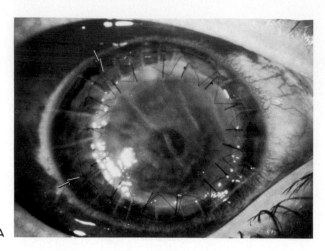
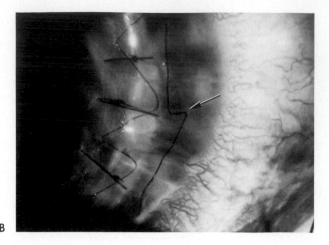

A

B

Figure 18-18
A, Penetrating keratoplasty for irregular astigmatism after radial keratotomy photographed on the day after surgery. Purse-string suture *(arrows)* was placed peripheral to the graph-host margin to decrease the chance of the radial incisions opening during trephination. Graft is centered over pupil. **B,** Close-up view of the wound shows the purse-string suture with a jog in it *(arrow)* along with interrupted and running sutures in the keratoplasty wound (see case report below).

Case Report: Penetrating Keratoplasty after Refractive Keratotomy

A 20-year-old man with mild congenital nystagmus underwent 16-incision radial keratotomy in 1985 in the left eye, followed 2 months later by the same procedure in the right eye. A detailed history was unavailable, but his myopia was approximately −8 D in his right eye and −6 D in his left. Because of an undercorrection, the patient underwent a repeated radial keratotomy 2 months later in his right eye and 4 months later in his left, with eight additional incisions in each eye. When seen at the Emory Eye Center approximately 2 years after surgery, he was still undercorrected: OD, −3.50 +1.00 × 10°; OS, −1.50 +1.00 × 170°. His main complaint, however, was severe glare.

Multiple attempts were made to fit him with rigid gas-permeable contact lenses to reduce his glare and myopia; all were unsuccessful. Therefore a penetrating keratoplasty was performed in his left eye on October 5, 1987, approximately 2 years after his radial keratotomy, using a 7.75-mm donor button in a 7.5-mm recipient bed. Because of the concern that the radial incisions in the recipient bed would spontaneously open during the surgical procedure, a running purse-string suture of 9-0 nylon was placed 360 degrees at the 9-mm diameter zone in the host cornea. None of the radial incisions opened during trephination, but the 2-year-old wounds in the host button could be separated easily with forceps. The donor was secured with the 16 interrupted 10-0 nylon sutures, and a running 11-0 nylon suture, the bites placed between the keratotomy scars. Postoperatively the patient noted a decrease in glare.

Four months postoperatively, the patient's refraction was −20.00 +9.00 × 10° for a visual acuity of 20/40. The keratometry readings were 42.50 × 95°/49.25 × 180°. Because it was believed part of the myopia was caused by the purse-string suture, it was removed without complications. Ten months postoperatively, the visual acuity in the left eye was 20/40 with −10.75 +2.25 × 05°. Keratometry readings were 42.50 × 95°/45.37 × 05°. The patient was fitted successfully with a rigid gas-permeable lens and has a corrected visual acuity of 20/30.

Comment: This case illustrates the length to which some patients will go to correct an undesirable result after refractive keratotomy and the time, energy, and money consumed in such cases. The final outcome certainly left the patient with more visual disability than he had before the original keratotomy surgery.

or corneal dystrophies. Problems with wound healing and allograft reactions seem minimal, but problems of regular and irregular astigmatism, as well as ametropia, can be severe.

Epikeratoplasty

Because the corneal endothelium generally functions well after radial keratotomy, a penetrating keratoplasty may be deemed excessive surgery and an epikeratoplasty more appropriate, with its ability to create a presumably more regular central corneal surface, without engendering the potential problems of intraocular surgery and allograft reaction. Unlike penetrating keratoplasty, epikeratoplasty also has the possibility of obtaining a further refractive correction by using a donor lenticule of known power.

The general surgical technique of epikeratoplasty is undergoing continual change.[24] As with penetrating keratoplasty after radial keratotomy, epikeratoplasty is more arduous under the circumstances. Interrupted or purse-string sutures should be used to reinforce the radial incision scars and to prevent them from being opened during the trephination. These sutures can be removed at the conclusion of the epikeratoplasty if the wounds have not pulled open, or the knots may be buried in the host tissue and the sutures left in place and removed selectively after surgery. If the ends of the radial wounds open during trephination, they should be sutured closed. To prevent the radial scars from being pulled open, the undermining is better done with a sharp instrument than with the usual dull spreader. An angled disposable knife easily accomplishes this. Interrupted sutures for the epikeratoplasty button are placed between the previous radial incision scars, and it may be necessary to use a single running suture to approximate the edges of the host tissue overlying the epikeratoplasty button if the radial keratotomy wounds splay apart.

Carlson and Goosey[4] have reported four eyes of three patients who underwent epikeratoplasty for

---

Case Report: Epikeratoplasty after Refractive Keratotomy

A 29-year-old man had undergone bilateral radial keratotomy and Ruiz trapezoidal keratotomy to correct myopic astigmatism. Preoperative history was not available. Postoperatively, the patient was intolerant of both spectacles and contact lenses and sought consultation at the Emory Eye Center. The refraction and keratometry readings were as follows:

Refraction and visual acuity	Keratometry measurements and mires
OD: +1.00 +4.00 × 160°, 20/50	38.37/39.25 × 180°, 3+ irregular
OS: −0.25 +5.50 × 150°, 20/80	37.12/37.25 × 165°, 3+ irregular

The patient received an epikeratoplasty with a +3.12 D lenticule in the right eye, the surgical procedure being complicated by wound gape in some of the radial incisions that required transverse suturing for closure.

During the first month after surgery, an epithelial plaque appeared at the interface and was treated by opening of the wound and scraping out the plaque. Nine months later, an epikeratoplasty was performed in the left eye. An epithelial plaque gradually appeared at the interface, requiring curettage 3 months after surgery.

At approximately 1 year after surgery in both eyes, the following values were obtained:

Refraction and visual acuity	Keratometry
OD: −9.25 +0.75 × 140°, 20/25	45.25 sphere
OS: −7.75 sphere, 20/50	41.50/44.00 × 75°

The patient was able to wear rigid gas-permeable contact lenses bilaterally. (Case history, courtesy of Drs. K. Carlson and J. Goosey.)

Comment: This case emphasizes that epikeratoplasty after radial keratotomy is a complex procedure that can result in significant postoperative complications and ametropia. It can, however, restore functional corrected vision to individuals who would otherwise experience great visual disability after radial keratotomy.

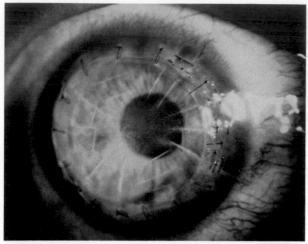

A

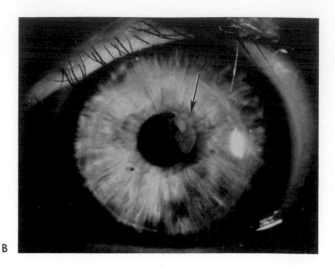

B

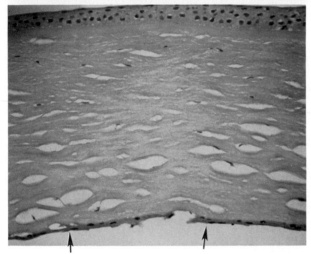

C

Figure 18-19
Epikeratoplasty after radial keratotomy. **A,** Epikeratoplasty button in place with radial sutures across the donor-host wound and transverse sutures across the radial incisions. The radial incisions are visible through the epikeratoplasty button. **B,** After all sutures were removed, an expanding plaque of implanted epithelium was present adjacent to the pupil *(arrow)*. **C,** The epikeratoplasty button was removed, and the epithelium identified on its posterior surface histopathologically *(arrows)*. (Courtesy Kent Carlson, MD, and John Goosey, MD.)

overcorrection after radial keratotomy. Two of the patients had anisometropia and one had high astigmatism. Each patient was contact lens– and spectacle-intolerant. In spite of suturing of the radial incisions before the time of trephination, all cases demonstrated some gaping of the radial wounds during surgery. In addition, all cases showed some epithelium in the lamellar interface after surgery, one lenticule being removed because of the glare and decreased vision produced by this epithelial plaque (Fig. 18-19). After surgery, irregular astigmatism required contact lens wear to obtain best-corrected visual acuity. Contact lens-fitting was facilitated by measurement of corneal topography.

Keates and colleagues[12] reported one case of epikeratoplasty done 18 months after a radial keratotomy had produced essentially no optical correction in an eye with a preoperative refraction of −8.75 +1.00 × 50°. Eight months after the myopic epikeratoplasty, the uncorrected visual acuity was 20/20 and the refraction was +0.75 D.[12]

McDonald and colleagues[32] have cited an unpublished series of approximately 20 epikeratoplasty cases done after radial keratotomy but have not published the results at the time of this writing.

Myopic keratomileusis

Radial keratotomy is most effective for myopia up to 5 or 6 D. Nevertheless, many patients with myopia greater than this have had radial keratotomy with unsatisfactory undercorrection. Some of these patients have then been treated with myopic keratomileusis using either a donor cornea or the patient's cornea for the lenticule.[22,28] Apparently the technical difficulty of the myopic keratomileusis is not increased by the presence of the radial keratotomy scars, although the corneas were found to be more flaccid by one author, and pathologic examination has demonstrated easy separation of the wounds.[22,28]

The proper calculations for grinding the lenticule are more difficult after radial keratotomy because the cornea is aspheric, a condition for which the computer programs were not designed. Nordan and Havins[22] recommended simply using the keratometry readings taken before the radial keratotomy for the keratomileusis calculations. They reported five cases of myopic keratomileusis after undercorrected radial keratotomy. The mean spherical equivalent refraction after the radial keratotomy was −6.50 D, with a range from −3.00 D to −11.00 D; the eyes had a corrected visual acuity of 20/40 or better. All five eyes had homoplastic keratomileusis. The reported outcomes varied from an overcorrection of +1.75 D to an undercorrection of −5.25 D.

GENERALITIES ABOUT REPEATED SURGERY AFTER RADIAL KERATOTOMY

From the few published reports and from personal experience, I offer a few generalities concerning repeated surgery after radial keratotomy.

1. Repeated radial and transverse keratotomy can further reduce myopia and astigmatism.
2. The second operation is less effective than the first, and there is no defined ratio between the effect of the first and second operations.
3. The technique of repeated keratotomy depends on the perceived cause of the undercorrection and the surgeon's own preference and experience.
4. Eyes with unacceptable overcorrection after radial keratotomy can be managed by opening and suturing the wounds.
5. The results of repeated surgery are less predictable than those of the primary operation.
6. Lamellar and penetrating keratoplasty after radial keratotomy should be performed only when no other therapeutic measures are available, and then with the patient's understanding that the outcome may be less than satisfactory.
7. Long-term follow-up of eyes with repeated surgery after radial keratotomy is needed.

UNFINISHED BUSINESS

The major unresolved problem in repeated refractive keratotomy is whether the operation should be intentionally staged. There are some studies by Salz and colleagues of an initial four incisions followed by an additional four incisions, but the more complex idea of tailoring the operation to the individual patient's refractive needs is not as well studied. Techniques such as selective deepening of incisions or selective lengthening of incisions in a repeated and titrated manner deserve further study to define the increase in predictability achieved by this approach as compared with a single operation. Inherent in such studies would be definitions of the most desirable method of repeated surgery: additional incisions, deepening, or lengthening. Can these repeated "touch-ups" be done at the slit-lamp microscope, or do they require another whole operation?

There is very little published information about other eye operations after radial keratotomy, and surgeons who perform cataract extraction, penetrating keratoplasty, retinal detachment surgery, eyelid tightening procedures, and glaucoma surgery should report their experience as compared to eyes without previous radial keratotomy. This will be particularly important in eyes receiving only four incisions, since they may be much more stable and tolerant of subsequent ocular surgery.

REFERENCES

1. Arrowsmith PN and Marks RG: Evaluating the predictability of radial keratotomy, Ophthalmology 1985;92:331-338.
2. Beatty RF, Robin JB, and Schanzlin DJ: Penetrating keratoplasty after radial keratotomy, J Refract Surg 1986;2:207-214.
3. Binder PS, Nayak SK, Deg JK, Zavala EY, and Sugar J: An ultrastructural and histochemical study of long-term wound healing after radial keratotomy, Am J Ophthalmol 1987;103(Part 2):432-440.
4. Carlson KA and Goosey JD: Epikeratoplasty following overcorrected radial keratotomy, Invest Ophthalmol Vis Sci 1988;29(suppl):390.
5. Chen R, Liang Y, Tsai J, and Wu F: Surgical results of second-attempt radial keratotomy, Ann Ophthalmol 1985;17:618-620.
6. Cowden JW, Lynn MJ, Waring GO, and the PERK Study Group: Repeated radial keratotomy in the Prospective Evaluation of Radial Keratotomy study, Am J Ophthalmol 1987;103:423-431.
7. Cowden JW and Weber B: Repeat radial keratotomy in monkeys, Ophthalmology 1983;909:251-256.
8. Franks S: Radial keratotomy undercorrections: a new approach, J Refract Surg 1986;2:171-173.
9. Fyodorov SN, Sarkizova MB, and Jurasova TP: Corneal biomicroscopy following repeated radial keratotomy, Ann Ophthalmol 1983;15:403-407.
10. Hofmann RF: Reoperations after radial and astigmatic keratotomy, J Refract Surg 1987;3:119-128.
11. Kaufman HE: Refractive surgery, Am J Ophthalmol 1987;103(Part 2):355-357.
12. Keates RH, Watson SA, and Levy SN: Epikeratophakia following previous refractive keratoplasty surgery: two case reports, J Cataract Refract Surg 1987;12:536-541.
13. Lindquist TD, Rubenstein JB, and Lindstrom RL: Correction of hyperopia following radial keratotomy: quantification in human cadaver eyes, Ophthalmic Surg 1987;10:432-437.
14. Lindquist TD, Williams PA, and Lindstrom RL: Management of overcorrection following astigmatic keratotomy, J Refract Surg 1988;4:218-221.
15. Lindstrom RL: Consultations in refractive surgery: reoperations, J Refract Surg 1987;3:64-66.
16. Lindstrom RL and Lindquist TD: Surgical correction of postoperative astigmatism, Cornea 1988;7:138-148.
17. Lynn MJ, Waring GO, and the PERK Study Group: Stability of refraction after radial keratotomy compared with unoperated eyes in the PERK study, Invest Ophthalmol Vis Sci 1987;28 (suppl):223.
18. Lynn MJ, Waring GO, Sperduto RD, and the PERK Study Group: Factors affecting outcome and predictability of radial keratotomy in the PERK study, Arch Ophthalmol 1987;105:42-51.
19. Mandelbaum S, Waring GO, Forster RK, Culbertson WW, Rowsey JJ, and Espinal ME: Late development of ulcerative keratitis in radial keratotomy scars, Arch Ophthalmol 1986;104:1156-1160.
20. McDonald MB and Morgan KS: Epikeratophakia for aphakia and myopia. In Kaufman HE et al, editors: The cornea. New York, 1988; Churchill Livingstone, pp 823-848.
21. Menezo JL, Cisneros AL, and Harto MA: Radial keratotomy: reoperations, J Refract Surg 1988;4:60-62.
22. Nordan LT and Havins WE: Undercorrected radial keratotomy treated with myopic keratomileusis, J Refract Surg 1985;1:56-58.
23. Robin JB, Beatty RF, Dunn S, Trusdale MD, Riffenburgh R, Rao N, and Smith RE: *Mycobacterium chelonei* keratitis after radial keratotomy, Am J Ophthalmol 1986;102:72-79.
24. Salz JJ, Villasenor RA, Elander R, Swinger C, and Reader AL: Four-incision radial keratotomy for low to moderate myopia, Ophthalmology 1986;93:727-733.
25. Sanders DR, Deitz MR, and Gallagher D: Factors affecting predictability of radial keratotomy, Ophthalmology 1985;92:1237-1243.
26. Spigelman AV, Williams PA, Nichols BD, and Lindstrom RL: Four-incision radial keratotomy, J Cataract Refract Surg 1988;14:125-128.
27. Starling JC and Hofmann RF: The new surgical technique for the correction of hyperopia after radial keratotomy: experimental model, J Refract Surg 1986;2:9-14.
28. Swinger CA and Barker BA: Myopic keratomileusis following radial keratotomy, J Refract Surg 1985;1:53-55.
29. Villasenor RA and Cox KC: Radial keratotomy: reoperations, J Refract Surg 1985;1:34-37.
30. Waring GO: Review: changing status of radial keratotomy for myopia: Part I. J Refract Surg 1985;1:81-86.
31. Waring GO: Review: changing status of radial keratotomy for myopia: Part II. J Refract Surg 1985;1:119-137.
32. Waring GO: Radial keratotomy. In Kaufman HE et al, editors: The cornea, New York, 1988, Churchill Livingstone, pp 849-896.
33. Waring GO, Lynn MJ, Culbertson W, and the PERK Study Group: Three-year evaluation of the Prospective Evaluation of Radial Keratotomy (PERK) study, Ophthalmology 1987;94:1339-1354.
34. Waring GO, Lynn MJ, Gelender H, et al: Results of the Prospective Evaluation of Radial Keratotomy (PERK) Study 1 year after surgery, Ophthalmology 1985;92:177-198.

Laser Corneal Surgery

Theo Seiler
Francisco E. Fantes
George O. Waring III
Khalil D. Hanna

BACKGROUND AND ACKNOWLEDGMENTS
My interest in laser corneal surgery commenced in 1983 when Stephen Trokel, MD, of Columbia University, and R Srinivasan, PhD, from IBM, published their initial observations on excimer laser keratectomy. The scope of the possibilities of laser corneal surgery became more clear when I met Khalil Hanna, MD, at the Forum Ophthalmologicum Centenarii sponsored by the Instituto Barraquer de America in 1984. Dr. Hanna is from Hotel Dieu Hospital in Paris, in the Department of Ophthalmology directed by Yves Pouliquen, MD. In one of those important chance conversations that peppers life with significant turning points, Dr. Hanna and I discussed the possibilities of using lasers for refractive surgery and for penetrating keratoplasty. Shortly thereafter, Trokel came to Emory University as a visiting lecturer and encouraged us to become active in this research; he has been a ready source of information and encouragement ever since. I visited the established laboratories of Hanna and Pouliquen in Paris; they visited Atlanta. That same year, with the support of the Department of Ophthalmology at Emory University, I established a laboratory for research in laser corneal surgery in collaboration with Dr. Hanna's laboratory at Hotel Dieu. Dr. Hanna became Associate Professor of Ophthalmology (part-time) at Emory. In 1986 I visited Theo Seiler, MD, PhD, at the Klinikum Charlottenburg at the Freie Universität in Berlin to observe his clinical use of excimer lasers. His training as a physicist and physician provided the broad knowledge that enabled him to carry out the first series of cases of excimer laser refractive corneal surgery, in collaboration with Thomas Bende, PhD.

We have collaborated with many individuals at the IBM Science Center in Paris. Mr. J.C. Chastang, Mr. Louis Asfar, and Mr. Jean Samson have applied their mathematical, engineering, and computer programming skills in the design of various delivery systems. At Hotel Dieu, we have collaborated with Drs. Yves Pouliquen, Gil Renard, Olivia Serdarevic, and Ms. Michelle Salvodelli.

At Emory University, four postdoctoral corneal fellows have diligently, consistently, and productively advanced work on this research—Drs. Francisco Fantes, Keith Thompson, Robert Maloney, and Ray Gailitis—with technical assistance of Mr. Dale Reddick and Quishi Ren, PhD. Immunohistochemical studies have been done by Nirmala SundarRaj, PhD, with the assistance of M.J. Geiss and S.C. Anderson at the University of Pittsburgh School of Medicine.

We have received research support from Coherent Radiation Corporation and its subsidiary Lambda Physik, Summit Technology, and the General Electric Corporation. Dr. Seiler and I are consultants for Summit Technology. Dr. Hanna and I have been consultants for General Electric.

Research has been supported by a grant to Dr. Waring from the National Eye Institute (EYO-7388).

The following individuals contributed to the section on terminology: Drs. Keith Thompson, Robert Maloney, John Marshall, Richard Lindstrom, and J.W. Koch.

This chapter is modified from a thesis previously published in the *Transactions of the American Ophthalmological Society*, and many of the figures are taken from that publication.[117]

All types of refractive keratotomy share one weakness—the inability to predict accurately the outcome of surgery for an individual patient. This defect results from variability in technique among surgeons and from variability in corneal biomechanical properties and wound healing among patients (Chapter 13, Predictability of Refractive Keratotomy; Chapter 20, Corneal Wound Healing and Its Pharmacologic Modification after Refractive Keratotomy).

The development of pulsed lasers, particularly the argon fluoride (193 nm) excimer laser, offers a potential solution to the first of these two problems because these lasers can create accurate and precise excisions of corneal tissue to an exact length and depth with minimal disruption of the remaining tissue. In addition, this minimal tissue disruption and the smooth edges may allow more uniform stromal wound healing. Laser surgery can also make cuts in almost any conceivable configuration, without touching the cornea. Using computers to control these lasers may create robotic refractive surgery, removing the art from the procedure and allowing the surgeon to perform the exact desired operation in case after case.[1,33,34,47]

Since 1983, when excimer lasers were first suggested as instruments for refractive surgery, researchers in numerous laboratories around the world have raced to define the conditions that might make this technology a clinical reality. Depending on one's perspective, progress has moved either rapidly—approximately five systems of varying sophistication are available for laboratory and clinical experimentation, or slowly—many fundamental technical and biologic questions about the process remain unanswered.

In this chapter we summarize selected aspects of excimer laser corneal surgery. After considering the terminology of this surgery and a few basic principles of lasers, we present the problems that face the creation of such a system: the selection of an appropriate laser, the design of an effective delivery system, the coupling of the delivery system to the eye, the interaction of the laser light with the cornea, the patterns of excisions to alter corneal curvature, and the effect of wound healing on these excisions.

Of the three types of excimer laser corneal surgery—photorefractive keratectomy (laser keratomileusis, surface area ablation), linear laser keratectomy, and laser therapeutic keratectomy—we discuss only the first two.

TERMINOLOGY FOR LASER CORNEAL SURGERY

The terminology used in laser corneal surgery can be confusing. Fundamental to all designations is the fact the pulsed laser light removes tissue from the cornea. Therefore a cut made with the laser is an excision—a keratectomy—that leaves a defect, not an incision—a keratotomy—that leaves only a dehiscence. A term such as "excimer laser radial keratotomy" is inaccurate. The fundamental effect of a pulsed excimer laser on tissue is a photochemical one, the breaking of molecular bonds with tissue fragments flying from the surface at supersonic speeds. This process has been designated photoablative decomposition—photoablation for short. This process contrasts with the more familiar photocoagulation of an argon laser and photodisruption of an Nd:YAG.[35]

The generic term "laser corneal surgery" can easily be modified to "laser refractive corneal surgery" or "laser therapeutic corneal surgery" to designate the two major categories. Since lasers remove tissue, the term "keratectomy" is used in the proposed terminology, and we think should be strictly adhered to in terms such as "laser refractive keratectomy" and "laser therapeutic keratectomy."

There are two types of laser refractive keratectomy: removal of a graded amount of tissue from the central cornea and the creation of linear excisions in a radial or transverse pattern. The term "photorefractive keratectomy" (PRK) has come to mean the central removal of a specific profile of Bowman's layer and anterior stroma to change the anterior curvature of the cornea. This is a good example of how the usage of language determines its meaning, since, strictly speaking, the term "photorefractive keratectomy" refers to all types of laser refractive corneal surgery. Nevertheless, photorefractive keratectomy has become the preferred term for what is otherwise called laser anterior keratomileusis, large area ablation, or reprofiling, or sculpting, of the cornea.

Designations of other refractive surgery techniques that involve the laser simply borrow preexisting terms preceded by "laser" or "excimer laser" to designate this new method of surgery, such as excimer laser keratomileusis (usage analogous to cryolathe keratomileusis and nonfreeze keratomileusis) and excimer laser keratomileusis-in-situ—both designating the removal of stromal tissue with a laser after a lamellar disc of cornea has already been removed.

Another surgical use of the laser is to modify a previous refractive surgical procedure to refine the result; we suggest simply using the term "photorefractive keratectomy" in conjunction with the original procedure, for example, PRK after myopic epikeratoplasty. If the modification is done on a synthetic epikeratoplasty, a new acronym, such as LASE (laser-adjustable synthetic epikeratophakia), may emerge.

Using a laser to make a linear cut is analogous to making cuts with a diamond knife, except that the cuts are excisions rather than incisions of tissue. There is no procedure called "laser radial keratotomy" be-

Table 19-1

Proposed Terminology for Laser Corneal Surgery

Type of procedure	Preferred term	Colloquial alternatives
I. General term	Laser corneal surgery	Laser keratoplasty Laser ablation of the cornea Laser keratectomy
II. Refractive	Laser refractive keratectomy	
A. Removal of central Bowman's layer and anterior stroma	Photorefractive keratectomy (PRK)	Laser anterior keratomileusis Large area ablation Reprofiling Sculpting En face ablation Tangential ablation
B. Linear keratectomy	Laser radial keratectomy Laser transverse keratectomy (straight, arcuate)	Laser RK
C. In conjunction with other techniques		
1. After removal of anterior lamellar disc (microkeratome)	Laser stromal keratomileusis Laser keratomileusis in-situ	Ablation of disc Ablation of bed
2. After previous refractive surgery	For example, PRK after radial keratotomy For example, PRK after epikeratoplasty	Laser adjustable synthetic epikeratoplasty (LASE)
D. Intrastromal laser surgery	Intrastromal photodisruption Intrastromal thermokeratoplasty	Intrastromal keratomileusis Intrastromal linear keratectomy Intrastromal "RK," "TK"
III. Therapeutic	Laser therapeutic keratectomy	
A. Removal of superficial corneal opacity	Phototherapeutic keratectomy (PTK)	Surface smoothing Superficial therapeutic keratectomy
B. Trephination	Laser circular or elliptical keratectomy	Laser penetrating keratoplasty Laser lamellar keratoplasty
IV. Removal of lamellar disc (replaces microkeratome)	Laser lamellar resection	Tangential lamellar resection

From Waring GO: Refract Corneal Surg 1990;6:318-320.
Type of laser to be specified (for example, excimer, argon fluoride.)

cause the laser actually creates a groove, or trough, in the tissue and does not merely sever the tissue; the proper term is laser radial (or transverse) keratectomy.

Using the laser to create a lenticule of corneal tissue, in the same way that a microkeratome or a manual lamellar dissection does, involves a lamellar cut tangent to the apex of the cornea, and therefore can be called a lamellar resection or a tangential resection. This is distinguished from a tangential ablation, in which the laser coming from the side ablates the tissue from the central anterior surface of the cornea, rather than cutting free a lamellar lenticule.

Laser therapeutic keratectomy comes in two varieties. The first involves the removal of a superficial corneal opacity or irregularity. Some have termed this "superficial keratectomy," which is an accurate but inadequate term because it also includes photorefractive

keratectomy, which is a type of superficial keratectomy. Again, usage dictates meaning, and the term "laser therapeutic keratectomy" generally means the removal of anterior diseased layers of the cornea.

However, there is a second type of laser therapeutic keratectomy, "laser trephination," which involves using a laser to make circular or elliptic incisions for penetrating or lamellar keratoplasty.

We have not mentioned some terms for procedures that are not yet in use, such as making a circular oblique keratectomy (as the bed for the wing of an epikeratoplasty) where the laser cut substitutes for the vertical trephination and lateral undermining. As new uses for the laser develop, there certainly will be new terms to describe them.

Table 19-1 presents a proposal for conventional terminology for laser corneal surgery.

PRINCIPLES OF LASERS

To understand the use of lasers in photorefractive keratectomy, it is helpful to review briefly the basic principles of lasers at a level suitable for ophthalmic clinicians. Details are presented in textbooks.[71,81] We use the argon fluoride excimer laser to illustrate these principles.[28,34,54,56,71] Light has both wave-like and particle-like properties. Wave-like properties explain optical phenomena such as refraction and interference; particle-like properties explain how tissues acquire and release energy—the absorption and emission of light by atoms and molecules. Therefore we use the terms "wave" and "photon" interchangeably, depending on the phenomena we want to explain.

The electromagnetic spectrum is composed of a broad range of wavelengths, from long radio waves to short gamma waves. Our interest is in the optical wavelengths in the invisible ultraviolet range (approximately 100 to 300 nm). Each wavelength of the electromagnetic spectrum interacts with the cornea in a specific way. The cornea absorbs well the ultraviolet and infrared radiation and transmits effectively the radiation between 300 and 1300 nm. Numerous wavelengths have been tested for photorefractive keratectomy: 193, 248, 2900, and 10,600 nm.

Specific characteristics of laser light as applied to corneal surgery

Monochromaticity. Light of a single wavelength forms a specific color in the visible spectrum and a specific invisible "color" outside that spectrum. Absolute monochromaticity is an unobtainable goal—even our best laser light is a mixture of some wavelengths. It is this characteristic that determines the amount of laser energy absorbed or transmitted by the cornea.

Directionality. Laser light is essentially collimated light that has a very small divergence, or spread, as it leaves the laser cavity. This characteristic allows laser light to be directed at a very small spot a relatively long distance from the laser itself and is the characteristic that allows laser light transmission through the delivery system to the eye. The directionality is measured by the full-angle beam divergence in radians. The typical laser beam increases in size for every meter of travel.

Brightness. The intense brightness of the laser light is an expression of the energy contained in the laser beam; because the energy is concentrated in a single wave train moving in one direction, the energies are extraordinarily high. This energy absorbed in the cornea is responsible for the ablation of tissue. The radiant energy is measured in joules; the radiant exposure of the tissue is measured in joules/cm^2; the radiant power is measured in watts; the irradiance is measured in watts/cm^2.

Coherence. Coherence occurs when the light waves in the laser are in phase and there is a predictable and constant correlation between the peak and the trough of the waves. The great regularity of coherence depends on the laser's monochromaticity and directionality and is measured by interferometry. Coherence is not a very important characteristic in the use of lasers for corneal or ophthalmic surgery, in which the major emphasis is on absorption of specific wavelengths and the energy of the beam. Coherence becomes important, however, in the use of lasers for communication, holography, and measurement. The coherence of an excimer laser beam is generally poor.

Mode structure. The distribution of energy in the laser beam is characterized as the mode of the beam, the energy distribution across the beam being called the transverse mode and that along the beam being called the longitudinal mode. The mode structure of the laser is important in determining its potential uses on the basis of the divergence and coherence of the beam. The transverse mode—more specifically, the transverse electromagnetic mode (TEM)—can have a number of patterns and configurations. When there is more power in the center of the beam than at the edge of the beam, the mode is designated TEM_{00}. If there is less power in the center and the distribution is bimodal, the designation is TEM_{01}. Depending on the resonant properties in the laser cavity, laser beams can acquire many different mode structures (multimode). Excimer lasers produce a multimode beam that is more difficult to render homogenous than are the beams of solid state or dye lasers. A homogeneous beam is an advantage in creating a smooth surface after photoablation.

Creation of laser light

To create laser light, three basic conditions must exist (Fig. 19-1). First, there must be an active medium—a collection of atoms, molecules, or ions that emit radiation in the optical part of the electromagnetic spectrum. The medium can be (1) a gas such as krypton, carbon dioxide, or those in an excimer, for example, argon fluoride; (2) a solid such as neodymium-doped yttrium-aluminum-garnet (YAG) crystal; or (3) a liquid, such as a dye laser. Second, there must be a source of energy for the laser, a pump that can cause a population of atoms to undergo the transition from their ground state to the higher energy level—a population inversion. The pumping may be achieved with an electrical discharge, as in an argon or excimer laser; by a flash lamp, as in an Nd:YAG laser; or by an optical source, as in dye lasers. The third necessary element is the optical resonator that allows the emitted light beam to feed back by being reflected between two mirrors, stimulating other atoms to a

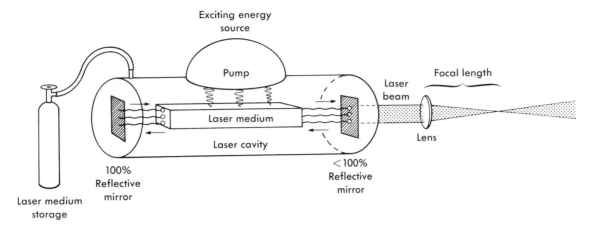

Figure 19-1
Basic configuration of excimer laser demonstrates the active laser medium as gas in the storage tank and in the laser cavity. The excited energy is pumped from a source illustrated as a bank of electrical capacitors whose discharge can create a population inversion in the laser medium. The laser cavity has mirrors at each end to amplify the laser beam before it is emitted through a delivery system containing lenses. (From Waring GO: Trans Am Ophthalmol Soc 1989;87:854-983.)

higher energy level in the process, thereby amplifying the light and creating a much more powerful beam. The number of feedback or resonating cycles varies greatly among lasers, from many in the argon to few in an excimer. A detailed examination of these three components provides a basis for understanding the development of a system for laser corneal surgery.

The active medium. The basis for understanding laser action is our current conception of how atoms behave. In an atom, the nucleus of protons and neutrons is surrounded by clouds of electrons at different energy levels—electron orbitals. An atom in its ground state of energy is at rest, but the addition of external radiation can induce it to make a transition to a higher energy level, the electrons being moved from their ground state inner orbital to a higher-energy outer orbital. This is a less stable condition, and the electron returns almost immediately to the less-energetic resting state, emitting a photon of surplus energy in the process (Fig. 19-2). This photon, with its specific wavelength, is the basis for creating laser light. When the photon is liberated spontaneously, the process is called spontaneous emission. In reality, however, the emission of photons is stimulated by the external energy source and the other photons that have been emitted in the active medium. Thus both the absorption of energy and the emission of energy by the atoms are stimulated, and the atoms undergoing stimulated emission radiate their photons of energy in phase with each other (coherence) so that the waves add energy to each other on a constructive basis, creating the

powerful laser light. This circumstance is the basis for the acronym LASER—Light Amplification by Stimulated Emission of Radiation. (Current commercial competition over the development of a clinically useful excimer laser led John Marshall to redefine the acronym LASER: Lucrative Acquisition Scheme and Expensive Research.)

Laser pumping and population inversion. To initiate the lasting process, an external source of energy must be pumped into the active medium so that the atoms can be excited to the higher energy state, a condition known as population inversion. Once this population inversion is achieved, the light amplification by stimulated emission can take place. Many sources of energy can be used. An electric discharge is commonly used in gas lasers. Electrons in the discharge are accelerated by the electric field between the two electrodes so that they collide with the atoms, ions, or molecules in the active medium, inducing transitions to higher energy states. In solid-state lasers, such as the Nd:YAG, the discharge is from a flash lamp. Dye lasers are optically pumped, usually by light from another laser that has a peak emission near the dye absorption band; this method creates a continuous wave dye laser. A flash lamp can be used as a pump to create a pulsed dye laser.

The transition of electrons from one energy level to another is not simple, and many transitions can occur in an atom, creating emissions of different wavelengths. Control of this process is part of the sophistication of laser design.

How a Photon is Formed

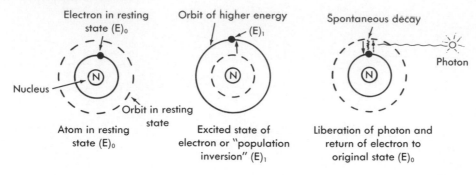

How the Laser Beam is Formed

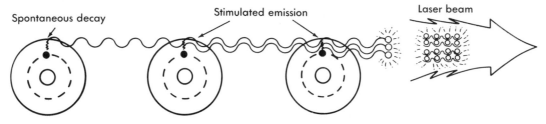

Figure 19-2
The process of photon formation and the stimulated emission of radiation from the active laser medium is illustrated here and explained in the text. (From Waring GO: Trans Am Ophthalmol Soc 1989;87:854-983.)

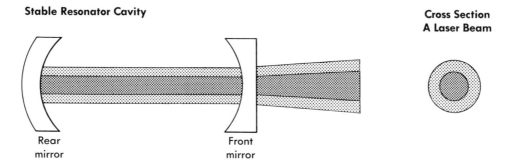

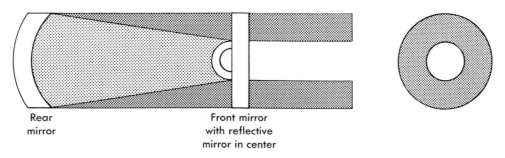

Figure 19-3
Stability conditions in the resonating chamber of a laser. In the stable configuration, two concave or a concave and planar mirror are used, resulting in a beam of higher power but more divergence. In an unstable configuration, the transmitting mirror has a convex mirror in the center of it, creating a beam with less power and less divergence and a less regular beam profile. (From Waring GO: Trans Am Ophthalmol Soc 1989;87:854-983.)

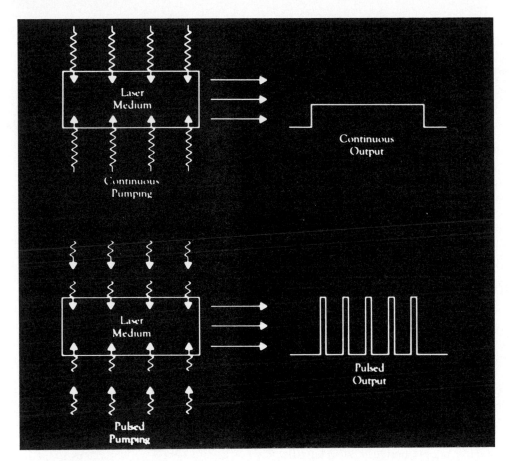

Figure 19-4
Pattern of cmission of laser light can be either a continuous wave from continuous
pumping of the laser medium or individual pulses from intermittent pumping of
the laser medium. (From Waring GO: Trans Am Ophthalmol Soc 1989;87:854-
983.)

***Optical feedback and amplification in a resonating
chamber.*** The active medium is contained within a
resonating chamber, into which the pumping energy
is discharged. The resonating chamber consists of mirrors at each end so that the stimulated emitted photons are reflected back and forth within the resonating
cavity. This increases the distance they travel and ensures the photons strike other atoms of the active medium and stimulate them to higher energy transitions,
with the production of more photons. This feedback
between the mirrors is the basis for the amplification
process that creates the great power of a laser beam.

The mirror at one end of the laser cavity is completely reflective, but the mirror at the other end is
only partially reflective, allowing the emission of the
laser beam. A laser with a 98% reflective mirror at the
emitting end has an effective length roughly 50 times
the actual separation distance between the mirrors.
The number of feedback trips varies from laser to laser. In an excimer, for example, the number of oscilla-
tions are very few because of the extremely high energy of the emitting photons.

The configuration of the mirrors at either end of the
resonating cavity determines the portion of the reflected waves that remain close to the optical axis of
the cavity and those that diverge from the axis.
Greater divergence creates lower power output. These
configurations are called "stability conditions" (Fig.
19-3). A stable resonator cavity has two concave mirrors or one concave and one planar mirror so that the
feedback paths are focused close to the optical axis.
An unstable resonator cavity has a central convex mirror at the partially reflective end, so much of the diverging beam emerges around this mirror. In a stable
cavity, less of the light within the cavity is used for the
lasing, but the emergent beam represents more of the
lasing light. In the unstable resonator, more of the reflected light is used for lasing within the cavity, but a
smaller percent of the total light is emitted in the
beam. These considerations become important in dealing with excimer lasers in corneal surgery, where
higher power outputs are more difficult to achieve.

Emission of laser light. Laser light is emitted either
continuously or in pulses (Fig. 19-4). With continuous

wave (CW) lasers, a constant pumping of the laser medium leads to a stationary emission of light, such as in the familiar argon laser. With pulsed lasers, excitation of the laser medium is achieved by single events, such as the flash from a flash lamp or an electrical discharge, leading to a single short emission of light—the laser pulse. This is familiar in the pulsed Nd:YAG laser. The power of a pulsed laser is on the order of 1000 to 1,000,000 times higher than that of a continuous wave laser. Only pulsed lasers are useful in refractive corneal surgery. The power emitted from a pulsed laser can be increased by ensuring that the longitudinal modes of the laser beam within the laser cavity are in phase and are emitted in brief spikes, for example, mode locking.

INTERACTION OF LASER LIGHT WITH THE CORNEA

There are four interactions that laser light may have with the cornea: transmission, scattering, reflection, and absorption (Fig. 19-5). Which of these four interactions occurs depends on the laser characteristics and the tissue characteristics, and most importantly, the amount of light energy that is absorbed by the molecules in the tissue—the chromophores.

Transmission of laser light through the normal human cornea generally occurs between wavelengths of 300 and 1600 nm.[34] Thus lasers such as the argon and the Nd:YAG pass through the cornea without difficulty. Laser light can also be scattered by the tissue if the beam is distributed over a large area, increasing the extension of thermal and other side effects and decreasing the efficiency of the laser. Reflection of the laser beam seldom occurs from the cornea.

The most important interaction is absorption of the laser energy by the cornea.

Absorption of laser light by the cornea

The higher the absorption, the more "opaque" the cornea to a given wavelength and the easier the process of surface ablation. Therefore the key to understanding the appropriate selection of lasers for keratectomy lies in the absorption spectrum of the corneal tissues (Figs. 19-6 and 19-7; Table 19-2).[5,47] The highest absorption in the cornea is by macromolecules, in the far ultraviolet region at wavelengths less than 300 nm, and by water, in both the middle infrared region near 3000 and 6000 nm and the far infrared region above 10,000 nm.

A good way to conceive of absorption is in terms of the penetration depth of the laser light: the greater the absorption, the less the penetration of a better potential for surface ablation and a decreased chance of thermal damage. Table 19-3 lists the penetration

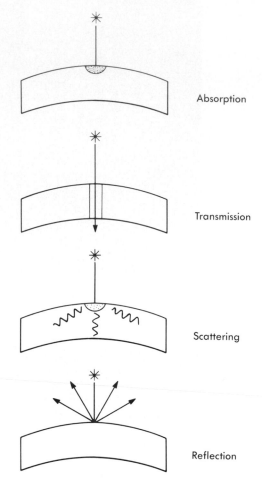

Figure 19-5
Four types of interaction of laser light with the cornea. (From Waring GO: Trans Am Ophthalmol Soc 1989; 87:854-983.)

depths of lasers that have been used for keratectomy and demonstrates that the argon fluoride excimer laser and the fifth harmonic Nd:YAG ultraviolet lasers have the smallest penetration depth and therefore are best suited for corneal surgery. The hydrogen fluoride and Er:YAG are also well absorbed. Wavelengths absorbed by nucleic acids may be mutagenic and therefore not appropriate for clinical use.

When laser light is absorbed by the cornea, there are three types of effects that can occur: (1) photothermal, (2) photodisruption, and (3) photochemical.

Photothermal effects. Photothermal effects occur when the energy absorbed by photons produces molecular vibration. This vibration produces heat and increases the temperature enough to break weaker bonds, such as hydrogen bonds, producing protein denaturation.

There are two types of thermal effects: photocoagulation and photovaporization. Photocoagulation is the

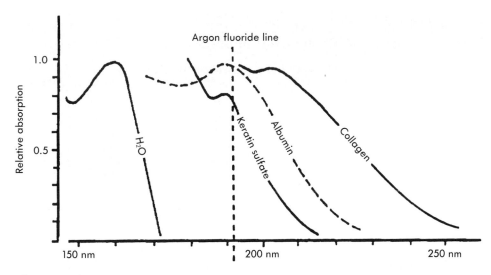

Figure 19-6
Absorption spectrum for molecules in the cornea. The x-axis indicates wavelength in nanometers. The y-axis indicates the relative absorption. The wavy dotted line shows the reference point for albumin. The vertical dotted line shows argon fluoride at 193 nm, where there is a relatively high absorption for collagen and keratin sulfate. (Courtesy Theo Seiler.)

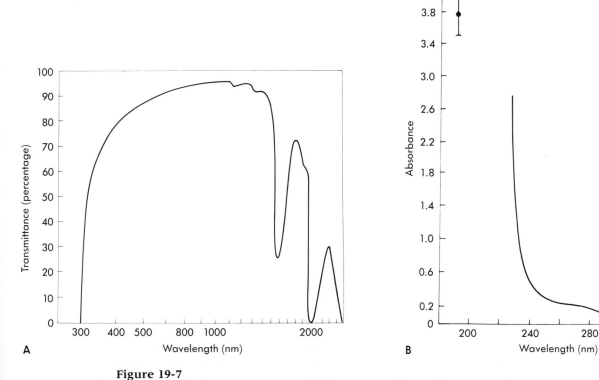

Figure 19-7
Transmission and absorption of light by the cornea. **A,** Transmission of light through the human cornea. **B,** Plot of absorbance versus wavelength in the far ultraviolet spectrum for a 32 μm thick section of bovine cornea. The point at 193 nm represents the average of laser transmission measurements made on eight different 32 μm thick samples. The error bar indicates one standard deviation. (**A** from Boettner EA: Invest Ophthalmol Vis Sci 1962;1:776-783; **B** from Puliafito CA et al: Ophthalmology 1985;92:741-748.)

Table 19-2

Absorption Bands for Components of Cornea

Cornea component	Absorption wavelength (nm)	Location of major concentration	Optimal radiation
Protein[5]	190	Stroma	Ultraviolet
GAG[105]	190	Stroma	Ultraviolet
Collagen[42]	240	Stroma	Ultraviolet
Nucleic acid[69]	248	Epithelium	Ultraviolet
Ascorbic acid[74]	250	Epithelium	Ultraviolet
Water[47]	2900	Stroma	Infrared
	10,000		

Table 19-3

Lasers Potentially Usable for Corneal Surgery

Laser	Wavelength (nm)	Pulse duration (nsec)	Penetration depth (μm)
Excimer (ArF)	193	10-20	2
Excimer (KrF)	248	10-20	10
Excimer (XeCl)	308	10-20	300
5th harmonic Nd:YAG	213	10	2
Holmium:YAG	2060	20,000	330
Hydrogen fluoride	2870-2910	50	1.5
Er:YAG	2940	20,000	0.75
ER:YSGG	2790	20,000	1.5
Raman shifted YAG	2800	10	1.5
CO_2 TEA	10,600		

most common use of CW lasers in ophthalmology, such as argon and krypton laser photocoagulation of the retina and choroid. The laser needs to elevate temperature only 10° to 20° C to coagulate the tissue. Variables set by the surgeon are power, duration of exposure, and spot size.

In photovaporization, very high radiant densities are used and tissue temperature rapidly reaches the boiling point of water, where both coagulation and excision of tissue occur. Photovaporization is the mechanism for keratectomy by the infrared lasers, such as HF and CO_2. The higher the irradiances, the greater the amount of tissue removed and the less the coagulation. For example, a CO_2 laser can ablate corneal tissue with less thermal damage if a pulsed rather than a CW laser is used.

Photodisruption effects. Photodisruption by means of ionization occurs at a very high irradiance, with pulse durations shorter than 20 nanoseconds. The high-energy density tears electrons from their atomic

orbitals and disintegrates the tissue into a collection of ions and electrons called plasma, a gas with the electrical properties of a metal. The effect produces mechanical shock waves. This is the mechanism used by the Nd:YAG laser and the pulsed dye laser.

Photochemical effects. Photochemical effects usually occur at shorter wavelengths, with low to moderate radiant exposures. There are two basic types of photochemical reactions: photoradiation and photoablation. Photoradiation is used in photoradiation therapy (PRT), in which a hematoporphyrin derivative is selectively taken up by active tumor cells and the laser radiation produces an excited state of the porphyrin, which triggers chemical reactions that destroy the cell.

The process most commonly used in refractive corneal surgery is ablative photodecomposition (photoablation for short) and is accomplished with ultraviolet radiation. The ultraviolet photons are almost completely absorbed by the surface of the cornea. They also have an extremely high photon energy (6.4 electron volts at 193 nm), an energy that is in excess of the intermolecular bond energy of approximately 3.5 ev. Thus the absorption of this energy at the surface breaks up the molecules with such energy that the fragments leave the surface at supersonic velocities of 1000 to 3000 m/sec. Thus the excess energy is carried off, and there is minimal thermal damage in the residual tissue.* This process is described in the following section.

LASERS USED FOR CORNEAL SURGERY

As laser refractive corneal surgery continues to develop and expand, an increasing number of lasers are being used for the process (see Table 19-3). Presently, numerous types of lasers are under active investigation.

Excimer lasers

Excimer lasers are discussed in detail in this chapter and are briefly defined here. In an excimer laser, the active medium is most commonly the excited combination of an excited rare gas atom (such as argon or krypton) with a diatomic halogen molecule (such as fluorine or chlorine). The laser is pumped by a high-voltage electrical discharge across the laser cavity and is emitted with megawatt intensity of ultraviolet light in the range of 190 to 350 nm, which is absorbed by the macromolecules (proteins, nucleic acids, proteoglycans) in the cornea. Excimer lasers have the potential advantage of precisely removing very small amounts of tissue with each pulse, leaving behind minimal thermal or acoustic damage.

Excimer lasers were first developed in 1975.[82,110] Extensive research on the excimer-polymer interactions was performed by Srinivasan, Sutcliffe, Dyer, and others,[11,41,96,101] who demonstrated that because the ultraviolet wavelengths were useful for etching silicones and other polymers,[94] they might be used for manufacturing microcircuits. Reed et al.[78] were the first to use the excimer laser on the cornea, and they demonstrated that the corneal epithelium is very sensitive to the wavelengths of krypton fluoride at 248 nm.

Their first application for refractive corneal surgery occurred when R. Srinivasan, IBM Research Center, Yorktown, N.Y., and Stephen Trokel, Columbia University, N.Y., reasoned that if excimer lasers could be used to etch and carve polymers, they might be used also to etch and carve the cornea. This resulted in their 1983 publication demonstrating exquisite linear excisions in the cornea and suggesting the use of these lasers for refractive corneal surgery[111] (Fig. 19-8).

*References 11, 32, 34, 41, 57-60, 77, 82, 94-97, 100-102, 111.

Carbon dioxide laser

In a carbon dioxide laser the lasing medium is a mixture of nitrogen, helium, and carbon dioxide. Pumping is usually accomplished by a high-voltage electric current that excites the nitrogen atoms, whose electrons are rapidly transferred to the carbon dioxide atoms. The excited carbon dioxide atoms decay, emitting infrared light, most commonly at a wavelength of 10,600 mm. This is amplified within the resonance cavity at high efficiency and can produce tremendous amounts of output power. Thermal interaction relies on water content to determine the effect produced by the CO_2 laser. The intracellular and extracellular water undergoes an abrupt phase change, creating steam and vaporizing the tissue. The dispersed energy can be absorbed by the tissue adjacent to the ablation, resulting in coagulation and carbonization of the remaining tissue. However, reducing the exposure time can minimize the thermal effect.

The features of the pulsed CO_2 laser that make it particularly suitable for corneal surgery are (1) CO_2 laser energy is strongly absorbed by water molecules and (2) the thermal relaxation time for water at the 10.6 μm wavelength is 200 μsec. Because the cornea is composed of 78% water, the corneal endothelium, as well as other portions of the eye, is protected from thermal damage from transmitted energy delivered with short exposure times. The thermal relaxation time of biologic tissue is different from that of water. However, with a pulse width shorter than 200 μsec, it should be possible to vaporize tissue without creating thermal damage to adjacent areas. A large amount of power will need to be delivered during the short-pulse duration, creating high-power densities. The poor hemostatic ability of the laser used in this fashion may be of concern in other tissues, but in an avascular tissue like the cornea, this is not relevant.

The first laser incisions in the cornea were made with a continuous wave carbon dioxide laser by Fine and colleagues in 1967.[15,16] The deep penetration of about 25 microns caused large zones of thermal damage adjacent to the incision, resulting in inflammation and corneal scarring, with a need for penetrating keratoplasty. Beckman and colleagues[6] used a pulsed carbon dioxide laser, reducing thermal damage to the cornea, but still leaving enough damage to render its use impractical for corneal surgery. Keates and colleagues[30] used a pulsed carbon dioxide laser and a specially designed delivery system to create a narrow cut into the cornea. The edges of the excised tissue were ragged compared with those achieved with an excimer laser. We have used a pulsed TEA carbon dioxide laser for experimental corneal surgery, as described later in this chapter.

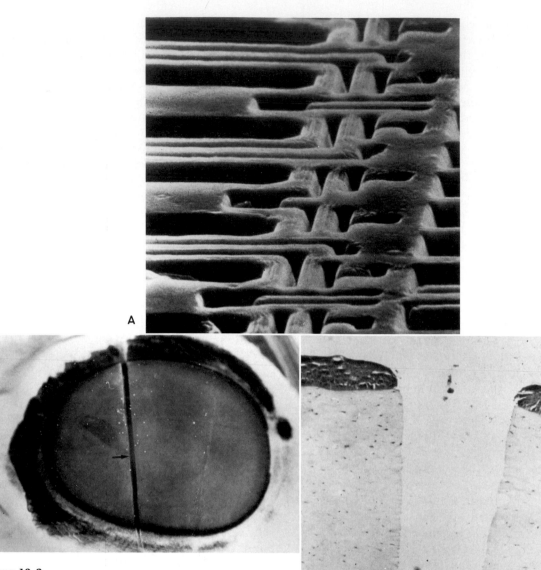

Figure 19-8

Early development of excimer laser corneal surgery stemmed from the use of excimers to etch surfaces in the manufacture of computer microcircuits. Trokel and Srinivasan applied the same concept to the "etching" of corneas to change their shape by linear keratectomy and by surface reprofiling (photorefractive keratectomy). **A,** Scanning electron micrograph of material prepared for a microcircuit by excimer laser etching (×12,626). **B,** Enucleated bovine cornea shows vertical linear keratectomy *(arrow)* extending from limbus to limbus—the first eye so treated by Stephen Trokel, MD. **C,** Light micrograph of the wide trough created by linear excimer laser incision in the bovine cornea showing a cut down to the level of Descemet's membrane *(arrow)* (H & E, ×4). (From Trokel S, Srinivasan R, and Braren BA: Am J Ophthalmol 1983;96:710-715.)

Hydrogen fluoride lasers

The lasing medium in a hydrogen fluoride laser consists of hydrogen and sulfurhexafluoride gases. The laser is pumped by an electrical discharge into vibrationally excited hydrogen fluoride molecules that have a number of emission lines, ranging from 2740 to 2960 nm. These wavelengths can be amplified in the stable resonator cavity and are emitted to be absorbed by the water in the cornea, with a penetration depth on the order of 1 micron.

Two groups have reported on the use of hydrogen fluoride lasers for surgery. Seiler and colleagues[89] observed that the excisions of tissue made with the laser created more thermal damage and a more irregular margin than those made with an argon fluoride (193-nm) excimer laser. However, with more careful design of the delivery system and more careful focusing of the laser, sharp-edged excisions with minimal remote thermal damage can be achieved.

Loertscher and co-workers[46,49] have used the hydrogen fluoride laser to perform laser circular trephinations using an axicon lens delivery system with a narrowly focused beam. Trephinations performed in eye bank eyes demonstrated a perfectly vertical incision with reasonably smooth edges, but not as smooth as those obtained with an argon fluoride excimer.

The experiments performed by these two groups have produced somewhat contradictory results. Seiler and co-workers[89] used lower radiant exposures of 100 mJ/cm^2, whereas Loertscher and colleagues[48] operated with higher fluences between 0.7 and 2.3 J/cm^2, identifying an ablation threshold of 400 mJ/cm^2 and an optimal radiant exposure to minimize thermal damage of 4 mJ/cm^2. Both groups have found thermal damage extending 10 to 30 microns laterally from the excision.

The advantages of a hydrogen fluoride laser are the simplicity of the laser itself and the greater possibility of creating delivery systems using fiberoptics.

Erbium:YAG laser

Very similar to the Nd:YAG laser, this type of solid-state laser uses a YAG crystal doped with erbium ions as a lasing medium. The emitted wavelength is 2.94 μm, near the maximal absorption of water. Commercial devices include a Q-switched mode that is able to create pulses with an energy of 100 mJ and a maximum pulse duration of 280 nsec and a non−Q switched mode with a pulse diameter at about 150 μsec. Only repetition rates of less than 10 Hz are available.

The advantages of this laser include its small size, its easy technical handling, and its transmission through optical fibers, making both direct application to the cornea and intraocular surgery possible. Manufacturing difficulties include the need for special optical elements that contain no absorbed water.

Pulsed holmium:YAG laser

Seiler and colleagues[90] used a pulsed holmium:YAG laser emitting at a wavelength of 2.06 μm to make focal thermokeratoplasty burns within the stroma, in an attempt to correct hyperopia by shrinking a paracentral ring of cornea and steepening the central cornea. The laser light was guided by a quartz fiber and focused by means of a handpiece. The beam was focussed about 400 μm in front of the handpiece. The pulse duration was approximately 200 msec. The output energy was maximally 35 mJ per pulse at a repetition rate of 4 Hz. The fluence at the cornea ranged from 10 mJ/cm^2 to 28 mJ/cm^2. For every coagulation, 30 pulses were applied. The studies were carried out in human cadaver eyes, demonstrating that a total energy delivered to the cornea of 15 to 20 mJ produced the maximal amount of correction. The smaller the diameter of the clear zone along which the burns were made, the greater the change in refraction. Histologically the coagulation formed a conical illusion, wider near the surface and tapered to approximately 50 μm in front of Descemet's membrane. In a series of four blind human eyes, corrections of approximately 3.00 to 5.00 D were achieved, with the values present at 1 month persisting to approximately 4 months.

Dye lasers

In general, lasers that emit visible light are not used for corneal surgery because they are not absorbed by the cornea. However, if a sufficiently high energy density can be applied in a short enough pulse, a keratectomy can be achieved by tissue disruption or ionization.

In a dye laser, an organic dye dissolved in a solvent is irradiated with a strong light source, such as an argon laser, which causes the dye to fluoresce over a broad spectrum of colors. A specific wavelength can be made to lase by inserting a birefringent crystal into the laser cavity. By turning this crystal, an appropriate angle can be found that will transmit only a narrow wavelength of light, allowing the operator to turn the crystal and dial the desired wavelength.

Troutman and colleagues[112] have used a pulsed dye laser to perform intrastromal keratectomies by focusing the laser in the center of the stroma. The rationale behind this approach to laser refractive surgery is to preserve an intact Bowman's layer and anterior corneal stroma so that the all-important anterior corneal surface is essentially undisturbed. The dye laser emitted a wavelength of 595 nm (yellow), which allowed the investigators to obtain radiances of up to 10^{15} watts/cm² when in focus, using picosecond pulses. Histologic examination of animal and human eye bank eyes showed creation of space within the stroma, with damage to the adjacent tissue extending 20 to 40 microns from the wound.

For such an approach to be successful, it must not only produce negligible stromal scarring and opacification from the intrastromal ablation, but it must also change the anterior corneal curvature. Because Bowman's layer and the anterior cornea are reasonably rigid compared with Descemet's membrane and the posterior cornea, and because there is a pressure differential across the cornea from the posterior side (the intraocular pressure exceeding atmospheric pressure), it seems more likely that the posterior layers of the cornea will collapse forward, leaving the anterior layers in their preoperative configuration, with minimal change in refraction. It seems that this approach will have more impact in linear excisions than in the central surface type of excisions.

Excimer lasers

Trokel[110] has summarized the early development of excimer laser technology. Two physical chemists, Velazco and Setser,[115] working at Kansas State University, noted in 1975 that certain physical properties of the metastable states of rare gas atoms resembled those of the alkali metals. They reported a similarity of the chemical properties of metastable xenon atoms (Xe) to the alkali metals in their ability to react with halogens (X) to produce an unstable compound, XeX. This compound rapidly dissociated to the ground state of the individual molecules with the release of an energetic ultraviolet photon. They inferred that the diatomic noble gas-halides were of special interest because "these bound-free emissions have considerable potential as ultraviolet laser systems for excitation of mixtures of xenon (or other rare gases) and halogen containing compounds." Within the few months following their suggestion that this metastable compound could be used as the basis of a laser, four molecules, XeF, XeCl, XeBr, and KrF, were observed to lase when they were excited in an electron beam under high pressure.

Nomenclature for these early ultraviolet lasers was mixed. The word "excimer" had been coined in 1960 as a contraction of "excited dimer" to describe an energized molecule with two identical components. When analyzing the action of these ultraviolet lasers, it was thought that the argon molecule formed an "excited dimer" during the preionization phase of its excitation. This was ultimately found not to be so, yet the common use of the term has persisted. Alternative names for these lasers include "rare gas-halide lasers," which describes the gas mixture in the cavity, and the name of the specific gas mixture, "argon fluoride laser," to describe a specific system. Another name was suggested when the actual lasing compound was recognized to be an "excited complex molecule" consisting of two different elements, the rare gas and the halide. Some workers suggested that this was best described as an "excited molecular complex," and the word "exciplex" was coined to describe the lasers. However, excimer stuck because of its simplicity.

Taboada[103,104] first reported that KrF (248 nm) exposure on the rabbit cornea produced either opacification or fluorescein staining that took the general shape of the laser beam distribution. He described a range of damage effects that varied with the energy distribution in the laser beam and observed that at exposures of 27.5 mJ/cm² or greater, an immediate indentation of the corneal surface appeared, taking the shape of the beam. Trokel interpreted this to mean that tissue was being removed, and he began research on excimer lasers to develop improved technology for radial keratotomy, reasoning that the technical limits of knife incision technology could be surpassed by using a laser that would create a perfectly predictable incision depth along the corneal curve. He also entertained the possibility that a direct laser keratomileusis could be done by removing tissue from the corneal surface to modify its curve and change its optics.

In collaboration with R. Srinivasan, a photochemist, who used the argon fluoride (ArF) excimer laser to ablate plastics and other organic materials at the IBM T.J. Watson Laboratories, Trokel used veal eyes to study the interaction of the laser beam with the cornea. The first eye done showed a crisply edged groove, made deeper in successive sections. They were able to remove a fraction of a micron of corneal tissue with each pulse of laser light. The resulting surfaces were extremely smooth and uniform, and there was no collateral damage to the adjacent unirradiated tissues. They could control the shape and pattern of tissue removed by adjusting the gradient of the incident beam. This commenced the effort to use ArF excimer lasers for human refractive corneal surgery.

Around the same time, Dr. Francis L'Esperance filed broad "method patents" that covered all types of laser corneal surgery using wavelengths less than 400 nm, including excimers. Trokel contended that he was the first person to come up with the idea of corneal laser surgery, and this led the Patent and Trademark Office to begin an "interference" legal proceeding to determine who was the first to create the idea. IBM joined the legal fray because it held a broad patent that covered the fundamental use of lasers in the far ultraviolet spectrum to remove human tissue. The issue between Trokel and L'Esperance[62,67] resolved when the two companies, in which both doctors held an interest (VISX and Taunton), amalgamated. But patent disputes among other parties will no doubt emerge.

Physics of excimer lasers

Lasing medium. Two gases in the laser resonating chamber, an inert gas (such as argon) and a diatomic halide gas (such as fluorine), left to their own devices, do not interact; but under the impact of the energy from a high-powered electrical discharge, the electrons are moved to a higher energy state and the atoms become excited and form an unstable molecule, such as argon fluoride. When the molecules decay, they emit highly energetic photons of ultraviolet light.[28]

Within the excimer laser cavity are three gases. The first is a buffer gas that simply mediates the transfer of energy. It is helium or neon and fills 88% to 99% of the cavity. The rare gas (argon, krypton, or xenon) constitutes 0.5% to 12% of the mixture. The halogen (fluorine or chlorine) contributes approximately 0.5% of the mixture. The combination of the rare gas and halogen gas produces photons of a specific wavelength (see Table 19-2). Modulation of the buffer gas and the addition of other gases, such as neon, affects the quality of the laser beam.

Electrical pumping. Pumping of the laser is produced by an electrical discharge—up to 5% of it being converted into laser energy. Electron beam pumping is achieved with a series of high-voltage potentials that accelerate electrons to high energies that are transmitted to the laser cavity at beam currents on the order of 100 kiloamperes. Lasing action is obtained parallel to the electrodes, perpendicular to the electric discharge path. With multiple uses, the gases deteriorate and need to be refilled frequently to maintain the high energy and the quality of the laser beam.

Optics and resonator cavity. If the gain produced by the population inversion is so large that lasing occurs without feedback between the mirrors, the laser is termed "superradiant." Excimer lasers are almost superradiant but still have a resonator configuration. The back mirror of the laser resonator cavity is completely reflective, and the front mirror has a reflectivity of about 4%, which is quite enough because of the high gain of the laser. The partial transmission of the front mirror allows the laser beam to escape in nanosecond pulses. The shape of the emergent beam is determined by stable or unstable configuration of the mirrors of the resonator cavity, as described earlier.

Effect of excimer laser on materials and tissue. The mechanism of ablative photodecomposition achieved by this laser is illustrated in Fig. 19-9. Puliafito and

colleagues[76,77] used high-speed photography to chronicle the ejection of fragments from the surface (Fig. 19-10).

Excimer laser variables

Many variables control the effect of an excimer laser on the cornea; the variables in the laser include wavelength, pulse duration, pulse energy, radiant exposure (fluence), and peak power. The variables the surgeon can easily change include the pulse repetition rate and the total number of pulses. The interaction between the laser and the tissue are determined by the depth of penetration of a pulse, the depth of ablation achieved by a single pulse, and the depth of the total excision of tissue. Table 19-4 lists the typical values for these variables. Table 19-5 summarizes the findings of selected early studies of the effect of these variables on the cornea.

Wavelength. Many ultraviolet wavelengths can be generated by excimer lasers (see Table 19-2); laboratory experiments and histopathologic studies have demonstrated that the argon fluoride laser emitting at 193 nm creates the most regular margin of excision with the least damage to residual tissue.[36,37,60,77,111] Presumably, this is because the shorter wavelengths have the higher photon energies and small penetration depths, and achieve a more purely photochemical process of ablative photodecomposition near the surface, whereas the longer wavelengths of krypton fluoride (248 nm) and xenon chloride (308 nm) have more energy dissipated in the adjacent tissue, causing thermal damage.

Specifically, Puliafito and colleagues[77] compared in human and bovine corneas the quality of the ablation achieved with argon fluoride at 193 nm and krypton fluoride at 248 nm. They found a better quality of ablation with the 193-nm laser. The zone of condensation and thermal damage was 0.1 to 0.3 μm thick with 193 nm, but it extended 2.5 μm for the 248 nm. The 248-nm wavelength also created more disorganization of the residual stromal tissue. They concluded the 193-nm excision was similar to the incision made with the diamond knife and that this was the preferred wavelength. Similar findings resulted from studies of Krueger[36] using 193-nm, 248-nm, and xenon chloride laser emitting at 308 nm. The walls of the remaining tissue at 193 nm showed only a thin layer of condensed tissue at the surface, but at 248 nm the residual tissue was irregular and vacuolated, and at 308 nm there was a wide area of cornea necrosis and coagulation, suggesting thermal damage. Similar findings were reported by Peyman and colleagues[78] using 308-nm excimer wavelength. Indeed, the 308-nm wavelength may pass through the cornea and damage intraocular structures. Marshall and colleagues[60] dem-

Text continued on p. 689.

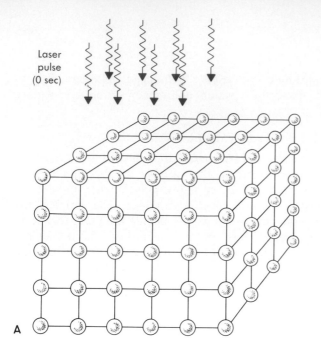

Laser
pulse
(0 sec)

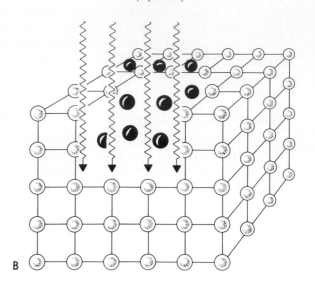

Ablative photodecomposition
(1 picosec)

Ejection of tissue fragments
(4 picosec)

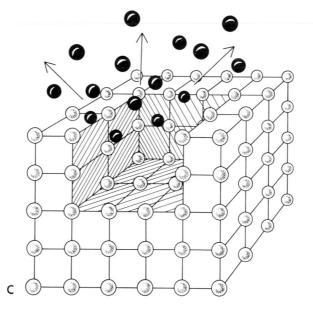

Figure 19-9
For legend see opposite page.

Termination of laser pulse and
tissue ablation (15 nanosec)

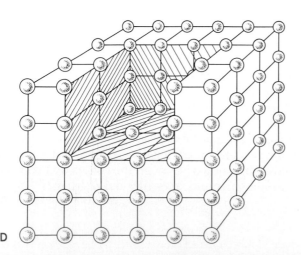

Repeated laser pulse and
photodecomposition

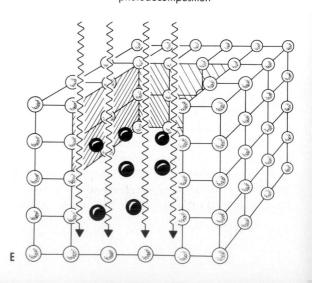

Table 19-4

Variables of Pulsed Lasers Used for Keratectomy

Variable	Dimension	Typical values
Variables in the laser		
Wavelength	nm	200 (UV)
		3000 (IR)
		10,000 (IR)
Pulse duration	nsec	10-50
Pulse energy	mJ	200-250
Fluence or radiant energy density	mJ/cm^2	100-300
Peak power	Watts	10^8
Beam profile and spatial regularity	Percent deviation from mean	±5% to 10%
Variables adjusted by the surgeon		
Repetition rate	Hz	5-50
Total number of pulses	N	50-5000
Laser-tissue interactions		
Penetration depth	μm	1-5
Ablation depth	μm/pulse	0.1-0.5 for UV
		0.1-2.0 for IR
Excision depth	μm	20-400

Figure 19-9
Model for the ablative photodecomposition of the cornea by argon fluoride (193 nm) laser ultraviolet radiation. **A,** The highly energetic (approximately 6.4 ev) ultraviolet photons head toward the organic material, with the intermolecular bond strength of approximately 3.5 ev. **B,** The photons break the intermolecular bonds, creating smaller molecular species, such as H^2, CO, CH$_3$, H$_2$. The entire laser pulse is absorbed in approximately 0.1 to 0.5 μm of the material. **C,** Because of the excess energy from the photons and the concentration of this energy in thin layers of material at the surface, there is an intense buildup of energy and pressure that ejects the fragments off the surface at speeds approximating 1500 meters per second. The fragments leave the tissue perpendicularly and clear the surface in times of picoseconds to a few nanoseconds. **D,** The laser pulse terminates at approximately 15 nanoseconds, leaving the surface clear of the effluent and allowing time for dissipation of any thermal energy that may have accumulated. **E,** Repeated laser pulses ablate successive layers of the material, requiring that the fragments travel farther to clear the surface and allowing fragments to fall back into the ablated area, possibly interfering with successive pulses if they are fired at a rapid rate. (Modified from Garrison BJ and Srinivasan R: Appl Phys Lett 1984;44:849-851. Also From Waring GO: Trans Am Ophthalmol Soc 1989;87:854-983.)

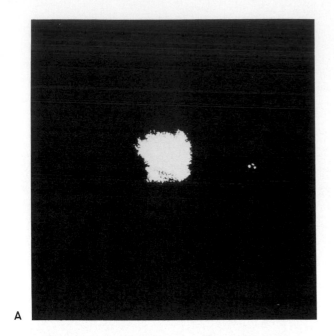
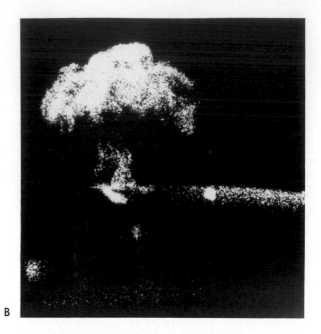
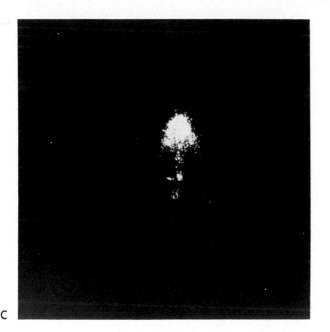
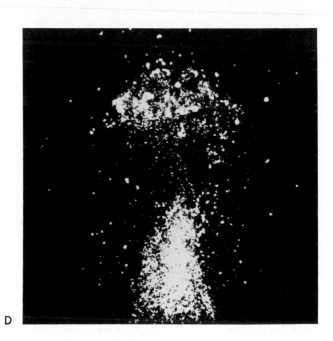

Figure 19-10
High-speed photography of the excimer laser ablation plume from cornea. Ablated fragments of tissue are leaving the surface in a vertical direction at speeds of approximately 2000 meters per second. **A,** Plume from 193-nm laser approximately 5 msec after ablation shows cloud of tissue fragments immediately above the surface. **B,** Plume from 193-nm laser approximately 50 msec after ablation resembles a nuclear mushroom cloud, with the fragments expanding away from the surface. **C,** Plume from 248-nm laser approximately 5 msec after ablation shows fragments farther from the surface with expansion into a larger cloud than that seen with 193 nm. **D,** Plume from 248-nm laser approximately 150 msec after ablation shows tissue fragments leaving the central cloud. Ablations with 193-nm laser were performed at 900 mJ/cm². Ablations with 248-nm laser were performed at 500 mJ/cm². (From Puliafito CA, Wong K, and Steinert RF: Lasers Surg Med 1987;7:155-159.)

Table 19-5

Summary of Selected Published Studies of ArF (193 nm) Excimer Laser Ablation of the Cornea

Author (year)	Fluence (mJ/cm²)	Repetition rate (Hz)	Findings
Trokel SL, Srinivasan R, and Braren B[111] (1983)	100-200	1-20	Defined 193 nm as preferable wavelength for corneal surgery; demonstrated discrete linear excisions; proposed laser keratomileusis.
Krueger RR and Trokel SL[36] (1985)	Range of fluences	NR	Ablation profile has sigmoidal shape with three different areas: (1) slow, (2) rapid increase, (3) level off. Threshold is >50 mJ/cm² Etching rate varies with fluence 100 mJ/cm² 0.1 mm 200 mJ/cm² 0.45 mm Most efficient fluence is 200 mJ/cm².
Marshall J et al.[58] (1985)	150 and 300	10	Description of "pseudomembrane" condensate on ablated surface, 20 to 100 nm thick. Endothelial cell damage beneath excision when 40 μm from the posterior surface.
Marshall J et al.[59] (1986)	150, 300, and 450	NR	Very smooth surface when compared with diamond knife incisions. No mention of difference of tissue quality with different parameters.
Seiler T and Wollensak J[91] (1986)	100-300	30	Uniform ablation up to 50 Hz, but less uniform at ≥60 Hz. Ablation depth proportional to exposure time (number of pulses).
Lieurance RC et al.[45] (1987)	15-30	NR	Good quality, clean lamellar keratectomies by histology, TEM, and SEM.
Puliafito CA, Wong K, and Steinert RF[76] (1987)	95,306 612	20	Levels ablation profile off approximately 600 mJ/cm²; Steinert suggested fluences above this level for less variation between pulses; TEM at 95, 306, and 612 mJ/cm² showed no difference among specimens.
Trentacoste J et al.[109] (1987)	3.5-13.4	1	Fibroblasts and tissue culture did not undergo transformation or mutagenesis after exposure to 193-nm radiation.
Munnerlyn CR, Kooms SJ, and Marshall J[66] (1988)	200 to 214	20	Calculation of depth of ablation required for optical correction of varying diameters of optical zone: 3 mm = 3 μm/D; 4 mm = 5.3 μm/D; 5 mm = 8.3 μm/D. Rotation of beam for spatial averaging.
Marshall J et al.[57] (1988)	140, 310	5-10	3-mm diameter ablation in monkeys 40-130 μm deep showed faint haze up to 6 months with later clearing grossly, but persistent haze biomicroscopically. Epithelium and epithelial basement membrane healed normally by 1 month. Subepithelial fibroplasia occurred with good remodeling by 8 months.
Serdarevic ON et al.[92] (1988)	110	15-20	Rotating slit excimer laser circular trephination wounds were more uniform in human eye bank eyes and in rabbits than those achieved with mechanical trephines. More endothelial damage occurred with mechanical trephination. There were no differences in rates of wound healing in rabbits up to 3 months.

Continued.

Table 19-5—cont'd

Summary of Selected Published Studies of ArF (193 nm) Excimer Laser Ablation of the Cornea

Author (year)	Fluence (mJ/cm²)	Repetition rate (Hz)	Findings
Hanna K et al.[24] (1988)	200	20	Each 4.5-mJ pulse ablated at 0.17 μm in stroma. Slit of calculated shape rotating at 0.03 Hz created minus lens surface contour.
L'Esperance FA et al.[44] (1989)	80-125	10	Eleven human beings with severe ocular disease had 3- to 5-mm diameter, 30- to 150-micron deep, circular superficial keratectomy. Slit-lamp examination showed fine fibrillar subepithelial haze. Delivery system using a rotating disc with circular apertures of varying sizes, a keratoscope imaging system, and a beam homogenizing and measuring system is described.
Goodman et al.[20] (1989)	160	5	DTAF staining demonstrated in rabbits showed new subepithelial connective tissue with more intense healing response after deeper ablations.
Gaster RN et al.[18] (1989)	23-178	10-40	Unmodified argon fluoride excimer beam used to ablate 6-mm diameter central area of rabbit corneas using a variety of radiant exposures, and repetition rates showed the laser beam to be nonuniform, and demonstrated best epithelial and stromal healing at a low fluence of 23 mJ/cm² and repetition rate of 40 Hz when examined up to 3 months after surgery.
Fantes FE et al.[12] (1990)	250	5	PRK in 29 monkey corneas with moving slit delivery system, 4-mm ablation zone 11 to 46 μm depth. Nine month follow-up. Clinical haze worst at 6 weeks and minimal by 9 months. Subepithelial fibroplasia maximum at 1 to 3 months with decrease by 9 months. Transient epithelial hyperplasia, none at 9 months.
SundarRaj N et al.[99] (1990)	250	5	Immunohistochemistry on eyes reported by Fantes[12] showed increased type III collagen, fetal antigen on fibroblasts, and keratan sulfate maximum at 6 months and persistent to 18 months, indicating new extracellular matrix as part of stromal wound healing. Transient increase in type VII collagen anchoring fibrils and fibronectin.
Seiler T et al.[88] (1990)	180	10	Blind (10) and sighted (13) human eyes treated with PRK, ablation zone diameter of 3.5 mm, maximum depth of 40 μm, and an ablation rate of approximately 0.2 u/pulse. Transient subepithelial haze. At 6 months 77% of eyes within ±1 D of emmetropia (preoperative = −1.50 to −7.00 D).

Table 19-5—cont'd

Summary of Selected Published Studies of ArF (193 nm) Excimer Laser Ablation of the Cornea

Author (year)	Fluence (mJ/cm²)	Repetition rate (Hz)	Findings
Bansal S et al.[4] (1990)	NR	NR	Linear excisions in human cornea followed with biopsies for 18 months. Wide wound gape and large persistent epithelial plug.
Malley DS et al.[55] (1990)	85	10	Subepithelial fibroplasia occurred with the deposition of type III collagen. The response to excimer laser keratectomy and mechanical keratectomy was similar up to 1 month.
Tuft S, Zabel RW, and Marshall JW[114] (1989)	100	10	DTAF staining in rabbits showed subepithelial connective tissue after laser and mechanical superficial keratectomy along with epithelial hyperplasia that tended to fill in the created defects. Intrastromal keratectomy showed much less scarring, emphasizing the role of epithelial stromal interactions in wound healing and subepithelial fibroplasia. Topical corticosteroids decreased the amount of scarring.

onstrated that 193 nm could create a smooth ablation surface in contrast to 248 nm, where edges and surface of the ablated zone were rougher with a 2- to 3-μm wide area of disruption of residual stromal tissue.

Thus the experience of all researchers seems consistent at this point: 193-nm argon fluoride lasers produce the most acceptable wounds in the cornea. As mentioned earlier, the proteins and proteoglycans of the cornea have a peak absorption at 190 nm, making the argon fluoride laser ideal. Collagen and nucleic acids have absorption at slightly higher wavelengths of 240 to 250 nm.

However, these wavelengths and their high energies impose limitations on the design of laser delivery systems. For example, excimer lasers cannot be transmitted through fiberoptic bundles, and they damage lenses and mirrors that do not have special nonabsorbing coatings.

Pulse duration. The duration of a single excimer laser pulse depends on the short lifetime of the excited dimer molecule—10 to 20 nanoseconds. The longer the wavelength, the shorter the pulse required to enhance the ablative action and minimize thermal effects. For example, at the 248-nm wavelength, a pulse duration as low as 300 femtoseconds can be achieved to improve the uniformity of the remaining surface.

Pulse energy. Interestingly, the total energy delivered in a single excimer laser pulse is not very great—usually a few hundred mJ. However, because the pulses are of such short duration, a high power is achieved, more than 10 million watts. This power may produce some plasma along with the ejected tissue fragments but is far below the threshold for optical breakdown. There must be a uniform energy in each pulse so that the total ablation of the tissue can be calculated and so that a uniform surface will result. Using a 193-nm excimer, the fluctuation of pulse energy is on the order of 5% to 10%,[28] a level too high to obtain refractive corrections of ±0.25 D accuracy. However, when using a pulse train of about 1000 pulses, this fluctuation averages out to less than ±0.3%.

Radiant exposure (fluence). Radiant exposure, or fluence, is a measure of the energy flux per unit area at the surface of the material ablated. It is usually expressed as millijoules per square centimeter (mJ/cm²). An ablation curve plots the amount of tissue removed and the cornea experiences only surface photochemical changes. Tissue removal begins at the ablation threshold, which is approximately 50 mJ/cm² for 193 nm in the cornea. The curve rises slowly as the radiant exposure increases, until it reaches a level-off point, at which point it flattens at approximately 600 mJ/cm². After this point, increasing fluences are not associated

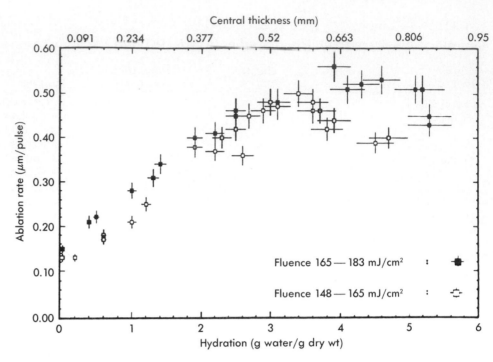

Figure 19-11
Effective corneal hydration on ablation rate demonstrates a marked effect is present below normal corneal thickness. In the range of normal corneal thickness from approximately 0.50 to 0.60, the ablation rate is reasonably constant. However, swollen corneas demonstrate some fall off the ablation rate, which can substantially alter the number of pulses needed to remove a specific amount of tissue to effect a given refractive change. (From Waring GO: Trans Am Ophthalmol Soc 1989;87:854-983.)

with increased tissue ablation.[3,37,60,76,95] The ablation threshold and the inflection on the curve vary with corneas from different species[3,59] (see Fig. 19-12, *A* and *B*). For example, Fantes, Waring, Hanna, et al. (unpublished data) determined the ablation curve for the rabbit cornea, measuring the thickness with an ultrasonic pachometer (1640 m/sec), using a Lambda Physik EMG103 laser with a repetition rate of 23 Hz and counting the number of pulses needed to perforate the cornea at seven fluences from 100 to 850 mJ/cm².

The rate of tissue ablation and consequently the location of the inflection point on the ablation curve vary with the hydration and thickness of the cornea (Fig. 19-11). This can be important in calculating the number of pulses used for a given refractive procedure in individuals with corneas of varying thickness and may have its greatest effect if excimer lasers are used in a therapeutic setting, such as the treatment of corneal infections or of superficial opacities, such as band keratopathy. Thus, in calibrating a laser on corneal tissue to determine its rate of ablation and the number of pulses necessary for a surgical procedure, the cornea must be dehydrated to a normal thickness.

As the radiant exposure increases, an optimal fluence is reached where, for a minimum exposure, tissue is most effectively removed. The exact location of this point is not known, although most studies have been done between 150 and 250 mJ/cm².[3,36,86,102] This is in the middle of the steepest part of the curve, but the value has been commonly derived from experiments on enucleated eyes, which may have been swollen. At this fluence, the laser ablates approximately 0.45 microns of tissue per pulse. It is difficult to work on this ascending part of the ablation curve at values of approximately 200 mJ/cm² because small differences in the energy density will create significant differences in the amount of tissue removed. Therefore, the beam must have a homogeneous energy profile and there must be uniform energy delivered from pulse to pulse. Variations in these factors will produce a rougher surface. On the other hand, working at higher fluences of 600 mJ/cm² or above may obviate this problem because in this flat part of the curve, the same amount of tissue is removed regardless of the energy density, so the technical demand for a homogeneous beam and a uniform pulse is not as great[34,66] (Fig. 19-12).

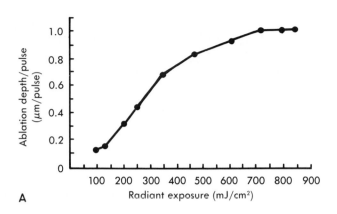

Rabbit

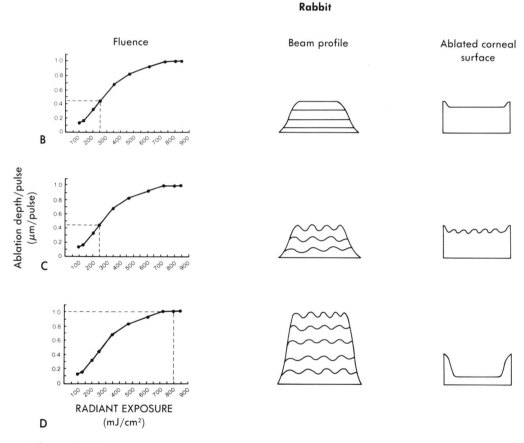

Figure 19-12

Theoretic effect of homogeneity of beam profile and radiant exposure on the rabbit cornea. **A,** Ablative curve for 193-nm excimer laser ablation of the cornea in living rabbits with the epithelium intact. The ablation threshold could not be determined in this system, but there was a gradual increase in the ablation depth per pulse with increasing radiant exposure up to approximately 700 mJ/cm^2 where a plateau occurred. **B,** A homogeneous beam profile at a fluence of 250 mJ/cm^2 will give a smooth ablated corneal surface. **C,** An inhomogeneous beam with variable pulse energy at 250 mJ/cm^2 will give an irregular surface because the ablation depth per pulse is markedly influenced by the radiant exposure. **D,** Working higher fluences on the order of 700 to 800 mJ/cm^2 creates a smooth surface in spite of inhomogeneities and variable pulse energy because the amount of tissue removed with each pulse does not depend on the radiant exposure at this level. (From Fantes FE and Waring GO: Lasers Surg Med 1989;9:533-542.)

Fantes and Waring[13] have studied the effect of radiant exposure on the smoothness of the ablated corneal surface using freshly enucleated rabbit eyes with the epithelium removed and using a converging lens system at radiant exposures of 50, 67, 104, 330, 500, and 850 mJ/cm² for each cornea, and a repetition rate of 10 Hz. When the ablated surfaces were examined by scanning electron microscopy, the investigators observed that increasing radiant exposure produced increasingly smooth surfaces (Figs. 19-13 and 19-14). Transmission electron microscopy showed a surface condensate (pseudomembrane) in all specimens with a slight increase in thickness corresponding to increasing radiant exposure. However, disruption of the underlying tissue increased minimally with increasing fluence, a finding also reported by Puliafito and colleagues.[76] Indeed, ablations of cornea tissue have been performed up to 30,000 mJ/cm², still showing minimal disruption of residual tissue.[45] A possible explanation for this lack of tissue damage at higher fluences is that the superficiality of the ablation allows heat to escape from the surface with the ejected tissue fragments, and a repetition rate slow enough allows time between pulses for the heat to dissipate so that it does not penetrate the remaining tissue. Using radiant exposure levels greater than 300 mJ/cm² is not practical with currently available lasers and delivery systems because so much energy is lost in the delivery system optics.

The fact the amount of tissue removed can be precisely determined for a single pulse at a given fluence is the basis for the exquisite accuracy and precision promised by excimer lasers for photorefractive keratectomy. However, accuracy may change under different surface conditions, such as humidity, or different degrees of corneal hydration—losing, therefore, the precision in excision depth.

Homogeneity of the laser beam and uniformity of the ablated surface. Beam uniformity is important because the energy profile of the beam is projected onto the surface of the cornea, leaving its "fingerprint." For example, if the beam has more energy concentrated in the center, the ablated area will have a central depression, whereas a beam with more energy concentrated at the periphery will create a doughnut configuration in the tissue. Because one of the goals of photorefractive keratectomy is to create as smooth a surface as possible, it is desirable to have as homogeneous a beam as possible. The laser beam at 193 nm is not homogeneous as it emerges from the resonating cavity, the energy density being greater in the center. The beam does not have a defined mode structure, and is therefore characterized only as a profile of energy density transversely and longitudinally. The beam profiles can change between pulses and have a tendency to become less uniform as the gases in the active medium degrade.

A number of technical adjustments can be made to increase the homogeneity of the beam, including configuring the laser cavity in the laser resonating cavity to use stable rather than unstable optics, aligning the mirrors in the cavity accurately with the assistance of a helium-neon laser, using an automated method to keep the mixture of laser gases in the cavity fresh and in the proper proportion (such as the intelligent laser control system in the Lambda Physik series, which monitors the emitted signal, stabilizes pulse energy in a preset level independent of gas contamination, and exchanges contaminated gas with fresh gas while the laser is operating), aligning the optics of the delivery system, using beam homogenizers within the delivery system as discussed later, using specially coated optical elements so that their surface will not become damaged by the excimer laser beam, conditioning the atmosphere over the surface of the cornea so that particles in the air or ejected from the surface do not block some of the laser beam, and the like.

There are few commercially available instruments to measure the energy distribution in the excimer laser beam. This is an extremely important variable, however, because the contour of the beam is imprinted on the tissue and the more irregular the beam, the more irregular the surface of the ablated cornea. Increasingly, manufacturers of delivery systems for excimer lasers are including methods to present a profile of the beam homogeneity to the user. One approach was developed by Fantes, Hanna, Waring, and Coherent Radiation (unpublished data), in which beam homogeneity was measured by imaging the beam on a fluorescent screen. The fluorescence emitted from this screen was proportional to the ultraviolet energy and was imaged with a television camera and frame grabber, then fed into a computer programmed with software to print out a graphic cross section and three-dimensional image of the beam configuration.

With a poorly adjusted laser and delivery system, the beam profile was irregular, showing 5% to 10% variability from one side to another (Fig. 19-15, *A*). After some of the adjustments described earlier, the homogeneity of the beam was greatly increased (Fig. 19-15, *B* and *C*).

Another way to visualize the creation of a smooth surface is to consider the beam homogeneous, but the surface itself irregular. The beam will then remove an equal amount of tissue over the exposed surface so that the high points and low points will be ablated at

Text continued on p. 697.

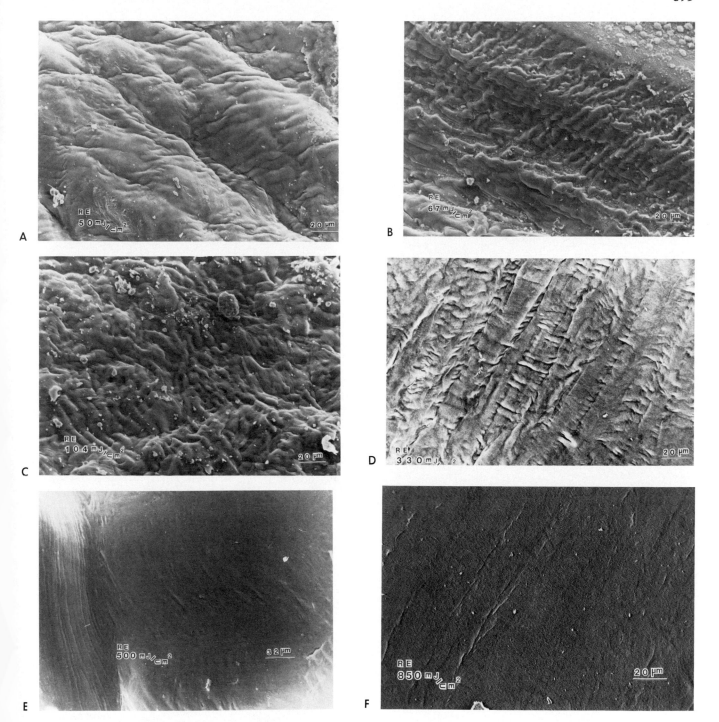

Figure 19-13

Comparison of the quality of the ablated surface as shown by scanning electron microscopy and the amount of disruption of corneal stromal tissue as shown by transmission electron microscopy with ablations at increasing radiant exposures (fluences). **A,** At 50 mJ/cm² the surface shows large corrugations and smaller ripples. **B,** At 67 mJ/cm² the surface is still, resembling a washboard. **C,** At 104 mJ/cm² the large corrugations and ripples have disappeared, but a finer surface roughness remains, resembling the surface of the sea on a choppy day. **D,** At 330 mJ/cm² there is a general smoothness of the surface, with finer irregularities resembling a plank of wood. **E,** At 500 mJ/cm² the surface is quite smooth with a few ripples near the edge of the ablated zone. **F,** At 850 mJ/cm² the surface is extraordinarily smooth, resembling a fine cloth with a few fine seams. (From Fantes FE and Waring GO: Lasers Surg Med 1989;9:533-542.)

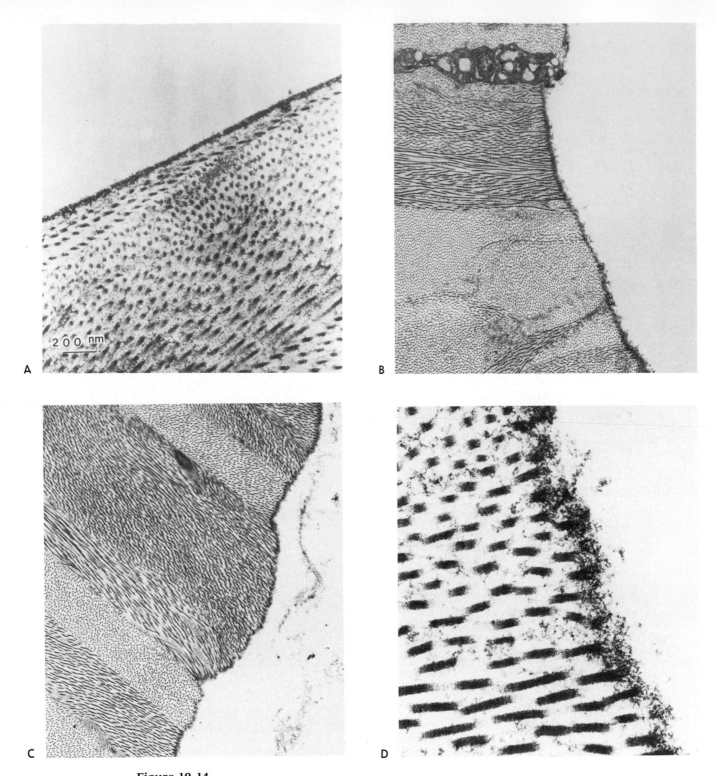

Figure 19-14

Effect of different radiant exposures on the surface of the ablated area in the human corneal stroma as examined by transmission electron microscopy. **A,** Exposure at 205 mJ/cm². Thin condensate lines the surface of the stroma. Underlying lamellar collagen architecture remains undisturbed. Vacuolated keratocyte is devoid of surface condensate (×1490). **B,** Exposure at 205 mJ/cm². Higher magnification reveals the surface condensate approximately 0.04 micron thick, with essentially no disruption of the underlying collagen stromal architecture (×9100). **C,** Exposure at 472 mJ/cm². The surface condensate is thicker and apparently bilayered, a thin layer remaining on the surface of the ablated margin and a thicker layer being detached. Underlying stromal collagen architecture remains undisturbed (×1490). **D,** Exposure at 472 mJ/cm². Higher magnification shows the residual surface condensate approximately 0.04 mm thick with essentially no disruption of the underlying stromal architecture (×9100).

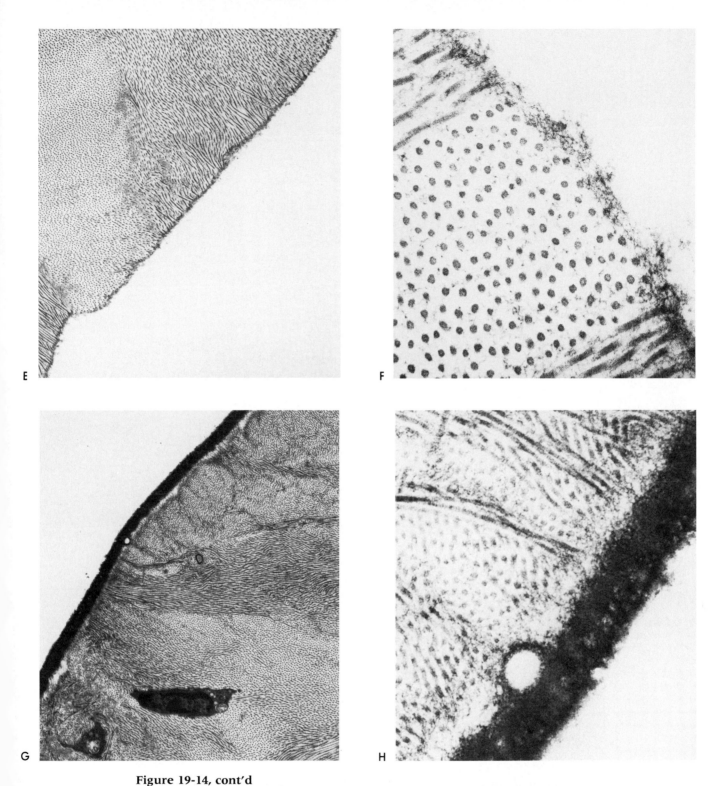

Figure 19-14, cont'd
E, Ablation at 841 mJ/cm². Surface condensate is present with minimal to no disruption of underlying stromal architecture (×1490). **F,** Ablation at 841 mJ/cm². Higher power shows surface condensate approximately 0.04 mm thick, with intact underlying stromal architecture. This finding represents the general appearance of this tissue (×9100). **G,** Ablation at 841 mJ/cm². Thick surface condensate is present, with an underlying lucent zone present approximately 0.05 micrometer thick (×1490). **H,** Thick surface condensate is approximately 0.2 micron thick, and there is an underlying zone of disrupted collagen approximately 0.05 mm thick. Beyond that, the architecture of the stroma seems intact (×9100). This thicker condensate was exceptional in this tissue.

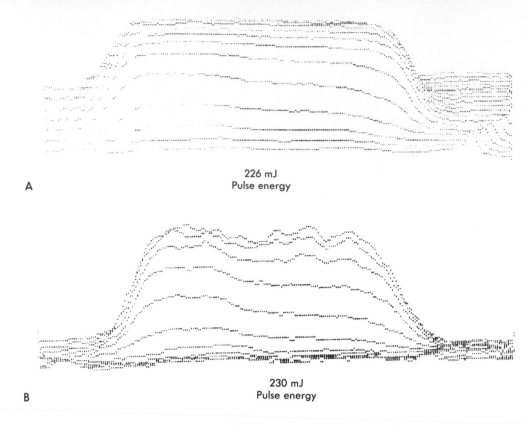

226 mJ
Pulse energy

A

230 mJ
Pulse energy

B

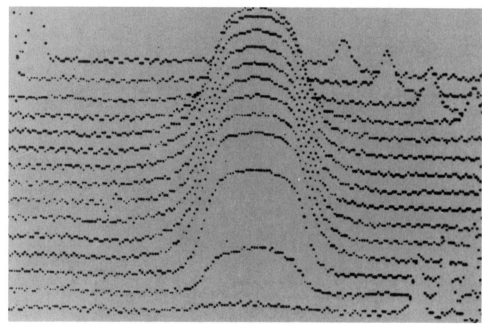

C

Figure 19-15

Configuration of one pulse of 193-nm argon fluoride excimer laser beam as it emerges from the resonating cavity as imaged on a fluorescent screen. Details of the method of imaging are explained in the text. **A,** With a pulse energy of 230 mJ, the beam profile shows longitudinal irregularity with hot spots (higher points on the profile) and cooler spots (lower points on the profile), as well as a sloping configuration on either end. **B,** After adjustment of the laser resonating cavity as described in the text, the beam profile at the same pulse energy is more uniform, showing a flattened top, although the edges still have a sloping configuration. **C,** Another view of the beam configuration after improved homogeneity shows a relatively uniform configuration across the width of the beam with slight sloping of the sides. Inserting a mask in the beam path can capture the uniform center of the beam, eliminating the sloping margins and creating a beam of uniform energy distribution that will create a smoother surface on the cornea after ablation with each pulse. (From Waring GO: Trans Am Ophthalmol Soc 1989;87:854-983.)

the same rate and the original surface contour will persist (Fig. 19-16).

Pulse repetition rate. The rate of delivery of the laser pulses to the cornea is measured as the number of pulses per second, expressed in Hertz (Hz). Ideally, laser corneal surgery should be completed as rapidly as possible to decrease the chances of patient movement and instrument malfunction. Therefore a higher repetition rate is most desirable. There are marked limitations, however, to the use of higher repetition rates (>60 Hz) with excimer lasers because the rapid sequence of pulses creates a thermal effect in the tissue and damages the optical components of the delivery system. In addition, the consistency of the pulse energy and beam profile may decline at higher rates.[91]

The time for diffusion of heat in the cornea is on the order of 1 second, and therefore repetition rates higher than 1 Hz allow heat to accumulate. In repetition rates higher than 20 Hz, the temperature may rise more than 10° C adjacent to the area of excision, depending on the fluence. In addition, pulses delivered in rapid succession may create an accumulation of ejected fragments that block the effectiveness of successive pulses.

Currently, repetition rates from 5 to 15 Hz are being used,* the most common being around 10 Hz.

Number of pulses. The most important factor the surgeon controls is the number of pulses, because this determines the amount of tissue removed. Potentially, this allows the surgeon to make a radial or transverse linear excision of an exact known depth, uniform from end to end, or perform photorefractive keratectomy by ablating a profile on the cornea of exact contour. The surgeon would compute the overall excision depth before surgery by multiplying the ablation depth per pulse times the total number of pulses. For example, if the surgeon wants to excise 100 μm of the cornea at 0.45 μm per pulse, a value of 222 pulses (100 × 0.45) would be entered into the operation terminal of the laser before surgery (Fig. 19-17).

The simplicity of these data is confounded by a number of problems. First, the consistency of the pulse energy and the spatial uniformity of the beam profile vary 5% to 10%, creating some inherent irregularity of the surface. Second, different tissues ablate at different rates; the epithelium slower than the stroma, for example. This would have been taken into consideration in preoperative calculations for the amount of tissue removed. Third, laser keratomileusis requires removal of different amounts of tissue in different areas of the cornea to create a new optical profile, and this presents a challenge in the design of the delivery system.

*References 23, 24, 60, 63, 77, 111.

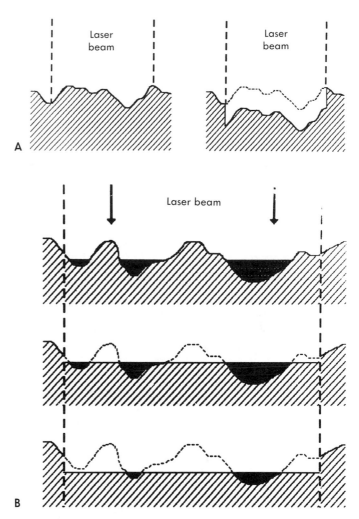

Figure 19-16
Effect of surface contour on pattern of ablation with a homogeneous excimer laser beam. **A,** As the laser beam encounters an irregular surface, it ablates an equal amount of tissue from the high points and low points of the surface so that the original contour of the surface remains. **B,** By applying a fluid to the surface to fill in the depressions, the elevations will be preferentially ablated, and as the fluid is also ablated and removed from the surface, it is possible to convert an irregular surface to a smooth one. Seiler and colleagues have used this method to smooth the corneal surface after pterygium surgery, putting methyl cellulose on the surface to fill in the depressions and then ablating the entire surface with a 193-nm excimer laser beam.

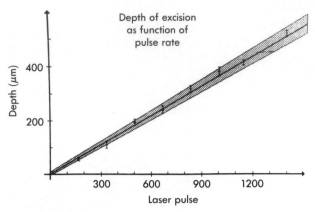

Figure 19-17
Graph demonstrates that the depth of excision of corneal tissue in microns is proportionate to the number of 193-nm excimer laser pulses. Y-axis indicates the depth in micrometers. X-axis indicates the number of laser pulses. Points with error bars indicate actual data from human eye bank eyes. Line shows best fit curve, and shaded area shows zone encompassing one standard deviation around the line of best fit. (From Seiler T and Wollensak J: Ophthalmologica 1986;192:65-70.)

Fourth, changes in conditions during the surgery, such as movement of the eye, variation in corneal thickness from changes in hydration, and contamination of the surface with fluid, make the exact determination of the amount of tissue removed more difficult.

EXCIMER LASER DELIVERY SYSTEMS

Between the time the laser beam emerges from the resonating cavity and the time it strikes the surface of the cornea, it must be directed, homogenized, and shaped by a delivery system. In general, the delivery systems required for excimer lasers are more complex than those needed for the more familiar continuous-wave argon or pulsed Nd:YAG lasers. This requires a combination of lenses, mirrors, masks, homogenizers, motors, computers, and detectors—all assembled in a clinically useful device that must be simple to use, versatile, and able to withstand the impact of the excimer beam itself (Fig. 19-18).[24,107] Numerous experimental and commercial delivery systems are in development (Fig. 19-19).

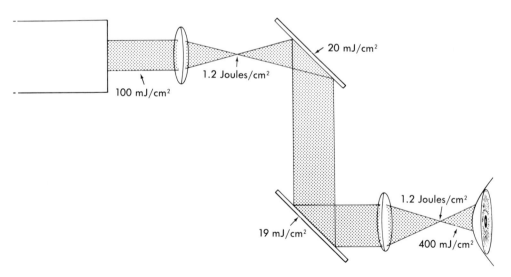

Figure 19-18
General depiction of the elements of an excimer laser delivery system. Cylindric and spheric lenses can shape the beam, and mirrors can direct the beam. In general, the optical elements should be placed at a distance from the focal point where the energy density is high to decrease the damage caused by the laser beam. Not depicted are other elements of a delivery system, such as the mask to shape the beam, prisms or mirrors that homogenize the beam, and detectors that measure the beam. (From Waring GO: Trans Am Ophthalmol Soc 1989;87:854-983.)

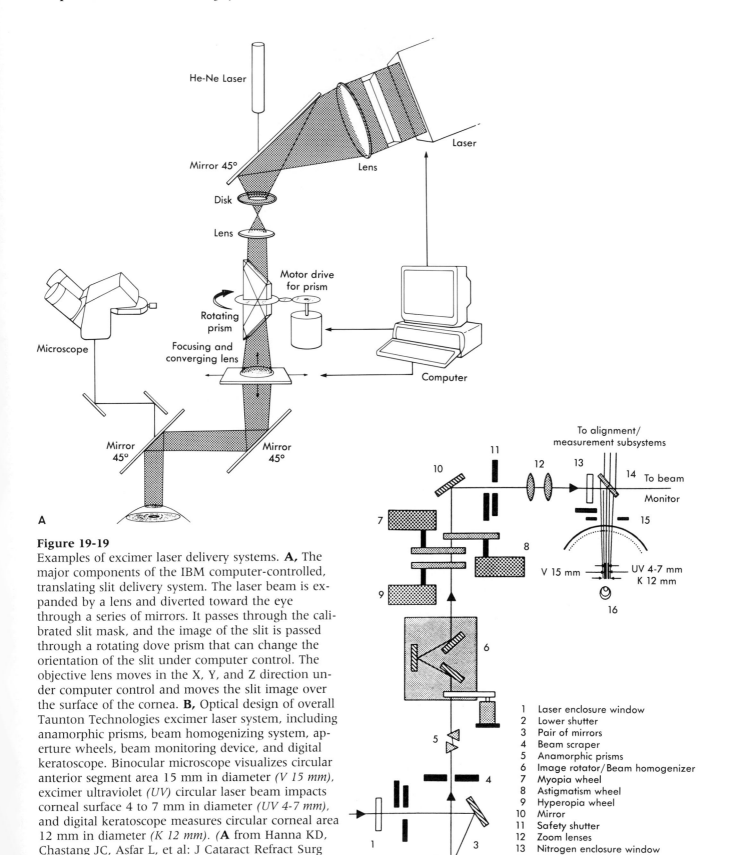

Figure 19-19

Examples of excimer laser delivery systems. **A,** The major components of the IBM computer-controlled, translating slit delivery system. The laser beam is expanded by a lens and diverted toward the eye through a series of mirrors. It passes through the calibrated slit mask, and the image of the slit is passed through a rotating dove prism that can change the orientation of the slit under computer control. The objective lens moves in the X, Y, and Z direction under computer control and moves the slit image over the surface of the cornea. **B,** Optical design of overall Taunton Technologies excimer laser system, including anamorphic prisms, beam homogenizing system, aperture wheels, beam monitoring device, and digital keratoscope. Binocular microscope visualizes circular anterior segment area 15 mm in diameter *(V 15 mm)*, excimer ultraviolet *(UV)* circular laser beam impacts corneal surface 4 to 7 mm in diameter *(UV 4-7 mm)*, and digital keratoscope measures circular corneal area 12 mm in diameter *(K 12 mm)*. (**A** from Hanna KD, Chastang JC, Asfar L, et al: J Cataract Refract Surg 1989;15:390-396; **B** from L'Esperance FA, Warner JW, Telfair WB, Yoder PR, and Martin CA: Arch Ophthalmol 1989;107:131-139.)

1   Laser enclosure window
2   Lower shutter
3   Pair of mirrors
4   Beam scraper
5   Anamorphic prisms
6   Image rotator/Beam homogenizer
7   Myopia wheel
8   Astigmatism wheel
9   Hyperopia wheel
10 Mirror
11 Safety shutter
12 Zoom lenses
13 Nitrogen enclosure window
14 UV mirror/Beam splitter
15 Upper shutter
16 Cornea of patient's eye

Continued.

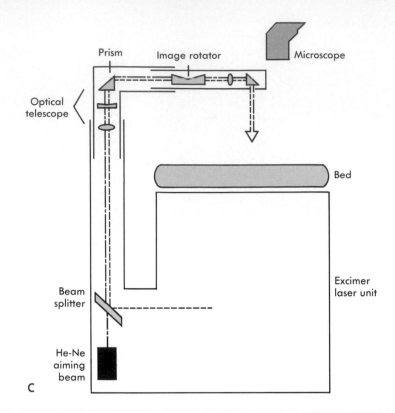

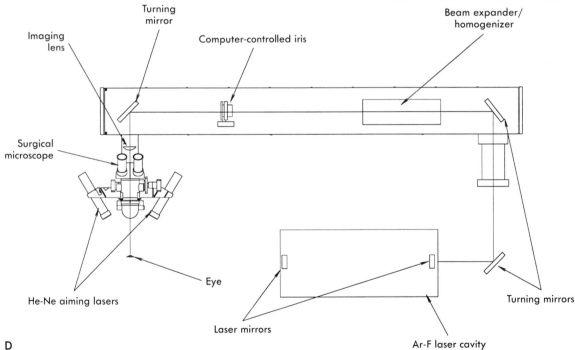

Figure 19-19, cont'd

C, A basic design of Meditec excimer laser system. The system consists of the excimer laser unit and the helium-neon laser aiming beam located in the bed beneath the patient. The delivery system consists of a beam splitter and optical telescope that transmits the laser beam to the image rotater that orients the beam on the eye. A final focusing lens and prism transmit the image to the eye, as viewed by an operation microscope. **D,** Summit Technology UV 200 Optical Delivery System. The excimer laser resonating cavity is shown below with its two mirrors. The beam enters the optical "rail" that is filled with nitrogen to decrease the interaction of the beam with air. The rectangular shape of the beam is made square by the beam expander, and the computer controlled iris determines the diameter of the circle of the beam that impacts the cornea. The helium-neon aiming lasers are used to focus the instrument before corneal ablation, which is observed through the surgical microscope. (**C** courtesy Meditec, Inc; **D** courtesy Summit Technology.)

Optical elements

The high-energy excimer laser will easily damage conventional lenses, mirrors, and prisms, even if made of quartz. To solve this problem, the optics should be coated with magnesium fluoride or calcium fluoride. In addition, the beam can be optically expanded so that the energy density is less at the optical interface, and then refocused by an objective lens at the end of the system. At every optical interface, some of the energy is lost, so the more complex the delivery system and the less efficient its components, the more powerful the laser required to deliver a beam of useful energy to the cornea, especially if there is a need to work at higher fluences along the upper part of the ablation curve.

The optical elements must be well aligned with the emergent beam and with each other for efficient transmission. The easiest "alignment system" is to transmit the beam through a fiberoptic bundle, but no optical fiber material is available that can withstand the high energies of the ultraviolet excimer laser. Helium-neon lasers are most commonly used for alignment.

Control of beam uniformity

The energy profile of the beam as it is emitted from the laser must be maintained or improved as it travels through the delivery system to present the best possible quality beam to the tissue. All optical elements must have smooth, nondegraded surfaces so that they do not disrupt the beam. Masking the peripheral part of the beam and using only its more homogeneous central part will enhance uniformity (Fig. 19-20). Using rotating prisms or lenses and spatial beam integrators can make the beam more homogeneous.

The beam homogenization is important because areas of higher and lower energy within the beam (hot spots and cold spots) will produce an irregular surface on the cornea. If portions of the beam are folded back into the beam by prisms, the hot spots and cold spots cancel each other out, producing a more homogeneous beam.

Shaping the beam for refractive ablation

The shape of the ablated area on the cornea is determined by the shape of the beam that strikes the cornea. The ideal shape is selected based on the ametropia to be corrected and the refractive surgical technique used.[116] A linear slit is used for radial and transverse linear keratectomy.

Two methods are available to shape the beam: masks and lenses. The principle of using a mask is to create an aperture that will ablate a desired configuration and profile on the cornea (Fig. 19-21). Lenses project a beam of desired configuration on the cornea.

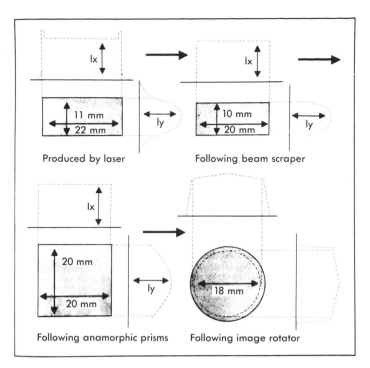

Figure 19-20

Cross section of excimer laser beam intensity distribution as it emerges from laser *(top left)* and after edges of beam are scraped away *(top right)*, which may contain irregular and high-intensity energy areas. Anamorphic prisms convert rectangular beam into square beam *(bottom left)*, which is then homogenized by image rotator into axisymmetric intensity distribution *(bottom right)*. (From L'Esperance FA, Warner JW, Telfair WB, Yoder PR, and Martin CA: Arch Ophthalmol 1989;107:131-139.)

Any moving mask system, whether slit diaphragm or disc, will require control of the rate of movement to govern the number of pulses that strike the cornea in a given area and to ensure an accurate ablation profile. This requires accurate mathematic calculations that take into account the configuration of the aperture in the mask, the rate of movement of the aperture over the surface of the cornea, the repetition rate of the laser, and the ablation per pulse.

Stationary slit masks. The simplest method of shaping the beam is a rectangular narrow slit to make a linear radial keratectomy to correct myopia or a linear transverse or arcuate excision to correct astigmatism. If enough energy is available, four or eight radial slits could be irradiated at the same time to make simultaneous radial excisions, but this would waste a lot of energy impacting the areas between the slits in the mask. Therefore a cylindrical lens can be used to shape the beam into a narrow rectangle that is then imaged onto one slit aperture in the mask, so that

Excimer Laser Mask Systems

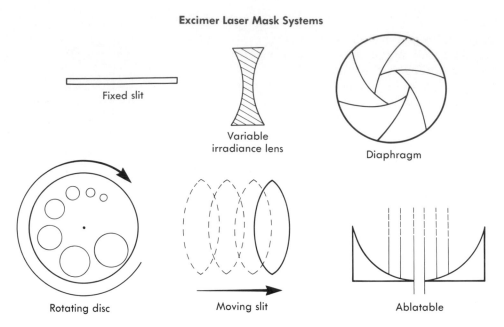

Figure 19-21

Types of masks to shape the excimer laser beam. The slit mask makes an elongated beam for radial or transverse keratectomy. A variable irradiance lens can distribute energy over the corneal surface in desired patterns. Diaphragm can expand or contract for myopic correction. Disc with multiple apertures rotates to create successively smaller or larger ablation zones. Moveable slit that is wider in the middle creates myopic correction. The ablatable mask is the shape of the desired tissue to be removed; as the mask ablates, the beam passes through to ablate the tissue.

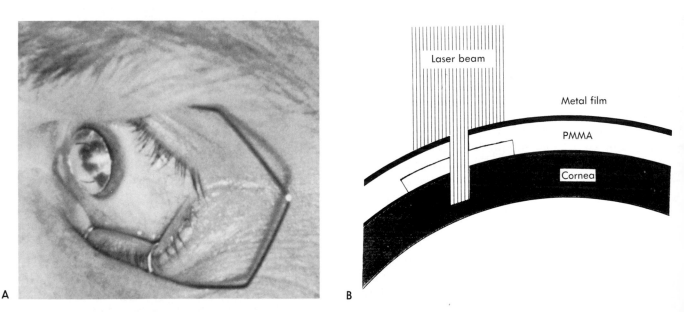

Figure 19-22

Contact lens mask for transverse linear keratectomy. **A,** Foil-coated contact lens is placed on the surface of the patient's cornea and the rectangular-shaped laser beam aligned with the slit aperture in the mask. The slit is 0.12 mm wide and 3.5 to 5.0 mm long. **B,** Drawing of the modifications of the PMMA contact lens shows the surface coat of metal film that blocks part of the laser beam, the slit in the contact lens allowing transmission of the laser beam, and the groove in the back of the contact lens to pull fluid away from the corneal surface in the area of the slit by surface tension.

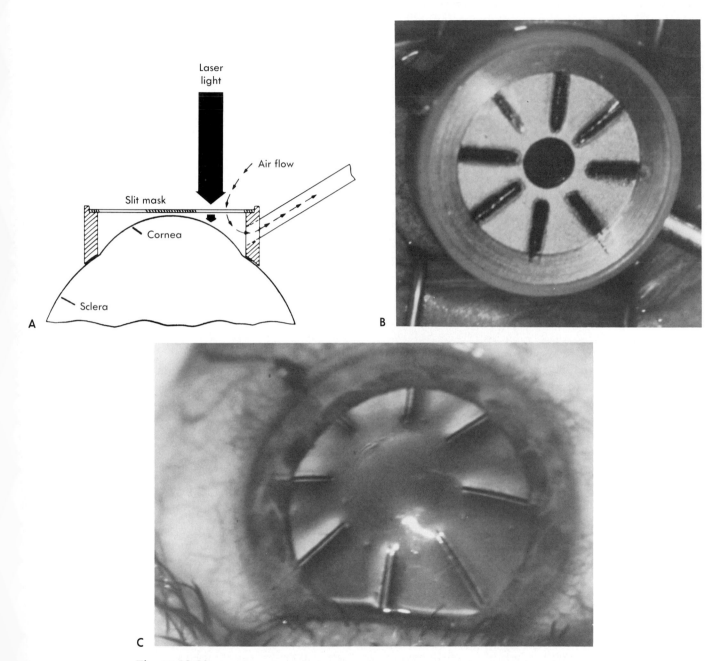

Figure 19-23

Suction ring slit mask used for radial linear excisions. **A,** Drawing shows a slit mask mounted in suction ring that is secured to the conjunctival limbus. Excimer laser beam passes through the slit to the cornea. Air flow removes photofragments and debris from over the cornea. **B,** Slit mask with eight radial slits mounted in the center of a suction ring secured to the conjunctival limbus. Tubes on either side of the ring allow suction of air through the central opening and slits to remove photofragments and debris. **C,** Eight radial slits in human cornea immediately after ablation using Meditec mask and suction ring. (**A** courtesy Meditec; **C** courtesy Alf Tenner, MD.)

each of the four or eight slits is irradiated in turn.

Seiler and colleagues[86] have used a PMMA contact lens with slits cut in it as a mask placed directly on the surface of the cornea, the slits being oriented in the desired direction of ablation. Two important modifications of the contact lens allow use with the excimer laser. The first is coating the anterior surface with a metal foil film that blocks the transmission of the beam in all areas except the slit. The second is to carve out a recess on the back of the lens in the area of the slit that pulls fluid and tears away from the slit area by surface tension, decreasing the amount of fluid present to absorb and quench the laser beam (Fig. 19-22). This method has been used particularly in making transverse incisions for the correction of astigmatism, as described later.

A slit mask can also be incorporated into a suction ring and suspended over the surface of the cornea, as done in the Meditec (Fig. 19-23).

Moving slit. For photorefractive keratectomy a slit image can move over the surface of the cornea, either rotating around the center or translating across the surface. The rotating slit is not ideal because the center ablation is not always smooth, and it is difficult to keep the eye aligned exactly in the center during ablation. The shape of the slit can be designed to correct a variety of ametropias. A slit wider near its central portion would ablate more tissue from the central cornea; one wider near its outer portion would ablate more of the paracentral cornea and correct hyperopia. Astigmatism could be corrected by varying the rate of movement of the slit so that one meridian was exposed to more pulses than another or by passing the slit more frequently over one meridian than the other. A moving slit system has been described by Hanna and colleagues[23,24,26] in the IBM system (Fig. 19-24; see Fig. 19-19, *A*).

Diaphragm mask. For photorefractive keratectomy a circular mask can be used. Obviously, if a simple disc-shaped mask is used, a circular depression with steep edges will appear without useful refractive effect. However, if a slowly constricting or dilating diaphragm is used to ablate a fixed circular area of the central cornea (for example, 5 mm in diameter), the outer portion of the ablation will be shallower than the continuously exposed inner portion. The profile of this ablation is controlled by the rate of movement of the diaphragm and the number of pulses delivered. This creates a minus lens effect on the surface of the cornea to treat myopia. The diaphragm can be controlled mechanically and linked to a feedback system for fine control. This approach has been used in the VISX and Summit[53] experimental excimer laser systems.[63]

Advantages of the diaphragm are its relative simplicity and ease of centration. Another advantage is the rapid rate at which an area ablation can be accomplished—less than 30 seconds. Disadvantages include the limitation of treating only myopia. In addition, the central cornea is exposed to all pulses, possibly elevating the temperature there and requiring that the ejected fragments be removed from the surface by suction or blowing air. The diaphragm steps are etched on the corneal surface, creating some irregularity; the more steps, the smoother the surface (Fig. 19-25).

Multiple disc masks. Another type of mask delivery system uses different sized apertures in a single circular disc. A sequence of circular apertures, from large (7 mm diameter) down to small (1 mm diameter) can be used to make a series of progressively constricting, stepped excisions of tissue by first exposing the large mask, then the next smallest, and so on. This creates a negative lens effect to correct myopia (Fig. 19-26). A similar approach can be used to correct hyperopia, using a translucent glass to mask the central unablated zone. A sequence of slits of different orientation could be used to create linear keratectomies. This system is used by Taunton Technologies.[43,44]

Optical shaping of beam. A number of optical methods can shape the beam. Spherical lenses that focus graded amounts of the laser beam across the optical zone can be fashioned to correct myopia and hyperopia, an approach currently under development in the Soviet Union. A cylindrical lens in the delivery system creates a linear beam configuration that ablates radial or transverse linear keratectomies in the cornea. This is one of the earliest methods used to test the different effect of wavelengths of excimer lasers.[77] A properly graded cylindrical lens probably can create an astigmatic correction.

Spherical lenses that transmit different amounts of energy in different areas of the lens can be used to modify the energy distribution over the surface of the cornea. This variable irradiance through an optical system can be achieved by a gas cell filter or by using lenses that absorb ultraviolet radiation selectively. Thus a lens thinner in the middle and thicker in the periphery will transmit more laser energy in the central portion than the periphery, creating a myopic correction on the cornea.

An axicon lens can be used to create a circular pattern. The axicon lenses are coin-shaped, and refract the laser light from the original central axis out to the edge of the ring-shaped lens, projecting a circle onto the cornea. This system has been used by Loertscher and colleagues[46-49] for circular corneal trephination (Fig. 19-27). This system could be modified to create two parallel surfaces that would image two transverse

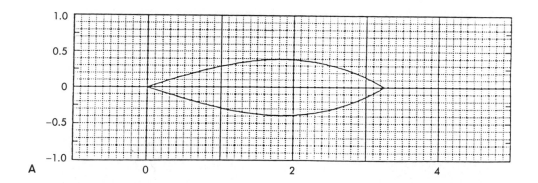

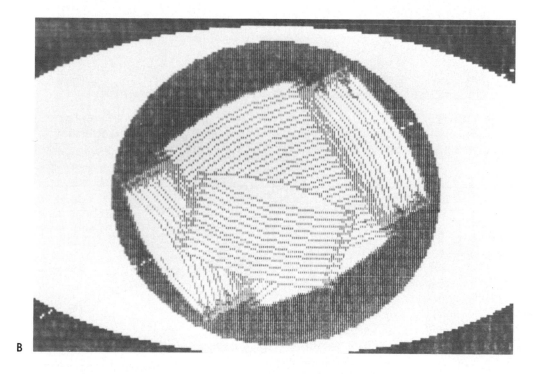

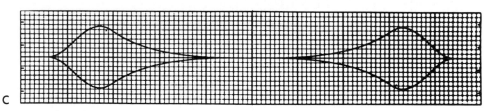

Figure 19-24
A, Configuration of slit for a laser myopic keratomileusis that can be rotated around the center point (00) or translated across the corneal surface. Units indicate only relative size. **B,** A diagram of ablated tissue shows images of pulses on cornea with translating slit system. **C,** Slit for hyperopic laser keratomileusis can be translated across the cornea in different meridians. (From Hanna KD, Chastang JC, Asfar L, et al: J Cataract Refract Surg 1989;15:390-396.)

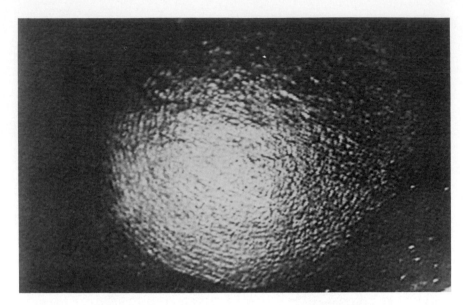

Figure 19-25
Photograph of surface of rabbit eye after ablation using a dilating diaphragm shows multiple small concentric ridges indicating the steps as the diaphragm opens.

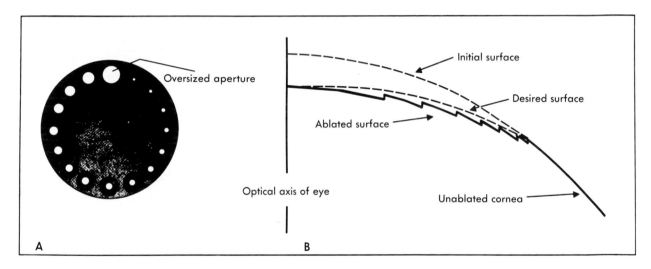

Figure 19-26
Taunton laser mask system. **A,** Aperture wheel that allows laser beam to ablate central cornea more deeply than peripheral cornea to flatten anterior surface curvature and increase anterior corneal surface radius of curvature, thereby reducing myopia. **B,** Exaggerated representation of stepped profile ablation of cornea to reduce myopia. (From L'Esperance FA, Warner JW, Telfair WB, Yoder PR, and Martin CA: Arch Ophthalmol 1989;107:131-139.)

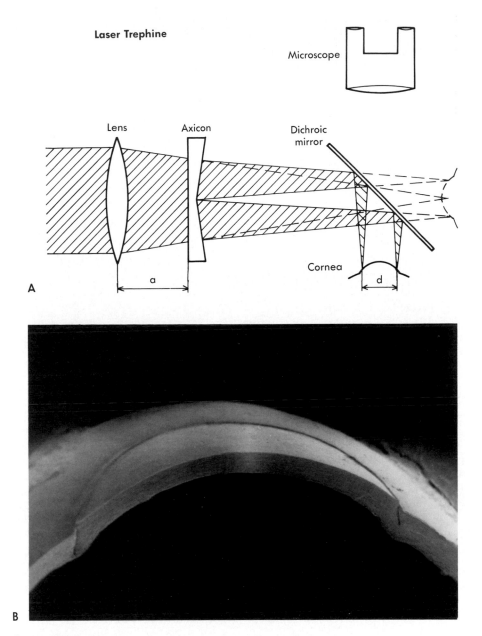

Figure 19-27
Axicon lens used for circular trephination with a hydrogen fluoride laser. **A,** Optical setup for the use of an axicon lens creates a circular pattern for the corneal trephination. The diameter of the annulus *(d)* can be varied by adjusting the distance between the axicon and the lens *(a)*. The cornea is observed using a microscope. **B,** Scanning electron microscopic cross-sectional view of an eye bank cornea after trephination shows asymmetric depths, approximately 90% of corneal thickness at 11 o'clock and 50% at 5 o'clock. The walls of trephination are parallel. (From Loertscher H, Mandelbaum S, Parel J-M, and Parrish RK: Am J Ophthalmol 1987;104:471-475.)

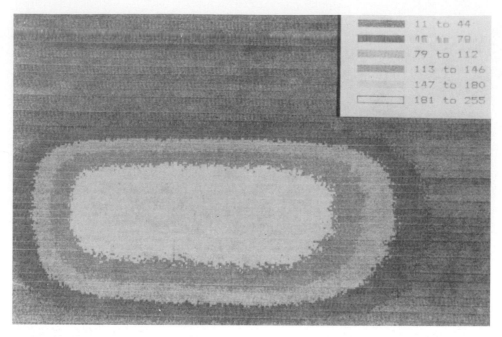

Figure 19-28
Profile of laser beam energy emerging from laser shows greater concentration of energy in the center and less at the periphery of the rectangular beam, as indicated in the grey scale of the photograph (mJ/cm^2). (Courtesy Questek, Inc.)

slits simultaneously for the correction of astigmatism.

Properly coated optical systems transmit more energy than masks that block considerable areas of the laser. If the beam is optically shaped to conform to the size of the mask aperture, less energy is wasted on the edge of the mask.

Delivery of the beam to the eye

Final focusing lenses are necessary to collect the expanded, homogenized, and shaped beam for delivery to the eye. The energy density at the surface of the cornea will be determined largely by the distance between the focal point of the objective lens and the corneal surface.

The excimer laser beam may be aimed parallel rather than perpendicular to the corneal surface to fashion a tangential cut and to excise a lenticule.[16,29] The tangential method can create clearer corneas with less damage to the endothelium in rabbit eyes.

Measuring the beam

All of the processes that modify the beam affect its energy profile. The surgeon needs the confidence that the pulse impinging on the cornea meets the calculated specifications. This requires detectors built into the system that can measure the final pulse energy, homogeneity, and shape (Fig. 19-28). Ideally, this detecting system would be linked to a computer-

controlled feedback mechanism that could modulate both the output from the laser and the beam management in the delivery system to ensure that each pulse meets exact specifications.

SYSTEMS TO COUPLE LASER AND EYE

Because laser corneal refractive procedures must be performed with micron accuracy, the demands for stability of the eye are greater than those required during other ophthalmic laser procedures. For example, during argon laser photocoagulation of the retina or Nd:YAG photodisruption of the posterior lens capsule, the eye can move between laser shots because the interaction between the laser and a single spot on the tissue is brief and because the location of the laser shot needs to be controlled only within tenths of a millimeter. In photorefractive keratectomy, even though interaction between the laser and the tissue lasts only nanoseconds, the train of pulses must be delivered to the same or exactly adjacent areas of the cornea during the entire 20- to 60-second procedure. The eye must therefore be kept in a fixed position with respect to the laser, using a coupling system.

Position of the patient

The first element in coupling is to have the patient comfortably in a stable position in front of the delivery system. Early attempts to accomplish this with the pa-

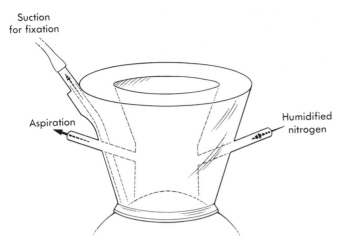

Suction
for fixation

Aspiration

Humidified
nitrogen

Figure 19-29
Drawing of suction cone coupling and surface conditioning system. Suction cone adheres to conjunctival limbus and can be connected mechanically to the end of the delivery system. The ablated debris and air are aspirated from the surface of the cornea as humidified nitrogen is blown across the surface. (From Waring GO: Trans Am Ophthalmol Soc 1989; 87:854-983.)

tient in a seated position before a slit-lamp apparatus achieved less control, so most systems now allow the patient to lie on a bed with the head stabilized beneath the overhanging delivery system.

Observation of the cornea

The surgeon should have visual control through an operation microscope of the ablation process to monitor its progress, viewing coaxially with the laser beam path.

Aiming the laser

Because the lasers used for photorefractive keratectomy have wavelengths outside the visible spectrum, an auxiliary aiming laser that is coaxial to the ablating laser is required to align and aim the laser. Helium-neon lasers are the standard for this. In automated systems, this is used only for initial alignment, but in manually controlled systems, it is used to align each location.

Stabilization of the eye

Eye movements during ablation create two problems. The first is ablation of undesired areas of the cornea so that linear ablations become wide, V-shaped troughs and surface area ablations have more irregular margins and surfaces. The second is inaccurate optical correction caused by aberrant pulses that deviate from the calculated amount of tissue ablation and disrupt the desired new corneal profile. The exact amount of eye movement allowable during ablation is unknown. Microsaccades that move the eye only a few microns may not be enough to disrupt the overall pattern of ablation, and the small movements may have an overall smoothing effect because they are somewhat random.

Manual stabilization. Early attempts at excimer laser corneal surgery used manual stabilization of the eye and manually directed micromanipulators to aim

the beam while the patient fixated a target. This can be adequate for therapeutic purposes, such as ablating the bed of an excised pterygium, but the level of control is far from that required for refractive purposes.

Contact lens mask. By having slits in a contact lens applied directly to the cornea, ablations remain in the same position. If the eye moves, the contact lens moves and the ablated area remains located beneath the opening in the mask. This approach was described earlier (see Fig. 19-22).

Fixation rings. The eye can be stabilized by a mechanical device. The simplest of these is a Thornton compression ring, as used in radial keratotomy. A suction ring, such as a Barraquer or Gelender suction ring, may also be used to stabilize the eye. Described earlier was the system of Meditec, in which a mask containing radial or transverse slits is held within a circular suction ring (see Fig. 19-23). Hanna and Parel have designed a conical suction ring that adheres to the limbus and contains ports for blowing humidified nitrogen over the surface and for aspirating air and debris from over the surface (Fig. 19-29).

Each of these devices can be held manually or can be attached mechanically to the end of the delivery system to help keep the eye properly aligned. The mechanism of attachment to the delivery system should have some flexibility to allow observation and manipulation of the position of the eye before ablation and to take up any compressive force that might be applied by moving the delivery system or the patient's head up and down during surgery.

Eye-tracking systems. The most elegant type of coupling system is an optical tracking system. Complex systems of eye tracking have been designed for research and military purposes and are just now being applied to laser corneal surgery. Tracking the eye in an x-y direction parallel to the corneal surface can be done by using infrared lights or other methods of creating two serial images on the ocular surface or at the pupil; these images are detected, their position related to computers, and the resulting electrical signal used to move mirror or lenses in the delivery system so that the laser beam will always hit the desired area of the cornea. The tracker could control firing of the laser so that it is fired only when the eye was in an acceptable position. Confocal microscopy can be used to track the eye in the z-plane, perpendicular to the corneal surface. Such an eye-tracking system has been integrated with a picosecond Nd:YLF laser system by Intelligent Laser Systems.

Environment over area of ablation

Even the most homogeneous and perfectly shaped laser beam that emerges from the delivery system must still traverse the distance between the condensing lens and the surface of the tissue. Things can happen here to disrupt the beam and make it less effective.

Tissue fragments ejected from the surface may interfere with successive pulses. Even though the fragments of tissue clear the area before the next nanosecond pulse arrives, the cumulative effect of this debris falling back onto the surface of the cornea or accumulating in the trough of a linear ablation may create an irregular surface and may absorb some of the energy, disrupting the exact calculations for the amount of tissue ablated. This problem can be decreased in part by blowing or sucking gas across the surface of the cornea so that the effluent is removed and does not accumulate in the area of ablation (see Fig. 19-10).

Ultraviolet excimer laser light is absorbed to some degree by particles in room air, and it is an advantage to remove this air from the delivery system and corneal surface and replace it with an inert gas such as nitrogen. However, blowing nitrogen gas across the surface will dehydrate and thin the cornea, disrupting the calculated tissue ablation. Therefore the area over the surface could be humidified, using very small water particles that will not absorb the laser beam.

Fluid on the corneal surface, whether from tears or irrigation, will also absorb the laser photons, so the surface must be kept dry during photoablation. This can be accomplished by using an eyelid speculum to prevent blinking, by mechanical drying, and by using grooves in a contact lens mask to wick away surface liquid.

Little information has been published concerning refinement of coupling systems and "conditioning" systems because researchers have concentrated their efforts on improving laser delivery systems and studying tissue interactions. Improvements in coupling will be forthcoming.

EXCIMER LASER INTERACTIONS WITH THE CORNEA
Ablative photodecomposition

The atomic and molecular events that occur when a pulse of excimer laser light strikes the cornea and the effects of different wave lengths of excimer lasers on the cornea are discussed in the preceding sections. The essential feature of this process is the ability of an argon fluoride (193-nm) excimer laser to remove a few molecular layers or portions of a single cell with each pulse, the total amount of tissue removed being determined by the pulse energy, the number of pulses, and the radiant exposure at the surface of the cornea.

Ablation of corneal epithelium and stroma

Different corneal tissues ablate at different rates, so the amount of tissue removed with each pulse varies. This is important in calculating the rate and amount of tissue removal to create an exact refractive change. Topical medications, both in the tears and absorbed into the stroma, theoretically can act as a dopant and change the ablation rates of corneal tissue. We have investigated the ablation rate of gels doped with cocaine, oxybuprocaine, proxymetacaine, and pilocarpine and found no change in ablation rates, although with fluorescein the ablation rate decreased from 0.30 to 0.18 μm/pulse.[35]

The corneal epithelium is an inhomogeneous structure and ablates at a faster rate than the corneal stroma. In a human donor eye model, the epithelium ablated at a rate of 0.68 $\pm$0.15 μm/pulse, whereas the stroma ablated at a rate of 0.55 $\pm$0.1 μm/pulse.[88] Within the epithelium the nuclei are more resistant than the cytoplasm to ablation (Fig. 19-30). The irregular ablation of the multilayered epithelium could create an irregular surface on the stroma, so the epithelium is simply mechanically scraped off before the ablation and calculations do not have to take the effect of the epithelium into account.

Bowman's layer ablates slower than the stroma. In a human donor eye model, the ablation rate was 0.38 $\pm$0.05 μm/pulse compared with the stromal rate of 0.55 $\pm$0.1 μm/pulse, at a radiant exposure of 205 mJ/cm^2.[88] This difference in ablation rate by a factor of 1.45 between stroma and Bowman's layer may create a difference in the calculations for photorefractive keratectomy. For example, using a 5-mm diameter ablation zone and allowing 39 μm of ablation to correct 4.0 D of myopia, an error of 12% is induced by using only the stromal ablation rate of 0.55 μm/pulse. Bowman's layer is 9 to 12 μm thick, so approximately 25 pulses are needed to ablate through Bowman's layer at a radiant exposure of 205 mJ/cm^2 [88] (Table 19-6).

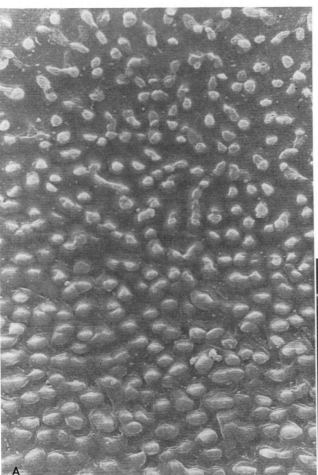

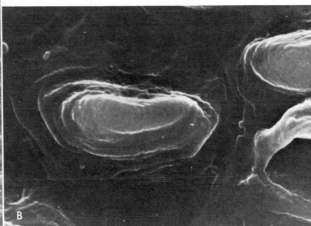

Figure 19-30
Scanning electron micrographs of ablated corneal epithelium in a human eye bank eye. **A,** Photograph at junction of more sparsely spaced polygonal cells (above) and more compact basal cells (below) demonstrate nuclei protruding from the surface of the surrounding cytoplasm (×500). **B,** Higher power view demonstrates a single nucleus with sloping ablated margins rising above the cytoplasm (×20,000). (Courtesy Gilles Renard, MD.)

Electron microscopic studies of the surfaces and edges of corneal stroma ablated at 193 nm emphasize three important findings (see Figs. 19-13 and 19-14). First, the surface is generally smooth but contains focal irregularities that result from inhomogeneities of the beam and surface irregularities of the tissue that are carried forward as "shadows" during the ablation process. The second observation is the frequent appearance on transmission electronmicroscopy of a layer of condensed material on the surface, sometimes called a "pseudomembrane." This tissue is approximately 0.02 to 0.05 micron thick and has a very smooth surface. Its composition is unknown. Presumedly it results from thermal effects at the surface. This condensed tissue is less permeable to water than normal stroma and can decrease stromal swelling. It may also provide a smooth surface over which epithelial cells can migrate, with the usual layer of fibronectin appearing in front of them. The third finding of electron microscopic studies is the general lack of disruption of remaining tissue. Beneath the pseudomembrane, a layer of slightly condensed and disrupted tissue, approximately 1 micron thick, is present in some areas, but beyond that disruption the tissue retains its normal ultrastructural configuration.

The clinical meaning of these three observations is being determined by continued investigation. One of the tacit assumptions of excimer laser corneal surgery is that a generally smooth surface, with minimal underlying tissue disruption, will allow rapid normal epithelial wound healing and will stimulate little or no stromal fibrosis and scarring. Unfortunately, biologic reality is not so simple; clinical and histopathologic reports in monkeys and human beings demonstrate a wide spectrum of tissue responses after excimer laser corneal surgery, especially photorefractive keratectomy. Epithelial hyperplasia and subepithelial scarring have occurred frequently, but technical refinements may be able to reduce their frequency and severity.[44,57]

Table 19-6

Histologically Determined Excision Depths in Human Donor Eyes at a Radiant Exposure of 205 mJ/cm²

Number of pulses	Excision depth (μm, mean, SD)	Original thickness (μm, mean)
Epithelium		
10	38	7 ±2
20	43	13 ±5
30	41	22 ±4
40	39	28 ±4
50	44	31 ±5
60	41	33 ±6
70	40	38 ±3
80	44	43 ±1
Bowman's layer		
5	No excision detected	
10	3.8 ±0.3	9.90
15	4.6 ±0.4	9.20
20	7.6 ±0.5	11.00
25	9.0 ±0.4	10.40
30	11.5 ±0.3	12.30

Stroma

Ablation rate = 0.55 ±0.1 μm/pulse

Modified from Seiler T, Kriegerowski M, Schnoy N, and Bende T: Refract Corneal Surg 1990;6:99-102.

Thermal effects

The cornea is a temperature-sensitive tissue, and corneal collagen extracts denature at approximately 40° C.

The time for heat diffusion in the cornea is on the order of 1 second, so heat accumulates when repetition rates higher than 1 Hz are used. To shorten the time required for a surgical procedure, repetition rates of 5 to 20 Hz are commonly used so that temperature increases adjacent to the area of ablation do occur. The gaseous mixture formed by the ablation process has a temperature of more than 1000° C, but most of this heat is dissipated as the fragments are ejected from the surface. The highest residual temperature is at the boundaries of the ablated tissue, and it declines logarithmically as the distance from the edge decreases. Seiler has measured a maximal temperature rise in the corneal tissue of 11° C adjacent to the trough, with a half value distance of 650 μm. Thus, the temperature at the edge of the ablation rises to approximately 45° C and, at a distance of 650 microns, it rises to approximately 40° C. On this basis, one would expect collagen denaturation, but the only evidence of thermal damage is the surface condensate (pseudomembrane) and slight disruption of tissue at a distance of 1 micron. Thus, clinical experience demonstrates that most of the heat energy is dissipated into the air, away from the tissues.

Mutagenesis induced by excimer lasers

Ultraviolet light is absorbed by DNA and therefore may have a mutagenic and carcinogenic effect on the rapidly multiplying corneal epithelium. The less active stromal fibroblasts are at less risk. It is well known that excimer laser radiation between 248 nm and 308 nm is mutagenic. The best experimental evidence shows that 193-nm radiation is not mutagenic.[61]

Skin fibroblasts irradiated in tissue culture with subablative fluences showed no more anaplastic change than controls and significantly less than cells exposed to x-ray.[109] Measurement of unscheduled DNA synthesis is a reflection of DNA damage, and when this was measured in the cornea after 193-nm ablation, it was no different from that found with a diamond knife, both showing much less unscheduled synthesis than radiation with 248-nm excimer and an ultraviolet germicidal lamp.[68] Green and colleagues[21,22] attributed the absence of unscheduled DNA synthesis after radiation of freshly excised human skin with a 193-nm argon fluoride laser to the shielding of DNA by the cellular interstitium, membrane, and cytoplasm. Human corneas ablated in vivo by Seiler and colleagues[91] have been observed for more than 4 years, with no signs of hyperproliferation or neoplastic change in the cornea. One experiment, using photoreactivation with yeast cells, revealed evidence of DNA damage in cells that are closer than 1 cm to the 193-nm excisions.[85] Perhaps vertebrate cells have different repair mechanisms from yeast cells.

Excimer laser keratectomy

Four different types of corneal laser surgery have been described: linear excisions, either radial to correct myopia or transverse to correct astigmatism*; photorefractive keratectomy (anterior keratomileusis, large area ablation) to correct myopia, hyperopia, and astigmatism[66]; circular trephination for corneal transplantation[46]; and superficial keratectomy for the removal of corneal scars and the smoothing of an irregular corneal surface.[46] We discuss here the first three (Fig. 19-31).

LINEAR EXCISIONS FOR MYOPIA AND ASTIGMATISM

When Trokel and colleagues[111] married the excimer laser to corneal surgery in 1983, their first

*References 2, 8, 24, 63, 86, 107.

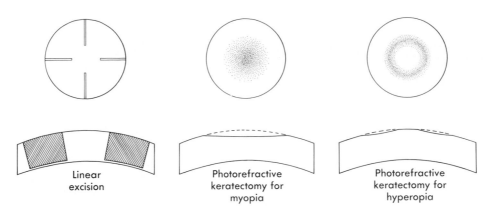

Figure 19-31
Drawing shows two basic types of laser keratectomy. Linear excisions can be done radially for myopia, transversely for astigmatism, or circularly for corneal trephination. Photorefractive keratectomy (anterior keratomileusis) can be done to correct myopia, hyperopia, and, potentially, astigmatism. (From Waring G: Trans Am Ophthalmol Soc 1989;87:855-983.)

thought was to use the laser as a substitute for the diamond knife—the light scalpel—in the performance of radial keratotomy for myopia (see Fig. 19-8). Puliafito and co-workers[77] compared a 193-nm laser with slits of different widths to diamond knife incisions. They showed comparability between the two, the major difference being the electron-dense condensate along the surface of the laser wound. Marshall and co-workers[59,60] demonstrated the superiority of cuts made with the 193-nm excimer laser when compared with diamond and steel knives because the edges were so much smoother.

Cotlier and colleagues[8] demonstrated a curvilinear correlation between the total laser output, the depth of excision, and the change in refractive power of the cornea in human eye bank eyes.

Using serial section of acute linear excisions, Seiler[91] has shown that a uniform depth of ablation can be achieved from one end of the incision to the other (Fig. 19-32).

Stern and colleagues[98] described a femtosecond optical ranging technique for measuring the depth of a corneal excision made with an excimer laser during the ablation process. The resolution limits were estimated to be 5 to 10 μm. Such a technique would be useful in attempting to control the exact level of a cut, a factor extremely important in determining the outcome of linear keratectomy surgery.

Laser radial keratectomy in humans

Tenner and colleagues[107] and Bansal and co-workers[4] performed radial keratotomies on blind eyes of human volunteers using the Meditec excimer laser system (see Fig. 19-33) and a peribulbar block for an-

esthesia and akinesia. The mask used in this study had eight slits, each 70 μm wide and 3.5 mm long. A total of eight radial excisions at approximately 50% to 60% of corneal thickness with a 5.0-mm central clear zone resulted in 1 to 2 D of corneal flattening, measured by the Zeiss ophthalmometer. Clinically the incisions appeared to heal well; however, they were more translucent than the radial keratotomy incisions made with a diamond knife with a railroad track configuration, with the two white areas of stromal scarring on either side bounding the central clearer epithelial plug.

Histologic study of biopsies of these wounds showed a wide separation of the ends of Bowman's layer (50 to 60 μm), and the wound filled with an epithelial plug that persisted up to 18 months. The epi-

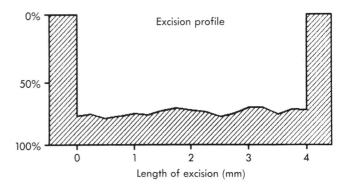

Figure 19-32
Uniformity of linear excision depth after excimer laser (193 nm) ablation. Drawing of the profile of a linear excision demonstrates consistent 80% depth across the entire 4 mm length of the excision. The depth varied only ±4%. (From Seiler T and Wollensak J: Ophthalmologica 1986;192:65-70.)

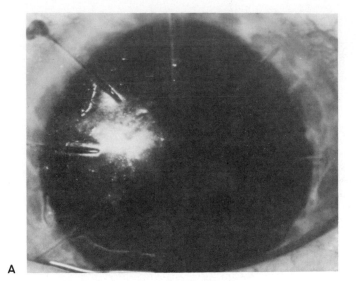

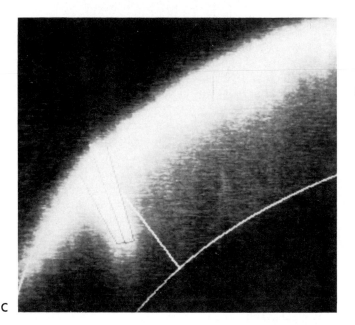

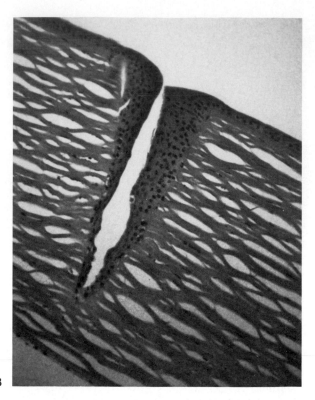

Figure 19-33

Excimer laser radial keratectomy in humans. **A,** Acute appearance immediately after treatment shows eight radial incisions with a 5-mm clear zone. **B,** Light micrograph of transverse excimer laser excision in human cornea 4 days after surgery. Epithelium has migrated down the sides of the wound but has not formed a complete epithelial plug to fill the wound. **C,** Confocal laser scanning image of a human cornea showing the outline of the excimer laser linear keratectomy (black trapezoid) 4 days after surgery. The wound is relatively wide. (**A** courtesy Alf Tenner, MD; **B** from Seiler T, Bende T, Wollensak J, and Trokel S: Am J Ophthalmol 1988;105:117-124; **C** courtesy of Josef Bille, PhD.)

thelial plug and the width of the stromal scar measured approximately 60 to 200 μm at various depths, much wider than the 10 μm usually seen after diamond knife radial keratotomy. Whether this wider stromal scar would produce meaningful differences in refractive outcome is unknown, but the wound gape theory of radial keratotomy suggests that a greater effect should result. Table 19-7 compares excimer laser and diamond knife cuts.

The published short-term follow-up[72] and the follow-up to 1 year indicate that the laser radial keratectomy wounds epithelialize rapidly and generally heal without difficulty. However, there is a major dif-

ference between these linear excisions and a standard radial keratotomy wound made with a diamond knife: the wider laser wounds filled with an epithelial plug that remains easily visible as a translucent clearer central zone in the wound for at least 1 year. An epithelial plug was persistently present for months to years in diamond knife radial keratotomy wounds, but it is visible with the slit-lamp microscope only under careful observation (see Chapter 20, Corneal Wound Healing and Its Pharmacologic Modification after Refractive Keratotomy). However, the epithelial plug after laser radial keratectomy is much more prominent (Fig. 19-33).

Table 19-7

Comparison of Excimer Laser and Diamond Knife Linear Corneal Cuts for Correction of Myopia and Astigmatism

	Excimer laser	Diamond knife
Type of cut	Excision	Incision
Control of depth	Excellent	Good
Control of shape	Excellent	Good
Versatility of shape	Excellent	Fair
Change in refraction per depth of cut	Possibly more	Standard
Wound healing	Epithelial plug larger and may persist longer	Spans approximately 4 to 5 years
Predictability of refractive outcome	Unknown	Fair-Good
Ease of technique	Good	Fair
Expense of instruments	High	Moderate

Transverse linear keratectomy for astigmatism in humans

The effect of different linear excision shapes—straight, concave, and convex—varied in enucleated human donor eyes under controlled conditions. The curved excision, with the concave side facing the center of the cornea, achieved approximately 60% more effect than straight or convex excisions, when the depth ranged from 70% to 80% (Fig. 19-34).

Seiler and colleagues[84] treated 13 eyes in 12 patients with transverse linear excisions for the treatment of astigmatism, using a 193-nm argon fluoride laser with a 15-nsec pulse and a fluence of 165 mJ/cm² at the corneal surface, repetition rate of 30 Hz, and the number of pulses necessary to create an approximately 80% depth. The ablation depth per pulse was calibrated on enucleated human eyes and corrected for the fact that the laser beam was not perpendicular to the surface throughout the cornea and that the peripheral cornea was thicker than the central cornea, so the thickness was increased by a factor of 1.18.[83] The contact lens mask system was described earlier (see Fig. 19-22). The ablation depth per pulse was established at approximately 0.32 μm, so the total number of pulses necessary to obtain a planned percentage of the corneal thickness, as measured by ultrasonic pachometry immediately before surgery, was calculated and was entered into the laser control terminal.

A pilot study in 20 patients with blind eyes indicated rapid epithelial healing with stabilization of corneal topography within 6 weeks of the transverse keratectomy, the stability lasting for more than 1 year. This led to experiments on sighted human eyes. The two parallel straight transverse excisions were made through the contact lens mask, with slits 4.5 mm long and 150 μm wide on either side of a 6-mm diameter zone. The ablation depth per pulse in the epithelium was approximately twice that obtained in the stroma, requiring two separate calculations to select the number of pulses needed to achieve the desired depth. Topical anesthesia was used and a corneal surface was kept dry during ablation using fixation with a Thornton compression ring. No microperforations occurred. Each of the slits was ablated separately, each lasting approximately 50 seconds.

In the first postoperative week, corneal astigmatism values fluctuated but tended to stabilize after 2 weeks. Slit-lamp microscopy on the first postoperative day showed stromal edema surrounding the excision sites, but by the third day epithelium had grown into the excisions, gradually filling the entire keratectomy site with an epithelial plug (Fig. 19-35). This process took up to 1 month in some eyes.

Once the wound healing had stabilized, slit-lamp microscopy demonstrated a railroad track configuration in each linear excision, with the center of the incision being clear (presumably because of the presence of the epithelial plug) and the edges of the excision and the sides of the excision being opaque (presumably because of stromal wound healing and remodeling). This configuration persisted throughout the first year of observation.

All 12 corneas flattened in the incised meridian,

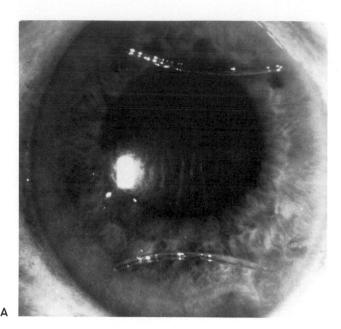

	Spherical change (diopters)	Astigmatic change (diopters)
n = 5	+0.11 ± 0.32	−5.0 ± 1.01
n = 5	−0.86 ± 0.24	−5.81 ± 0.77
n = 5	−0.92 ± 0.3	−8.6 ± 1.56

A

B   Optical zone, 6 mm; excision depth, 75%; excision length, 4.5 mm

Figure 19-34
Effect of configuration of linear laser transverse keratectomy. **A,** Human eye bank eye demonstrates a pair of convex linear excisions in the vertical meridian. **B,** Results of three different patterns of transverse excisions demonstrate that the concave excision (bottom) achieves a greater change in astigmatism than the straight or convex patterns.

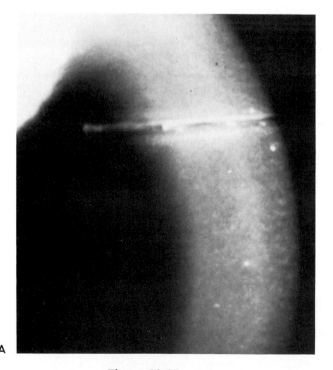

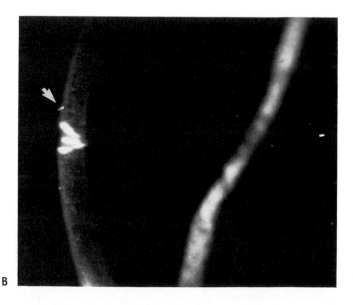

A

B

Figure 19-35
Slit-lamp microscope appearance of human excimer laser transverse keratectomy. **A,** A few days after surgery the width of the wound is apparent. **B,** Approximately 2 months after surgery the railroad track configuration of the wound is apparent with a clearer center and **V**-shaped opaque edges. The white curved line on the right side of the figure is the surface of the iris. (Arrow is above the keratectomy.)

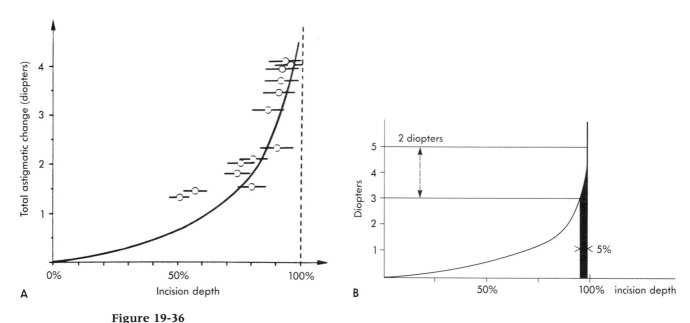

Figure 19-36

Relationship between depth of transverse laser keratectomy and total change in astigmatism. **A,** Open circles represent actual values. The line represents the theoretic curve calculated from biomechanical formulas. The excision depths were determined from slit-lamp photographs. The measurement error was measured to be ±8%. **B,** Schematic drawing of similar information emphasizes the large effect of the deepest 5% of the excision. This information emphasizes the importance of accurate incision depth in refractive keratotomy. (**A** From Seiler T, Bende T, Wollensak J, and Trokel S: Am J Ophthalmol 1988;105:117-124.)

with a range of 0.21 D to 2.78 D (see Table 19-7). In general, the refraction remained stable after approximately 1 month (Fig. 19-36). The temporal course of the refractive effect after linear laser excision was different from that after a diamond knife incision. The maximum change in refraction after a diamond knife incision occurs immediately, followed by a regression, whereas the maximum change after laser linear keratectomy occurred over 1 month. Long-term follow-up (reported at the German Ophthalmology Society Meeting, Heidelberg, October 1989) of 42 eyes with naturally occurring astigmatism reported an average decrease in astigmatism of 2.3 ±1.1 D at 6 months to 2 years postoperatively. The refractive change was stable after 2 months, with a regression of less than 0.50 D up to 2 years.

Seven eyes with high astigmatism after penetrating keratoplasty (range 7.5 to 19.5 D, average 12.5 D) were treated in a somewhat different manner. Only one excision was performed at 90% depth, perpendicular to the steepest semimeridian defined by photokeratographs. After 3 weeks a second excision was made in the remaining steepest semimeridian, again taking into account that the mechanical stress pattern inside the button is not regular, so the second cut was not performed necessarily in the exact opposite semi-

meridian as the first cut. In three eyes a third cut was necessary. The average decrease of astigmatism was 8.4 ±4.7 D, resulting in a final astigmatism of 2.7 ±1.6 D.

There was a close correlation between the intended excision depth and the verified excision depth (error of ±8%), as measured from slit-lamp microscope photographs. Having demonstrated that the excision depth is proportionate to the number of pulses, Seiler computed the incision depth for each case. There was a curvilinear relationship between the incision depth and the magnitude of astigmatic change, the amount of change increasing markedly as the incisions got deeper than 80%. Incisions from 50% to 85% depth generally accomplished 1.5 to 2.5 D of change in astigmatism, but incisions from 85% to 95% depth accomplished 3 to 4 D change. This observation was modeled using biomechanical principles so that the amount of astigmatic change could be predicted for given transverse linear excisions (Fig. 19-37). These findings emphasize the extreme importance of accurate incision depth in refractive keratotomy and help explain some of the variability seen in radial keratotomy performed with a diamond knife (see Chapter 13, Predictability of Refractive Keratotomy).

An unexpected finding was the pattern of steepen-

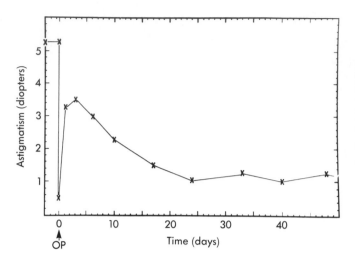

Figure 19-37
Change in astigmatism over time after excimer laser transverse keratectomy in one patient. Refractive equilibrium was obtained after 1 month. The rapid changes within the first postoperative days probably result from stromal edema. The refractive result remained reasonably stable during the second and third months. (From Seiler T, Bende T, Wollensak J, and Trokel S: Am J Ophthalmol 1988;105:117-124.)

ing in the meridian parallel to the linear excision. In general, with a diamond knife creating a straight transverse incision, the amount of flattening perpendicular to the incision is approximately equal to the amount of steepening in the meridian parallel to the incision.[80] However, with transverse laser keratectomy in human beings, there was always more steepening in the meridian parallel to the excision, sometimes with values two to three times the amount of flattening 90 degrees away.

In Chapter 36 we discuss the biomechanics of transverse incisions of the cornea. A theoretic biomechanical model predicts that there should be a twofold to threefold greater flattening of the meridian perpendicular to the transverse incisions than steepening in the meridian parallel to the incisions. However, the clinical data showed the proportion to be nearly the opposite. This discrepancy may result from the failure of the theoretic model to take into account the influence of the corneal lamellae that do not cross the center, but instead are oriented more parallel to the corneal scleral limbus.

The overall conclusion drawn from this series of eyes is that transverse laser keratectomy for astigmatism, and presumably radial laser keratectomy for myopia, differ in their results from the more familiar diamond knife keratotomy. Although the overall outcome is similar, the amount of change varies between the two techniques in a way that has yet to be defined.

Clinical usefulness of linear keratectomy

There is little laboratory or clinical investigation of the use of radial or transverse linear keratectomy to correct myopia and astigmatism. There are three major reasons for this. The first reason is the fact that this technique actually makes a V-shaped trough in the cornea. It is not possible to make the thin linear cut that is possible with a diamond knife. Although the depth of the cut can be reasonably well measured, techniques have not yet been refined to allow for different depths along the length of an excision to allow for regional differences in corneal thickness, although this technology is theoretically possible. The second reason is that the cornea is weakened by a deep keratectomy, and corneal wound healing plays a major role in determining the outcome, the same problems that plague diamond knife radial keratotomy. Indeed, wound healing may play even a larger role because of the excised trough. The third reason is expense. A diamond knife and associated instruments cost approximately $2000; current clinical models of excimer lasers cost approximately $400,000. Table 19-7 compares laser and diamond knife techniques. Thus the clinical utility of this technique is in doubt, and the major research effort has turned to photorefractive keratectomy (anterior keratomileusis).

PHOTOREFRACTIVE KERATECTOMY

The concept of directly reshaping the curvature of the cornea with a laser was propounded before the excimer laser entered the ophthalmic field when Keats[30] proposed the use of a carbon dioxide laser. Marshall and colleagues[60] recognized the exquisite qualities of the wounds made by an excimer laser and proposed in 1986 the direct carving of the cornea into a different radius of curvature to change its optical power, a technique dubbed photorefractive keratectomy (PRK). The major advantage of photorefractive keratectomy over linear keratotomy or keratectomy is the ability to achieve a direct optical correction rather than depending on the indirect biomechanical effects of the paracentral and peripheral cuts. However, the idea that

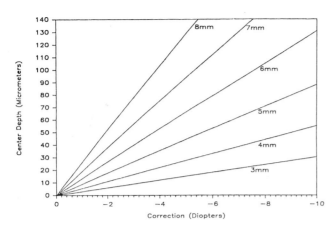

Figure 19-38
Plot of the center depth of tissue removed against the myopic correction achieved for ablation zones of 3 to 8 mm in diameter. As the diameter gets larger, an increasingly deep excision is required to achieve a specific correction. (From Munnerlyn CR, Kooms SJ, and Marshall J: J Cataract Refract Surg 1988;14:46-52.)

there would be minimal stromal wound healing without opacification and a rapidly achieved stable refraction has not been supported by laboratory and clinical experience. Corneal wound healing does occur. The major disadvantage of this technique is one that accompanies all lamellar refractive keratoplasty surgery: The operation is done across the visual axis and any surgical error or problem with healing that creates scarring or irregular astigmatism degrades visual function.

Optical calculations

The optical calculations for the acute change in corneal curvature are simple enough, derived from the elementary geometry used for the manufacture of contact lenses. Munnerlyn and colleagues[66] performed these calculations assuming that the posterior surface of the cornea remains fixed and that only the anterior surface of the cornea is modified (Fig. 19-38). Therefore a true index of refraction of 1.376 was used, not the keratometric index of 1.3375. An estimate of the amount of tissue that needs to be removed centrally can be made by using the following formula:

$$\text{Thickness of tissue removed } (\mu m) = \frac{\text{Refractive change (D)}}{3} \times \left(\frac{\text{Diameter of ablated zone (mm)}}{}\right)^2$$

Unfortunately, wound healing limits somewhat the value of these ideal optical calculations.

Although the diameter of the ablation zone can be well defined, the optically effective part of that zone is smaller. That is, the ablation zone consists of a central optical zone and a peripheral transition zone. The contour of these curves and the rate at which one area blends into another will have an important effect on both corneal wound healing and the postoperative optics and quality of vision.

Laboratory studies of photorefractive keratotomy

One of the advantages of the excimer laser is its ability to create a very smooth wound bed. Theoretically, this leads to less opacification. Thus great efforts have been made to create a very homogeneous laser beam emerging from the delivery system without hot spots and to create surface contours that have very smooth transitions to foster minimal wound healing with opacification.[45,60] The surface irregularities in the stromal bed should be minimal, dependent only on the steps created by the variable iris diaphragm or the moving slit. There may be some inevitable roughness that would be created by the retraction of the dissected corneal lamellae, which are under tension by the intraocular pressure. Marshall and colleagues[60] and Kerr-Muir and colleagues[31] demonstrated in rabbits and primates that epithelial healing occurred rapidly, completely, and apparently without difficulty. The authors reported the use of an early model instrument in 12 monkeys with 24 months of follow-up.[57] Immediately after epithelialization the anterior cornea was clear, but 1 to 6 months after surgery, subepithelial haze appeared, which gradually cleared but persisted out to 24 months. McDonald and co-workers[63] reported similar findings.

We have described the clinical, histologic, and immunohistochemical findings during a 12- to 18-month follow-up in rabbits and monkeys.[12,25,99] The clinical course was highly variable in the rabbits. Four animals (eight eyes) were followed for more than 21 days, half of the corneas remaining clear and the other half developing a subepithelial ground-glass haze that diminished but never completely cleared. The results were also variable in 29 monkeys' eyes, with the appearance of a subepithelial haze of a 2+ density in the majority of corneas by 6 weeks, but some of the corneas

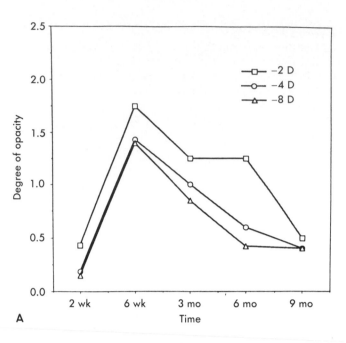

A

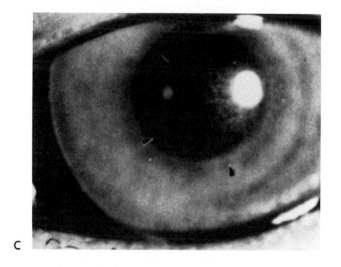

C

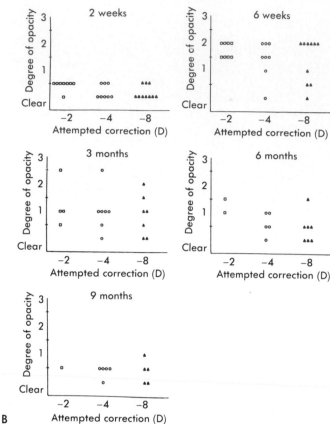

B

Figure 19-39

Central subepithelial corneal haze in monkeys after myopic photorefractive keratectomy. **A,** Graphic representation of the average density of corneal haze in each ablation group (−2, −4, and −8 D) at different time intervals. **B,** Scattergrams of the density of haze of individual corneas according to each group of attempted correction (−2, −4, and −8 D) and at different time intervals after ablation. The opacities were graded 0 to 4+. **C,** Slit-lamp photograph of the rhesus monkey cornea after ablation. Grade 1+ opacity *(arrowheads)* could be easily seen by direct diffuse illumination. (From Fantes FE, Hanna KD, Waring GO, Pouliquen Y, Thompson KP, and Savoldelli M: Arch Ophthalmol 1990;108:665-675.)

remaining clear. The density of the haze gradually diminished, so by 6 to 9 months, 12 of 13 surviving corneas (92%) were either completely clear (four corneas) or trace hazy (eight corneas) (Fig. 19-39).

All histologic studies of both rabbit and primate eyes after photorefractive keratectomy have demonstrated subepithelial fibroplasia, with the deposition of a new layer of extracellular connective tissue that contains type III collagen, type VII collagen, and newly produced keratan sulfate and that is highlighted by the absence of staining with DTAF, which stains only the preexisting stroma.[20,25,55,99,114] The newly produced tissue begins to appear approximately 1 month after ablation, corresponds to the onset of subepithelial haze, and gradually becomes remodeled with associated decreasing haze clinically. The changes are highly variable from one cornea to another; some corneas become completely clear and others remain slightly hazy. The histologic changes persist for at least 18 to 24 months, which is the longest reported animal series.[27,61,99] The fibroblastic response can be decreased with topical steroids,[114] and therefore intensive post-

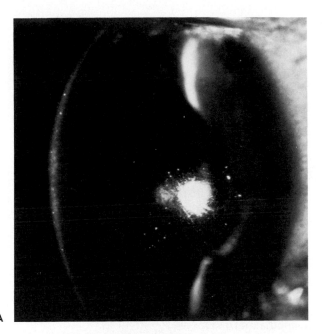

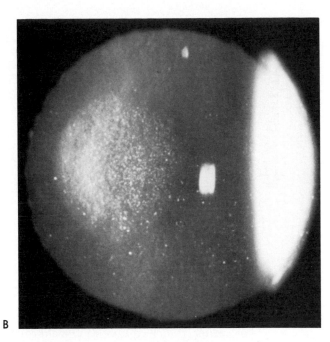

Figure 19-40
Slit-lamp photomicrograph of human cornea 4 weeks after −6.00 D myopic photorefractive keratectomy shows trace subepithelial haze **(A)** and ablated zone visible
in retroillumination **(B)**.

operative topical corticosteroids have been used clinically. How much the subepithelial fibroplasia affects
the refractive outcome is not completely clear. It probably accounts for some of the initial loss of effect seen
in the first 3 months after surgery, but how it affects
the final outcome remains to be defined.

Photorefractive keratectomy in humans

Studies to date in humans can be divided into two
time periods, the early, more experimental period
when the technology was being improved and corticosteroids were used infrequently, and the more recent, refined period when the lasers and delivery systems had passed through a series of design improvements and corticosteroids were used intensively after
surgery.

The early experience was reported by Taylor and
colleagues,[106] who treated 11 blind human eyes and
observed normal reepithelialization but also the general persistence of mild to moderate subepithelial haze
within the few months after surgery. Aron-Rosa and
co-workers[2] described subepithelial opacification 14
days after ablation in one eye. In a series of nine blind
eyes, McDonald and colleagues[64] demonstrated the
ability to achieve a myopic refractive correction with
only moderate subepithelial haze. They described an
initial regression of effect and poor predictability.

Seven of the nine eyes developed 1+ haze and one
eye 2+ haze. There was a gradual clearing of the haze,
and by 6 months only 30% of the eyes were completely clear, although the remaining haze was interpreted as not clinically significant (Fig. 19-40). No
postoperative corticosteroids were used. A refractive
correction of between +1.75 and +11.00 D was attempted, and at 1 month all eyes but one were within
3.00 D of the desired correction. However, by 3
months only five of the eyes were within 3.00 D, and
considerable variability in the regression of effect was
noted (Fig. 19-41). The keratometric and video keratographic findings correlated with the refractions, and
the topography had generally smooth contours. Some
of the variability in this series can be attributed to attempts to refract blind eyes.

In the more recent experience, Seiler and colleagues[87] have reported results in 10 blind and 13
sighted human eyes. All eyes showed mild subepithelial haze that resolved to a barely perceptible level by 6
months in all but one eye. Topical steroids were used
postoperatively five times a day for 1 month and twice
a day for another month with gradual tapering. Preoperative refraction ranged from −1.50 to −5.90 D. A
spherical equivalent refraction of ±1.00 D was
achieved in eight of 13 eyes (62%) at 1 month, in
92% at 3 months, and in 77% at 6 months (Fig. 19-42

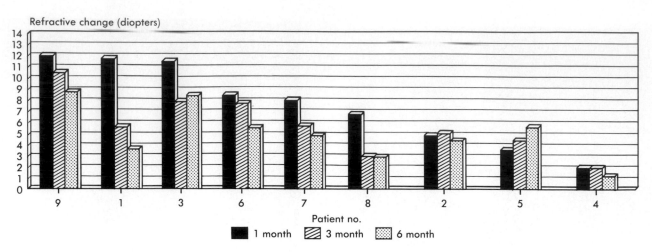

Figure 19-41

Bar graph shows the changes in refraction in individual blind eyes after myopic photorefractive keratectomy. Loss of effect is characteristic, and there is considerable variability in the change in refraction among individual eyes. Accurate refractive measurements in blind eyes are difficult, and results in sighted eyes may be better. (Modified from McDonald MB et al: Arch Ophthalmol 1990;108:799-808.)

and Table 19-8). The authors made a series of important observations:

1. The programmed correction entered into the computer algorithm was 0.50 to 1.50 D greater than that desired clinically, an adjustment necessary to compensate for the early regression of effect.

2. Eyes with smaller corrections, particularly those with less than 2.00 D of correction that are likely to have had their ablation confined to Bowman's layer, showed the most stability. Eyes with 5.00 D or more of correction showed the largest regression of effect over 6 months, as emphasized by Wilson[119] in a subsequent letter. This suggests that photorefractive keratectomy may be more useful in the same range than is diamond knife radial keratotomy, between approximately −1.50 and −5.00 D. The refractive results achieved by Seiler in his paper are similar to those reported for radial keratotomy in the same range (see Chapter 21, Published Results of Refractive Keratotomy).

3. Postoperative topical corticosteroids play an integral role in decreasing the subepithelial fibroplasia, therefore decreasing the postoperative haze and increasing the postoperative stability of refraction. In fact, the corticosteroids can be used to crudely modulate the response, increasing steroids being used to treat an undercorrection and decreasing steroids being used to treat an overcorrection.

4. The balance between depth of excision and diameter of ablated zone requires further study. Whereas a larger diameter of the ablated zone is desirable to decrease optical aberrations over the pupil, it requires a deeper excision, which may be associated with more subepithelial haze and less refractive stability. The authors preferred excisions shallower than 40 μm with a maximum ablation zone of 3.5 mm.

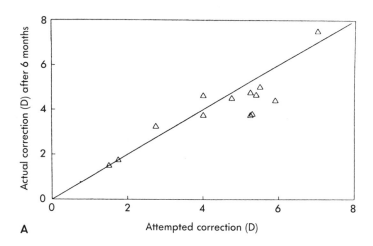

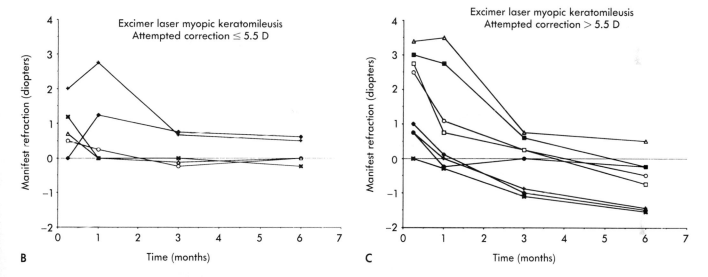

Figure 19-42
Results of photorefractive keratectomy for myopia in 13 sighted human eyes 6 months after surgery. **A,** The attempted correction on the x-axis is compared with the actual change in manifest refraction on the y-axis. **B** and **C,** Change in manifest refraction over time in eyes divided according to preoperative myopia. Eyes with less than 5.00 D of preoperative myopia **(B)** appear to be more stable than eyes with more than 5.00 D of myopia **(C).** (**A** from Seiler T, Kahle G, and Kriegerowski M: Refract Corneal Surg 1990;6:165-173; **B** and **C** from Wilson SE: Refract Corneal Surg 1990;6:383-385.)

Table 19-8

Excimer Laser Myopic Photorefractive Keratectomy in Sighted Human Eyes: Refractive* Results (D) Using the Summit Excimed Clinical Instrument

Patient (sex and age)	Before surgery	Desired goal	After surgery				Deviation
			1 mo	3 mo	6 mo	9 mo	
M, 40	−2.25	0.0	+2.25	0.0	+0.5	0.0	0.0
M, 30	−5.25	0.0	+1.1	+0.1	+0.25	+0.5	+0.5
W, 44	−7.0	0.0	+3.5	−0.1	+0.75	+0.5	+0.5
M, 27	−1.75	0.0	+0.25	−0.25	+0.3	+0.1	+0.1
W, 37	−5.0	0.0	+2.0	+2.75	+0.1	−0.5	−0.5
W, 25	−2.5	0.0	+0.75	−0.25	0.0	−0.25	−0.25
W, 44	−5.25	0.0	+0.5	−0.25	−0.5	−0.5	−0.5
W, 23	−4.25	0.0	+1.0	−0.5	−2.0	−0.9	−0.9
W, 30	−5.9	−0.5	0.0	−0.25	−0.6	−1.0	−0.5
W, 32	−4.75	0.0	+2.25	−0.5	−0.9	−1.2	−1.2
M, 62	−5.25	−1.25	+0.25	−1.0	−2.25	−2.25	−1.0
M, 25	−4.0	0.0	0.0	0.0	†	−1.5	−1.5
M, 33	−2.25	0.0	+1.0	+0.5	0.0	−0.25	−0.25
W, 31	−6.0	0.0	+1.0	−1.0	0.0	−0.75	−0.75
M, 27	−1.4	0.0	+0.75	+0.25	+0.25	0.0	0.0
W, 37	−5.25	0.0	+0.25	−0.9	−0.65	−0.75	−0.75
M, 39	−4.75	0.0	−0.7	−1.0	−1.7	−2.1	−2.1
W, 41	−5.4	0.0	+0.75	+0.25	−1.0	−0.75	−0.75
W, 42	−4.0	0.0	+1.25	+0.75	+0.25	−0.1	−0.1
W, 28	−2.75	0.0	+2.75	+1.0	0.0	0.0	0.0
W, 29	−4.9	0.0	+1.5	0.0	−0.75	−1.0	−1.0
M, 39	−2.6	0.0	+3.1	+1.25	+1.35	+1.0	+1.0
W, 28	−6.9	0.0	+1.0	−0.5	−1.0	−1.25	−1.25
M, 57	−9.25	−2.0	+3.0	+0.75	†	−1.4	+0.6
W, 30	−4.25	0.0	+1.6	+1.1	+0.4	0.0	0.0
W, 39	−3.75	0.0	+3.0	+1.0	−0.25	−0.5	−0.5

*Spherical equivalent of the manifest refraction.
†Value not determined in the time specified.
(From Seiler T, Kahle G, Kriegerowski M: Refract Corneal Surg 1990;6:165-173.)

In the early 1990s numerous reports of photorefractive keratectomy in humans will be published. In the United States the use of excimer lasers in humans is under the control of the Food and Drug Administration (FDA), which has set clear guidelines for the gradual employment of the laser for refractive keratectomy and phototherapeutic keratectomy.[70] Verbal presentations have generally indicated that corrections under 5.00 D myopia can achieve reasonable stability after approximately 3 months with minimal corneal haze if topical corticosteroids and modern technical improvements are used. However, eyes with a refraction of over 5.00 D tend to lose effect gradually, presumably because the surface contours and depth of the incisions trigger more wound healing response with filling in of the ablation. New techniques are being developed to improve results in eyes with greater myopia. One advantage of the FDA regulation in the United States is that investigators are required to report detailed data on the cases according to prescribed guidelines, so the quality of information resulting from these studies will be reasonably high. There is less regulation outside the United States, and numerous reports will be coming forth from investigators. We hope the information will be detailed with a high percentage of follow-up and a thorough analysis of clinical and refractive data.

CORNEAL TREPHINATION

One of the major challenges in penetrating keratoplasty is the creation of a perfectly round donor and host with uniformly shaped edges, on the premise that uniform wounds will decrease the amount of astigmatism after the sutures are removed.[9] The ability of lasers to cut a perfectly round circle with perfectly vertical edges could be an advantage in corneal transplantation, especially if tissue adhesives could be used to close the wound without distorting the tissue.

Using the axicon lens system as described above, Loertscher and colleagues[46,49] have used an infrared laser to create circular trephination wounds. The diameter of the annulus could be varied from 5 to 7 mm by altering the position of the axicon along the longitudinal beam axis. At the focal plane of the annulus the width varied from 100 to 150 μ over 340°, and narrowed to 50 μ for 20° at the 5 o'clock position. Using a hydrogen fluoride (HF) laser and the axicon lens optical delivery system, rapid noncontact trephination of the cornea was performed. The HF laser was run at a fixed repetition rate of 10 Hz and delivered an average radiant exposure to the cornea of 200 mJ/cm². Seventy-five to 85 pulses were required to penetrate the cornea. Due to nonuniformities in both beam homogeneity and corneal thickness, it is not possible to trephine the cornea at full thickness for 360°. Instead, corneal perforation occurs at one point corresponding to the thinnest area of cornea or the highest rated exposure. Immediately following perforation the wound fills with aqueous, impairing further trephination.

Serdarevic et al.[92] have used the rotating slit delivery system to create circular full thickness trephination wounds in rabbits, with a description of clinical and histopathologic wound healing up to 3 months. The delivery system was configured with a mask containing three arcs 100° in length, 0.5 mm wide, with a radius of 3.5 mm. As the mask rotated, a circular cut was made. The laser variables employed were a radiant exposure of 200 mJ/cm², repetition rate of 10 Hz, and a rotation rate of the slit of 1 Hz. It took 0.5 to 3 minutes to penetrate the anterior chamber. Once aqueous filled the perforation of Descemet's membrane, the ablation stopped immediately, since the laser energy was absorbed by the aqueous humor. The authors compared this type of wound with that created by manual trephination (Figs. 19-43 and 19-44).

Lang and associates[38-40] have proposed using the

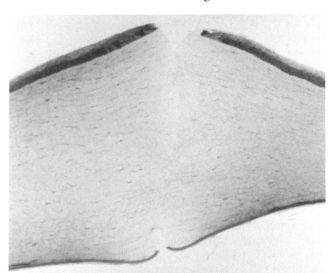

Figure 19-43
Full thickness ArF excimer laser trephination of a rabbit cornea. Light micrograph demonstrates appearance of full thickness laser trephine wound. (Courtesy Olivia Serdarevic, MD. From Waring GO: Trans Am Ophthalmol Soc 1989;87:854-983.)

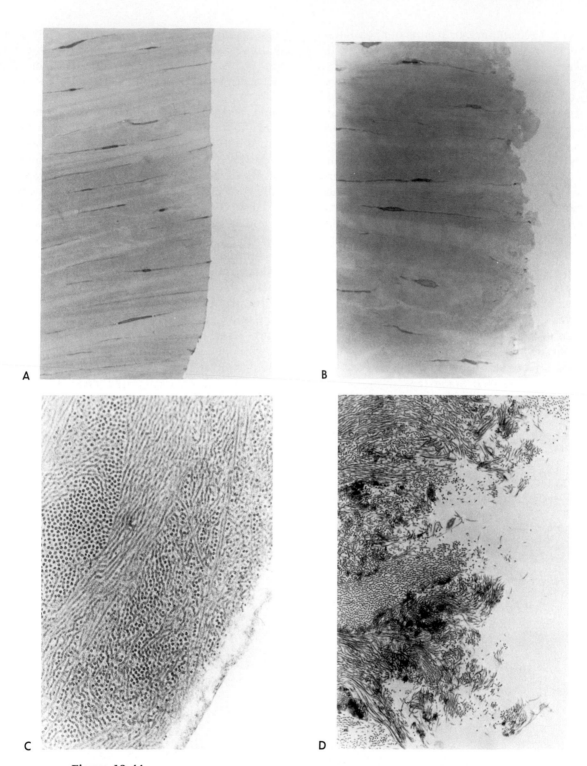

Figure 19-44
Comparison of trephine wound made by ArF excimer laser and manual circular razor blade of the corneal wound in rabbit cornea. **A,** After laser trephination the edge of the corneal wound is smooth and regular with minimal disruption. **B,** After manual trephination the edge of the corneal wound is ragged and disrupted (toluidine blue, ×500). **C,** After excimer laser trephination the surface of the wound is covered by a slightly detached pseudomembrane, and the underlying collagenous stroma is minimally disrupted (×14,000). **D,** Transmission electron micrograph after manual trephination shows fragmented wound margin (×4000). (Courtesy Olivia Serdarevic, MD. From Waring GO: Trans Am Ophthalmol Soc 1989;87:854-983.)

excimer laser to make an elliptic donor and host wound for penetrating keratoplasty. This is accomplished by placing a mask over the surface of the donor and host corneas, and ablating along the edge to cut an elliptic partial thickness button that is removed with scissors. Since the anterior corneal limbus forms an elliptic shape, wider horizontally than vertically, the elliptic graft keeps the donor equidistant from the host vessels and may decrease allograft rejection. In addition, the fit of the elliptic donor and host might be more exact, with less graft rotation, decreasing postoperative astigmatism. Whether either of these theories works will require studies of the technique. These penetrating keratoplasty wounds are wider, more wedge-shaped, and represent the excision of tissue in contrast to those made with trephine.

EFFECT OF CORNEAL WOUND HEALING ON PHOTOREFRACTIVE KERATECTOMY

Corneal wound healing can affect the outcome of refractive corneal surgery in general and excimer laser photorefractive keratectomy in particular. The general principles of corneal stromal wound healing and the healing of linear keratotomy are discussed in Chapter 20, Corneal Wound Healing and Its Pharmacologic Modification after Refractive Keratotomy. The healing of linear excimer laser keratectomies follows the same general principles, except for the wider gap and larger epithelial plug,[107,108] as described earlier in this chapter.

The extent of wound healing can affect the results of surgery to three different degrees:

1. *None.* Presently, all refractive corneal surgery procedures are affected by wound healing. Corneal wound healing after refractive keratectomy has been described by a number of investigators,* and the information presented here summarizes these findings. The histochemical studies of SundarRaj and colleagues[99] help explain the time course of changes in the basement membrane and anterior stromal zones (Fig. 19-45 and Table 19-9).

2. *Limited.* Wound healing that produces changes in corneal clarity or refraction that are transient and reasonably anticipated can be considered as part of the morbidity of the surgical procedure itself.

3. *Persistent.* Prolonged effects of wound healing that do not have a known time of termination can represent a significant problem.

One of the underlying assumptions in the early development of excimer laser photorefractive keratectomy was that the laser could remove corneal stroma accurately and gently enough that a wound

*References 12, 24, 25, 52, 57, 65, 99, 114, 121.

Table 19-9

Summary of Wound Healing Findings after Argon Fluoride Excimer Laser Myopic Photorefractive Keratectomy (PRK) in Monkey Corneas

| | | | Severity grade* by time after PRK | | | | |
| | | | 2-3 mo | | 6 mo | | |
	7 d	**21 d**	**Haze**	**Clear**	**Haze**	**Clear**	**9 mo**
Epithelial thickening	2	1	0	0	0	0	0
Dark basal epithelial cells	2-3	2-3	2	2	1	1	0
Epithelial detachment	0	0	2	1	0	0	0
Subepithelial vacuolization	1	1	2-3	1-2	1-2	1	0-0.5
Basement membrane disruption	1-2	1-2	2-3	1-2	1-2	1	0-0.5
Activated anterior stromal fibrocytes	2	3	2	1	2	0-0.5	0-0.5
Clumps of extracellular stromal microfibrils	1	1-2	2-3	1-2	2	0-0.5	0-0.5

From Fantes FE, Hanna KD, Waring GO, Pouliquen Y, Thompson KP, and Savoldelli M: Arch Ophthalmol 1990;108:665-675.
*The severity grades follow: 0 indicates normal; 1, nearly normal; 2, moderately abnormal; and 3, highly abnormal. The clinical grades follow: haze was defined as corneas with grade 1 or more opacity; clear, corneas with grade 0.5 or less opacity.

Figure 19-45
Wound healing of anterior cornea after excimer laser photorefractive keratectomy in monkeys (250 mJ/cm^2, depth 11 to 46 μm) depicted with immunohistochemical techniques. (From SundarRaj N, Geiss MJ, Fantes F, Hanna K, Anderson SC, Thompson K, Thoft RA, and Waring GO: Arch Ophthalmol 1990;108:1604-1610.)

Monoclonal antibody*	Normal control	Acute	7 days
A. Type VII collagen (Ab 185, globular domain)			
B. Fibronectin (gelatin-binding region)			
C. Type III collagen (Ab 175, bacterial collagenase-resistant region)			
D. Keratan sulfate (J10, J19, J35, J38, Surfactal epitopes)			
E. Fetal antigen in fibroblast (intermediate filament associated protein, IFAP 130)			
F. Phase contrast micrograph (for histologic orientation)			

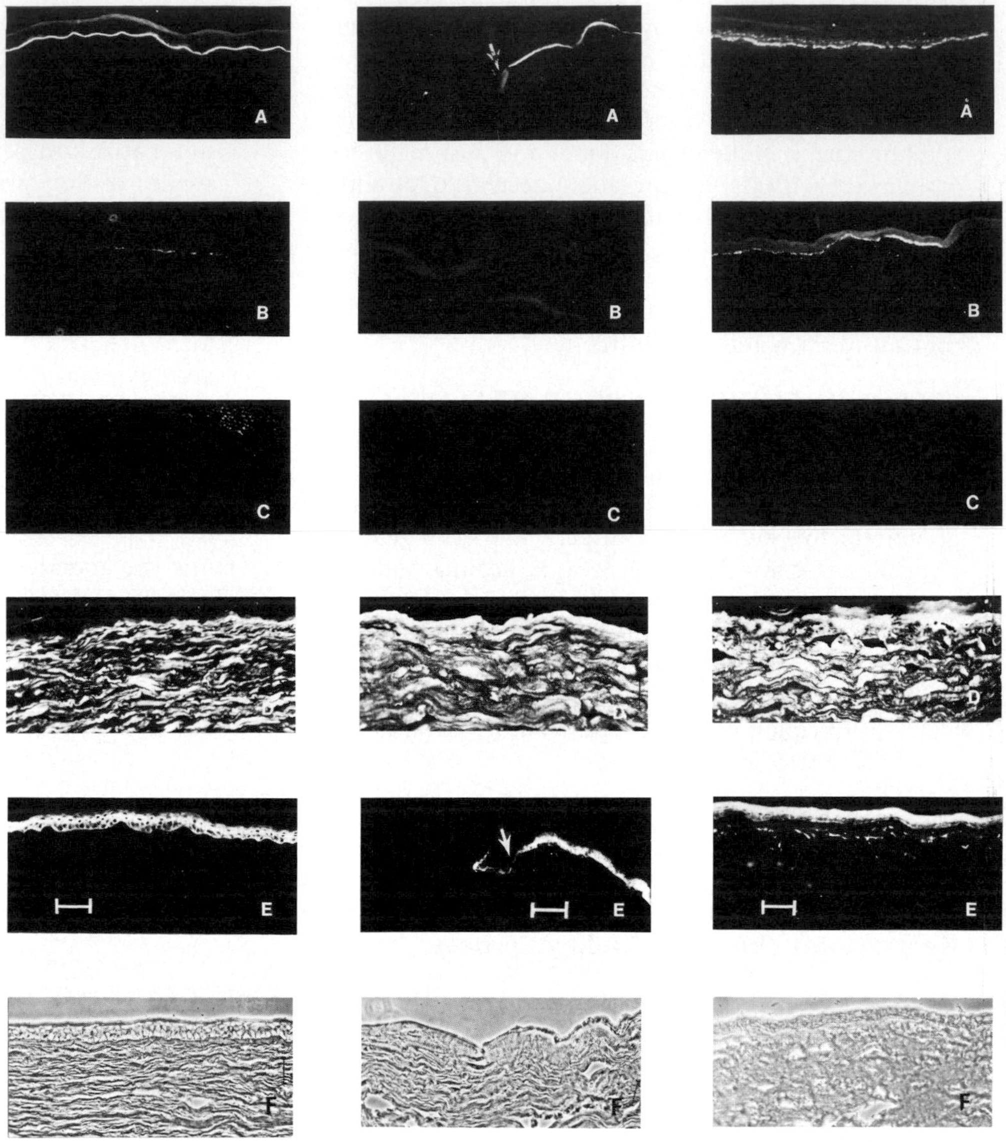

*Indirect fluorescein conjugated antibody technique, bar = 100 μm

Type VII collagen (**A**) localizes in the basement membrane zone where the anchoring fibrils are. Keratan sulfate (**B**) is distributed in a lamellar pattern throughout the stroma. There is no significant straining for fibronectin (**B**), type III collagen (**C**), or fetal antigen (**E**).

Both type VII collagen (**A**) and fetal antigen in the epithelium (**E**) stop abruptly at the edge of the ablated zone. There is no significant staining for fibronectin (**B**), type III collagen (**C**) or fetal antigen (**E**).

Type VII (**A**) and fibronectin (**B**) form linear concentrations in the basement membrane zone. Some fetal antigen is being expressed by fibroblasts in the anterior stroma (**E**). No type III collagen (**C**) or new keratan sulfate (**D**) is present.

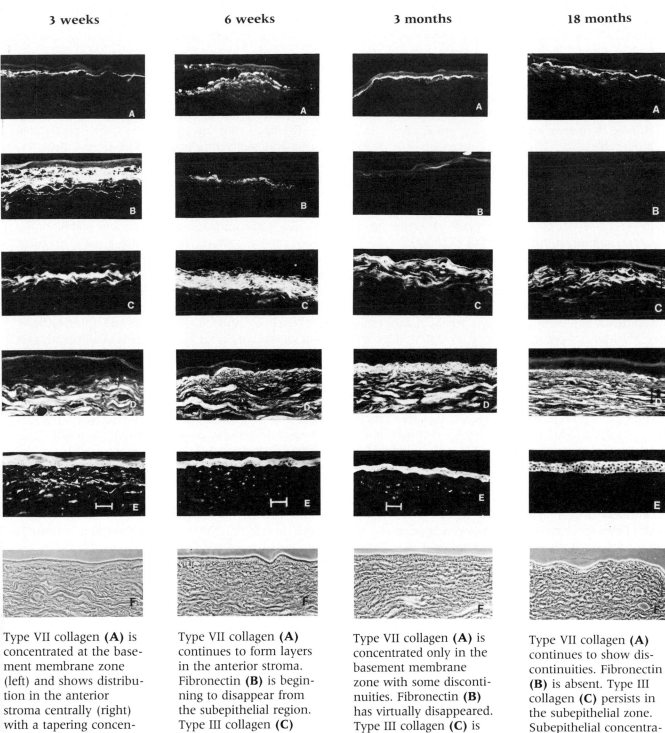

3 weeks · **6 weeks** · **3 months** · **18 months**

Type VII collagen **(A)** is concentrated at the basement membrane zone (left) and shows distribution in the anterior stroma centrally (right) with a tapering concentration to the unablated zone. There is an intense reaction for fibronectin **(B)**. Type III collagen **(C)** has begun to appear beneath the epithelium. Keratan sulfate **(D)** is absent from the subepithelial new stroma. Large numbers of fibroblasts are expressing fetal antigen **(E)**.

Type VII collagen **(A)** continues to form layers in the anterior stroma. Fibronectin **(B)** is beginning to disappear from the subepithelial region. Type III collagen **(C)** shows a layer of more intense subepithelial staining. New keratan sulfate **(D)** has been produced in the subepithelial zone. The number of fibroblasts expressing fetal antigen **(E)** is decreasing.

Type VII collagen **(A)** is concentrated only in the basement membrane zone with some discontinuities. Fibronectin **(B)** has virtually disappeared. Type III collagen **(C)** is still present in the anterior stroma. Keratan sulfate **(D)** shows a higher density of staining beneath the epithelium. The number of fibroblasts **(E)** is decreasing.

Type VII collagen **(A)** continues to show discontinuities. Fibronectin **(B)** is absent. Type III collagen **(C)** persists in the subepithelial zone. Subepithelial concentrations of keratan sulfate **(D)** persist. There are no fetal antigens seen in fibroblasts **(E)** in the anterior stroma.

healing response would not be mounted once the epithelium had resurfaced the defect. Unfortunately, this has proved to be incorrect; subepithelial fibroplasia produces corneal haze and alters the refractive result. If the cornea behaved like plastic, excimer laser reprofiling of the surface could be done with great accuracy. However, if hyperplastic epithelium or newly secreted extracellular matrix fills in part of the ablated zone, the refractive effect will be decreased and the outcome rendered less predictable.

Time course of corneal wound healing

The temporal response of the cornea to photorefractive keratectomy can be divided into three phases: acute (1 to 3 weeks), intermediate (3 weeks to 6 months), and long term (6 months or more).

During the acute phase the cornea mounts its initial response to epithelial removal and photoablation. Fibronectin, a glycoprotein that facilitates the adhesion among cells and molecules, is not normally present in the epithelial basement membrane area, but after excimer ablation it appears as the epithelium slides in, presumably serving as an attachment molecule to assist its migration. Once the epithelium is healed the fibronectin disappears. The epithelium migrates and divides to resurface the cornea, begins to produce attachment complexes, and undergoes a transient period of hyperplasia. The anterior stroma becomes transiently acellular and is repopulated by fibroblasts. This corresponds to a clinical appearance of general corneal clarity.

In the intermediate phase, the epithelium remodels itself to a normal thickness if the surface contours are gradual and regular. Type VII collagen is produced as part of the anchoring fibril complex and new basement membrane is secreted, both components showing spotty production and fragmentation as they are remodeled. Large numbers of fibroblasts populate the anterior stroma and secrete new extracellular matrix of type III collagen (which is not present in the normal cornea) and new keratan sulfate proteoglycan. This corresponds to a clinical phase of subepithelial haze and loss of initial refractive effect.

In the long-term phase the subepithelial stroma remodels itself, the fibroblasts reverting to a more normal complement of quiescent keratocytes, and the stromal type VII and type III collagens gradually disappear over 18 to 24 months. Clinically, this corresponds to a phase of decreasing corneal haze and increasing refractive stability. The duration of this phase is unknown.

Epithelial wound healing

The epithelium is removed mechanically or chemically in most cases before photoablation, and it must resurface the central cornea, a task it accomplishes in a manner similar to that of any epithelial abrasion. Cells at the leading edge flatten and migrate over the defect, and once the defect is closed, mitosis becomes more important and the epithelium undergoes a transient, overreactive hyperplastic thickening (Fig. 19-46). The basal cells are adaptive to their new stromal surface and conform to small surface irregularities, reducing irregular astigmatism, like asphalt smoothing over a gravel driveway (Fig. 19-47). This results in a smooth epithelial surface with a smooth refracting tear-air interface. These variations in epithelial thickness may have some effect on refractive stability after surgery. If the surface contours are grossly irregular, creating depressions that the epithelium senses must be filled in, persistent hyperplasia will result with facet formation (Fig. 19-47). The basement membrane zone remodels for at least 6 months and possibly longer, as manifested by areas of thickened and thinned basement membrane, areas of absent basement membrane, and a zone of type VII anchoring fibril collagen that can extend some 30 μm into the newly produced subepithelial stroma. After months of remodeling the basement membrane area returns to a normal configuration of focal hemidesmosomes and type VII collagen anchoring fibrils with a reasonably uniform basal lamina consisting of a lamina lucida and a lamina densa (Fig. 19-48).

In spite of these active changes the epithelium remains securely attached to the stroma throughout the healing process, so recurrent erosions and persistent epithelial defects occur rarely, unless the procedure is complicated by some untoward event. No drugs are available to modulate the healing of the epithelium.

Response of Bowman's layer

Once the acellular Bowman's layer is ablated, it does not regenerate. The edges may have a tapered appearance as a result of the graded ablation. Ablations confined to Bowman's layer are rare, but theoretically can induce a refractive change of up to 2 D. Whether ablations confined to Bowman's layer induce subepithelial fibroplasia is unknown.

Anterior stromal wound healing

The earliest response of the anterior stroma to an epithelial scrape injury or to photoablation is disappearance of the keratocytes in approximately the anterior 40 μm. The cause for this is unknown. After a

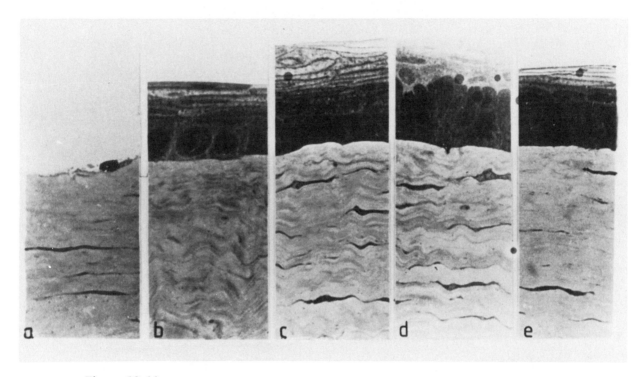

Figure 19-46
Light micrographs of epithelium and anterior stroma after photorefractive keratectomy in rabbits. **A,** Day 0. The acutely ablated surface showed cellular debris. The
anterior stroma demonstrated normal fibrocytes. **B,** Day 3. The surface was epithelialized with six to seven layers, the basal cells showing mitotic figures. The anterior
stroma (approximately 45 μm) was acellular. **C,** Day 7. The epithelium was thickened with 10 to 12 differentiated layers. The subepithelial stroma was being repopulated by fibrocytes of normal appearance. **D,** Day 21. The epithelium was of normal
thickness with a tall basal layer. The intermediate and superficial layers were well
differentiated. The subepithelial stroma has been repopulated by apparently normal
fibrocytes. **E,** Day 100. The anterior stroma appeared normal with no sign of subepithelial fibrosis. (From Hanna KD, Pouliquen Y, Waring GO, Savoldelli M, Cotter J,
Morton K, and Menasche M: Arch Ophthalmol 1989;107:895-901.)

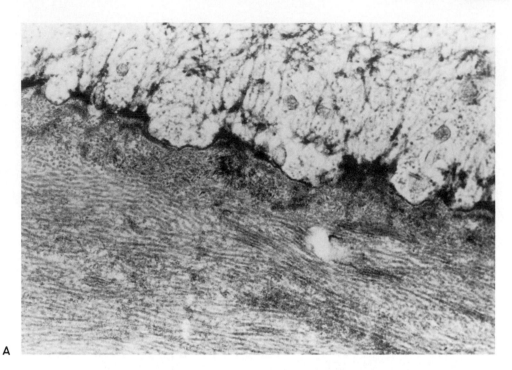

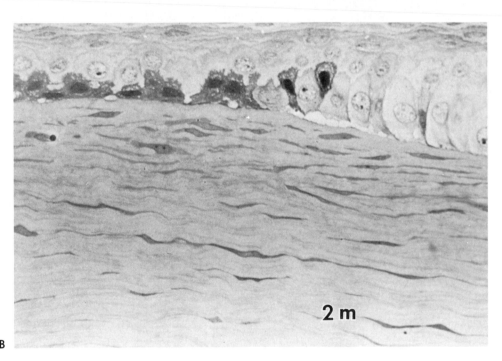

Figure 19-47
Epithelial healing 2 months after excimer laser keratomileusis in the rhesus monkey.
A, Ablated zone demonstrates focal hemidesmosome formation with only spotty se-
cretion of epithelial basement membrane. Bowman's layer is absent. The underlying
collagenous stroma has a generally lamellar configuration (×20,000). **B,** At 2
months the epithelium showed a generally smooth surface and a thickness of approximately five cells, although some zones of hyperplasia (right side of figure) were
apparent. Numerous dark basal cells were present, interspersed with lighter basal
cells. The vacuolated zone between the epithelium and stroma persisted. The underlying stroma was densely populated with active fibroblasts. Some newly secreted extracellular matrix was present in a generally lamellar array (hematoxylin-PAS,
×200). (From Waring GO: Trans Am Ophthalmol Soc 1989;87:854-983.)

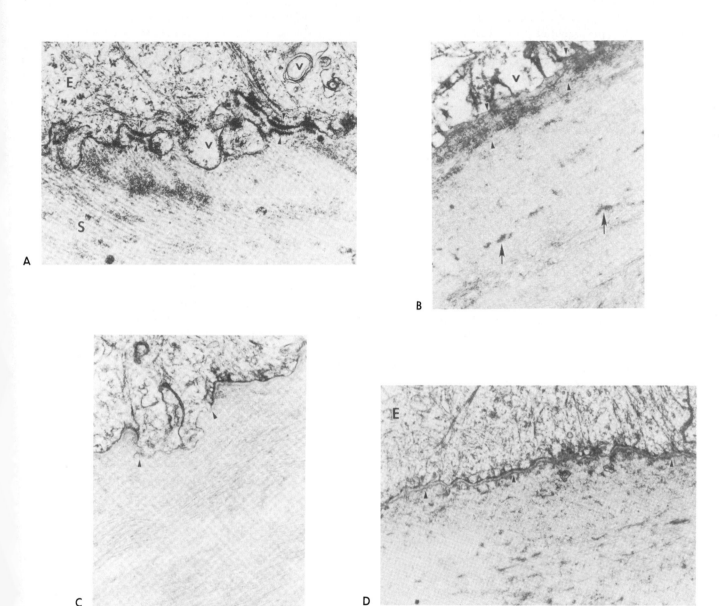

Figure 19-48

Healing of epithelial basement membrane zone after photorefractive keratectomy in monkeys as shown by transmission electron micrography. **A,** Seven days after ablation there is focal formation of the basement membrane with hemidesmosomes and laminodensa (between arrowheads). Intraepithelial *(E)* and subepithelial vacuoles *(V)* are present. *S,* Stroma (×55,400). **B,** Six months after ablation, cornea with a clinical density of 1.5$^+$ shows extensive thickening of basement membrane (between arrowheads), marked vacuolization of the epithelial-stromal junction *(V),* and focal accumulations of electron-dense deposits throughout the anterior stroma *(arrows)* (×28,000). **C,** At 6 months a cornea graded with a trace clinical density shows basal epithelial cells well approximated to the stroma and focal disruptions in the basement membrane *(arrowheads)*. The underlying stroma appears normal (×33,000). **D,** Nine months after ablation the basal epithelial cells *(E)* appear normal with normal basement membrane *(arrowheads)* consisting of a lamina lucida and a lamina densa, with an occasional focal disruption. Anterior stroma has electron-dense deposits not normally present (×33,000). (From Fantes FE, Hanna KD, and Waring GO: Arch Ophthalmol 1990;108:665-675.)

scrape injury the fibrocytes repopulate this area without secreting a clinically visible, new extracellular matrix. However, after excimer laser ablation the keratocytes are converted to fibroblasts that repopulate the subepithelial stroma within the first week (Fig. 19-49). By approximately 3 to 6 weeks after ablation the subepithelial zone is filled with fibroblasts exhibiting rough endoplasmic reticulum and staining positively for fetal antigen (Fig. 19-49). These cells are engaged in the production of a new extracellular matrix characteristic of typical corneal stromal wound healing. Type III collagen, not normally present in the corneal stroma, occupies a zone some 40 μm thick and increases the volume of tissue in the subepithelial area. There is also an increased amount of keratan sulfate proteoglycan. During this time clinical subepithelial haze appears as a result of the disrupted structure of the anterior stromal lamellae. This process reaches its maximum intensity between 6 weeks and 3 months after surgery. The new material is laid down between the epithelium and the ablated stromal surface, as evidenced by the appearance of type VII collagen anchoring fibrils throughout this 20 to 40 mm thick zone of new tissue. Tuft and colleagues[113] have demonstrated this with fluorescein staining (DTAF) in rabbits. The anchoring fibrils are secreted by the epithelium and could be present only at sites that were once adjacent to the basal epithelial cells themselves. The density and distribution of new tissue determine the clinical appearance of the subepithelial haze and the final refractive change. In general, the haze occupies the entire ablated zone and is present in all eyes after ablation.

From approximately 3 months to 1 year after surgery, one of two processes occurs. Most commonly, the subepithelial zone remodels, with disappearance of the fibroblasts and the type III and type VII collagen and the reemergence of a reasonably normal lamellar stromal structure occupied by scattered keratocytes. This corresponds clinically to a decrease in subepithelial haze, which usually occurs in a spotty, irregular pattern. Sometimes, however, the new subepithelial extracellular matrix consolidates into scar tissue, creating a dense layer of apparent type I irregularly arranged fibrous tissue histologically and a circular corneal scar clinically (Fig. 19-50).

Tuft and co-workers[114] demonstrated in rabbits a dramatic decrease in extracellular matrix production after photorefractive keratectomy followed by the use of topical corticosteroids.

Endothelium and Descemet's membrane

Theoretically the ultraviolet radiation from an excimer laser is absorbed within a few microns of the surface, and damage should not occur 500 μm away in the endothelium. However, secondary phenomena such as shock waves, fluorescence, secondary irradiation, and posterior migration of toxic by-products all might affect the endothelium. Fortunately, laboratory and clinical experience have not shown any clinically meaningful changes in the endothelium, but experimental studies have shown that the endothelium can be affected.

Linear laser keratectomy extending 90% deep into the cornea can produce endothelial cell loss and ridges between the endothelial cells.[58,77,93] Even following anterior stromal large area ablation, changes can occur in the endothelium. Zabel and colleagues[121] measured the pressure produced by shock or acoustic waves near the posterior surface of the bovine cornea during 193-nm excimer laser ablation. The pressure was approximately 100 atmospheres during ablation of the superficial stroma, but endothelial disruption did not appear until 85% to 90% of the corneal thickness had been removed. Marshall and colleagues[58] used a radiant exposure of 1,000 mJ/cm^2, which might be expected to create a larger acoustic effect from the photoablation. Dehm and colleagues[10] demonstrated similar disruption along a linear line underlying deep linear laser ablations and diamond knife incisions. Koch and colleagues[33] used a radiant exposure of 750 mJ/cm^2 in rabbits and observed no endothelial cell damage at incisions 80% or less of corneal thickness, minimal disruption at 90% deep incisions, and focal disruption at the area of perforation in 100% deep excisions. The endothelium healed over the perforation site with the formation of rosettes, multinucleated giant cells, and the production of a fibrillar posterior collagenous layer. The endothelial wound was healed by 6 months after surgery.

In our study of rabbits we did not identify disruption of the endothelial monolayer histologically, but we did observe an amorphous fibrillogranular material that appeared in Descemet's membrane in the central zone beneath the ablation (Fig. 19-51). This 1 μm thick layer of material migrated forward in Descemet's membrane during the healing period over the next 3 months without associated thickening of Descemet's membrane. We think this might have occurred from the shock wave impacting the endothelium and stimulating it transiently to produce extracellular matrix, "endothelial sweat," that then migrated anteriorly in Descemet's membrane along the gradient of the fluid leak from the aqueous. The nature of this material is unknown, but immunohistochemical staining of Descemet's membrane and the posterior stroma after ablation in rabbits showed increased amounts of type IV collagen (particularly in the posterior stroma), lami-

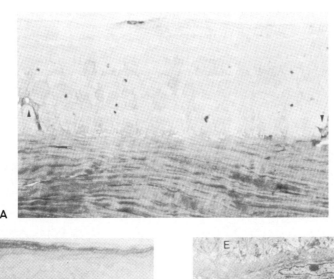

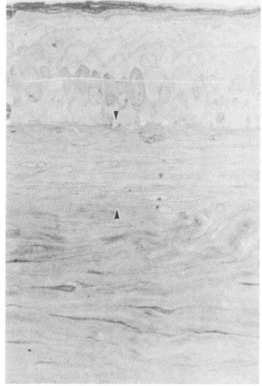

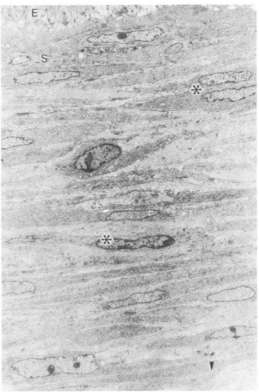

Figure 19-49
Healing of corneal epithelium after keratectomy in monkeys. **A,** Light micrograph of cornea 7 days after ablation demonstrates thickened epithelium with approximately 10 layers, demonstrating loss of orderly maturation. Epithelium is approximately 60 μm thick. Dark cells, presumably active, occupy approximately 10% of the basal area *(arrowheads)*. The epithelial-stroma junction shows small areas of vacuolization. Fibrocytes are scattered throughout the stroma (toluidine blue, ×40). **B,** Cornea 3 weeks after ablation. Light micrograph shows epithelium with a generally normal pattern of maturation but continued thickening (approximately 50 μm). There is a mild vacuolization of the epithelial-stromal junction. The anterior 50 to 60 μm of the stroma *(between arrowheads)* shows a striking increase in active fibrocytes (toluidine blue, original magnification ×40). **C,** Transmission electron micrograph shows mild vacuolization beneath the epithelium *(E)* and the stroma *(S)*. The anterior stroma is almost completely occupied by active fibroblasts *(asterisks)* with poorly organized, presumedly newly secreted, extracellular matrix between them. There is a fairly sharp zone of demarcation *(arrowhead)* between this streaming layer of fibrocytes and more normal lamellar collagen structure (original magnification ×3500). (From Fantes FE, Hanna KD, Waring GO, Pouliquen Y, Thompson KP, and Savoldelli M: Arch Ophthalmol 1990;108:665-675.)

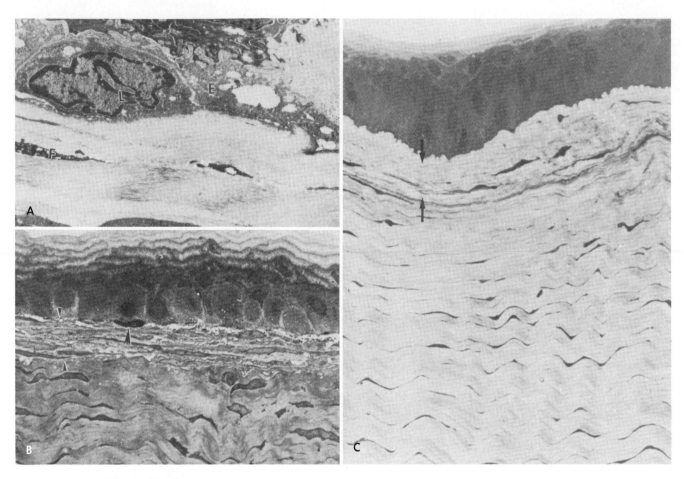

Figure 19-50
Histopathologic findings of anterior stromal scarring after excimer laser ablation in rabbits. **A,** Four days after ablation, lymphocyte *(L)* is interdigitated between healing vacuolated epithelium *(E)* and residual stroma that contains activated fibrocytes *(F)* (×13,400). **B,** At 21 days the epithelium is slightly hyperplastic with delayed maturation. Lymphocyte *(large arrowhead)* lies between epithelium and underlying connective tissue. Layer of hypercellular, loosely organized scar tissue *(between small arrowheads)* lies beneath epithelium. Remaining stroma shows active keratocytes with generally compact lamellar architecture (toluidine blue, ×200). **C,** At 100 days there is normal stratified epithelium with tall basal cells and layer of compact subepithelial scar tissue (between arrows) approximately 20 μm thick with transition zone leading to corneal stroma with generally normal architecture (toluidine blue, ×200). (From Hanna DK, Pouliquen Y, Waring GO, et al: Arch Ophthalmol 1989;107:895-901.)

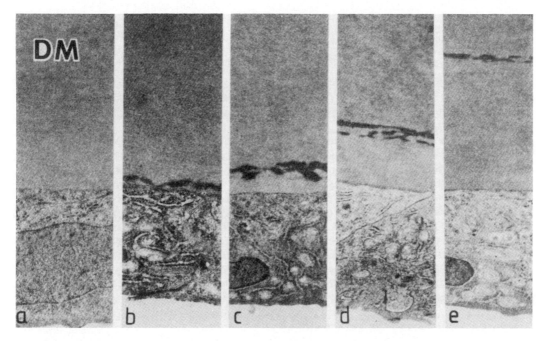

Figure 19-51
Transmission electron micrographs of Descemet's membrane *(DM)* and endothelium from 6 hours to 100 days after photorefractive keratectomy in rabbits. Discontinuous layer of fibrillogranular material had moved anteriorly in DM. **A,** Control. **B,** 7 days. **C,** 14 days. **D,** At 21 days the endothelial structure was generally normal with slight dilation of mitochondria. Discontinuous layer of fibrillogranular material migrated farther anteriorly in DM. **E,** At 100 days the endothelial structure was normal. Discontinuous layer of amorphous fibrillogranular material migrated farther forward in DM (×12,500). (From Hanna KD, Pouliquen Y, Waring GO, et al: Arch Ophthalmol 1989;107:895-901.)

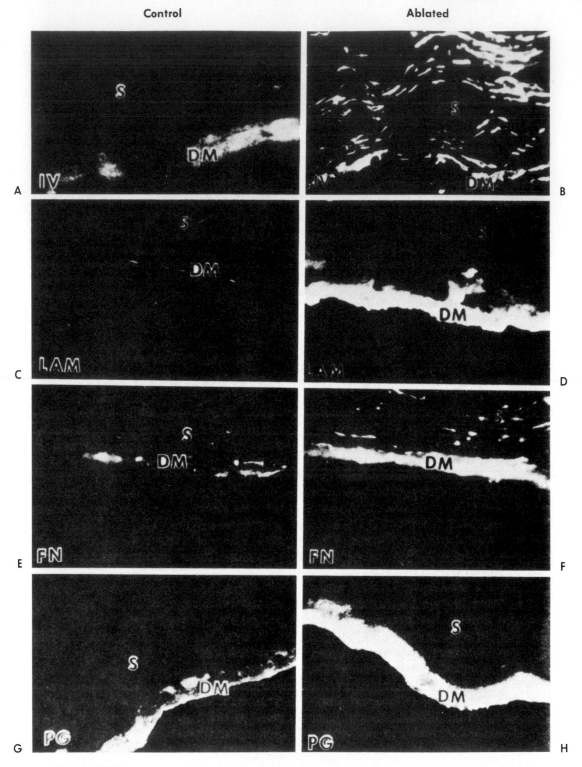

Figure 19-52

Immunohistochemical staining of endothelium, Descemet's membrane *(DM),* and posterior stroma *(S)* for extracellular matrix components at 6 days after photorefractive keratectomy in rabbits. *Left,* column shows nonablated control cornea. *Right,* column shows area beneath zone of ablation. **A** and **B,** Type IV collagen *(IV).* **C** and **D,** Laminin *(LAM).* **E** and **F,** Fibronectin *(FN).* **G** and **H,** Proteoglycans *(PG).* All four types of molecules show minimal to mild staining in controls and marked staining results in areas of ablation. Increased fibronectin is also deposited in the stroma, apparently near keratocytes. Increased synthesis of these molecules probably results from transient damage to the posterior stroma and endothelium during ablation. (From Hanna KD, Pouliquen Y, Waring GO, et al: Arch Ophthalmol 1989;107:895-901.)

nin, fibronectin, and proteoglycans in Descemet's membrane (Fig. 19-52), all suggesting activation of the endothelium and posterior keratocytes from the effect of the ablation. Indeed, transmission electron microscopy showed transient activation of posterior stromal keratocytes in rabbits in the few weeks after ablation.[18,25] We have not observed similar phenomena in monkey corneas.[12]

REPEATED PHOTOREFRACTIVE KERATECTOMY

If an initial photorefractive keratectomy was unsuccessful, because of either persistent subepithelial scarring or inaccurate refractive correction, it would be theoretically possible to repeat the surgery either to remove the scar or to refine the refractive change. Little is published on this, but we have observed that repeated ablations in monkeys with the goal of removing a previous subepithelial opacity caused only further scarring.[27] However, it is possible that refinements in technology may allow successful repeated ablations in the future. Poole and colleagues[75] also found scarring after repeated ablation in rabbits, but it did not appear worse than that from the primary ablation either clinically or histopathologically.

LASER-ADJUSTABLE SYNTHETIC EPIKERATOPLASTY (LASE)

Lack of adjustability is a major drawback for all types of refractive corneal surgery. Thompson and colleagues[108] have proposed a novel solution to the problem of adjustability. A synthetic epikeratoplasty lenticule could be attached to the corneal surface either by inserting it into a standard circular keratotomy or by securing it with a biologic adhesive. The lenticule would be designed to correct the existent refractive error in the eye. Should the correction turn out to be inaccurate or should changes in refraction occur, it would be possible to remove the epithelium and perform photorefractive keratectomy on the acellular lenticule, which should have a more predictable response to the ablation because of the absence of a cellular response. Multiple repeated ablations could be achieved until the lenticule becomes too thin. Even then, it would be possible to remove the lenticule and apply another, making the LASE concept reversible as well as adjustable. There are many unsolved problems with this experimental approach, but the feasibility of the concept has been identified by Thompson and colleagues (unpublished data) (Fig. 19-53).

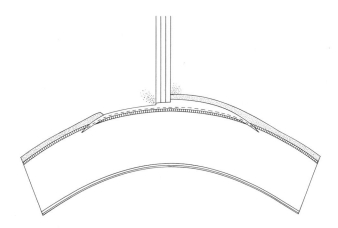

Figure 19-53
Laser-adjustable synthetic epikeratoplasty (LASE) consists of the placement of a synthetic epikeratoplasty lenticule with appropriate corrective power on the cornea.[108] If adjustment of the refractive power is necessary, an excimer laser keratomileusis can be performed, repeatedly if necessary, without damaging the patient's central cornea and without concerns about stromal wound healing. There are, however, the challenges of achieving successful attachment of the lenticule and persistent epithelial wound healing over a synthetic surface. (From Waring GO: Trans Am Ophthalmol Soc 1989;87:854-983.)

INTRASTROMAL LASER SURGERY

A number of strategies are being investigated to use lasers to remove tissue from within the stroma or to make intrastromal incisions to flatten the central cornea. The advantage of this approach is that the epithelium and Bowman's layer are not removed. This leaves the anterior surface of the cornea smoother, although it does not ensure that the surface contours will be uniformly acceptable. It also eliminates the contact between the keratocytes and the epithelium and leukocytes; theoretically, this should decrease the fibroblastic response of the keratocytes and decrease stromal scarring.

One approach is to use a dye laser-pumped neodymium-YLF (yttrium-lithium-fluoride) solid-state laser to generate picosecond pulses delivered at megahertz rates. Under these circumstances, the laser behaves like a continuous wave laser delivering large amounts of energy in a small spot size. The laser is focused approximately 50 μm below the corneal surface where it creates small cavities and gas bubbles that disappear in 30 to 60 minutes. Presumably the volume of tissue that is removed can be controlled so that the anterior cornea will collapse in the space created by the ablated tissue and will therefore flatten to decrease myopia. This is the approach taken in the instrument being designed by Intelligent Laser Systems. A similar approach involves the use of a frequency-doubled Nd:YAG laser emitting at 532 nm, with nanosecond pulses emitted at a repetition rate of 50/sec. This system for intrastromal ablation has been devised by the Phoenix Corporation.

An alternative to intrastromal area ablation is the use of a neodymium YAG laser transmitted through a fiber optic hand-held tip that is placed directly on the surface of the cornea. This creates a 1-μm spot with an energy of 10 mJ lasting 100 ns. By focusing the laser in the posterior stroma, the beam can be used as an intrastromal scalpel. As the tip is pulled across the corneal surface along radial lines, the laser makes an intrastromal radial keratotomy, weakening the stromal structure from within.

Numerous questions remain to be answered with intrastromal ablation. Where do the ablation products go? Are they toxic to the stroma? Do shock waves or secondary radiation damage the endothelium? At what layer of the cornea should the ablations be placed for maximum effect? How much of the stroma needs to be ablated to create the response? And of course, can the response be accurately and precisely achieved with good predictability and stability?

SCOPE OF LASER CORNEAL SURGERY

The scope of laser corneal surgery is illustrated in the montage of Fig. 19-54, which emphasizes the technical demands of the laser, the delivery system, and the coupling system (Fig. 19-55), as well as the variety of types of surgery that can be done with the laser. Whether the excimer laser itself will remain the primary surgical tool or whether other, less cumbersome, less expensive, and more user-friendly lasers will be developed requires future research. Measurement of the topography and optics of the cornea after photorefractive keratectomy is an essential feature of the study of this new technology, which is certainly opening windows to the future.

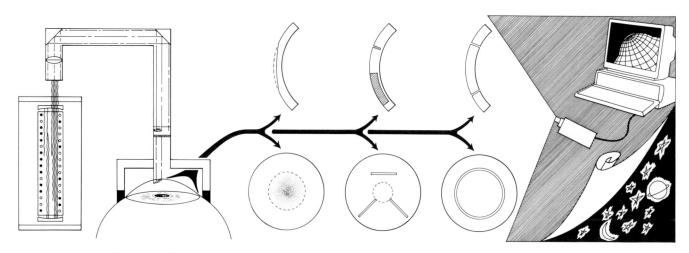

Figure 19-54
The scope of laser corneal surgery is illustrated in a composite montage, read from left to right. An appropriate laser passes through an effective delivery system that is coupled to the eye. Interaction of the laser with the corneal tissue sets the stage for wound healing. Patterns of photorefractive keratectomy include photorefractive keratectomy (surface area ablation) for all ametropias, transverse linear keratectomy for astigmatism, radial keratectomy for myopia, and circular trephination for corneal transplantation. Measurement of the topography and thickness of the cornea allows computation of the effect of refractive surgery, and in conjunction with biomechanical data, computer simulation of surgery. The future is bright, but like the exploration of space, fraught with technical challenges and the unknown. (From Waring GO: Trans Am Ophthalmol Soc 1989;87:854-983.)

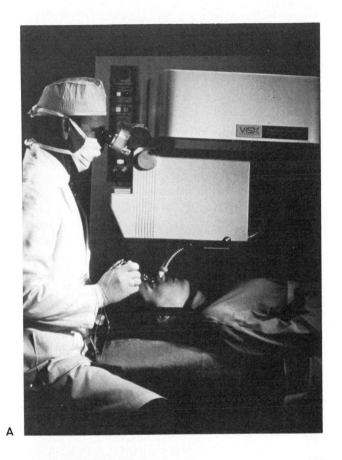

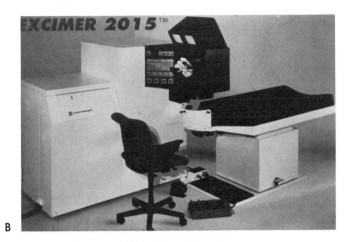

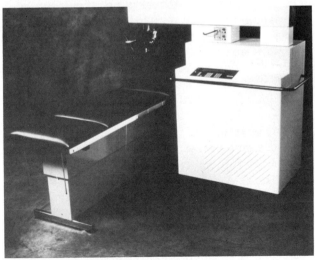

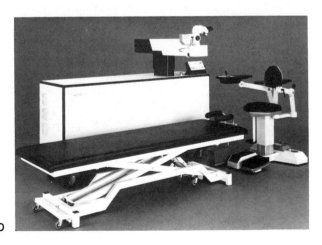

Figure 19-55
Clinical excimer laser consoles available in early 1990. **A,** VISX Twenty/Twenty Excimer Laser System. **B,** Taunton Excimer 2015 Laser. **C,** Summit Eximed UV200 Laser. **D,** Meditec Excimer Laser.

UNFINISHED BUSINESS

The whole field of laser technology remains, in a sense, unfinished business. Improvement in the technologic aspects of excimer lasers and delivery systems is a major challenge. New types of lasers emerge frequently, and applying this technology to corneal surgery is always fruitful research. For example, instead of using the large, expensive, relatively unfriendly excimer laser, more compact, less expensive, easier to control lasers might be considered, such as a fifth harmonic Nd:YAG. Meanwhile, improvement in the quality of excimer lasers and delivery systems used for corneal surgery is a major technical challenge; improved laser beam quality, optical elements, beam homogenizers, beam shapers, mechanical or optical coupling systems, and beam measurement systems are all necessary. But even with a perfectly homogeneous laser beam with the exact desired shape and energy, interactions with the tissue must be better defined. Does a homogeneous beam mean a smooth ablation? Does a smooth ablation give a better optical result? How can ablation rates for individual corneas be accurately calculated? Can aspheric and radially asymmetric corrections be created by advanced delivery systems?

A refinement of the laser parameters to improve the quality of ablation includes definition of optimal radiant exposure (particularly higher fluences), accurate definition of ablation rate per pulse, careful definition of allowable depth of ablation and whether deeper ablations create more subepithelial scarring, definition of the optimal diameter of the ablation zone and whether smaller zones create greater visual distortion and glare, a definition of the maximum achievable correction with a combination of ablation depth and diameter, characterization of the optimal rate of ablation, and definition of optimal surface contours within and at the edge of the ablation zone.

There must be control of subepithelial fibrosis by improving the quality of the laser beam that impacts the cornea and by pharmacologic manipulation with corticosteroids and other drugs. Careful definition of the effect of corneal wound healing on the refractive outcome is still needed, especially to define whether laser keratectomy can achieve results superior to that of radial keratotomy.

Creating hyperopic and astigmatic corrections with photorefractive keratectomy is apparently more difficult than achieving myopic corrections; the variables that affect hyperopic correction must be better defined.

Exploration of other laser technologies, such as the holmium-YAG thermokeratoplasty to correct hyperopia, requires further research.

The U.S. Food and Drug Administration (FDA) clinical trials of excimer laser photorefractive keratectomy should be carried out according to the principles of prospective formal clinical trials. The FDA has encouraged manufacturers to use common standards so that results can be readily compared.[70] The development of excimer laser corneal surgery requires active collaboration among business, industrial, and clinical interests. In this context, all agree that patient benefit must take precedence over profit and prestige.

Further research on the use of lasers to make linear cuts in the cornea is needed to test the premise that the excimer laser can create cuts of a known depth and configuration that are superior to those made manually with a diamond knife. The difference in effect between a diamond knife radial keratotomy and an excimer laser radial keratectomy should be better defined.

Clinicians using excimer lasers outside the United States where regulatory controls are less stringent are encouraged to report results on consecutive series of eyes with a high percentage of follow-up and prospectively designed clinical measurements.

REFERENCES

1. Absten GT and Joffe SN: Lasers in medicine, New York, 1985, Chapman Co.
2. Aron-Rosa DS, Boerner CF, Bath P, et al: Corneal wound healing after laser keratotomy in a human eye, Am J Ophthalmol 1987;103:444-464.
3. Aron-Rosa DS, Boulnoy JL, Carre F, et al: Excimer laser surgery of the cornea: qualitative and quantitative aspects of photoablation according to the energy density, J Cataract Refract Surg 1986;12:27-33.
4. Bansal S, Salz JJ, Tenner A, Rao N, and McDonnell PJ: Clinicopathologic study of healing excimer laser radial excisions, Refract Corneal Surg 1990;6:188-192.
5. Beaver GH and Holiday ER: Ultraviolet absorption spectrum of protein and aminoacids, Adv Prot Chem 1952;7:319-386.
6. Beckman H, Rota A, and Barraco R: Limbectomies, keratectomies, and keratotomies performed with a rapid-pulsed carbon dioxide laser, Am J Ophthalmol 1971;71:1277-1283.
7. Bende T, Kriegerowski M, and Seiler T: Photoablation in different ocular tissues performed with an Erbium:YAG laser, Laser Light Ophthalmol 1989;2:263-269.
8. Cotlier AM, Shubert HD, Mandel E, et al: Excimer laser keratotomy, Ophthalmology 1985;92:206-208.
9. Cotton KL and Tripoli NK: Tissue fit and corneal shape after transplantation, Invest Ophthalmol Vis Sci 1987;28(suppl):276.
10. Dehm EJ, Puliafito CA, Adler CM, and Steinert RF: Corneal endothelial injury in rabbits following excimer laser ablation at 193 nm and 248 nm, Arch Ophthalmol 1986;104:1364-1368.
11. Dyer PE and Srinivasan R: Nanosecond photoacoustic studies on ultraviolet laser ablation of organic polymers, Appl Phys Lett 1986;48:445-447.
12. Fantes FE, Hanna KD, Waring GO, Pouliquen Y, Thompson KP, and Savoldelli M: Wound healing after excimer laser keratomileusis (photorefractive keratectomy) in monkeys, Arch Ophthalmol 1990;108:665-675.
13. Fantes FE and Waring GO: Effect of excimer laser radiant exposure on uniformity of ablated surface, Laser Surg Med 1989;9:533-542.
14. Fine BS, Feigen L, and McKeen D: Corneal injury threshold to carbon dioxide laser radiation, Am J Ophthalmol 1986;1:1-15.
15. Fine BS, Fine S, Peacock GR, et al: Preliminary observations on ocular effects of high power, continuous CO_2 laser irradiation, Am J Ophthalmol 1967;2:209-222.
16. Fouraker BD, Holme RJ, and Schanzlin DJ: A comparison of en face and tangential wide-area excimer surface ablation in the rabbit, Invest Ophthalmol Vis Sci 1990;31(suppl):476.
17. Garrison BJ: Microscopic model for the ablative photodecomposition of polymers by far-ultraviolet radiation (193 nm), Appl Phys Lett 1984;9:44.
18. Gaster RN, Binder PS, Coalwell K, et al: Corneal surface ablation by 193-nm excimer laser and wound healing in rabbits, Invest Ophthalmol Vis Sci 1989;30:90-98.
19. Gibson IK: Hemidesmosome formation in vitro, J Cell Biol 1983;97:849.
20. Goodman GL, Trokel SL, Stark WJ, Munnerlyn CR, and Green WR: Corneal healing following laser refractive keratectomy, Arch Ophthalmol 1989;107:1799-1803.
21. Green H, Bold J, Parrish JA, et al: Cytotoxicity and mutagenicity of low intensity, 248- and 193-nm excimer laser radiation in the mammalian cell, Cancer Res 1987;47:410-423.
22. Green HA, Margolis R, Bold J, et al: Unscheduled DNA synthesis in human skin after in vitro ultraviolet excimer laser ablation, J Invest Dermatol 1987;89:201-204.
23. Hanna K, Chastang JC, Pouliquen Y, et al: A rotating slit delivery system for excimer laser refractive keratoplasty, Am J Ophthalmol 1987;103:474.
24. Hanna K, Chastang JC, Pouliquen Y, et al: Excimer laser keratectomy for myopia with a rotating slit delivery system, Arch Ophthalmol 1988;106:245-250.
25. Hanna KD, Pouliquen Y, Savoldelli M, Cotter J, Waring GO: Corneal stromal wound healing in rabbits after 193-nm excimer laser surface ablation, Arch Ophthalmol 1989;107:895-901.
26. Hanna KD, Chastang JC, Asfar L, et al: Scanning slit delivery system, J Cataract Refract Surg 1989;15:390-396.
27. Hanna KD, Pouliquen YM, Savoldelli M, et al: Cornal wound healing in monkeys 18 months after excimer laser keratomileusis (photorefractive keratectomy), Refract Corneal Surg 1990;6:340-345.
28. Hecht J: Excimer laser update, Lasers Applications 1983;12:43-48.
29. Reference deleted in galleys.
30. Keates RH, Pedrotti L, Weichel H, et al: Carbon dioxide laser beam control for corneal surgery, Ophthalmic Surg 1981;12:117-122.
31. Kerr-Muir MG, Trokel SL, and Marshall J: Ultrastructural comparison of conventional surgical and argon fluoride excimer laser keratectomy, Am J Ophthalmol 1987;103:448-453.
32. Keyes T and Clarke RH: Theory of photoablation and its implication for laser phototherapy, J Chem Phys 1985;89:4194-4196.
33. Koch JW, Lang GK, and Naumann GOH: Endothelial reaction to perforating and non-perforating excimer laser excisions in rabbits, Refract Corneal Surg (in press).
34. Krauss JM, Puliafito CA, and Steinert R: Laser interactions with the cornea, Surv Ophthalmol 1986;31:37-53.
35. Kriegerowski M, Bende T, and Seiler T: Do eye drops influence ablation rate during laser keratomileusis? Invest Ophthalmol Vis Sci 1990;31(suppl):478.
36. Krueger RR and Trokel SL: Quantitation of corneal ablation by ultraviolet laser light, Arch Ophthalmol 1985;103:1741-1742.
37. Krueger RR, Trokel SS, and Shubert H: Interaction of UV light with the cornea, Invest Ophthalmol Vis Sci 1985;26:1455-1464.
38. Lang GK, Koch JW, Naumann GOH, and Yanoff M: Lamellar excimer laser keratoplasty, Suppl Ophthalmology 1989;96:122-126.
39. Lang GK, Schroder E, Koch JW, Yanoff M, and Naumann GOH: Excimer laser keratoplasty. Part 1: basic concepts, Ophthalmic Surg 1989;20:262-265.
40. Lang GK, Schroder E, Koch JW, Yanoff M, and Naumann GOH: Excimer laser keratoplasty. Part 2: elliptical keratoplasty, Ophthalmic Surg 1989;20:342-346.
41. Lazare S and Srinivasan R: Surface properties of polyethylene terephthalate films modified by far-ultraviolet radiation at 193 nm (laser) and 185 nm (low intensity), J Phys Chem 1986;90:2124-2132.
42. Lee I, Bourow JR, Gould BS, et al: Studies on the ultraviolet absorption spectra of collagen, Arch Biochem 1949;22:406-411.
43. L'Esperance FA, Taylor DM, and Warner JW: Human excimer laser keratectomy: short-term histopathology, J Refract Surg 1988;4:118-124.

44. L'Esperance FA, Warner JW, Telfair WB, et al: Excimer laser instrumentation and technique for human corneal surgery, Arch Ophthalmol 1989;107: 131-141.

45. Lieurance RC, Patel AC, Wan WL, et al: Excimer laser cut lenticules for epikeratophakia, Am J Ophthalmol 1987;103:475-476.

46. Loertscher H, Mandelbaum S, Parel JM, et al: Noncontact trephination of the cornea using a pulsed hydrogen fluoride laser, Am J Ophthalmol 1987;104:471-475.

47. Loertscher H, Mandelbaum S, Parrish RK, et al: Preliminary report on corneal incisions created by a hydrogen fluoride laser, Am J Ophthalmol 1986;102:217-221.

48. Loertscher H, Parel JM, Parrish RK, et al: Effect of selected beam parameters on corneal incisions produced with a hydrogen fluoride laser, Am J Ophthalmol (in press).

49. Loertscher H, Parel JM, Parrish RK, et al: Laser trephination of the cornea, Am J Ophthalmol (in press).

50. MacDonald IM, Zabel RW, Chen V, Choi KY, Skeinik D, and Lindstrom RL: Corneal astigmatism: generation and correction using a fiberoptic-delivered holmium laser, Invest Ophthalmol Vis Sci 1990;31(suppl):476.

51. Macruz R, Ribeiro M, Mauro J, et al: Laser surgery in enclosed spaces, Lasers Surg Med 1985;5:199-218.

52. Magnante DD, Kornmehl EW, Steinert RF, Gregory WA, and Puliafito CA: Immunohistochemical analysis of rabbit corneal wound healing following excimer laser linear keratectomy, Invest Ophthalmol Vis Sci 1989;30 (suppl):217.

53. Mainster MA: Finding your way in the photo forest: laser effects for clinicians, Ophthalmology 1984;91:886-888.

54. Mainster MA: Ophthalmic applications of infrared laser-thermal considerations, Invest Ophthalmol Vis Sci 1979;18:414-420.

55. Malley DS, Steinert RD, Puliafito CA, and Dobi ET: Immunofluorescent study of corneal wound healing after excimer laser anterior keratectomy in the monkey eye, Arch Ophthalmol 1990;108:1316-1322.

56. March WF: Ophthalmic lasers, Thorofare, NJ, 1984, Slack, Inc.

57. Marshall J, Trokel SL, Rothery S, and Krueger RR: Long-term healing of the central cornea after photorefractive keratectomy using an excimer laser, Ophthalmology 1988;95:1411-1421.

58. Marshall J, Trokel S, Rothery S, et al: An ultrastructural study of corneal incisions induced by an excimer laser at 193 nm, Ophthalmology 1985;92: 749-758.

59. Marshall J, Trokel S, Rothery S, et al: A comparative study of corneal incisions induced by diamond and steel knives and two ultraviolet radiations from an excimer laser, Br J Ophthalmol 1986;70:482-501.

60. Marshall J, Trokel S, Rothery S, et al: Photoablative reprofiling of the cornea using an excimer laser: photorefractive keratotomy, Lasers Ophthalmol 1986;1:21-48.

61. Matchette LS, Waynant RW, Royston D, et al: Induction of lambda prophage near the site of focused UV laser radiation, Photochem Photobiol 1989;49: 161-167.

62. McDonald M: The future of R and D jeopardized, J Refract Surg 1987;3: 207.

63. McDonald MB, Beuerman R, Falzoni W, et al: Refractive surgery with excimer laser, Am J Ophthalmol 1987; 103:469.

64. McDonald MB, Frantz JM, Klyce SD, et al: Central photorefractive keratectomy for myopia: the blind eye study, Arch Ophthalmol 1990;108:799-808.

65. McDonald MB, Frantz JM, Klyce SD, et al: One-year refractive results of central photorefractive keratectomy for myopia in the nonhuman primate cornea, Arch Ophthalmol 1990;108: 40-47.

66. Munnerlyn R, Kooms SJ, and Marshall J: Photorefractive keratectomy: a technique for laser refractive surgery, J Cataract Refract Surg 1988;14:46-52.

67. News commentary: Patent fight erupts over excimer laser corneal surgery, Refract Corneal Surg 1989;5:3.

68. Nuss RC, Puliafito CA, and Dehm E: Unscheduled DNA synthesis following excimer laser ablation of the cornea in vivo, Invest Ophthalmol Vis Sci 1987;28:287-294.

69. O'Brien WJ: Measurement of DNA content, Invest Ophthalmol Vis Sci 1979;18:518-543.

70. Office of Device Evaluation, Division of Ophthalmic Devices, Food and Drug Administration: Draft clinical guidance for the preparation and contents of an investigational device exemption (IDE) application for excimer laser devices used in ophthalmic surgery for myopic photorefractive keratectomy (PRK), Refract Corneal Surg 1990;6:265-269.

71. O'Shea DC, Callen WR, and Rhodes WT: Introduction to lasers and their applications, Reading, Mass, 1977, Addison-Wesley Publishing Co, Inc.

72. Parker P, Zabel RW, Maguire LJ, Chen V, Choi KY, and Lindstrom RL: Computed topographic analysis following myopic excimer laser photorefractive keratectomy, Invest Ophthalmol Vis Sci 1990;31(suppl):480.

73. Peyman GA, Kuszak JR, Weckstrom K, et al: Effects of Xe excimer laser on the eyelid in anterior segment structures, Arch Ophthalmol 1986;104: 118-122.

74. Pirie A: Ascorbic acid content of cornea, Bio Chem J 1946;40:96-100.

75. Poole TG, Goodman GL, Munnerlyn C, Gottsch JD, and Stark WJ: Excimer laser photorefractive keratectomy: the effect of reablation, Invest Ophthalmol Vis Sci 1990;31(suppl):477.

76. Puliafito CA, Wong K, and Steinert RF: Quantitative and ultrastructural studies of excimer laser ablation of the cornea at 193 and 248 nanometers, Lasers Surg Med 1987;7:155-159.

77. Puliafito CA, Steiner RF, Deutsch TF, et al: Excimer laser ablation of the cornea and lens, Ophthalmology 1985; 92:741-748.

78. Reed RD, Taboada J, and Midsell JW: Response of the corneal epithelium to krypton fluoride excimer laser, Health Phys 1981;40:677-683.

79. Rhodes CK: Excimer lasers, New York, 1984, Springer Verlag.

80. Sanders DR, editor: Radial keratotomy surgical techniques, Thorofare, NJ, 1986, Slack, Inc, pp 99-130.

81. Scientific American Readings: Lasers and light, San Francisco, 1969, WH Freeman.

82. Searles SK and Hart GA: Stimulated emission at 281 nm XC, Br Appl Phys Lett 1975;27:243-245.

83. Seiler T: Laser Chirurgie der Kornea: Habilitations Schrift, Berlin, 1987, Freie Universitat Berlin, pp 134-137.

84. Seiler T, Bende T, Wollensak J, and Trokel S: Excimer laser keratectomy for correction of astigmatism, Am J Ophthalmol 1988;105:117-124.

85. Seiler T, Bende T, Winckler K, et al: Side effects in excimer corneal surgery—DNA damages as a result of 193-nm excimer laser radiation, Graefes Arch Clin Exp Ophthalmol 1988;266:273-276.

86. Seiler T, Berlin M, Bende T, et al: Transverse keratectomy: laboratory and clinical experience, Ophthalmology (in press).

87. Seiler T, Kahle G, and Kriegerowski M: Excimer laser (193 nm) myopic keratomileusis in sighted and blind human eyes, Refract Corneal Surg 1990;6:165-173.

88. Seiler T, Kriegerowski M, Schnoy N, Bende T: Ablation rate of human corneal epithelium and Bowman's layer with the excimer laser (193 nm), Refract Corneal Surg 1990;6:99-102.

89. Seiler T, Marshall J, Rothery S, et al: The potential of an infrared hydrogen fluoride laser or corneal surgery, Lasers Ophthalmol 1986;1:49-60.

90. Seiler T, Matallana M, and Bende T: Laser thermokeratoplasty by means of a pulsed holmium:YAG laser for hyperopic correction, Refract Corneal Surg 1990;6:335-339.

91. Seiler T and Wollensak J: In vivo experiments with excimer lasers—technical parameters and healing processes, Ophthalmologica 1986;192:65-70.

92. Serdarevic O, Hanna K, Gribomont A, et al: Excimer laser trephination in penetrating keratoplasty: morphologic features in wound healing, Ophthalmology 1988;95:493-505.

93. Shimada H, Barraquer E, Bosio P, Lowery JA, and Parel J-M: Vital staining analysis of endothelial cell damage and excision depth following laser cuts, Invest Ophthalmol Vis Sci 1990;31(suppl):479.

94. Srinivasan R: Ablation of polymers and biological tissue by ultraviolet lasers, Science 1986;234:559-565.

95. Srinivasan R, Dyer PE, and Braren B: Far-ultraviolet laser ablation of the cornea: photoacoustic studies, Lasers Surg Med 1987;6:514-519.

96. Srinivasan R, Braren B, Dreyfus RW, et al: Mechanism of ultraviolet laser ablation of polymethylmethacrylate at 193 and 248 nm: laser-induced fluorescence analysis, chemical analysis, and doping studies, J Opt Soc Am 1986;3:785-791.

97. Srinivasan R, Braren B, Seeger DE, et al: Photochemical cleavage of a polymeric solid: details of the ultraviolet laser ablation of pol (methymethacrylate) at 193 nm and 248 nm, Macromolecules 1986;19:916-920.

98. Stern D, Lin W, Puliafito CA, et al: Femtosecond optical ranging of corneal incision depth, Invest Ophthalmol Vis Sci 1989;30:99-104.

99. SundarRaj N, Geiss MJ, Fantes F, et al: Healing of excimer laser ablated monkey corneas: an immunohistochemical evaluation, Arch Ophthalmol 1990;108:1604-1610.

100. Sutcliffe E and Srinivasan R: Dynamics of UV laser ablation of organic polymer surfaces, J Appl Phys 1986;60:3315-3322.

101. Sutcliffe E and Srinivasan R: Dynamics of the ultraviolet laser ablation of corneal tissue, Am J Ophthalmol 1987;103:470-471.

102. Sutcliffe E and Srinivasan R: Time-dependent analysis of the UV laser ablation of corneal tissue, Lasers Ophthalmol 1987;2:1201-1208.

103. Taboada J and Archibald CJ: An extreme sensitivity in the corneal epithelium to far UV ArF excimer laser pulses. Proceedings of the Scientific Program of the Aerospace Medical Association, San Antonio, Tex, 1981.

104. Taboada J, Mikesell GW, and Reed RD: Response of the corneal epithelium to KrF excimer laser pulses, Health Phys 1981;40:677-683.

105. Tapazto I and Vass Z: Alteration in muchopolysacchalios compounds of tea and that of corneal epithelium caused by ultraviolet radiation, Ophthalmologica 1969; 5B(Suppl):343-347.

106. Taylor DM, L'Esperance FA, Del Pero RA, et al: Human excimer laser lamellar keratectomy, Ophthalmology 1989;96:654-663.

107. Tenner A, Neuhann T, Schroder E, et al: Excimer laser radial keratotomy in the living human eye: a preliminary report, J Refract Surg 1988;4:5-8.

108. Thompson KP, Hanna KD, and Waring GO: Emerging technologies for refractive surgery: laser-adjustable synthetic epikeratoplasty, Refract Corneal Surg 1989;5:46-48.

109. Trentacoste J, Thompson K, Parrish RK, et al: Mutagenic potential of an 193-nm excimer laser on fibroblasts in tissue cultures, Ophthalmology 1987;94:125-129.

110. Trokel SL: Development of the excimer laser in ophthalmology—a personal perspective, Refract Corneal Surg 1990;6:357-362.

111. Trokel SL, Srinivasan R, and Braren BA: Excimer laser surgery of the cornea, Am J Ophthalmol 1983;96:710-715.

112. Troutman RC, Veronneau-Troutman S, Jakobiec FA, et al: A new laser for collagen wounding in cornea and strabismus surgery: a preliminary report, Trans Am Ophthalmol Soc 1986;84:117-332.

113. Tuft S, Marshall J, and Rothery S: Stromal remodeling following photorefractive keratectomy, Lasers Ophthalmol 1987;1:177-183.

114. Tuft S, Zabel RW, and Marshall JW: Corneal repair following keratectomy: a comparison between conventional surgery and laser photoablation, Invest Ophthalmol Vis Sci 1989;30:1769-1777.

115. Velazco JE and Setser DW: Bound-free emission spectra of diatomic zenon halides, J Chem Phys 1975;62:1990-1991.

116. Waring GO: Development and evaluation of refractive surgical procedures. Part I. Five stages in the continuum of development, J Refract Surg 1987;3:142-157.

117. Waring GO: Development of a system for excimer laser corneal surgery, Trans Am Ophthalmol Soc 1989;87:854-983.

118. Waring GO and Rodrigues MM: Patterns of pathologic response in the cornea, Surv Ophthalmol 1987;31:262-266.

119. Wilson SE: Excimer laser (193 nm) myopic keratomileusis in sighted and blind human eyes, Refract Corneal Surg 1990;6:383-385 (letter).

120. Yariv A: Optical electronics, ed 3, New York, 1985, Holt, Rinehart & Winston, Inc.

121. Zabel R, Tuft S, and Marshall J: Excimer laser photorefractive keratectomy: endothelial morphology following area ablation of the cornea, Invest Ophthalmol Vis Sci 1988;29(suppl):390.

Results

Corneal Wound Healing and Its Pharmacologic Modification after Refractive Keratotomy

Richard A. Eiferman
Gregory S. Schultz
Robert E. Nordquist
George O. Waring III

Two major variables determine the outcome of refractive keratotomy: the surgical technique and corneal wound healing. Although surgeons can continually refine their surgical plans and techniques (see Chapter 13, Predictability of Refractive Keratotomy, Chapter 14, Computerized Predictability Formulas for Refractive Keratotomy, and Section IV, Surgery), control of corneal wound healing is beyond practical clinical application. Presumably, individual corneas heal at different rates and with different tensile strengths, based on the intrinsic biomechanical properties of that cornea, the depth and pattern of the incisions made, the age and sex of the patient, and the individual patient's health and metabolic status.

BACKGROUND AND ACKNOWLEDGMENTS
The desire to use pharmacologic agents to modulate the effect of refractive keratotomy by controlling corneal wound healing has led to the collaboration between basic scientists and clinicians. In this chapter the basic science information provided by researchers Gregory Schultz and Robert Nordquist adds a molecular biologic dimension to our knowledge of corneal wound healing.

Dr. Eiferman has collaborated with these basic scientists for many years, and their combined talents have produced substantive advancements in our knowledge of corneal wound healing. I appreciate the time and effort they invested in this chapter. Perry Binder, M.D., also has contributed material and advice. Some of this chapter was published in a previous form as "Corneal Wound Healing After Radial Keratotomy" in Beuerman RW, Crosson CE, and Kaufman HE, editors: *Healing Processes in the Cornea*, Houston, 1989, Gulf Publishing Co., a book that provides more in-depth information for the interested reader.

In this chapter, we outline briefly normal corneal wound healing, wound healing after refractive keratotomy, and some of the drugs that may be used to modulate this wound healing.

NORMAL HEALING OF CORNEAL WOUNDS—LABORATORY STUDIES

Most studies of normal corneal wound healing have been carried out in the rabbit, so the findings may not be applicable to humans. Fewer studies have been done in nonhuman primates. Binder[7] has summarized normal corneal wound healing in detail.

Refractive keratotomy has provided a unique opportunity to study corneal wound healing because the surgery consists of regular partial thickness incisions in an anatomically normal cornea and because the wounds are not sutured, in contrast to those of penetrating keratoplasty, which are performed in a diseased cornea and are sutured. Designations of refractive keratotomy wound healing as "delayed" or "abnormally slow" are appropriate only in comparison to the standard sutured corneal wound; the rate of wound healing after a keratotomy incision should be considered normal for that circumstance.

Epithelial wound healing

Incisions or abrasions that involve only the corneal epithelium induce the epithelial cells immediately adjacent to the damage to flatten, shed their microvilli, and develop pseudopodeal extensions.[30] After about a 1-hour delay, the cells actively slide along the underlying tissue until the defect is covered.

This migration is associated with a complex interaction of intracellular and extracellular molecules. The actin component of the microfilament system within the epithelial cytoplasm becomes prominent in the extended pseudopod. The actin molecule is connected to the glycoprotein vinculin within the cytoplasm. Vinculin attaches to transmembrane proteins, the integrins, which in turn attach to the extracellular glycoprotein fibronectin that is found ubiquitously on the surface of connective tissues in front of healing epithelium. The fibronectin has numerous binding domains that attach to extracellular matrix molecules such as fibrin, collagen, and proteoglycans. The glycoprotein laminen also may play a role in surfacing the extracellular matrix in front of the migrating epithelium.

If the wound extends into the stroma, the epithelial cells migrate down the walls of the defect until they meet their counterparts from the opposite side. All wounds are initially filled with an epithelial plug of cells recruited from the wound margins.[31,44] These epithelial cells spread in waves toward the defect.[71]

When an intact monolayer of epithelium is reestablished over the wound, the cells multiply and the daughter cells enlarge until a normal thickness epithelium is established. Mitosis of the surface epithelium is almost entirely confined to a radius of 3 to 5 mm from the injury. There is an inherent leveling of the corneal epithelium that tends to eliminate irregularities of the surface; the epithelial layer will be thicker where underlying tissue is absent and thinner over stromal elevations. This creation of a smooth epithelial surface has the teleologic purpose of providing a smooth air-tear interface for optimal image formation. The factors that control epithelial "leveling" are unknown.

Stromal wound healing

As soon as the epithelial barrier is broken by the incision, the stroma begins to imbibe fluid and becomes edematous adjacent to the wound. This process is enhanced if the wounds are irrigated. The edema persists until the tight zonula occludens junctions of the surface squamous epithelial cells are reconstituted over the wound, after which the endothelial pump gradually removes the edema from the area of the wound.

The severed, acellular Bowman's layer does not heal; the cut ends remain retracted or overlapped and discontinuities are filled in by the overlying epithelium.

Healing in the corneal stroma is considerably slower than in most other connective tissues, presumably because of the lack of blood vessels.[9,10] Immediately after an injury, numerous chemoattractant inflammatory mediators are released that attract polymorphonuclear leukocytes from the tear film. These leukocytes invade the stroma where they elaborate proteases and engulf and eliminate debris.[59] Severed keratocytes retract and assume a stellate configuration. In the rabbit, a fibrin plug initially fills the wound and is quickly invaded by inflammatory cells. In about 2 hours most undamaged keratocytes within 500 μm of the incision are activated, begin intense metabolic activity, and transform into fibroblasts; the surrounding tissues appear unaffected. At 24 to 48 hours after the incision in rabbits, fibroblasts begin to migrate into the fibrin plug that fills the wound and initiate synthesis of proteoglycans and collagen to regenerate an extracellular matrix and heal the wound.[64] New connective tissue fibrils are produced to bridge the gap. These primitive collagen fibrils are thicker than normal and do not run in parallel bundles.[42,70] During the next 6 months (and even during the next few years) the collagen is progressively remodeled into a more normal configuration of layers parallel to the surface.[28] The stromal scar persists indefinitely, and the incision never regains the clarity or tensile strength of the original tissue, remaining a potential site for traumatic rupture, as in penetrating keratoplasty.[6]

In humans the epithelial plug persists in place of

the fibrin plug seen in rabbits. Thus there is no scaffolding across which the fibroblasts can migrate, and the wound gradually fills in with cicatricial tissue from the bottom, as the epithelial plug recedes toward the surface. This epithelial plug is a normal occurrence; it has sometimes been referred to as epithelial ingrowth, a misleading term more properly applied to the spread of epithelium into the anterior chamber.

The epithelium that fills the wound persists for months to years and secretes a thin basement membrane along the edges of the wound. The epithelial plug plays an active role in corneal stromal wound healing, similar to the epithelial-mesenchymal interactions that have been described in the cornea during normal maturation. The interactions are a delicate balance between synthesis of new collagen and proteoglycans with its assembly in a more normal pattern and the degradation of extracellular matrix to allow the restoration of more normal structure. The epithelium can produce both inhibitory cytokines that keep the stromal fibroblast at rest and stimulatory cytokines related to plasminogen activation that can affect the release of collagenase and other proteases as well as inhibitors of collagenase. Thus a carefully balanced molecular feedback cycle is established to allow the corneal stroma to remodel itself into as clear and uniform a structure as possible, a process that takes years. Direct cell contact or close proximity between the epi-

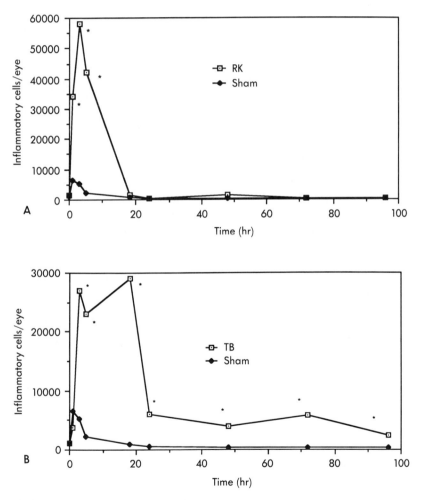

Figure 20-1
The number of inflammatory cells in the tear film after radial keratotomy and thermal burns in rabbits. **A,** After radial keratotomy (RK) in six eyes, the number of inflammatory cells rises markedly and falls quickly. In the sham (nonincised) eyes there is no significant change. **B,** After a thermal burn (four eyes) there is a marked rise in inflammatory cells that follows within 4 days, but never to the normal levels indicated in the sham-operated eyes. Asterisks indicate a statistically significant difference from the sham-operated values at the level of *P* < 0.05. (From Anderson JA, Murphy JA, and Gaster R: Refract Corneal Surg 1989;5:21-26.)

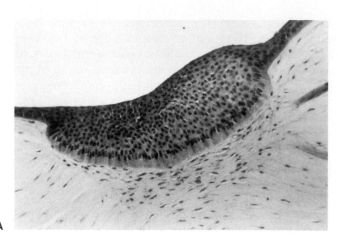
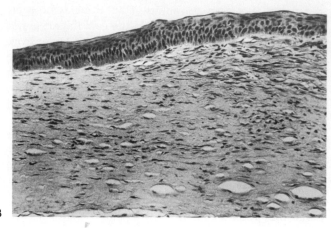

Figure 20-2
Comparison of radial keratotomy and thermal burns 3 to 4 weeks after injury in the rabbit eye. **A,** After radial keratotomy, an epithelial plug is present and is surrounded by fibroblastic cells. Note polymorphonuclear leukocytes are present (H & E) (×50). **B,** After a thermal burn, a thickened layer of epithelial cells covers the surface of the wound, and fibroblasts and newly synthesized extracellular matrix lie in the anterior stroma, with a heavy infiltration of leukocytes (H & E) (×50). (From Anderson JA, Murphy JA, and Gaster R: Refract Corneal Surg 1989;5:21-26.)

thelial and stromal cells enhances stromal collagenase production in rabbit organ cultures.[39,40] Collagenases play an important role in cleaning up and remodeling stromal wounds. In addition, corneal epithelium stimulates the synthesis of glycosaminoglycans by stromal cells[17] and may affect the synthesis of collagen as well. Therefore the epithelial plug is not a passive bystander, but an active participant in corneal stromal wound healing.[46] Some stromal wounds seem to remain filled with an epithelial plug. This is seen commonly in clinical practice after superficial injuries, such as a focal foreign body injury, or microbial corneal ulcers covered by thickened epithelium, commonly known as an epithelium facet, that level stromal defects.

The fibroblasts secrete a new extracellular matrix consisting of both normal components of the corneal stroma (type I collagen, chondroitin sulfate, and keratan sulfate proteoglycans) in addition to the transient presence of other macromolecules (such as types II and III collagen and some dermatan sulfate and heparan sulfate proteoglycans).

Anderson and colleagues[1] have shown that after radial keratotomy incisions in rabbits, polymorphonuclear leukocytes appear in large numbers in the tear film but disappear within 20 hours after wounding. The epithelial plug remains in place for a few weeks, and there is only slight stromal scarring at the edges of the wound. These findings are in contrast to deep thermal burns in the rabbit cornea, which elicit a large

polymorphonuclear leukocyte response in the tears that lasts many days longer and is much more intense than that of the simple keratotomy incision. In addition, the stromal wound healing occurs much more rapidly, with ejection of the epithelial plug from the wound and filling in of the wound with fibrous scar tissue. Thus the wounds of keratotomy incisions are somewhat atypical, in that they are unsutured, elicit a minimal inflammatory response, and show persistence of the epithelial plug, in contrast to surgical wounds in diseased corneas, accidental wounds, and corneal infections and inflammations, where the inflammatory response is more intense and the wounds tend to heal with scarring much more rapidly (Figs. 20-1 and 20-2).

The role of the myofibroblast has been reviewed by numerous authors.[66] It is a participant in wound healing. During early wound healing fibroblasts in the area of the wound acquire characteristics that distinguish them from typical fibroblasts, specifically increased bundles of microfilaments of actin and myosin as well as desmosomal intercellular junctions. Early wound contraction may be mediated by the contraction of these myofibroblasts. Randa and colleagues[62] demonstrated in rabbits that the initial presence of myosin and alpha-actinin at day 14 after the incision appeared to correlate with contraction of the wound as demonstrated by a reduction in wound gape from 7 to 14 days. The subsequent, more chronic phase of wound healing is characterized by the deposition and cross-linking of collagen as well as by the production of other components of the extracellular matrix. The collagen cross-linking also may produce contraction in the wound.[26] Moorhead and colleagues[52] have suggested that interruption of the activity of the myofibroblasts or collagen cross-linking might be used to enhance the effect of surgery by diminishing the postoperative wound contraction.[27]

Gradually the inflammatory cells recede, the active fibroblasts begin to resemble keratocytes, myofibroblasts are present, and wound remodeling proceeds apace. The scar seems to contract. The residual stroma adjacent to the scar gradually assumes the structure of more normal stroma with the 20 nm diameter, normal collagen fibrils being separated by the proteoglycans to form a more evenly spaced lamellar structure that is transparent to light. On the other hand, the area of the incision scar itself never remodels enough to regain transparency because the variable size collagen fibrils arranged in a nonuniform pattern scatter light and create the opaque appearance of the scar.

Normal endothelial wound healing

In the adult human, damage to the corneal endothelium is repaired by means of cellular reorganization, enlargement, and migration. Mitosis can occur, but it is a rare event.[13,19,75] Damaged endothelial cells probably desquamate into the anterior chamber. Adjacent viable cells disconnect their intracellular junctions, become flattened and attenuated, develop extensive filopodial cytoplasmic processes, activate the actin-containing terminal web, and migrate into the wounded area.[8,15]

Contact among cells inhibits further migration, and the junctional complexes reform to establish the endothelial monolayer. Cells that have been involved in the healing process become larger than those in the undamaged area.[67,80] Even with larger cells and reduced endothelial cell density, the human cornea can maintain its clarity, presumably because individual cells can increase the number of fluid pump sites.

WOUND HEALING AFTER RADIAL KERATOTOMY—LABORATORY STUDIES
Healing of keratotomy in rabbits

A study of radial keratotomy in rabbits by Yamaguchi and colleagues[79] over a 3-year period (Fig. 20-3) demonstrated that the wound was epithelialized by 24 hours and fibroblastic cells were present adjacent to the incision. By 3 months the epithelial plug had disappeared, but the epithelial layer was thin. Unique to the rabbit was the finding that by 6 months the stromal wound had widened considerably and that between 1 and 3 years after surgery the wound became

even wider, creating an indentation that was filled by a thickened epithelial facet. The elastic rabbit cornea seemed to stretch out and thin in the area of the incisions. By 3 years the anterior stromal area near the epithelium was not yet healed, but continued to widen. The study indicates that the rabbit is a poor model for studying keratotomy wounds as applied to refractive surgery because the rabbit cornea has no Bowman's layer and wound healing in rabbits does not closely resemble that in humans.

Seiler and colleagues have carried out linear radial keratectomy using an argon fluoride (193 nm) excimer laser (see Chapter 19, Laser Corneal Surgery). Figure 20-4 shows the wide V-shaped excision filled with a large epithelial plug and some cicatricial tissue, demonstrating the tendency of rabbit corneal wounds to spread open and fill with a large flat epithelial plug.

Palkama et al.[57] identified nerve damage adjacent to the wound and absence of epithelial sodium and potassium ATPase over a 6-month study.

Recupero and colleagues[63] studied radial keratotomy in rabbits, using a double-edged diamond knife and incisions of 70% depth to avoid direct damage to the endothelium. They emphasized findings in the endothelium, observing swelling of mitochondria and increased numbers of microplicae, 7 to 14 days after surgery. Thereafter the endothelium was normal, up to 30 days after surgery.

Healing of keratotomy in monkeys

Jester and colleagues[36] carried out a detailed histopathologic and ultrastructural study of radial keratotomy wound healing in the owl monkey. The acute wound showed sharply demarcated edges and minimal epithelial damage. Polymorphonuclear leukocytes migrated into the wound in the first 24 hours, followed by surface epithelium that migrated to the depth of the wound by 48 hours. Polymorphonuclear leukocytes and macrophages showed active organelles. Endothelial cell changes were minor. By 1 week the epithelial plug completely filled the wound and fibroblastic activity had begun at the wound margins. By 2 weeks the epithelial plug was replaced by active fibroblasts and new extracellular matrix that contained a few collagen fibrils. Endothelial cells under the area of the incisions showed vacuolization and retraction with some cell death. The wound had contracted by 3 months, and its width was less than that when it filled with the epithelial plug. The wound contracture was correlated with the steepening of the corneal curvature. By 3 to 6 months the fibroblastic reaction had resolved, the scar contained an increased number of keratocytes, and an epithelial basement membrane had formed over the scar. The irregularly

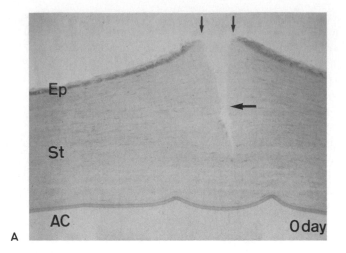

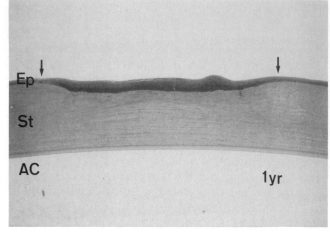

Figure 20-3
Time course of healing of radial keratotomy wound in rabbits. Incisions were made with a metal blade approximately 60% of corneal thickness, using 4 to 16 incisions per eye, a 3-mm clear zone, and a centrifugal direction. **A,** Appearance immediately after incision shows the wound separation *(between small arrows)* and the absence of inflammatory or fibroblastic cells at the margin of the wound *(large arrow)*. **B,** One year after surgery the anterior cornea has stretched *(between arrows)*, leaving an epithelial facet and a thin layer of cicatricial tissue. Note the slight thinning of the cornea in the area between the corneal stroma and the area between the arrows. **C,** At 3 years after surgery the stretched area of the cornea is still apparent *(between arrows)* with a persistent but less thick epithelial facet and persistent subepithelial scarring. *EP,* Epithelium; *ST,* stroma; *AC,* anterior chamber. (Courtesy T. Yamaguchi, M.D.)

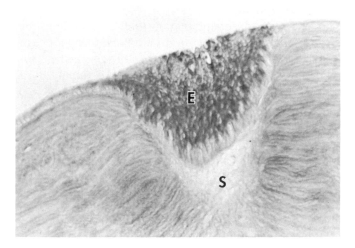

Figure 20-4
Histologic secton through a rabbit cornea 6 weeks after linear keratectomy with an argon fluoride (193 nm) excimer laser shows the wide V-shaped wound, large epithelial plug, and scar tissue deep in the wound. The wide wound results from both the excision of tissue by the laser and the tendency of rabbit corneal wound to spread open during healing. *E,* Epithelial plug; *S,* stromal scar. (Courtesy Theo Seiler, M.D.)

arranged collagen fibrils had a diameter of approximately 600 nm, about two to three times that of the normal fibrils. In a separate study, Jester et al.[37] demonstrated the presence of myofibroblasts in the wound and attributed the contracture of the wound to the activity of these cells.

WOUND HEALING AFTER REFRACTIVE KERATOTOMY IN HUMANS
Clinical observations in uncomplicated cases

Slit-lamp microscopic study of keratotomy wounds has shown continued and dynamic changes over 4 to 5 years. These changes were described in detail by Waring and colleagues[76] in 84 eyes of 51 consecutive patients in the Prospective Evaluation of Radial Keratotomy (PERK) study; Fyodorov and colleagues[25] described "fleecy, fringed, and fimbriated" scars after repeated keratotomy.

The appearance of the scars for each of the postoperative periods is shown in Figs. 20-5 and 20-6. At 24 to 48 hours after surgery the corneal incision appeared as a dark space or line surrounded by diffuse gray edema. Two weeks after surgery a dense, gray, cloudy, diffusely marginated opacity extended approximately 0.1 mm from each side of the entire incision. This cloudy opacity had no observable substructure and the incision stood out as a straight black line. By 3 months after surgery the gray cloudy zone around the incision had become less dense and was filled with discrete, fine gray spicules that protruded approximately 0.1 mm into the adjacent stroma at a variety of angles, and some spicules appeared to bifurcate. Each incision appeared to be festooned with a sheet of fine ice crystals. In some areas the gray cloudiness had receded enough for the tips of the spicules to extend into the adjacent clearer stroma, so the margins resembled the edge of a feather. Careful examination of the central part of the scar showed a lucent area extending at variable depths into the wound, corresponding to the epithelial plug.

The gray cloudiness had completely disappeared 6 months after surgery, so the spicules stood out discretely. In most wounds the spicules had begun to disappear from the anterior half of the paracentral portion of the wound adjacent to the central clear zone, leaving behind the focal gray incision scar. The lucent epithelial plug was visible in some incisions. By 1 year after surgery the spicules had disappeared from the anterior portion of the incision, with most remaining in the posterior two thirds. In some incisions a layer of longer spicules occupied the deepest part of the incision. The focal gray scar of the incision itself also became narrower and less dense. Some incisions showed the pattern of an inverted T, the scar forming the stem

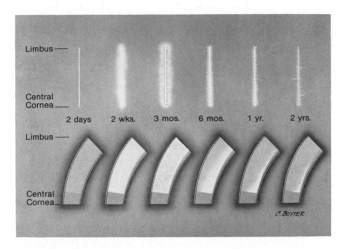

Figure 20-5
Changes in slit-lamp microscope appearance of corneal wound from 2 days to 2 years after radial keratotomy in man. At 2 days the incision is present as a discrete line surrounded by faint edema. By 2 weeks a diffuse, cloudy, gray haze surrounds both sides of the incision. By approximately 3 months fine, discrete spicules appear within the cloudiness. By 6 months the cloudiness has disappeared and the spicules appear to be more distinct, imparting a feathered appearance to the incision. Spicules begin to disappear from the anterior portion of the incision. At 1 year the density of the spicules has diminished and they occupy primarily the deep portion of the incision. By 2 years only a few discrete spicules extend from the incision, mostly in the deep stroma; these disappear by 3 to 4 years. (From Waring GO, Steinberg EB, and Wilson LA: Am J Ophthalmol 1985;100:218-224.)

of the T and the remaining spicules the top. Two years after surgery the incision scar itself was fainter but easily recognizable with both a penlight and the slit-lamp microscope. The feathered edge also was fainter, but many incisions demonstrated residual spicules in the posterior peripheral part. Three to four years after surgery (unpublished data), the incision scar continued to become fainter, and only a few spicules were present in the deepest part of the incision, spread along its base.

Clinical observations in complicated cases

Numerous types of inclusions can be seen within the scars: globular yellow deposits from residual degenerated blood, discrete round epithelial inclusion cysts,[37] and small foreign bodies, such as talc or fine threads. Fyodorov[25] compared the refractive results in corneas with wounds that healed without inclusions with refractive results in corneas that healed with

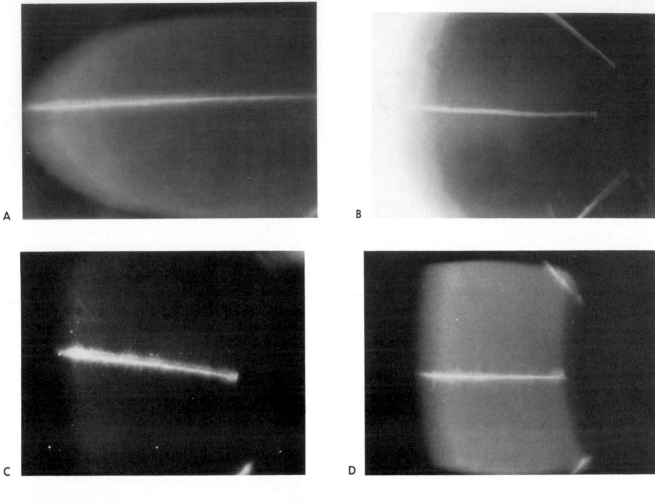

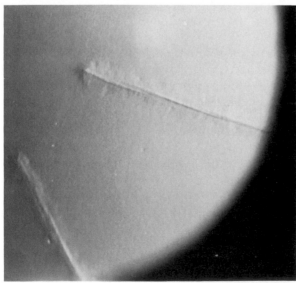

Figure 20-6
Slit-lamp photomicrographs of radial keratotomy incisions in man. **A,** At 2 weeks after surgery the wound shows diffuse gray cloudiness around the white incision line. **B,** At 3 months after surgery the wound shows a decrease in the cloudy haze and the emergence of faint small spicules adjacent to the incision. **C,** At 6 months after surgery the wound shows fine spicules extending along both sides of the incision, imparting a feathered, fuzzy appearance. **D,** At 1 year after surgery longer, fainter spicules extend from the sides of the incision. **E,** In retroillumination, 1½ years after surgery the central incision line is still bounded by the fine feathered spicules on each side. (From Waring GO, Steinberg EB, and Wilson LA: Am J Ophthalmol 1985;100:218-224.)

beads and pearls, finding that the wounds with inclusions produced less effect.

In areas of corneal perforation, slit-lamp microscopy demonstrates a focal, gray, diffusely marginated scar at the level of Descemet's membrane. Histopathologic studies[6] have shown that a fibrocellular posterior collagenous layer (retrocorneal membrane) results in this area, either from metaplasia of the corneal endothelium or from migration of stromal fibroblasts through the wound. This tissue increases the density of the scar, but probably has little other effect.

Keratotomy wounds are sutured in cases of large corneal perforations or decrease overcorrection. The only published clinical study of healing sutured corneal wounds and their evolution over time is that of Mathers and Lemp.[50] In 75 eyes the authors described the slit-lamp microscopic appearance of the corneal wounds after penetrating keratoplasty from 0 to 100 months, observing an overall decrease in fibrosis. Most of the fibrosis occurred in the anterior stroma and particularly subepithelially around the areas of the sutures. This precluded a detailed examination of the underlying stromal scar itself, about which very little is known, as a basis for comparing sutured penetrating keratoplasty wounds with unsutured refractive keratotomy wounds.

Intersecting transverse and radial incisions, such as those performed in the early 1980s to correct astigmatism (Ruiz procedure, combined circular trephination and radial incisions, and grouped radial and transverse incisions) produce excessive wound gaping at the points of intersection. In these areas, dense proliferative stromal scarring can occur, spreading out as subepithelial fibrosis (see Chapter 23, Complications of Refractive Keratotomy).

Clinical observations of excimer laser excisions

Slit-lamp microscopic examination of linear keratectomy wounds (the laser removes tissue, so the linear wound is a keratectomy, not a keratotomy) made by an excimer laser demonstrate the prolonged presence of a large epithelial plug. The wounds resemble a railroad track, with a clear zone separating two gray parallel edges—the clear zone presumably corresponding to the wide, deep epithelial plug and the parallel gray lines the scar of the adjacent stroma. This configuration can persist up to 1 year. It is possible that the distance between the two sides of the laser keratectomy is too great to be bridged by the fibroblasts, and the epithelial plug may persist indefinitely as a deep facet[73] (see Chapter 19, Laser Corneal Surgery).

Histology of human refractive keratotomy wounds

Table 20-1 summarizes the histopathologic and ultrastructural findings in human corneas studied after refractive keratotomy (Figs. 20-7 to 20-14).

Epithelial healing. The most striking finding is the persistence of the epithelial plug for approximately 4 to 5 years after surgery.[6,18] The size and depth of the epithelial plug vary greatly from one wound to another in a single eye and from one eye to another, reflecting the great variability in healing of individual wounds. The plug causes increased wound gape and increased effect. Clearly, the stromal scar cannot form across a wound as long as the epithelial plug is in place, so the wounds are less strong and probably less stable as long as the epithelial plug is present. The epithelium within the wound forms a basement membrane along the wound margin. Epithelial inclusion cysts are randomly identified within these wounds as epithelial-lined spaces containing debris. The epithelium over the incision also may thicken to form a facet that smooths the corneal surface.

It is possible that the surface epithelial cells over a plug may turn over more actively and may have more irregularities. In many of the histopathologic reports, scanning electron microscopy delimits a ridge of epithelium over the wound that shows a swirling pattern and disruption of epithelial continuity and microvilli. The area between the incisions is slightly indented, forming a location for a stellate iron line. Theoretically the elevated cells over the incision might form small defects that serve as points of attachment for microorganisms, possibly explaining the occurrence of late, spontaneous bacterial keratitis in keratotomy wounds.[49]

Once the epithelial plug extrudes and the stromal wound closes, the epithelium forms a continuous basement membrane over the defect in Bowman's layer.

Stromal healing. Because Bowman's layer does not heal, the cut edges are often malopposed; however, the surface irregularity created is filled in by epithelial hyperplasia and does not seem to create an optical or functional problem.

The stromal wound undergoes slow healing. Corneas removed within the first year after radial keratotomy show fibroblasts aligned parallel to the wound with some histocytes still present, a pattern seen in early wound healing in experimental animals. The wound fills with extracellular matrix that is disorganized—compared with the normal lamellar corneal structure—and is populated by active fibroblasts.

Table 20-1

Summary of Pathology of Human Corneas after Refractive Keratotomy

Author, year	Age/sex	Initial diagnosis	Keratotomy surgery	Reason for tissue procurement	Time after last surgery (months)
Stainer[72] 1982	42M	Penetrating keratoplasty, keratoconus	Radial (8) + transverse (5)	Repeat penetrating keratoplasty	5
Ingraham[35] 1985	36M	Myopia	Radial (8)	Death—gunshot wound	17 to 18
Yamaguchi[78] 1985	31M	Myopia	OD: Radial (11) OS: Radial (8)	Death	3
Deg[18] 1985	46M	Keratoconus	Radial (8)	Penetrating keratoplasty	6
	43M	Myopia	Radial (16+16 additional 4 months later)	Penetrating keratoplasty	43
	43M		Radial (8+8 additional 2 months later)	Homoplastic myopic keratomileusis	19
Binder[5] 1987	33F	Myopia	Radial (16+8 additional 55 months later)	Homoplastic myopic keratomileusis	11 (66 after first keratotomy)
	33M	Keratoconus	Radial (8+4 additional 6 months later)	Penetrating keratoplasty	65
Binder[6] 1988	24F	Myopia	OS: Radial (16)	Motor vehicle accident; traumatic rupture-repair + penetrating keratoplasty	24
	27M	Myopia	Radial (OD 4, OS 8)	Death, motor vehicle accident; OD: Traumatic rupture, OS: Intact	12
Binder[5] 1987	25M	Myopia	OU, Radial (8)	—	—
	36M	Myopia	Radial (4)	—	—
	73M	Penetrating keratoplasty, astigmatism	"L"	—	44
	73M	Penetrating keratoplasty, astigmatism	Ruiz trapezoidal	—	9
	77M	Penetrating keratoplasty, astigmatism	Ruiz trapezoidal	—	10
	70M	Keratophakia, astigmatism	Trapezoidal	—	10
	??	Keratoconus	Radial (8) + transverse	—	24

Table 20-1—cont'd

Summary of Pathology of Human Corneas After Refractive Keratotomy—cont'd

Histologic depth of incisions	Epithelial plug	Epithelial basement membrane	Bowman's layer	Stromal scar	Descemet's membrane (DM); endothelium
16% to 77%	15 cells thick	In plug	—	Fibroblasts	Ridges in DM; no endothelial damage
83% to 93%	13% to 37%, all incisions	In plug	Closely apposed	No new collagen across wound	Linear disruption of endothelium
48% to 98%	All incisions, inclusion cysts	In plug	Malapposed	Fibroblasts, histiocytes	Ridges under incisions: linear disruption of endothelium
77% to 90%	Anterior	In plug	—	Slight fibroplasia	No ridges in DM
58% to 71%	Anterior	In plug	Malapposed	Slight fibroplasia	Ridges in DM
—	—	—	—	Gaping incisions	—
—	None at 66 months	Continues across scar surface	Malapposed	Mild fibroplasia	—
36% to 58%	Slight	Continues across scar surface	Malapposed	Active fibroblasts	Ridges in DM
50% to 100%	0% to 33%	—	—	—	—
60%	Yes	—	—	Minimal fibroplasia	—
—	Small	—	—	Closed	—
—	Large	—	—	Closed	—
—	Small	—	—	—	—
—	Large	—	—	—	—
—	Absent	—	—	Gaping	—
—	Absent	—	—	Gaping	—
—	Large	—	—	—	—

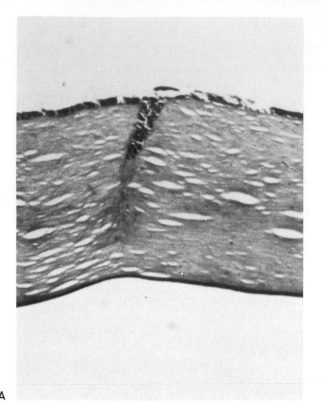
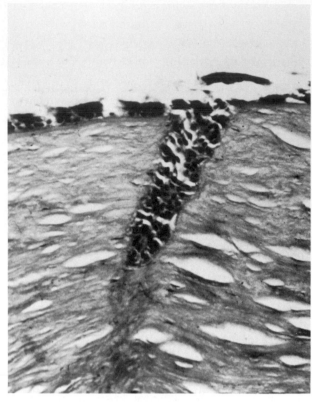

A

B

Figure 20-7
Histopathology of human radial keratotomy wound 18 months after surgery. **A,** Incision scar extends 80% of corneal thickness, and epithelial plug extends 36% of corneal thickness (periodic acid–Schiff, ×40). **B,** Higher power magnification shows epithelial plug over stromal scar (periodic acid–Schiff, ×100). (From Ingraham HJ, Guber D, and Green WR: Arch Ophthalmol 1985;103:683-688.)

Figure 20-8
Epithelial plug fills anterior part of human keratotomy wound many months after surgery (periodic acid–Schiff, ×100). (Courtesy Perry Binder, M.D.)

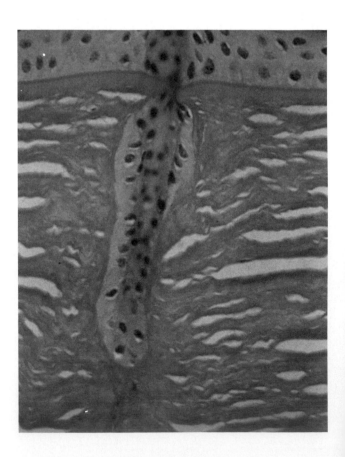

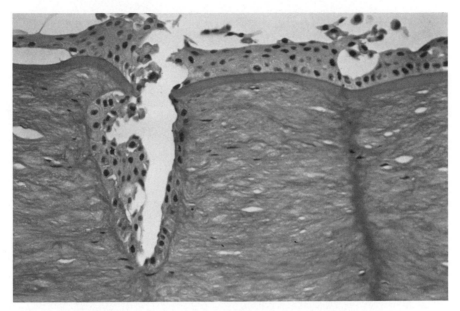

Figure 20-9
Two keratotomy wounds in one section. *Left wound,* 11 months after surgery. *Right wound,* 66 months after surgery. The anterior part of the left wound contains an epithelial plug that is disrupted from surgical removal or histologic processing. The right wound shows advanced healing with no epithelial plug and no hypercellularity (periodic acid–Schiff, ×100). (Courtesy Perry Binder, M.D.)

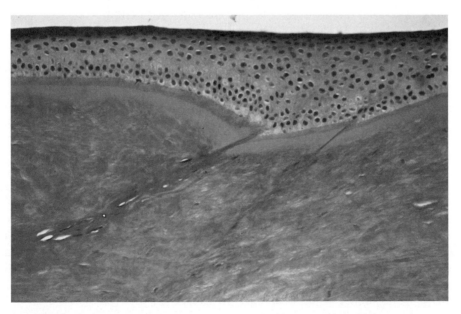

Figure 20-10
Human cornea 43 months after keratotomy demonstrates epithelial facet over an oblique keratotomy wound, the hyperplastic epithelium filling in the indentation in the stroma to create a smoother surface (periodic acid–Schiff, ×100). (Courtesy Perry Binder, M.D.)

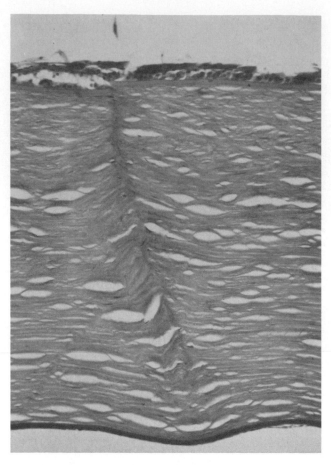

Figure 20-11
Human cornea 18 months after successful radial keratotomy shows 80.7% depth scar with no epithelial plug and no increased cellularity (periodic acid–Schiff, ×100). (Courtesy Herbert J. Ingraham, M.D.)

Even the specimens studied approximately 5 years after keratotomy show hypercellularity and continued disorganization within the scar, suggesting that even though the epithelial plug has been extruded, there is continued remodeling of the scar itself.[5] Binder and colleagues[5] used lectins to identify glycosaminoglycans within the cornea, identifying varying patterns of keratan sulfate.

No clear histopathologic explanation has been offered for the continued increase in effect of surgery in approximately 20% of eyes after radial keratotomy. Presumably, the wounds stretch enough to produce more corneal flattening.

Endothelial healing. Scanning electron microscopy of the posterior cornea shows alterations and ridges in Descemet's membrane beneath the corneal scars in many studies, some also showing mild disruption of endothelial cells. This reinforces the findings in animal studies of mild endothelial damage. A detailed study of the corneal endothelium in these human specimens is difficult because many specimens have been subjected to uncontrolled handling and preservation. Nevertheless, it seems certain that refractive keratotomy incisions of at least 70% to 80% of corneal thickness have a mild, acute, disruptive effect on the endothelium. There are no reports, however, of gross endothelial defects, of large numbers of abnormally shaped cells, or of a posterior collagenous layer in these human specimens, indicating that endothelial recovery from the surgical insult is good, as well as suggesting that persistent endothelial disruption is absent.

The studies of human pathology therefore indicate prolonged wound healing for at least 5 years and have not identified the time when the stromal scar is completely remodeled and quiescent.

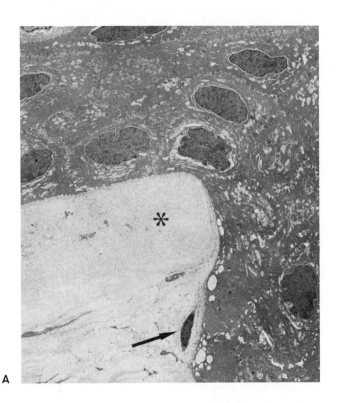

A

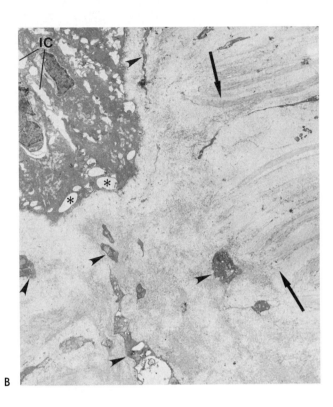

B

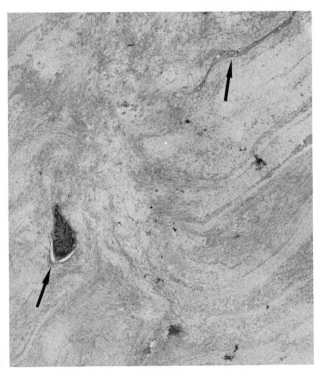

C

Figure 20-12

Transmission electron micrograph of human radial keratotomy wound 18 months after surgery. Figure shows different portions of wound. **A,** Anterior. **B,** Base of epithelial plug. **C,** Bottom of stromal wound. Anterior edge of wound **(A)** shows Bowman's layer (*) with an epithelial plug extending past it into the anterior portion of the wound. Beneath Bowman's layer at the edge of the epithelial plug are the basement membrane, randomly oriented collagen fibrils, and a fibroblast *(arrow)* oriented parallel to the wound (×3000). **B,** The area of greatest extent of epithelium into the wound shows epithelial cells with numerous intracellular (*) and intercellular *(IC)* edematous vacuoles. Normally arranged stromal collagen lamellae *(right of arrows)* are disrupted *(left of arrows)* in the wound site. Within the wound, randomly oriented fibers, granular material, and fibroblasts *(arrowheads)* are present. Collagen bundles at the margin are separated (×3000). **C,** At the deepest extent of the corneal wound, there are rare fibrocytes *(arrows)* and randomly oriented collagen fibrils that measure 25 to 28 nm in diameter (×4200). (From Ingraham HJ, Guber D, and Green WR: Arch Ophthalmol 1985;103:683-688.)

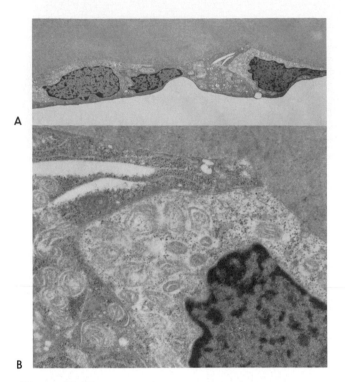

Figure 20-13

Transmission electron micrograph of endothelium subjacent to radial scar in a human 18 months after radial keratotomy. **A,** There is irregularity of spacing and staining of the endothelium (×2000). **B,** A higher power view shows lighter staining of the cytoplasm of an apparently swollen endothelial cell (×20,000). (From Ingraham HJ, Guber D, and Green WR: Arch Ophthalmol 1985;103:683-688.)

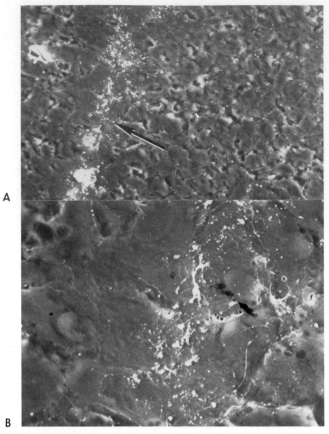

Figure 20-14

Scanning electron micrograph of endothelium beneath radial scar in a human 18 months after radial keratotomy. **A,** The endothelial surface shows linear abnormality *(arrow)* beneath the radial wound (×420). **B,** Higher power view shows the endothelium to be intact, but some endothelial cells are larger and smoother than surrounding cells. There is also a loss of cellular apposition and a reduced number of characteristic nuclear bulges (×1500). (From Ingraham HJ, Guber D, and Green WR: Arch Ophthalmol 1985;103:683-688.)

TRAUMATIC RUPTURE OF THE CORNEA AFTER RADIAL KERATOTOMY

There are two common types of corneal wounds made by surgeons: refractive keratotomy wounds that are unsutured and not treated by prolonged doses of topical corticosteroids and penetrating keratoplasty wounds that are sutured and are often treated with chronic topical corticosteroids. In both types of wounds, the corneal scars do not regain normal tensile strength; the scars are always weaker than the unincised cornea.

The following are three types of studies and reports of wound strength after corneal surgery:

1. Laboratory studies of acute or healing wounds after radial keratotomy or penetrating keratoplasty
2. Accidental trauma after radial keratotomy or penetrating keratoplasty
3. Secondary surgical procedures after an initial radial keratotomy procedure

Luttrull and colleagues[48] studied the effect of depth of keratotomy incisions that extended across the limbus in enucleated porcine eyes. They demonstrated that when incisions exceeded 70% of corneal depth, there was an increased incidence of rupture of the cornea throughout the incisions after blunt trauma. They also observed that incisions traversing the limbus increased the incidence of corneoscleral rupture.

Larson and colleagues[45] observed that 98% of the wound ruptures in rabbit eyes after an eight-incision radial keratotomy procedure occurred in one or more of the incisions, with patterns that connected one incision to the other extending out into the sclera and forming stellate wounds. They observed that the blunt force required to rupture the globe after radial keratotomy within 90 days of healing was approximately half that of unoperated control eyes; those eyes with intraoperative corneal perforations required even less force to rupture.

Rylander et al.[65] studied the effect of radial keratotomy on the rupture strength in a porcine model. They concluded that ruptures most frequently occurred at the equator in normal eyes and through the cornea in radial keratotomy eyes. The radial keratotomy eyes ruptured at less force than the paired normal eyes in eight of nine experiments.

The effect of accidental trauma on corneal wounds is determined by the amount of direct trauma to the globe itself. There is no way this can be quantified because the force impacting the globe is a capricious combination of events that depends on the severity of the wound, the amount of force absorbed by the periocular structures, and the amount of force absorbed by the globe itself. Thus reported cases of ocular trauma span a spectrum from severe periorbital trauma with an intact globe to severe trauma directly to the globe with rupture and subsequent enucleation.

John and Schmitt[38] reported one case of severe blunt trauma to an eye 6 months after an eight-incision radial keratotomy procedure with a 4-mm optical clear zone. No mention was made of achieved incision depth. The patient sustained a blow to the left side of his face that produced a corneal abrasion and a 75% hyphema. The vision without correction returned to 20/50. Twelve months after the radial keratotomy and 6 months after the injury, the uncorrected visual acuity was 20/15. The keratometric astigmatism had increased from 42.12/43.25 to 41.25/43.37. The only remaining abnormality was an enlarged fixed pupil. Spivak[69] reported a case of a male who had facial trauma from a plane crash 4 months after a 16-incision radial keratotomy and 2 months after a reoperation for residual astigmatism. Despite bilateral orbital floor fractures, a severe nasofrontoethmoid discontinuity and a Le Fort 2 maxillary fracture, no corneal rupture occurred and the patient regained 20/20 uncorrected visual acuity. McDonnell and colleagues[51] reported the rupture of a cornea caused by blunt trauma after a hexagonal keratotomy. Unfortunately, this patient required several surgical procedures for repair of the corneal wound and for a retinal detachment associated with retinoschisis. Simons and Linsalata[68] and Forstot and Damiano[24] have reported several cases of blunt trauma to the globe after radial keratotomy, resulting in various complications.

Binder and colleagues[6] reported on wound healing after accidental traumatic corneal rupture in two patients (three eyes) who had previously undergone successful radial keratotomy procedures. One patient required penetrating keratoplasty to recover 20/50 visual acuity. The second patient died, sustaining bilateral ruptured corneas and extensive intraocular injuries. Histologic and ultrastructural studies showed incomplete healing of the radial keratotomy wounds in the three corneas. The authors concluded that individuals who have had radial keratotomy are at increased risk of corneal rupture after direct ocular trauma (see Chapter 23, Complications of Refractive Keratotomy).

Most studies of corneal wound healing have been done with a penetrating keratoplasty model. Histopathologically, the fibrin plug within the corneal stromal wound is replaced with collagenous tissue by 6 months.[7] In rabbit corneas, the tensile strength of a central corneal wound has reached 50% of the tensile strength of the intact tissue by 3 months.[28] After penetrating keratoplasty, surgeons know that wounds may slip when sutures are removed even 1 to 2 years postoperatively, although wounds are more likely to slip and separate when sutures are removed less than 1 year after surgery.[4] Calkins and colleagues[12] used holograms taken of corneas after penetrating keratoplasty to demonstrate structurally weak areas in the wound. They demonstrated that even 1 year after penetrating keratoplasty when vascularization was present in the wound, weak areas were present.[4] Considering the studies of corneal wound healing after penetrating keratoplasty, it is no surprise that blunt trauma can cause reopening of the wound months to years after surgery, with or without the presence of intact sutures.[22]

In radial keratotomy, in contrast to penetrating keratoplasty, there are two factors that theoretically predispose to better wound strength: incisions that are not of full thickness and not using topical corticosteroids for prolonged periods. Nevertheless, corneal wounds after radial keratotomy pose a hazard because the cornea probably does not recover full tensile strength of normal tissue in the areas of the incisions. Although it is not known exactly when the wounds of radial keratotomy heal, evidence suggests that even 5 years after surgery, the wounds may not be fully healed.[5]

Karr et al.[41] reported wound gape and persistent epithelial defects in a radial keratotomy case that had a combined radial and transecting circumferential incision. Girard et al.[29] described a case of radial keratotomy incisions that reopened 6 months postoperatively during subsequent transverse keratotomy incisions to correct residual astigmatism. Binder[3] reported a single case of presumed epithelial ingrowth after a microperforation at surgery.

PHARMACOLOGIC MANIPULATION OF CORNEAL WOUND HEALING

Because of the prolonged corneal wound healing after refractive keratotomy, it would be ideal to develop drugs that could control this process. Drugs that could either speed or retard wound healing might help the surgeon adjust overcorrections and undercorrections and then cement the final desirable result as a stable correction. Unfortunately, this ideal is not yet a clinical reality.

With the advent of genetic engineering, bioactive mitogenic agents can be produced commercially in large quantities. The role of growth factors in refractive corneal surgery will depend on the development of successful drug delivery systems. It is possible to use these agents as topical eyedrops or ointments. Clinical effectiveness will probably require formulations that produce prolonged exposure time, such as liposomes, collagen contact lens delivery systems, macromolecular conjugates of epithelial growth factor (EGF), or thin films containing EGF and other mitogens, which can be put into keratotomy wounds.

A combination of extracellular matrix components including fibronectin, collagen, chondroitin sulfate, and epidermal growth factor might be useful in promoting wound healing after radial keratotomy, particularly if it could be delivered in a vehicle such as a gel or film that could hold the keratotomy wound in the desired configuration during healing (see Fig. 20-23, *B*).

For the clinician to modulate the shape of the cornea pharmacologically after keratotomy, drugs must be available that retard wound healing, as well as stimulate it. This would be particularly useful in patients who are undercorrected, in whom slower, less efficient, less strong wound healing might be desirable to enhance the effect of the surgery.

Growth factors

Biochemistry of growth factors. What is a "growth factor"? These polypeptide hormones secreted by cells can stimulate repetitive cycles of cell division. This definition distinguishes growth factors from simple nutritional substances such as vitamins, amino acids, or cofactors, which can reduce cell growth if their concentration becomes too low. It also excludes substances such as lectins or antibodies to membrane proteins, which can stimulate a single cycle of cell division by artificially perturbing cell membrane structure. It also excludes chemicals, radiation, and viruses, which permanently transform cells.

Researchers have screened extracts of many fluids and tissues for potential new growth factors. If a promising activity is detected, the substance is purified and fractionated by standard biochemical techniques such as size exclusion gel chromatography, ion exchange chromatography, and, more recently, high-pressure liquid chromatography. As the crude samples are separated into many smaller fractions by these techniques, those that contain growth factor activity are identified by assaying each fraction for biologic activity, such as incorporation of tritiated thymidine in human corneal fibroblasts in tissue culture.

The nomenclature of growth factors is very confusing, since researchers have often isolated the same bioactive hormones from different tissues. For example, "retinal-derived growth factor (RDGF)," which was discovered in homogenates of bovine retina, and "endothelial cell growth factor," which was found in extracts of bovine pituitary glands, appear to be identical to "fibroblast growth factor," which was originally isolated from bovine hypothalamus. The list of bona fide growth factors probably will be limited to about a dozen polypeptides, and only about half of those may actually have activity toward corneal cells. A list of polypeptide growth factors that have been rigorously characterized biochemically and that may have significant effects in cornea is presented in Table 20-2. Reviews of growth factors as applied to the cornea have been published.[23,74]

Production of growth factors. The quantity of polypeptide growth factors present in homogenates of animal tissue is extremely low; in vivo, only nanomolar amounts (10^{-9} M) are required to generate a biologic response. Consequently the isolation of polypeptide growth factors from animal tissue sources is not practical for producing the amounts of factors needed on a commercial level. Furthermore, the amino acid sequence of human growth factors differs by varying degrees from the amino acid sequence of corresponding growth factors from lower mammals. Thus there al-

Table 20-2

Properties of Biochemically Characterized Growth Factors and Their Receptors

Growth factor	Approximate molecular weight (daltons)	Possible corneal target cells	Biochemical structure	Receptor properties
Epidermal growth factor (EGF)	6,000	Epithelial cells, stromal fibroblasts, endothelial cells	Single chain with three disulfide bonds	170,000 dalton tyrosine, kinase
Transforming growth factor-alpha (TGF-α)	6,000	Epithelial cells, stromal fibroblasts, endothelial cells	Structure similar to EGF	170,000 dalton tyrosine, kinase
Platelet-derived growth factor (PDGF)	31,000	Stromal fibroblasts	Heterodimer with two disulfide bridges	180,000 dalton tyrosine, kinase
Fibroblast growth factor (FGF)	16,000 to 19,000	Stromal fibroblasts, endothelial cells	A family of single-chain polypeptides that bind heparin	145,000 dalton tyrosine, kinase
Connective tissue activator peptide (CTAP)	9,300	Stromal fibroblasts	Single chain	Uncharacterized
Insulin (I)	6,000	Stromal fibroblasts	Heterodimer with two disulfide bridges	350,000 dalton tyrosine, kinase, oligomeric $(\alpha\beta)_2$
Insulin-like growth factor I	6,000	Stromal fibroblasts	Structurally similar to insulin	350,000 dalton tyrosine, kinase, oligomeric $(\alpha\beta)_2$
Transforming growth factor-beta (TGF-β)	24,000	Epithelial cells, stromal fibroblasts, endothelial cells	A family of growth factors; homodimer of two identical subunits linked by disulfide bonds	Three membrane-binding proteins (not kinases) 50 kDa 130 kDa 250 kDa

ways is a potential for an immune reaction to be generated against the animal sequence protein. Fortunately, with the advent of recombinant DNA technology, it is now possible to genetically engineer yeast or bacteria to synthesize large amounts of the desired human sequence polypeptide growth factors that can then be purified for clinical use.

Genetic engineering of growth factors. Production of biosynthetic polypeptide growth factors is individualized to some extent for each hormone because of unique problems posed by their differing structures. The strategy used for manufacturing an individual polypeptide growth factor will involve several common steps, including isolation of the correct sequence of DNA for the growth factor from a "gene library" or chemical synthesis of the correct sequence of DNA using a "gene machine." The gene is inserted into a DNA vector, which is transfected into bacteria or yeast cells. Transfected cells are selected, then screened for cells that synthesize and secrete the correct product. Fi-

nally, the desired transfected cells are cloned to ensure homogeneity of product. Using this approach biosynthetic EGF, TGF$_\alpha$, PDGF, FGF, CTAP, insulin, and IGF-I (Table 20-2) have all been successfully expressed by genetically engineered cells. Adequate amounts of growth factors may be produced by these methods for evaluation of their clinical usefulness.

The general strategy can be illustrated by the production of human epidermal growth factor (h-EGF). H-EGF is a relatively small polypeptide whose 53 amino acid sequence is known (Fig. 20-15). Using solid-phase DNA synthesis techniques, the entire DNA sequence was assembled from shorter sequences that, when the triplet codons were precisely transcribed to mRNA, coded for the correct amino acid sequence. The synthetic gene was then purified by selecting DNA of the correct size by polyacrylamide gel electrophoresis.

The newly constructed gene was then inserted into another segment of DNA that served as the vector to

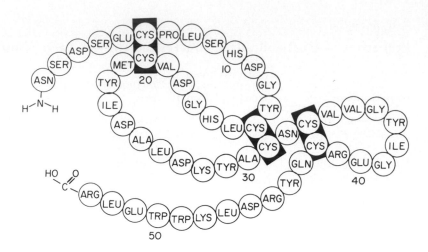

Figure 20-15
Structure of human epidermal factor (EGF). The primary amino acid sequence of EGF, a single-chain 53 amino acid polypeptide, is characterized by three disulfide bonds that give the molecule exceptional stability. EGF shares substantial sequence homology with transforming growth factor alpha (TGF-α) and vaccina growth factor (VGF).

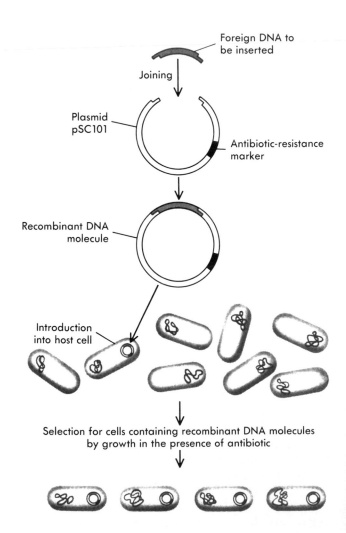

Figure 20-16
Cloning of a gene in a plasmid. The DNA coding for the gene is inserted into an antibiotic-resistance plasmid that has been constructed to have "sticky ends" that will base pair with the complementary sequence of bases at the ends of the gene. The plasmid and gene are then joined permanently by the action of DNA ligase (producing site-specific genetic recombination molecule). Cells (bacteria or yeast) are then transfected with the plasmid and grown under conditions that allow only the transfected cells to survive, such as in antibiotics. The transfected cells are then cloned by limiting dilution and screened to identify those clones that are expressing the desired gene's protein. (From Watson JD, Tooze J, and Kurtz DT: Recombinant DNA: a short course, New York, 1983, WH Freeman Co.)

deliberately carry (transfect) the gene into baker's yeast or bacterium (Fig. 20-16). The transfection was accomplished by mixing the vector DNA containing the desired gene with yeast or bacteria in a solution containing elevated calcium ions. The cells nonspecifically engulfed the vectors. Transfected cells carrying the extra DNA were isolated by growing the cells in solutions that killed the nontransfected cells and left the transfected cells alive. This was accomplished by choosing a vector that contained additional genes coded for proteins that make transfected cells resistant to the selection medium. A topical system could incorporate the desired gene as well as the gene for resistance to tetracycline; hence, the nontransfected cells would be eliminated by growing cells in a tetracycline-containing solution. Transfected cells then can be cloned to ensure that a homogenous produce is manufactured. "Promotion regions" and specific amino acid sequencers are typically added to the growth factor gene to optimize maximal production of the new gene product.

A different approach to production of growth factors is used for large peptides such as platelet-derived growth factor (PDGF) (MW 36,000), since these genes are too large to be synthesized accurately by present day solid-phase DNA technology. The gene must be isolated from the natural DNA within cells. Although this task at first may seem to be insurmountable because of the enormous number of genes in human cells, hundreds of human genes already have been cloned and sequenced. The process starts by taking the total DNA of a human cell, cutting it into fragments by restriction enzymes that can recognize a specific, short sequence of bases. Human DNA fragments produced by the restriction endonuclease are incorporated into plasmid vectors that contain DNA fragments cut by the same restriction enzymes and thus have "sticky ends" that are complementary to the ends of the human DNA fragments. Vectors carrying the human genes are then transfected into bacteria or yeast generating a "gene library." The next problem is to screen all of the transfected cells of the gene library and identify only those that carry the desired gene. This is usually accomplished by preparing a radioactive "probe" that has a base sequence that is complementary to a part of the entire gene. Bacteria or yeast are cloned and their DNA is replica-plated onto nitrocellulose filters. The filters are incubated with the radioactive probe that recognizes only the desired gene. By using autoradiography, positive colonies can be isolated, picked, and expanded. In an ideal situation, the entire gene coding for the growth factor is present in the DNA fragment cloned in the selected bacteria. If not,

partial sequences of the gene isolated from different clones can be isolated and subsequently united to generate the full length gene.

Mechanisms of action of growth factors. Although the complete story is not known, polypeptide growth factors share many common aspects of their cellular biology (Fig. 20-17). All known growth factors initially interact with their target cells by binding to specific, high-affinity, receptor proteins in the plasma membrane. This is quite different from the action of steroid or thyroid hormones, which must actually enter the cytoplasm of target cells and bind to receptor proteins present in the nucleus and possibly in the cytoplasm. Within minutes of binding, isolated growth factor/receptor complexes begin to aggregate into clusters and very rapidly a basketlike structure composed of the specialized protein called clatherin begins to form on the cytoplasmic surface of the membrane underlying the clusters of growth factor receptors. These "coated pits" continue to become internalized and, once inside the cells, the endocytic vesicles lose their clatherin coating and fuse with organelles, such as lysosomes, that degrade the hormone-receptor complex. Some of the receptors may recycle to the cell's plasma membrane or fuse with the nuclear membrane.

At the molecular level, an event that occurs within seconds of the exposure of cells to a growth factor (for example, EGF, PDGF, insulin, and IGF-I) is activation of each receptor's kinase activity. This is a specific process. The receptors for these growth factors stimulate phosphorylation only of tyrosine residues in proteins. In contrast, cyclic AMP–dependent protein kinase specifically phosphorylates serine or threonine residues. Thus growth factors stimulate phosphorylation of a unique amino acid that is distinctly different from those phosphorylated by hormones that act through the more common cyclic AMP cascade system. Presumably, activation of this specific receptor-kinase activity is important in mediating some of the actions of growth factors on cells.

Two important cellular proteins, lipocortin and calpactin, which are phosphorylated in response to EGF, have been identified. Lipocortin is involved in regulating the activity of phospholipase A_2, a key enzyme in prostaglandin production. Calpactin is part of the submembrane cytoskeletal complex of proteins and interacts with actin presumably to influence cellular shape.

While phosphorylation of these cellular proteins is probably important in the sequence of events following EGF binding to its receptor, we do not have a complete understanding of the mechanism of action of EGF. It is most probable that activation of DNA syn-

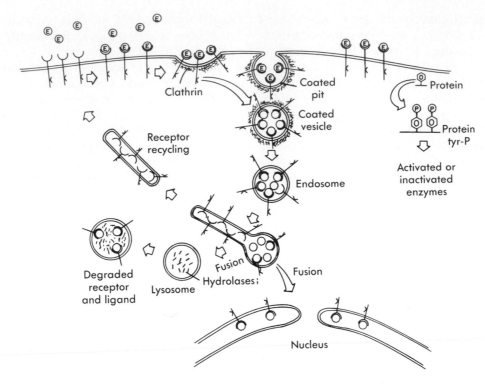

Figure 20-17

Interaction of EGF with cells. Within seconds after EGF binds to its receptor in the plasma membrane, the receptor's kinase is activated and begins phosphorylating proteins on tyrosine residues. Presumably the activities of the proteins are altered by this phosphorylation. Within minutes after EGF binds to its specific receptors on the surface of cell, the randomly dispersed receptors become clustered in specialized regions of plasma membrane, which are associated with the cytoplasmic protein clathrin. These coated pit regions then internalize and lose their clathrin coating. Some EGF-receptor complexes present in endosomes may fuse with other intracellular organelles, such as the nuclear membrane of lyosomes, where they are degraded, or the EGF-receptor complexes may dissociate and segregate with the receptor recycling to the plasma membrane.

thesis by EGF and other polypeptide growth factors will not be a simple single-step process involving a single "second messenger" and that multiple "messengers" are probably required to initiate and complete mitosis. For example, EGF must be in contact with target tissues for prolonged periods (6 to 12 hours) to induce mitosis, which may explain some of the early failures of topical applications of EGF to stimulate wound healing.[14] When EGF was applied as a mist to a thermal skin burn and then wiped off, it had no effect. Only when EGFd was applied in a cream that maintained exposure to the hormone was healing accelerated.[10] Thus a key aspect in using EGF clinically will be to develop formulations and regimens that allow adequate exposure time of cells to EGF.

In tissue culture, when keratocytes demonstrated specific receptors for EGF and when incubated with EGF, these cells increase their synthesis of DNA. When applied clinically, we believe EGF stimulates epithelium and keratocytes to divide and secrete more collagen and other biochemical mediators.

Effect of epidermal growth factors in full-thickness rabbit corneal wounds. Can biosynthetic growth factors actually accelerate or modify normal corneal wound healing? Results have been reported from several preclinical animal studies modeling human corneal disease and a limited number of clinical evaluations in humans using mouse EGF.[33]

In our laboratory, topical applications of EGF significantly increased the tensile strength of full-thickness, nonsutured incisions in rabbit corneas. Using a strain gauge to pull the wound apart, we found

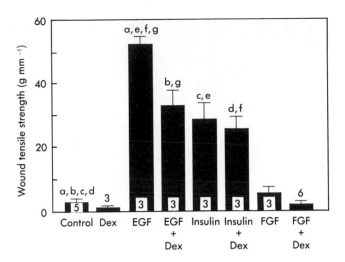

Figure 20-18

Comparison of effect of drug treatments on the tensile strength of perforating incisions in the center of rabbit corneas. The incisions were treated with two drops three times a day for 5 days with the following drugs: no medication *(control)*, dexamethazone 1 mg/ml *(dex)*, epidermal growth factor 0.5 mg/ml *(EGF)*, epidermal growth factor plus dexamethasone *(EGF + dex)*, insulin 0.5 mg/ml, insulin plus dexamethasone, fibroblastic growth factor 20 mg/ml (FGF), and fibroblastic growth factor plus dexamethasone. *a, b, c, d, p* less than 0.001; *e, f, p* less than 0.01; *g, p* less than 0.025. Epidermal growth factor produced the greatest tensile wound strength. (From Woost PG, Brightwell J, Eiferman RA, and Schultz GS: Exp Eye Rcs 1985;40:47-60.)

EGFR increased tensile strength approximately tenfold compared with a saline control. The addition of topical corticosteroids along with EGF only slightly depressed the tensile strength but still resulted in approximately a sevenfold increase over control eyes[77] (Fig. 20-18). Similar results were found with nonsutured incisions in primates treated topically with EGF and corticosteroids (Fig. 20-19). Histologic evaluation of incisions in primate corneas revealed that in untreated eyes the epithelial plug extended the full depth of the incision with minimal signs of stromal healing, while eyes with EGF treatment had a smaller epithelial plug that extended approximately one third of the depth of the incision and new collagen production with more extensive scar formation. Liebowitz and colleagues[47] reported an increase in wound strength in full-thickness wounds in rabbit corneas 9 days after wounding with the use of topical mouse and human epidermal growth factor. The wounds were 2 to 2½ times as strong with a twice daily administration of 10 mg/ml of human epidermal growth factor.

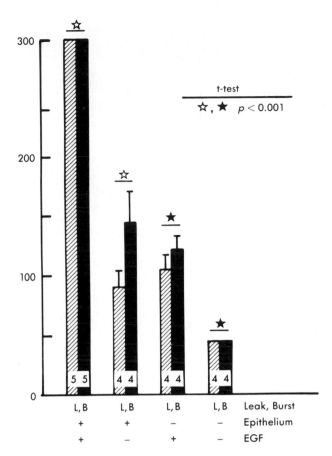

Figure 20-19

Effect of epidermal growth factor *(EGF)* on strength of corneal wounds in monkeys. A full-thickness corneal laceration 5 mm long was made in the center of the cornea. Corneal epithelium was left adjacent to the incision and allowed to heal (+) or was removed by n-octanol and scraping (−). Left eyes were treated with two drops three times daily of hEGF (0.1 mg/ml) in neomycin-dexamethasone (NeoDecadron) solution, and the right eyes received the same treatment with NeoDecadron alone. After 9 days of treatment a cannula was inserted into the anterior chamber and the pressure was increased and measured with an aneroid manometer. The pressure that caused the wound first to leak *(L)* and then to burst *(B)* was measured. The numbers of corneas tested for each circumstance are shown inside the bars. The values plotted are the means with the standard error of the means. Mean bursting pressures for corneas under the open stars (or closed stars) were compared for statistically significant differences by the paired *t* test. Corneas with an intact epithelium treated by epidermal growth factor withstood pressures up to 300 mm Hg (higher pressures were not tried), whereas those wounds with either absent epithelium or absent EGF burst at much lower pressures. This indicates that both the epithelium and the epidermal growth factor contribute to the rate and strength of stromal wound healing. (From Brightwell JR, Riddle SL, Eiferman RA, et al: Invest Ophthalmol Vis Sci 1985;26:105-110.)

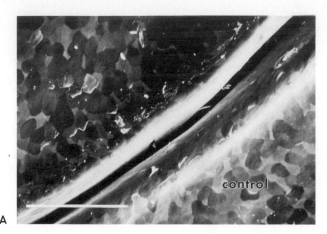

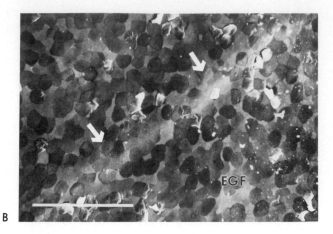

Figure 20-20
Scanning electron micrographs of a partial-thickness radial keratotomy in the cat cornea 7 days postoperatively. **A,** After treatment with phosphate-buffered saline, the wound gaped open with some epithelium growing down the sides of the wound. **B,** After treatment with epidermal growth factor (EGF), the wound bed *(arrows)* filled completely and was covered by well-differentiated epithelium (bars = 250 μm).

Epidermal growth factor and radial keratotomy in cats and monkeys. The effect of EGF on radial keratotomy was studied in the cat. Slit-lamp microscope examination showed that all animals treated with EGF appeared to heal faster than controls. The surface of a cornea treated for 7 days with saline revealed wide, unhealed incisions, but the surface of the opposite eye treated topically with EGF at 10 hg/ml revealed only a slight depression covered by an intact epithelial layer (Fig. 20-20). Transmission electron microscopy of the cornea treated with phosphate buffered saline (PBS) showed the epithelium had migrated down the sides of the radial keratotomy incision, but a wide gap remained between the cut edges of the stroma (Fig. 20-21). In contrast, the tract of the radial keratotomy incision treated with EGF was filled with an epithelial plug and with keratocytes that contained marked amounts of rough endoplasmic reticulum, suggesting active synthesis protein (including collagen) and other extracellular matrix material. The epithelium was healed over the wound, with a continuous basement membrane containing hemidesmosomes. Photokeratography showed central corneal flattening as much as 19 D in the EGF-treated eyes, as opposed to 2 or 3 D in the controls.

Clinical use of growth factors in refractive surgery. With the advent of genetic engineering, bioactive mitogenic agents can be produced commercially in large quantities. We think there is an important clinical role for these molecules, since they are naturally occurring hormones that are not carcinogenic, mutagenic, or teratogenic. They may prove to be useful in promoting wound healing in all areas of ophthalmic surgery, but as of 1991, none has shown clinical applicability.

Fibronectins

The ubiquitous presence of fibronectins in the body has spawned widespread study, creating a field of research that is changing rapidly and has been summarized in books and monographs.[16,34]

Fibronectin is an adhesive protein that acts as a biologic organizer by holding cells in position and guiding their migration. It is a glycoprotein that is one of the components of the extracellular matrix. Discovered in 1948, fibronectin (L. *fibra,* fiber + *nectere,* to connect) is synthesized by a variety of cells including fibroblasts, vascular and corneal endothelium, and macrophages. It is found in particularly high concentration in areas of cell migration, in basement membranes, and in loose connective tissue. Chemically, plasma fibronectin is a dimer of two similar polypeptides connected at one end by disulfide bonds (Fig. 20-22). Along each of the molecules, specific domains have been characterized as binding specific extracellular components, including domains for fibrin, collagen, cell receptors, and heparin. Fibronectin's role in mediating cell migration and adhesion occurs because of its ability to attach to both cells and components of the extracellular matrix.

In addition to enhancing cell migration and attach-

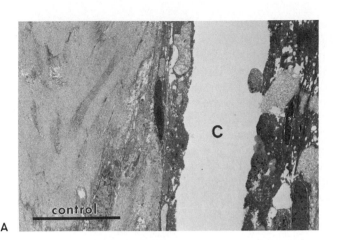

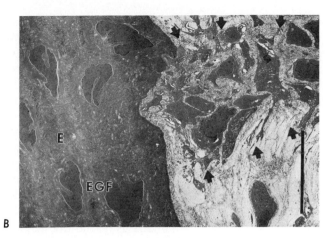

Figure 20-21

Transmission electron micrographs of a radial keratotomy incision in a cat cornea 7 days postoperatively. **A,** After treatment with phosphate-buffered saline (control), the unhealed incision demonstrated a clear zone *(C)* with an epithelial layer on each edge. The adjacent stroma had minimal keratocyte activity and no new collagen had been synthesized. **B,** After treatment with EGF, the wound was filled with epithelial cells *(E)* and the adjacent stroma contained many fibroblasts and new extracellular matrix *(between arrows)* (bar = 10 μm).

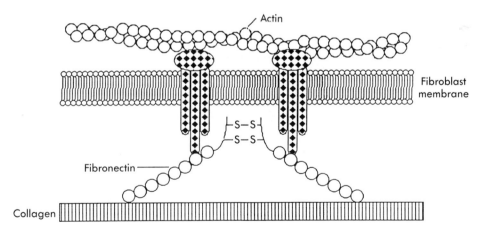

Figure 20-22

Illustration of the role of fibronectin in cellular migration and attachment. The specific binding domains on the fibronectin molecule attach the fibroblast to the extracellular collagen. Attachment to the fibroblast is mediated by a transmembrane protein known as integrin *(long ovals with diamonds)* that connects to an intracellular protein known as vinculin *(short ovals with diamonds),* that attaches to the contractile actin molecule. (Courtesy Chiron Ophthalmics.[16])

ment, fibronectin serves as a chemotactic agent for endothelial cells, fibroblasts, and epithelial cells—all important in corneal wound healing after keratotomy. The molecular domains responsible for this activity are less well defined.

Fibronectin is found throughout the cornea, concentrated most densely in the epithelial basement membrane and the anterior portion of Descemet's membrane, but also being present in the stroma, Bowman's layer, and the endothelium. Apparently the corneal epithelium itself does not synthesize fibronectin, and its presence in the epithelium basement membrane may be from the tears. During wound healing the amount of fibronectin increases within the wound. However, as the epithelium spreads over these wounds, the fibronectin falls to much lower levels, largely disappearing when wound healing is complete. The cells producing fibronectin during corneal healing have not been accurately identified, but stromal keratocytes seem likely. Ohashi and colleagues[56] showed that one day after the application of a heated brass rod in the center of the rabbit cornea, keratocytes had completely disappeared from the burned region and fibronectin could be detected only in the anterior and posterior stromal surfaces. As keratocytes began to migrate into the stromal lesion by day 3, fibronectin was present at the margin of the lesions as well as on both sides of Descemet's membrane. The mechanisms of degradation and removal of fibronectin may involve the plasminogen activator–plasmin system, since plasmin can degrade fibronectin.

Currently, fibronectin is isolated from both human and animal plasma, being purified by chromotography, after which it is heated to inactivate potential viral contaminates, including HIV.

Falcone and colleagues[21] demonstrated that exogeneous fibronectin can increase wound strength and the amount of force required to break wounds in the skin between 7 and 21 days after incisions, the amount of force required to break the fibronectin-treated wounds being about 30% greater than that of the untreated controls. Fibronectin has been used therapeutically to treat nonhealing epithelial defects in humans, often with a result in reepithelization of these wounds that had lain dormant for weeks to months[54]; however, it has not been approved by the United States FDA for clinical use as of 1991.

Berkeley has reported results of a multicenter, single-masked, randomized, controlled trial of topical recombinant DNA–synthesized fibronectin in human radial keratotomy cases. Patients used two drops of fibronectin solution four times daily for the first 7 days after surgery. At one day there was a difference in the mean keratometric power between the two groups, the control group showing a larger initial effect with an average keratometric power of 39.6 D compared with 41.1 D in the fibronectin group. However, no statistical differences in average keratometric readings were seen between the two groups at any of the study intervals. There was a suggestion that the fibronectin-treated eyes remained more stable throughout the 3 months of follow-up than the placebo group. Further studies are needed to determine whether fibronectin will become a clinically useful drug after refractive keratotomy.

Corneal mortar

Combinations of extracellular matrix components including fibronectin, chondroitin sulfate, and epidermal growth factor might be useful in promoting wound healing after radial keratotomy, particularly if they could be delivered in a vehicle such as a biodegradable film that could hold the keratotomy wound in the desired configuration during healing. Such a product has been labeled corneal mortar and has undergone testing in owl monkeys. The mortar is inserted into the keratotomy wound immediately after surgery with the purpose of keeping the wound spread open and providing continuous contact between the drugs and the tissues; this would stimulate wound healing and provide a scaffolding in which wound healing can occur.

We placed corneal mortar into the radial keratotomy incisions in owl monkeys. The photokeratographs taken 2 weeks after surgery indicated a substantial flattening of the cornea, approximately 9 D in ring 1 and 4.4 D in ring 2. These changes were stable for several weeks. Histopathologic examination demonstrated that the base of the incisions treated with corneal mortar was much wider than controls (Fig. 20-23) and that a substantial number of active fibroblasts populated the scar with the abundant production of new extracellular matrix (Fig. 20-24). In contrast, the control keratotomy incisions were narrow and contained few keratocytes and scant extracellular matrix.

Although these early experiments have been encouraging, their transition to clinical experimentation has been very slow. The Food and Drug Administration does not allow the initial testing of combination drugs, so each of the components of corneal mortar must be tested individually first, as done for fibronectin in the Berkeley study of fibronectin mentioned previously. Thus it will be many years before a practical combination of wound healing drugs will be developed for use in refractive keratotomy.

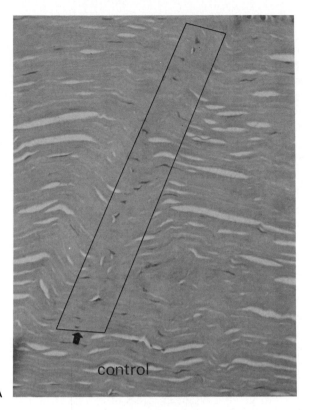 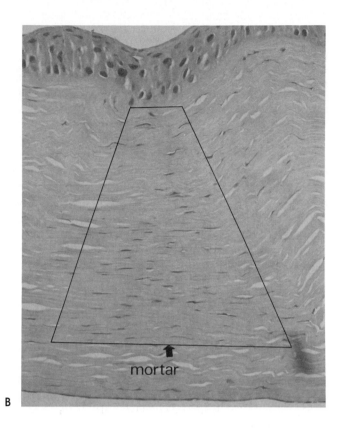

Figure 20-23

Effect of corneal mortar on stromal wound healing after radial keratotomy in the owl monkey at 170 days after surgery. The wound margins are outlined in the boxes; the depth of the wounds is indicated by an arrow. **A,** In an untreated incision the wound is narrow, with only a slight increase in fibroblasts and scar tissue. **B,** The wound filled with corneal mortar has the shape of an inverted pyramid, wider in the posterior stroma and narrower near the epithelial side. The wound is filled with numerous fibroblasts and newly produced extracellular matrix (hematoxylin and eosin, ×200).

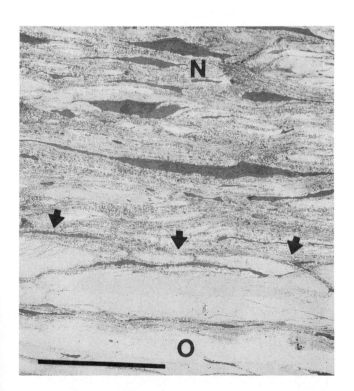

Figure 20-24

Transmission electron micrograph taken from the base of the corneal wound treated with corneal mortar. The original, unincised stroma *(O)* is sparsely populated with keratocytes, whereas the newly produced scar in the mortar-filled keratotomy wound *(N)* is densely packed with fibroblasts and horizontally arranged new collagen and extracellular matrix. The arrows indicate the junction between these two zones (bar = 10 μm).

Drugs that decrease corneal wound healing

For the clinician to modulate pharmacologically the shape of the cornea after keratotomy, drugs must be available that retard wound healing, as well as stimulate it. This would be particularly useful in patients who are undercorrected, where slower, less efficient, less strong wound healing might be desirable to enhance the effect of the surgery.

Glucocorticosteroids. A description of the structure and function of corticosteroids is far beyond the scope of this chapter. Even its role in wound healing, which has been extensively described in the literature, is complex enough to preclude a thorough review here. We summarize the salient facts as might be applied to keratotomy.

Topical corticosteroids slow normal corneal wound healing. Gasset and colleagues[28] showed that topical dexamethasone decreased the tensile strength of full-thickness corneal wounds in rabbits, demonstrating a dose-response effect and clarifying previous contradictory studies about the effect of steroid treatment on corneal wound healing. For example, dexamethasone 0.1% given every hour for 12 hours for 11 days after wounding allowed the 5-mm wounds to rupture with 58 ±8 g of force, whereas the untreated controlled eyes required 102 ±11 g of force. Phillips and colleagues[60] demonstrated the effectiveness of both prednisolone and medroxyprogesterone on the strength of healing corneal wounds in rabbits. One week after 3-mm linear perforating wounds, topical 1% prednisolone given six times daily suppressed the wound tensile strength by 20%, and medroxyprogesterone suppressed it by 11%. In addition, after full-thickness trephination, drug administered for 14 days decreased collagen formation in the scar buttons by 43% in the prednisolone-treated group and 39% in the medroxyprogesterone-treated group.

Durant and colleagues[20] have reviewed the factors involved in the control of fibroblast proliferation by glucocorticoids. Glucocorticoids tend to decrease proliferation of in vitro cultures of human fibroblasts, but the effects differ greatly according to the species, age, and tissue origin of the cells. By using an in vivo model more relevant to corneal wound healing, Polack and Rosen[61] demonstrated that topically applied dexamethasone decreased the number of labeled fibroblasts twofold following central transcorneal freezing in rabbit corneas. The specific effect of glucocorticoids on myofibroblast is unknown. Glucocorticoids have less effect on healing corneal epithelium than on the fibroblasts and keratocytes of the stroma.

At the molecular level, corticosteroids influence the genetic regulation of collagen synthesis by reducing the formation for procollagen messenger RNA. The molecular control of collagenases in stromal melting and in normal wound remodeling is also affected by glucocorticoids, but the interactions are complex.[20]

Some surgeons use topical corticosteroids for a few weeks after surgery to decrease the postoperative inflammation and to enhance the effect of the surgery. The only published study of topical corticosteroids on the results of keratotomy is the abstract by Hayes and colleagues.[32] They studied 41 eyes that were part of the PERK study and were treated postoperatively with only topical gentamicin drops four times daily for 2 weeks and 50 eyes that were operated by a different surgeon in a similar manner, which received subconjunctival gentamicin and betamethasone at surgery followed by topical dexamethasone 0.1% with neomycin and polymixin (Maxitrol) for a few weeks. In eyes with a 3.0-mm clear zone, the average change in refraction at 6 months was +3.99 D in the untreated PERK group and +5.26 D in the steroid-treated group. In the 3.5-mm clear zone groups, the change at 6 months in the untreated PERK group was +3.07 D and in the treated group +3.67 D. The difference was statistically significant in the 3.0-mm group but not in the 3.5-mm group. Whether short-term topical corticosteroids affect the final outcome of radial keratotomy remains to be determined.

Betaaminopropionitrile. Betaaminopropionitrile (BAPN) is a compound that irreversibly inhibits the enzyme lysil hydroxylase, preventing the cross linking of collagen.[53] It has been used to decrease scarring in conjunctival alkali burns in rabbits and in human urethral strictures.[58]

Topical BAPN significantly decreases the tensile strength of full-thickness corneal incisions in rabbits, presumably by decreasing the cross-linking of the newly produced collagen. However, the experimental evidence about the effect of topically applied BAPN to the outcome of radial keratotomy incisions is inconsistent. Moorhead and colleagues[53] postulated that topical BAPN would increase the flexibility of the keratotomy scar and reduce wound contraction and regression after radial keratotomy, enhancing the effect. At 6 to 8 weeks after surgery in rabbits, the BAPN-treated group showed a mean reduction of 1.85 ±0.13 D in corneal curvature compared with 1.18 ±0.08 D in the control group. A study of the compliance and strength of the corneas demonstrated that the BAPN-treated corneas changed curvature more than the controls at the same pressures. Another preliminary report showed a 20% enhancement of radial keratotomy in rabbits.[43] Contrary findings were demonstrated by Busin and colleagues,[11] who observed that rabbits treated with topical BAPN or d-penicillamine three times daily for 6 weeks had similar mean changes in keratometric power readings at 6 weeks (BAPN, 5.81 D; control, 6.58 D) and 4 months (BAPN, 6.81 D;

control, 7.35 D) after surgery. It has been well demonstrated, however, that the rabbit cornea is a poor model for studying keratotomy. In addition, it is extremely hard to obtain refractive, keratometric, or keratographic data from rabbits. BAPN has found no clinical use in refractive keratotomy.

Garret and colleagues[27] studied the effect of a topical smooth muscle antagonist, thiphenamil, to inhibit wound contracture in the cornea by inhibiting the myofibroblasts. Slit-lamp microscope examination and light microscopy suggested that transient inhibition of wound contracture lasted approximately 1 week.

ROLE OF CORNEAL WOUND HEALING IN REFRACTIVE KERATOTOMY

Corneal wound healing is a major determinant of the outcome of refractive keratotomy. Even if surgical techniques could be designed that were absolutely accurate and repeatable, once the wounds are made in the cornea, the surgeon and the patient must simply wait for the somewhat random results of wound healing to determine the final outcome. To date, no drugs are available for use clinically to modify these events predictably.

In the early wound healing phase, there is a loss of the initial refractive effect in almost all eyes, probably resulting from a decrease in the stromal edema as the epithelial barrier is reconstituted and from contraction of the wound scar by myofibroblasts and by collagen cross-linking. Once this acute process is concluded, long-term instability has been demonstrated in approximately 20% of eyes, most of these showing a continuing increase in the effect of the surgery, which suggests that the wounds are not completely healed and that there is slight spreading of the keratotomy scar tissue over time. A few eyes show a progressive loss of the effect of the surgery, which might suggest prolonged wound contracture (see Chapter 24, Stability of Refraction after Refractive Keratotomy). Stabilizing the wounds pharmacologically would improve the predictability of refractive keratotomy.

Permanent weakening of the cornea results from severing the stromal collagen fibrils that normally extend from limbus to limbus and substituting less strong scar tissue. This may allow rupture of the cornea in the case of direct severe trauma to the globe. Pharmacologic agents that create stronger wounds might decrease this complication.

UNFINISHED BUSINESS

Without doubt, the most difficult factor to measure and control after refractive keratotomy is corneal wound healing. Even if a perfectly replicable surgical technique were available, the presumed variability in corneal wound healing among different patients would interfere with the predictability of outcome in an individual case. Two aspects of wound healing need research: (1) the measurement of the wounds and wound healing strength and stability and (2) drugs to predictably modulate the wound healing process—both tall orders. To measure the configuration of a wound, an imaging device based on the principles of the slit-lamp microscope that could create cross sections of a wound and measure its volume would be useful. To measure wound strength and stability, an in vivo method such as holography[12] could be used but is technically very difficult. Such a device might also be used to measure the stress in the normal unincised cornea to give an indication of how different corneas might respond to the same amount of surgery. To speed wound healing, drugs that increase the formation and migration of fibroblasts and increase the synthesis and assembly of collagen and proteoglycans are required. Such substances could be placed in the keratotomy wound at the time of surgery or used topically postoperatively, although their effect on the normal unincised cornea would have to be controlled. The molecules currently known to be active in corneal wound healing, such as laminin, fibronectin, vinculin, and growth factors, form a good basis for research.

Accelerating corneal wound healing may not always be desirable, and drugs that interfere with corneal wound healing should be developed. Corticosteroids are currently the only practical drugs available. They play a valuable role in reducing corneal healing and scarring after photorefractive keratectomy (see Chapter 19, Laser Corneal Surgery) but do not provide a controlled or a predictable method of "setting" keratotomy wounds.

REFERENCES

1. Anderson JA, Murphy JA, and Gaster RN: Inflammatory cell responses to radial keratotomy, Refract Corneal Surg 1989;5:21-26.

2. Binder PS: Optical problems following refractive surgery, Ophthalmology 1986; 93:739-745.

3. Binder PS: Presumed epithelial ingrowth following radial keratotomy, CLAO J 1986;12:247-255.

4. Binder PS, Able R, Polack FM, et al: Keratoplasty wound separations, Am J Ophthalmol 1975;80:105-111.

5. Binder PS, Nayak SK, Deg JK, Zavala EY, and Sugar J: An ultrastructural and histochemical study of long-term wound healing after radial keratotomy, Am J Ophthalmol 1987;103:432-440.

6. Binder PS, Waring GO, Arrowsmith PN, and Wang C: Histopathology of traumatic rupture of the cornea after radial keratotomy, Arch Ophthalmol 1988; 106:1584-1590.

7. Binder PS, Wickham MG, Zavala EY, and Arens PH: Corneal anatomy and wound healing. In Symposium on medical and surgical diseases of the cornea, St Louis, 1980, Mosby–Year Book, Inc, pp 1-35.

8. Binder RF and Binder HF: Regenerative processes in the endothelium of the cornea, Arch Ophthalmol 1957;57:11-13.

9. Brightwell JR, Riddle SL, Eiferman RA, Valenzuela P, Barr PJ, Merryweather JP, and Schultz GS: Biosynthetic human EGF accelerates healing of NeoDecadron-treated primate corneas, Invest Ophthalmol Vis Sci 1985;26 (suppl):105.

10. Brown G, Brightwell J, Curtsinger L, Polk H, Merryweather J, Valenzuela P, and Schultz G: Enhancement of epidermal regeneration by biosynthetic growth factor, J Exp Med 1986; 163:1319-1322.

11. Busin M, Uyau CW, Yamaguchi T, McDonald MB, and Kaufman HE: The effect of collagen cross-linkage inhibitors on rabbit corneas after radial keratotomy, Invest Ophthalmol Vis Sci 1986;27:1001-1005.

12. Calkins JL, Hochheimer BF, and Start WJ: Corneal wound healing: holographic stress-test analysis, Invest Ophthalmol Vis Sci 1981;21:322-324.

13. Capella JA: Regeneration of endothelium in diseased and injured corneas, Am J Ophthalmol 1972;74:810-817.

14. Carpenter G and Cohen S: Epidermal growth factor, Annu Rev Biochem 1979;48:193-216.

15. Chi HH, Teng CC, and Katzin HM: Healing process in the mechanical denudation of the corneal endothelium, Am J Ophthalmol 1960;49:693-703.

16. Chiron Ophthalmics: Epidermal growth factor, monograph published by Chiron Ophthalmics, 15A Marconi, Irvine, CA 92718, 14 pp.

17. Clintworth GK and Smith CF: A comparative study of extracellular sulfated glycosaminoglycans synthesized by rabbit corneal fibroblasts in organ and confluent cultures, Lab Invest 1976;35: 258-263.

18. Deg JK, Zavala EY, and Binder PS: Delayed corneal wound healing following radial keratotomy, Ophthalmology 1985;92:734-740.

19. Doughman DJ, Van Horn D, Rodman WP, et al: Human corneal endothelial layer repair during organ culture, Arch Ophthalmol 1976;94:1791-1796.

20. Durant S, Duva D, and Homo-Delarche R: Factors involved in the control of fibroblast proliferation by glucocorticoids, Endocr Rev 1986;7:254-269.

21. Falcone PA, Bonaventure AM, Turner DC, and Fromm D: The effect of exogenous fibronectin on wound breaking strength, Plast Reconstr Surg 1984;74: 809-812.

22. Farley MK and Pettit TH: Traumatic wound dehiscence after penetrating keratoplasty, Am J Ophthalmol 1987; 104:44-49.

23. Feldman ST: The effect of epidermal growth factor on corneal wound healing: practical considerations for therapeutic use, Refract Corneal Surg (in press).

24. Forstot SL and Damiano RE: Trauma following radial keratotomy (RK), Ophthalmology 1988;95:833-835.

25. Fyodorov SN, Sarkizova MB, and Kurasovat P: Corneal biomicroscopy following repeated radial keratotomy, Am J Ophthalmol 1983;15:403-407.

26. Gabbiani G, Hirschel BJ, Ryan BG, et al: Granulation tissue as a contractile organ: a study of structure and function, J Exp Med 1972;135:719-734.

27. Garrett C, Pressley E, Prager TC, and Moorhead LC: The use of thiphenamil hydrochloride (Trocinate) to control wound contraction after radial keratotomy, Ophthalmic Surg 1986;18:428-431.

28. Gasset AR and Dohlman CH: The tensile strength of corneal wounds, Arch Ophthalmol 1968;79:595-602.

29. Girard LJ, Rodriguez L, Nino N, et al: Delayed wound healing after radial keratotomy, Am J Ophthalmol 1985;99:485-486.

30. Haik BG and Zimny ML: Scanning electron microscopy of corneal wound healing in the rabbit, Invest Ophthalmol Vis Sci 1977;16(suppl):787.

31. Hanna K: Proliferation and migration of epithelial cells during cornea wound repair in the rabbit and the rat, Am J Ophthalmol 1966;61:55-62.

32. Hayes JC, Rowsey JJ, and Balyeat H: Effect of postoperative steroids on the refractive results of radial keratotomy, Invest Ophthalmol Vis Sci 1985;26 (suppl):150.

33. Ho P and Elliott J: Kinetics of corneal epithelial regeneration: epidermal growth factor and topical corticosteroids, Invest Ophthalmol Vis Sci 1975; 14:630-634.

34. Hynes RO: Fibronectins, Sci Am 1986; 254:42-51.

35. Ingraham HJ, Guber D, and Green WR. Radial keratotomy—clinical pathologic case reports, Arch Ophthalmol 1985; 103:683-688.

36. Jester JV, Steele D, Salz J, et al: Radial keratotomy in non-human primate eyes, Am J Ophthalmol 1981;92:153-161.

37. Jester JV, Villasenor RA, and Miyashiro J: Epithelial inclusion cysts following radial keratotomy, Arch Ophthalmol 1983;101:611-615.

38. John ME Jr and Schmitt TE: Traumatic hyphema after radial keratotomy, Ann Ophthalmol 1983;15:930-932.

39. Johnson-Muller B, and Gross J: Regulation of corneal collagenase production: epithelial stromal cell interactions, Proc Natl Acad Sci USA 1978;75:4417.

40. Johnson-Wint B: Regulation of stromal cell collagenase production in an adult rabbit cornea: in vitro stimulation and inhibition by epithelial cell products, Proc Natl Acad Sci USA 1980;77:5531.

41. Karr DJ, Grutzmacher RD, and Reeh MJ: Radial keratotomy complicated by sterile keratitis and corneal perforation: histopathologic case report and review of complications, Ophthalmology 1985; 92:1244-1248.

42. Kitano S and Goldman JN: Cytologic and histochemical changes in cornea wound repair, Arch Ophthalmol 1966; 76:345-354.

43. Kogan LL and Katzen L: Enhancement of radial keratotomy by chemical inhibition of collagen cross-linkages: a preliminary report, Ann Ophthalmol 1983;15:842-845.

44. Kuwabara T, Perkins DG, and Cogan DG: Sliding of the epithelium in experimental corneal wounds, Invest Ophthalmol 1976;15(suppl):4.

45. Larson BC, Kremer FB, Eller AW, et al: Quantitated trauma following radial keratotomy in rabbits, Ophthalmology 1983;90:660-667.

46. Leonardy NJ, Smith CF, Brown CF, and Clintworth GK: Intercellular relationships in the synthesis of macromolecules by organ cultures of corneas, Invest Ophthalmol Vis Sci 1985;26:1216-1222.

47. Liebowitz HM, Morello S, Stern M, and Kupferman A: Effect of topically administered epidermal growth factor on corneal wound strength, Arch Ophthalmol 1990;108:734-737.

48. Luttrull JK, Jester JV, and Smith RE: The effect of radial keratotomy on ocular integrity in an animal model, Arch Ophthalmol 1982;100:319-320.

49. Mandelbaum S, Waring GO, Forster RK, Culbertson WW, Rowsey JJ, and Espinal ME: Late development of ulcerative keratitis in radial keratotomy scars, Arch Ophthalmol 1986;104:1156-1160.

50. Mathers WE and Lemp MA: Corneal scarring: the evolution of scarring following penetrating keratoplasty. In Cavanagh DW, editor: The cornea: transactions of the World Congress on the Cornea, New York, 1988, Raven Press, pp 373-375.

51. McDonnell PJ, Lean JS, and Schanzlin DJ: Globe rupture from blunt trauma after hexagonal keratotomy, Am J Ophthalmol 1987;103:241-242.

52. Moorhead LC: Inhibition of collagen cross linking: a new approach to ocular scarring, Curr Eye Res 1981;9:77-83.

53. Moorhead LC, Carroll J, Constance G, et al: Effects of topical treatment with beta-aminopropionitrile after radial keratotomy in the rabbit, Arch Ophthalmol 1984;102:304-307.

54. Nishida T, Nakagawa S, and Manabe R: Clinical evaluation of fibronectin eye drops on epithelial disorders after herpes keratitis, Ophthalmology 1985;92:213-216.

55. O'Day DM, Feman SS, and Elliot JH: Visual impairment following radial keratotomy: a cluster of cases, Ophthalmology 1985;92:72-76.

56. Ohashi Y, Nakagawa S, Nishida T, Suda T, Watanabe K, and Manabe R: Pairs of fibronectin rabbit cornea after thermal burn, Jpn J Ophthalmol 1983;27:547-555.

57. Palkama A, Uusitalo R, Lehtosalo J, and Uusitalo H: Histochemical analysis of wound healing in radial keratotomy, Invest Ophthalmol Vis Sci 1987;28 (suppl):223.

58. Peacock EE and Madden JW: Administration of beta-aminopropionitrile to human beings with urethral strictures: a preliminary report, Am J Surg 1978; 136:600-605.

59. Pfister RR: The healing of corneal epithelial abrasions in the rabbit: a scanning electron microscope study, Invest Ophthalmol 1975;14(suppl):648.

60. Phillips K, Arffa R, Cintron C, Rose J, Miller D, Kublin CL, and Kenyon KR: Effects of prednisolone and medroxyprogestrone on corneal wound healing, ulceration, and neovascularization, Arch Ophthalmol 1983;101:640-643.

61. Polack FM and Rosen PN: Topical steroids and titrated thymidine uptake, Arch Ophthalmol 1967;77:400-404.

62. Randa MR, Garana W, Petroll M, Fend W, Cavanagh HD, and Jester JV: Cell biology of corneal wound fibroblasts: mechanism of wound contraction in radial keratotomy (RK), Invest Ophthalmol Vis Sci 1990;31(suppl):3.

63. Recupero SM, Feher J, and Contestabile MT: Radial keratotomy: histopathological changes in rabbits, Ital J Ophthalmol 1989;3:77-80.

64. Robb RM and Kuwabara T: Corneal wound healing. II. An autoradiographic study of the cellular components, Arch Ophthalmol 1964;72:401-408.

65. Rylander HG, Welch AJ, and Fremming B: The effect of radial keratotomy in the rupture strength of pig eyes, Ophthalmic Surg 1983;14:774-779.

66. Seemayer TA, Lagace R, Schurch W, et al: The myofibroblast: biologic, pathologic and theoretical considerations. In Sommers W, editor: Pathology annual, New York, 1980, Appleton-Century Crofts, pp 443-470.

67. Sherrard ES: The corneal endothelium in vivo: its response to mild trauma, Exp Eye Res 1976;22:347-357.

68. Simons KB and Linslata RP: Ruptured globe following blunt trauma after radial keratotomy: a case report, J Refract Surg 1988;4:132-135.

69. Smelser GK and Ozanics V: Reaction of the cornea to injury and wound healing: symposium on the cornea, Transactions of the New Orleans Academy of Ophthalmology, St Louis, 1972, Mosby–Year Book, Inc.

70. Spivak L: Case report: radial keratotomy incisions remain intact despite facial trauma from plane crash, J Refract Surg 1987;3:59-60.

71. Srinivasan BD, Worgul BV, Iwamoto T, and Eakins KE: The reepithelialization of rabbit cornea following partial and complete epithelial denudation, Exp Eye Res 1977;25:343-351.

72. Stainer GA, Shaw EL, Binder PS, et al: Histopathology of a case of radial keratotomy, Arch Ophthalmol 1982;100: 1473-1477.

73. Tenner A, Neuhann T, Schroder E, Salz JJ, and Maguen E: Excimer laser radial keratotomy in the living human eye: a preliminary report, J Refract Surg 1988;4:5-8.

74. Tripathi BJ, Kwait PS, and Tripathi RC: Corneal growth factors: a new generation of ophthalmic pharmaceuticals, Cornea 1990;9:2-9.

75. Van Horn DL, Sendelee DD, Seideman S, et al: Regenerative capacity of the corneal endothelium in the rabbit and cat, Invest Ophthalmol Vis Sci 1977; 16:597-613.

76. Waring GO, Steinberg EB, and Wilson LA: Slit-lamp microscopic appearance after corneal wound healing, Am J Ophthalmol 1985;100:218-224.

77. Woost PG, Brightwell JR, Eiferman RA, and Schultz GS: Effect of growth factors with dexamethasone on healing of rabbit corneal stromal incisions, Exp Eye Res 1985;40:47-60.

78. Yamaguchi T, Tamaki K, Kaufman HE, et al: Histologic study of a pair of human corneas after anterior radial keratotomy, Am J Ophthalmol 1985;100: 281-292.

79. Yamaguchi T, Tamaki K, Nakata S, Nakajima A, and Kaufman HE: Long-term histologic evaluation of wound healing after anterior radial keratotomy in rabbits, Invest Ophthalmol Vis Sci 1988;29(suppl):391.

80. Yano M and Tanishima T: Wound healing in rabbit corneal endothelium, Jpn J Ophthalmol 1980;24:297-309.

Results of Refractive Keratotomy

George O. Waring III
Katherine K. Lindstrom

Since Fyodorov's first report of anterior radial keratotomy was published in English in 1979 numerous clinical studies of radial keratotomy have been reported. The type and quality of these reports vary widely. There are preliminary observations on small series, series done and reported in books published by the author without peer review, series with 30% or more loss to follow-up, series in which analysis is extensive but confusing, large series presented with anecdotal summary statistics, informal trials with long follow-up, and one formal multicenter trial. Each such study has something to offer, sometimes early information that was later validated or shown to be incorrect and at other times valuable insights and observations that influenced the execution of radial keratotomy. One thing is clear: the studies cannot be pooled. They are too disparate. On the other hand, to survey the results of all the studies gives a general impression of the outcome of radial keratotomy.

TWO GROUPS OF STUDIES

To summarize the published studies we have resorted to presentation in tabular form and have divided the studies into two groups. The first group consists

BACKGROUND AND ACKNOWLEDGMENTS
The profusion of reports of case series of refractive keratotomy by authors from around the world threatened to overwhelm us as we attempted to summarize the extant literature. After attempting various types of narrative and integrative summaries, which invariably ended up as a seemingly endless, numbing recitation of figures, we elected a tabular format to summarize the published results of these studies. The topics that we included are those we believe should be covered in all publications regarding refractive surgery. Of course, not all articles contain all of the information, and sometimes the method of presenting the information was not easy to summarize in a tabular manner. Thus we have had to interpret and interpolate in some places, and we take responsibility for any errors or inadvertent misrepresentations that may have resulted. In some instances we contacted the authors directly for clarification. The interpretative comments by Dr. Waring represent his point of view, not necessarily that intended by the original authors. These comments have not been submitted to peer review.

We acknowledge and thank all the authors not only for their original publications but also for their help in making this summary as accurate and intelligible as possible. We apologize to those whose work we have omitted.

of the 5-year results of the PERK study, the 5-year results of Arrowsmith and Marks, and the 1-year results of Deitz and Sanders. These are the best published studies of radial keratotomy for the following reasons: (1) they are prospective; (2) data were analyzed independently by a biostatistician at a different institution than that of the surgeon; (3) the surgeons in all three groups have published multiple articles analyzing their experience with radial keratotomy, including information on long-term stability and predictability of outcome, all in peer-review journals; (4) the surgeons have long experience with radial keratotomy, stemming from 1980; and (5) the studies involved collaboration between ophthalmologists in private practice and those in university centers. Of course, there are many differences among the three studies, including variable surgical techniques and different loss to follow-up rates. Interestingly the general conclusions and results from the three studies are quite similar and taken together provide a good picture of the results of refractive keratotomy.

The second grouping of studies presents an extensive listing of published articles that report results of a series of refractive keratotomy cases. Annotations within each table are intended to clarify the information presented. More thorough discussion of clinical testing is found in Chapter 4, of variables affecting outcome in Chapter 26, of surgical instruments in Chapter 15, of surgical techniques in Chapters 17 and 32, of stability in Chapter 24, and of complications in Chapter 23.

SELECTION CRITERIA FOR REPORTED SERIES

The purpose of publishing the results of these many studies is to display in one place the comparative methodologies and outcome of studies of refractive keratotomy. Of necessity, the studies included have been selected, since there is not room to present every single report of clinical results that has been published. The criteria used for selection of reports are summarized in the box above. We have modeled the table after one in Curtis Meinert's book, *Clinical Trials: Design, Conduct, and Analysis,* New York, Oxford University

---

Criteria for Selection of Articles on Refractive Keratotomy

1. Minimum follow-up of 6 months
2. Omission of "preliminary reports"
3. Data presented in a manner that can be compared with other reports.
4. Published in peer-reviewed journal (some exceptions)

Press, 1986, pp. 327-346. We have selected articles from peer-reviewed journals primarily, with an occasional article from a non–peer reviewed source. Exceptions are made in two instances where material was published in book form that had not appeared in the periodical literature. We have selected articles that present a series of cases with a reasonable follow-up. Some reports simply represented so little information that a comparison with the results of others was almost meaningless, and these have been omitted as well.

Two major aspects of each study are emphasized: (1) *study design,* which reflects the quality of the information and results being presented, and (2) *study results,* conveyed in terms of refraction and visual acuity. We have omitted results of keratometric measurements because we do not think they are directly relevant to the management of refractive keratotomy patients, but we have indicated whether or not keratometric measurements were reported.

We have omitted most listings of complications, particularly in terms of glare, fluctuating vision, and endothelial cell counts, because the methods by which this information was collected are so widely variable as to make comparison meaningless. These complications are discussed in detail in Chapter 23, Complications of Refractive Keratotomy, where individual reports are summarized. We have presented the reported perforation rate and the reported loss of best-corrected visual acuity. We have selected the results reported at the last follow-up in each study and have not tried to present the changes over time as reported. Changes over time are discussed in detail in Chapter 24, Stability of Refraction after Refractive Keratotomy. For studies in which there is a series of papers reporting the outcome on the same group of patients, we have included the most recent publication, citing the references of the previous ones.

Many of the studies reported in this chapter have used combinations of radial and astigmatic keratotomy techniques, and therefore it is not possible to report separately the results of the pure radial keratotomy cases from those of the combined radial and astigmatic keratotomy cases. Therefore in this chapter we present results of published studies that emphasize primarily the correction of myopia. In Chapter 31, Keratotomy for Astigmatism, we present the results of studies that emphasize primarily the correction of astigmatism.

TYPES OF REPORTS NOT PUBLISHED

What is missing from the literature is a prospective series of cases that uses the techniques in current practice in the late 1980s and early 1990s and is analyzed by independent biostaticians. This series would include specific adjustment for the preoperative nomogram and surgeon's technique, patient age, use of intraoperative ultrasonic pachometry and diamond knives calibrated with a compound microscope and reticule at magnifications of 150 to 200×, intentional undercorrection at the level of −0.50 to −1.00 D, use of four primary incisions with the addition of four more incisions or the opening and deepening/lengthening of the original four incisions to fine tune the results, calculation of the 90% (or 95%) confidence interval, and documentation of stability of refraction in individual eyes over time. The articles by Salz and colleagues and by Spigelman and colleagues present some of this more contemporary information.

It would be interesting to do a formal metaanalysis on the published data from refractive keratotomy series. The comparative tables presented here allow the reader to gain a general overall impression of surgical outcome, but a formal, more quantitative treatment would facilitate a better interpretation of the world's literature. The inconsistency of information gathered here emphasizes the need for adherence to conventional standards of reporting results of keratotomy.

NEED FOR STANDARDS FOR REPORTING

Many types of refractive corneal surgery are being investigated in laboratory studies, informal clinical tests, and formal clinical trials (see Chapter 4, Development and Classification of Refractive Surgical Procedures). Ophthalmologists, researchers, patients, insurance companies, and regulatory agencies are comparing the results of approximately 15 different techniques now being performed on human beings, attempting to decide which technique is the most effective, safe, predictable, stable, and modifiable. Comparisons are difficult because there are no conventional standards for reporting results.

For example, in studies of radial keratotomy the definition of "overcorrection" differs, some defining it as a refractive error greater than +1.00 D, some as more than +2.00 D, and some as "symptomatic hyperopia." The formats for scattergrams of the refractive outcome differ. Some plot baseline refraction (x-axis) versus change (y-axis); others plot baseline refraction (x-axis) versus final refraction (y-axis); still others plot baseline refraction (y-axis) versus final refraction (x-axis). A significant loss of best spectacle-corrected visual acuity is one or more Snellen lines in some studies, two or more in others. How can we compare these different reports?

The solution is simple: create a set of conventional standards on which most refractive surgeons agree; publish these standards in a clear and useful form that serves as a guide and checklist; adopt these conventions formally through societies, such as the International Society of Refractive Keratoplasty; and encourage authors through editorial policy to use these guidelines in their publications (see box on pp. 784 and 785). Such standards do not truncate creativity, restrict freedom, or force conformity. Authors simply agree to report results according to common criteria in addition to whatever other formats they desire. Such standards are no different from the accepted conventions of "20/20" as the norm for "good" visual acuity and of "20/200" as the norm for "legal blindness."

Minimal Essential Standards for Reporting Studies of Refractive Surgical Procedures

Methods

Population studied	Original total number of patients and eyes
Population reported at follow-up interval	Number of eyes (percent of original population) studied at each specific follow-up interval
Surgical technique; number of surgeons	Detailed description that allows replication by trained surgeon; number of surgeons in this report
Examination technique	Description of who examined the patients and how the measurements were made
Baseline refraction groups	Number (percent) of eyes with preoperative refraction* in the following categories (either myopic or hyperopic):

$$0 \text{ to } -1.50$$
$$-1.62 \text{ to } -3.00 \text{ D}$$
$$-3.12 \text{ to } -6.00 \text{ D}$$
$$-6.12 \text{ to } -10.00 \text{ D}$$
$$-10.12 \text{ to } -15.00 \text{ D}$$
$$-15.12 \text{ to } -20.00 \text{ D}$$
$$-20.12 \text{ or more}$$

These seven categories can be grouped as lower, middle, higher, and highest amounts of ametropia, using different distributions for different studies. For example, the "lower" group for three operations could differ as follows:

a. Transverse keratotomy for naturally occurring astigmatism, 1.00 to 1.50 D

b. Radial keratotomy for myopia, -1.62 to -3.00 D

c. Epikeratoplasty for aphakia, $+6.12$ to $+10.00$ D

From Waring GO: Refract Corneal Surg 1989;5:285-287.
*Spherical equivalent of the cycloplegic or manifest refraction; for studies of astigmatism, the absolute amount of residual refractive or keratometric astigmatism is reported.

Minimal Essential Standards for Reporting Studies of Refractive Surgical Procedures—cont'd

Efficacy

Refractive outcome

Number (percent) of eyes with refraction* in the following categories (either myopic or hyperopic):

0 to   −0.50 D
−0.62 to   −1.00 D
−1.12 to   −2.00 D
−2.12 to   −3.00 D
−3.12 to   −6.00 D
−6.12 to −10.00 D
>−10.00 D

In addition, the mean, standard deviation, and range of the refraction for the population can be reported.

Visual acuity

Number (percent) of eyes with uncorrected visual acuity in four categories:
20/20 (1.0) or better
20/40 (0.5) or better
20/50 (0.4) to 20/100 (0.2)
20/200 (0.1) or worse

Safety

Loss of best spectacle corrected visual acuity

Number (percent) of eyes losing two or more Snellen lines

Vision-threatening complications

Number (percent) of eyes that experienced adverse events that potentially or actually reduced best spectacle corrected visual acuity

Predictability

Range of final refraction* around the preoperative predicted outcome which contained 90% of the eyes; or the 90% confidence interval

Stability

Number (percent) of eyes with a change in refraction* of 1.00 D or more between 6 months and a specified follow-up time

SECTION I: Detailed Summary of Three Major Studies of Refractive Keratotomy

Authors	Arrowsmith PN and Marks RG	Waring GO, Lynn MJ, and the PERK Study Group	Deitz MR, Sanders DR, and Raanan MS
Article title and citation	Visual, Refractive, and Keratometric Results of Radial Keratotomy: 5-Year Follow-up, Arch Ophthalmol 1989;170:506-511.	Results of the Prospective Evaluation of Radial Keratotomy (PERK) Study 5 Years after Surgery for Myopia, Ophthalmology 1991;98:1164-1176.	A Consecutive Series (1982-1985) of Radial Keratotomies Performed with the Diamond Blade, Am J Ophthalmol 1987;103:417-422.

Comment: To merit publication in peer-reviewed journals, an article must pass the rigors of critical assessment by experts in refractive keratotomy.

| Other publications | Arrowsmith PN, Sanders DR, and Marks RG: Visual, Refractive, and Keratometric Results of Radial Keratotomy, Arch Ophthalmol 1983;101:873-881.
Arrowsmith PN and Marks RG: Visual, Refractive and Keratometric Results of Radial Keratotomy; 1-Year Follow-up, Arch Ophthalmol 1984;102:1612-1617.
Powers MK, Meyerowitz BE, Arrowsmith PN, and Marks RG: Psychosocial Findings in Radial Keratotomy Patients 2 Years after Surgery, Ophthalmology 1984;91:1193-1198.
Arrowsmith PN and Marks RG: Evaluating the Predictability of Radial Keratotomy, Ophthalmology 1985;92:331-338.
Arrowsmith PN and Marks RG: Visual, Refractive, and Keratometric Results of Radial Keratotomy: a 2-Year Follow-up, Arch Ophthalmol 1987;105:76-80.
Arrowsmith PN and Marks RG: Four-Year Update on Predictability of Radial Keratotomy, Refract Surg 1988;4:37-45. | Waring GO, Moffitt SD, Gelender H, et al, and the PERK Study Group: Rationale for and Design of the National Eye Institute Prospective Evaluation of Radial Keratotomy (PERK) Study, Ophthalmology 1983;90:40-58.
Waring GO, Lynn MJ, Gelender H, et al, and the PERK Study Group: Results of the Prospective Evaluation of Radial Keratotomy (PERK) Study 1 Year after Surgery, Ophthalmology 1985;92:177-198.
Bourque LB, Cosand BB, Drews C, et al, and the PERK Study Group: Reported Satisfaction, Fluctuation of Vision, and Glare among Patients 1 Year after Surgery in the Prospective Evaluation of Radial Keratotomy (PERK) Study, Arch Ophthalmol 1986;104:356-363.
Waring GO, Lynn MJ, Culbertson W, et al, and the PERK Study Group: Three-Year Results of the Prospective Evaluation of Radial Keratotomy (PERK) Study, Ophthalmology 1987;105:42-51.
Lynn MJ, Waring GO, Sperduto RD, et al, and the PERK Study Group: Factors Affecting Outcome and Predictability of Radial Keratotomy in the PERK Study, Arch Ophthalmol 1987;105:42-51. | (Some information not contained in the published papers was verbally provided by Dr. Deitz June 1988.)
Deitz MR, Sanders DR, and Marks RG: Radial Keratotomy: an Overview of the Kansas City Study, Ophthalmology 1984;91:467-478.
Deitz MR and Sanders DR: Progressive Hyperopia with Long-term Follow-up of Radial Keratotomy, Arch Ophthalmol 1985;103:782-784.
Sanders DR, Deitz MR, and Gallagher D: Factors Affecting Predictability of Radial Keratotomy, Ophthalmology 1985;92:1237-1243.
Deitz MR, Sanders DR, and Raanan MG: Progressive Hyperopia in Radial Keratotomy: Long-term Follow-up of Diamond Knife and Metal Blade Series, Ophthalmology 1986;93:1284-1289.
Deitz MR, Sanders DR, and Raanan MG: A Consecutive Series (1982-1985) of Radial Keratotomies Performed with the Diamond Blade, Am J Ophthalmol 1987;103:417-422. |

Authors	Arrowsmith PN and Marks RG	Waring GO, Lynn MJ, and the PERK Study Group	Deitz MR, Sanders DR, and Raanan MS
		Santos VR, Waring GO, Lynn MJ, et al, and the PERK Study Group: Relationship between Refractive Error and Visual Acuity in Operated and Unoperated Eyes in the Prospective Evaluation of Radial Keratotomy (PERK) Study, Arch Ophthalmol 1987;105:86-92.	
		Santos VR, Waring GO, Lynn MJ, et al: Morning-to-Evening Change in Refraction, Corneal Curvature, and Visual Acuity 2 to 4 Years after Radial Keratotomy in the PERK Study, Ophthalmology 1988;95:1487-1493.	
		Lynn MJ, Waring GO, Nizam A, et al, and the PERK Study Group: Symmetry of Refractive and Visual Acuity Outcome in the Prospective Evaluation of Radial Keratotomy (PERK) Study, Refract Corneal Surg 1989;5:75-81.	
		Waring GO, Lynn MJ, Fielding B, et al, and the PERK Study Group: Results of the Prospective Evaluation of Radial Keratotomy (PERK) Study 4 Years after Surgery for Myopia, J Am Med Assoc 1990;263:1083-1091.	
		Lynn MJ, Waring GO, and the PERK Study Group: Stability of Refraction after Radial Keratotomy Compared with Unoperated Eyes in the PERK Study, Am J Ophthalmol 1991;111:133-144.	

Comment: All three studies have published a series of articles reporting the outcome of surgery at different time intervals and reporting on other aspects, such as predictability. The PERK Study Group published approximately 25 peer-reviewed articles.

Dates of Surgery	December 1980 to August 1981	March 1982 to October 1983	January 1982 to May 1985

Comment: The Arrowsmith and Marks series was the first conducted and therefore uses the oldest surgical techniques. The PERK study was designed in 1981, and the surgery spanned approximately 18 months in 1982 and 1983, overlapping with Deitz's diamond knife series. The Deitz series extended to 1985, allowing use of preoperative nomograms and surgical techniques based on previous experience.

Authors	Arrowsmith PN and Marks RG	Waring GO, Lynn MJ, and the PERK Study Group	Deitz MR, Sanders DR, and Raanan MS
Funding source (*Major source)			
National Institutes of Health	Yes	Yes*	Yes
Private	Yes*	Yes	Yes*
Industry	Yes	Yes	Not reported

Comment: The PERK Study was supported in a large part by a grant from the National Institutes of Health (NIH), but all participating institutions and all participating investigators donated their facilities and time without charge to either the patient or the NIH. The grant has been renewed to allow a 10-year follow-up in 1993. The Arrowsmith and Deitz studies received a small grant given initially to the Analysis of Radial Keratotomy (ARK) group, and the biostatisticians obtained some support from their universities, but the major funding source was the private practices of the surgeons. Some instruments and services were donated by industry.

Study design			
Prospective	Yes	Yes	Yes
Sample size calculation	No	Yes	No
Selection criteria specified	Yes	Yes	Yes
Consecutive eyes	Yes	Yes	Yes

Comment: All three studies were prospective with a specified cohort of consecutive eyes. The PERK study published a manual of procedures that standardized all aspects of the trial. The Arrowsmith and Deitz studies were conducted informally.

Investigators and number of surgeons			
Study centers	1	9	1
Surgeons	1	10	1
Independent physician examiners	No	Yes	No
Independent technician examiners	Yes	Yes	No
Independent monitors	No	Yes	No
Independent biostatistician	Yes	Yes	Yes

Comment: All three studies were collaborative efforts between ophthalmologists with private practices and individuals employed by universities. The PERK study was a multicenter clinical trial carried out at nine different centers with ten different surgeons. Analysis of the results from the nine different centers showed no statistically significant differences, so the data were pooled. The other two studies were carried out in individual private practices. An independent biostatistician working at a different location than the surgeons managed the data in all three studies—a strength in the study designs. In the PERK study the surgeon gathered none of the preoperative or postoperative data, which were procured by independent physician examiners and specially trained clinical coordinators. In addition, independent monitors from outside the study centers made site visits to ensure adherence to the protocol. A separate data and safety monitoring board periodically reviewed the course of the study and the results. Although both Arrowsmith and Deitz employed independent examiners in the early phases of their studies, independent examiners were not part of the Arrowsmith and Deitz studies reported here.

Disclosure of financial interest	No disclosure (the surgeon and biostatistician had a financial interest in the AMARK Company, which sells radial keratotomy computer programs and data base management systems).	Disclosure (one investigator had a financial interest in the Villasenor ultrasonic pachometer).	No disclosure (the surgeon and biostatistician had a commercially available radial keratotomy software program—the DRS program).

Comment: Two of the three studies made no disclosure of financial interests, an important omission that may mask possible bias.

Authors	Arrowsmith PN and Marks RG	Waring GO, Lynn MJ, and the PERK Study Group	Deitz MR, Sanders DR, and Raanan MS
Clinical examination conditions			
Office practice	Yes	No	Yes
Standardized	No	Yes	No

Comment: Examination conditions were standardized in the PERK study so that the same examiners used the same instruments and the same room under the same conditions for all examinations, as specified in the protocol. New personnel were required to pass a PERK certification site review and examination. When a patient was examined at more than one PERK center, the same protocol was followed. The Arrowsmith and Deitz studies used procedures similar to those used in office practice, but with special care to record the needed information for the study.

Data analysis			
Informal (tables, graphs)	Yes	Yes	Yes
Arithmetic (mean, standard deviation, range	Yes	Yes	Yes
Statistical (regression analysis, confidence limits)	Yes	Yes	Yes

Comment: All three studies used similar types of data analysis, although the methods differed. For example, in graphically plotting the outcome the PERK study compared the final refractive results with the baseline refraction, whereas the other two studies plotted the change in refraction versus the baseline refraction. The Arrowsmith and Deitz studies quantified predictability in terms of the R^2 factor, whereas the PERK study also computed confidence intervals.

Patient population			
Number of patients	101	435	458
Number of eyes	123 (79% of original population)	793	972
Withdrawals/exclusions accounted for	Yes	Yes	Yes
Age; mean(range)	30 yr (18 to 76 yr)	33.5 yr (21 to 58 yr)	34.2 yr (18 to 62 yr)
Sex, % female	44%	48%	56%

Comment: Deitz had the largest population, followed by PERK and then Arrowsmith. The 5-year PERK study differed from the PERK reports published at 1, 3, and 4 years because it included all operated eyes: two eyes of each patient, eyes that had received repeated surgery, and eyes that had worn contact lenses. Thus, whereas the previous reports presented "pure" results from the standardized PERK surgical technique, the 5-year report presented the overall "real life" clinical outcome for the entire population. All three studies accounted somewhat for the patients lost to follow-up or excluded from the study. The similarity in mean age and sex ratio is striking.

Repeated operations (% of eyes)	11%	12%	None (personal communication)
Included in results	Yes	Yes	Not reported
Technique	Not reported	Eight additional incisions between original ones	Not reported
Postoperative corticosteroids	Yes	No	Yes

Comment: Arrowsmith and PERK included the outcome of repeated operations in the results to reflect the outcome of the total surgical effort in the population. Deitz did not define how many eyes were reoperated in his published study, but indicated in a personal communication that none was reoperated.

Follow-up			
Mean (range)	5 yr	5.2 yr (36 to 78 mo)	1 yr (83% between 9 to 15 mo)
Percentage of original population at follow-up	79% (123 of 156)	95%(757 of 793)	68%(656 of 972)

Authors	Arrowsmith PN and Marks RG	Waring GO, Lynn MJ, and the PERK Study Group	Deitz MR, Sanders DR, and Raanan MS

Comment: The PERK study had the largest population reported—757 eyes. The Deitz follow-up was the shortest, spanning only the first year after surgery. The Arrowsmith and PERK follow-up were each 5 years. A major difference among the studies was the percentage of patients followed. The PERK study followed 95% of the eyes, whereas the other 2 followed 68% to 79%. Clearly, the larger the loss to follow-up is, the less representative are the results. A 10-year follow-up in the PERK study has been funded by the National Eye Institute for 1993.

Surgical protocol

Formal, replicable	No	Yes	No
Informal, not replicable	Yes	No	Yes

Comment: The surgical protocol varied greatly among the three studies; Deitz reported essentially no surgical protocol. Arrowsmith presented a very complex protocol that probably is not replicable by other investigators and reflected the changing state of surgical techniques at that time. The PERK protocol was standardized and easily replicable but not customized for each patient.

Patient variables used to determine surgical plan

Basis for surgical plan	Fyodorov equation and personal informal relationships used to determine corneal thickness	Clear zone diameter based on refraction; depth (100%) and number of incisions (8) constant	Deitz, Retzlaff, Sanders (DRS) program and personal informal relationships
Myopia	Yes	Yes	Yes
Age	No	No	Yes
Sex	Yes	No	Yes
Corneal thickness	Yes	Yes	Yes
Keratometry reading	Yes	No	Yes
Intraocular pressure	Yes	No	Yes
Ocular rigidity	Yes	No	No
Corneal diameter	Yes	No	No

Comment: The PERK study used only two patient variables (refraction and corneal thickness) to design the surgical plan; Arrowsmith and Deitz used multiple variables in "predictability equations" to attempt to tailor the operation to the individual patient. At the time the Arrowsmith and PERK protocols were designed, it was not known that the age of the patient affected the outcome; Deitz used an age factor. All three studies related preoperative refraction to clear zone diameter, and corneal thickness to knife blade extension. How much the outcome was influenced by the formal use of preoperative variables and how much it was influenced by biologic variability and surgical artistry is unknown.

Measurement of corneal thickness

Optical	No	No	No
Ultrasonic (speed of sound, m/sec)	Yes (1610)	Yes (1640)	Yes (1640)
Preoperative	Yes	No	Yes
Intraoperative	No	Yes	No
Location of measurement used for blade setting	Paracentral	Paracentral	Central

Comment: All three studies used ultrasonic pachometry. An analysis from the PERK study demonstrated a difference between preoperative and intraoperative ultrasonic pachometry measurements of 30 to 80 μm in 13% of eyes. Therefore they elected to use intraoperative pachometry.

Anesthesia

Topical	Yes	Yes (0.5% proparacaine)	Yes (personal communication)
Retrobulbar	Yes (Plus O'Brien)	No	No

Authors	Arrowsmith PN and Marks RG	Waring GO, Lynn MJ, and the PERK Study Group	Deitz MR, Sanders DR, and Raanan MS
	Comment: The PERK and Deitz studies used topical anesthesia only. Arrowsmith used retrobulbar and peribulbar nerve blocks, largely because surgery in this series was performed early in the development of radial keratotomy when surgeons were more cautious about controlling patients' ocular movements.		
Knife blade and handle			
Metal blade	Yes	No	No
Diamond blade	No	Yes (single edge)	Yes (double edge)
Cutting edge	Vertical	Oblique	Oblique
Micrometer handle	Yes	Yes	Yes
Blade length; percentage of corneal thickness	83% to 98% of paracentral readings at clear zone	100% of thinnest paracentral reading at clear zone	108% of central thickness
Calibration block	Yes	Yes	Yes
	Comment: All three studies used a micrometer knife handle and verified blade length on a calibration block. Arrowsmith used a metal blade, a technique now outmoded, whereas the PERK study used a single-edged diamond and Deitz a double-edged diamond. Variations in knife style affect the outcome.		
Clear zone			
Range of diameters	3.0 to 5.0 mm	3.0, 3.5, and 4.0 mm	2.7 to 6.0 mm
Circular (%)	82%	100%	100%
Elliptical (%)	12%		
	Comment: Arrowsmith used elliptical clear zones to manage astigmatism, a technique now obsolete.		
Incisions			
Number of radial (% of eyes)	Not reported	8 (100%)	8 (89%) 16 (6%) Other (5%)
Direction of incisions			
Clear zone to limbus	No	Yes	Yes
Limbus to clear zone	Yes	No	No
Technique (% of eyes)			
Single pass	42%	100%	Majority
Peripheral deepening	57%		Yes
Recut; same blade length	0%		> 6.00 D
Freehand dissection	1%		No
Across limbus	0%		No
	Comment: Eight incisions were used most commonly in all three studies. Arrowsmith and Deitz used 16 in eyes with higher amounts of myopia. The PERK study and Deitz cut centrifugally (the "American" technique), whereas Arrowsmith cut centripetally (the "Russian" technique). The technique of incisions was simple in the PERK study (a single pass), more complex in the Deitz study (a single pass plus a second pass in a more myopic eye), and quite complex in the Arrowsmith study (three zones of peripheral deepening were used).		
Achieved incision depth			
Method of measurement	Slit-lamp microscopy, visual inspection with average estimate	Formal protocol for visual inspection with slit-lamp microscopy in at least three locations in 3204 incisions	Optical pachometry in the middle of the incisions
Depth as percentage of corneal thickness (% of eyes)	75% to 100% in 95% of eyes	76% to 100% in 66% of eyes 51% to 75% in 28% of eyes 26% to 50% in 6% of eyes	85% to 98% in 82% of eyes
Transverse incisions for astigmatism (% of eyes)	Approximately 0.6%	0%	16% (personal communication)

Authors	Arrowsmith PN and Marks RG	Waring GO, Lynn MJ, and the PERK Study Group		Deitz MR, Sanders DR, and Raanan MS

Comment: It is difficult to estimate the depth of the incisions, as discussed in Chapter 13, Predictability of Refractive Keratotomy. Deitz used optical pachometry, a more reliable but time-consuming method than the visual inspection used by the other two studies. The PERK depth estimates were given in quartiles, so a 75% and 100% incision were classified together; thus the eye with the deepest incision scar in the PERK study was graded as 87% (between 75% to 100%). This made comparisons more difficult. The incisions in the PERK study were shallower than those in the other two studies. This may have accounted in part for the higher undercorrection rate in PERK. Only Dietz used a significant number of transverse incisions to correct astigmatism.

Perforations (% of eyes)	35%	2%		Not reported

Comment: The high perforation rate in the Arrowsmith study reflected the early stage of development of radial keratotomy. The low perforation rate in the PERK study reflected the fact that the incisions were generally made shallowly, but with a margin of safety.

Baseline refraction groups (range in diopters)

		Original categories and clear zone diameter		
Lower	1.50 to 2.90	2.00 to 3.12(4.0 mm)		0.60 to 3.00
Middle	3.00 to 5.90	3.25 to 4.37(3.5 mm)		3.10 to 6.00
Higher	6.00 to 9.90	4.50 to 8.00(3.0 mm)		6.10 to 11.90
Highest	10.00 to 16.00	Adjusted categories for comparison with two studies		
		2.00 to 3.00		
		3.12 to 6.00		
		6.12 to 8.00		

Comment: All studies divided the eyes according to the amount of preoperative myopia. We recalculated the PERK data according to the ranges of Arrowsmith and Deitz so that reasonably direct comparisons could be made. The PERK study used different categories based on the diameter of the central clear zone as indicated in parentheses. Outcomes for the PERK study are presented for both their original and adjusted refraction groups.

Refraction results

Refraction technique				
Cycloplegia	Yes	Yes		Yes
Manifest	No	No		No
Percentage of eyes ±1.00 D		Original categories	Adjusted categories	
All eyes	53%	64%	64%	76%
Lower group (1.50 to 3.00 D)	75%	76%	76%	90%
Middle group (3.10 to 6.00 D)	50%	67%	61%	76%
Higher group (6.12 to 9.00 D)	38%	49%	46%	53%
Highest group (>10.00 D)	38%			
Overcorrected > 1.00 D (%)	33%	17%		13%
Undercorrected > 1.00 D (%)	13%	19%		12%
Figure	Fig. 21-1 (p. 798)	Fig. 21-3 (p. 799)		—

Comment: All three studies used cycloplegic refraction, an important factor in longitudinal studies in which the influence of the patient's accommodation is unknown. The overall refractive results were disappointing: only half of the eyes in the Arrowsmith and PERK studies fell within 1 D of emmetropia, whereas 75% of the eyes in the Deitz study fell within this range. All studies reported best results in the lower refraction group (−1.50 to −3.00 D) and fair results in the middle group (−3.00 to −6.00 D). The worst results were in the higher myopia group. Because of this most surgeons restrict radial keratotomy to eyes with approximately less than 7.00 D of myopia, allowing some exceptions. The startlingly high overcorrection rate (33%) in Arrowsmith's series emphasizes the need for a more accurately modulated surgical technique, preferably one that undercorrects intentionally to achieve a result of −0.50 to −1.00 D, which compensates somewhat for both presbyopia and the long-term trend toward hyperopia in some eyes. The fact that one out of three of Arrowsmith's patients will be prematurely presbyopic and may require optical correction for both distance and near

Authors	Arrowsmith PN and Marks RG	Waring GO, Lynn MJ, and the PERK Study Group	Deitz MR, Sanders DR, and Raanan MS

is unacceptable. The high rate of overcorrection may have occurred because of the special effort made to achieve very deep incisions. The high undercorrection rate of approximately 25% of both the Arrowsmith and PERK studies derives largely from the eyes in the higher refractive groups. We reemphasize that the surgical plans and some of the surgical techniques used in all of these studies have greatly improved in the past decade. The fact that these surgical techniques are somewhat outmoded does not detract from the usefulness of the reports, which serve as standards against which progress can be measured. The best results of the three studies were those of Dietz, probably because he used age as a predictive factor and used improved surgical instruments and predictability formulas based on his previous experience. Unfortunately, Dietz did not describe his surgical technique in detail, so we do not know how the results were achieved. His findings emphasize that improved surgical techniques can improve the refractive outcome.

Predictability

Reference	Arrowsmith PN and Marks RG: Four-Year Update on Predictability of Radial Keratotomy, J Refract Surg 1988;4:37-45.	Lynn MJ, Waring GO, Sperduto RD, and the Perk Study Group: Factors Affecting Outcome and Predictability of Radial Keratotomy in the PERK Study, Arch Ophthalmol 1987;105:42-51.	Sanders D, Deitz M, and Gallagher D: Factors Affecting Predictability of Radial Keratotomy, Ophthalmology 1985;92:1237-1243.

Population
Number of eyes	157	793	972
Percentage follow-up	74%	86%	57%
Time after surgery	4 yr	4 yr	2 yr
Blade	Metal	Diamond	Diamond
90% confidence interval (D)	Not reported		Not reported
All eyes		4.42	
Low group		3.27	
Middle group		4.45	
High group		5.26	

Factors that affect outcome (yes, no, or ranked 1 to 5, 1=highest, 5=lowest)
Method of study	Regression analysis	Regression analysis	Regression analysis
Clear zone diameter (linked to baseline myopia)	Yes	1	1
Patient age	Yes	2	5
Depth of incision	Yes	3	2
Number of incisions	Yes	Eight only	3
Average central keratometry	Yes	No	4
Number of zones	Yes	Not used	Not used
Patient sex	No	No	No
Intraocular pressure	No	No	No
Corneal thickness	No	No	No
Ocular rigidity	Not reported	No	No
R^2 for all eyes	57%	44%	73%

Comment: There was remarkable concordance among the three studies for factors that affect outcome. All demonstrated a greater effect associated with a smaller clear zone diameter (invariably linked to a larger amount of preoperative myopia), deeper incisions (including secondary and tertiary deepening incisions as well as perforations), increased number of incisions (except for PERK, which used eight only), and increasing patient age (approximately 0.7 to 1.0 D per decade). Arrowsmith and Deitz found a very small role for average central keratometry (Deitz, steeper corneas have more effect; Arrowsmith, flatter corneas have more effect). Thus the overall conclusion is that one or two patient factors can be used to help design the preoperative plan: patient age and the preoperative refraction (always linked to clear zone diameter in current surgical plans). Corneal thickness is adjusted for by setting the knife blade based on thickness measurements. Equally consistent are the negative findings, including an absence of correlation with patient sex, preoperative intraocular pressure, central corneal thickness, corneal diameter, and ocular rigidity (PERK). Only the PERK study used confidence intervals as a measure of predictability; it is regrettable that the other two studies reported only the R^2 value, which may have usefulness in statistical analysis, but which does not translate into clinically meaningful terms.

| Authors | Arrowsmith PN and Marks RG | | Waring GO, Lynn MJ, and the PERK Study Group | | | | Deitz MR, Sanders DR, and Raanan MS | |

The 90% prediction range (the range of refraction around the predicted outcome value within which 90% of the eyes fell) was remarkably wide, 4.50 D ($\pm$ 2.25) in PERK. Given the fact that spectacles and contact lenses can be fitted in a range of $\pm$ 0.50, the outcome of radial keratotomy is not as predictable as surgeons and patients would want for an individual eye. The discussion by Arrowsmith and Marks of incision depth in both their 5-year metal blade clinical series and their 2-year diamond blade predictability series is particularly thought provoking. The authors compared their depth of incision information to that reported in Sawelson's study, in which the incisions were more shallow, and to that reported in Deitz's study, in which a larger number of the incisions were very deep. Two observations arose from this information. First, 33% of eyes in Arrowsmith were overcorrected by more than 1.00 D (yes, with a metal blade, probably because of the very deep incisions). Second, deeper incisions (those of 90% or greater depth) are probably responsible for the increasing effect of the surgery over time because Sawelson had the least progressive change, Arrowsmith an intermediate amount, and Deitz the most. Furthermore, Arrowsmith and Marks found a quadratic relationship between incision depth and change in refraction, so incisions greater than 90% depth (including perforations) will exponentially increase the effect and also the error in prediction. The conclusion is speculative but substantive enough to encourage surgeons to aim for an incision depth of 80%-90% and not "99%." They also suggest that predictability increases with fewer incisions and a larger clear zone diameter. Achieving a consistent 85% depth is a difficult clinical challenge for this manual surgical technique.

Both Arrowsmith and Deitz used the regression analysis of their initial series of cases to refine their surgical plan and surgical technique for a subsequent series of cases, showing improvement in the results. For example, Arrowsmith and Marks found a difference between the observed and predicted change in the spherical equivalent refraction in their first and second series: 85% of the eyes in their first series fell within 2.00 D of the predicted values, whereas in the second series of eyes 92% fell within 2.00 D of the predicted value. Both Arrowsmith and Deitz also reported predictability analysis of metal blade cases, but they are not included here. Similarly, Sanders and Dietz (Sanders DR, Dietz MR, and Gallagher D: Factors affecting predictability of radial keratotomy, 1985; Ophthalmology 92:1237-1243) studied a series of initial cases done with a metal blade. The regression equation derived from this was fitted to data from a subsequent series of cases done with a diamond knife blade. Using the initial regression equation as applied to the second group of eyes, the predicted outcome for the spherical equivalent refraction was within 1.5 D of the actual refractive outcome in 93% of eyes, suggesting that the experience derived from the first series of patients had positively influenced the surgical technique and the outcome of the second group.

Visual acuity results	≥ 20/40	≥ 20/20	Original categories		Adjusted categories		≥ 20/40	≥ 20/20
			≥ 20/40	≥ 20/20	≥ 20/40	≥ 20/20		
Lower (0.00 to 3.00 D)			95%	75%	92%	75%	96%	65%
Middle (3.12 to 6.00 D)	Not reported		89%	63%	86%	57%	89%	44%
Higher (6.12 to 9.00 D)			79%	43%	72%	29%	77%	30%
Highest (> 10 D)								
All eyes	76%	37%			88%	60%	88%	47%

Comment: In all three studies the visual acuity results for the lower refractive group were quite satisfying, 90% or more seeing 20/40 uncorrected and approximately 70% seeing 20/20 or better. In the middle refractive group the vast majority of eyes could see 20/40 or better. As with refraction, the results are less satisfactory for the higher group. The results of Deitz were superior to those of PERK and Arrowsmith, especially in the higher myopia group. Striking is the similarity among the three studies in the uncorrected visual acuity of 20/40 or better for all eyes: 75%, 75%, and 88%. When one considers that the visual acuity in almost all eyes was 20/80 or worse before surgery, the number of eyes seeing 20/40 or better is remarkable.

Authors	Arrowsmith PN and Marks RG	Waring GO, Lynn MJ, and the PERK Study Group	Deitz MR, Sanders DR, and Raanan MS
Intermediate-term (6 mo to 5 yr) stability of refraction			Fig. 21-2 (p. 798)
Time interval	1 to 5 yr	6 mo to 3-6 yr	1 to 4 yr
Increased minus power = 1.00 to 2.50 D		2%	2%
Change < 1.00 D	Not reported	76%	67%
Decreased minus power = 1.00 to 4.00 D		22%	31%
Mean change (D)	+0.7 D	−0.41 D	−0.53 D

Comment: During the 5 years after surgery interval the majority of eyes (70% to 80%) had a change in refraction of less than 1.00 D and therefore were considered stable. Most of the remaining 25% showed a continued increase in surgical effect; that is, a continued decrease in the minus power with a shift in refraction in the hyperopic direction. Few eyes showed mild regression of effect. Deitz and colleagues and the PERK study have published a detailed analysis of stability of refraction, but Arrowsmith and Marks have not. When Arrowsmith and Marks analyzed the differences in these studies, they speculated that the depth of the incision might explain the differences, since Deitz reported the deepest incisions and PERK the shallowest. Unfortunately, it is not possible to identify ahead of time eyes that will stabilize and those that will exhibit a continued surgical effect. It is therefore wise to aim for a slight undercorrection for most individuals (see Chapter 24, Stability of Refraction after Refractive Keratotomy).

Authors	Arrowsmith PN and Marks RG	Waring GO, Lynn MJ, and the PERK Study Group	Deitz MR, Sanders DR, and Raanan MS
Loss of spectacle-corrected visual acuity			
Loss of one Snellen line	18 of 122 eyes (15%)	106 of 752 (14%)	Not reported
Loss of two or more Snellen lines	Not reported	25 of 752 (3%)	0.5%

Comment: Three percent or less of all eyes lost two or more lines of spectacle-corrected visual acuity in all three studies; seven lines of best-corrected visual acuity was the most lost. This indicates good safety for the procedure and suggests that patients with a less than optimal refractive outcome have the option of wearing spectacles again and recovering their original Snellen visual acuity.

Authors	Arrowsmith PN and Marks RG	Waring GO, Lynn MJ, and the PERK Study Group	Deitz MR, Sanders DR, and Raanan MS
Vision-threatening complications			
Delayed bacterial keratitis	None	Two eyes	One eye (personal communication)

Comment: The only vision-threatening complication that occurred in these three series was delayed bacterial keratitis in the PERK and the Dietz studies. The eyes were treated successfully, with the return of 20/16 spectacle-corrected visual acuity. This small number of vision-threatening complications bodes well for the safety of refractive keratotomy. However, Arrowsmith has reported serious complications outside the original series listed above. In addition, with one out of every three or four patients lost to follow-up in the Deitz and Arrowsmith series, some long-term complications may have gone unrecognized (see Chapter 23, Complications of Refractive Keratotomy).

Authors	Arrowsmith PN and Marks RG	Waring GO, Lynn MJ, and the PERK Study Group	Deitz MR, Sanders DR, and Raanan MS
Ruptured globe	None	None	None
Non−vision threatening complications			
Epithelial erosion	None	One eye	None
Moderate to severe glare	0%	0%	Not reported
Moderate to severe subjective fluctuation of vision	1%	33% at 1 year	Not reported

Authors	Arrowsmith PN and Marks RG	Waring GO, Lynn MJ, and the PERK Study Group	Deitz MR, Sanders DR, and Raanan MS

Comment: It is difficult to quantify subtler, non–vision threatening complications of refractive keratotomy, particularly when subjective assessment is involved. Different methods of eliciting information from patients and the highly variable subjective assessment on the part of patients make this softer information to garner. In general, the subjective symptoms are worse within the first few months after surgery and gradually diminish over a few years. These factors can lead to widely disparate results, such as the report from the PERK study of significant trouble with fluctuating vision in one third of the patients 1 year after surgery, whereas Arrowsmith reported no moderate to severe fluctuating vision at 1 year after surgery and one at 5 years after surgery. Unfortunately, the Dietz study reported no data on such complications.

Patient satisfaction			Not reported
Level of overall satisfaction (%)			
High	71%	49%	
Average	14%	41%	
Low	15%	6%	
Reference	Powers MK, Meyerowitz BE, Arrowsmith PN, and Marks RG: Psychosocial Findings in Radial Keratotomy Patients 2 Years after Surgery, Ophthalmology 1984;91:1193-1198.	Bourque LB, Cosand BB, Drews C, Waring GO, Lynn M, Cartwright C, and PERK Study Group: Reported Satisfaction, Fluctuation of Vision, and Glare among Patients 1 Year after Surgery in the Prospective Evaluation of Radial Keratotomy (PERK) Study, Arch Ophthalmol 1986;104:356-363.	
Percentage of patients who would undergo repeat surgery	8%	95%	Not reported

Comment: The patient's subjective satisfaction with the results of surgery is an important variable that is difficult to measure. The objective clinical measurements of outcome, such as the final refractive error and corrected visual acuity, form the basis for evaluating the effectiveness of keratotomy. However, in the operational world of clinical practice, overall personal satisfaction with the results is the main criterion by which patients make a final judgment about the outcome. The fact that only 50% to 70% of patients were highly satisfied with the results suggests that patients make their own critical assessments of surgical outcome. Indeed, the patient's subjective evaluation may surprise the surgeon. For example, an individual with −8.00 D of myopia before surgery who postoperatively has −2.00 D of myopia with an uncorrected visual acuity of 20/40 may judge the surgery a rousing success, even though the patient elects to wear spectacles for driving and watching television. On the other hand, a patient with a preoperative refraction of −4.00 D who saw 20/10 with contact lenses may be dissatisfied with the postoperative refraction of −0.75 D that gives an uncorrected visual acuity of only 20/20. Among the probable factors that determine a patient's subjective satisfaction are their preoperative expectations (which should be guided as realistically as possible by the surgeon), their postoperative visual needs, the experiences of friends with keratotomy, and ultimately their own personality.

Authors	Arrowsmith PN and Marks RG	Waring GO, Lynn MJ, and the PERK Study Group	Deitz MR, Sanders DR, and Raanan MS
Symmetry of refractive outcome	Not reported		Not reported
Number of patients		346	
Mean difference between two eyes		0.93 D	
Percentage of patients with a difference of	Not reported		Not reported
1.00 D or less		51%	
2.00 D or less		88%	
3.00 D or greater		4%	

Comment: The only published report giving data about the symmetry of outcome in two eyes of the same patient is from the PERK study. The fact that over 88% of the patients had 2.00 D or less of refractive anisometropia is quite encouraging. This may reflect to some degree the PERK study's design, in which the outcome in the first eye was used to help plan the surgery in the second eye. However, 14% of the patients had four to eight Snellen lines difference in the uncorrected visual acuity between their two eyes (only 1% had such a difference before surgery), emphasizing that induced asymmetry of refraction is a potential clinical problem for some patients (see Chapter 22, Bilateral Results of Refractive Keratotomy).

Authors	Arrowsmith PN and Marks RG	Waring GO, Lynn MJ, and the PERK Study Group	Deitz MR, Sanders DR, and Raanan MS
Visual function score	Not reported		Not reported
Qualitative outcome		Excellent Good Fair Poor	
Percentage of eyes		39% 29% 20% 12%	

Comment: Lynn and colleagues (Lynn MJ, Waring GO, and Carter JT: Combining Refractive Error and Uncorrected Visual Acuity to Assess the Effectiveness of Refractive and Corneal Surgery, Refract Corneal Surg 1990;6:103-112) revised the visual function index of Nordan and colleagues (Nordan LT, Bores L, Brent S, et al: Meaningful Evaluation of Refractive Surgery (letter), J Cataract Refract Surg 1988;14:99-100) to devise a visual function score that related both the uncorrected visual acuity and the spherical equivalent refractive error after surgery. This method gives a more realistic assessment of the outcome of refractive corneal surgery and particularly guards against labeling overcorrected eyes with residual hyperopia as having an excellent result on the basis of the visual acuity alone. For example, a 25-year-old man with a preoperative refraction of -3.00 D who has a postoperative refraction of $+2.00$ D and sees 20/20 would have an excellent outcome on the basis of the visual acuity, but the hyperopic overcorrection represents only a fair result. Combining the excellent visual acuity and the fair refractive result would give him an overall good outcome.

Authors	Arrowsmith PN and Marks RG	Waring GO, Lynn MJ, and the PERK Study Group	Deitz MR, Sanders DR, and Raanan MS
Percentage of eyes requiring no spectacle or contact lens correction	60%	65%	Not reported

Comment: On a very pragmatic level, the overall effectiveness of refractive keratotomy can be judged by whether or not the patient stops wearing an optical correction. Although this is a useful criterion, it does not take into account those patients who are able to go without optical correction most of the time, but use glasses for driving, theater, or close work. Also, there needs to be a clear distinction made between distance and near correction, since most patients in the presbyopic age range who had successful radial keratotomy will need reading glasses. Finally, even those patients who still must wear glasses after surgery, but whose glasses are much thinner and lighter than before, can express considerable satisfaction with the surgery. The fact that approximately two thirds of the patients in the Arrowsmith and PERK studies went without glasses is probably an underestimate of what can be achieved with current techniques.

Figure 21-1   Arrowsmith and Marks: 5-Year Refractive Results

Scattergram at 5 years after refractive keratotomy shows change in spherical equivalent refraction after surgery compared with preoperative values. Note the wide scatter and the tendency for overcorrection. Only 85 dots are present of the 123 eyes in the study. Some dots must represent more than one eye. An ideal result is one that falls on the diagonal emmetropia line. (From Arrowsmith PN and Marks RG: Visual, refractive, and keratometric results of radial keratotomy, Arch Ophthalmol 107:506, 1989.)

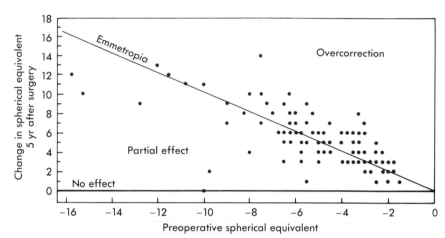

Figure 21-2   Deitz, Sanders, and Raanan: Stability over 2 Years

Change in mean spherical equivalent refraction from beginning to end of three time intervals after radial keratotomy. Metal blade cases represent 165 eyes (73% of total) between 12 and 48 months. Diamond blade cases represent 77 eyes (26% of total) between 12 and 24 months. There is an increasing effect of the surgery with a trend in the hyperopic direction. (From Dietz MR, Sanders DR, and Raanan MG: Progressive hyperopia in radial keratotomy, Ophthalmology 93:1284, 1986.)

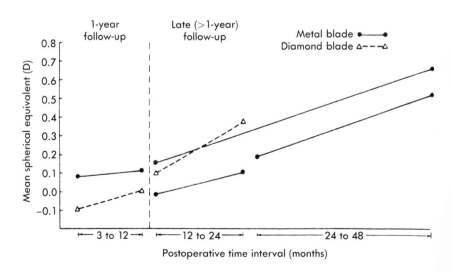

Figure 21-3   Waring, Lynn, and the PERK Study Group: 5-Year Refractive Results

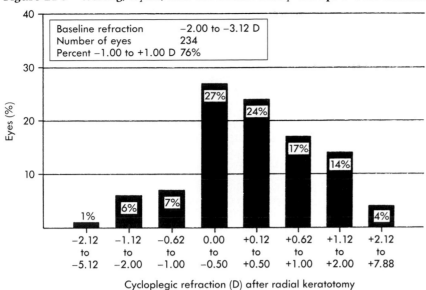

Baseline refraction   −2.00 to −3.12 D
Number of eyes   234
Percent −1.00 to +1.00 D 76%

Cycloplegic refraction (D) after radial keratotomy

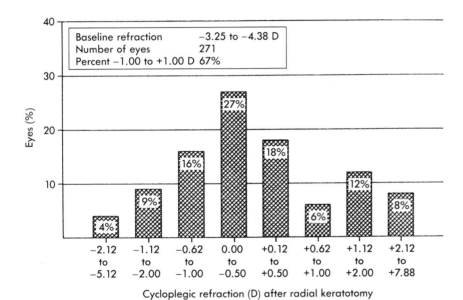

Baseline refraction   −3.25 to −4.38 D
Number of eyes   271
Percent −1.00 to +1.00 D 67%

Cycloplegic refraction (D) after radial keratotomy

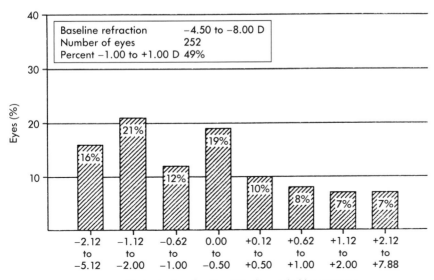

Baseline refraction   −4.50 to −8.00 D
Number of eyes   252
Percent −1.00 to +1.00 D 49%

Cycloplegic refraction (D) after radial keratotomy

The spherical equivalent of the cycloplegic refraction at 5 years after radial keratotomy in the three baseline refraction groups; lower group *(top)*, middle group *(center)*, and higher group *(bottom)*. The height of the bars represents the percentage of eyes in each range of refraction. The percentage of eyes between +1.00 and −1.00 D is given in the inset.

SECTION II: Summary of Published Studies of Refractive Keratotomy in Chronological Order

Authors	Waring GO, Lynn MJ, and the PERK Study Group	Bauerberg J, Sterzovsky M, and Brodsky M	Sawelson H and Marks G
Article title and citation	Results of the Prospective Evaluation of Radial Keratotomy (PERK) Study 4 Years after Surgery for Myopia, JAMA 1990;263:1083-1091.	Radial Keratotomy in Myopia of 6 to 12 Diopters Using Full-Length Deepening Incisions, Refract Corneal Surg 1989;5:150-154.	Five-Year Results of Radial Keratotomy, Refract Corneal Surg 1989;5:8-20.
Other publications	See Section I, pp. 786-787.	Brodsky M, Bauerberg J, and Sterzaovzky M: Quertotomia Radial Analisis Global de Nuestros Primeros 380 Ojos, Arch Oftal Buenos Aires, 1986;61:74-78.	Sawelson H and Marks G: Two-Year Results of Radial Keratotomy, Arch Ophthalmol 1985;103:505-510. Sawelson H and Marks G: Three-Year Results of Radial Keratotomy, Arch Ophthalmol 1987;105:81-85. Sawelson H, Marks G: Two-Year Results of Reoperations for Radial Keratotomy, Arch Ophthalmol 1988;106:497-501.
Dates of Surgery	March 1982 to October 1988	April 1985 to April 1988	October 1980 to July 1981
Funding source			
National Institutes of Health	Yes	No	Yes
Private	Yes	Yes	Yes
University	Yes	No	No
Industry	Yes	No	No
Study design			
Prospective	Yes	Yes	
Retrospective	No	No	Yes
Consecutive eyes	Yes	Yes	Yes
Sample size calculation	Yes	No	No
Selection criteria specified	Yes	Yes	No
Participants and number			
Study centers	9	1	1
Surgeons	10	3	1
Independent physician examiners	Yes	Not reported	No
Independent technician examiners	Yes	Not reported	No
Independent monitors	Yes	Not reported	No
Biostatistician	Yes	Not reported	Yes
Disclosure of financial interest	No disclosure; one investigator had a financial interest in the Villasenor pachometer	Not reported	Not reported
Patient population			
Number of patients	435	364	Not reported
Number of eyes	435	409	134 (68% of original 198)
Reoperations included	No	No	Yes (18%)
Withdrawals/exclusions accounted for	Yes	Yes	Yes
Age; mean (range)	33.5 yr (21 to 58 yr)	35.77 yr (22 to 64 yr)	Not reported (19 to 65 yr)
Sex; % female	48%	59%	Not reported

Authors	Waring GO, Lynn MJ, and the PERK Study Group	Bauerberg J, Sterzovsky M, and Brodsky M	Sawelson H and Marks G
Clinical examination conditions			
Office practice	No	No	Yes
Standardized	Yes	Yes	No
Data analysis			
Informal (tables, graphs)	Yes	Yes	Yes
Arithmetic (mean, standard deviation, range)	Yes	Yes	Yes
Statistical (regression analysis, confidence limits)	Yes	No	Yes
Follow-up			
Mean (range)	4 yr (45 to 56 mo)	Not reported	4.85 yr (3.0 to 6.3 yr)
Percentage of original population of follow-up	92% (401 of 435)	65% at 6 mo; 41% at 12 mo	68%
Surgical protocol			
Formal, replicable	Yes	Yes	No
Informal, not replicable	No	No	Yes
Patient variables used to determine surgical plan			
Refraction	Yes	Yes	Yes
Age	No	Not reported	No
Sex	No	Not reported	No
Keratometry readings	No	Not reported	Yes
Intraocular pressure	No	Not reported	Yes
Ocular rigidity	No	Not reported	Yes
Corneal diameter	No	Not reported	Yes
Corneal thickness	Yes	Yes	No
Measurement of corneal thickness			
Optical	No	No	No
Ultrasonic (speed of sound, m/sec)	Yes (1640)	Yes (1720)	Yes (1550)
Preoperative	No	Yes	Yes
Intraoperative	Yes	Yes	No
Location of measurement	Paracentral	Central	Central
Anesthesia			Not reported
Topical	Yes (0.5% proparacaine)	Yes (0.5% proparacaine)	
Retrobulbar	No	No	
Knife blade and handle			
Metal blade	No	No	Beaver 57, Sputnik
Diamond blade	Yes (single edge)	Yes	No
Blade holder	Yes	Yes	Yes
Micrometer handle	Yes	Yes	No
Blade length; percentage of corneal thickness	100% of thinnest paracentral reading at clear zone	110% of central reading for initial incisions; 115% of central for deepening	80% to 90%, paracentral
Calibration block	Yes	Yes	Bores

Authors	Waring GO, Lynn MJ, and the PERK Study Group		Bauerberg J, Sterzovsky M, and Brodsky M	Sawelson H and Marks G
Clear zone				Not reported
Range of diameters	3.0, 3.5, and 4.0 mm		Not reported	
Circular (%)	100%		100%	
Elliptical	No		No	
Incisions				
Number (%) of radial	8 (100%)		8 (100%)	8, 16
Transverse	No		No	No
Direction				
Clear zone to limbus	Yes		Yes	No
Limbus to clear zone	No		No	Yes
Technique				
Single pass	100%		No	Yes
Peripheral deepening	No		0%	Yes
Recut; same blade length	No		100% recut using full-length deepening incisions	No
Freehand dissection	No		0%	No
Across limbus	No		0%	No
Reoperations (%) included in results	No		No	18%
Baseline refraction groups (range in diopters)	Original categories and clear zone diameter	Adjusted categories for comparison with other studies		
Lower	2.00 to 3.12 (4.00 mm)	0.60 to 3.00	Group I, −6.0 to −8.0	−1.50 to 2.88
Middle	3.25 to 4.37 (3.5 mm)	3.10 to 6.00	Group II, −8.1 to −12.0	−3.00 to 5.88
Higher	4.50 to 8.00 (3.0 mm)	6.10 to 11.90		−6.00 to 10.38
Highest				
Postoperative corticosteroids	Yes		Yes	Not reported
Achieved incision depth				
Method of measurement	Formal protocol for visual inspection with slit-lamp microscopy in at least three locations in 3204 incisions		Not reported	Slit-lamp microscopy
Depth as percentage of corneal thickness	76% to 100% in 66% 50% to 75% in 28% 26% to 50% in 6%		Not reported	75% to 90% in 67%; 90% in 17%
Perforations (%)	2%		Not reported	Not reported
Refraction results				
Cycloplegic	Yes		No	No
Manifest	No		Yes	Yes
Percentage ± 1.00 D, all eyes	55%		58%	56%
	Original	Adjusted		
Lower	73%	76%	65% at 6 mo; 69% at 1 yr	
Middle	58%	55%	39% at 6 mo; 33% at 1 yr	
Higher	39%	21%		
Overcorrected > 1.00 D	17%		3% at 6 mo	22%
Undercorrected > 1.00 D	26%		Not reported	18%
Figure	Fig. 21-5 (p. 805)		—	Fig. 21-4 (p. 805)

Authors	Waring GO, Lynn MJ, and the PERK Study Group		Bauerberg J, Sterzovsky M, and Brodsky M	Sawelson H and Marks G	
Uncorrected visual acuity results					
Acuity category	≥ 20/40	≥20/20	≥ 20/40	≥20/40	≥20/20
Total	76%	52%	38%	62%	
Lower	94%	76%	48% at 1 yr	75%	11%
Middle	79%	53%	14% at 1 yr	65%	7%
Higher	58%	32%	—	36%	0%
Loss of best-corrected visual acuity					
Loss of one Snellen line	Not reported		25%	Not reported	
Loss of two or more Snellen lines	11 of 433 eyes (2.5%)		Not reported	10%	
Figure	Fig. 21-6 (p. 805)		—	—	
Predictability			Not reported	Not reported	
Prediction or confidence interval (D)	4.42 for all eyes (3.27 for lower group, 4.45 for middle group, and 5.26 for higher group)				
Factors affecting outcome					
Method of study	Regression analysis		Clinical experience		
Clear zone diameter	Yes		Not reported		
Refraction	Yes		Yes		
Patient age	Yes		Yes		
Depth of incision	Yes		Yes		
Number of incisions	8 only in this study		8 only with full-length deepening		
Average central keratotomy	No		Not reported		
Patient sex	No		Not reported		
Topography	Not used		Not reported		
Intraocular pressure	No		Not reported		
Corneal thickness	No		Not reported		
Number of zones	Not used		Not reported		
Stability of refraction (Change in minus power)			Not reported		
Time interval	6 mo to 4 yr			18 mo to 5 yr for 123 eyes	
Increased myopia = 1.00 to 2.50 D	4%			5%	
Change = < 1.00 D	73%			78%	
Decreased myopia = 1.00 to 2.50 D	1.00 to 1.87 = 21%			17%	
Mean change	−0.41			+0.20 D	
Vision-threatening complications					
Present series	No		No	Two eyes of one patient showed stromal haze	
Additional reports by same author	No		No	No	
Delayed bacterial keratitis	Two eyes		No	No	
Ruptured globe	No		No	No	
Patient satisfaction			Not reported	Not reported	
Percentage satisfied (low, medium, high)	Low, 6%; Med, 41%, High, 49%				
Percentage of patients who would undergo repeat surgery	9.5%				
Figure	Fig. 21-7 (p. 806)		—	—	

Authors	Waring GO, Lynn MJ, and the PERK Study Group	Bauerberg J, Sterzovsky M, and Brodsky M	Sawelson H and Marks G
People wearing lenses after surgery		Not reported	Not reported
Total polled (%)	64% required no spectacle or contact lens correction		
Percentage of patients wearing glasses/contact lenses part-time	Not reported		
Percentage of patients wearing glasses/contact lenses full-time	Not reported		

| **Comment** | The fact that the article presenting the 4-year results of the PERK study was chosen to be the lead article in the *Journal of the American Medical Association* attests to the broad interest in radial keratotomy among the medical community. At 91% follow-up rate the PERK study has the highest follow-up of any reported radial keratotomy series. The 4-year study was the last study to report one eye of each patient and to omit patients that had repeated operations, so it gives a picture of what was achieved with a single operation using a standardized technique. In the discussion the authors outlined changes in surgical technique that occurred since the PERK study was designed. The PERK study is the only study to report 90% prediction intervals to quantify the "predictability" of radial keratotomy. At 4 years the prediction interval is 4.50 D wide, which the authors conclude qualifies as "unpredictable." The authors found patient age to be the only patient characteristic that affected surgical outcome. The operation is considered safe, since only two eyes were not correctable to 20/25 or better after surgery, and only 2.5% of the eyes lost two or more lines of best-corrected visual acuity. | Although surgeons commonly state that radial keratotomy is most useful up to approximately 6.00 D of myopia, Bauerberg and colleagues have demonstrated that it can be effective in eyes with 6.00 to 12.00 D of myopia. The follow-up at 6 months was only 65%, so one third of the eyes remain unaccounted for. They achieved a residual refractive error at 6 months within 2.00 D of emmetropia in 90% of eyes from −6.00 to −8.00 D preoperatively and in approximately 80% of eyes with −8.00 to −12.00 D of myopia preoperatively. These results were achieved by a double-pass technique, in which the blade was extended an extra 5% of the paracentral corneal thickness and a full-length second pass incision was made centrifugally. The frequency of perforations was not reported. However, their overall results of 58% of eyes within ±1.00 D of emmetropia and 38% of eyes seeing 20/40 or better uncorrected are not outstanding, but certainly useful. A psychometric test to determine patient satisfaction in this group would be most interesting. The authors provided a useful table summarizing eight articles in which surgery was done for eyes with more than −6.00 D of myopia. | These authors, a private practice clinician and a university biostatistician, have reported in a series of four articles, detailed long-term follow-up on patients receiving keratotomy performed with metal blades in 1980-1981. Although the follow-up is only 68% at 5 years, the reports are extremely important because they are among the few that present 5-year data on a single cohort of patients. The lack of a replicable surgical protocol is of little consequence, since the techniques used are now out-of-date. In general the results tend toward undercorrection, only 15% of the eyes showing an overcorrection of +1.00 D or greater at 5 years. This is in marked contrast to the metal blade series of Arrowsmith, in which overcorrections occurred in almost one third of eyes and is similar to the 16% overcorrection achieved in the PERK study at 3 years. Most significant is the identification of a continued effect of the surgery, 17% of the eyes showing a 1 D or greater change between 18 months and 5 years. Their analysis suggests that the continued effect stops at 3 years, but the data that support that contention are not convincing. The authors conclude that radial keratotomy is "effective for the vast majority of patients," but only half of the eyes had a refraction within ±1.00 D of emmetropia. |

Figure 21-4 Sawelson and Marks

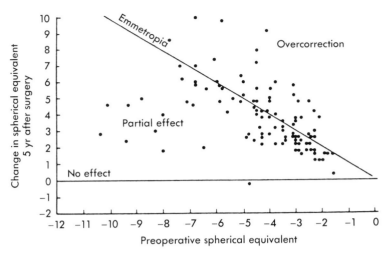

Scattergram demonstrates the change in refraction spread after radial keratotomy at 5 years. There is considerable spread in the results; particularly, there is a trend toward undercorrection in eyes with −7.00 D or more of myopia. Eyes with −4.00 D or less cluster reasonably well around the line of emmetropia. (From Sawelson H and Marks G: Five-year results of radial keratotomy, Refract Corneal Surg 1989;5:8-20.)

Figures 21-5 and 21-6 Waring, Lynn, and the PERK Study Group

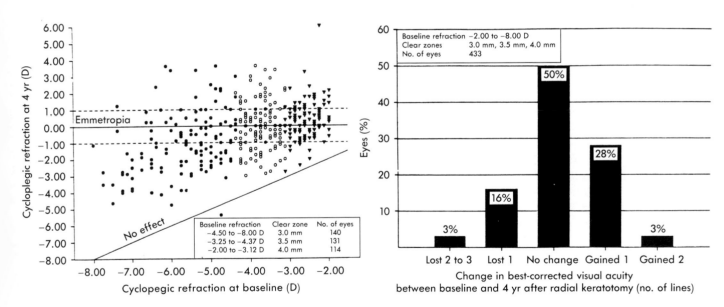

Figure 21-5
The spherical equivalent of the cycloplegic refraction at 4 years after radial keratotomy compared with the refraction at baseline. The three symbols indicate the three baseline refraction groups *(inset)*. There was a wide spread of results, with a particular weighting toward undercorrection in eyes with −6.00 D or more of myopia. Dotted lines indicate +1.00 and −1.00 diopters (D). (From Waring GO, Lynn MJ, Fielding MS, et al: Results of the Prospective Evaluation of Radial Keratotomy (PERK) study 4 years after surgery for myopia, JAMA 1990;263:1083.)

Figure 21-6
The change in spectacle-corrected visual acuity between baseline and 4 years after radial keratotomy. The change is expressed as a gain or loss of Snellen lines. The authors considered a change of one Snellen line clinically insignificant; they regarded only the 3% of eyes that lost two to three Snellen lines as having a meaningful change in best spectacle-corrected visual acuity. (From Waring GO, Lynn MJ, Fielding MS, et al: Results of the Prospective Evaluation of Radial Keratotomy (PERK) study 4 years after surgery for myopia, JAMA 1990;263:1083.)

Figure 21-7 Waring, Lynn, and the PERK Study Group

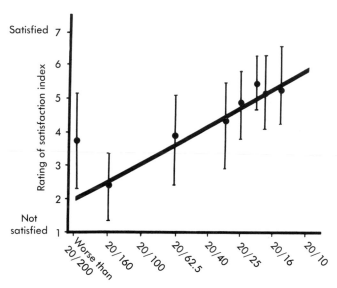

Regression of reported satisfaction index scores and unaided visual acuity shows linear relationship between the two. Persons with better visual acuity 1 year after surgery on one eye were more satisfied. Exceptions were three persons whose unaided visual acuity after surgery remained worse than 20/200. Although uncorrected visual acuity remains poor for these three patients, their visual ability when measured with spherical equivalent cycloplegic refractions is significantly better than it was before surgery. The small size of this group and marked improvement in their vision explain their status as outliers. (From Bourque LB, Cosand BB, Drews C, et al: Reported satisfaction, fluctuation of vision, and glare among patients 1 year after surgery in the Prospective Evaluation of Radial Keratotomy (PERK) study, Arch Ophthalmol 1986;104:356.)

SECTION II: Summary of Published Studies of Refractive Keratotomy in Chronological Order—cont'd

Authors	Spigelman AV, Williams PA, and Lindstrom RL	Kim JH	Salz JJ and Salz MS
Article and journal citation	Further Studies of Four-Incision Radial Keratotomy, Refract Corneal Surg 1989;5:292-295.	A Prospective Clinical Study of Radial Keratotomy in Koreans, J Korean Ophthalmol Soc 1988;2:13-21.	Salz JJ, Salz JM, Salz M, and Jones D: Ten Years' Experience with Conservative Approach to Radial Keratotomy, Refract Corneal Surg 1991;7:12-22.
Other publications	Spigelman AV, Williams PA, Nichols BD, and Lindstrom RL: Four-Incision Radial Keratotomy, J Cataract Refract Surg 1988;14:125-128.	Kim JH: Clinical Experiences of Radial Keratotomy for Reduction of Myopia, J Kor Ophthalmol Soc 1983;24:735. Kim JH, and Ham TS: A Prospective Clinical Study of Radial Keratotomy: report 2. J Kor Ophthalmol Soc 1986;27.	Salz JJ and Salz MS: Results of Four- and Eight-Incision Radial Keratotomy for 6 to 11 Diopters of Myopia, J Refract Surg 1988;4:46-50. Salz JJ, Villasenor RA, Elander R, et al: Four-Incision Radial Keratotomy for Low to Moderate Myopia, Ophthalmology 1986;93:727-738.
Dates of surgery	Before September 1986	February 1982 to December 1986	September 1980 to June 1990
Funding source			
National Institutes of Health	No	No	No
Private	No	No	Yes
University	Yes	Yes	Yes
Industry	No	No	No
Study design			
Prospective	No	Yes	No
Retrospective	Yes	No	Yes
Consecutive eyes	Yes	Not reported	No
Sample size calculation	No	No	No
Selection criteria	Not reported	No	No
Participants and number			
Study centers	1	1	1
Surgeons	Not reported	1	1
Independent physician examiners	No	Not reported	No
Independent technician examiners	No	Not reported	No
Independent monitors	No	Not reported	No
Biostatistician	No	Not reported	No
Disclosure of financial interest	Yes	Not reported	Yes
Patient population			
Number of patients	30	246	135
Number of eyes	52	348	225
Reoperations included	No	Yes (two patients—two eyes)	Yes
Withdrawals/exclusions accounted for	Yes	No	Not reported
Age: Mean(range)	Not reported	26 yr (16 to 44 yr)	36 yr (20 to 73 yr)
Sex, % female	Not reported	47%	45%

Authors	Spigelman AV, Williams PA, and Lindstrom RL	Kim JH	Salz JJ and Salz MS
Clinical examination conditions			
Office practice	Yes	Yes	Yes
Standardized	No	No	No
Data analysis			
Informal (tables, graphs)	Yes	Yes	Yes
Arithmetic (mean, standard deviation, range)	Yes	Yes	Yes
Statistical (regression analysis, confidence limits)	No	No	No
Follow-up			
Mean (range)	62% at 1 yr (1 to 3 yr)	12 mo (6 mo to 4 yr)	3 to 12 mo (100%)
Percentage of original population at follow-up	62%	Not reported	24 to 110 mo (44%)
Surgical protocol			
Formal, replicable	No	No	No
Informal, not replicable	Yes	Yes	Yes
Patient variables used to determine surgical plan			
Refraction	Yes	Yes	Yes
Age	Yes	No	Yes
Sex	No	No	No
Keratometry reading	No	No	Yes
Intraocular pressure	No	No	No
Ocular rigidity	No	No	No
Corneal diameter	No	No	No
Corneal thickness	No	No	No
Measurement of corneal thickness			
Optical	No	No	No
Ultrasonic (speed of sound, m/sec)	Yes (1640)	Yes	Yes (1640)
Preoperative	Yes		No
Intraoperative	No		Yes
Location of measurement	Central and at 3, 6, 9, and 12 o'clock around optical zone	Center, mid-periphery, and periphery	Paracentral
Anesthesia			
Topical	Yes	Yes	Yes
Retrobulbar	No	No	No
Knife blade and handle			
Metal blade	No	Yes	No
Diamond blade	Yes	Yes	Yes
Blade holder	No	Yes	No
Micrometer handle	Yes	Yes	Yes (PERK style)
Blade length; thickness	100% to 115% of thinnest paracentral	95% of mid-periphery	100% to 110% of thinnest paracentral
Calibration block	Coin gauge	Yes	Not reported
Clear zone			
Range of diameters	3.0 to 5.0 mm	3.0 to 4.0 mm	3.0 to 4.0 mm
Circular (%)	100%	Yes	100%
Elliptical (%)	No	Yes	No

Authors	Spigelman AV, Williams PA, and Lindstrom RL	Kim JH		Salz JJ and Salz MS
Incisions				
Number (%) of radial	4 (100%)	8 (92%)		4 (51%)
		16 (5%)		8 (45%)
		> 30 (3%)		6, 10, 12 (4%)
Transverse	No	Yes		Yes
Direction				
Clear zone to limbus	Yes	No		Yes
Limbus to clear zone	No	Yes		No
Technique				
Single pass	Yes	Yes		Yes
Peripheral deepening	No	Yes		No
Recut; same blade length	No	No		No
Freehand dissection	No	No		No
Across limbus	No	No		No
Reoperations (%) included in results technique	No	Yes		Yes (15%)
Baseline refraction groups (range in diopters)				
Lower	−1.50 to −4.75	−1.75 to −2.75		−1.25 to −3.00
Middle	—	−3.00 to −5.75		−3.10 to −5.80
Higher	—	> −6.00		−6.00 to −11.60
Highest	−8.37 (one eye)	—		Not reported
Postoperative corticosteroids	Yes (if uncorrrected)	Yes		Yes
Achieved incision depth				Not reported
Method of measurement	Not reported	Slit-lamp microscopy		
Depth as percentage of corneal thickness	Not reported	80% to 85%		
Perforations(%)	4%	3%		3.5%
Refraction results				
Cycloplegic	Yes	Yes		No
Manifest	No	Yes		Yes
Percentage ±1.00 D	91%	Not reported		73% (total all eyes)
Lower	Not reported			97%
Middle				81%
Higher				45%
Highest				
Overcorrected > 1.00 D (%)	Not reported	2%		3%
Undercorrected > 1.00 D (%)	3%	1%		24%
Figure	—	Fig. 21−8 (p. 812)		Fig. 21−9 (p. 812)
Uncorrected visual acuity results				
Acuity category	≥20/40	≥20/40	≥20/20	≥20/40
Total	—	56%	22%	69%
Lower	88%	79%	47%	100%
Middle	—	73%	36%	73%
Higher	—	34%	50%	47%
Highest	—			
Loss of best-corrected visual acuity		Not reported		
Loss of one Snellen line	—			Four eyes
Loss of two or more Snellen lines	0%			—

Authors	Spigelman AV, Williams PA, and Lindstrom RL	Kim JH	Salz JJ and Salz MS
Predictability		Not reported	Not reported
Prediction or confidence interval	Not reported		
Factors affecting outcome			
Method of study	Regression analysis		
Clear zone diameter	Yes		
Refraction	Yes		
Patient age	Yes		
Depth of incision	Yes		
Number of incisions	No		
Average central keratometry	No		
Patient sex	No		
Topography	No		
Intraocular pressure	No		
Corneal thickness	No		
Number of zones	Not reported		
Stability of refraction		Not reported	
(Change in minus power)			
Time interval	1 to 3 yr (five eyes)		50 eyes—12 to 60 mo (48 to 110 mo)
Increased myopia = 1.00 to 2.50 D	0		6%
Change = < 0.87 D	3		72%
Decreased myopia = 1.00 to 2.50 D	2		22%
Mean change	+0.72 D		Not reported
Vision-threatening complications			
Present series	No	None	No
Additional reports by same author	No	No	No
Delayed bacterial keratitis	No	—	No
Ruptured globe	No	—	No
Patient satisfaction	Not reported		Not reported
Percentage of patients satisfied (low, medium, high)		61% high 29% medium 10% not satisfied	
Percentage of patients who would undergo repeat surgery		Not reported	
People wearing lenses after surgery	Not reported		Not reported
Total polled (%)		90% stated postoperative vision allowed them to work without glasses	

Authors	Spigelman AV, Williams PA, and Lindstrom RL	Kim JH	Salz JJ and Salz MS
Comments	This is one of the few published studies limited to the results of four-incision radial keratotomy. Unfortunately the retrospective study follows only 69% of the eyes from 6 to 12 months. The most remarkable finding is the refractive results, with 91% within 1 D of emmetropia and only two eyes overcorrected, a tribute to the relatively low preoperative refractive range of -1.50 to -4.75 D. Regression analysis identified only two patient variables as predictors: age and refraction. The authors advocate staging the operation; the seven eyes had a second procedure, but were excluded from this four-incision-only report.	The article is thoroughly done and presents a reasonably comprehensive analysis of an apparent consecutive series of eyes. A strength of the article is the display of information in the tables and graphs, which lay out the results in low, moderate, and high myopia groups in a very thorough manner so that they can be reasonably compared with the results of other studies. A weakness of the series is that a large number of different operative procedures were used, and although 92% of the eyes had eight incisions, deepening incisions were used where needed and steroid drops were used postoperatively, so the exact methods of obtaining the results are not clear. The techniques, however, reflect the realities of clinical practice and are quite acceptable. The author describes at least a 1-year follow-up but does not state how many total eyes were operated between 1982 and 1986, so the total percentage of follow-up is unknown. Bridle sutures were used on the superior and inferior rectus muscles. Endothelial microscopy done on 6% of the eyes showed approximately a 5% cell loss centrally. Twelve percent of eyes had an increase in refractive astigmatism of 1.00 D to approximately 3.00 D. Eight percent of eyes had a decrease in refractive astigmatism in that range. A subjective questionnaire yielded patients reporting symptoms of fluctuation of vision during the day (52%), glare at night (39%), photophobia (25%), and diplopia (5%). Unfortunately there were no baseline data to which these postoperative percentages could be compared.	The authors report on a heterogeneous group of patients who underwent keratotomy over a 10-year period, representing a "conservative approach" in both patient selection and surgery. Approximately half the operations were performed using four incisions only, most of those being performed for the more recent patients. The authors favor the concept of titrating surgery by starting with four incisions and then adding more as necessary, with the overall goal of eliminating overcorrection. For example, the authors emphasize that eyes with 3.00 D or less preoperative myopia numbered only 15% in this study, as compared with 70% in the Deitz diamond-knife study and 47% in the PERK study. They had only eyes with a hyperopic postoperative correction of only $+0.10$ D or greater. They emphasize that radial keratotomy can be "disconcertingly unpredictable" for individual patients and illustrate this with case examples. The authors emphasize the improvements that have been made in radial keratotomy in a table comparing earlier studies, and point out that a residual refraction within ±1.00 D of emmetropia was achieved in 55% of eyes in the PERK study and 70% in the Deitz study, both earlier studies, whereas it was achieved in 93% in the previous four-incision study by Salz, 92% in Spigelman, and 80% in the present study, which actually spanned 10 years.

Figure 21-8   Kim

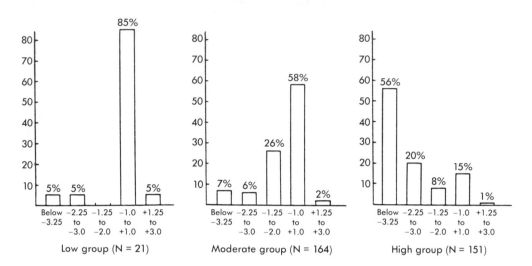

Low group (N = 21)   Moderate group (N = 164)   High group (N = 151)

Spherical equivalent refraction at 1 year or more after radial keratotomy in three refractive groups: low, −1.75 D to −2.75 D; moderate, −3.00 D to −5.75 D; high, −6.00 D and greater. (From Kim JH: A prospective clinical study of radial keratotomy in Koreans, Kor J Ophthalmol 1988;2:13.)

Figure 21-9   Salz and Salz

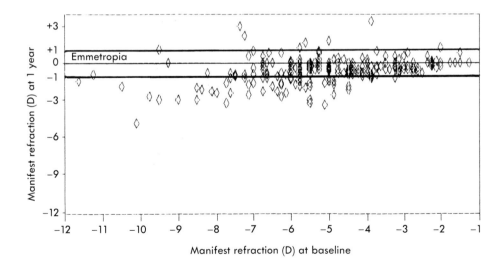

Scattergram displays a spherical equivalent refraction at 3 months to 1 year after radial keratotomy as compared with the baseline refraction in 225 eyes. The bold lines indicate +1.00 and −1.00 D. Between −1.00 and −5.00 D the eyes clustered generally within the ± 1.00 D range. From −5.00 to −7.00 D, undercorrections began to appear. At greater than −7.00 D, most of the eyes were undercorrected. (From Salz JJ, Salz JM, Salz M, and Jones D: Ten years' experience with a conservative approach to radial keratotomy, Refract Corneal Surg 1991;7:12-22.)

SECTION II: Summary of Published Studies of Refractive Keratotomy—cont'd

Authors	Arne JL and Bourdiol AM	Lavery FL	Menezo JL, Cisneros A, and Harto M
Article title and citation	Results of 350 Anterior Radial Keratotomies in Myopia: Postoperative Follow-up of More Than 1 Year, Implant Refract Surg 1987;5:94-103.	Comparative Results of 200 Consecutive Radial Keratotomy Cases Using Three Different Nomograms, J Refract Surg 1987;3:88-91.	Cirugia de la Myopia Analysis Bioestadistico de la Queratotomia Radial, 1986, Barcelona, Salvat Editores.
Other publications	None	None	None
Dates of surgery	1983 to 1984	Not reported	Not reported
Funding source		Not reported	Not reported
National Institutes of Health	No		
Private	Yes		
University	No		
Industry	No		
Study design			
Prospective	No	No	No
Retrospective	Yes	Yes	Yes
Consecutive eyes	Not reported	Yes	No
Sample size calculation	No	No	No
Selection criteria	No	No	No
Participants and number			
Study centers	1	1	Not reported
Surgeons	Not reported	1	Not reported
Independent physician examiners	No	Not reported	No
Independent technician examiners	No	Not reported	No
Independent monitors	No	Not reported	No
Biostatistician	No	Not reported	Yes
Disclosure of financial interest	Not reported	Not reported	Not reported
Patient population			
Number of patients	198	Not reported	Not reported
Number of eyes	350	200	820
Reoperations included	Yes	No	Not reported
Withdrawals/exclusions accounted for	Not reported	Not reported	Not reported
Age; mean (range)	Not reported (20 to 41 yr)	Not reported	24 to 40 yr
Sex, % female	Not reported	Not reported	43%
Clinical examination conditions			
Office practice	Yes	Yes	Yes
Standardized	No	No	No
Data analysis			
Informal (tables, graphs)	Yes	Yes	Yes
Arithmetic (mean, standard deviation, range)	Yes	No	Yes
Statistical (regression analysis, confidence limits)	No	No	Yes

Authors	Arne JL and Bourdiol AM	Lavery FL	Menezo JL, Cisneros A, and Harto M
Follow-up			
Mean (range)	1 yr (not reported)	6 mo	1 yr
Percentage of original population at follow-up	Not reported	100%	Not reported
Surgical protocol			
Formal, replicable			
Informal, not replicable	Yes	Yes	Yes
Patient variables used to determine surgical plan			
Refraction	Yes	Sawelson, Ellis, Thornton nomograms used to determine surgical parameters	Yes
Age	Yes		Yes
Sex	No		No
Keratometry reading	No		Yes
Intraocular pressure	No		No
Ocular rigidity	No		No
Corneal diameter	No		No
Corneal thickness	No		No
Measurement of corneal thickness			
Optical	No	Yes	No
Ultrasonic (speed of sound, m/sec)	Yes (1640)	Not reported	Yes
Preoperative	Not reported	Not reported	Not reported
Intraoperative	Not reported	Not reported	Yes
Location of measurement	Central, peripheral	Not reported	Not reported
Anesthesia	Not reported		Not reported
Topical			
Retrobulbar		10% (retrobulbar or periorbital)	
Knife blade and handle			Variable
Metal blade	No	No	
Diamond blade	Yes	Yes	
Blade holder	No	Not reported	
Micrometer handle	Yes	Yes	
Blade length; percentage of corneal thickness	100% of central	Central optical pachometer thickness plus 15%	
Calibration block	Yes	Not reported	
Clear zone			
Range of diameters	3 to 4 mm	Not reported	2.75 to > 4.50 mm
Circular (%)	100%	Not reported	100%
Elliptical (%)		Not reported	
Incisions			
Number (%) of radial	4,8 (not reported)	4 to 16	1 to 8 (40%) 9 to 12 (14%) 13 to 24 (29%) 25 to 32 (11%) > 33 (6%)

Authors	Arne JL and Bourdiol AM	Lavery FL	Menezo JL, Cisneros A, and Harto M
Incisions			
Transverse	No	Yes	Yes
Direction			
Clear zone to limbus	Yes	Yes	Yes
Limbus to clear zone	No	No	No
Technique			Not reported
Single pass	Yes	Yes	
Peripheral deepening	Yes	Yes	
Recut—same blade length	No	No	
Freehand dissection	No	No	
Across limbus	No	No	
Reoperations (%)	7%	No	16%
Included in results	Yes		Yes
Technique	Recut original incisions without opening		Not reported
Baseline refraction groups (range in diopters)			Not reported
Lower	1.50 to 3.00	−1.50 to −3.00	
Middle	3.25 to 4.50	−3.25 to −4.50	
Higher	4.75 to 6.00	−4.75 to −9.75	
Highest			
Postoperative corticosteroids	Not reported	Yes	Not reported
Achieved incision depth	Not reported		Not reported
Method of measurement		Not reported	
Depth as percentage of corneal thickness		90% to 95%	
Perforations (%)	2%	3% during primary incisions; 6% during deepening	Not reported
Refraction results			
Cycloplegic	Yes	Yes	Not reported
Manifest	No	Not reported	Not reported
Percentage ±1.00 D			
Total	Not reported	Not reported	40%
Lower	Not reported	70% to 92%	Not reported
Middle	Not reported	77% to 100%	Not reported
Higher	Not reported	27% to 70%	Not reported
Highest			Not reported
Overcorrected > 1.00 D (%)	Not reported	Lower: 0% to 25% Middle: 0% to 10% Higher 10% to 18%	18%
Undercorrected > 1.00 D (%)	Not reported	Lower: 0% to 8% Middle: 0% to 15% Higher: 15% to 55%	33%
Uncorrected visual acuity results			
Acuity category	≈20/30	≥ 20/40 ≥ 20/20	≥ 20/20 ≥ 20/40
Total (all groups)	Not reported	25% to 44% 39% to 57%	45% 89%
Lower	89%	69% to 100%	Not reported
Middle	68.5%	54% to 75%	Not reported
Higher	14%	Not reported 30% to 44%	Not reported
Highest			Not reported

Authors	Arne JL and Bourdiol AM	Lavery FL	Menezo JL, Cisneros A, and Harto M
Loss of best-corrected visual acuity	Not reported	Not reported	
Loss of one Snellen line			7.5%
Loss of two or more Snellen lines			Not reported
Predictability		Not reported	
Prediction or confidence interval	Not reported		90%, 3 D at 12 mo
Method of study	Clinical experience		Not reported
Factors affecting outcome			Not reported
Clear zone diameter	Yes		
Refraction	Yes		
Patient age	No		
Depth of incision	Yes		
Number of incisions	Yes		
Average central keratometry	Yes		
Patient sex	No		
Intraocular pressure	Not reported		
Corneal thickness	Not reported		
Number of zones	Not reported		
Stability of refraction			Not reported
(Change in minus power)			
Time interval	1 to 4 yr	Baseline to 1 yr; "85% suggest a stable result"	
Increased myopia = 1.00 to 2.50 D	Not reported	Not reported	
Change = < 0.87 D	Not reported	Not reported	
Decreased myopia = 1.00 to 2.50 D	Not reported	Not reported	
Mean change	+0.50 D	Not reported	
Vision-threatening complications		Not reported	
Present series	No		0.5%
Additional reports by same author	No		No
Delayed bacterial keratitis	No		0.5%
Ruptured globe	No		No
Patient satisfaction	Not reported	Not reported	Not reported
People wearing corrective lenses after surgery	Not reported	Not reported	Not reported

Authors	Arne JL and Bourdiol AM	Lavery FL	Menezo JL, Cisneros A, and Harto M
Comments	This is a retrospective study of 350 eyes with a nonreplicable surgical protocol. It is one of the early papers to report the use of four incisions, although the effect of four versus eight incisions is not studied. The authors state that keratometric power and patient sex affect the outcome. The uncorrected visual acuity results in patients with lower myopia resembles those of other studies, but in the higher group of 4.75 to 6.00 D, only 14% of the patients could see 20/30 uncorrected, an unusually low number. Quite interesting is the observation from endothelial cell counts of an average cell loss of approximately 7% at 1 year, of 12% in eyes that had repeated operations, and of 27% in eyes with perforations. Glare in 25% of patients and daily fluctuation of vision in 95% of patients occurred in the first 6 months. The authors discourage reoperations.	This is the only published article that compares systematically different surgical plans performed by the same surgeon in similar groups of patients. Unfortunately the cases were apparently done in sequence, using the Sawelson plan in the first group, the Ellis plan in the second group, and the Thornton plan in the third group, rather than randomizing the patients among the different plans. Therefore the surgeon's experience and other changes in knowledge and technique might influence the results. Since the author found that the Thornton nomogram gave slightly superior results, this could have been a function of the author's increased experience. Unequivocally, in eyes with a refraction of between −4.75 and −9.75 D the Sawelson nomogram gave much poorer results than the other two. The author concludes that all three nomograms showed "satisfactory predictability" 6 months after surgery but does not quote any quantitative predictability figures, an important fact, since the goal for surgery was different in the first eye and the second eye of each patient, the second eye being scheduled for undercorrection. The results do not appear "satisfactory" when the Ellis nomogram produced more than 1.00 D of overcorrection in 25% of the lower group and when the Sawelson nomogram produced 55% undercorrection in the higher group.	This study is presented as a single chapter in the 1985 book by the author, J.L. Menezo, who discusses all aspects of radial keratotomy in Spanish. The data reported represent a retrospective study involving numerous surgeons performing numerous techniques of radial keratotomy, and this approach may explain the overall refractive outcome of 40% of the eyes falling within ±1 D at least 1 year after surgery. Interestingly, approximately 15% of the eyes had more than 24 incisions. The predictability was calculated at 12 months, and the range within which 90% of the eyes fell was 3 D wide, similar to that in other reports. The study makes a useful contribution to the growing worldwide literature on radial keratotomy.

SECTION II:　Summary of Published Studies of Refractive Keratotomy—cont'd

Authors	Shepard DD	Vaughan ER	Vaughan ER and Paschall WJ
Article title and citation	Radial Keratotomy: Analysis of Efficacy and Predictability in 1058 Consecutive Cases. Part I: Efficacy. Part II: Predictability, J Cataract Refract Surg 1986;12:632-643; 1987;13:32-34.	The Four-Cut Radial Keratotomy in Low Myopia, Refract Corneal Surg 1986;2:164-169.	A Statistical Analysis of Radial Keratotomy Results, Ann Ophthalmol 1985;17:275-283.
Other publications	None	Vaughan ER and Paschall WJ: A Statistical Analysis of Radial Keratotomy Results, Ann Ophthalmol 1985;17:275-283.	Vaughan ER: The Four-Cut Radial keratotomy in Low Myopia, J Refract Surg 1986;2:164-169.
Dates of surgery	November 1980 to January 1985	July 1981 to March 1985	July 1980 to June 1983
Funding source			
National Institutes of Health	No	No	No
Private	Yes	Yes	Yes
University	No	No	No
Industry	No	No	No
Study design			
Prospective	No	No	No
Retrospective	Yes	Yes	Yes
Consecutive eyes	Yes	Yes	Yes
Sample size calculation	No	No	No
Selection criteria	Yes	No	No
Participants and number			
Study centers	1	1	1
Surgeons	1	1	1 or 2
Independent physician examiners	No	No	No
Independent technician examiners	No	No	No
Independent monitors	No	No	No
Biostatistician	Yes	Yes	Yes
Disclosure of financial interest	Not reported	Yes	Not reported
Patient population			
Number of patients	Not reported	Not reported	557
Number of eyes	1058	86	557
Reoperations included	Yes (19%)	One eye	Yes (2.5%)
Withdrawals/exclusions accounted for	Yes	Not reported	Not reported
Age; mean (range)	32.4 yr (17 to 78 yr)	35 yr (9 to 50 yr)	Not reported
Sex, % female	43.5%	Not reported	Not reported

Authors	Shepard DD	Vaughan ER	Vaughan ER and Paschall WJ
Clinical examination conditions			
Office practice	Yes	Yes	Yes
Standardized	No	No	No
Data analysis			
Informal (tables, graphs)	Yes	Yes	Yes
Arithmetic (mean, standard deviation, range)	Yes	Yes	Yes
Statistical (regression analysis, confidence limits)	Yes	No	No
Follow-up			
Mean (range)	5.33 mo (not reported)		1 yr (not reported)
Percentage of original population at follow-up	90.9%	58% (6 mo); 34% (12 mo)	1 yr: 15.6% (88/557) 6 mo: 51% (286/557)
Surgical protocol			
Formal, replicable	No	No	No
Informal, not replicable	Yes (72% simultaneous, bilateral surgery)	Yes	Yes
Patient variables used to determine surgical plan			
Refraction	Yes	No	Yes
Age	Yes	Yes	Yes
Sex	No	Yes	No
Keratometry reading	Yes	Yes	Yes
Intraocular pressure	Yes	No	No
Ocular rigidity	No	No	No
Corneal diameter	No	No	No
Corneal thickness	Yes	No	No
Measurement of corneal thickness			Yes; type not specified
Optical	No	No	No
Ultrasonic (speed of sound, m/sec)	Yes (1550, 1640, 1970)	Yes	Yes
Preoperative	Yes	Not reported	Yes
Intraoperative	No	Yes	No
Location of measurement	Central, paracentral		Central
Anesthesia			
Topical	Yes	Yes	Yes
Retrobulbar	Yes (100%)	No	No
Knife blade and handle			Not reported
Metal blade	15 cases	No	
Diamond blade	1043 cases	Yes	
Blade holder	15 cases	No	
Micrometer handle	1043 cases	Yes	
Blade length; percentage of corneal thickness	90% of central	90%, central	100% of central
Calibration block	Coin gauge	Not reported	Not reported

Authors	Shepard DD	Vaughan ER	Vaughan ER and Paschall WJ
Clear zone			
Range of diameters	2.75 to 5.00 mm	4.00 to 5.00 mm	2.75 to 5.00 mm
Circular (%)	100%	100%	100%
Elliptical (%)	No	No	No
Incisions			
Number (%) of radial	4(4.5%) 8(53.5%) 12 to 16 (22%) 20 to 32 (20%)	4 (100%)	16 (100%)
Transverse	Yes	No	Not reported
Direction			
Clear zone to limbus	Yes	Yes	Yes
Limbus to clear zone	No	No	No
Technique	Not reported		
Single pass		Yes	Yes
Peripheral deepening		No	No
Recut—same blade length		No	No
Freehand dissection		No	No
Across limbus		No	No
Reoperations (%)	21.6%	Not reported	2.5%
Included in results	Yes		Yes
Technique	Not reported		Not reported
Baseline refraction groups (range in diopters)			
Lower	0.12 to 3.00	Mean = −1.06 (−0.75 to −2.87)	1.00 to 2.75
Middle	3.12 to 6.00		3.00 to 4.75
Higher	6.12 to 13.50		5.00 ≥ 6.00
Highest			
Postoperative corticosteroids	Not reported	Yes	Yes
Achieved incision depth	Not reported	Not reported	Not reported
Method of measurement			
Depth as percentage of corneal thickness			
Perforations (%)	7%	One eye	3.9%
Refraction results		Not reported	
Cycloplegic	No		No
Manifest	Yes		Yes
Percentage ±1.00 D		±0.50 ±1.00	
Total	76%	6 mo 87% 100%	Not reported
Lower	Not reported	1 yr 86% 97%	(results presented as decrease in myopia)
Middle	Not reported		
Higher	Not reported		
Highest			
Overcorrected >1.00 D(%)	7.7%	Not reported	Not reported
Undercorrected >1.00 D(%)	11.3%		Not reported
Uncorrected visual acuity results			
Acuity category	≥ 20/40	20/20	≥20/40
Total (all groups)	86.1%	6 mo 100% 12 mo 23%	Not reported
Lower	Not reported	Not reported	95%
Middle	Not reported	Not reported	79%
Higher	Not reported	Not reported	31%
Highest			
Figure	—	—	Fig. 21-10 (p. 822)

Authors	Shepard DD	Vaughan ER	Vaughan ER and Paschall WJ
Loss of best-corrected visual acuity	Not reported	None	Not reported
Loss of one Snellen line			
Loss of 2 or more Snellen lines			
Predictability		Not reported	Not reported
Prediction or confidence interval	Not reported		
Method of study	Regression analysis		
Factors affecting outcome			
Clear zone diameter	Yes		
Refraction	No		
Patient age	Yes		
Depth of incision	No		
Number of incisions	Yes		
Average central keratometry	Yes		
Patient sex	No		
Intraocular pressure	Yes		
Corneal thickness	No		
Number of zones	Not reported		
Stability of refraction	Not reported	Not reported	
(Change in minus power)			
Time interval			3 to 12 mo
Increased myopia = 1.00 to 2.50 D			Not reported
Change < 0.87 D			Not reported
Decreased myopia = 1.00 to 2.50 D			Not reported
Mean change			−0.25 D
Vision-threatening complications	Not reported	None	None
Present series			
Additional reports by same author			
Delayed bacterial keratitis			
Ruptured globe			
Patient satisfaction	Not reported	Not reported	44% polled (at 6 mo)
Percentage of patients satisfied (low, medium, high)			97.2% glad, 2.4% maybe, 0.4% no
Percentage of patients who would undergo repeat surgery			Not reported
People wearing corrective lenses after surgery	Not reported		
Total polled (%)		94%	51% polled (at 6 mo)
Percentage of patients not wearing lenses		Not reported	65%
Percentage of patients wearing lenses part time		67%	25%
Percentage of patients wearing lenses full-time		0%	15%

Authors	Shepard DD	Vaughan ER	Vaughan ER and Paschall WJ
Comments	This is the largest consecutive series of radial keratotomy eyes reported, 1058. It represents the cumulative experience of the author and a variety of changing surgical techniques. A large amount of data is presented. A regression analysis identified the variables that affect the outcome. Distinctive features of this pair of papers include the use of more than 16 incisions in 19% of the eyes, the conclusion that depth of incision is not an important variable in surgical outcome (the author does not think it can be accurately achieved or measured), and the performance of bilateral surgery at the same sitting in 72% of cases. These distinctive approaches fostered a vigorous critical correspondence (Salz JJ: Radial keratotomy: a different point of view, J Cataract Refract Surg 1987;13:574-578 and Shepard DD: [reply to above letter to editor], J Cataract Refract Surg 1987;13:578-580). He selected a group of eyes with preoperative refractions similar to those in the PERK study and reported the number of eyes within 1.00 D of emmetropia. The results were similar in the lower group (PERK, 84%, Shepard, 90%), and were better in the middle (PERK, 62%, Shepard, 82%) and higher (PERK, 38%, Shepard, 70%) groups. A major drawback of this paper is the mean follow-up time of 5 months, which means that half of the patients were followed for less than this time. If many of the examinations reported were conducted early in the follow-up, regression of effect could have taken place, diminishing the reported good results. The problem is that it is not possible to determine how Shepard achieved his results because of the wide variety of surgical techniques employed. The author used astigmatic techniques, and reported that parallel radial incisions do not effectively reduce astigmatism, but that transverse incisions do.	This is the first report of four-incision radial keratotomy results in a population with less than 3.00 D of myopia. Although the follow-up is poor (only 58% of the patients were followed for 6 months), the results are outstanding, 100% of the eyes being within 1.00 D of emmetropia and seeing 20/20 uncorrected at 6 months. Although published in 1986, the first 4-incision cases in this study were done in 1981, emphasizing that this technique had an early introduction into the United States.	This is one of the first series in which eight instead of sixteen incisions were used. The reasonably large patient population of 557 and the use of a statistician to help analyze the results are strengths undermined by the poor follow-up, 51% at 6 months and 16% at 1 year. The authors do not report the refractive outcome. The author rightly observes that the results are much better in the low group of less than 3 D of myopia than in the middle group of 3.25 to 6.00 D or the higher group of greater than 6.25 D. Approximately two thirds of the patients were not using corrective lenses 6 months after surgery.

Figure 21-10 Vaughan and Paschall

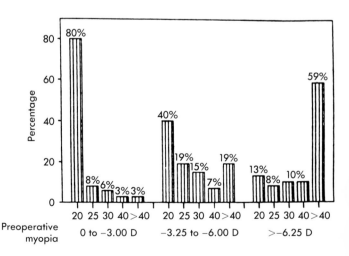

Uncorrected visual acuity 6 months after radial keratotomy in 286 eyes. Percentage of eyes is indicated on the y-axis. Eyes are divided into three groups. On the x-axis the Snellen fraction is indicated beneath each bar. (From Vaughan ER and Paschall WJ: A statistical analysis of radial keratotomy results, Ann Ophthalmol 1985;70:275-283.)

SECTION II: Summary of Published Studies of Refractive Keratotomy—cont'd

Authors	Singh P, Grewal SPS, and Kumar N	Smith RS and Cutro J	Hoffer KJ, Darin JJ, Pettit TH, Hofbauer JD, Elander R, and Levenson JE
Article title and citation	Anterior Radial Keratotomy Experience in 600 Cases of Myopia, Ann Ophthalmol 1984;16:757-761.	Computer Analysis of Radial Keratotomy, CLAO J 1984;10:241-248.	Three years' Experience with Radial Keratotomy: The UCLA Study, Ophthalmology, 1983;90:627-636.
Other publications	None	None	Hoffer KJ, Darin JJ, Pettit TH, Hofbauer JD, Elander R, and Levenson JE: UCLA Clinical Trial of Radial Keratotomy, preliminary report, Ophthalmology 1981;88:729-736.
Dates of surgery	January 1979 to December 1981	December 1980 to October 1983	1979 to 1982
Funding source			
National Institutes of Health	No	No	No
Private	No	No	No
University	Yes	Yes	Yes
Industry	No	No	No
Study design			
Prospective	No	Yes	Yes
Retrospective	Yes	No	No
Consecutive eyes	Not reported	Yes	Yes
Sample size calculation	No	No	No
Selection criteria	Not reported	Yes	Yes
Participants and number			
Study centers	1	1	1
Surgeons	Not reported	1	3
Independent physician examiners	No	No	Yes
Independent technician examiners	No	No	No
Independent monitors	No	No	No
Biostatistician	No	No	Yes
Disclosure of financial interest	Not reported	Not reported	No
Patient population			
Number of patients	600	263	69 (16 incision) 47 (8 incision)
Number of eyes	1200	263	81 (16 incision) 62 (8 incision)
Reoperations included	No	Not reported	No
Withdrawals/exclusions accounted for	Not reported	Not reported	Yes
Age; mean (range)	25 yr (8 to 40 yr)	Not reported (85% between 20 to 35 yr)	Not reported
Sex, % female	60%	53%	Not reported

Authors	Singh P, Grewal SPS, and Kumar N	Smith RS and Cutro J	Hoffer KJ, Darin JJ, Pettit TH, Hofbauer JD, Elander R, and Levenson JE
Clinical examination conditions			
Office practice	Yes	Yes	Yes
Standardized	No	No	No
Data analysis			
Informal (tables, graphs)	Yes	Yes	Yes
Arithmetic (mean, standard deviation, range)	No	Yes	Yes
Statistical (regression analysis, confidence limits)	No	No	No
Follow-up			
Mean (range)	Minimum of 6 mo	1 to 24 mo	16 incisions: 24.7 mo (21 to 30 mo) 8 incisions: 9.4 mo (2 to 21 mo)
Percentage of original population at follow-up	Total done not reported	44% at 1 yr 14% at 2 yr	58% (16 incision); not reported (8 incision)
Surgical protocol			
Formal, replicable	No	No	No
Informal, not replicable	Yes	Yes	Yes
Patient variables used to determine surgical plan	Not reported	Not reported	Not reported
Refraction			
Age			
Sex			
Keratometry reading			
Intraocular pressure			
Ocular rigidity			
Corneal diameter			
Corneal thickness			
Measurement of corneal thickness	Not reported		
Optical		Yes	Yes (1979 protocol)
Ultrasonic (speed of sound, m/sec)		No	Yes (1981 protocol)
Preoperative		Yes	Yes
Intraoperative		No	No
Location of measurement		Central, paracentral	Not reported
Anesthesia			Not reported
Topical	"Local"	Yes	
Retrobulbar			
Knife blade and handle	Not reported		
Metal blade		Beaver 76-A	Beaver 76A (1979)
Diamond blade		Sputnik Yes	Yes (1981)
Blade holder		Yes	Yes (1979)
Micrometer handle		Yes	Yes (1981)
Blade length; percentage of corneal thickness		Thinnest paracentral thickness −0.08 mm	0.55 mm
Calibration block		Bores	Kremer gauge

Authors	Singh P, Grewal SPS, and Kumar N	Smith RS and Cutro J	Hoffer KJ, Darin JJ, Pettit TH, Hofbauer JD, Elander R, and Levenson JE
Clear zone			
Range of diameters	3.00 mm	2.75 to 4.00 mm	3.0 to 4.0 mm
Circular (%)	100%	100%	Most
Elliptical (%)			
Incisions			
Number (%) of radial	16 or 12 incisions	16	8 (second series) 16 (first series)
Transverse	Not reported	Not reported	Not reported
Direction			
Clear zone to limbus	Yes	Yes	Yes
Limbus to clear zone	No	No	No
Technique	Not reported		
Single pass		No	Freehand deepening
Peripheral deepening		Yes (100%)	Often (16 incision); no (8 incision)
Recut—same blade length		No	No
Freehand dissection		No	No
Across limbus		No	To limbus (16 incision) Into sclera (some) 1 mm from limbus (8 incision)
Reoperations (%)	No	Not reported	No
Included in results			
Technique			
Baseline refraction groups (range in diopters)		1.75 to 11.0	
Lower	−1.00 to −3.00		> 5.00 (16 incision) < 5.00 (8 incision)
Middle	−3.25 to −5.00		
Higher	−5.50 or above		
Highest			
Postoperative corticosteroids	Yes	Not reported	Yes
Achieved incision depth	Not reported	Not reported	Not reported
Method of measurement			
Depth as percentage of corneal thickness			
Perforations (%)	Yes (percentage not reported)	Initial eyes, 12%; final eyes, 5%	16 incision: 11 (19%) 8 incision: No
Refraction results		Not reported	
Cycloplegic			Yes
Manifest			
Percentage ±1.00 D			Not reported
Total	Mean correction = 1.90 D (range, 0.00 to 5.00 D)		
Lower			
Middle			
Higher			
Highest			
Overcorrected >1.00 D (%)	Not reported		13% (16 incision) 3% (8 incision)
Undercorrected >1.00 D (%)	Not reported		Not reported
Figure	—	Fig. 21-11 (p. 828)	—

Authors	Singh P, Grewal SPS, and Kumar N	Smith RS and Cutro J	Hoffer KJ, Darin JJ, Pettit TH, Hofbauer JD, Elander R, and Levenson JE
Uncorrected visual acuity results			
Acuity category	≥ 20/30	≥ 20/40	≥20/40
Total	55.5%	72.5%	50% (16 incision)
			65% (8 incision)
Lower	Not reported	Not reported	Not reported
Middle	Not reported	Not reported	Not reported
Higher	Not reported	Not reported	Not reported
Highest	—	—	—
Loss of best-corrected visual acuity	Not reported	Not reported	Not reported
Loss of one Snellen line			
Loss of two or more Snellen lines			
Predictability			Not reported
Prediction or confidence interval	No	No	
Factors affecting outcome			
Method of study	Clinical experience	No statistical evaluation	
Clear zone diameter	Not reported	Yes	
Refraction	No	No	
Patient age	No	Not reported	
Depth of incision	Not reported	Yes	
Number of incisions	Not reported	Not reported	
Average central keratometry	No	Not reported	
Patient sex	Not reported	Not reported	
Intraocular pressure	Not reported	Not reported	
Corneal thickness	Not reported	Not reported	
Number of zones	Not reported	Not reported	
Stability of refraction	Not reported		Not reported
(Change in minus power)			
Time interval		1 mo to 2 yr	
Increased myopia = 1.00 to 2.50 D		Not reported	
Change = < 0.87 D		Not reported	
Decreased myopia = 1.00 to 2.50 D		Not reported	
Mean change		Not statistically significant	
Vision-threatening complications			
Present series	No	No	One case bacterial corneal ulcer
Additional reports by same author	No	No	No
Delayed bacterial keratitis	No	No	No
Ruptured globe	No	No	No
Patient satisfaction	Not reported	Not reported	Not reported
People wearing corrective lenses after surgery	Not reported	Not reported	Not reported

Authors	Singh P, Grewal SPS, and Kumar N	Smith RS and Cutro J	Hoffer KJ, Darin JJ, Pettit TH, Hofbauer JD, Elander R, and Levenson JE
Comments	This article reports relatively early experience in radial keratotomy done in 1979 to 1981 and illustrates the problems with making incisions superficially. The author reports cutting the anterior two thirds of the cornea, and obtaining 20/30 uncorrected visual acuity or better in approximately half the eyes. This is probably why the authors concluded, "we have found radial keratotomy to be suitable for patients with simple myopia, around 2 diopters." The authors observed almost prophetically, "One major drawback of the procedure is the unpredictable change in refraction and lack of consistent and reproducible results." The large number of cases reported is undermined by the lack of detailed description of the surgical methods and the absence of refractive outcome. Two conclusions in the article can now be seen as erroneous: age does not affect the outcome, and the refraction is stable by 6 weeks.	This prospectively designed study that used statistical analysis based on computer programs suffers from poor follow-up, 44% at 1 year. Observations made by the authors include the increased glare with a 2.75-mm clear zone, the superior quality incision of a diamond blade over a metal blade, and the slight trend for a continued effect of the surgery 1 to 2 years after the operations, some patients showing a late change of 1 to 2 D. This may have been the first citation of "progressive hyperopia." Endothelial cell counts done at 6, 12, or 24 months in 38 eyes showed no statistically significant decrease. For example, in the patients examined 2 years after surgery, the mean cell count was 2561 $\pm$241 cells/mm^2, and the 2-year cell count was 2429 $\pm$353 cells/mm^2. The author included only one eye per patient, thus avoiding the "double dose" so common to radial keratotomy series.	This study was an early attempt to garner reliable information about radial keratotomy, and therefore it included incisions across the limbus, freehand dissection, and a setting of the metal blade to a fixed length. Regrettably, no refractive outcome is reported, only refractive change for the group. The achievement of visual acuity of 20/40 or better in only 69% of eyes with less than 5.00 D of myopia reflects the results of these early techniques. The study employed independent examiners, which increases its veracity. An important aspect of the study is the endothelial cell counts that were done for 48 eyes at 3 months after surgery with a loss of 9 $\pm$ 6.8%. Forty-six of these had repeat cell counts at two years, which showed an increase of $\pm$4.3% from the 3-month time. The authors concluded that there is not continued endothelial cell loss. The study emphasizes the difficulty in getting follow-up. Even with the employment of a full-time secretary to track patients and call them in for the 2-year examination, only 54% of the patients were able to return and fulfill the criteria for a 2-year postoperative examination. Within the study, there was considerable improvement between the early 16-incision cases and the later 8-incision cases, with no perforations and only two eyes overcorrected more than 1.00 D in the 8-incision group. Nevertheless, only 65% of the eyes could see 20/40 or better at an average of 9 months after surgery. One acute bacterial corneal ulcer occurred, but the patient recovered with a refractive error of +0.13 D and an unaided visual acuity of 20/20. At 2 years 5% of patients complained of severe glare and 12% of severe variable vision.

Figure 21-11　Smith and Cutro

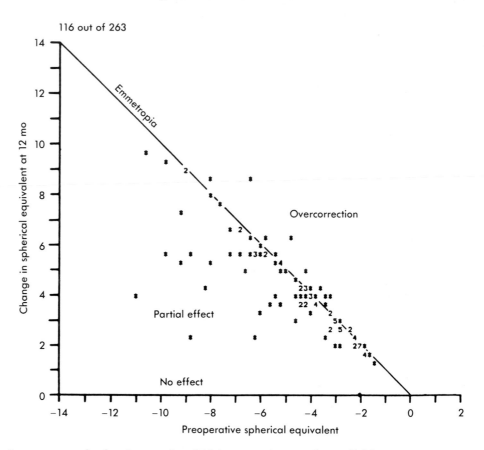

Scattergram of refractive results of 116 eyes at 1 year after radial keratotomy. Spherical equivalent refraction is indicated preoperatively on the x-axis, and the change in the spherical equivalent refraction from baseline to 12 months is indicated on the y-axis. Numbers in the scattergram indicate the number of eyes at that location. At approximately −2.00 to −5.00 D the eyes clustered around the line of emmetropia. The number of eyes with undercorrection increased as the amount of preoperative myopia increased. (From Smith RS and Cutro J: Computer analysis of radial keratotomy, CLAO J 1984;10:241-248.)

SECTION II: Summary of Published Studies of Refractive Keratotomy—cont'd

Authors	Kremer FB and Marks RG	Neumann AC, Osher RH, and Fenzl RE	Nirankari VS, Katzen LE, Karesh JN, Richards RD, and Lakhanpal V
Article and journal citation	Radial Keratotomy: Prospective Evaluation of Safety and Efficacy, Ophthalmic Surg 1983;14:925-930.	Radial Keratotomy: A Clinical and Statistical Analysis, Cornea 1983;2:47-55.	Prospective Clinical Study of Radial Keratotomy, Ophthalmology 1983;90:637-641.
Other publications	Kremer FB and Steer RA: Stability of Refractive Correction with Radial Keratotomy, Ann Ophthalmol 1985;17:660-663. Kremer FB and Steer RA: Stability of Refraction following Radial Keratotomy over 4 Years, J Refract Surg 1986;2:217-220.	Neumann AC, Osher RH, and Fenzl RE: Radial Keratotomy: A Comprehensive Evaluation, Doc Ophthalmol 1984;56:275-301.	Nirankari VS, Katzen LE, Karesh JW, Richards RD, and Lakhanpal V: Ongoing Prospective Clinical Study of Radial Keratotomy, Ophthalmology 1983;90:637-641.
Dates of surgery	July 1980 to July 1981	March 1980 to November 1980	Not reported
Funding source			
National Institutes of Health	No	No	No
Private	Yes	Yes	No
University	Yes	No	Yes
Industry	No	No	No
Study design			
Prospective	Yes	Yes	Yes
Retrospective	No	No	No
Consecutive eyes	Yes	Yes	Yes
Sample size calculation	No	No	No
Selection criteria	Yes	Yes	Yes
Participants and number			
Study centers	1	1	1
Surgeons	1	1	Not reported
Independent physician examiners	No	Yes	Yes
Independent technician examiners	No	Not reported	No
Independent monitors	No	Not reported	No
Biostatistician	Yes	Not reported	No
Disclosure of financial interest	No	No	No
Patient population			
Number of patients	69	123 patients (24 excluded)	83
Number of eyes	105	147	58
Reoperations included	Yes (one eye)	Yes	Yes (six eyes)
Withdrawals/exclusions accounted for	No	Yes	No
Age; mean (range)	Not reported	32.7 yr (18 to 58 yr)	32 yr (19 to 57 yr)
Sex, % female	34%	54%	30%

Authors	Kremer FB and Marks RG	Neumann AC, Osher RH, and Fenzl RE	Nirankari VS, Katzen LE, Karesh JN, Richards RD, and Lakhanpal V
Clinical examination conditions			
Office practice	Yes	Yes	Yes
Standardized	No	No	No
Data analysis			
Informal (tables, graphs)	Yes	Yes	Yes
Arithmetic (mean, standard deviation, range)	Yes	Yes	Yes
Statistical (regression analysis, confidence limits)	Yes	Yes	No
Follow-up			
Mean (range)	Not reported (12 to 19 mo)	17 mo (14 to 21 mo)	19 mo (6 to 38 mo)
Percentage of original population at follow-up	91% at 1 yr	Not reported	100% at 6 mo
Surgical protocol			
Formal, replicable	No	No	No
Informal, not replicable	Yes	Fyodorov technique	Yes
Patient variables used to determine surgical plan		Not reported	Not reported
Refraction	Yes		
Age	No		
Sex	No		
Keratometry reading	No		
Intraocular pressure	No		
Ocular rigidity	No		
Corneal diameter	No		
Corneal thickness	No		
Measurement of corneal thickness			Not reported
Optical		Specular microscope	
Ultrasonic (speed of sound, m/sec)	Yes	Yes	
Preoperative	Yes	Yes	
Intraoperative	No	Not reported	
Location of measurement	Not reported	Central, paracentral	
Anesthesia			
Topical	Yes	Yes	Yes
Retrobulbar	No	Majority	No
Knife blade and handle			
Metal blade	Beaver 76A, Feather	Razor blade	Beaver 76A, Feather, Sputnik
Diamond blade	No	No	Yes
Blade holder	Yes	No	Yes
Micrometer handle	No	Yes	Yes
Blade length; percentage of corneal thickness	Not reported	95% of paracentral	100% depth of central
Calibration block	Kremer gauge	Fyodorov gauge	Bores gauge
Clear zone			
Range of diameters	3.0 to 5.0 mm	3.0 to 4.5 mm	3.0 mm only
Circular (%)	100%	Majority	100%
Elliptical (%)		Yes	

Authors	Kremer FB and Marks RG	Neumann AC, Osher RH, and Fenzl RE	Nirankari VS, Katzen LE, Karesh JN, Richards RD, and Lakhanpal V
Incisions			
Number (%) of radial	8 (69%)	8, 16	8 (24%)
	16 (30%)		16 (76%)
	20 (1 case)		
Transverse	Yes (1 case)	No	Not reported
Direction			
Clear zone to limbus	Yes	No	Yes
Limbus to clear zone	No	Yes	No
Technique			
Single pass	Yes	Yes	Yes
Peripheral deepening	Yes (≥ -5.00 D)	Yes	Yes
Recut; same blade length	No	No	No
Freehand dissection	No	No	No
Across limbus	First five cases	No	Yes (some)
Reoperations (%) included in results technique	Yes (one case)	13 eyes (8%)	Yes (six eyes)
Baseline refraction groups (range in diopters)			
Lower	< 3.00	1.75 to 2.75 (6%)	< 5.00
Middle	3.00 to 5.90	3.00 to 5.75 (60%)	
Higher	6.00 to 9.90	6.00 to 11.75 (34%)	> 5.00
Highest	> 10.00		
Postoperative corticosteroids	Not reported	Yes	Yes
Achieved incision depth			
Method of measurement	Slit-lamp microscopy	Slit-lamp microscopy	Slit-lamp microscopy
Depth as percentage of corneal thickness	Not reported	85% (68 eyes); 65% (10 eyes)	Each cut was of a different depth and varied from 30% to 80% of corneal thickness; mean, approximately 50%.
Perforations (%)	One case	35 eyes (26%)	No
Refraction results			
Cycloplegic	No		Not reported
Manifest	Yes	Yes	
Percentage ±1.00 D	39%	Not reported	43%
Lower	75%		Not reported
Middle	58%		
Higher	18%		
Highest	0%		
Overcorrected > 1.00 D (%)	4%	18%	Not reported
Undercorrected > 1.00 D (%)	37%	46%	61%
Figure	Fig. 21-12 (p. 834)	Fig. 21-13 (p. 834)	—

Uncorrected visual acuity results

Acuity category	Kremer FB and Marks RG	Neumann AC, Osher RH, and Fenzl RE				Nirankari VS, Katzen LE, Karesh JN, Richards RD, and Lakhanpal V	
		20/20 to 20/25	20/30 to 20/40	20/50 to 20/100	≥20/200	≥20/50	≥20/40
Total	Not reported					64%	48%
Lower		89%	100%			93%	< 5.00 65%
Middle		60%	84%	16%		82%	> 5.00 19%
Higher		44%	68%	22%	10%	45%	
Highest						0%	

Authors	Kremer FB and Marks RG	Neumann AC, Osher RH, and Fenzl RE	Nirankari VS, Katzen LE, Karesh JN, Richards RD, and Lakhanpal V
Loss of best-corrected visual acuity	Not reported		Not reported
Loss of one Snellen line		No	
Loss of two or more Snellen lines		No	
Predictability			Not reported
Prediction or confidence interval	Not reported	Not reported	
Factors affecting outcome			
Method of study	Regression analysis	"Efficiency quotient"	
Clear zone diameter	Yes	Yes	
Refraction	Yes	Yes	
Patient age	Yes	Yes	
Depth of incision	Yes	Not reported	
Number of incisions	No	No	
Average central keratometry	No	No	
Patient sex	Yes	Yes	
Intraocular pressure	Yes	No	
Corneal thickness	No	Yes	
Number of zones	Not reported	Not reported	
Stability of refraction		Not reported	Not reported
(Change in minus power)			
Time interval	1 to 4 yr		
	1-2 yr 2-3 yr 3-4 yr		
Increased myopia = 1.00 to 2.50 D	4% 2% 0%		
Change = < 0.87 D	76% 88% 95%		
Decreased myopia = 1.00 to 2.50 D	9% 9% 5%		
Mean change	−0.32 D		
Vision-threatening complications	Not reported		
Present series		No	No
Additional reports by same author			No
Delayed bacterial keratitis			No (three eyes with central erosion and scarring)
Ruptured-globe			No
Patient satisfaction	Not reported		Not reported
Percentage of patients satisfied (low, medium, high)		High (72%) Medium (11%) Low (17%)	
Percentage of patients who would undergo repeat surgery		Not reported	
People wearing lenses after surgery			
Total polled (%)	Not reported	73% wore glasses or contact lenses	Not reported

Authors	Kremer FB and Marks RG	Neumann AC, Osher RH, and Fenzl RE	Nirankari VS, Katzen LE, Karesh JN, Richards RD, and Lakhanpal V
Comments	This prospective report on 105 consecutive eyes has a commendable 91% follow-up at 1 year. This is an early study in which metal blades were used, possibly accounting for the predominance of undercorrections. The surgical technique is not described in enough detail to be replicated. The authors observed an average greater change in refraction than in corneal curvature in many eyes. Zone cutting was used but not reported in enough detail to be replicated. In 19 cases the mean central endothelial cell count was 2940 cells/mm^2, and postoperatively it was 2810 cells/mm^2, a decrease of 4.5%. It is remarkable that the authors concluded that the procedure was "predictable" when only 39% of the eyes had a refraction at 1 year between + 1.00 and −1.00 D. In the study of stability between 1 and 4 years, average values were used, which is not a very useful method, the actual change in individual eyes being more pertinent. Although there was an overall trend for a continued surgical effect with the average value showing a continued decrease in myopia, these differences did not reach statistical significance, and the authors claimed to have demonstrated that "progressive hyperopia" did not exist in this population. Unfortunately, only 17% of 250 eyes were consistently followed during the 4 years.	This is the only study that reported results of centripetal incisions made from the limbus to the clear zone. Surgical techniques were early in development and involved multiple metal knife blades on a micrometer knife. This is one of the few places in which the surgeon documents his learning curve. After 21 cases results were consistent. Two novel approaches to reporting results are presented, the efficiency quotient and the total excursion. Since no other author has used these, they are not very meaningful for the assessment of the results. The authors concluded that preoperative central keratometry readings and intraocular pressure did not play a role in predicting the outcome. However, experience with a patient's first eye led to a better outcome in the second. The incision scar entered the optical zone in 9 of 64 eyes, most of them early cases. The high perforation rate of 26% may also reflect the early development of techniques in this report. An independent physician examiner was used. The authors found that older patients had an increased effect from the surgery, but there was marked scatter in this observation.	This article presents a variety of surgical techniques with the advantage of independent examination and a 100% follow-up of 6 months in a small group of eyes. The authors experienced great difficulty using a metal blade to obtain a desired incision depth from one end to the other of an incision and from one incision to another, with a range varying from 30% to 80% (average, 50%), which explains the complete absence of microperforations and overcorrections. This would also explain the average reduction in myopia of 2.7 D. The authors found no differences in surgical outcome between 8 and 16 incisions.

Figure 21-12   Kremer and Marks

The graph represents the time course of the mean spherical equivalent refraction at different intervals after radial keratotomy in approximately 105 eyes. The initial overcorrection was followed by a loss of effect up to 6 months after surgery on the average. No ranges or standard deviations were indicated on the graph. (From Kremer FB and Marks RG: Radial keratotomy: prospective evaluation of safety and efficacy, Ophthalmic Surg 1983;14:925-930.)

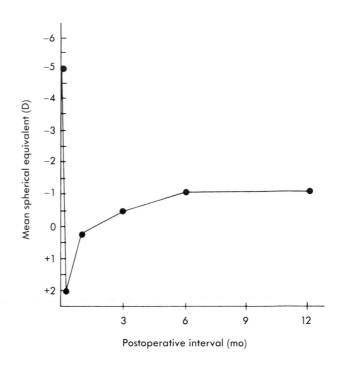

Figure 21-13   Newmann, Osher, and Fenzl

Scattergram compares the preoperative spherical equivalent refraction to that achieved at 1 year. A linear regression line is drawn through the data corresponding to the formula on the plot. The 18% overcorrected and 46% undercorrected eyes are apparent from the scattergram. (From Neumann AC, Osher RH, and Fenzl RE: Radial keratotomy: a clinical and statistical analysis, Cornea 1983;2:47-55.)

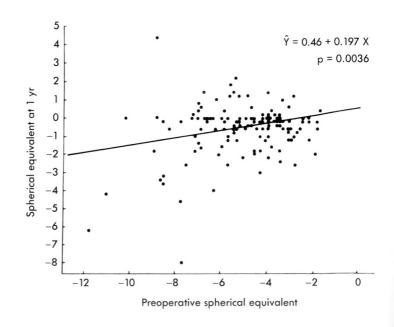

SECTION II: Summary of Published Studies of Refractive Keratotomy—cont'd

Authors	Ranga Reddy P	Rowsey JJ, Balyeat HD, Rabinovitch B, Burns TE, and Hays JC	Cowden JW
Article title and citation	Anterior Keratotomy: Follow-up Results, Indian J Ophthalmol 1983;31:888-889.	Predicting the Results of Radial Keratotomy, Ophthalmology 1983;90:642-654.	Radial Keratotomy: A Retrospective Study of Cases Observed at the Kresge Eye Institute for 6 Months, Arch Ophthalmol 1982;100:578-580.
Other publications	Reddy PS and Reddy PR: Anterior Keratotomy, Ophthalmic Surg 1980;11:765-767. Reddy PS and Gupta M: Anterior Keratotomy, Indian J Ophthalmol 1981;29:217-220.	Rowsey JJ and Balyeat HD: Preliminary Results and Complications of Radial Keratotomy, Am J Ophthalmol 1982;93:437-455. Rowsey JJ and Balyeat HD: Radial Keratotomy: Preliminary Report of Complications, Ophthalmic Surg 1982;13:27-35.	None
Dates of surgery	Not reported	Not reported	July 1979 to December 1979
Funding source			
National Institutes of Health	No	No	No
Private	No	Yes	No
University	Yes	Yes	Yes
Industry	No	No	No
Study design			
Prospective	No	Yes	No
Retrospective	Yes	No	Yes
Consecutive eyes	Not reported	Yes	Yes
Sample size calculation	No	No	No
Selection criteria	Not reported	Yes	Yes
Participants and number			
Study centers	1	1	1
Surgeons	1	Not reported	1
Independent physician examiners	Not reported	Not reported	1
Independent technician examiners	Not reported	Not reported	Yes
Independent monitors	Not reported	Not reported	No
Biostatistician	Not reported	Not reported	No
Disclosure of financial interest	No	Not reported	No
Patient population			
Number of patients	Not reported	Not reported	36
Number of eyes	200	112	25
Reoperations included	Not reported	Yes	No
Withdrawals/exclusions accounted for	Not reported	No	Yes

Authors	Ranga Reddy P	Rowsey JJ, Balyeat HD, Rabinovitch B, Burns TE, and Hays JC	Cowden JW
Age; mean (range)	Not reported (16% children)	> 18 yr	Not reported
Sex, % female	74%	Not reported	Not reported
Clinical examination conditions			
Office practice	Yes	Yes	Yes
Standardized	No	No	No
Data analysis			
Informal (tables, graphs)	Yes	Yes	Yes
Arithmetic (mean, standard deviation, range)	No	Yes	Yes
Statistical (regression analysis, confidence limits)	No	Yes	No
Follow-up			
Mean (range)	Not reported (2 to 5 yrs)	1 yr	6 mo
Percentage of original population at follow-up	70%	45% (112 or 251)	Not reported
Surgical protocol			
Formal, replicable	No	No	No
Informal, not replicable	Yes	Yes	Yes
Patient variables used to determine surgical plan	Not reported		Not reported
Refraction		Yes	
Age		No	
Sex		No	
Keratometry reading		No	
Intraocular pressure		No	
Ocular rigidity		No	
Corneal diameter		No	
Corneal thickness		No	
Figure	—	Fig. 21-14 (p. 839)	—
Measurement of corneal thickness	Not reported		Not reported
Optical		No	
Ultrasonic (speed of sound, m/sec)		Yes	
Preoperative			
Intraoperative		Not reported	
Location of measurement			
Anesthesia		Not reported	
Topical			Yes
Retrobulbar	Yes (majority)		Two eyes
Knife blade and handle	Not reported		
Metal blade		Yes	Razor blade
Diamond blade		Yes	No
Blade holder		Yes	Yes
Micrometer handle		Yes	No
Blade length; percentage of corneal thickness		90% of central	0.05 to 0.10 mm less than central corneal thickness
Calibration block		Line gauge	Bores gauge
Clear zone			
Range of diameters	Not reported	3.0 to 4.0 mm	2.5 to 5.0 mm
Circular (%)	Not reported	100%	Yes
Elliptical (%)	12%		

Authors	Ranga Reddy P	Rowsey JJ, Balyeat HD, Rabinovitch B, Burns TE, and Hays JC	Cowden JW
Incisions			
Number (%) of radial	16 (majority)	8 16	16 (100%)
Transverse direction	Not reported	No	No
Clear zone to limbus		Yes	Yes
Limbus to clear zone		No	
Technique	Not reported		
Single pass		Yes	Yes
Peripheral deepening		No	Yes
Recut; same blade length		No	No
Freehand dissection		No	No
Across limbus		First 13 cases (12%)	No
Reoperations (%) included in results	Not reported	Yes	Four eyes (11%); not included in results
Baseline refraction groups (range in diopters)	Not reported	Not reported	Not reported
Lower			
Middle			
Higher			
Highest			
Postoperative corticosteroids	Not reported	Yes	Yes
Achieved incision depth	Not reported	Not reported	Not reported
Method of measurement			
Depth as percentage of corneal thickness			
Perforations (%)	Not reported	Not reported	Two eyes
Refraction results			Not reported
Cycloplegic	Not reported	Yes	
Manifest	Not reported	No	
Percentage ±1.00 D	Eyes returned to original myopic correction after surgery	Scattergram only in terms of clear zone (3.00, 3.5, 4.0)	
Lower			
Middle			
Higher			
Highest			
Overcorrected > 1.00 D (%)	Not reported	Not reported	
Undercorrected > 1.00 D (%)	All eyes undercorrected	Not reported	
Uncorrected visual acuity results			
Acuity category	≥20/40	≥20/40	≥20/60
Total	7%	63% of total with optical zone of 3.5 to 4.0 mm	48%
Lower			
Middle		82% of total with optical zone of 3.0 mm	
Higher			
Highest			
Loss of best-corrected visual acuity	Not reported	Not reported	
Loss of one Snellen line			—
Loss of two or more Snellen lines			12%

Authors	Ranga Reddy P	Rowsey JJ, Balycat IID, Rabinovitch B, Burns TE, and Hays JC	Cowden JW
Predictability	Not reported		
Prediction of confidence interval		Not reported	Not reported
Factors affecting outcome			
Method of study		Not reported	Clinical observation
Clear zone diameter		Yes	Yes
Refraction		Yes	Not reported
Patient age		Yes	Yes
Depth of incision		No	Not reported
Number of incisions		No	Yes
Average central keratometry		No	Not reported
Patient sex		"Corneal shape factor"	Not reported
Topography		No	Not reported
Intraocular pressure		No	Not reported
Corneal thickness		No	Not reported
Number of zones		No	Not reported
Stability of refraction	Not reported	Not reported	Not reported
(Change in minus power)			
Time interval			
Increased myopia = 1.00 to 2.50 D			
Change = < 0.87 D			
Decreased myopia = 1.00 to 2.50 D			
Mean change			
Vision-threatening complications	Not reported	Not reported	None
Present series			
Additional reports by same author			
Delayed bacterial keratitis			
Ruptured globe			
Patient satisfaction	Not reported	Not reported	
Percentage satisfied (low, medium high)			80% patients benefited from surgery
Percentage of patients who would undergo repeat surgery			Not reported
People wearing lenses after surgery	Not reported	Not reported	Not reported
Comments	This paper reflects the discouraging experience with radial keratotomy in India in the late 1970s. We know from personal communication that the incisions were made extremely shallowly, explaining why 60% of the eyes had no change in refraction and the maximum change achieved was approximately 2 D. Peripheral corneal vascularization with calcium and	Rowsey and colleagues detail the factors that affect radial keratotomy. The initial group of patients had incisions across the limbus, a surgical technique that was stopped after 13 patients. The transition from metal blades to diamond blades was also made. The authors are careful to describe their patients in terms of clear zone diameter and number of incisions, so the	This article reports the results of the earliest performed cases of radial keratotomy in the United States, the surgery being done in 1979. The surgeon is not identified, and the author is the observer. By modern standards the results are discouraging, only 48% of the patients seeing 20/60 or better uncorrected 6 months after surgery. The case series straddles the time when sur-

Authors	Ranga Reddy P	Rowsey JJ, Balyeat HD, Rabinovitch B, Burns TE, and Hays JC	Cowden JW

cholesterol deposits occurred, probably because many of these corneas were already vascularized from previous disease. This paper greatly tempers the results from the same authors published in 1980 on the same series of cases where, even though the outcome was extremely poor by modern standards, a claim of 40% of patients maintained 20/20 acuity from 3 to 22 months after surgery.

results can be related to a group of patients that had a specific type of surgery. The major contribution here is the demonstration of a correlation between change in refraction and the patient's age, the first thorough demonstration of this fact. The regression analyses for the different groups of patients shows an increased effect of approximately 0.6 to 1.0 D per decade, a range that corresponds to subsequent measurements by others. The authors also emphasize the similarity of effect between 8 and 16 incisions and did not think that increasing the number of incisions from 8 to 16 increased the overall effect of the surgery. They also describe the change in corneal shape based on keratometric readings, observing that corneas have a positive shape factor preoperatively (steeper in the center and flatter toward the periphery), and a negative shape factor postoperatively. This formed the basis for the authors' subsequent study of corneal topography and refractive surgery.

geons stopped cutting across the limbus and started making peripheral deepening incisions. The complications are reported candidly, including two complaints from patients who could not drive at night because of glare. This is one of the first documentations of daily fluctuation of vision that occurred at 6 months, with vision being better in the morning than in the evening for most patients. The authors observed, "Because of the mutiple variables that were altered during the study, a valid relationship between the technique used and the results achieved cannot be made."

Figure 21-14   Rowsey, Balyeat, and Rabinovitch

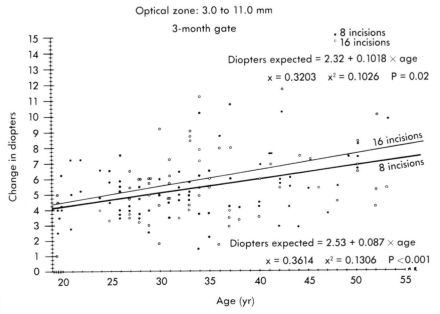

Optical zone: 3.0 to 11.0 mm

3-month gate

• 8 incisions
○ 16 incisions

Diopters expected = 2.32 + 0.1018 × age

x = 0.3203   x² = 0.1026   P = 0.02

16 incisions

8 incisions

Diopters expected = 2.53 + 0.087 × age

x = 0.3614   x² = 0.1306   P <0.001

Refractive change of radial keratotomy (3.0-mm optical zone) as a function of patient age 3 months after surgery. The intercept for an 8-incision radial keratotomy at age zero would be 2.53 D *(lower regression line)*, compared with an intercept for a 16-incision operation of 2.32 D *(upper regression line)*. (From Rowsey JJ, Balyeat HD, and Rabinovitch B: Predicting the results of radial keratotomy, Ophthalmology 1983;90:642.)

SECTION II: Summary of Published Studies of Refractive Keratotomy—cont'd

Authors	Fyodorov SN and Agranovsky AA	Grady FJ	Schachar RA, Black TD, and Huang I
Article title and citation	Long-term Results of Anterior Radial Keratotomy, J Ocular Therapy Surg Vol I:217-223, 1982.	Experience with Radial Keratotomy, Ophthalmic Surg 1982;13:395-399.	Understanding Radial Keratotomy, Denison, Tex, 1981, LAL Publishing.
Other publications	Fyodorov SN, Ivashina AI, Gudechkov VB, and Iatsenko IA: Characteristics of the Surgical Technique in Anterior Radial Graduated Keratotomy or High Myopia, Vest Oftalmol 1983;5:20-22. Fyodorov SN, Sarkizova MG, and Kurasova TP: Corneal Biomicroscopy following Repeated Radial Keratotomy, Ann Ophthalmol 1983;15:403-407.	None	Schachar RA, Black TD, and Huang T: Surgical Implications of the Theory of Radial Keratotomy. In Schachar RA et al: Radial Keratotomy, Denison, Tex, 1980, LAL Publishing. Black TD, Schachar RA, and Huang T: Optical Correction Following Radial Keratotomy. In Refractive Modulation of the Cornea, Denison, Tex, 1981, LAL Publishing.
Dates of surgery	Not reported	Not reported	Not reported
Finding source			Not reported
National Institutes of Health	No	No	
Private	Yes	Yes	
University	No	No	
Industry	No	No	
Study design			
Prospective			
Retrospective	Yes	Yes	Yes
Consecutive eyes	Not reported	Not reported	No
Sample size calculation	No	No	No
Selection criteria	Not reported	Age only	No
Participants and number	Not reported		
Study centers		1	1
Surgeons		1	2
Independent physician examiners		No	No
Independent technician examiners		No	No
Independent monitors		No	No
Biostatistician		No	Yes
Disclosure of financial interest	No	No	No
Patient population			
Number of patients	Not reported	Not reported	148
Number of eyes	500	198	244
Reoperations included	Not reported	Not reported	37
Withdrawals/exclusions accounted for	Not reported	No	Not reported
Age; mean (range)	Not reported (18 to 56 yr)	Not reported (19 to 40 yr)	Not reported (18 to 49 yr)
Sex, % female	Not reported	Not reported	44%

Authors	Fyodorov SN and Agranovsky AA	Grady FJ	Schachar RA, Black TD, and Huang I
Clinical examination conditions			
Office practice	Yes	Yes	Yes
Standardized	No	No	No
Data analysis			
Informal (tables, graphs)	Yes	Yes	Yes
Arithmetic (mean, standard deviation, range)	No	No	Yes
Statistical (regression analysis, confidence limits)	No	No	Yes
Follow-up			
Mean (range)	4.5 to 5 yr	10 mo (5 to 16 mo)	Not reported (1 to 2 yr)
Percentage of original population at follow-up	48% (242 of 500)	Not reported	Total population not reported
Surgical protocol			
Formal, replicable	No	No	No
Informal, not replicable	Yes	Yes	Yes
Patient variables used to determine surgical plan			
Refraction	Yes	Yes	Yes
Age	No	No	No
Sex	No	No	No
Corneal thickness	Yes	Yes	Yes
Keratometry reading	Yes	Yes	Yes
Intraocular pressure	yes	No	No
Ocular rigidity	Yes	No	No
Corneal diameter	Yes	No	No
Measurement of corneal thickness	Not reported		
Optical		Yes	Yes
Ultrasonic (speed of sound, m/sec)		No	No
Preoperative		Yes	Yes
Intraoperative		No	No
Location of measurement		Central	Central, paracentral
Anesthesia			
Topical	Yes	Yes	Yes
Retrobulbar	No	No	No
Knife blade and handle			
Metal blade	Yes (Group A)	Super blade	Yes
Diamond blade	Yes (Group B)	No	No
Blade holder	Yes (Group A)	Yes	Not reported
Micrometer handle	Yes (Group B)	No	Not reported
Blade length; percentage of corneal thickness	Not reported	0.02 mm less than central thickness	83% paracentral thickness
Calibration block	Not reported	Kremer or Schachar gauge	Not reported
Clear zone	Not reported		
Range of diameters		2.80 to 4.25 mm	2.5 to 5.0 mm
Circular (%)		100%	97%
Elliptical (%)			3%

Authors	Fyodorov SN and Agranovsky AA		Grady FJ	Schachar RA, Black TD, and Huang I
Incisions				
Number (%) of radial	Not reported (probably 16)		8 (90%)	8 (87%)
			16 (10%)	16 (13%)
Transverse	Not reported		10% intersecting transverse	Yes
Direction			Not reported	
Clear zone to limbus				
Limbus to clear zone				Yes
Technique	Not reported		Not reported	
Single pass				Yes
Peripheral deepening				Yes
Recut; same blade length				No
Freehand dissection				No
Across limbus				No
Reoperations (%) included in results	Not reported		Yes (3%)	Yes (15%)
Baseline refraction groups (range in diopters)				
Lower	1.00 to 3.00		1.50 to 2.00	1.00 to 4.00
Middle	3.25 to 6.00		2.25 to 3.50	4.25 to 6.00
Higher	6.25 to 9.50		3.75 to 5.00	> 6.25
Highest			> 5.00	
Postoperative corticosteroids	Not reported		Yes	No
Achieved incision depth	Not reported		Not reported	Not reported
Method of measurement				
Depth as percentage of corneal thickness				
Perforations (%)	Not reported		19%	10% (12% sutured)
Loss of best-corrected visual acuity	Not reported		Not reported	Not reported
Loss of one Snellen line				
Loss of two or more Snellen lines				
Refraction results			Not reported	Scattergram
Cycloplegic	Not reported			
Manifest				
Percentage ±1.00 D	Group A	Group B		
Lower	68% (±0.50)	77% (±0.50)		
Middle	37% (±1.00)	63% (±1.00)		
Higher	0%	57%		
Highest	0%			
Overcorrected > 1.00 D (%)	0%			
Undercorrected > 1.00 D (%)	19%			
Figure	—		Fig. 21-15 (p. 844)	Fig. 21-16 (p. 844)
Uncorrected visual acuity results				
Acuity category	≥20/20		≥20/40	≥20/40
Total	Group A	Group B	94%	71%
Lower	98%	100%	100%	86%
Middle	97%	100%	100%	47%
Higher	39%	100%	94%	24%
Highest			87%	71%

Authors	Fyodorov SN and Agranovsky AA	Grady FJ	Schachar RA, Black TD, and Huang I
Predictability or confidence interval reported		Not reported	
Prediction interval	Not reported		Not reported
Factors affecting outcome			
Method of study	Math formula		Not reported
Refraction	Yes		No
Clear zone diameter	No		Yes
Patient age	Yes		No
Depth of incision	Yes		Yes
Number of incisions	No		No
Average central keratometry	No		No
Patient sex	No		No
Intraocular pressure	Yes		Yes
Corneal thickness	No		No
Number of zones	Not reported		No
Stability of refraction	Not reported	Not reported	Not reported
Vision-threatening complications	Not reported		
Present series		Perforations with suture, 1% Induced astigmatism, 10% Recurrent erosion, yes	No
Delayed bacterial keratitis		No	No
Ruptured globe		No	No
Patient satisfaction	Not reported	Not reported	Not reported
People wearing lenses after surgery	Not reported	Not reported	Not reported
Comments	This was the second of Fyodorov's papers published in English, both colloquial reports. The authors make three major points. First, the surgeon can improve the results by using multiple variables to determine the operative procedure and by using a micrometer diamond-bladed knife. Second, the results are approximately stable over 5 years; even though no actual stability data are presented, the over-all stability of the results is documented. Third, the results claimed are spectacular for the lower group (100% are within 1 D of emmetropia and have 20/30 uncorrected visual acuity), and for the middle group (98% are within 1 D of emmetropia and 100% see 20/40 uncorrected). These results were not duplicated by other investigators until the late 1980s.	This article presents results of surgery performed with a metal knife blade and emphasizes the great scatter of results. The author is suprised at the large number of patients with good visual acuity and speculates that radial keratotomy makes "the normal aspheric corneal curvature even more aspheric." So, "the patient selects a point on the curvature from which he gets his best vision."	This book published by the author details a number of interesting aspects about radial keratotomy done before 1981 with metal blades, with a thoughtful and detailed analysis. The authors found a wide spread in the results and observed that patient age (between 18 and 49 years) did not have any relationship to the result, a conclusion since discredited. Preoperative keratometry and preoperative intraocular pressure between 12 and 18 mm Hg also did not affect the results. The authors state that transverse incisions for astigmatism give disappointing results when intersecting the radius and favor freehand dissection to Descemet's membrane along the steep meridian. They performed radial keratotomy on four patients with keratoconus, with generally poor results. They document the problems with the keratotomy scars when doing a penetrating keratoplasty.

Figure 21-15   Grady

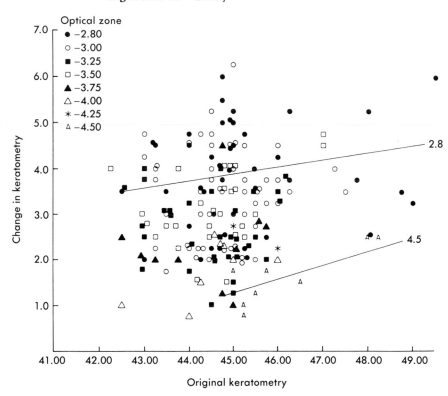

Comparison of original average central keratometric power with the change in keratometric power for different diameter clear zones. There is considerable scatter, and although the author's lines drawn on the table suggest an increasing surgical effect in corneas with a steeper preoperative curvature, the overall spread of the results suggests that there is no clinically meaningful relationship between preoperative keratometric power and the change in keratometric power. (From Grady FJ: Experience with radial keratotomy, Ophthalmic Surg 1982;13:395-399.)

SECTION II: Summary of Published Studies of Refractive Keratotomy—cont'd

Authors	Bores LD, Myers W, and Cowden J	Fyodorov SN and Durnev VV
Article and journal citation	Radial Keratotomy: An Analysis of the American Experience, Ann Ophthalmol 1981;13:941-948.	Operation of Dosaged Dissection of Corneal Circular Ligament in Cases of Myopia of Mild Degree, Ann Ophthalmol 1979;11:1885-1890.
Other publications	None	See p. 840
Dates of surgery	Group 1: April 1979 to October, 1979 Group 2: November 1979 to December 1980	Not reported
Funding source		
National Institutes of Health	No	No
Private	Yes	Yes
University	Yes	No
Industry	No	No
Study design		
Prospective		
Retrospective	Yes	Yes
Consecutive eyes	No	No
Sample size calculation	No	No
Selection criteria	Yes	No
Participants and number		
Study centers	1	1
Surgeons	1	1
Independent physician examiners	No	Not reported
Independent technician examiners	No	Not reported
Independent monitors	No	Not reported
Biostatistician	No	Not reported
Disclosure of financial interest	No	No
Patient population		
Number of patients	223	30
Number of eyes	400 (Group 1, 97 eyes; Group 2, 303 eyes)	60
Reoperations included	Not reported	Not reported
Withdrawals/exclusions accounted for	No	No
Age; mean (range)	Not reported	Not reported (17 to 43 yr)
Sex, % female	Not reported	Not reported
Clinical examination conditions		
Office practice	Yes	Yes
Standardized		
Data analysis		
Informal (tables, graphs)	Yes	Yes
Arithmetic (mean, standard deviation, range)	Yes	No
Statistical (regression analysis, confidence limits)	No	No
Follow-up		Not reported
Mean (range)	Minimum 12 mo (not reported)	

Authors	Bores LD, Myers W, and Cowden J	Fyodorov SN and Durnev VV
Percentage of original population at follow-up	Total operated not reported	
Surgical protocol		
Formal, replicable	No	Yes
Informal, not replicable	No	Yes
Patient variables used to determine surgical plan	Not reported	Not reported
Refraction		
Age		
Sex		
Keratometry reading		
Intraocular pressure		
Ocular rigidity		
Corneal diameter		
Corneal thickness		
Measurement of corneal thickness		Not reported
Optical	Yes	
Ultrasonic (speed of sound, m/sec)	No	
Preoperative	Yes	
Intraoperative	No	
Location of measurement	Paracentral	
Anesthesia		
Topical	Yes	Yes
Retrobulbar	No	No
Knife blade and handle		
Metal blade	Beaver 76A	Razor blade
Diamond blade	No	No
Blade holder	Yes	Yes
Micrometer handle	No	No
Blade length; percentage of corneal thickness	Group 1: 75% of paracentral; Group 2: subtract 0.05 mm from paracentral	"Approached 75%"
Calibration block	Bores gauge	No
Clear zone		
Range of diameters	Not reported	3.0 to 4.5 mm
Circular (%)	Not reported	100%
Elliptical (%)	Not reported	No
Incisions		
Number (%) of radial	16 (100%)	16 (100%)
Transverse	No	No
Direction		
Clear zone to limbus	Yes	Yes
Limbus to clear zone	No	No
Technique		
Single pass	Yes	Yes
Peripheral deepening	Yes	No
Recut; same blade length	No	No
Freehand dissection	No	Yes
Across limbus	No	Not reported
Reoperations (%) included in results technique	No	Not reported

Authors	Bores LD, Myers W, and Cowden J	Fyodorov SN and Durnev VV
Baseline refraction groups (range in diopters)	−2.00 to −11.00	Not reported
Lower		
Middle		
Higher		
Highest		
Postoperative corticosteroids	Yes	Not reported
Achieved incision depth		Not reported
Method of measurement	Not reported	
Depth as percentage of corneal thickness	Not reported	
Perforations (%)	Group 1 6%	
	Group 2, 17%	
Refraction results		Not reported
Cycloplegic	Yes	
Manifest	No	
Percentage ±1.00 D	±0.50; Group 1, 25%; Group 2, 59%	
Lower		
Middle		
Higher		
Highest		
Overcorrected > 1.00 D (%)	>0.50 D	
	Group 1, 3%	
	Group 2, 0%	
Undercorrected > 1.00 D (%)	> 0.50 D	
	Group 1, 72%	
	Group 2, 41%	
Uncorrected visual acuity results		
Acuity category	20/20 to 20/25 20/30 to 20/40	≥20/50
Total	40% 16%	98%
Lower	25% (Group 1) 4% (Group 1)	
	45% (Group 2) 20% (Group 2)	
Middle		
Higher		
Highest		
Loss of best-corrected visual acuity	Not reported	Not reported
Loss of one Snellen line		
Loss of two or more Snellen lines		
Predictability	Not reported	
Prediction or confidence interval		
Factors affecting outcome		
Method of study		Clinical experience
Clear zone diameter		Yes
Refraction		Not reported
Patient age		Not reported
Depth of incision		Not reported
Number of incisions		Not reported
Average central keratometry		Not reported
Patient sex		Not reported
Intraocular pressure		Not reported
Corneal thickness		Not reported
Number of zones		

Authors	Bores LD, Myers W, and Cowden J	Fyodorov SN and Durnev VV
Stability of refraction	Not reported	
(Change in minus power)		No change after 3 mo
Time interval		
Increased myopia = 1.00 to 2.50 D		
Change = < 0.87 D		
Decreased myopia = 1.00 to 2.50 D		
Mean change		
Vision-threatening complications		Not reported
Present series	No	
Additional reports by same author		
Delayed bacterial keratitis		
Ruptured globe		
Patient satisfaction	Not reported	Not reported
People wearing lenses after surgery	Not reported	Not reported
Comments	This paper reports the results of the earliest cases of radial keratotomy done in the United States by Dr. Bores, who introduced the procedure from the Soviet Union. The early nature of this series is reflected in the fact that in the first group, only 29% of the eyes saw 20/40 or better 1 year or more after surgery, and that group 2 improved considerably to 65% seeing 20/40 or better. The difference is explained largely by deeper incisions in Group 2. The diameter of the central clear zone was not reported, and cannot be evaluated. The authors concluded that the refraction stabilizes between 3 and 6 months for individual cases and remains permanently stable thereafter, a conclusion that did not anticipate the continued effect of the surgery found in later studies with longer follow-up. The authors conclude that "this procedure is obviously in no way intended to replace glasses or contact lenses," but is for patients who are contact-lens intolerant or have occupation-related indications.	This was the first paper published in English about modern anterior radial keratotomy; at best it qualifies as a colloquial report. Nevertheless, it kicked off the radial keratotomy craze in the United States. Fyodorov first used freehand dissection for all of his incisions and later in the series went to a guarded blade holder. He preferred the freehand dissection, using "visual control through the operating microscope." That 98% of these eyes saw 20/50 or better is indeed astounding. A brief addendum reports a total of 676 additional procedures summarized as follows: Group A, 130 eyes, −0.75 to −3.00 D, 78% emmetropic, 100% 20/50 or better uncorrected; Group B, 546 eyes −3.25 to −6.00 D, 21% emmetropic, 80% 20/50 or better uncorrected. The surgical technique included centrifugal incisions ("American" technique) that theoretically were to cut the circular ligament of the cornea (Kokott), leading to peripheral bulging and compensatory central flattening of the cornea under the influence of the intraocular pressure. Current thinking now holds that the paracentral part of the incision achieves the most effect, not the peripheral part.

Bilateral Results of Radial Keratotomy

Azhar Nizam

Michael J. Lynn

Michael H. Kutner

George O. Waring III

Since most patients who undergo radial keratotomy have symmetric myopia before surgery, it is important to know how often bilateral radial keratotomy preserves a relatively symmetric refraction and results in clinically meaningful asymmetry. For patients who receive unilateral surgery, it is of interest to know the amount of surgically induced refractive asymmetry and patients' motivations for not having bilateral surgery.

The importance of reporting the results in both eyes of a single patient can be appreciated from a simple example. A patient who has an uncorrected visual acuity after surgery of 20/25 bilaterally would be considered successful. However, such an individual could have a refraction of -1.50 D in one eye and $+2.00$ D in the other,[12] with bothersome anisometropia.

In this chapter we discuss the definition of anisometropia and what levels of anisometropia are thought to be clinically acceptable. We also report the refractive and visual acuity results in both eyes of 269 patients who received bilateral surgery in the PERK study, as well as the results for 81 PERK patients who had surgery in only one eye.

TERMINOLOGY: ANISOMETROPIA AND ANISEIKONIA

Anisometropia refers to asymmetry of refractive error in a patient's two eyes; aniseikonia refers to asymmetry of the retinal image size; anisophoria refers to asymmetric alignment of both eyes stemming from an unequal refraction, which is usually induced by wearing spectacles that produce unequal prismatic effects on vertical and lateral gaze.

BACKGROUND AND ACKNOWLEDGMENTS

Most of the material in this chapter originates from the Statistical Coordinating Center of the Prospective Evaluation of Radial Keratotomy (PERK) study. I am not aware of reported information about symmetry of outcome after refractive keratotomy other than the paper by Lynn et al.[9] This chapter is a modification of that paper, with the addition of previously unpublished material.

Limits for clinically acceptable anisometropia

It is difficult to establish a cutoff value for clinically acceptable asymmetry of refraction after radial keratotomy because many factors determine whether a patient will develop symptoms from surgically induced anisometropia. These factors include the following:

1. The magnitude of the difference in the spherical equivalent refraction between the two eyes
2. The magnitude of meridional anisometropia induced by asymmetric astigmatism, especially in the vertical meridian
3. The type of optical correction worn, especially spectacles
4. The rate of onset of the anisometropia, with the acute, surgically induced type usually being more bothersome than that of gradual onset
5. The patient's age, with presbyopes having more difficulty
6. The type of refractive error in each eye, with bilateral myopia or hyperopia usually being more tolerable than myopia in one eye and hyperopia in the other
7. The types of daily visual demands made on the individual
8. The patient's adaptability to the asymmetry, based on both physiologic central nervous system plasticity and psychologic tolerance

Anisometropia produces symptoms through two mechanisms: differences in retinal image size (aniseikonia) and prismatic displacement of images by spectacle lenses (anisophoria), which is particularly bothersome in the vertical meridian. In general, intraocular lenses produce less aniseikonia than contact lenses or spectacles; spectacles create the most troublesome situation because they induce prismatic displacement of the image on paracentral and peripheral gaze.

From approximately 1940 to 1960, researchers performed detailed and meticulous measurement of anisometropia and aniseikonia using the sensitive space eikonometer. This led to a high detection rate of small amounts of aniseikonia that were considered responsible for patients' symptoms, such as eye strain, double vision, headaches, and nausea. For example, Thill[13] has cited a 0.75% difference in image size between a patient's two eyes as a clinically meaningful cutoff value. However, experience with contact lenses and more recently with intraocular lens implants after cataract surgery has shown that patients tolerate aniseikonia better, with approximately 5% to 8% disparity in retinal image size.[3,5-8,10,11] For example, Hillman and Hawksell[5] studied the postoperative refraction and eikonometry of 50 patients who had unilateral cataract extraction with implantation of an intraocular lens and found that, despite aniseikonia of up to 7.8%, no diplopia was present. Similarly Huber[6] examined 20 patients with a monocular intraocular lens implant, using a television-based method of measuring retinal image size and subjective stereo acuity tests. They found that up to 6% aniseikonia was compatible with excellent stereo acuity. As explained in the following discussion, this corresponds to anisometropia of approximately 3.00 to 4.00 D.

Spectacle lenses produce approximately 1.5% change in retinal image size for each diopter of correction at a vertex distance of 10 mm, assuming a refractive and not an axial cause of the ametropia. If one postulates conservatively that after radial keratotomy most myopic patients can tolerate a 5% aniseikonia, then more than 3.00 D of anisometropia would be considered clinically meaningful. In general, spectacle wearers become symptomatic when approximately a 4.00 vertical prism diopter disparity exists between the two eyes. This corresponds to a difference in spectacle correction power of approximately 3.00 D, depending on the amount of eccentric gaze. Such image displacement can be particularly bothersome if the patient with anisometropia is hyperopic in one eye and myopic in the other, because of the anisophoria produced by the peripheral images moving in opposite directions as the head and eyes move.

On the basis of these observations, we have selected a 3.00 D cutoff value for meaningful spherical equivalent and meridional anisometropia after radial keratotomy.

SYMMETRY OF OUTCOME AFTER RADIAL KERATOTOMY IN THE PERK STUDY
Surgical protocol

The surgical protocol for the second eye incorporated the refractive outcome of the first eye in the preoperative planning for the second in patients with symmetrical refractions in each eye. If the first eye had a postoperative refraction within 1.00 D of emmetropia, the second eye received the same clear zone as the first eye. If the first eye was overcorrected or undercorrected by more than 1.00 D after surgery, the diameter of the clear zone for the second eye was 0.5 mm larger or smaller, respectively, than that used in the first eye. However, a clear zone smaller than 3.0 mm was not used. Patients whose first eye was undercorrected with a 3.0 mm clear zone also had a 3.0 mm clear zone for the second eye, but the blade length was set at 110% rather than 100% of the thinnest paracentral corneal thickness reading.

If the preoperative refractions of a patient's two eyes were not similar, the diameter of the clear zone used for the second eye was based only on the preoperative refractive error measured in the second eye, as just specified. Details are reported by Lynn and colleagues.[9]

Methods of analysis

The uncorrected visual acuity and the cycloplegic refraction for both the first and the second surgically treated eye of each patient were studied. Baseline measurements on both eyes were determined at the clinical visit preceding initial surgery. These values served as the reference point. The follow-up time when both eyes were measured was the visit approximately 1 year after surgery on the second eye, a time at which the first eye was approximately 2 to 3 years after surgery.

The symmetry of the refractive outcome in the patients' two eyes was evaluated using two measures. The first measured the difference in the spherical equivalent refraction of the two eyes. The second measured the net contribution of the refractive cylinder in the vertical (90-degree) meridian, calculated as sphere + (cylinder $\times \cos^2$ [axis]). We elected to use this vector analysis method instead of the absolute amount of refractive or keratometric astigmatism because power differences between a patient's two eyes in the vertical meridian are more important for visual function than the absolute amount of astigmatism irrespective of axis.

Uncorrected visual acuity was measured as the total number of letters read, which was converted to Snellen lines.[15] The refractive and visual acuity results in the two eyes were compared by taking the absolute value of the difference, that is, ignoring the plus or minus sign between the two eyes.

Study population

Of the 435 patients in the PERK study, 354 had had radial keratotomy on both eyes at the time of this analysis. Of these 354 patients, 52 had a repeat procedure on at least one of their eyes by 1 year after surgery on the second eye. These patients were not included in the analysis because the repeat surgery pre-

Table 22-1

Clear Zone Diameter for First and Second Eyes: Number of Patients with Each Clear Zone Combination*

First eye	Second eye				
	4.5 mm	4.0 mm	3.5 mm	3.0 mm	3.0 mm at 110%
4.0 mm	8	64	19	3	
3.5 mm		22	52	17	
3.0 mm		1	13	42	21

From Lynn MJ, Waring GO, Nizam A, et al: Refract Corneal Surg 1989;5:75.
*Seven patients had other procedures. All eyes had eight centrifugal incisions with the knife blade set at 100% of thinnest paracentral corneal thickness.

Figure 22-1
Bar graph demonstrates the differences, at baseline and 1 year after surgery on the second eye, between the spherical equivalents of the cycloplegic refractions of the two eyes of 269 patients. (From Lynn MJ, Waring GO, Nizam A, et al: Refract Corneal Surg 1989;5:3.)

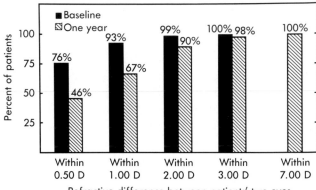

vented our analyzing the effects of a single procedure on each eye. Follow-up data were missing for 33 additional patients. As a result, 269 patients were included in the analysis of the symmetry of outcome (Table 22-1).

The time after surgery at which the analysis was done was: second eye, mean 11 months (range, 6 to 18); first eye, mean 26 months (range, 22 to 53).

Symmetry of spherical equivalent refraction at baseline and at 1 year

At the baseline examination the median difference between the refractive errors in the 269 patients' two eyes was 0.25 D (range, 0 to 2.37 D); all patients had a difference of 3.00 D or less (Fig. 22-1). At 1 year after surgery on the second eye, this median difference was 0.62 D (range, 0 to 6.87 D); 90% of the patients had a difference of 2.00 D or less (Fig. 22-1). Six patients (2%) had refractive differences between their two eyes that were greater than 3.00 D: three with a 3.25 D difference and three with 4.25 to 6.87 D difference.

Change in symmetry of spherical equivalent refraction from baseline to 1 year

After surgery on both eyes the disparity between the refractive error of the two eyes increased as compared with baseline values. On the average, a 0.51 D increase in the difference between the refractive errors in the two eyes occurred (SD = 0.98, p < 0.01). For 26% of patients, the difference between the refractions of their two eyes was 1.00 to 6.87 D greater at 1 year than at baseline. For 2% of patients, the difference in refraction between their two eyes was 1.00 to 1.37 D less after surgery than at baseline.

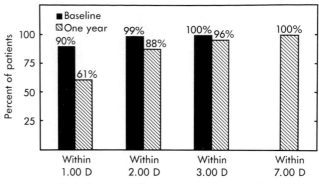

Table 22-2

Refractive Error in Each Eye at 1 Year after Surgery on Second Eye

Spherical equivalent of cyloplegic refraction	Percentage of 269 patients
Both eyes ± 1.00 D	55
One eye ± 1.00 D; other undercorrected > −1.00 D	21
One eye ± 1.00 D; other overcorrected > +1.00 D	12
Both eyes undercorrected > −1.00 D	8
Both eyes overcorrected > +1.00 D	2
One eye undercorrected > −1.00 D; other overcorrected > +1.00 D	2

From Lynn MJ, Waring GO, Nizam A, et al: Refract Corneal Surg 1989;5:75.

Figure 22-2
Bar graph demonstrates the differences, at baseline and 1 year after second eye surgery, between the refractive powers in the vertical (90 degree) meridian of the two eyes of 269 patients. (From Lynn MJ, Waring GO, Nizam A, et al: Refract Corneal Surg 1989;5:3.)

Spherical equivalent refractive error in both eyes of each patient

As shown in Table 22-2, 55% of the patients had a residual refractive error in both eyes within 1.00 D of emmetropia. In 10% of patients, both eyes were either overcorrected or undercorrected by more than 1.00 D. For 33% of patients, one eye was within 1.00 D of emmetropia, whereas the other eye was either overcorrected or undercorrected by more than 1.00 D. In 2% of patients, one eye was overcorrected by more than 1.00 D and the other undercorrected by more than 1.00 D.

Symmetry of astigmatic refractive power in vertical meridian at baseline and at 1 year

The effect of astigmatism on the symmetry of the refractive error was evaluated by comparing the power in the vertical meridian in the patients' two eyes. At baseline the median difference between the powers in the vertical meridian in the two eyes was 0.50 D (range, 0 to 2.33 D); one patient had a difference greater than 2.00 D (Fig. 22-2). At 1 year after surgery on the second eye, this median difference was 0.73 D (range, 0 to 6.48 D); 96% of patients had a difference of 3.00 D or less.

Change in symmetry of astigmatic refractive power in vertical meridian from baseline to 1 year

After surgery on both eyes, the difference between the power in the vertical meridian in the patients' two eyes was greater as compared with baseline. On the average, a 0.52 D increase in the difference between the vertical refractive powers in the two eyes occurred (SD = 1.00, p < .01). For 25% of patients, the difference between the refractions of their two eyes was 1.00 to 6.24 D greater at 1 year than at baseline. For 2% of patients, the difference in refraction between their two eyes decreased by 1.00 to 1.50 D after surgery.

Interpretation of results

One year after surgery on the second eye, 98% of patients had a spherical equivalent anisometropia of 3.00 D or less, and 96% had a calculated astigmatic anisometropia in the vertical meridian of 3.00 D or less. Adopting more stringent criteria, 90% had 2.00 D or less of spherical equivalent anisometropia, and 88% had 2.00 D or less of vertical astigmatic anisometropia. The PERK study group concluded that the induction of an asymmetric refraction was not a major complication, although visual complaints could occur in a minority of patients, as the case report emphasizes. If one eye is overcorrected and the other eye undercorrected, spectacles will induce significant anisophoria; accommodative effort in the overcorrected eye will render the undercorrected eye even more myopic.

Symmetry of uncorrected visual acuity at baseline and at 1 year

At baseline, 85% of patients had no significant difference (one Snellen line or less) in the uncorrected visual acuity of their two eyes (Table 22-3); many patients (33%) could not read the first line on the chart (20/200) with either eye. At 1 year after surgery on the second eye, most patients (60%) had a difference of one Snellen line or less in the uncorrected visual acuity of their two eyes; 14% were highly asymmetric, showing a difference of four or more Snellen lines.

Table 22-3

Symmetry of Uncorrected Visual Acuity at Baseline and at 1 Year After Surgery on Second Eye

Difference in Snellen lines read by first and second eyes	Baseline (269 eyes)	1 year (266 eyes)
0 to 1	85%	60%
2 to 3	14%	26%
4 to 8	1%	14%

From Lynn MJ, Waring GO, Nizam A, et al: Refract Corneal Surg 1989;5:75.

Characterization of uncorrected visual acuity in highly asymmetric patients

Among the 38 patients with four or more Snellen lines of asymmetry of uncorrected visual acuity, the amount of refractive anisometropia was 0.50 to 0.75 D in 2 patients (5%), 1.12 to 3.00 D in 31 patients (82%), and 3.12 to 6.87 D in 5 patients (13%). We noted that in 33 (87%) of these 38 patients, the more myopic eye was undercorrected by 1.00 to 4.00 D. Therefore the asymmetry of uncorrected visual acuity depended not only on the amount of anisometropia, but also on the level of the refractive error.

For example, of the 82 patients with 1.00 to 3.00 D of anisometropia, 42 were undercorrected by more than 1.00 D in their more myopic eye. Of these 42 patients, 62% had four or more Snellen lines of asymmetry of visual acuity. Of the remaining 40 patients, who were not undercorrected, 13% had four or more Snellen lines of asymmetry of visual acuity.

It was difficult to measure accurately the baseline asymmetry of uncorrected visual acuity, since almost all patients saw 20/50 or worse and 33% could not see any letters on the chart. Assuming that patients who saw worse than 20/200 had symmetric visual acuity, only 1% had four Snellen lines or more of asymmetric visual acuity before surgery, whereas 14% had a four− to eight−Snellen line difference in uncorrected acuity between the two eyes after surgery. Asymmetry of uncorrected visual acuity depended on the level of refractive error, as well as the amount of anisometropia. Patients with 1.00 to 3.00 D of anisometropia were more likely to have asymmetry of visual acuity if one eye was undercorrected by more than 1.00 D. We do not know if symptoms result from asymmetry of visual acuity in the absence of significant anisometropia.

SYMMETRY OF CHANGE IN REFRACTION AFTER RADIAL KERATOTOMY IN THE PERK STUDY

If a surgeon performs the same surgical technique on both eyes of the same patient, will the refractive results in the two eyes be similar? How predictable is the outcome of the second eye as compared with that of the first?

The design of the PERK study provides answers to these questions because 136 patients had radial keratotomy on each eye by the same surgeon, who used the same surgical instruments and followed the same protocol. In addition, preoperative and postoperative examinations were done in the same clinical lane by (in most cases) the same technician and independent examining physician.

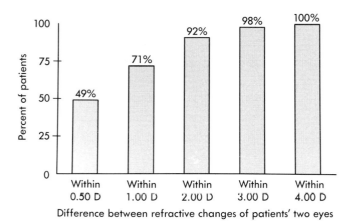

Figure 22-3
Bar graph demonstrates the difference between the refractive changes, from baseline to 1 year after second eye surgery, of the two eyes of 136 patients. (From Lynn MJ, Waring GO, Nizam, et al: Refract Corneal Surg 1989;5:3.)

Under these controlled circumstances we examined the change in refraction induced by the surgery in each eye. The baseline examination was performed at different times for the first and second eye to document accurately the refraction and visual acuity just before surgery. The postoperative time when each eye was examined was the visit closest to 1 year after the surgery on that eye. The absolute value of the difference between the refractive changes was calculated, and the percentage of patients with differences of 1.00 D or less, 2.00 D or less, and so on was determined.

The median difference between the refractive changes obtained in the patients' two eyes was 0.62 D (range, 0 to 3.62 D). For 71% of the patients, the changes in refraction in the two eyes were within 1.00 D of each other (Fig. 22-3); the remaining 29% had differences between the changes in refraction ranging from 1.12 to 3.62 D. Thus the change in the second eye was considerably different than that in the first for almost one-third the patients.

Two reasons exist for not achieving identical results when presumably identical surgery was performed:

1. The surgical technique was not executed identically in the two eyes. This fact is well known to surgeons and well documented by slit-lamp microscopy of the incisions' depth, which shows variability from one incision to another.

2. Although one would expect similar wound healing in two corneas of the same individual, histopathologic studies[1] have demonstrated that the epithelial plug extrudes from wounds in the same eyes at different rates. Thus an intrinsic variability exists in healing from one incision to another in the same eye in the same patient.

These observations emphasize the difficulty in accurately predicting the outcome of radial keratotomy for a single eye.

PATIENTS WITH ONE EYE OPERATED IN THE PERK STUDY

Eighty-one of the 435 patients (19%) in the PERK study elected not to have surgery on the second eye.

Motivations for having unilateral surgery

In interviews with these 81 patients, 46% stated dissatisfaction with the results of the first surgery as the main reason for not having surgery on their second eye. Complaints included overcorrection, undercorrection, fluctuating vision, and glare. Of the remaining patients, 28% stated that they preferred their current asymmetric state; 10% were still considering surgery for the second eye; 4% had contraindications to surgery, including glaucoma, cataracts, and basement membrane dystrophy; 6% cited other reasons, such as unrelated health problems; and 6% could not be interviewed.

Timing of examinations

The cycloplegic refraction and uncorrected visual acuity were studied for both eyes of each patient. Postoperative measurements were taken from the most recent visit at which both eyes were examined. For 77% of the patients, this was the 4-year follow-up visit; for 15%, the 3-year visit; for 1%, the 2-year visit; and for 4%, the 1-year visit. Three percent of patients could not be found for follow-up.

Symmetry of spherical equivalent refraction

At the baseline examination the median difference between the spherical equivalent cycloplegic refractive error in the 81 patients' two eyes was 0.25 D, with the difference between 0.00 and 2.62 D for 100% of patients (Fig. 22-4).

Postoperatively for 79 patients, the median difference was 3.75 D (range, 0.62 to 9.12 D); 37% had a difference of 3.00 D or less; 54% had a difference of 4.00 D or less; 72% had a difference of 5.00 D or less; and 85% had a difference of 6.00 D or less (Fig. 22-4). Of the remaining 15% (12 patients), nine patients had differences ranging from 6.12 to 7.87 D, and the other three had differences of 8.25, 8.75, and 9.12 D.

Figure 22-4
Bar graph demonstrates the differences, at baseline and postoperatively, between the spherical equivalent cycloplegic refractions of the operated and unoperated eyes of 81 patients. (From Lynn MJ, Waring GO, Nizam A, et al: Refract Corneal Surg 1989;5:3.)

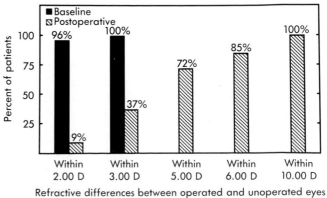

Refractive differences between operated and unoperated eyes

Symmetry of astigmatic refractive power in vertical meridian

At baseline the median difference between the refractive power in the vertical meridian in the two eyes was 0.47 D (the range was 0.00 to 2.60 D).

After surgery in 78 patients, the median difference was 3.95 D (the range was 1.07 to 9.44 D); only 36% had differences of 3.00 D or less, and approximately 50% had differences of more than 4.00 D.

Symmetry of uncorrected visual acuity

Of the 81 patients, 85% had a difference of one Snellen line or less in the visual acuities of their two eyes at baseline; 12% had a difference of two to three Snellen lines; and 3% had a difference of four Snellen lines (Table 22-4).

After surgery for 76 patients, only 8% had a difference of one Snellen line or less; 9% a difference of two to three Snellen lines; 18% a difference of four to seven Snellen lines; 64% a difference of eight to 12 lines; and 1% a difference of 13 lines.

Table 22-4

Symmetry of Uncorrected Visual Acuity for Patients with Only One Eye Operated in the PERK Study

Difference in Snellen lines read by operated and unoperated eyes	Baseline (81 patients)	Postoperative (76 patients)
0 to 1	85%	8%
2 to 3	12%	9%
4 to 7	3%	18%
8 to 13		65%

Optical correction for monocularly treated patients

To cope with the surgically induced anisometropia, most of the 81 patients who had unilateral surgery wore spectacles or contact lenses. Only 15% did not wear any correction at all; 11% wore contact lenses in both eyes; and 28% used spectacle correction for both eyes. Thirty percent wore no correction for the treated eye but wore contact lenses in the untreated eye, and 3% wore no correction for the treated eye with spectacle correction of the untreated eye. Seven percent used spectacle correction for the treated eye while wearing a contact lens in the untreated eye. Correction information was not available for 6% of the patients.

OBSERVATIONS ABOUT ANISOMETROPIA AFTER RADIAL KERATOTOMY

That one of five patients in the PERK study elected to have surgery on only one eye is a strong testimony to individuals' willingness and ability to tolerate moderately severe anisometropia and these patients' capacity to decide what they consider best for their ocular health care.

Special factors might affect the adaptation of patients in the PERK study to any induced anisometropia, including the following:

1. The anisometropia was surgically induced and therefore acute, making it more likely to be clinically bothersome.

Case Report: Anisometropia after Bilateral Radial Keratotomy

The following case report illustrates the possible complications of anisometropia after radial keratotomy. A 36-year-old white male entered the PERK study and had surgery on his left eye in January 1983 and in his right eye in May 1984. Table 22-5 summarizes his preoperative and postoperative course, which was characterized by anisometropia, anisophoria, and asthenopia.

During his routine follow-up examination in 1988, the patient complained of persistent double vision when wearing his glasses, as well as an inability to focus at distance. For these reasons he wore his glasses only 5 to 6 hours per week. Although the uncorrected visual acuity of the right eye was 20/50, the patient complained of blurring of the first line of Snellen letters (20/200).

The cause of these symptoms became apparent during clinical examination. When the occluder was removed from the right eye during the manifest refraction, the patient demonstrated 30 prism diopters of esotropia. A cover test revealed a variable intermittent esotropia of 20 to 25 prism diopters. As Table 22-5 indicates, no change occurred in the refraction of the right eye with cycloplegia. However, the refraction of the left eye increased by +2.50 D. The patient apparently was accommodating to clear the vision of the left eye; this not only induced blurring of the right eye but also caused esotropia and diplopia. The patient was given the option of wearing a contact lens on the right eye or having repeated surgery; he elected surgery. Early in the postoperative period, his refraction was almost symmetric.

Table 22-5

Clinical Data on 36-Year-Old Man with Anisometropia after Bilateral Radial Keratotomy

Preoperative refraction	Right eye −4.25 +0.25 × 180°	Left eye −4.00 +0.50 × 065°
First surgery		
Dates	May 1984	January 1983
Number of incisions	Eight centrifugal	Eight centrifugal
Clear zone diameter	4.0 mm	3.5 mm
Depth of incisions (% of paracentral thickness)	100	100
Date of last follow-up	January 1989 (4½ years)	September 1988 (5½ years)
Uncorrected visual acuity	20/50	20/20+
Manifest refraction (D)	−2.00 +1.00 × 175°	+0.50 +0.75 × 180°
Cycloplegic refraction (D)	−2.00 +1.00 × 175°	+3.00 +0.75 × 175°
Symptoms	Blurring	Diplopia
Second surgery		
Date	January 1989	
Number of incisions	Four centripetal	
Clear zone diameter	4.0 mm	
Depth of incision (% of paracentral thickness)	95	
Uncorrected visual acuity at 1 month	20/30	
Postoperative refraction at 1 month	−0.50 +0.50 × 180°	

From Lynn MJ, Waring GO, Nizam A, et al: Refract Corneal Surg 1989;5:75.

2. These patients were required by the protocol to wait 1 year between surgery on the first and second eyes; 95% complied. Thus they had a prolonged experience with moderate to severe anisometropia and might have been less likely to have difficulty with the residual anisometropia after both eyes were treated.

3. The anisometropia was refractive and therefore less severe than that accompanying surgically induced axial aniseikonia, as sometimes occurs after monocular retinal detachment surgery with scleral buckling.

4. In the PERK population, 64% of the patients with both eyes treated stated that they wore no optical correction at 4 years after surgery[16]; thus they would be expected to experience minimal symptoms from aniseikonia. The 32% who wore spectacle correction some of the time would be at greater risk for symptoms if they were anisometropic.

5. Patients entering the PERK study were highly motivated to avoid the use of corrective lenses and therefore might have been more tolerant of induced anisometropia than the average myopic individual.

INTENTIONAL MONOVISION AFTER RADIAL KERATOTOMY

Some surgeons have advocated correcting one eye near emmetropia and intentionally leaving one eye 1.00 to 1.50 D myopic to offset symptomatic presbyopia. This technique is known as *monovision* and is often used when fitting contact lenses for individuals in their early 40s. The nondominant eye is usually undercorrected for near vision. The success of this technique depends on two major variables. The first is the patient's ability to tolerate the intentional anisometropia. If the anisometropia is about 1.00 to 2.00 D and the patient does not wear spectacles; most individuals should be able to tolerate the anisometropia. However, based on the experience with contact lens monovision, some persons cannot make this adjustment. With contact lenses a simple solution exists: change the lenses. With radial keratotomy the solution is not so simple and would probably require repeat surgery in an attempt to gain further correction in the undercorrected eye.

The second problem with surgically created monovision is the unpredictability of radial keratotomy for individual eyes. The 90% prediction interval in the PERK study was 4.00 D wide, which is not accurate enough to allow fine adjustments of refraction such as needed for monovision. However, improvements in preoperative planning and surgical technique have increased the predictability, especially in the range of −2.00 to −5.00 D. Each surgeon must analyze his or her own results to see whether they are accurate enough to allow monovision to be achieved.

Mild intentional undercorrection is the general goal of radial keratotomy, which leaves the patient with a refractive error of −0.50 to −1.00 D. Under these conditions, patients see better than expected without correction,[12] so this represents a reasonable safety zone to aim for in attempting surgical monovision.

OTHER REPORTS OF ANISOMETROPIA AFTER RADIAL KERATOTOMY

No other systematic reports exist on large series of radial keratotomy patients concerning binocular refractive error, visual acuity, or visual function.

Duling and Wick[4] have presented a detailed, instructive analysis of four patients with binocular vision complications after radial keratotomy, emphasizing the variety of complaints and adaptability among individuals. A law student who had a resulting refractive error in the right eye of +0.50 −0.50 × 105°, and in the left eye of +2.75 −2.25 × 75°, with a bilateral near addition of +1.50 D.

The approximate difference in meridional magnification in the two eyes was 6.25% × 60°. After 6 months' adjustment to conventional spectacle lenses, the patient remained asymptomatic, so an aniseikonic correction was not required. Two other patients were reported with only one eye operated, each with an overcorrection. The postoperative refractive error in the first patient was OD, +1.25 −0.25 × 175°, and OS, −8.00 −0.75 × 160°; and in the second patient OD, +7.25 −2.50 × 80°, and OS, −1.25 −0.25 × 90°. Both were successfully fit with contact lenses and became asymptomatic.

Duling and Wick emphasized the following alternatives available in the management of anisometropia after radial keratotomy:

1. A careful explanation to patients of the cause of their symptoms and the implications of different types of management with the hope of successful adaptation
2. Contact lens fitting if the patient will accept it on one or both eyes
3. Fitting of regular spectacles with a supportive period of adjustment
4. Fitting of asymmetric iseikonic spectacles, which is rarely done
5. Management of preexisting binocular disorders, such as convergence insufficiency
6. Repeat refractive corneal surgery to decrease the anisometropia in cases that cannot be handled optically or in which the patient insists on further surgery. Surgery may include repeat keratotomy for residual myopia or astigmatism; opening and suturing of wounds for residual hyperopia; or an epikeratoplasty, keratomileusis, or penetrating keratoplasty in severe cases (see Chapter 18, Repeated Surgery for Residual Myopia and Hyperopia after Refractive Corneal Surgery).[2,14]

UNFINISHED BUSINESS

The obvious need in understanding a patient's visual function after refractive keratotomy is for further study of bilateral results and overall visual success. This requires that authors report not only the results on individual eyes, but also the percentage of patients with varying amounts of anisometropia in the following categories: within 0.50 D, 1.00 D, 2.00 D, 3.00 D, 4.00 to 6.00 D, and greater than 6.00 D. These are simple numbers to procure from a review of cases and should be part of the data reported from any series of cases. In addition, there is a need for refinement of fundamental studies of anisometropia and aniseikonia to define the functional limits in modern terms. Much of this information will probably come from patients who have had cataract extraction with intraocular lens implantation, as the interest in the quality of visual function in these individuals, both monocular and binocular, increases.

There is no published series of patients who have had refractive keratotomy with intentional monovision. Such a series would report the preoperative intended refraction in each eye with the intended amount of anisometropia and that achieved postoperatively, as well as the patient's adaptation and adjustment to this surgical monovision.

REFERENCES

1. Binder PS, Nayak SK, Deg JK, Zavala EY, and Sugar J: Ultrastructural and histochemical study of long-term wound healing after radial keratotomy, Am J Ophthalmol 1987;103:432-440.

2. Cowden JW, Lynn MJ, Waring GO, et al: Repeated radial keratotomy in the prospective evaluation of radial keratotomy study, Am J Ophthalmol 1987;103:423-431.

3. Crone RA and Leuridan OMA: Unilateral aphakia and tolerance of aniseikonia, Ophthalmologica 1975;171:258-263.

4. Duling K and Wick B: Binocular vision complications after radial keratotomy, Am J Optom Physiol Opt 1988;65:215-223.

5. Hillman JS and Hawkswell A: The control of aniseikonia after intraocular lens implantation, Trans Ophthalmol Soc UK 1985;104:582-585.

6. Huber C: Aniseikonia in lens implantation, Am Inst Barraquer 1988;20:367-369.

7. Huber C and Binkhorst CD: Iseikonic lens implantation in anisometropia, Am Intra-Ocular Implant Soc J 1979;5:194-202.

8. Huber C, Meier U, and Hess F: Klinischer Wert der Iseikonie bei der Korrektur des aphaken Auges, Klin Monatsbl Augenheilkd 1983;182:379-382.

9. Lynn MJ, Waring GO, Nizam A, et al: Symmetry of refractive and visual acuity outcome in the Prospective Evaluation of Radial Keratotomy (PERK) study, Refract Corneal Surg 1989;5:75-81.

10. Miyake S, Awaya S, and Miyake K: Aniseikonia in patients with a unilateral artificial lens measured with Aulhorn's phase difference haploscope, Am Intra-Ocular Implant Soc J 1981;7:36-39.

11. Nolan J and Hawkswell A: Clinical aspects of unilateral aphakia, Trans Ophthalmol Soc UK 1974;94:480-486.

12. Santos VR, Waring GO, Lynn MJ, et al: Relationship between refractive error and visual acuity in the Prospective Evaluation of Radial Keratotomy (PERK) study, Arch Ophthalmol 1987;105:86-92.

13. Thill EZ: Theory and practice of spectacle correction of aniseikonia. In Dwayne TE and Jagger EA: Clinical ophthalmology, Philadelphia, 1987, JB Lippincott Co, pp 1-13.

14. Waring GO: Repeated keratotomy for residual myopia in PERK. In Spaeth G and Katz L, editors: Current therapy in ophthalmic surgery, Philadelphia, 1989, BC Decker, Inc, pp 71-77.

15. Waring GO, Lynn MJ, Gelender H, et al: Results of the Prospective Evaluation of Radial Keratotomy (PERK) study one year after surgery, Ophthalmology 1985;92:177-199.

16. Waring GO, Lynn MJ, Fielding B, and the PERK Study Group: Results of the Prospective Evaluation of Radial Keratotomy (PERK) study four years after surgery for myopia, JAMA 1990;263:1083-1091.

Complications of Refractive Keratotomy

Edward R. Rashid
George O. Waring III

When ocular surgery is done to prevent a blinding disease, such as advanced cataract or uncontrolled glaucoma, the periodic occurrence of complications can be understood in terms of the risk-benefit ratio: if the surgery had not been performed, the patient would go blind, so the small risk is worth taking. In the case of myopia, optical correction is available and the surgery is elective; therefore the standards for safety, including predictability of outcome, must be higher than those for operations that correct blinding disorders. The surgeon must take unusual precautions to prevent all possible complications.

Unfortunately, this attitude of extreme caution is sometimes lost in the clinical practice of refractive keratotomy because the operation can be performed very quickly on an outpatient basis (sometimes simply in a room in the physician's office) with minimal equipment. Although advertisements may condition patients to expect a quick, painless procedure with rapid recovery of visual function, they almost never mention complications (see Chapter 10, Patient Educational Materials for Refractive Keratotomy). Thus both patient and surgeon can be lulled into questionable practices that might increase the probability of complications, a consequence that must be guarded against by the most rigorous application of ophthalmic practice and surgical principles.

The very low rate of complications for keratotomy improves the risk-benefit ratio, so a partial correction or even an overcorrection is more acceptable. Individuals who are undercorrected after the surgery can reason, "I'm a lot less nearsighted now than before, and if I need to see well, I can simply put my glasses on for a while." There is no doubt that an individual functions better with a refraction of −2.00 D than with −7.00 D.

BACKGROUND AND ACKNOWLEDGMENTS
This description of the complications of refractive keratotomy was previously published in the *Survey of Ophthalmology* (Rashid ER and Waring GO: Complications of radial and transverse keratotomy, Surv Ophthalmol 1989;34:73-106). The information is drawn from the published literature and personal experience. Some nonpublished case histories were contributed by Perry Binder. Other contributions are acknowledged in the text. Our goal in this chapter is not only to describe the complications of refractive keratotomy, but also to emphasize methods of preventing them.

The reports of refractive keratotomy from 1979 through 1981 indicated few problems.[26,28,53,71,72] However, the subsequent decade saw hundreds of thousands of patients undergo refractive keratotomy and witnessed a wide spectrum of complications (see box below). However, it has been difficult to document the incidence of many of these complications (see Chapter 21, Published Results of Refractive Keratotomy).

Complications and Sequelae of Refractive Keratotomy

I. Complications resulting from errors before surgery
  A. Inaccurate refraction
  B. Incorrect surgical plan
II. Complications of anesthesia
  A. Uncooperative patient
  B. Systemic sedation
  C. Topical anesthesia
  D. Retrobulbar anesthesia
    1. Retrobulbar hemorrhage
    2. Optic nerve damage
    3. Perforation of the globe
  E. Peribulbar anesthesia
III. Operative complications
  A. Corneal perforations
    1. Small
    2. Large
  B. Decentered clear zone
  C. Incisions across the visual axis
  D. Incorrect number of incisions
  E. Incorrect meridian of incisions
  F. Incisions across the limbus
IV. Early postoperative course
  A. Pain
  B. Photophobia
  C. Epithelial defects
  D. Fluctuating vision and corneal edema
V. Reduced best-corrected visual acuity
VI. Refractive complications
  A. Overcorrection
  B. Undercorrection
  C. Anisometropia
  D. Astigmatism
    1. Residual regular
    2. Induced regular
    3. Irregular
  E. Premature presbyopia
VII. Visual acuity
  A. Unstable visual acuity
    1. Diurnal fluctuation
    2. Unstable visual acuity over time
  B. Glare
    1. Starburst pattern
    2. Disability glare
  C. Changes in contrast sensitivity
  D. Color vision
  E. Diminished night vision
  F. Monocular diplopia

VIII. Corneal complications
  A. Bacterial or fungal keratitis
    1. Early postoperative
    2. Delayed
  B. Sterile nonhealing corneal defects
  C. Herpes simplex keratitis
  D. Endothelial cell loss
  E. Stellate epithelial iron line
  F. Epithelial basement membrane changes
  G. Epithelial erosions
  H. Abnormal incisions and scars
    1. Intersecting incisions
    2. Multiple scars from repeated operations
    3. Hypertrophic scar
    4. Posterior plaque at perforation site
    5. Limbal scarring
    6. Irregular incisions
    7. Vascularization of scars
    8. Epithelial inclusion cysts
    9. Debris and deposits
IX. Intraocular and eyelid complications
  A. Endophthalmitis
  B. Cataract
  C. Traumatic rupture of keratotomy scars
  D. Epithelial ingrowth
  E. Iridocyclitis
  F. Elevated intraocular pressure and glaucoma
  G. Retinal detachment
  H. Ptosis
X. Ocular surgery following keratotomy procedures
  A. Cataract extraction
  B. Penetrating keratoplasty
  C. Myopic keratomileusis
  D. Epikeratoplasty
  E. Retinal detachment and vitreous
XI. Contact lens fitting problems

SOURCES OF INFORMATION ON COMPLICATIONS OF KERATOTOMY

Reliable statistics on the incidence of complications of keratotomy for myopia and astigmatism in the United States are not readily available. One source is the PERK study. It has reported a low incidence of vision-threatening complications over a 4-year follow-up (Table 23-1). But one would expect a low complication

---

Table 23-1

Change in Spectacle-Corrected Visual Acuity after Radial Keratotomy in the PERK Study

Number of Snellen lines changed	Years after surgery and number (%) of eyes		
	One (N = 411)	Three (N = 435)	Four (N = 435)
Gain two	7(1.7)	17(4)	12(2.8)
Change zero to one	401(97.6)	412(94.6)	412(94.7)
Lose two or three	3(0.7)	6(1.4)	11(2.5)

---

rate in such a monitored, standardized study involving specially trained corneal surgeons. The incidence of complications can be expected to be higher when the procedure is performed in general office practice by surgeons of varying training and skill.

This pattern is familiar in other studies. Examples include the increase in microbial keratitis associated with use of extended-wear soft contact lenses and the increase in complications following the use of closed-loop anterior chamber intraocular lenses. Both of these were shown to be safe and effective in short-term monitored trials but demonstrated serious problems in general use. Thus there is a need to document all cases with a loss of best-corrected visual acuity after refractive keratotomy. Studies of a limited number of cases, such as those of Arrowsmith and colleagues[6-9] and Neumann and colleagues,[160-162] give the frequency of complications in that small population, but larger scale epidemiologic studies are required to detect the number of complicated cases in the larger population of operated eyes.

Salz[186] conducted an informal survey, combining 935 eyes from the PERK study and 680 from the private practices of R. Lindstrom, Salz, and Villasenor, to estimate the incidence of complications within 5 years after surgery. Only three vision-threatening complications occurred in this series, all late-onset bacterial keratitis. In addition, all eyes had a spectacle-corrected visual acuity of 20/30 or better at the last follow-up examination. Salz concluded that a properly performed refractive keratotomy is an extremely safe operation.

Three registries in the United States were established between 1980 and 1986 for the reporting of results and complications. The Radial Keratotomy Complications Registry was established at the Center for Clinical Research and Anterior Segment Surgery at the Illinois Eye and Ear Infirmary. Data forms were published in an ophthalmic newspaper that was sent weekly to most American ophthalmologists. Unfortunately, few were returned and the project was abandoned. The Keratorefractive Society[145] reported their data on complications after sending a questionnaire to 200 refractive keratotomy surgeons. Unfortunately, in many instances the extremely low complication rates reported do not agree with most other published papers on this subject. Thus the information in this chapter is drawn from the published literature and our personal experience. We discuss the normal sequelae and the complications after refractive keratotomy following a basic outline: definition, description, reports in the literature, prevention, management, and illustrative case summaries. Intraoperative complications are discussed in Chapter 17, Atlas of Surgical Techniques of Radial Keratotomy, Chapter 18, Repeated Surgery for Residual Myopia and Hyperopia after Refractive Corneal Surgery, Chapter 31, Keratotomy for Astigmatism, and Chapter 32, Atlas of Astigmatic Keratotomy.

COMPLICATIONS RESULTING FROM ERRORS BEFORE SURGERY

Planning refractive keratotomy surgery has been discussed in Chapter 12, Patient Selection and Preoperative Examination, and Chapter 13, Predictability of Refractive Keratotomy. We emphasize here that an inaccurate refraction and an incorrect surgical plan are preoperative complications that will certainly affect the postoperative outcome.

Inaccurate refraction

A cycloplegic refraction should be part of the routine preoperative examination. Careful refinement of the cylinder axis will ensure better alignment of astigmatism surgery. Stability of the refraction should be confirmed by reference to previous records or by neutralization of previous spectacles. Cessation of contact lens wear for 2 weeks to 6 months will help ensure a stable corneal shape.

Case Report: Unstable Preoperative Refraction

A 38-year-old man who had worn hard contact lenses for 25 years experienced unplanned orthokeratology with flattening of the cornea, which was unappreciated before refractive keratotomy surgery. Minimal myopia and mild astigmatism existed at the time of contact lens wearing. The myopia increased some after the contacts were removed. Properly planned and executed refractive keratotomy surgery did not decrease the myopia or astigmatism significantly, and the surgeon thought the contact lens–induced flattening of the cornea was still reversing itself at the time of surgery. The keratometric and refractive measurements demonstrate the minimal effect of the surgery: Such patients should go at least 6 months without contact lenses to determine the full amount of uncorrected myopia.

Time and events	Right eye		Left eye	
	Keratometry	Refraction	Keratometry	Refraction

August 1985
  Corneal warpage
  Contacts removed
	40.12 × 178°
	43.00 × 88°
		−0.50 −1.00 × 180°	40.12 × 177°
			43.50 × 88°
				−0.50 −3.50 × 180°

October 1986
  Preoperative
  measurements
	41.62 × 177°
	43.87 × 87°
		−1.75 −1.75 × 180°	41.75 × 178°
			44.75 × 88°
				−2.00 −2.00 × 180°

Surgery	October 1986—right eye Four radial—4-mm clear zone One transverse—5-mm clear zone		January 1987—left eye Four radial—4-mm clear zone Two transverse—5-mm clear zone	

December 1987
  Postoperative
  measurements
  (little change)
	40.50 × 160°
	43.00 × 20°
		−0.125 −0.75 × 132°	41.87 × 163°
			41.50 × 73°
				−1.25 −2.00 × 120°

Courtesy Perry Binder, M.D., personal written communication, July 1988.

Incorrect surgical plan

Designing the surgical plan is an art that requires experience based on individual surgical techniques and instruments, as discussed in Chapter 13, Predictability of Refractive Keratotomy, and Chapter 14, Computerized Predictability Formulas for Refractive Keratotomy. The surgical plan should be devised before the day of surgery, double-checked the morning of surgery, and posted in the operating room in an easily viewed and clearly defined form to minimize errors.

Of course, the proposed surgical technique may be flawed, as were Sato's posterior keratotomy, Fyodorov's intersecting radial and transverse incisions for astigmatism (Chapter 31), Gills's combined radial and circumferential keratotomy,[80] and Ruiz's connecting trapezoidal keratotomy. Unfortunately, such flawed surgical techniques are often disseminated by a common pattern: early, apparently successful experience by the innovator, premature dissemination of results before careful analysis and adequate follow-up, adoption by colleagues who want to offer the latest advances to their patients, delayed recognition of the problems, and abandonment of the technique only after damage has occurred to more eyes than necessary.

COMPLICATIONS OF ANESTHESIA

Preoperative patient management and methods of administering anesthesia are discussed in Chapter 17, Atlas of Surgical Techniques of Radial Keratotomy.

Uncooperative patient

There are two reasons why patient cooperation is more important in keratotomy surgery than in standard intraocular surgery: increased accuracy and precision in making the incisions is necessary, since patient movement during an incision can cause the diamond knife to go astray, and less anesthesia is usually used for keratotomy, many surgeons using topical anesthesia alone without systemic sedation or intraorbital anesthesia, so the patient's voluntary cooperation plays a greater role in the surgery.

The patient may become uncooperative for many reasons, the two most common being internal psychologic fear and their response to an external problem, such as claustrophobia beneath the drapes. The surgeon can decrease the patient's anxiety and fear before surgery by reassuring conversation, clearly explaining the surgical procedure, and using a gentle touch with both the patient and his or her family and friends. Preparation and draping by the surgeon will reassure and calm the patient, particularly with the addition of practical hypnotic suggestion and a clear explanation about what the patient can expect next. If patient preparation is delegated to an assistant surgeon or to operating room personnel who are not skilled in patient management or whom the patient does not know, the strangeness of the situation may increase the patient's inherent anxiety.

Specifically avoiding certain maneuvers may reduce the patient's discomfort and anxiety. Intravenous lines cause additional pain and anxiety and are unnecessary for a healthy patient undergoing a procedure under topical anesthesia. Surgeons should avoid having the patient's blood pressure and vital signs taken during the procedure, especially with an automatic blood pressure cuff that inflates and may startle the patient. The patient should be assured that a simple request for "more air" will produce a greater flow of air through the mask or cannula beneath the drapes.

Particularly anxious patients can be reassured by having an operating room staff person seated by the bedside and holding the patient's hand throughout the procedure. In cases of extreme uncooperation, the surgeon should terminate the operation and complete it at a later date.

Systemic sedation

Providing oral, intramuscular, or intravenous sedation may calm the patients, but oversedation will reduce their ability to cooperate if they become disoriented or groggy. An appropriate amount of fear may be a positive factor, making them more alert, controlled, and cooperative.

Topical anesthesia

Most refractive keratotomy surgeons use only topical anesthesia and are well aware that excess application of tetracaine, lidocaine, or proparacaine to the cornea will roughen and soften the epithelium. Therefore one or two applications to the cornea is all that is necessary, but multiple applications to the limbus and conjunctiva with a moist cellulose sponge may be necessary to give good anesthesia for adequate fixation of the globe. Topical cocaine produces significant corneal epithelial damage and should be avoided.[17]

Immediate toxic reactions to local anesthetics on the cornea have been described by Theodore.[221] He reported several instances in which a single drop of proparacaine led to pain and clouding of the epithelium in 30 minutes, progressing to swelling of the cornea and wrinkling of Descemet's membrane. These are rare occurrences. A patient with a history of "allergy" to topical local anesthetic is probably not cross-allergic to all topical anesthetics. A careful history may help define the problem.[98] Patients sensitive to topical anesthetics may show punctate epithelial keratopathy, conjunctival hyperemia, slight lid swelling, pain, and profuse tearing.[98] Management with topical corticosteroids may help slightly, but the symptoms may not abate for 24 hours.

Retrobulbar anesthesia

A regional intraorbital block with a blunt needle offers several advantages over topical anesthesia.[164,238] The patient gets a more prolonged anesthetic effect that will increase comfort after surgery and the surgeon has better control of the position of the eye.[192] Unfortunately, complications of retrobulbar injections can produce severe loss of vision,[45,173] so most surgeons do not use retrobulbar anesthesia during keratotomy procedures.

Retrobulbar hemorrhage. Posterior orbital hemorrhages from retrobulbar anesthetics have been reported in patients undergoing refractive keratotomy. A severe orbital hemorrhage produces increasing proptosis, tightness of the lids, conjunctival ecchymosis, elevated intraocular pressure,[118] and, most tragically, occlusion of the central retinal artery. Management includes immediate cessation of the surgical procedure and a lateral canthotomy to decrease orbital pressure, maintain retinal circulation, and prevent retinal anoxia. Cross and Head[43] cite unpublished reports of seven significant retrobulbar hemorrhages following refractive keratotomy, three apparently resulting in significant and permanent decrease in visual acuity.

Optic atrophy. All reported cases of optic atrophy following refractive keratotomy were associated with retrobulbar anesthetic injections.[27,164] The probable cause is impalement of the optic nerve with a retrobulbar needle and perineural or intraneural injection of the anesthetic. This complication also has been reported after retrobulbar injection for cataract surgery.[238] Unfortunately, there is no effective treatment.

Perforation of the globe. A myopic eye, which may be longer than normal with a thinner posterior sclera, is more likely to be perforated during retrobulbar anesthesia. Several cases of this complication have been reported during refractive keratotomy. In one case, a double perforation was noted, and in another case, a retinal detachment followed the perforation and useful vision was lost.[135,192]

Case Report: Optic Nerve Damage from Retrobulbar Anesthesia

A 36-year-old man underwent refractive keratotomy in his left eye with retrobulbar anesthesia. The day after surgery, visual acuity was hand motions. Examination 2 years later by another physician revealed a visual acuity of hand motions, an atrophic optic disc (Fig. 23-1), and a large central scotoma on visual field examination. Ptosis and exotropia developed on the affected side with an afferent pupillary defect.

From O'Day DM, Feman SS, and Elliott JH: Ophthalmology 1986;93:319-326.

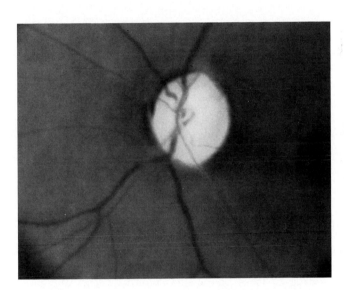

Figure 23-1
Optic atrophy with severe pallor of the disc after damage to the optic nerve from a retrobulbar injection for radial keratotomy. (Courtesy Dennis O'Day.)

The best prevention is to avoid orbital anesthesia or to use a peribulbar technique. Management includes termination of the procedure, dilation of the pupil with careful indirect ophthalmoscopy, and appropriate retinal repair.

Peribulbar anesthesia. In peribulbar anesthesia,[45,46,81] the injections are made adjacent to the globe and optic nerve, without trying to enter the muscle cone to prevent damage to the posterior globe and optic nerve. Disadvantages are potentially poorer akinesia and anesthesia, a longer time until onset of anesthesia, and the requirement for a larger volume. However, some advantages exist for refractive keratotomy because the globe is pushed forward as a result of increased volume, slightly increasing intraocular pressure and making the globe recoil less if a compression fixation ring (Thornton ring) is used.

The rates of globe perforation are low for both peribulbar and retrobulbar anesthesia. In one series of 4000 cases of retrobulbar anesthesia, three globe perforations were reported.[173] In another report of 1600 cases of peribulbar anesthesia, no apparent complications were reported.[46] There is at least one case report of a globe perforation after peribulbar injection for cataract surgery.[128] An immediate vitreous hemorrhage developed, and at exploration the sclera demonstrated a single, small, pre-equatorial laceration at the 11:30 position. The patient underwent a successful pars plana lensectomy, vitrectomy, cryopexy, and scleral buckling.

OPERATIVE COMPLICATIONS

Complications during surgery are described here and are illustrated in Chapter 17, Atlas of Surgical Techniques of Radial Keratotomy, and Chapter 32, Atlas of Astigmatic Keratotomy.

Corneal perforations

Corneal perforations during the incisions can be subdivided into small perforations (microperforations) and large perforations (macroperforations). A microperforation is small enough to produce the loss of one or two drops of aqueous humor and allows continuation of the operation. A macroperforation is large enough to produce shallowing of the anterior chamber depth and may terminate the procedure or require closure with sutures.

Small perforations. The incidence of small punctures of Descemet's membrane in refractive keratotomy generally varies between 0.006% and 35%.[5,145,192,198-200,230] More recent reports indicate a rate of 2% to 10%.[145] This reduction results from more accurate pachometry and improved surgical knives. The PERK study reported a 2.3% microperforation rate; none of the perforations was large enough to require suturing or termination of surgery, but one leaked for 5 days. This low perforation rate was achieved by setting the diamond knife blade at 100% of the thinnest paracentral corneal thickness reading, as measured by calibrated intraoperative ultrasonic pachometry that was set for a speed of sound of 1640 meters per second and by not deepening the incisions after the first pass of the knife.[232]

Case Report: Corneal Perforation with Persistent Aqueous Leak

A 19-year-old man with a refraction in the left eye of $-4.50 +1.75 \times 95°$ underwent refractive keratotomy with a 3-mm diameter clear zone, eight centrifugal incisions, and blade length of 100% of the thinnest paracentral thickness. A perforation occurred in the 3 o'clock incision with shallowing of the anterior chamber. On the first day after surgery, fluorescein stain showed persistent aqueous leakage from the perforation. The anterior chamber was deep, however, and the eye was pressure patched. Leakage from the perforation continued for 3 days, so the patient was taken back to the operating room where two interrupted 10-0 nylon sutures closed the wound. Three weeks later, the sutures loosened spontaneously and were removed. Eight months after surgery, his cycloplegic refraction was +0.50 D.

Microperforations occur more frequently in the inferior and temporal cornea because of the relative thinness in these areas,[178,179,192] but they may appear in any location[179] (Fig. 23-2).

Prevention of corneal perforation is a combination of science and art, the science requiring accurate measurements of corneal thickness[174] and accurate setting of the length of the knife blade,[105] and the art requiring the surgeon's knowledge of how deep to make the incisesion in the cornea with the given knife and a given technique. Thus one surgeon may set a knife blade at 95% of the measured corneal thickness, whereas another may set the knife blade at 115% of the measured corneal thickness, neither perforating.

Factors that increase the chance of corneal perforation include an unfamiliar knife blade, centripetal incisions, greater elevation of intraocular pressure during incisions, recutting incisions to make them deeper, tilting the knife off the perpendicular and sweeping the tip more deeply (especially paracentrally in patients with deeply set orbits and a high brow),[57,179] allowing prolonged dehy-

Perforations

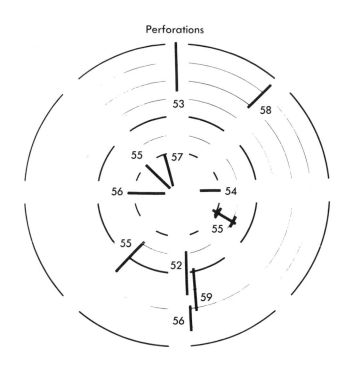

Figure 23-2
Location and length of corneal perforations. The numbers indicate the central corneal thickness readings determined by ultrasonic pachometry. The figure indicates that perforations can occur in almost any location and in corneas across a full range of corneal thickness. (From Rowsey JJ and Balyeat HD: Ophthalmic Surg 1982;13:27-35.)

dration and thinning of the cornea intraoperatively[192,226] (a problem seldom encountered in practice), inaccurate corneal thickness measurement (especially when using a new pachometer), sudden movements of the patient, and sliding of the footplate into a previously made incision during deepening.[192] From this list of problems, the steps to prevention are obvious.

The management of small perforations includes stopping the incision, drying the surface and the knife, and completing the incision with a slightly retracted knife blade or slightly less pressure on the knife. More than one microperforation indicates the knife blade is set too long and the blade should be retracted. As long as the chamber retains normal depth, the operation can be continued. If the perforation occurs in the thicker superonasal cornea, care should be taken in the inferotemporal thinner cornea. Some surgeons give a subconjunctival injection of antibiotics (for example, 20 mg of gentamicin), the pain of which can be diminished by a small injection of anesthetic before the antibiotic. Postoperative topical broad-spectrum antibiotics (for example, gentamicin or neomycin-bacitracin-polysporin) given at least four times daily for 5 days is reasonable prophylaxis.

The complications of a small or large perforation of the cornea include damage to the endothelium (Fig. 23-3) with the production of a scar in Descemet's membrane (a posterior collagenous layer or retrocorneal membrane), iridocorneal adhesions if the chamber remains flat,[92] laceration of the lens if the incision is carried deeply after the perforation, and the rare development of endophthalmitis and epithelial ingrowth, all discussed in subsequent sections. Whether corneal perforations produce greater amounts of astigmatism after surgery has not been well documented but remains a reasonable hypothesis.[9,179] Some incisions are so deep that they leave only Descemet's membrane uncut. It is possible to see a small seepage of aqueous humor from the wound in such cases, without the actual production of drops indicating a perforation. Barraquer[14] described production of a descemetocele with a knuckle of Descemet's membrane protruding up through a radial keratotomy incision.

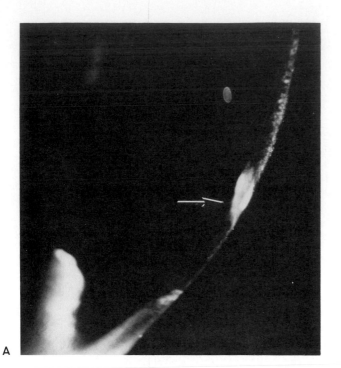

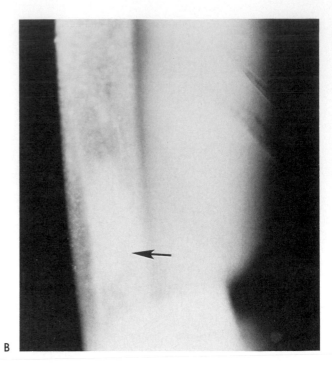

Figure 23-3
Deep stromal and Descemet's membrane scarring from corneal perforation. **A,** Slit
view shows full-thickness corneal scar with dense plaque posteriorly *(arrow).* **B,**
Broader slit beam shows deep stromal and Descemet's membrane scar *(arrow).*
(From Rashid ER and Waring GO: Surv Ophthalmol 1989;34:73-106.)

Large perforations. The frequency of large perforations varies from 0 to
0.45%,[145,179,192,196,200] although there is one report of a macroperforation rate
of 13%.[13] The most important factor in preventing large perforations is the
prompt recognition of a small perforation, usually betrayed by the appearance of
a drop of aqueous around the knife blade and footplates. This emphasizes the
importance of drying the knife blade and footplates before making an incision so
that fluid around the knife is not misinterpreted as coming from a small perforation. Immediate cessation of an incision when a drop of aqueous appears will
prevent the extension of the laceration of Descemet's membrane.

At the conclusion of surgery, if the anterior chamber is well formed and there
is no active leak of aqueous from a perforation, the eye can simply be patched
and examined the next day. If the aqueous leak persists on the first postoperative day, continued patching or the application of a flat-fitting, high water content soft contact lens will help seal the wound. Shallowing of the anterior chamber and persistent leakage for more than 2 or 3 days are indications for suturing
the wound shut with one or two 10-0 nylon sutures tied loosely enough just to
approximate the wound. The sutures should be left in place for only 2 or 3
weeks in most cases and then removed to decrease the amount of scarring that
would result from the sutures themselves.

Decentered clear zone

Centering of corneal surgical procedures is discussed in Chapter 16, Centering
Corneal Surgical Procedures. The frequency of a decentered clear zone is not reported in the literature. The smaller the clear zone the greater the effect of decentration, with increased glare and irregular astigmatism (Fig. 23-4).

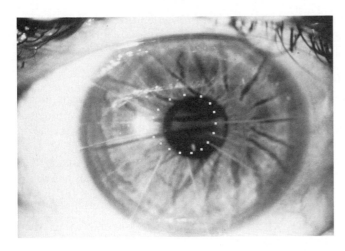

Figure 23-4
Decentered optical clear zone. Dotted line outlines ends of incisions. (From Rashid ER and Waring GO: Surv Ophthalmol 1989;34:73-106.)

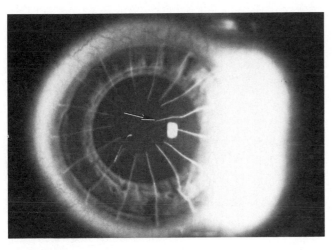

Figure 23-5
Incision at 2 o'clock passing into the clear zone *(arrow)*. (From Rashid ER and Waring GO: Surv Ophthalmol 1989;34:73-106.)

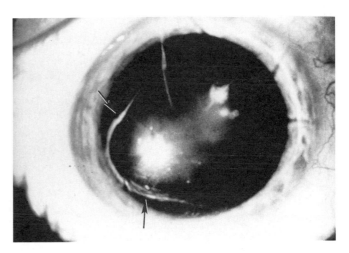

Figure 23-6
Irregular, curvilinear incision *(arrow)* caused by patient movement during radial keratotomy. (Courtesy Robert Hofmann.)

The surgeon can prevent decentration by making at least two optical marks to identify the center of the clear zone and then, after marking the clear zone, comparing its location with the margin of the pupil, which should be concentric.

Incisions across the visual axis

An incision that extends into the clear zone or across the visual axis disrupts vision by producing scarring, irregular astigmatism, and glare (Fig. 23-5) and usually occurs with incisions made from the limbus toward the optical zone or when a double-bladed knife is used for centrifugal incisions and inadvertently moves toward the center of the cornea.

Factors that predispose to this include sudden movement of the patient (Fig. 23-6), sudden Bell's reflex, an awkward position of the surgeon's hand, an unfamiliar knife or fixation forceps, and a very dry corneal surface, over which the knife does not slide smoothly. Optimal anesthesia, full patient cooperation, and adequate practice by the surgeon will help prevent this rare complication. Most reported cases of incisions into the clear zone occurred in the early 1980s with the use of blade fragments in a blade holder that proceeded through the tissue in a jerky, less controlled fashion. Diamond blades and smooth footplates make control of the knife much easier.

Incorrect number of incisions

It is possible for the surgeon to place too many or too few incisions in the cornea (Fig. 23-7). The chance of this occurring increases with the number of incisions used, and because four to eight incisions are used most commonly, an incorrect number is a rare event. Poor cooperation between patient and surgeon can cause omission of some incisions. The complication can be decreased with a corneal incision marker. Surprisingly, the addition or omission of one or two incisions may not make a great difference in the outcome because most of the effect of the surgery is obtained with the first four incisions.[188,192,225] If an extra incision is made and the surgeon notices it during the case, the placement of an additional symmetric incision is not indicated.[192]

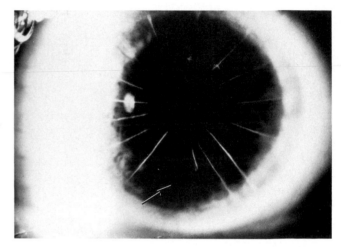

Figure 23-7
Incomplete and missing incisions at 6:00 *(arrow)* in radial keratotomy. (Courtesy Robert Hofmann.)

Incorrect orientation of incisions

Placing transverse keratotomy incisions for astigmatism in the improper axis can cause significant refractive problems. This complication can occur if the surgeon does not clearly understand astigmatism surgery, but it is more likely to occur simply because of momentary disorientation. The incisions for astigmatism will always be made in the steepest meridian, which will be 90° from the axis of the minus cylinder refraction.[192] A corneal sketch showing an anatomic landmark (for example, iris nevus, limbal vessel), the axes of greatest and least curvature, and the proposed surgery should be hung in easy view of the surgeon.

Management of an improperly placed transverse incision includes: (1) explaining the event to the patient so that future problems in astigmatism care will be understood, (2) suturing the wound to decrease its effect if the error is recognized during the operation, (3) opening, cleaning, and suturing the wound if the error is not recognized until later, and (4) treating residual astigmatism in an appropriate manner with further surgery, contact lenses, or corrective spectacle lenses after 3 to 6 months of healing.

Case Report: Incorrect Location of Transverse Incisions

A 27-year-old man could not wear contact lenses or spectacles on his assembly-line job. His cycloplegic refraction was $-1.50 +1.00 \times 180°$. He underwent a four-incision radial keratotomy. The transverse cuts for astigmatism were inadvertently placed at 90° meridian instead of 180°. On the first postoperative day, the patient's refraction was $-0.50 +1.50 \times 150°$. Three days after surgery, the transverse incisions were sutured, and 5 months later the sutures were removed. Two months after suture removal, the patient had a cycloplegic refraction of $-2.50 +2.75 \times 180°$ in the right eye. A reoperation was performed 9 months after the original operation. Two transverse incisions were made at a zone of 5 mm across the 180° meridian (Fig. 23-8). Two months later, the cycloplegic refraction showed persistent induced oblique astigmatism of $-1.25 +2.50 \times 75°$. The patient elected to have no further surgery.

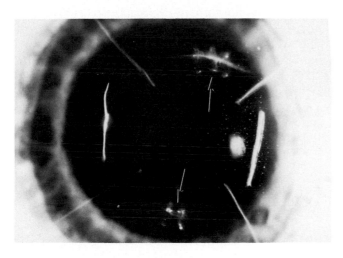

Figure 23-8
Patient with four transverse incisions in addition to four radial incisions. Incisions were erroneously placed in the vertical meridian (the flat meridian) and were sutured (note suture scars—*arrows*). Several months later the correct horizontal transverse incisions were made across the horizontal meridian. (From Rashid ER and Waring GO: Surv Ophthalmol 1989;34:73-106.)

Curvilinear incisions

The ideal radial incision is straight, but a curved, S-shaped, or slightly irregular incision can occur, especially when a very thin double-edged knife, or an unfamiliar knife, is used; patient movement during surgery and interrupted and subsequently completed incisions are other causative factors. There is no published evidence to indicate that a curvilinear incision has a different effect from a straight incision on the overall refractive outcome of the procedure.

Incisions across the limbus

The surgeon should not extend the incision into the limbus, since this does not enhance the effect of the surgery, causes bleeding into the wound, and may stimulate a triangular vascularized limbal scar.[57] Vessels are more likely to grow into the wound, especially if the patient wears a soft contact lens. It is sometimes difficult to see the end of the incision when cutting centrifugally because the footplate blocks visualization, but experience and controlled movement will stop the knife at the end of the vascular arcade. The surgeon should not use cautery to attain hemostasis because it may distort the peripheral wound and induce vascularization into the scar. Bleeding can be stopped with direct pressure.

EARLY POSTOPERATIVE SEQUELAE

The normal consequences of refractive keratotomy for the first few days after surgery include pain, light sensitivity, and fluctuating vision, all of which gradually decrease in the days to weeks after surgery. Patients should be informed of these events before surgery, particularly because refractive keratotomy is often advertised as being a painless procedure that allows patients to return to their work the same day.

Pain

For 24 hours following keratotomy, most patients experience a moderate throbbing, aching pain that is usually controllable by oral analgesics such as acetaminophen or codeine. However, some patients experience severe ocular pain that lasts 12 hours to 2 days and requires oral narcotics such as hydromorphone (Dilaudid), 2 to 4 mg every 4 hours, and (in rare cases) intramuscular analgesics. A mild oral sedative such as 15-mg flurazepam (Dalmane) or 0.125-mg triazolam (Halcicon) will help patients sleep better the first night or two.

In the PERK study, patients were initially patched for 12 to 24 hours after surgery, but when it was found that the patch increased postoperative pain, the surgeons stopped using it.[228,230]

Some surgeons think that irrigation of the incision increases postoperative pain, but no published data verify this impression. Irrigation of blood and epithelial cells from the wound is the generally accepted approach in the early 1990s.

Case Report: Severe Postoperative Pain

A 29-year-old man who was contact lens–intolerant underwent a four-incision refractive keratotomy in his right eye, complicated by one small perforation. On the following day the patient reported severe pain that was not reduced by oral hydromorphone (Dilaudid). Examination at that time showed normal mild edema around the incisions and trace iritis. The patient was given cycloplegic drops and topical antibiotics, but the pain continued and he required oral and intramuscular Demerol for the next 48 hours to relieve his discomfort.

Photophobia

Photophobia and glare occur commonly for several weeks after surgery. This probably results from epithelial incisions and abrasions, mild stromal edema, inflammation, and minimal iridocyclitis.[57] Sawelson and Marks[197] reported that one third of their patients had intermittent burning and itching after surgery, similar to the symptoms of patients with dry eyes, which resolved with lubricating drops by 6 weeks. Epithelial filaments developed along the incisions between the seventh and fourteenth postoperative day in approximately 10% of their patients.

An ophthalmologist[240] who underwent refractive keratotomy observed:

My lacrimation, pain, and upper lid swelling were worse right after getting up each morning. Self-administration of the antibiotic drop was harder than I had imagined; sometimes a painful self-perpetuating blepharospasm was triggered. The eye was very tender to the slightest touch, and I certainly could not sleep on that side. Occasionally, I cheated and used a drop of topical anesthetic. Photophobia made dark sunglasses with side shields mandatory outside. I noted a starburst effect and blurred vision, which changed a little with each blink.

Epithelial defects

The epithelium covers the incisions in 24 to 48 hours and shows some pooling of fluorescein for a few weeks. Periodically, punctate fluorescein stain appears in the epithelium over the wound.

Punctate epithelial keratopathy was noted in 95% of Kremer's cases, but by 1 week the incidence had decreased to 16% and by 1 year to 1%.[130] Epithelial abrasions may occur during surgery, leaving epithelial defects in the area of the incisions that usually heal in approximately 48 hours without difficulty. Artificial tears will decrease the foreign body sensation.

Fluctuating vision and corneal edema

Diurnal fluctuation of refraction and vision is discussed in Chapter 24, Stability of Refraction after Refractive Keratotomy. Most patients experience daily fluctuation in vision in the first few weeks after surgery. The cornea is usually flatter upon arising, producing better uncorrected visual acuity for the undercorrected patient and worse acuity for those overcorrected. Many influences may produce this. Stromal edema around the incisions occurs in all cases, enhancing the effect of the surgery. It is difficult to quantify this phenomenon because there is no way to measure the amount of localized stromal swelling, but the edema decreases gradually as the epithelium reestablishes its surface barrier of zonule occludens and as the endothelium recovers from mild injury. It is probably this disappearance of stromal swelling that accounts for the loss of initial effect that occurs in almost all eyes. Other factors contributing to fluctuation in vision are the corneal edema that occurs during sleep, external pressure from the eyelids, which may change the shape of the weakened cornea, and possibly, diurnal variations in intraocular pressure.[192,228]

REDUCED BEST SPECTACLE-CORRECTED VISUAL ACUITY

The most important indicator of the safety of refractive keratotomy is no change in spectacle-corrected visual acuity from before to after surgery. In the PERK study, a loss of two or more Snellen lines was selected as being clinically meaningful because a change of one line (three to five letters) can occur from one examination to another in unoperated eyes,[230] especially when acuities of 20/10, 20/12, and 20/16 are being tested. (See Chapter 12, Examination and Selection of Patients for Refractive Keratotomy. In the PERK study, 3% of eyes lost two or three lines of spectacle-corrected visual acuity (see Table 23-1 and Fig. 23-9) at 4 years. This indicates that vision-threatening complications occurred rarely.[230] In an informal survey that included approximately 63,000 cases of refractive keratotomy, the incidence of reduced spectacle-corrected visual acuity was 0.91%.[145]

The causes for visual loss fall into three main categories: corneal complications from the keratotomy procedure (such as an incision across the visual axis), noncorneal complications from the keratotomy itself (such as laceration of the lens), and events outside the keratotomy procedure (such as damage to the optic nerve by retrobulbar anesthesia).

The most common cause of loss of spectacle-corrected acuity is probably irregular astigmatism, usually occurring after a repeated operation, as discussed in a subsequent section.

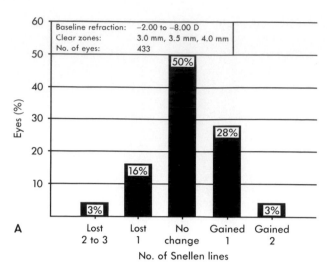

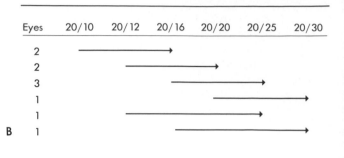

Figure 23-9

Change in spectacle-corrected visual acuity between baseline and 4 years after radial keratotomy in the PERK study. **A,** Bar chart shows change, expressed as a gain or loss of Snellen lines. **B,** Loss of visual acuity is confined to changes between 20/10 and 20/25 in most eyes. (From Waring GO, Lynn MJ, Fielding B, et al: JAMA 1990;263:1083-1091.)

REFRACTIVE COMPLICATIONS

The most frequent refractive complication is an inaccurate outcome: overcorrection, undercorrection, and increased astigmatism. In general, these inaccuracies stem from the inherent surgical and biologic variability of refractive keratotomy, discussed in Chapter 13, Predictability of Refractive Keratotomy. Prevention of these refractive complications requires that the surgeon design a surgical plan that takes into account the idiosyncrasies of his or her own surgical instruments and artistic technique, as well as the idiosyncrasies of individual patient response during long-term wound healing. Until ophthalmologists can account for these, overcorrections, undercorrections, and other refractive complications will remain.

Refractive results reported in published studies are tabulated in Chapter 21, Published Results of Refractive Keratotomy.

Overcorrection

The conversion of a myopic refractive error to a hyperopic one is one of the most significant complications of refractive keratotomy. Myopic patients seem to adapt better if they remain undercorrected than if they become overcorrected.[192] Milder and Rubin[156] state that the myopic individual who becomes hyperopic in an abrupt, sudden fashion (that is, overcorrected by refractive keratotomy or by a new pair of spectacles) has extra accommodative demand produced by the sudden change. The young uncorrected hyperopic individual has learned from childhood to effect a comfortable balance between the accommodation required to see clearly and the vergence necessary to maintain fusion. At infinity the hyperopic person had to accommodate but not converge, using fusional divergence to counter the convergence that normally accompanied this accommodation. These individuals usually have a slow decrease in hyperopia during adolescence, so the demand for fusional divergence diminishes gradually; these hyperopic persons become comfortable because of the slow, long adaptation time. The situation is different for the suddenly overcorrected myopic individual. In the first and second decades, people with myopia are often undercorrected by their spec-

---

Case Report: Eleven Diopter Overcorrection

A 68-year-old woman with a preoperative refraction of −2.00 +1.00 × 90° in the right eye and −4.00 +1.00 × 120° in the left eye underwent a 16-incision radial keratotomy in her right eye in July 1980. The procedure was done with an unguarded, metal super blade and the postoperative measurement of the clear zone diameter was between 3 and 4 mm horizontally.

On the first postoperative visit, she was noted to be overcorrected by +5.00 D, gradually progressing over the next several weeks to +11.00 D. She was placed on a regimen of prednisolone drops on and off for several weeks postoperatively. She was then fitted with a +11 D soft contact lens, which she has worn as an extended wear lens.

Four years later, the refraction over her soft contact lens was plano −1.50 × 130°, with a best visual acuity of 20/200, and her refraction without the soft contact lens in the right eye was +11.50 D, with a spectacle-corrected visual acuity of 20/200. Her best visual acuity in the right eye with a hard contact lens, however, was 20/40. Keratometry in the right eye was 36.00/36.00 with distorted mires. Keratographs demonstrated a large central ring, with considerable distortion of the inferior circles in the right eye, confirming the flat cornea. Corneal endothelial cell counts were 1680 cells/mm^2 in the operated right eye and 3250 cells/mm^2 in the unoperated left eye.

From Salz JJ: Ophthalmic Surg 1985;16:579-580.

---

tacles because of the progression of the myopia. Therefore the accommodative demand is less than normal, and fusional convergence is required to maintain binocular vision. When the myopic person is suddenly overcorrected (even by +0.75 D), there is an abrupt demand for increased accommodation with the accompanying accommodative-convergence of the near reflex, so fusional divergence must be used to maintain binocularity. This sudden stress on the vergence system probably produces more symptoms than the sudden demand for more accommodation. The greater the refractive overcorrection the greater the symptoms, especially if the patient has a high accommodative convergence/accommodation (AC/A) ratio.

Presbyopia is discussed in a later section.

The definition of overcorrection varies: (1) the literal definition is any hyperopic refractive error, (2) a refraction greater than +1.00 D (used in the PERK study),[9,196,197,230] and (3) the inadequate definition of Sawelson and Marks—hyperopia that generates patient complaints.[196] The definition of greater than +1.00 D is reasonable because the accuracy of clinical refraction is on the order of 0.50 to 1.00 D in successive examinations and because 1.00 D of hyperopia produces symptomatic presbyopia in individuals in the presbyopic age group.

Depending on the definition of overcorrection, the incidence of this complication is between 0.82% and 33%.* The PERK Study Group reported a 17% prevalence of overcorrection at 4 years.[231] Arrowsmith and Marks[8] reported that 33% of patients were overcorrected by more than 1 D at 5 years, a substantial increase over the 20% that were overcorrected 1 year after surgery. These authors attribute the overcorrection rate to the overuse of small diameter clear zones. In a review of refractive keratotomy, Barker and Swinger[13] noted that overcorrections of greater than 1.00 D occurred in 1% to 24% of patients, greater than 1.50 D in 0.8% to 2%, and greater than 2.00 D in 0% to 6%.

*References 9, 145, 184, 192, 196, 197, 230.

There are four circumstances in which overcorrections occur. The first is in the immediate postoperative period, when corneal edema and the effects of the incisions themselves cause excessive wound gaping and greater flattening of the central cornea.[214] This can be minimized by reducing the amount of wound irrigation at the end of the case and possibly by using some hypertonic topical solutions postoperatively, although it disappears spontaneously in a few weeks to months as the wounds begin to heal. The second circumstance is incorrect surgery for an individual patient, such as using too small a clear zone or too deep incisions in an older patient, depending on the surgeon's technique. Using four incisions for an initial refractive keratotomy decreases the number of overcorrections. For example, Salz[164] achieved a 4% overcorrection rate in his initial study of four-incision refractive keratotomy, and Spigelman and colleagues[188] reported no refraction greater than +1.00 D 6 months or more after four-incision refractive keratotomy in 38 eyes.[211]

The third circumstance in which overcorrection occurs is the unexplained "overresponder," who had surgery correctly performed on the basis of the surgeon's previous experience but in whom a large overcorrection developed. The cause of this response is unclear, but using four incisions when possible reduces its occurrence. This is a good reason for allowing 4 to 12 weeks between surgery on the first and second eyes so that the patient might not be rendered bilaterally hyperopic. Fyodorov has suggested a corneal biopsy to identify the ultrastructure of corneal collagen as a method of predicting overresponders,[74] but he does not specify the characteristics of such collagen. The fourth reason is the well-documented continued effect of the surgery for a few years, such that a person who is emmetropic 6 months after surgery might end up with a significant overcorrection 3 to 5 years after surgery,* as discussed in Chapter 24, Stability of Refraction after Refractive Keratotomy. Thus the true long-term incidence of overcorrection is not known.

The management of overcorrected patients after refractive keratotomy falls into two categories: medical and surgical. The simplest medical approach is to provide appropriate spectacles or contact lenses, including a reading correction for presbyopic patients. Antiglaucoma medications that reduce intraocular pressure have been advocated to decrease overcorrections,[33,192] but no published data document their usefulness. Although there is no doubt that intraocular pressure is the motive force that causes changes in corneal shape, lowering the intraocular pressure a few millimeters of mercury with topical beta blockers or with miotics is unlikely to alter the refractive outcome significantly, particularly because the wounds take years to heal. Maloney et al.[122] have shown in cadaver eyes that fluctuations in refractive error after refractive keratotomy are not caused by fluctuations in intraocular pressure. They concluded that the action of the intraocular pressure is necessary for central corneal flattening, but that the refractive effect of refractive keratotomy is insensitive to changes in intraocular pressure in the physiologic range. Miotics have other possibly beneficial effects in addition to lowering intraocular pressure, such as causing accommodative spasm (which would reduce the residual hyperopia) and also causing miosis (which would promote a greater depth of field). Andrade and colleagues[2] demonstrated that pilocarpine can induce a myopic shift on the order of 1.50 D, which overcorrected patients may find advantageous. In addition, it induces myosis, which can decrease glare and improve contrast sensitivity, except under direct glare conditions at night. However, miotics also produce brow ache, and phospholine iodide has the potential of causing retinal detachment and iris pigment epithelial cyst formation, so this type of management may be unsuccessful.[164]

*References 50, 52, 90, 137, 197, 201, 230.

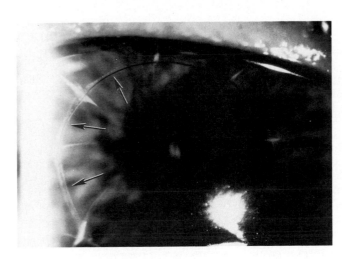

Figure 23-10
Purse-string suture *(arrows)* used in a case of overcorrection following radial keratotomy. (Courtesy Robert Hofmann.)

Using orthokeratology to steepen the cornea with a gas-permeable hard contact lens has been advocated without supporting evidence.[104]

The second approach to managing overcorrections is to suture the wounds closed, as discussed in detail in Chapter 18, Repeated Surgery for Residual Myopia and Hyperopia after Refractive Corneal Surgery. Starling and Hofmann[214] proposed a purse-string suture for correcting hyperopia (Fig. 23-10), and Lindquist and colleagues[137] advocated reopening the incisions, cleaning out the epithelial plug, and closing them with interrupted 10-0 nylon sutures, a technique that seemed to work in a laboratory eye bank model. The degree to which resuturing keratotomy incisions will change the final refraction in clinical circumstances remains to be determined.

A homoplastic hyperopic keratomileusis or epikeratoplasty could be used to treat overcorrection as well.

Undercorrection

Undercorrection is usually more acceptable than overcorrection because the patient is accustomed to being myopic, because repeated operations can be used to further decrease the myopia, and because the patient has the option of wearing glasses or contact lenses similar to those used preoperatively.[228] The incidence of undercorrection varies widely; each study has its own definition. As would be expected, undercorrections occur more frequently in higher myopic individuals. In the PERK study, at 4 years approximately 28% of the patients were undercorrected greater than 1.00 D,[231] a figure in general agreement with other major clinical studies.* Deitz and colleagues[53] reported a prevalence at 1 year of 11.8% in 656 eyes.

Undercorrections occur in four clinical circumstances. The first occurs a few months after surgery, when a patient who has apparently had a good outcome with emmetropia or a slight hyperopia regresses to myopia once again. After refractive keratotomy the majority of patients show a regression of the initial effect, but whether it produces undercorrection depends on the amount of regression. The second is a simple miscalculation in which insufficient surgery is done based on the surgeon's and patient's preoperative variables. Such undercorrections are more likely to occur in young patients. The third circumstance is the patient who remains undercorrected in spite of apparently proper surgery. The

*References 6, 7, 51, 196, 197, 230.

Case Report: Persistent Undercorrection

A 43-year-old man with a refraction of $-6.50 +0.75 \times 150°$ underwent an eight-incision refractive keratotomy using the PERK protocol in his right eye only. A 3-mm diameter clear zone was used. One day postoperatively, the patient's uncorrected visual acuity was 20/125, with a refraction of $+4.00$, which yielded a visual acuity of 20/40. Two weeks after surgery, the uncorrected visual acuity was 20/20, and his refraction was $-0.75 +0.75 \times 180°$, 20/16. Six months postoperatively, the patient's uncorrected visual acuity was 20/100, with a refraction of $-2.00 +0.75 \times 160°$, 20/16.

Five years postoperatively, the uncorrected visual acuity was 20/50 and his spectacle-corrected visual acuity was 20/20−, with a refraction of $-2.75 +1.00 \times 145°$. The patient never requested surgery in his second eye because of his undercorrection and fluctuations in his vision.

---

variables that affect this type of undercorrection are unknown. Although some observers have postulated that patients with low intraocular pressure and flatter corneas will have less response to the surgery,[57,192] no objective quantitative information documents these speculations. Fyodorov has gone so far as to make a small test incision in the peripheral cornea and observe the healing over 7 months, abandoning the future refractive keratotomy if marked scarring occurs.[57] The fourth circumstance is the patient who regresses over a long period, which is exceptional after refractive keratotomy.

Management of patients with undercorrected vision includes both medical and surgical means. Spectacles and contact lenses remain the mainstay of management. Postoperative topical corticosteroids will delay wound healing and may increase intraocular pressure, thus enhancing the surgical effect (as discussed in Chapter 20, Corneal Wound Healing and Its Pharmacologic Modification after Refractive Keratotomy) but their effect needs further study.[83,170] Moorhead and colleagues[158] have observed that the use of betaaminopropionitrile to decrease collagen cross-linking and retard wound healing may decrease the amount of regression that usually follows the initial refractive keratotomy, but these findings could not be replicated in an animal model by Busin and colleagues.[34]

Surgical management of undercorrection may include repeated operations, as described in Chapter 18, Repeated Surgery for Residual Myopia and Hyperopia after Refractive Corneal Surgery. In exceptional cases, myopic keratomileusis or myopic epikeratoplasty[22,192] may be indicated.

Anisometropia

Anisometropia is a difference in the refractive error of the two eyes; it can cause asthenopia. Anisometropia occurs in most patients who have refractive keratotomy in one eye and not in the other and is a common condition between surgery on the first eye and second eye. A thorough explanation to the patient beforehand of this temporary imbalance allows patients to adjust easier after surgery. Symmetry of refractive outcome is discussed in Chapter 22, Bilateral Results of Radial Keratotomy.

The PERK study created an interesting clinical experience with anisometropia, since 95% of the patients waited 1 year between surgery on the first and second eye, as required by the protocol. Techniques for managing this temporary anisometropia included: (1) wearing a contact lens on the unoperated eye, (2) wearing spectacles with a plano glass over the operated eye and a full correction over the unoperated eye, (3) wearing no correction and using only the operated eye for distance vision, and (4) occluding one eye with an opaque spectacle lens. Some surgeons operate on both eyes on the same day or within the same week to reduce the inconvenience of anisometropia. In so doing, they sacrifice the information that might be obtained from a study of the outcome in the first eye in planning surgery on the second. A patient who has undergone the procedure in one eye may decide not to have any further surgical intervention on the other eye. In the PERK study, at 4 years after surgery approximately 20% of the patients had elected not to have surgery on their second eye, some because they were completely satisfied with their monocular result and others because they were dissatisfied with the outcome in the first eye.[231]

Anisometropia can occur after bilateral surgery. The PERK study also demonstrated a refractive difference of more than 1 D in 33% of patients who had bilateral surgery.[230]

Astigmatic errors, either preexisting or induced by refractive keratotomy, can complicate anisometropic difficulties, especially when only one eye is astigmatic or when both eyes have differing astigmatic axes or powers.[135]

Many uncorrected anisometropic myopic and antimetropic eyes (one eye is myopic, the other hyperopic) escape asthenopia completely by simply alternating fixation and making no attempt at all to fuse.[156] Some patients have symptoms associated with panoramic eye movements—nausea, vertigo, or motion sickness.[156] Most patients are able to fuse the images in both eyes only if the difference is smaller than 3 D, but others with 7 or 8 D differences are not bothered by the disparity.[156] Many other factors determine the patient's tolerance for anisometropia, including age, fusion capability, and previous spectacle history.[156] Significant anisometropia from refractive keratotomy can sometimes unmask a latent phoria and cause symptomatic heterotropia.[146]

Management of each case must be individualized but should include consideration of special spectacle prescriptions, contact lenses, and further refractive surgery. Milder and Rubin[135] have addressed this problem comprehensively.

Some surgeons advocate surgical "monovision," purposefully undercorrecting one eye approximately 1.00 D to decrease symptomatic presbyopia while trying to make the other eye emmetropic. Such fine tuning of refractive keratotomy is very difficult, given the unpredictability of the operation for an individual eye. Nevertheless, the functional advantage of monovision can be great, as demonstrated by the intentional undercorrection of a contact lens in one eye of presbyopic individuals.[145]

Astigmatism

Residual astigmatism. Residual refractive astigmatism is defined as preexisting astigmatism not corrected by the surgical procedure (see Chapter 18, Repeated Surgery for Residual Myopia and Hyperopia after Refractive Corneal Surgery). Surgeons in the PERK study made no attempt to correct existing corneal astigmatism because all patients had 1.50 D or less,[233] but at 4 years after surgery 16% of the eyes had a decrease in the preexisting astigmatism of 0.50 to 1.25 D.[231]

Induced astigmatism. By induced astigmatism we mean an increase after surgery. In the PERK study at 4 years, 36% of the eyes had an increase in refractive astigmatism of 0.50 to 2.75 D from the radial incisions, more than 1.00 D.[230]

After repeated operations in 59 eyes in the PERK study[38] the amount of induced astigmatism increased, 19% having 0.50 D or more. Interestingly, 15% of

Case Report: Induced Irregular Astigmatism

A 57-year-old female librarian underwent bilateral keratotomy surgery to correct myopia. Preoperative spectacle correction was approximately −7.00 D bilaterally. In 1981 she underwent a 16-incision radial keratotomy with a 360-degree circular keratotomy in her right eye. Several months later she had a similar procedure in her left eye. Because of an undercorrection in her right eye, she then underwent a reoperation. A few years after surgery, her cycloplegic refraction was −6.00 −2.75 × 15° in the right eye, and −4.00 +2.50 × 180° in the left. Slit-lamp microscope examination of both eyes revealed the radial and circumferential keratotomy scars in both eyes. Many of the radial incisions were of variable length and depth. In addition, some partial-length incisions were noted. Keratographs demonstrated significant irregular astigmatism centrally in both eyes. She had severe glare in the sunlight and always wore her prescription sunglasses. Her discomfort disrupted her reading and driving, and she had to retire from her job. She filed a malpractice lawsuit against the surgeon, and the jury acquitted the surgeon.

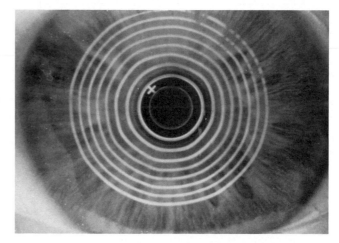

Figure 23-11
Keratograph 2 years after uncomplicated radial keratotomy. The two inner rings are smooth, and the outer rings are slightly irregular because of the scars. (From Rashid ER and Waring GO: Surv Ophthalmol 1989;34:73-106.)

the eyes had more than 1.50 D of astigmatism after the initial and repeated operation, compared with no patients before surgery. Three eyes (5.0%) had 2.25 to 2.50 D of astigmatism after the two operations.

The true amount of surgically induced astigmatism must be calculated vectorally, as described in Chapter 30, Optics and Topography of Corneal Astigmatism. We do not report vectorally corrected values here.

Irregular astigmatism. Irregular astigmatism exists when the two major cylindric axes are not orthogonal to each other, or when an irregular change in curvature from the center to the peripheral cornea exceeds the changes found in the normal aspheric cornea. All corneas after refractive keratotomy have some irregular astigmatism, which can be detected on keratographs, where the regular, smooth circular configuration of the inner two mires over the clear zone contrast with the slightly irregular outer mires over the incisions (Fig. 23-11). This irregular astigmatism probably causes the stellate epithelial iron line. Fortunately, this minimal irregular astigmatism seems to have little effect on visual function under daylight conditions, presumably because it is outside of the optically important central cornea. When the pupil dilates, more glare and distortion result, usually reported as a starburst phenomenon.

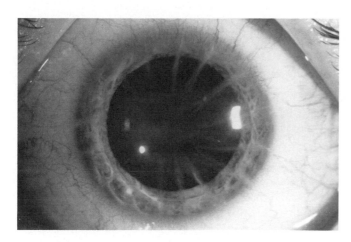

Figure 23-12
Multiple, repeated keratotomy procedures in the same areas have produced large scars with significant irregular astigmatism. (From Rashid ER and Waring GO: Surv Ophthalmol 1989;34:73-106.)

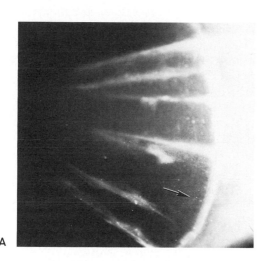

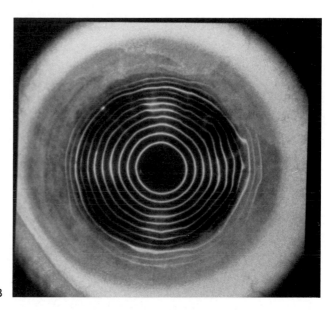

A   B

Figure 23-13
Combined radial and circular keratotomy with irregular astigmatism. **A,** Patient had radial incisions and circumferential trephination *(arrow)* followed by a repeated operation for undercorrection (close-up photograph shows attempt to jump the radial incisions over the circumferential one). **B,** Keratograph shows irregular astigmatism that produced spectacle-corrected visual acuity of 20/50. (From Rashid ER and Waring GO: Surv Ophthalmol 1989;34:73-106.)

Functionally significant irregular astigmatism occurs most commonly in eyes that have had repeated operations (Fig. 23-12) or "creative keratotomy," consisting of intersecting radial and transverse incisions, combined radial and circumferential incisions (Fig. 23-13), or incisions that extend too close to the line of sight.[5,91,228] Such irregular astigmatism can greatly reduce visual function, not only decreasing spectacle-corrected visual acuity, but also producing glare and light sensitivity. High-quality ultraviolet-infrared filtering sunglasses help treat the associated glare. Mild to moderate astigmatism can be masked by a rigid, gas-permeable contact lens, but if severe, particularly if a contact lens cannot be fit, a patient may experience great visual disability. Such a case is presented in Chapter 25, The Patient Speaks: Testimonials after Refractive Keratotomy.

If contact lens fitting is unsuccessful and the patient's visual disability warrants, a penetrating keratoplasty or lamellar refractive keratoplasty (keratomileusis, epikeratoplasty) may be required.

Premature presbyopia

Individuals with minimal refractive error after refractive keratotomy will lose their ability to see objects up close without correction as their accommodative reserve drops with increasing age. Those who are overcorrected will become symptomatically presbyopic prematurely because of their hyperopia. Few data have been published about the effect of refractive keratotomy on the onset of presbyopia, but many individuals may begrudge the earlier use of reading glasses. Patients in the presbyopic age range who are interested in radial keratotomy for myopia must be counseled carefully about the instant dependence they will acquire for a reading correction should they be emmetropic or hypermetropic after the surgery.[228] On the other hand, many patients would rather depend on reading glasses a few hours a day than on a myopic correction all the time. There is a need for clinical and psychometric studies of the effect of presbyopia on refractive keratotomy patients.

One approach to the preoperative planning of middle-aged patients receiving radial keratotomy is to leave one eye emmetropic and the other 0.75 to 1.50 D myopic. This technique of monovision could free patients from spectacle correction most of the time.[75] Making four incisions in older patients will help decrease overcorrection.

Management of presbyopia consists of a near spectacle or contact lens correction.

VISUAL ACUITY PROBLEMS
Unstable visual acuity

Problems of diurnal fluctuation of vision and unstable vision over time are discussed in detail in Chapter 24, Stability of Refraction after Refractive Keratotomy. We summarize them here.

Diurnal fluctuation. After the first few months, vision continues to fluctuate during the day, from 1.9% to 60% of reported cases.[6,9,51,102,201] Undercorrected patients see better in the morning than in the evening because the cornea progressively steepens, resulting in an increase in myopia during the day, a change that may be as much as 1.5 D.[201] The most vivid descriptions of diurnal variation and the most detailed documentation come from ophthalmologists who have had refractive keratotomy and who refracted themselves throughout the day.[176,240]

Although a noticeable and sometimes bothersome problem, the amount of fluctuation is seldom enough to warrant multiple pairs of spectacles. No effective method exists to control this fluctuation, other than waiting for the cornea to heal and stabilize.

Unstable visual acuity over time. As the unsutured corneal wounds heal, the cornea changes shape, producing changes in refraction and visual acuity. Such instability has been reported up to 4 years after surgery.* Between approximately 1 and 4 years after surgery, 10% to 30% of eyes experience changes from 1 to 3 D. The majority of unstable eyes show a continued flattening of the central cornea, resulting in either a decrease in myopia or an increase in hyperopia. The time at which the corneal wounds heal and refraction stabilizes in all eyes remains to be determined, but the continued increase in the effect of the surgery can last up to 7 years.

---

*References 29, 49-51, 90, 137, 197, 201, 230, 234.

Glare

A major concern about refractive keratotomy has been that the residual corneal scars would scatter light and increase glare.

Definition and subjective estimates of glare. Light that is scattered from opacities or irregularities in the eye can lower the contrast of the retinal image, an effect called "veiling glare,"[8] the type of glare that follows refractive keratotomy. Unfortunately, it is difficult to measure glare clinically and reports of the prevalence and severity of glare therefore vary widely, both in assessment of patients' subjective responses and in attempted objective clinical measurement.

In a broad sense it is helpful to define glare as nondisabling or disabling, particularly when discussing the subjective response after refractive keratotomy. Detailed subjective assessment of glare should not only contain elements of control and formality but also require the patient to specify conditions under which glare is or is not a problem and how much the perceived glare disrupts daily living.

Subjective assessment is usually conducted by way of an informal patient questionnaire, most commonly asking a patient to assess the amount of glare as none, mild, moderate, or severe—an inexact approach. For example, Arrowsmith and Marks[5] asked patients to rate the severity of glare. One year after surgery, 93% had no glare or occasional glare, 7% mild to moderate, and none severe; 5 years after surgery, 98% had no glare to occasional glare, 2% mild, and none moderate or severe.

More formal methods of subjective testing include the creation of psychometric instruments (formal detailed questionnaires) with a broader grading scale (for example, 1 to 7) for glare severity and with multiple questions in different contexts about glare as part of an overall subjective assessment.[29] The results can be startling. For example, on the PERK psychometric test *before* radial keratotomy surgery, 40% of the patients reported "a lot" of glare. Testing with the same questionnaire 1 year after surgery showed no significant increase. Imagine what would have happened if the baseline measurements had not been carried out carefully and an assessment was done only after surgery. Grossly misleading conclusions might have resulted: "A startling 40% of PERK patients had a lot of glare after surgery! Radial keratotomy clearly creates severe visual difficulties."

Case Report: Persistent Glare after Repeated Refractive Keratotomy

A 32-year-old female secretary was seen in consultation because of variable vision after three refractive keratotomy operations in each eye. In May 1980 she gave the following history:

After her left eye was operated on in March 1979, she experienced good, uncorrected vision and was extremely satisfied. In April 1979 the right eye was operated on, and extra incisions were made in the left eye because of "slippage" of the initial effect. Once again, she enjoyed good, stable vision and was excited enough to call her brother and extol the virtues of this surgery.

A second reoperation was performed on the left eye a few months later, followed by intense photophobia that forced her to stay at home in a dark room. Even though the light sensitivity persisted for months, she returned for a reoperation on the right eye in July 1979. This time, unfortunately, she perceived no improvement in vision and experienced persistent, moderate glare. She stopped driving at night. She had to squint at work when bright lights were on and wear sunglasses indoors.

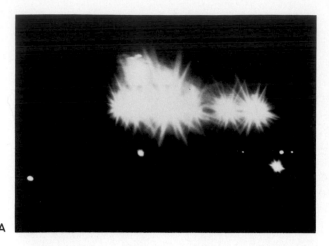

A

Figure 23-14
Glare after refractive keratotomy. **A,** Simulation of moderate starburst pattern glare (flare) as seen at night. **B,** Simulated disability glare. Control conditions show peripheral glare sources well defined and central test targets not obscured by glare. **C,** An eye experiencing glare sees the test lights enlarged and blurred and the central test targets obscured by the light scatter. (**A** courtesy Michael Deitz; **B** and **C** courtesy Vistech Consultants, Inc.)

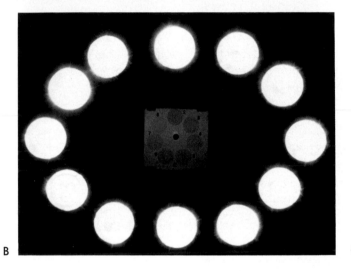

B

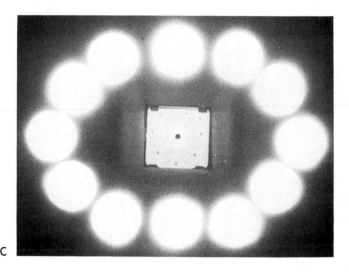

C

Other reports of the incidence of glare in the first 3 to 6 months after radial keratotomy range from 30% to 50%,[6,64,179] and after 1 year from 0% to 4%.[6-8,22,102,196]

Glare testers. The use of glare testers to measure glare clinically is in its infancy. Such instruments include the Miller-Nadler glare tester, the Holladay-Mentor brightness acuity tester (BAT), the Ginsburg-Vistech contrast sensitivity glare tester, and more formal contrast sensitivity testing itself, as discussed in Chapter 12, Patient Selection and Preoperative Examination.

Causes of glare. Factors that increase glare after surgery include a smaller diameter clear zone, wider scars, increased numbers of incisions, and increased irregular astigmatism.[102,157,192,222,230] These factors underscore the reasonableness of establishing the center of the pupil as the center of refractive keratotomy surgery. An inadvertent stray incision into the clear zone will increase glare. Patients commonly describe a decrease in glare when they wear contact lenses after refractive keratotomy, presumably because the irregular astigmatism has been eliminated, even though the amount of opacity in the cornea is the same. No published data have correlated the amount of scar opacity with the amount of glare.

The larger the diameter of the pupil the more glare can be expected, particularly when the pupil is larger than 5 mm.[178,222] Thus most patients after refractive keratotomy report more glare at night or under dim lighting than under conditions of normal lighting.

Starburst pattern. The most commonly reported, nondisabling type of glare is the starburst pattern, flare, or halo effect. Patients report this most commonly when looking at point sources of light at night, such as headlights or street lights. They often report the rays of light "looking like" the scars in their cornea[9] (Fig. 23-14). In general, patients acknowledge this visual phenomenon and say it is not disruptive to their daily living. In fact, many say it is no different from the patterns they noticed with their contact lenses or dirty spectacles before surgery. Thus most do not seek any treatment for this starburst effect and consider it a bothersome but acceptable side effect of the surgery.

Disability glare. By definition, disability glare is light scattering that disrupts visual function and daily living. After refractive keratotomy, this occurs most commonly at night. This can be a problem even when refractive keratotomy has been performed in only one eye. Some patients have voluntarily stopped driving at night because they thought it was too dangerous. Assessment of this difficulty is subjective, sporadic, and in need of more careful clinical study.[208] Disability glare can severely disrupt a patient's life.

The problems of glare after refractive keratotomy hit the national news when a *20/20* television news magazine story featured a radial keratotomy patient who complained bitterly about the glare, filming him in his home with blankets covering the windows to keep the light out. The dramatization overstated the problem of glare but served as a caution to emphasize that complications can occur after refractive keratotomy.

Management of glare. Management of patients with glare from refractive keratotomy is no different from that of patients with glare from any opacity in the cornea or lens. High-quality sunglasses with ultraviolet and infrared filters[205] greatly reduce glare under daytime conditions. Night glare is much more difficult to manage.

Wearing contact lenses may decrease the glare from irregular astigmatism (see Chapter 25, The Patient Speaks: Testimonials after Refractive Keratotomy). The opacity around the scars decreases markedly in the first 12 to 24 months after surgery and gradually becomes fainter over 4 or 5 years as the scars remodel. Whether this is associated with the clinical reduction in glare is unknown.

In one laboratory study[147] in rabbits, tattoo dyes were placed in the corneal incisions and decreased the amount of light scattering from the scars when examined in retroillumination. Such management is not practical in human beings.

Changes in contrast sensitivity

Scholarly treatises and papers have been written on contrast sensitivity testing.[58,83-87] The use of contrast sensitivity for testing vision is analogous to using multiple tone frequencies to test hearing. Audiologists describe auditory capability with loudest threshold measurements of pure tones over a wide sound frequency range, resulting in a loudness sensitivity curve (an audiogram). Contrast sensitivity to sine wave grating is analogous to loudness sensitivity to a range of pure tones; the contrast sensitivity curve is the visual analogue of the audiogram.[83,95] Contrast sensitivity gratings are superior to the high-contrast Snellen chart letters at estimating visual task performance, such as target detection by pilots in simulators[87] and under field conditions,[85] such as highway sign discrimination,[58] especially under low-contrast conditions of twilight, nighttime, fog, or rain. Numerous studies of contrast sensitivity following radial keratotomy have been carried out* to see whether the scars or irregular astigmatism of refractive keratotomy reduced contrast sensitivity.

Ginsburg and colleagues[89] took advantage of the unique design of the PERK

---

*References 11, 29, 150, 157, 168, 179, 223, 229-231.

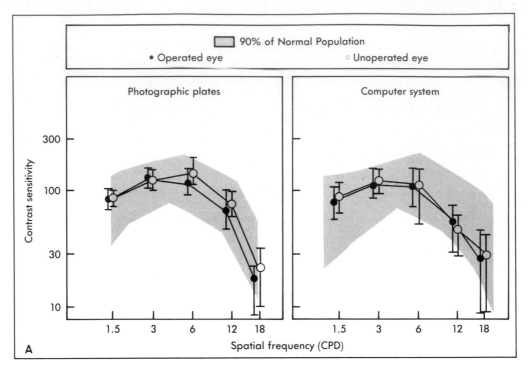

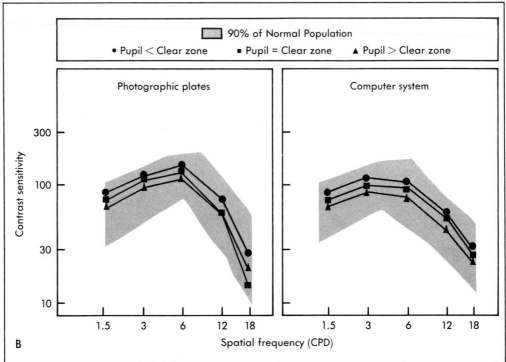

Figure 23-15
A, Contrast sensitivity curves show mean and standard deviation of the values for operated and unoperated eyes of the same 69 patients in the PERK study, a mean of approximately 1 year after surgery. Testing was done under photopic conditions. Photographic plates are from the Vistech vision contrast test system, and the computer system is the Nicolet Optronix 200 computer-video system. Gray zone indicates the previously reported range for a normal population. Small differences appeared at higher spatial frequencies, but all mean values fell within the normal range of contrast sensitivity. **B,** Mean contrast sensitivity scores for 69 eyes with radial keratotomy comparing the diameter of the pupil to the diameter of the central clear zone. When the pupil was larger than the clear zone, contrast sensitivity decreased. Testing was done under photopic conditions. (From Ginsburg AP, Waring GO, Steinberg EB, et al: Refract Corneal Surg 1990;6:82-91.)

study, in which patients waited at least 1 year between operations on their first and second eyes. This allowed contrast sensitivity testing on both the operated and unoperated eyes of the same patient with full spectacle correction at 6 months or more (mean, 13.8 months) after surgery. The unoperated eye served as an excellent control for the operated eye. Testing was done only under photopic conditions with normal pupil diameter. Two test systems were used, a set of photographic plates and a computerized presentation of sine wave gratings. In general, neither of the two test systems demonstrated a clinically meaningful loss of contrast sensitivity in the operated eyes. There was a small, statistically significant difference at the middle spatial frequencies, but this was not just clinically meaningful because all values were within the range of previously published normal populations[82,86] and because the small decrease in higher spatial frequencies could be associated with the myopia.[88] The average contrast sensitivity differences between the operated and unoperated eyes were not judged to affect visual performance. The authors did not find a statistically significant correlation between the diameter of the central clear zone and the contrast sensitivity function. However, they did find that when the diameter of the pupil was the same as or greater than the diameter of the central clear zone, contrast sensitivity fell significantly, but never to values outside the previously established normal range (Fig. 23-15).

The three examples on p. 892 of individual contrast sensitivity data from the PERK study show the great variation that can occur after radial keratotomy (Fig. 23-16). Refraction is presented as the spherical equivalent of the cycloplegic refraction.

Krasnov and colleagues[129] studied contrast sensitivity after radial keratotomy in 44 eyes using a television system with horizontal and vertical patterns. They observed a statistically significant drop in contrast sensitivity compared with baseline values during the first month after surgery, minimal differences at 2½ months to 4 months after surgery, and no differences at 10 to 12 months after surgery. Trick and Hartstein[223] used a video test system to compare contrast sensitivity in six patients who had had radial keratotomy in one eye, the other eye being unoperated. They found no statistically significant difference between the operated and unoperated eyes at approximately 6 weeks after surgery under photopic conditions.

Atkin and colleagues[11] studied 15 patients with unilateral radial keratotomy with two test systems, low spatial frequency contrast sensitivity gratings and higher frequency unpatterned field flicker targets, presented against a diffuse background glare source, comparing the results both with and without the glare. They found that both operated and unoperated eyes showed losses of contrast sensitivity with the glare on and that the radial keratotomy eyes showed a larger glare loss for flicker, but a smaller glare loss for gratings than that demonstrated by the unoperated eyes. Eyes with larger pupil diameters had greater glare loss after radial keratotomy. They could not correlate these findings with a questionnaire index of glare complaints or with the score obtained with the Miller-Nadler glare tester.

Applegate[3] has emphasized the importance of pupil diameter in assessing visual function after radial keratotomy. Further testing of patients with dilated pupils or under scotopic conditions will be necessary to define contrast sensitivity function more broadly after radial keratotomy.

Hemenger and colleagues[100] postulated that the loss in contrast sensitivity after radial keratotomy is caused by the change in spherical aberration in the cornea. Using photokeratoscope pictures, they calculated the change in image contrast based on the modulation transfer function induced by the change in spherical aberration, finding that their theoretical calculations corresponded to clinical measurements in some eyes but not others. In a follow-up study[101] they refined

---

*Case Reports of Contrast Sensitivity Measurements
after Refractive Keratotomy*

Contrast sensitivity the same in operated and unoperated eyes

A 32-year-old man had a baseline refraction of -3.50 D in his right eye and -3.00 D in his left eye. Ten months after radial keratotomy in the right eye, the refraction was -0.50 D and the corrected visual acuity 20/20. The contrast sensitivity curves for the operated and unoperated eyes overlapped and were similar. He had no subjective complaints about the operated eye and elected to have radial keratotomy on the other eye (Fig. 23-16, *A*).

Contrast sensitivity higher in operated eye

A 32-year-old woman had a baseline refraction of -4.50 D in her left eye and -5.00 D in her right eye. Five months after her second radial keratotomy in the left eye (eight incisions placed between the initial eight at 14 months after the first operation) she had a refraction of -1.50 D in the operated eye. Her contrast sensitivity curve was much higher at the three highest frequencies (42%, 39%, and 94% for 6, 12, and 18 cycles per degree, respectively). Although she complained of glare and night vision problems, she decided to have the surgery on the other eye (Fig. 23-16, *B*).

Contrast sensitivity lower in operated eye

A 44-year-old woman had a baseline refraction of -3.00 D in her right eye and -2.75 D in the left. Fifteen months after radial keratotomy the right eye had a refraction of $+1.00$ D with a corrected visual acuity of 20/20 and showed considerably less contrast sensitivity in four of the five spatial frequencies. The greatest differences in sensitivity were at 12 cycles per degree (44% difference) and 18 cycles per degree (98% difference). This patient elected to have radial keratotomy performed on her other eye, despite complaints of moderate glare difficulties at night in her right eye (Fig. 23-16, *C*).

From Ginsburg AP, Waring GO, Steinberg EB, et al: Refract Corneal Surg 1990;6:82-91.

---

this approach, using a sixth order polynomial. They found that for large pupil diameters, the induced spherical aberration of some corneas produced a second distinct focus about 1.5 D in front of the primary focus, predicting that contrast sensitivity would be reduced with pupillary dilation.

Color vision after refractive keratotomy

Color vision does not appear to be affected by keratotomy incisions. One study that used the Gunkel Chromagraph to test color vision 6 to 24 weeks after refractive keratotomy detected no defects in color vision.[150]

Diminished night vision

Reduced night vision in myopic individuals is very common and results from a change in the focal point of light at night when the pupil is dilated. This can be corrected by adding approximately 0.50 D of minus correction in spectacle lenses, which may help improve driving at night.[156] The effect of refractive keratotomy on this physiologic night myopia has not been studied.

After refractive keratotomy, visual function at night is complicated by glare.[11,154,179] For example, in the PERK study three patients (0.6%) who had bothersome glare at night reduced their night driving and refused surgery on their second eye.[232] Other series have reported similar findings.[51]

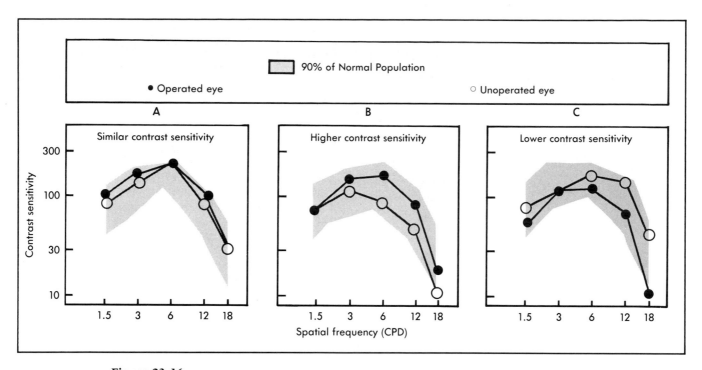

Figure 23-16
Three examples of contrast sensitivity testing under photopic conditions in the PERK study. Values on the x-axis indicate the spatial frequency in cycles per degree. Values on the y-axis are contrast sensitivity. **A,** Contrast sensitivity is similar in operated and unoperated eyes. **B,** Higher contrast sensitivity in the eye with radial keratotomy that had repeated surgery with 16 incisions as compared with the unoperated eye. **C,** Lower contrast sensitivity in the eye with radial keratotomy as compared with the unoperated eye. (From Ginsburg AP, Waring GO, Steinberg EB, et al: Refract Corneal Surg 1990;6:82-91.)

The following testimonial from an ophthalmologist who underwent refractive keratotomy highlights some of the phenomena of night vision.[240]

Still, several months after my operation, I found night driving difficult. The left eye had purposely been set for near [objects at close distance], and my dominant right eye was still myopic by 0.75 diopters. Oncoming headlights seemed to sharpen vision, possibly by miosis. Starburst effect from taillights made judging distance much more difficult and left me unable to distinguish small distant bright objects on a black background. Reflections from mudflaps on trucks appeared to be showers of sparks from a fire under the vehicle. More than once I mistakenly thought a muffler had come loose. Luminous markings on the road seemed to be projecting upward. But, by a little miracle, about 8 months after the single RK on the right eye, there was a very distinct improvement in night vision.

The following letter was received by the authors on March 6, 1990. It is presented slightly abridged.

Last week I saw part of your interview on one of the morning television talk shows. I normally don't write this sort of letter, but the basic subject of your interview struck home. If your study of the effects and the efficacy of the radial keratotomy operation had included my records, you would have found that my eyes went from 20/200 to 20/20. No one, however, has been able to convince my eyes of that.

For my first postoperative examinations, my complaints and questions were ignored or

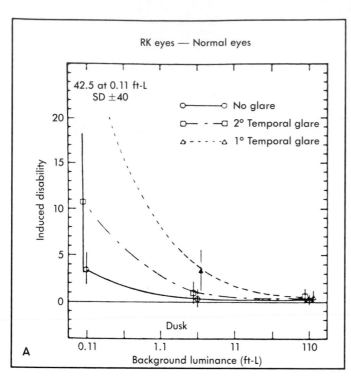

A

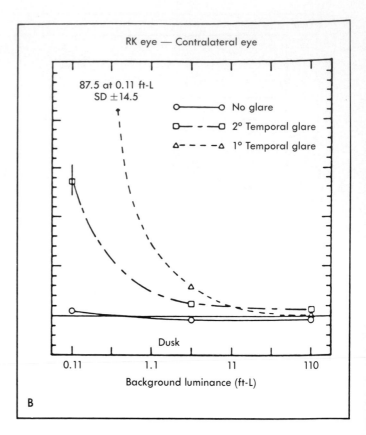

B

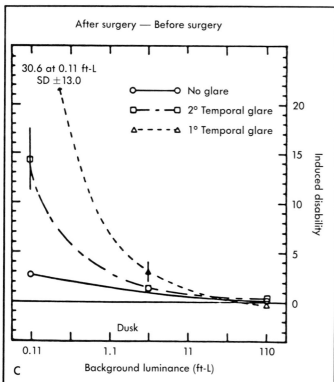

C

Figure 23-17

Surgery-induced disability as a function of background luminance for three experimental conditions: no glare, a point glare source located 2 degrees temporal to the test disc, and a point glare source located 1 degree temporal to the test disc. **A,** Group data comparing radial keratotomy eyes (seven eyes, four patients) to normal eyes (ten eyes, five age-matched controls). **B,** Individual data comparing the operated eye with the contralateral unoperated eye. **C,** Individual data comparing the same eye before and after surgery. The 1 degree temporal glare data point for the 0.11 ft-L background luminance level plots off the graph in each panel. The values for these points and their standard deviation appear in the upper left corner of each panel. Test conditions labeled with an asterisk were significant at *p* < 0.01. (Courtesy Ann Ophthalmol 1987;8:296.)

passed off with "that will correct itself over time." It's been 7 years and my eyes are worse. The astigmatism is so great in one eye that my choice of glasses is limited by the ability of the lens maker. During my eye examinations, the top big "E" was not clear because there were three sharply defined images superimposed on each other but off slightly. I could understand that happening if there were only two such images and both eyes were being used, but there were three and one eye was covered! I consider my operation to be the worst mistake of my life. I had been wearing glasses since I was 5 years old and I hated them. I saw that operation as a chance to rid myself of them. Was I ever wrong! I used to read a book a day and used to peer at the stars through a telescope. Now reading gives me a headache and I see far too many stars. Night driving is a danger with multiple images and streaks radiating from light sources. Glasses make it so that I can survive but they do not correct fully. Before my operation, they did.

Don't go by a doctor's records, for they are written by a biased observer. Find out how the operations went with the people.

Guillon and colleagues[95] compared 50 eyes of 26 patients who had had radial keratotomy with a variety of techniques with 17 eyes of nine patients with similar demographics. They found a high degree of subjective overall satisfaction among the patients who had radial keratotomy surgery. However, the objective analyses of visual function demonstrated poorer function among the radial keratotomy patients than among the controls. Specifically, radial keratotomy patients reported greater difficulties with nighttime visual performance, particularly driving. The best spectacle visual acuity was statistically significantly lower in the operated eyes, and the difference between the operated and control eyes was increased under reduced luminance and lower contrast. The authors concluded that radial keratotomy patients, even those who report subjective satisfaction, should be warned of their decreased visual performance, particularly under nighttime conditions.

Applegate and colleagues[4] measured disability glare in a series of operated and unoperated eyes. They demonstrated that under high luminance conditions, there was only a slight difference in glare between the operated and unoperated eyes. However, under conditions of lower luminance with the pupil dilated, large amounts of disability could be induced by introducing a glare source in the radial keratotomy eyes (Fig. 23-17).

There are two possible sources for the diffusive blur that produces glare and decreases contrast sensitivity under nighttime conditions with a pupil dilated: spherical aberration from the cornea and intraocular light scattering from the scars. Although the scattering of light from the scars has classically been considered the major cause, it is likely that the aberrations produced by the front surface of the cornea might be the most disturbing factor in radial keratotomy patients. Reasons for this include the demonstration of paracentral steepening in these corneas that might produce multiple points of focus, and improved visual acuity with contact lenses as opposed to spectacles after surgery, indicating that it is the more irregular surface that decreases the acuity. The multifocal cornea and the spherical aberration after radial keratotomy are discussed in detail in Chapter 3, Optics and Topography of Radial Keratotomy.

Monocular diplopia

Reports of monocular double vision or ghost images may indicate the incisions are too close to the visual axis, the optical clear zone is decentered, there is asymmetry of scarring, or there are more than one effective power areas in the central cornea (multifocal cornea). A decentered visual axis in keratomileusis, keratophakia, and epikeratoplasty also may be implicated in this complaint.[17]

Another cause for monocular diplopia after refractive keratotomy is a multifocal cornea, discussed in detail in Chapter 3, Optics and Topography of Radial Keratotomy. The following is a summary of the report of Peter Wyzinski, MD, an ophthalmologist who had radial keratotomy without complications in the left eye but with monocular diplopia in the right.

Case Reports: Monocular Diplopia

Case 1

A 51-year-old man with a cycloplegic refraction of −5.75 +0.75 × 090°, 20/16, in the right eye and −4.00 +0.25 × 130°, 20/20 in the left, underwent bilateral eight-incision radial keratotomy 1 year apart in the PERK study.

Five years after the first surgery, the patient had uncorrected visual acuity of 20/160 in the right eye and 20/40 in the left. He reported fluctuating, blurred, and double vision in the right eye. His cycloplegic refraction was +3.50 +1.00 × 130°, 20/25 in the right eye, and +1.75 + 0.50 × 70°, 20/12 in the left. Slit-lamp microscope examination revealed a hypertropic dense keratotomy scar in the 7:30 position (Fig. 23-18).

This was confirmed by the photokeratograph, which showed an irregular surface in the same location. The patient also described his double vision by drawing the way the letter "T" appeared to him from the right eye.

A revision of the 7:30 incision was performed. The scar was gently teased open with a cyclodialysis spatula. No epithelium was found in the wound. A diamond knife was used to excise a narrow strip of the scar tissue. Attempts to scrape the scar tissue free of the wound were unsuccessful. The wound was closed with three 10-0 nylon sutures.

Seven months postoperatively, the patient's vision was still fluctuating during the day, but the double vision was much improved. His uncorrected visual acuity in the right eye was 20/100. His refraction was +3.00 +0.75 × 105°, 20/20.

Case 2

A 38-year-old ophthalmologist had a refraction in the right eye of −4.50 −0.75 × 28°, 20/20. A 12-incision radial keratotomy with a 3.5-mm clear zone using centrifugal incisions was done on the right eye. Because of an unexpected upward rotation of the right eye just as the surgeon was beginning the 12 o'clock incision, a 1 mm long superficial extension was made into the central clear zone. Four years after surgery, the patient was carrying on his usual activities completely independent of corrective lenses. The vision in the right eye was not perfect under all circumstances. When very high−contrast objects were presented in dim light, a ghost image was seen. This phenomenon was more apparent with white objects on a black background than with black objects on a white background. The false image was about one third as bright as the true image. The subjective midday refraction of the right eye postoperatively yielded two quite different results, each providing a visual acuity of 20/20+. Refraction for a bright high-contrast image obtained a result of +1.00 −1.00 × 180°, whereas a refraction as determined to push plus power to the maximum obtained a result of +3.25 −2.25 × 95°. The refraction, reported as streak retinoscopy along the horizontal meridian, showed the curvature relatively constant across the cornea; in the vertical meridian a prominent scissoring reflex was observed. A color-coded map of corneal topographic power from a video keratograph revealed a horizontal oval of relative flattening of about 37 D located below a somewhat larger central region with a power of approximately 40 D. We thought the larger, superiorly located refractive zone gave a visual acuity of 20/20 uncorrected, whereas the smaller, inferiorly located refractive zone produced a ghost image. This was confirmed by covering parts of the cornea with the edge of a piece of paper. As the inferior cornea was progressively covered, the ghost image progressively faded. When the cornea was progressively covered from its superior aspect the true image reached the ghost image when approximately 60% of the cornea was covered. The ghost image was present only when viewing high-contrast objects under low light conditions, and confusion of the true and false images never occurred during regular daily activities. However, there was a loss of contrast in the right eye.

From Wyzinski P and O'Dell L: Ophthalmology 1989;86:108-111.

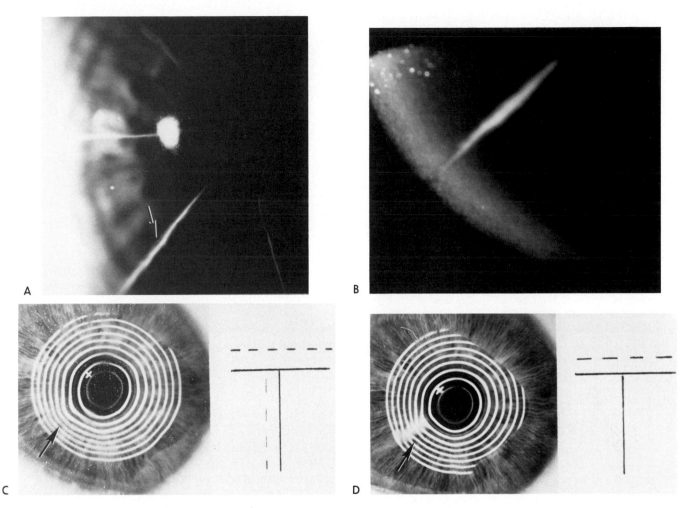

Figure 23-18
Focal hypertrophy of radial keratotomy scar 5 years after surgery. **A,** Increased density of keratotomy scar at 7:30 o'clock *(arrow).* **B,** Close-up showing hypertrophic scar at 7:30 o'clock. **C,** Left: Keratograph shows irregular astigmatism in 7:30 hemi-meridian *(arrow).* Right: Drawing made by patient shows monocular diplopia. **D,** Left: Three months after revision of scar, keratograph shows persistent irregular astigmatism *(arrow).* Right: Patient's drawing of decreased monocular diplopia. (From Rashid ER and Waring GO: Surv Ophthalmol 1989;34:73-106.)

CORNEAL COMPLICATIONS
Bacterial or fungal keratitis

Bacterial or fungal keratitis may occur at two distinct times after refractive keratotomy: shortly after surgery, as might be expected from any operative incision, or after 1 to 3 years, probably because of continued remodeling of the corneal epithelium.

Early postoperative keratitis

Numerous cases of bacterial corneal infections have been reported after refractive keratotomy* (Figs. 23-19 and 23-20). One registry reported two infections in 62,814 cases of refractive keratotomy.[145] In a survey by Lewicky and Salz[135] of 24 corneal refractive surgeons, five cases of bacterial keratitis were reported, one requiring a penetrating keratoplasty. The location of the infiltrate

*References 41, 102, 135, 142, 164, 187, 230, 236.

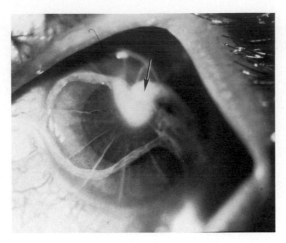

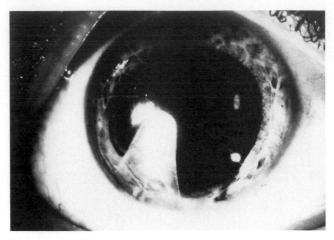

Figure 23-19
Severe suppurative keratitis invading the central cornea after radial keratotomy *(arrow)*. A therapeutic soft contact lens is in place. A strand of mucus lies on the corneal surface. (From Rashid ER and Waring GO: Surv Ophthalmol 1989;34:73-106.)

Figure 23-20
Scar following bacterial corneal ulcer after radial keratotomy. Patient had initial four-incision radial keratotomy followed by a repeated four-incision radial keratotomy. One of the repeated wounds became infected in the immediate postoperative period and left a dense scar between the two wounds. (Courtesy R. Doyle Stulting.)

Case Report: Early Postoperative Bacterial Keratitis

A 33-year-old atopic woman underwent eight-incision radial keratotomy in the right eye. A 1.5-mm microperforation occurred in the inferior incision. Ten days postoperatively, a suppurative stromal keratitis developed in the area of the previous perforation site. Topical cefazolin 5% eyedrops were administered every half hour. All cultures grew *Staphylococcus aureus.*

Twenty-four hours after antibacterial therapy was begun, the stromal infiltrate became more circumscribed, but the linear perforation site gradually opened with shallowing of the anterior chamber. A therapeutic bandage lens was applied, but the leak persisted and the anterior chamber shallowed. In the operating room 10 days after her admission, epithelium was debrided from the wound and tissue adhesive applied to the perforation site. The contact lens was reapplied and the patient treated with oral acetazolamide for 5 days. The topical antibiotics were tapered and discontinued; vascularization of the inferior corneal stroma was gradually increased.

The glue extruded 20 days postoperatively without leakage of aqueous humor. Residual scarring produced 3.00 D of with-the-rule astigmatism. Visual acuity stabilized at 20/25 without correction 4 months after the gluing.

From Wilhelmus KR and Hamburg S: Cornea 1983;2:143-146.

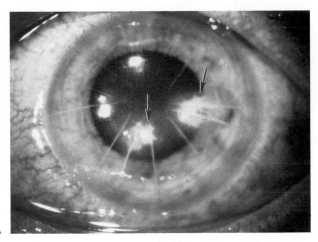
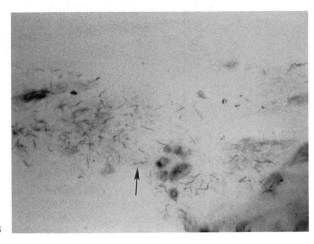

Figure 23-21
Mycobacterium chelonei keratitis after radial keratotomy. **A,** Focal infiltrates in the area of radial keratotomy wounds *(arrows).* Surgery was done in an office setting with cold sterilization of the instruments. **B,** Corneal scraping shows acid-fast bacteria *(arrow).* (**A** from Robin JB, Beatty RF, Dunn S, et al: Am J Ophthalmol 1986;102:72-79; **B** courtesy Jeff Robin.)

was usually within a refractive keratotomy incision. Causative organisms included *Pseudomonas, Staphylococcus aureus,* and *Staphylococcus epidermititis.*

The frequency of microbial keratitis occurring shortly after surgery may be reduced by prophylactic topical antibiotics, such as neomycin-polymycin-bacitracin or gentamicin, until the incisions are epithelized. The management of ulcerative keratitis in these patients should follow standard guidelines,[15] including corneal scrapings, Gram stains, and cultures, followed by frequent topical fortified antibiotics with broad-spectrum coverage initially and later adjustment based on culture and sensitivity results.

Robin and colleagues[177] reported two cases of *Mycobacterium chelonei* keratitis from the same surgeon's office in which outpatient refractive keratotomy had been performed using cold-sterilized instruments (Fig. 23-21). Symptoms and signs developed in both cases approximately 2 weeks after surgery. The corneal lesions consisted of white irregular infiltrates with radiating projections at all levels of the stroma with overlying epithelial defects. Cultures from scrapings were negative, and both cases required corneal biopsy for diagnosis. Both patients were treated with topical fortified amikacin. In one patient medical therapy cleared the infection. The other patient had a recurrence of the infiltrate and required therapeutic corneal transplantation, resulting in an uncorrected visual acuity of 20/40.

Delayed bacterial and fungal keratitis

An unanticipated complication of keratotomy has been the late development of ulcerative keratitis.[41,142,203] Cottingham et al.[41] reported a series of 14,163 corneal refractive procedures in which six cases of delayed infectious keratitis were reported. This is an incidence of about one in 2400. Mandelbaum and colleagues[142] described ulcerative keratitis that developed in three patients 7 months to 2½ years after uncomplicated refractive keratotomy. All the infiltrates occurred in the keratotomy scars. One patient was wearing an extended wear soft contact lens for the correction of residual myopia; ulcers developed in the other two spontaneously.

Speculation about the cause of delayed infection has centered around the persistent epithelial plug in the keratotomy wounds. As the epithelium gradually

---

Case Report: Delayed Postoperative Bacterial Keratitis

A 35-year-old woman underwent an eight-incision refractive keratotomy in her right eye. Seven and one half months after surgery, the patient noticed irritation of the eye while she was vacuuming at home, with no recognizable trauma or injury. The following morning she awoke with pain, discharge, and severe photophobia.

Examination of the right eye demonstrated an uncorrected visual acuity of 20/60. There was mild right-lid edema, conjunctival injection, and mucopurulent discharge adhering to the inferotemporal cornea (Fig. 23-22). The peripheral area of the 7:30-o'clock scar had a 3-mm diameter epithelial and stromal ulcer with dense stromal infiltrate. The cornea had splayed open along the refractive keratotomy incision, thinning in some regions to about 20% of normal corneal thickness.

The ulcer was cultured and the patient treated with subconjunctival and high-dose topical antibiotics. *Pseudomonas aeruginosa* was the causative organism. Gradually the infiltrate resolved, the cornea thickened, the ulcer epithelized, and a small peripheral vascularized scar remained. Fourteen months after the keratitis, the uncorrected visual acuity was 20/16 OD.

From Mandelbaum S, Waring GO, Forster RK, et al: Arch Ophthalmol 1986;104:1156-1160.

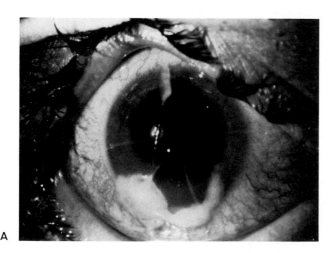

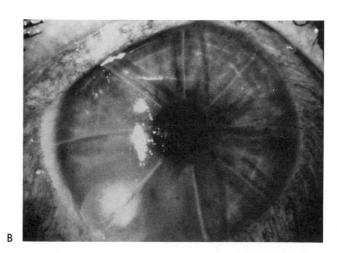

A

B

Figure 23-22
A, Delayed ulcerative keratitis secondary to *Pseudomonas aeruginosa* occurring 7½ months after radial keratotomy. **B,** Same eye after 4 days of intensive antibiotic therapy. (**A** from Mandelbaum S, Waring GO, Forster RK, et al: Arch Ophthalmol 1986;104:1156-1160; **B** courtesy Sidney Mandelbaum.)

extrudes, surface irregularities appear where bacteria could attach and, under the proper conditions, produce an active keratitis. The redistribution of the tear film over the slightly irregular cornea might also affect these epithelial irregularities. This hypothesis is supported by the research of Stern et al.,[217] who demonstrated that bacteria can adhere in large numbers to injured epithelial cells, whereas few organisms attach to an intact epithelium or bare stroma, a phenomenon important in keratitis after penetrating keratoplasty[97] and with extended wear soft contact lenses.

Delayed bacterial and fungal keratitis occurs so rarely that long-term prophylactic antibiotics would be inappropriate. However, patients should be warned about this potential complication and instructed to consult their ophthalmologist at the earliest sign of persistent blurred vision or redness of the eye.

Geggel[77] reported an unusual case in which sterile keratitis involving four adjacent nasal incisions occurred 34 months after a 16-incision radial keratotomy. Multiple cultures and biopsies failed to show a pathogen. The keratitis was confined to the incisional area without involvement of the intervening stroma. The histopathological studies demonstrated only delayed corneal wound healing and wounds filled with inflammatory cells consisting primarily of macrophages and lymphocytes. No pathogenic organisms were identified.

Nonhealing sterile corneal defects

A severe sterile keratitis with progressive corneal thinning and perforation occurred in a 35-year-old physician after combined radial and intersecting circumferential incisions.[123] A wound gape appeared at the intersecting incisions, resulting in a persistent epithelial defect and stromal melting that required a patch graft and, 4 months later, a penetrating keratoplasty. Histopathology of the recipient cornea revealed epithelial plugs in the incisions, deep and superficial stromal vascularization, endothelial cell loss, and inflammatory cell infiltration at all levels of the cornea. Postoperatively, the patient had 20/200 vision and an early cataract.

Avoiding intersecting incisions is now a basic tenet of keratotomy surgery.

Herpes simplex keratitis

Recurrent herpes simplex keratitis can be stimulated by numerous exogenous insults to the eye, including sunlight, fever, minor accidental trauma, contact lenses, and menstruation.[146] The trauma of keratotomy surgery can be added to the list. Not only might the trauma stimulate recurrence of the viral infection, but the hypesthetic cornea from herpes simplex keratitis might decrease wound healing. Patients with a history of herpes simplex keratitis should not undergo refractive keratotomy.

Several cases of herpes simplex keratitis have been reported after refractive keratotomy.[192-195] In one of these patients, a 30-year-old woman with no medical history of herpes simplex keratitis, a typical dendritic epithelial ulcer developed on the second day after refractive keratotomy. Unfortunately, no scrapings or viral cultures were obtained to document the presumed diagnosis.

Endothelial cell loss

The effect of keratotomy on the corneal endothelium has been a subject of great interest and debate, arguments often clouded by the experience of Sato (see Chapter 6, Development of Radial Keratotomy in Japan, 1939-1960). Because Sato made multiple incisions (up to 40) in the posterior cornea, severe endothelial damage occurred during surgery.[1,19,242] Because most of the patients were young, the endothelium recovered, only to decompensate with resultant corneal edema 20 years or later after surgery. This has led some individuals to

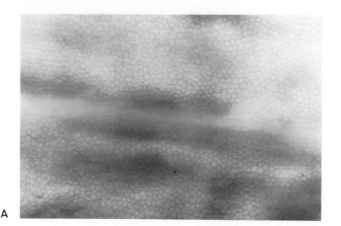

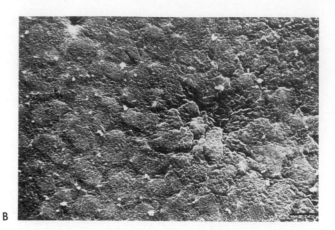

Figure 23-23
A, Wide-field endothelial specular photomicrograph demonstrates horizontal incision scar *(white line)* and moderate variation in cell size and shape. The patient had worn contact lenses for many years before surgery, and therefore it is not known whether the changes in the endothelium are from contact lens wear or radial keratotomy. **B,** Scanning electron micrograph of the corneal endothelium of a monkey 1 year after radial keratotomy demonstrates a focal area of damage in the area of the incisions. (**A** courtesy Scott McRae; **B** courtesy Tatsuo Yamaguchi.)

exaggerate the possible long-term damage to the endothelium from anterior keratotomy. Clearly, four to eight anterior keratotomy incisions made with a diamond knife will not damage the endothelium in the same way that 40 anterior and 40 posterior incisions made with a metal knife blade did 40 years ago.

Laboratory experiments in animal eyes have documented acute damage to the endothelium just beneath the incisions. Apparently, the cornea and Descemet's membrane are stretched, and endothelial cells in that area show disruption of cell borders and rupture of some cells. For example, Yamaguchi and colleagues performed anterior radial keratotomy in rhesus monkeys and showed significant endothelial changes using scanning and transmission electron microscopy.[119] Swollen endothelial cells were seen at the central cornea in 33% of the eyes. Linear protrusions on the posterior cornea, beneath and parallel to refractive keratotomy incisions, were seen in all cases. In eight of nine eyes, damaged endothelial cells were seen with invading inflammatory cells. The authors suggest that cuts in Bowman's layer and in the stroma may cause stretching of the cornea and create instability, which could later result in continuing mild injury to the endothelium, a speculation needing verification. Binder has shown similar changes in a laboratory model.[24] The question remains: Do these mild acute changes significantly affect the endothelium, and are they chronically progressive? No evidence of progressive damage has been published.

One confounding variable in the studies of the corneal endothelium after refractive keratotomy is the influence of preexisting contact lens wear, which can produce morphologic changes in the corneal endothelium.[107-115] This emphasizes the importance of preoperative and postoperative measurements. Without preoperative measurements, it would not be known whether postoperative endothelial abnormalities resulted from many years of contact lens wear or from the surgery itself (Fig. 23-23).

The study of the endothelium in humans after refractive keratotomy centers on clinical specular microscopy; two points should be emphasized. First, keratotomy is done in the paracentral and peripheral cornea. Therefore, central corneal endothelial measurements are less likely to detect endothelial damage than measurements adjacent to and beneath the incisions themselves. The most meaningful studies of the endothelium will include preoperative and postoperative measurements in the same eyes taken from the same area of the paracentral cornea. Second, in addition to measurements of cell density (cell/mm^2), the more sensitive indices of coefficient of variation in cell area (polymegathism) and changes in cell shape expressed as the percentage of hexagonal cells (pleomorphism) should be studied.[207]

In the past decade, numerous studies have reported average central corneal endothelial cell loss of 4% to 10% in the first several years after radial keratotomy.* The endothelial loss has been shown to be more significant in the first months following the procedure and not progressive on later examinations.[54,102,119,178] The study suggests that more surgery produces more damage. For example, Rowsey and colleagues[180] have shown that a second refractive keratotomy on the same eye produces an average additional cell loss of 14.6% at 2 years and 9.8% at 3 years.

It is common sense that a corneal perforation will damage the endothelium more in that area. Chiba and colleagues[38] showed more endothelial cell loss in the central cornea of eyes that had microperforations than in those that did not. They performed morphometric analysis of the central corneal endothelium on 24 eyes after refractive keratotomy. They found a statistically significant decrease in mean cell density, increase in mean cell perimeter and mean side length, but no statistically significant change in the coefficient of variation of cell area, the number of hexagonal cells, or the change in cell shape. They identified significant endothelial cell damage associated with microperforations and with clear zone diameters less than 3.5 mm. The variables for microperforations were the following:

Cell density: microperforation = increase of 14.3%
                  no microperforation = increase of 1.6%

Cell perimeter: microperforation = increase of 7.9%
                  no microperforation = increase of 1.1%

Side length: microperforation = increase of 7.7%
                  no microperforation = increase of 1%

Eyes with clear zone diameters of 3.75 to 4.50 showed no changes in these parameters, but eyes with clear zone diameters of 3.0 to 3.5 mm showed statistically significant damage in all three of the forementioned parameters.

There have been case reports of severe endothelial cell loss in patients who have undergone extensive keratotomy with multiple incisions and repeated operations.[183,185] Some of these patients were elderly. Corneal edema after refractive keratotomy has also occurred.[213]

The most encouraging studies of the corneal endothelium after keratotomy have been morphometric analyses.[38,140] McRae and colleagues[140] showed a 3.3% decrease in central endothelial density, but no statistically significant change in cell size or shape in either the central or the peripheral endothelium 1 year after refractive keratotomy in a small number of eyes. When these eyes were reexamined 2 years after surgery, there was no significant decrease in central cell density from preoperative measurements, and still no significant morphometric changes centrally or peripherally. Similarly, Asbell and colleagues[7]

---

*References 51, 102, 132, 161, 178, 180.

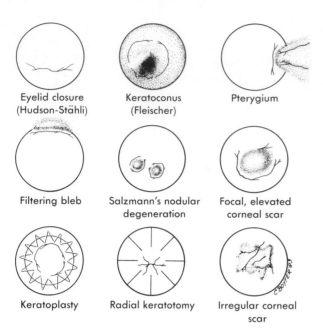

Figure 23-24

Nine different patterns of iron lines in the corneal epithelium. (From Steinberg EB, Wilson LA, Waring GO, et al: Am J Ophthalmol 1984;98:416-421.)

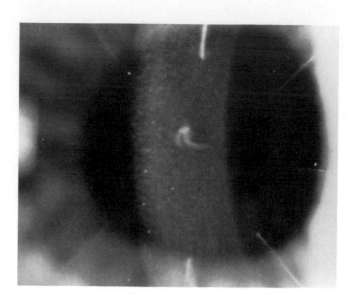

Figure 23-25

A central stellate iron line in an eye with radial keratotomy shows a dense central nodule and a whorl-shaped pattern with arms radiating out between the incisions. (From Rashid ER and Waring GO: Surv Ophthalmol 1989;34:73-106.)

studied the endothelium between and beneath the incisions and found no statistically significant decrease in endothelial cell density when compared with preoperative levels.

Uncertainties linger about the effect of anterior refractive keratotomy on the endothelium. Further studies are needed of the endothelium in the area of the incisions over long periods. There is no question that the mechanical structure of the cornea is weakened by keratotomy, and it is theoretically possible that a small increase in the bending of the cornea, with blinking or rubbing of the eyes, could produce a slow cumulative rate of increased endothelial cell loss over many years, a speculation that has never been documented. It is unknown whether the mild endothelial damage from refractive keratotomy would affect the cornea's resistance to future endothelial insult, either from intraocular surgery or from primary diseases such as Fuchs' endothelial dystrophy.[228]

Stellate epithelial iron lines

A brown stellate epithelial iron line appears in the majority of eyes after refractive keratotomy. This line is similar to the epithelial iron line that appears in any disorder producing a persistent irregularity in the corneal epithelium (Fig. 23-24). After refractive keratotomy, the deposit varies from a faint, tan horizontal line in the same location as the Hudson-Stahli line (Fig. 23-25), studded with small branches, to a dense, yellow-brown deposit, with eight radiating arms that extend out between the eight incisions (Fig. 23-26). The density and extent of the deposit vary greatly from one eye to another.[47,216,229]

In the PERK study, stellate epithelial iron lines appeared in 13 of 16 eyes

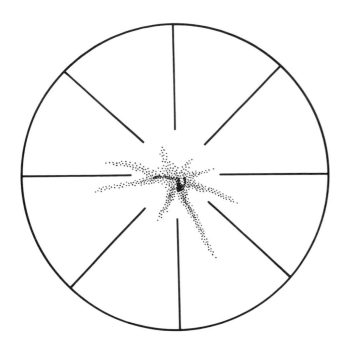

Figure 23-26
A corneal epithelial iron line after radial keratotomy located at the junction of the middle and inferior thirds of the cornea and the stellate configuration, in which the inferior branches are usually longer and more prominent than the superior branches. (From Steinberg EB, Wilson LA, Waring GO, et al: Am J Ophthalmol 1984;98:416-421.)

(81%) examined 6 months after surgery and in 43 of 50 eyes (86%) 1 year after surgery. We have now extended these observations (unpublished data) and find the iron line did not change its appearance after 3 years' follow-up in 68 of 91 eyes (75%), but progressed in 18% and regressed in 8%.

The pathogenesis of the stellate iron line after refractive keratotomy is similar to that of other corneal iron lines—the iron is eluted by an unknown mechanism from the tears and is deposited in the epithelium in depressions on the corneal surface. After refractive keratotomy such depressions occur centrally in the flattened area and between the slightly elevated scars. In the PERK study, an analysis of the configuration of the iron lines showed that eyes with a greater flattening in the central cornea had more prominent iron lines. Davis et al.[47] reported that iron lines were more frequent in eyes with higher amounts of myopia, more surgery, and more central flattening.

The iron lines apparently do not reduce visual acuity and therefore do not need management.

Epithelial basement membrane changes and epithelial erosions

Corneal epithelial basement membrane changes are described in terms of their clinical appearance as maps, fingerprint lines, and dots.[159] Changes in the epithelial basement membrane after refractive keratotomy were studied in 71 eyes at one PERK center.[159] Corneal epithelial opacities, similar to those seen in epithelial basement membrane dystrophy, appeared in 46.5% of eyes after surgery. They had a map-dot configuration over less than one eighth of the corneal surface and tended to be transient, persisting less than 3 months in 75.3% of the eyes. Three of the eyes had changes that persisted for 12 months. One eye had transient visual blurring attributed to the basement membrane changes, but there were no episodes of recurrent epithelial erosion in this group of patients.[232]

The cause of the epithelial basement membrane changes is unknown. Presumably, the epithelium is disrupted during surgery and may secrete excess basement membrane during healing. Why some eyes develop the map-dot

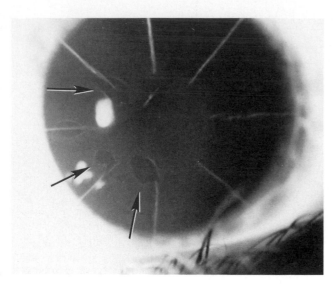

A

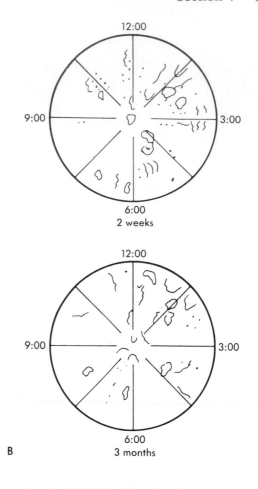

12:00

9:00   3:00

6:00
2 weeks

12:00

9:00   3:00

6:00
3 months

B

Figure 23-27
Epithelial basement membrane changes after radial
keratotomy. **A,** Map-shaped changes *(arrows)* appear in
the area of the incisions. **B,** Map-dot-fingerprint changes
in the epithelium after radial keratotomy show a dynamic course, changing their configuration and gradually disappearing. (**A** courtesy J. Daniel Nelson; **B** from
Nelson JD, Williams P, Lindstrom RL, and Doughman
DJ: Ophthalmology 1985;92:199-205.)

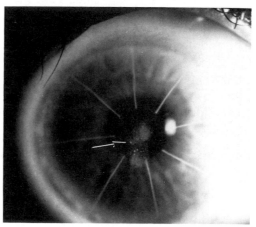

Figure 23-28
Central corneal epithelial erosion with epithelial cysts
and edema that recurred for a few months after radial
keratotomy and then resolved with topical lubricants.
(From Rashid ER and Waring GO: Surv Ophthalmol
1989;34:73-106.)

changes and others do not is unknown[94, 159] (Fig. 23-27).

Recurrent epithelial erosions after refractive keratotomy occur rarely. Four
patients in the PERK study experienced symptoms of corneal epithelial erosion;
three were associated with epithelial basement membrane map-shaped changes.
These occurred 1 to 7 months after surgery and disappeared after topical therapy, except in one patient who required treatment with a therapeutic soft contact lens that induced the growth of blood vessels in five incisions[232] (Fig. 23-
28).

Prevention of this complication should include questioning the patient for a
history of corneal erosions and a meticulous, preoperative slit-lamp microscope

---

Case Report: Epithelial Erosion after Refractive Keratotomy

A 37-year-old woman was seen 4 years after undergoing a unilateral refractive keratotomy in her left eye. No records of her preoperative examination or surgical procedure were available. She stated that she had a severe reaction to the topical anesthetic, with loss of most of her corneal epithelium, which took several weeks to heal. She reported fluctuating vision, chronic irritation, and significant glare at night only in the eye that had been operated on, and therefore declined surgery on her right eye. Her examination revealed a visual acuity of OD:20/20, with a refraction of −6.00 D, and OS:20/25, with a refraction of −1.50 +1.75 × 180°. The left cornea demonstrated 15 healed, radial, corneal scars and marked map-dot-fingerprint changes between each scar, sparing the central 2-mm clear zone. The right cornea demonstrated a 0.5-mm epithelial map in the inferior nasal area. This patient probably had a subclinical case of epithelial basement membrane dystrophy that was aggravated by the refractive keratotomy surgery.

---

search for epithelial basement membrane changes. Of the patients who request refractive keratotomy because of contact lens intolerance, some may have epithelial problems that would make contact lens wear difficult. Whether epithelial abrasions during surgery caused by dull blades, rough footplates, or excessive topical anesthesia lead to recurrent erosions is unknown, but these operative problems should be prevented.[179,192]

Management of recurrent corneal epithelial erosions after refractive keratotomy is similar to that in other circumstances: topical hyperosmotic agents (5% sodium chloride, colloidal dextran), lubricating ointments, pressure patching, therapeutic bandage lenses, epithelial scraping, and epithelial micropuncture.

Abnormal incisions and scars

Keratotomy converts a structurally normal cornea to a structurally abnormal one. When uncomplicated, the incision scars undergo a natural, predictable course of healing. However, surgical errors and disorders in wound healing after surgery can produce clinical problems.

Intersecting incisions. Although it is now well known that intersecting incisions produce severe wound gapes and larger amounts of scarring, they were commonly advocated in the early 1980s, particularly to correct astigmatism: the TL procedure of Fyodorov, the Ruiz trapezoidal keratotomy, combined circular and radial keratotomy of Gills, "flag" transverse incisions, and the like.* The greater the number of intersecting incisions and the closer they are to each other, the greater the resulting abnormality of the scars.

These abnormalities fall into two categories: wound gaping and creation of a corneal flap. Intersecting incisions, particularly radial and transverse, create a wound gape at the area of intersection that becomes large and fills with abundant stromal scarring (Fig. 23-29), sometimes accompanied by extensive subepithelial scarring spreading out from the wound. Such scars not only create irregular astigmatism but also increase the light scattering and glare. The amount of scarring is unpredictable; some intersecting wounds heal nicely, others with exuberant cicatrization. When transverse incisions intersect two radial incisions, a flap of cornea is created that may protrude forward, become edematous, and heal slowly over a period of months (Fig. 23-30). Intersection of a transverse incision to only one side of a radial incision (flag T cuts) produces less wound

---

*References 57, 66, 70, 73, 80, 104, 123, 192.

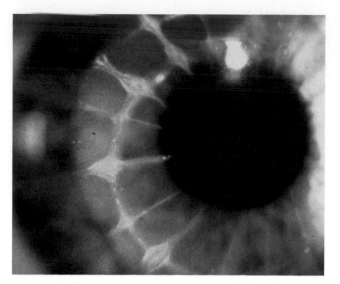

Figure 23-29
Combined circular and radial keratotomy for myopia. The 16 radial incisions intersect the two circular incisions leaving large diamond-shaped scars at the intersection with multiple epithelial inclusions. (Courtesy Richard Villasenor.)

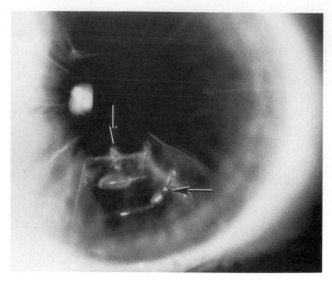

Figure 23-30
A Ruiz trapezoidal keratotomy was performed in this cornea to treat astigmatism, the two semiradial incisions being joined at their central ends with a transverse incision. This created an elevated flap of corneal stroma, which required suturing *(arrows)*. (Courtesy Robert Hofmann.)

gaping and scarring than transverse incisions that go completely across a radial incision.

Management of wound gapes in inadvertent intersections includes a circular purse-string suture to close the wound and prevent excessive scarring.

Multiple scars from repeated operations. One technique of repeated refractive keratotomy involves a second set of incisions in the same location as the first, trying to follow the course of the initial incisions, a difficult technical task that usually results in two interwoven scars (Fig. 23-31). Residual astigmatism has been treated by placing transverse incisions across previously healed radial scars.[192] In these circumstances, the previously healed scars usually seldom open up, so wound gaping is not a problem. The additive effect of two corneal scars in the same area, however, increases the amount of irregular astigmatism and glare (Fig. 23-32).

More detailed discussion is presented in Chapter 18, Repeated Surgery for Residual Myopia and Hyperopia after Refractive Corneal Surgery, and a case example is presented in Chapter 25, The Patient Speaks: Testimonials after Refractive Keratotomy.

Hypertrophic scar. In some instances, an apparently normal, uncomplicated, single-pass radial incision may heal in a hypertrophic fashion, whereas other incisions in the same eye heal normally in patients with no history of keloid formation. Such a case has been reported in the PERK study,[230] and discussed in the section on irregular astigmatism (see Fig. 23-15). Whether the patients who form keloids in skin incisions do so in corneal incisions is unknown.

Posterior plaque at perforation site. Damaged corneal endothelium tends to produce excess extracellular matrix in the form of a posterior collagenous layer,

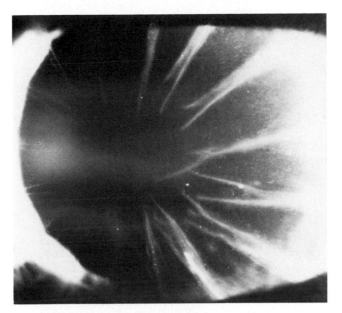

Figure 23-31
Repeated 16-incision radial keratotomy with the first set of incisions made in the region of the second set. All incisions have a double contour, indicating that the second set of incisions was not made exactly on top of the first set. The patient developed irregular astigmatism but could not wear a contact lens. (From Rashid ER and Waring GO: Surv Ophthalmol 1989;34:73-106.)

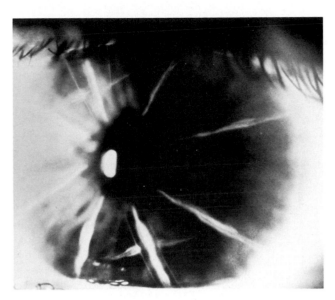

Figure 23-32
Radial scars in an eye after reoperations show excessive scarring with very wide opacities. (Courtesy Robert Hofmann.)

commonly referred to as a thickened or duplicated Descemet's membrane. This material appears as a gray plaque at the level of Descemet's membrane.[227] Corneal perforation during refractive keratotomy damages the endothelium, which during healing produces a focal scar in Descemet's membrane and the posterior stroma, which appears as a focal, gray plaque with feathered edges (Fig. 23-3).

Limbal scarring. When a keratotomy incision extends into or across the corneal limbus, the adjacent conjunctival and scleral tissue sometimes heals with increased scarring, often forming a wedge-shaped finger of tissue that extends 0.5 to 1.0 mm into the cornea. This is a rare occurrence now that incisions usually stop short of the limbal vascular arcade.

Irregular incisions. A wiggling knife during the incision will create an irregular, serpentine scar. This is most likely to occur when: (1) the globe shifts with single-point fixation, (2) the surgeon is nervous or inexperienced, (3) a new style knife is tried, (4) knife blades are thin or double edged, (5) the incision is made from the limbus toward the central clear zone, and (6) the surgeon stops an incision partway through and then completes it with a second cut. Although such irregular incisions may be an aesthetic affront to the surgeon, they seem to have little effect on the outcome of the operation, unless the irregularity is extreme (see Fig. 23-6).

Vascularization of incision scars. Most refractive keratotomy scars heal without vascularization. Events that stimulate vascularization of the scar include incisions across the limbus, wearing of contact lenses—particularly extended wear soft lenses, cautery at the limbus, and inflammation or infection in the scars.[57,192]

Contact lens wear with its associated corneal hypoxia is the most common

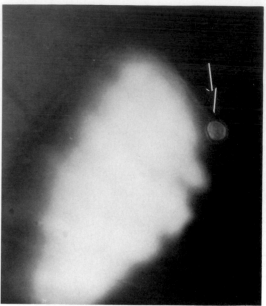

Figure 23-33
High-power slit-lamp photograph demonstrates a single epithelial inclusion *(arrow)* in a keratotomy scar. (From Rashid ER and Waring GO: Surv Ophthalmol 1989;34:73-106.)

cause of vascularization, particularly since surgeons now no longer cut across the limbus, as demonstrated in both animal studies and clinical experience.* In the PERK study 1 year after surgery, 1.5% of the incisions demonstrated vascularization, not extending more than 1 mm,[232] but after 3 years, progression of vascularization was noted in 16 eyes (3.6%), extending 5% to 50% of the length of the incisions. All but three of these patients had worn a contact lens.[230]

The vessels themselves increase the density of the corneal scar, but there are no published reports of secondary hemorrhage or lipid deposition from the vessels after refractive keratotomy.

Prevention of vascularization includes avoidance of incisions across the limbus, cautery at the limbus, and the fitting of contact lenses after surgery. Specifically, extended wear soft contact lenses should be avoided, and daily wear soft lenses fit only when necessary. The most desirable contact lens is a rigid gaspermeable daily wear lens, as discussed in a later section. In an animal model, Katz and colleagues[124] have shown a significant inhibition of corneal neovascularization with flurbiprofen after contact lens fitting. Whether the appearance of neovascularization of the scars is a sufficient basis to require cessation of contact lens wear requires further study.

Most vascularization of the wounds occurs subepithelially, but if a stromal vascularization is induced, the patient may be at a higher risk of allograft reaction if a penetrating keratoplasty is needed in the future.

Epithelial inclusions. The unsutured keratotomy wounds heal in the initial stages by being filled with a normal epithelial plug (not "epithelial ingrowth") that is gradually extruded during wound healing.

Careful examination of normal keratotomy scars with a narrow slit-lamp microscope beam demonstrates a lucent area in the center of the incision scar—a narrow epithelial plug. Clinical and histologic examinations have shown that this plug can persist for 4 or 5 years after surgery.[48,117,244]

However, if nests of epithelial cells remain trapped within the scar, they produce discrete, round, refractile bodies known as inclusion cysts—a misnomer

*References 124, 125, 178, 179, 181, 185, 192, 230.

Case Report: Epithelial Inclusion Cysts and Vascularization of Scars

A 32-year-old aviation electronics technician in the United States Navy underwent bilateral refractive keratotomy in 1980. The patient's preoperative refraction was approximately −8.00 D in each eye, and his cycloplegic refraction 7 years later was −2.50 +0.75 × 180° in the right eye and −3.00 sphere in the left. For optical correction, the patient was wearing CSI soft contact lenses daily wear, approximately 17 hours a day, with a visual acuity of 20/20 bilaterally. Lenses were cleaned with a hydrogen peroxide chemical system daily and an enzyme cleaner weekly.

Slit-lamp microscope examination revealed 32 radial keratotomy scars in the right eye and 16 in the left. Some incisions contained epithelial inclusion cysts. All incisions contained superficial blood vessels that extended approximately 60% along the length of the incision. There were no lipid deposits from the vessels.

because this is not a cystic structure, but rather a solid collection of epithelial cells (Fig. 23-33). Just how such inclusions form is unknown.[48,120,175]

In the PERK study at 1 year, deposits and epithelial inclusions occurred in approximately 7% of the scars.[232] Jester and colleagues[120] reported an epithelial inclusion in an incision of a 26-year-old woman with radial and circumferential incisions. One of the epithelial inclusions began to enlarge at the junction of the radial and circumferential incision. A 2-mm excisional biopsy of superficial stroma and epithelium was performed to remove the enlarging inclusion.

These epithelial inclusions make the scar more dense but do not seem to cause clinical problems within the wound. Whether irrigation of the incisions at the conclusion of surgery prevents epithelial inclusions is not clear. Irrigation may indeed remove epithelial cells that are implanted during surgery, but because the entire wound fills with epithelium anyhow, irrigation may not reduce the incidence of inclusions.

Debris and deposits. One type of deposit that has been noted, especially when incisions are made across the limbus, is multiple, discrete, round, yellowish, pearl-like inclusions within the wound (Fig. 23-34). Fyodorov et al.[74] reported these corneal incision opacities in addition to plaques and bubble-like changes in the healing wound, especially in patients who had undergone a second set of radial incisions that were on top of or adjacent to the original radial cuts. Some of these inclusions were probably epithelial, but others may have represented degeneration of blood that was retained in the incision. Such deposits are less common now because incisions are not extended across the limbus and the blood is routinely irrigated from the wound.

Fyodorov and colleagues[74] described two groups of eyes that had undergone these reoperations. The first group consisted of 24 eyes in which the incision healing occurred with the formation of a delicate scar without inclusions. The second group consisted of 36 eyes with the formation of a wider scar that contained circular inclusions. The first group had two times more reduction in myopia than the second. No relationship could be demonstrated between the initial degree of myopia and the corneal healing type.[102]

Particulate debris including fibers, metal fragments, and fine particles is sometimes seen in keratotomy scars but have not been noted to have any apparent untoward effect.

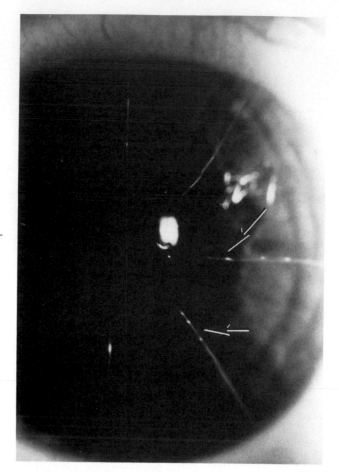

Figure 23-34
Epithelial inclusions *(arrows)* scattered along the keratotomy scars, as shown in sclerotic scatter illumination.

INTRAOCULAR COMPLICATIONS

Complications that involve intraocular structures, such as endophthalmitis, cataract, epithelial ingrowth, and rupture of the globe through the keratotomy incisions, pose a great threat to vision. They are even more onerous after refractive keratotomy than after surgery performed for potentially blinding diseases because refractive keratotomy is an elective procedure. Fortunately, the incidence of these severe complications is exceedingly low, but for each patient to whom they happen, the consequences may be tragic.

Endophthalmitis

The three published case reports of endophthalmitis after refractive keratotomy are strikingly similar. All three patients developed discomfort in an eye that had been operated on 8 to 10 days previously. All developed a small hypopyon, and the cultured organism was *Staphylococcus epidermidis.* One patient underwent a diagnostic and therapeutic vitrectomy, whereas the other two were treated medically. All patients had excellent visual outcome several months later.[78,143,164] Cross and Head[43] cite nine unpublished cases of endophthalmitis, including cases caused by *Pseudomonas* and *Serratia marcescens,* and estimate the incidence of endophthalmitis, based on an approximation of the total cases of refractive keratotomy performed in the Houston area, as 1:8300.

Endophthalmitis following keratotomy presumably begins with the introduction of the infectious agent into the eye through a corneal perforation during or shortly after surgery.[9,57,190,192] Pathogenic organisms probably come from the

Case Report: Endophthalmitis after Refractive Keratotomy

A 47-year-old man underwent refractive keratotomy on his right eye in an office operating room under sterile conditions. At the fifteenth incision, in the mid-periphery a small perforation occurred with a slight loss of aqueous. On the first postoperative day, there was no aqueous leak at the site of the perforation. On the seventh postoperative day, conjunctival injection and a mild discharge were present. On the ninth postoperative day, the patient awoke with significant pain and decreased vision in the right eye. The visual acuity was 3/200 best corrected. The patient had prominent conjunctival injection, a ciliary flush, no corneal infiltrates, a marked cell and flare, and a 5% hypopyon. There was a marked cellular reaction in the vitreous, with white, fluffy balls layering the inferior and posterior vitreous. The retina was attached.

During the emergency pars plana vitrectomy, a central core vitrectomy was performed and invitreal antibiotics injected. Cultured aqueous and vitreous specimens grew *Staphylococcus epidermidis*.

Treatments with intravenous and topical antibiotics and oral prednisolone were gradually tapered. Several months later, the corrected visual acuity was 20/30.

From Gelender H, Flynn HW, and Mandelbaum SH: Am J Ophthalmol 1982;93:323-326.

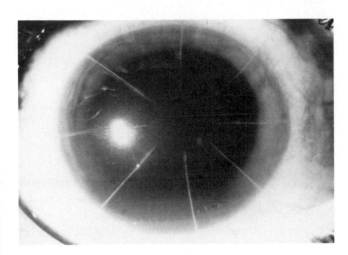

Figure 23-35
Twenty-nine-year-old female had an eight-incision radial keratotomy and developed staphylococcal epidermis endophthalmitis postoperatively. Appropriate antibiotic treatment eliminated the infection, but the patient developed a retinal detachment and vitreous hemorrhage. The detachment was successfully repaired, but the patient developed preretinal fibrosis, which was treated with a vitrectomy and membranectomy. The most recent visual acuity was 20/200. (Courtesy Sidney Mandelbaum.)

lids, lashes, conjunctiva, and lacrimal apparatus, although contaminated air, instruments, or surgical field may also be sources. Therefore strict adherence to sterile technique is mandatory.[61]

The clinical severity of acute postoperative endophthalmitis depends on the pathogenicity of the infectious agent and the eye's response. Management includes early diagnosis, anterior chamber aspiration and culture, vitreous aspiration and culture if the vitreous is involved, topical, intraocular, and systemic antibiotics, and possibly therapeutic vitrectomy[61] (Fig. 23-35).

Cataract

Most of the lens opacities occurring after refractive keratotomy have resulted from direct laceration of the lens at the time of a corneal perforation* (Fig. 23-36). This is one time when the diminutive term "microperforation" takes on a

*References 12, 79, 164, 192, 213, 228.

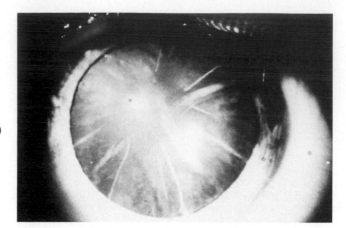

Figure 23-36
Opaque lens caused by laceration of anterior lens capsule during radial keratotomy. (Courtesy Walter Stark.)

Case Report: Postoperative Cataracts Unrelated to Refractive Keratotomy

A 46-year-old man underwent bilateral refractive keratotomy. Before surgery, his best-corrected vision was 20/20 in each eye. Postoperatively, his vision fluctuated widely and he was placed on topical 0.1% Decadron to both eyes four times a day. Treatment in the left eye was discontinued after 6 months, when he reported that the vision had become "smokey." He was examined 14 months after surgery, and bilateral posterior capsular cataracts were present, with best-corrected visual acuity of 20/30 in the right eye and 20/70 in the left.

From MacRae SM, Matsuda M, and Rich LF: Am J Ophthalmol 1985;100:538-542.

---

more onerous meaning. This complication was not only limited to the early 1980s when metal-bladed knives and cruder techniques were used; we are aware of cases in the late 1980s. Direct laceration of the lens is most likely to occur when the surgeon uses new techniques or instruments that cause deeper incisions in the cornea, when the surgeon is careless or in a hurry, when the patient moves inadvertently in the midst of an incision, and during deepening incisions. Other causes of cataracts after keratotomy surgery include endophthalmitis[123,192] and prolonged topical corticosteroid use.[192]

One unusual case[79] occurred in a 31-year-old man in whom an intumescent cataract developed 3½ months after refractive keratotomy. The operation had been complicated by a microperforation of the cornea, but there was no loss of the anterior chamber during the procedure or postoperatively, and no damage to the lens capsule was ever observed. The authors theorized that the cause of this cataract may have been direct mechanical trauma to the lens during the sudden decompression.[79]

Naturally occurring cataracts may appear after refractive keratotomy, presumably unrelated to the procedure. For example, in the PERK study a patient who preoperatively was noted to have a few small cortical flecks in the lens had radial keratotomy in one eye only. Postoperatively, cataracts developed symmetrically in each eye, requiring surgical removal. If radial keratotomy had been performed in both eyes, the progression of the cataracts might have been incorrectly attributed to the radial keratotomy surgery.[230]

Prevention of cataracts following refractive keratotomy includes accurate corneal incisions without perforation and minimal use of postoperative topical corticosteroids. Management of cataracts that reduce visual function is discussed in a subsequent section.

TRAUMATIC RUPTURE OF KERATOTOMY SCARS

Once an incision is made in the cornea, whether from refractive keratotomy, penetrating keratoplasty, or accidental trauma, the resultant scar does not have as much tensile strength as the original cornea. The collagen fibrils do not heal end to end and do not reestablish the strong cables that span the entire cornea, but the cornea heals by the creation of a new extracellular matrix that cements together the two sides of the incision, resulting in an opaque, weaker scar (see Chapter 20, Corneal Wound Healing and Its Pharmacologic Modification after Refractive Keratotomy). Thus after refractive keratotomy the cornea is permanently weaker than its normal state and therefore increases its risk of rupture from direct ocular trauma.[147]

Five laboratory studies of wound strength after refractive keratotomy have been published. Luttrull and colleagues[138] studied the effect of the depth of keratotomy incisions that extended across the limbus in enucleated porcine eyes. They demonstrated that when achieved incision depth exceeded 70%, there was an increased incidence of corneal rupture through the incisions after blunt trauma. They also observed that incisions transversing the limbus increased the incidence of corneal scleral rupture.

Larson and colleagues[133] observed that 98% of the wound ruptures in rabbit eyes following an eight-incision refractive keratotomy procedure occurred in one or more of the incisions with patterns that connected one incision to the other and that extended out into the sclera, forming stellate wounds. They observed that the blunt force required to rupture the globe after refractive keratotomy within 90 days of healing was approximately half that required to rupture the control eyes not operated on; those eyes with intraoperative corneal perforations required even less force to rupture.

Rylander and colleagues[182] studied the effect of refractive keratotomy on the rupture strength in a porcine model. They concluded that ruptures most frequently occurred at the equator in normal eyes and through the cornea in eyes after refractive keratotomy. The refractive keratotomy eyes ruptured at less force than the paired normal eyes in eight of nine experiments.

Darakjian and Marchese[44] demonstrated that rabbit eyes, 9 to 12 months after refractive keratotomy, ruptured at a pressure of 60 lbs per square inch through the sclera, not through the cornea. With support of the sclera, however, the refractive keratotomy wounds burst at a mean pressure of 90 to 110 lbs per square inch, whereas the unincised corneas remained intact. It is important to keep in mind species differences in studies of refractive keratotomy.

McKnight and colleagues[153] investigated BB gun injuries with calibrated force on the corneas of cats that had undergone eight-incision radial keratotomy. Their investigation showed that the eyes that underwent radial keratotomy ruptured much more readily than an unoperated control group.

Studies on the strength of full-thickness corneal wounds indicated little healing in the first week, an early, rapid rise to about 30% of normal strength by the first month, then a slow rise until the strength was about 50% of normal at 3 to 6 months.[40,76] Studies longer than 6 months have not been carried out.

Therefore much of our information about long-term corneal wound strength comes from reports of accidental trauma in humans. Of course, it is not possible to quantify the amount of trauma received by the globe under accidental circumstances because the history of trauma does not allow a clear measure of the

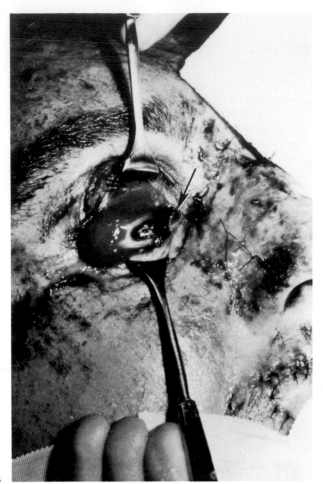

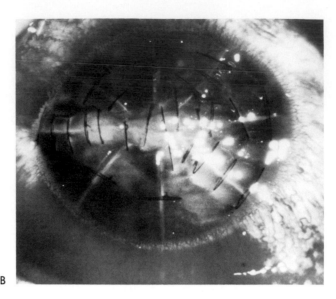

Figure 23-37
Traumatic rupture of globe after refractive keratotomy.
A, A patient who had radial keratotomy 2 years previously was involved in a motor vehicle accident and suffered severe facial injuries that resulted in death. The photograph shows the eyelids being retracted to reveal a cornea rupture through the radial keratotomy incisions with central iris prolapse *(arrow).* **B,** Postoperative photograph of an eye that sustained significant trauma during a fight. The patient had undergone radial keratotomy in this eye 1 year before the injury. (**A** courtesy Dennis O'Day; **B** courtesy Richard L. Lindstrom.)

amount of force absorbed by the periocular structure and the amount of force absorbed by the globe itself.

Examples of ocular trauma without rupture of the keratotomy wounds have been reported. John and Schmitt[121] reported one case of severe blunt trauma to an eye 6 months after an eight-incision radial keratotomy procedure that produced a corneal abrasion and a 75% hyphema without rupture of the keratotomy scars. Spivak[212] reported a similar case, in which a patient experienced facial trauma in a plane crash 4 months after a 16-incision refractive keratotomy and 2 months after a reoperation for residual astigmatism. In spite of bilateral facial fractures, no rupture of the cornea occurred, and the patient recovered 20/20 uncorrected visual acuity.

Forstot and Damiano[62] emphasized the variable visual outcome of six patients who had refractive keratotomy with subsequent accidental trauma. They reported two patients with direct severe trauma to the globe that separated an incision and produced a flat chamber. In both cases, successful treatment with a soft contact lens restored the corneal integrity. Four other cases with mild to severe periocular injury did not display rupture of the keratotomy wounds. None of their six cases exhibited significant visual or ocular sequelae from the trauma.

Other reports, however, document severe ocular damage from rupture of the cornea after refractive keratotomy (Fig. 23-37). Binder and colleagues[25] reported three eyes with corneal rupture after motor vehicle accidents. One woman, 2 years after a 16-incision refractive keratotomy, sustained a stellate rupture of the

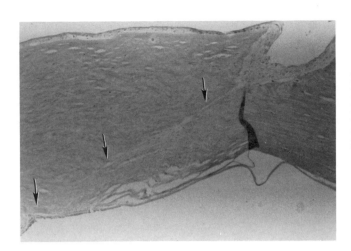

Figure 23-38
Histopathologic section of a cornea ruptured through radial keratotomy wounds from blunt trauma in a motor vehicle accident. After primary repair, penetrating keratoplasty was performed, producing this specimen. The oblique, partially healed full-thickness traumatic wound is indicated by the arrows. (Courtesy Perry S. Binder.)

Case Report: Traumatic Rupture of Refractive Keratotomy Scars

In 1981, a 24-year-old woman underwent a 16-incision radial keratotomy procedure in the left eye. The details of her refraction and surgery are not available. Two years later she experienced blunt trauma to her head in a motor vehicle accident, with loss of consciousness. In the intensive care unit, visual acuity was light perception in the left eye, and a stellate rupture of the cornea and sclera connected the two vertical refractive keratotomy scars. In addition, a horizontal rupture of the cornea occurred in the 9:00 o'clock keratotomy scar, extending to the center of the cornea, connected to the vertical rupture. The lens and the iris were totally avulsed, and vitreous extruded from the wound. A dense vitreous hemorrhage obscured view of the retina. The right eye was normal.

On the day of the accident, the corneoscleral wounds were repaired, but in spite of an anterior vitrectomy, a dense vitreous hemorrhage persisted, with light perception visual acuity. One month after surgery, ghost cell glaucoma developed, requiring a posterior vitrectomy. Corneal edema developed subsequently, and penetrating keratoplasty was performed. Eight months after surgery, the visual acuity was 20/50 with a contact lens.

Histopathologic examination of the excised button demonstrated original refractive keratotomy scars that were not ruptured and extended perpendicularly in the cornea from 50% to 100% of full corneal thickness, and larger oblique, more recent, partially healed wounds that resulted from the rupture and subsequent repair, extending the full thickness through the cornea (Fig. 23-38).

---

cornea and sclera with avulsion of the lens and iris as recounted in the following case history. The second case involved a man, approximately 1 year after undergoing bilateral refractive keratotomy, who was involved in a motor vehicle accident, sustained severe head trauma, and died 7 days later. The right cornea sustained a corneal scleral rupture through the keratotomy wounds.

McDonnell and colleagues[151] reported corneal rupture following blunt trauma after a hexagonal keratotomy. The patient required several surgical procedures for repair of the corneal wound and a retinal detachment. Simmons and Linsalata[209] reported a case of blunt trauma caused by an elbow approximately 2 weeks after refractive keratotomy with rupture of the cornea followed by primary repair and subsequent enucleation.

That traumatic dehiscence of keratotomy wounds may occur should come as no surprise. Penetrating keratoplasty wounds, with their attendant corticosteroid therapy, are known to slip 1 or 2 years after surgery when the sutures are removed.[23] Calkins and colleagues[35] used holograms taken of corneas after penetrating keratoplasty to demonstrate structurally weak areas in the wound even 1 year after keratoplasty in the face of vascularization. Traumatic rupture of penetrating keratoplasty wounds has been reported by numerous authors, including two cases by Friedman[68] 4 and 5 years after surgery, 12 cases by Raber et al.,[172] including three at 14, 17, and 18 months postoperatively, four cases by Topping et al.,[222] one 6 years after surgery, and 14 cases by Farley and Pettit,[59] one 13 years after surgery.

Refractive keratotomy wounds can open not only after accidental trauma, but also during surgical trauma. Girard et al.[90] described a case in which the incisions reopened 6 months after the original refractive keratotomy while transverse incisions were being made to correct residual astigmatism. Beatty et al.[18] described in detail the difficulties of corneal transplantation when the relatively unhealed corneal wounds separate. Techniques such as a continuous purse-string suture or interrupted sutures across the refractive keratotomy wounds before or after trephination can be used to reinforce the radial wounds in these cases. Swinger and Barker[220] have reported the successful use of keratomileusis after undercorrected or overcorrected refractive keratotomy procedures and observed that the keratotomy wounds separate easily in the excised lenticule.

Accidental trauma may occur to anyone after refractive keratotomy, not only to individuals involved in high-risk activities or with pugnacious natures. Therefore patients must be warned that their corneas are permanently weakened by the procedure. Of course, there is little caution that can be truly taken by such individuals because most persons seeking refractive keratotomy are in an active age group. Indeed, many have the surgery so that they can pursue vigorous sporting and recreational activities. Individuals who have had refractive keratotomy and who participate in sports such as racquetball, squash, and basketball, in which severe direct trauma to the globe is more likely to occur, should wear protective eye wear. But it does little good to warn people to stay out of car wrecks because their eye might get hurt.

Epithelial ingrowth

Binder[22] has reported the only case of presumed epithelial ingrowth following refractive keratotomy (Fig. 23-39). The corneal epithelium grows into the anterior chamber through a microperforation.[22,103]

Case Report: Epithelial Ingrowth through a Microperforation

A single microperforation occurred when a peripheral deepening incision was performed as part of a refractive keratotomy procedure. A postoperative wound leak at the site of the perforation closed spontaneously following occlusive pressure patching. Four months after surgery, a flat, refractile plaque appeared on the posterior cornea in the area of the perforation. The lesion grew five times in size over the next 5 months, had all of the clinical characteristics of an epithelial ingrowth, and reduced the best-corrected visual acuity to 20/100. The lesion was treated with full-thickness corneal cryotherapy and within 96 hours retracted off the cornea. It disappeared spontaneously from the anterior chamber. The patient's vision improved to 20/30 without correction (Fig. 23-39).

From Binder PS: CLAO J 1986;12:247-250.

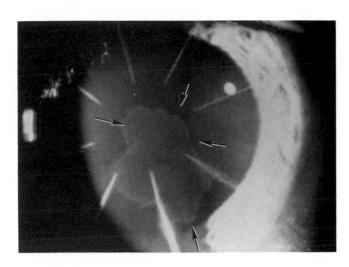

Figure 23-39
Epithelial ingrowth after radial keratotomy forms a dense plaque on the posterior cornea *(arrows)*. Details of this case are given in the text. Interestingly, this was the first corneal perforation during radial keratotomy that occurred for the surgeon. (From Binder PS: CLAO J 1986;12:247-250.)

Prevention of epithelial ingrowth following refractive keratotomy includes minimizing corneal perforation and avoiding injection of an irrigating stream through a perforation. Management depends on the extent of the ingrowth.[103]

Iridocyclitis

After refractive keratotomy, most patients have mild anterior chamber cell and flare, which usually disappears over 1 to 3 weeks.[232] However, severe postoperative iridocyclitis has been reported in several patients.[31,192,215] Brodsky et al.[31] reported two patients in whom a marked anterior chamber reaction developed. Both had microperforations, and the authors believed the iritis was directly attributable to the instillation of 0.25% fluorescein drops (Grant's solution) on the first day postoperatively.

Delayed iridocyclitis of unknown cause occurred in a 36-year-old patient 6 months after refractive keratotomy.[215]

Elevated intraocular pressure

Intraocular pressure is the driving force behind the changes in corneal shape that occur after refractive keratotomy, as discussed in the chapter on factors that affect outcome (Chapter 26) and in the chapters on biomechanical modeling (Chapters 27 to 29, 33, and 34). We discuss here the effect of elevated intraocular pressure on refraction and visual acuity after refractive keratotomy.

Elevated intraocular pressure produces further flattening of the central cornea, with further decrease in minus power of the refractive correction. Thus an undercorrected patient will probably have better visual acuity when the pressure rises and an emmetropic or overcorrected patient will have worse acuity, depending on his or her ability to accommodate.

Deitz et al.[53] documented the effect of topical corticosteroids in a nurse who was a steroid responder and was undercorrected from her radial refractive keratotomy. When she used the topical steroids in the immediate postoperative period to decrease inflammation, her pressure rose into the 30s, her residual myopia decreased, and her visual acuity improved. When she stopped the corticosteroids at her physician's instruction, the pressure fell and she became more undercorrected. She commenced the topical corticosteroids again on her own accord, raising the intraocular pressure, decreasing her myopia, and improving her visual acuity.

Topical corticosteroids are used after refractive keratotomy for three reasons: (1) to decrease the postoperative mild inflammation of the cornea, a use that can

Case Report: Delayed Iridocyclitis

A 36-year-old female underwent an eight-incision, 3.0 optical zone refractive keratotomy procedure on her right eye, and 13 months later had an identical procedure on her left eye. The surgery in both eyes was uncomplicated. Her uncorrected visual acuity 2 months later was 20/20 in both eyes. Her refraction in the right eye was −0.25 sphere and in the left eye −0.50 +0.50 × 180°.

Five months after surgery on the left eye, pain, photophobia, and decreased visual acuity developed. Her uncorrected vision was now 20/20 OD and 20/200 OS, correctable to 20/20 with +3.50 +0.75 × 180°. A moderate inflammatory reaction was noted in the left anterior chamber, with fine keratitic precipitates and intraocular pressures of 16 mm Hg in the right eye and 21 mm Hg in the left. The patient was 5 months pregnant. She was treated with topical mydriatics, corticosteroids, and hypertonic agents. One week later her visual acuity had dropped to 20/400 without correction in the left eye, correctable only to 20/100. Central corneal thickness was 0.65 mm, compared with 0.58 mm preoperatively. The intraocular pressure had returned to its normal preoperative measurement of 16 mm Hg. The iridocyclitis was worse with mutton-fat keratic precipitates. The posterior segment appeared clear. Laboratory tests, including CBC, sedimentation rate, fungal serologies, VDRL, toxoplasmosis titer, serological titers for herpes simplex and cytomegalic viruses, as well tuberculosis skin tests, were negative or normal.

On intensive topical steroid therapy, the inflammation gradually subsided, and by 2 months from the onset of the inflammation her uncorrected vision had returned to 20/20, correctable with a +0.25 D sphere. All medications were discontinued. There has been no recurrence (Fig. 23-40). Whether the iridocyclitis was caused by the refractive keratotomy or some other etiology is unknown.

From Starling J and Hofmann R: J Refract Surg 1986;2:96-98.

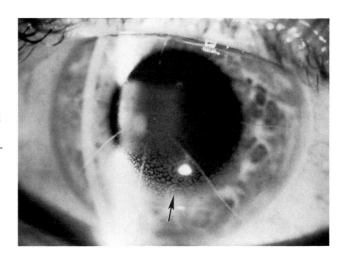

Figure 23-40
Severe iridocyclitis with mutton-fat keratic precipitates *(arrow)* developed 5 months after uncomplicated radial keratotomy in the left eye of a pregnant woman who had bilateral radial keratotomy. The case history is presented in the text. (From Starling J and Hofmann R: J Refract Surg 1986;2:96-98.)

be effective within less than a week, at which time the steroids should be stopped; (2) to enhance the effect of the surgery by presumably retarding wound healing in patients who retain normal intraocular pressure, a use that has been supported by one report[99]; and (3) to enhance the effect of the surgery by elevating the intraocular pressure, an effect that is clearly demonstrative on the short term, but the long-term benefit has never been documented.* Surgeons

*Carlucio Andrade, MD, personal communication, Sept 1987.

Case Report: Reversal of Overcorrection after Hyperbaric Oxygen

A 56-year-old woman with a cycloplegic refraction of −2.87 D in her right eye had refractive keratotomy in the PERK study. Her left eye remained unoperated on. Two years after surgery, she was overcorrected with a refraction of +4.00 D in the operated right eye, corrected by a contact lens. Approximately 3 years after surgery, she had a Morton's neuroma removed from her foot and the surgical incision would not heal. She took five hyperbaric oxygen treatments down to 30 feet for 3 hours on each of 5 consecutive days to enhance the healing of the foot wound. After the third treatment, she noticed blurred vision in her right eye while wearing her contact lens; when she took the contact lens off, her visual acuity without correction was remarkably good. The foot wound did not heal. At her 3-year PERK examination approximately 3 months later, her refraction was +0.25 D and her uncorrected visual acuity was 20/20, findings that remained unchanged at the time of her 4-year PERK examination. The causal relationship between the hyperbaric oxygen treatments and the decrease in the patient's hyperopia is not established, but the proximity of time suggests that the hyperbaric oxygen affected the shape of her cornea.

From Waring GO, Lynn MJ, Culbertson W, et al: Ophthalmology 1987;94:1339-1354.

---

should guard against the chronic use of topical corticosteroids to affect the outcome of refractive keratotomy because of the danger of optic nerve damage from elevated intraocular pressure and of the induction of posterior subcapsular cataracts.

Busin and colleagues[29] describe a case in the PERK study of the reverse phenomenon. The patient's intraocular pressure increased spontaneously and for unknown cause—presumably the onset of chronic open-angle glaucoma—from 12 to 26 mm Hg 2 years after refractive keratotomy, with flattening of the central cornea and a change in refraction from +2.00 to +5.75 D. Topical 0.5% timolol twice daily decreased the intraocular pressure to 10 mm Hg, with subsequent steepening of the cornea and lessening of the overcorrection to +1.75 D. After subsequent cessation of the timolol, the intraocular pressure rose again to 20 mm Hg and the refractive error again increased to +5.00 D. Thus patients in whom chronic, open-angle glaucoma or elevated intraocular pressure from other causes develops are in danger of marked fluctuations in refraction and visual acuity within a few years after refractive keratotomy. Whether this will occur many years after surgery, when the cornea is presumably more completely healed, remains to be determined.

An interesting anecdotal observation raises questions about the effect of atmospheric pressure on the outcome of refractive keratotomy.

Glaucoma

When incisions were made across the limbus and possibly damaging Schlemm's canal, development of glaucoma was theoretically possible, but no cases have been reported. This problem is no longer a consideration because incisions are confined to the cornea.

A similar observation has been made by Dr. Lawrence Spivak,* who has managed overcorrected patients in Denver, Colorado, observing that the effect of the surgery was reduced and the refraction changed toward emmetropia when

---

*Lawrence Spivak, personal communication, March 1987.

they moved to lower elevations such as Florida, where atmospheric pressure is greater. One ophthalmologist who was overcorrected tried hyperbaric oxygen therapy to reduce the overcorrection without success (see Chapter 25: The Patient Speaks: Testimonials after Refractive Keratotomy).

The significance of these observations remains to be determined.

Retinal detachment and maculopathy

Individuals with myopia, especially those with lattice degeneration of the retina,[218] have an increased risk of retinal detachment. Some reports indicate that 75% of persons with myopia have some form of lattice degeneration.[164] Although no cases of retinal detachment after refractive keratotomy were encountered in the PERK study, several cases have been reported in the literature.[106,164,192,230] In one case, retinal detachment was a direct result of a double perforation during the retrobulbar block.[134,164] In two other cases,[106,164] strong miotics were used postoperatively in overcorrected eyes to improve the visual acuity by miosis and by increasing accommodation. The cause of these detachments may have been related to the increased ciliary muscle activity induced by the miotics, which may exert traction on the peripheral retina and cause a retina to tear, with subsequent detachment.[17,216] Strong miotics should be avoided in cases of overcorrection.

No evidence indicates that the surgical trauma of refractive keratotomy predisposes a patient to retinal detachment. However, all myopes scheduled for refractive keratotomy should have a dilated peripheral fundus examination and appropriate management of any retinal pathology. Surgeons participating in the Houston study waited at least 6 weeks after cryopexy or laser retinal repair before refractive surgery was undertaken.[192]

Management of retinal detachment in patients who have undergone refractive keratotomy may be complicated,[106,192] as discussed in a subsequent section.

As with any procedure using the operating microscope, prolonged exposure of the eye to the microscope light during surgery can produce a photic maculopathy. This can occur during radial keratotomy, particularly if the procedure is prolonged.[155] The result is a central or paracentral scotoma, which can be detected on visual field testing or Amsler grid testing. An area of pigmentary disruption in the macular region can be seen on ophthalmoscopy, and fluorescein angiography usually reveals a hyperfluorescent round or oval zone in the macula. The burn is usually permanent, thereby nullifying treatment. The light-induced maculopathy can be prevented by using infrared filters and the lowest intensity of the microscope light, keeping the pupil small, and performing the operation quickly. The case described by Menezo and colleagues[155] lasted approximately 7½ minutes.

PTOSIS

Blepharoptosis has been reported after refractive keratotomy.[37] Linberg and colleagues[136] documented unilateral postoperative ptosis in approximately 10% of the patients who only had one eye operated on at one PERK clinical center. Interestingly, five of these patients chose refractive keratotomy in the opposite eye; four developed mild ptosis in the second eye. In their series of seven cases, all followed for a minimum of 6 months, only one patient showed significant spontaneous improvement over 30 months.[136] Cross[39] reported that seven of 16 cases resolved within 6 months.

The pathogenesis of acquired ptosis after ocular surgery is unknown.[16,59,166] Most authors propose that ptosis results from a dehiscence of the levator palpebrae superioris aponeurosis. On examination, these patients generally have mild ptosis with excellent levator function.[166] Since the refractive keratotomy proce-

---

Case Report: Ptosis after Refractive Keratotomy

A 30-year-old woman underwent refractive keratotomy in her left eye in 1983. The surgery was uncomplicated and there were no postoperative problems. The patient did not use topical medications or a contact lens, but noticed a mild narrowing of her lid fissure on the left side.

Six months after surgery, the lid fissures measured 10 mm in the right eye and 9 mm in the left. Levator palpebrae superioris function was normal (14 mm) in each eye.

Refractive keratotomy of the right eye was performed in 1984, and again there were no operative or postoperative complications. After the second procedure, the lid fissures were symmetric. Measurements of 8.5 mm in the right eye and 9.0 mm in the left suggested that symmetry was caused by bilateral ptosis rather than resolution of the acquired ptosis in both eyes[117] (Fig. 23-41).

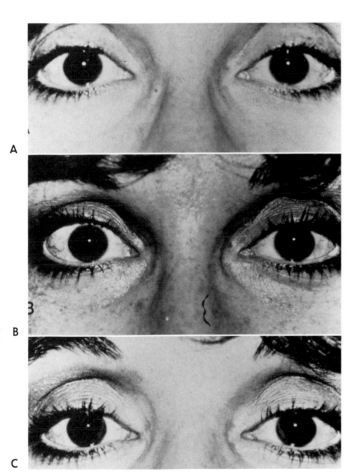

A

B

C

Figure 23-41
Acquired ptosis after radial keratotomy. **A,** Preoperative appearance. Fissures measure 10 mm in the right eye and 10 mm in the left eye. **B,** Six months after radial keratotomy in the left eye. Mild ptosis present in the left eye. Fissures measure 10 mm in the right eye and 9 mm in the left eye. **C,** After radial keratotomy in both eyes. Nearly symmetric fissures with mild ptosis in both eyes. Fissures measure 8.5 mm in the right eye and 9 mm in the left eye. (From Linberg JV, McDonald M, Safir A, and Googe JM: Ophthalmology 1986;93:1509-1512.)

dure that was done under the protocol of the PERK study did not use anesthetic injections or superior rectus sutures, the most likely cause was damage to the levator aponeurosis by the eyelid speculum. A solid, rigid Knapp eyelid speculum was used in the cases reported by Linberg, and he suggested that a gentle wire speculum might be less likely to induce ptosis.

If the mechanism of trauma to the lids after refractive keratotomy is similar to other forms of ocular surgery, then management should include advancement of the levator muscle.[16,65] None of the reported cases of ptosis after refractive keratotomy had surgical repair. Therefore direct observation of a levator aponeurosis disinsertion has not been made.[37,136] Surgical repair should be delayed until both eyes have had refractive keratotomy and an adequate period has elapsed to allow for spontaneous recovery.

OCULAR SURGERY AFTER REFRACTIVE KERATOTOMY

Refractive keratotomy causes permanent structural alterations in the cornea that may complicate subsequent surgery. Penetrating keratoplasty, epikeratoplasty, and myopic keratomileusis after refractive keratotomy are discussed in Chapter 18, Repeated Surgery for Residual Myopia and Hyperopia after Refractive Keratotomy.

Cataract surgery

Several cases of cataract extraction after refractive keratotomy with and without intraocular lens implantation have been reported, most without corneal wound rupture or other complications.[12,79,144,192] Markovits[144] reported a case of extracapsular cataract extraction with a posterior chamber intraocular lens implant, done in a patient 18 months after a 32-incision refractive keratotomy, who was placed on topical prednisolone acetate four times a day for 8 months after refractive keratotomy. He reported: (1) a variation in lens power calculations, primarily resulting from variation in axial length measurements; (2) low corneal rigidity causing some problems with nuclear expression; and (3) fluctuating and poor postoperative visual acuity for 3 months. In another case, a successful phacoemulsification with an intraocular lens implant and an excellent visual recovery has been reported.[192]

Because keratometric readings are not stable for months (and sometimes years) after refractive keratotomy, calculation of intraocular lens power is more difficult.

Retinal detachment/vitrectomy

One informal report describes a patient who underwent a pars plana vitrectomy for endophthalmitis after refractive keratotomy, and no specific problems with the keratotomy incisions were encountered.[78]

In another case report of retinal detachment after refractive keratotomy, no difficulties were noted with the retinal examination, laser therapy, or scleral buckling procedure.[106]

Case Report: Retinal Detachment after Refractive Keratotomy

A retinal detachment developed in a 29-year-old man 24 months after bilateral 32-incision refractive keratotomy. Preoperatively the refractive error was approximately −10 D OD and −12 D OS, with 20/20 vision with contact lenses. Two years after the refractive keratotomy, the patient's refraction was plano −1.25 × 30°, 20/20, in the right eye and −6.00 D in the left, corrected with a contact lens. Vision decreased in his left eye and the patient had multiple retinal tears and nearly 270 degrees of lattice degeneration involving both eyes. The highly elevated retinal detachment in the left eye involved the macula and had fixed folds. When the surgeon performed a scleral depression, he noted temporal leaking of aqueous from three or four of the corneal incision scars. During the operative procedure, four of the incisions opened were before the scleral buckling, and gaped during the buckling. Postoperatively the patient obtained a left visual acuity of 20/40, a refraction of −6.00 D that was corrected with a soft contact lens.

CONTACT LENS FITTING PROBLEMS AFTER KERATOTOMY

The fitting and caring for contact lenses after refractive keratotomy is more difficult than that in normal eyes for two reasons. The first is the psychologic aspect, that most patients who choose refractive keratotomy do so to avoid corrective lenses. For example, Bourque and colleagues[30] found in the PERK study that 58% of men and 73% of women desired refractive keratotomy to achieve independence from lenses. The second reason is the change in corneal topography, with flattening of the central cornea that makes conventionally designed lenses more difficult to fit.[107,206]

The prevalence of patients who wear contact lenses after refractive keratotomy is unknown. In a series of 1100 consecutive refractive keratotomies, Shivitz and colleagues[206] reported that 4% had visually significant refractive errors that were corrected with contact lenses. In the PERK study, 34% of the patients with bilateral surgery required use of some type of corrective lenses, at least part of the time, 4 years after surgery.[231]

Indications for contact lens fitting include not only undercorrection and overcorrection, which also could be managed with spectacles, but also residual astigmatism, anisometropia, and irregular astigmatism, for which contact lenses are better suited. Additional refractive surgery can manage some of these problems, either with repeated keratotomy (as described in Chapter 18) or with epikeratoplasty or keratomileusis in selected cases. Nevertheless, many patients will require fitting with contact lenses for full visual rehabilitation.

Anatomic and physiologic problems in contact lens fitting

Epithelial changes, such as map-dot-fingerprint basement membrane abnormalities and persistent punctate epithelial keratopathy in the area of the healing incisions, may give rise to surface abnormalities that cause chronic irritation with contact lenses.[39,130,159] A careful examination with the slit-lamp microscope will detect these problems before fitting. Keratotomy can produce slight decreases in corneal sensation, particularly if transverse incisions have been used. This may make the symptomatic fitting of contact lenses easier.[20,192,204,208]

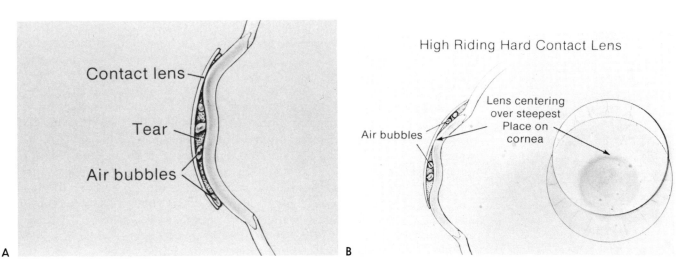

Figure 23-42
Drawings demonstrate problems in contact lens fitting after radial keratotomy. **A,** Flat central cornea and relatively steeper paracentral cornea create a bulge over which the lens rides, so it is easily displaced eccentrically. **B,** Air bubbles can accumulate in the relative depression in the central cornea beneath the contact lens. (Courtesy Joseph W. Soper.)

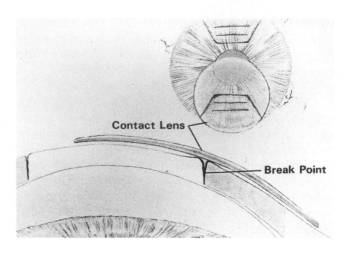

Figure 23-43
Contact lens fitting after astigmatic keratotomy using Ruiz incisions demonstrates poor centration of the lens over the areas of the incisions. (From Hofmann RF, Starling JC, and Masler W: J Refract Surg 1986;2:155-162.)

The corneal topographic changes seen after refractive keratotomy have created a new, unique problem in the fitting of contact lenses. The regular aspheric topography of the cornea is significantly modified with central flattening and paracentral steepening (Fig. 23-42) (see Chapter 3, Optics and Topography of Radial Keratotomy). The corneal contour is also affected by each of the corneal scars. Surface irregularities caused by intersecting keratotomies are most prone to mechanical abrasion.[192]

History and examination of the contact lens candidate

Most refractive keratotomy patients have previously worn or attempted to wear contact lenses, and some have long histories of contact lens intolerance and problems. Special attention should be given to the types of lenses worn previously, the reasons for discontinuing contact lenses wear, and past problems with the lens care regimen. The fitter should obtain the patient's preoperative keratometric readings because they will be useful in selection of the first trial lens. In addition to the standard clinical examination, keratographs should be taken to show the corneal topography. A detailed slit-lamp microscope search for epithelial and wound abnormalities, including vascularization, helps the fitter anticipate problems. A careful drawing should be placed in the patient's record.

Fitting problems

A contact lens fit after refractive keratotomy produces a fluorescein pattern of central tear pooling, paracentral contact bearing, and peripheral edge lift. The lens pivots over the paracentral "break points," often decentering supernasally or inferotemporally[107] (Fig. 23-43). Centration may be more difficult to maintain if transverse incisions are present. The tear lens is thicker and creates more plus power, which must be offset by adding extra minus power in the lens nearly equal to the original myopia.[107] This large tear pool probably turns over more slowly, creating fluid stagnation that can result in hypoxia with stromal and epithelial edema.

Subjectively, patients notice fluctuating vision. Sliding of the lens over the break points may create irritation and foreign body sensation as a result of epithelial breakdown. The edge lift can produce both easy dislocation and increased awareness of the lens.[107] In addition, edge lift allows drying of that local area of the cornea, causing punctate epithelial keratopathy.

Techniques of contact lens fitting

The most successful lenses fit in patients after refractive keratotomy have been rigid, large-diameter, highly gas-permeable lenses, with thin edges fit using a trial-and-error system.[107,157,158,205,206] Fitting is more difficult and time consuming than normal.

The initial trial lens for both rigid and soft lenses should have a base curve similar to the preoperative flatter central keratometry measurement.[206] The flattened central corneal curvature created by the refractive keratotomy does not correlate with the base curve of the final contact lens because the lens rides on the paracentral and peripheral cornea. Trial lenses fit with a base curve similar to the postoperative central keratometry measurement often have excessive movement and decenter. Because the contact lens base curve is relatively steep compared with the new central corneal curvature, air bubbles can accumulate. Fenestrated lenses may solve this problem.[107,206]

Larger diameter lenses are more likely to center, so the diameter is selected first. Adjustment of the base curve is then made to provide the best fit. Overrefraction then determines the lens power.[206] Interestingly the power of the contact lens fit after refractive keratotomy may be similar to that of the preoperative lens because of the optical effect of the positive central tear meniscus.[107] The newly created aspheric surface may require the use of contact lenses, such as Soper or Maguire series.

Toric lenses may be necessary to correct residual astigmatism. Prism or hyperflange edge design may help center a superiorly decentered lens. A mild flange edge or decreasing the diameter of the lens (which will decrease the weight) may be useful to center an inferiorly positioned lens.[205]

We do not advocate the use of extended wear soft contact lenses after refractive keratotomy because vascularization of the wounds occurs frequently in this patient population.

All wearers of soft contact lenses, daily or extended, should be counseled about the risk of corneal infection with these optical devices. Numerous cases of microbial keratitis occurring in soft contact lens wearers after refractive keratotomy have been reported.*

Therapeutic uses of contact lenses after keratotomy

A few authors[51,104] have advocated the use of hard and soft contact lenses to promote additional corneal refractive changes after refractive keratotomy—a form of orthokeratology.† Although unproven, these authors believe an improved result after an undercorrection or an overcorrection can be achieved through the use of contact lenses.

Therapeutic contact lenses have been advocated immediately after surgery to reduce discomfort, treat epithelial defects, and manage perforations.[192] Such therapeutic lenses should be placed under sterile conditions.

Results of contact lens fitting after keratotomy

In the study by Hofmann and colleagues,[107] 56% of patients were successfully fitted with rigid gas-permeable lenses. Patients fitted with a daily wear soft contact lens had only a 37% success rate at 1 year. Fitting of custom toric soft lenses had a success rate of 33%. The overall success rate was 41%. Hofmann reviewed the patients' preoperative history of contact lens success or failure. Of the 18 patients who were contact lens failures preoperatively, 13 (72%) were still contact

---

*References 41, 102, 135, 142, 164, 169, 202, 230, 236.
†Ira Shivitz, personal communication, August 1987.

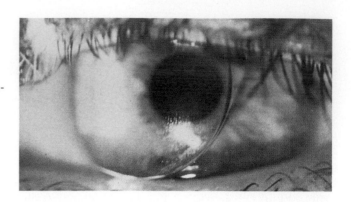

Figure 23-44
Transverse incisions create a break point in the topography, which causes the contact lens to decenter easily. (From Hofmann RF, Starling JC, and Masler W: J Refract Surg 1986;2:155-162.)

lens failures after surgery. For all those patients who were contact lens successes before refractive keratotomy, the chance of success was only 50% after refractive keratotomy.

Patient age and the residual refractive error also are important factors in success. Hofmann et al.[107] analyzed results by age and found a successful fit in 75% of patients under 40 years of age and 36% of patients older than 40. The chance of success for a patient with residual myopia was 55% and 34% with hyperopia, regardless of age. Those patients in whom astigmatic variations were performed with the refractive keratotomy—such as the interrupted transverse or Ruiz trapezoidal procedure—had only an 18% success rate with all types of contact lens attempts (Fig. 23-44). In Hofmann's study, the most common reasons cited for failure were: (1) variable vision, (2) irritation, (3) increased neovascularization, and (4) increased hyperopia.

Shivitz et al.[205,206] also reported on contact lens fitting after refractive keratotomy. These authors reported on 44 eyes of 31 patients that were fitted from a total of 1100 cases (4.0%). In this group, 58.2% were fitted with rigid gas-permeable lenses, 25.5% with daily wear soft lenses, 12.7% with extended wear lenses on a daily wear basis, and 3.6% with silicone lenses. Eleven eyes required refitting; corneal vascularization developed in six eyes with soft lenses, and were subsequently fitted with rigid lenses; and five eyes were changed to soft lenses because of intolerance to rigid lenses. Wearing of contact lenses was discontinued in nine eyes (20.4%) because of poor comfort, inadequate vision, or the desire to have a reoperation. The only complication in this study of contact lens wear after refractive radial keratotomy was corneal neovascularization.[206]

Complications of contact lens wear after keratotomy

The most significant corneal complication has been neovascularization of the incision scars, which occurs in 33% to 61% of patients fitted with soft contact lenses,[107,192,205,206] and rarely with daily wear, rigid, gas-permeable lenses. The mechanisms by which contact lenses induce corneal neovascularization are not well understood. Possibilities include corneal hypoxia, mechanical trauma with metabolic changes, release of chemical mediators from inflammatory cells or injured ocular tissue, and direct toxic effects of the contact lens material.[125] Eyes with incisions made up to or across the limbus are more susceptible to vessel ingrowth, especially if there is epithelial damage at the limbus.[192]

Management of significant corneal vascularization can be a difficult problem. Total cessation of contact lens wear is usually indicated. However, in some patients, changing the contact lens parameters may solve the problem. Attempts should be made to fit a rigid gas-permeable contact lens, where the incidence of neovascularization is quite low. If the fitter is unable to get a satisfactory fit with a rigid contact lens, another soft contact lens with a higher oxygen permeability or better fitting characteristics should be attempted. Recent animal studies have shown that flurbiprofen, an antiinflammatory agent, inhibits contact lens–induced corneal neovascularization in rabbits.[124]

Endothelial cell damage is another area of concern in patients wearing contact lenses after refractive keratotomy. A number of studies have shown changes in the endothelial cells in normal patients wearing hard polymethylmethacrylate and extended wear soft contact lenses.* Contact lenses and refractive keratotomy together might have an additive effect damaging the endothelium. This could be a combination of the initial insult of the refractive keratotomy plus the ongoing hypoxic or toxic insult of the contact lens, with a possible addition of increased mechanical flexing of the cornea after refractive keratotomy beneath the contact lens. These are speculative concerns now and need clinical and experimental documentation before they can be stated as true clinical problems.

Contact lenses, both hard and soft, can induce corneal warpage in normal corneas, and because the cornea after radial keratotomy is more malleable than normal, one might expect an increased incidence of induced astigmatism and varying spherical refractive error. Little has been written about this, and there is a need for documentation of this potential problem. It will be difficult to distinguish normal fluctuation of vision and instability of refraction from the refractive keratotomy itself from that induced by contact lenses. However, the daily fluctuation of vision is seldom more than 1.50 D, and changes over 1 to 4 years seldom exceed 2 D, so larger fluctuations of this sort in the face of contact lens wear might be attributed in part to the contact lens.

Contact lens fitting in patients after keratotomy procedures is a new and unique situation for ophthalmic practitioners. Patients contemplating refractive keratotomy should be strongly counseled that their chances of tolerating contact lenses after the procedure are less than their chances before surgery. Those who are successful contact lens wearers should be encouraged to continue with those contact lenses.[107]

*References 55, 107-114, 132, 140, 154, 165, 170, 224, 237, 245.

UNFINISHED BUSINESS

Better prevention is the major unfinished business concerning complications after refractive keratotomy. Development of improved instruments and algorithms to make the surgery more standardized and predictable will diminish the problems of undercorrection and overcorrection, the frequency of unwanted corneal perforations, and the like. Continued reporting of complications, particularly those occurring many years after surgery, is important to establish the overall risk-benefit ratio for refractive keratotomy.

Studies of patients' experience with presbyopia after radial keratotomy for myopia have not been published; there is a need for documentation of patients' attitudes toward the swapping of dependence on distance glasses for dependence on reading glasses. Especially needed is information on intentionally leaving patients with mild residual myopia and on how possible it is for individuals in the early presbyopic age range to retain good, uncorrected distance and near acuity.

More detailed studies of contrast sensitivity after refractive keratotomy are necessary, particularly after four-incision radial keratotomy, during which the degradation of contrast sensitivity might be diminished. Similarly, studies of glare sensitivity after surgery should be done using modern glare-testing apparatus. All such studies should be carried out with the pupil of normal diameter and also with the pupil dilated, or under controlled mesoic and scotopic testing conditions.

Most important, long-term follow-up of a cohort of refractive keratotomy patients, such as those in the PERK study, must be carried out for 10 to 20 years to identify late, unanticipated complications. The experience of Sato is an example: corneal edema did not occur in his patients until 20 years or more after surgery. Long-term studies can identify instability of refraction and visual acuity (particularly the continued increased effect of the surgery), lipid leakage from vessels in the radial keratotomy wounds, occurrence of late bacterial or fungal keratitis, frequency of corneal rupture with late trauma, long-term loss or damage to the corneal endothelium, and the like.

Such studies also will identify overall patient satisfaction and the frequency of wearing of corrective lenses.

REFERENCES

1. Akiyama K, Tanaka M, Kanai A, and Nakajima A: Problems arising from Sato's radial keratotomy procedure in Japan, CLAO J 1984;10:179-184.

2. Andrade HA, Megeed MA, McDonald M, and Guinsbury A: Changes in contrast sensitivity and refraction after application of 0.5% pilocarpine solution in over- and under-corrected radial keratotomy patients with symptoms of glare and starbursts, Invest Ophthalmol Vis Sci 1990;31(suppl):29.

3. Applegate RA and Gansel KA: The importance of pupil size in optical quality measurements following radial keratotomy, Refract Corneal Surg 1990;6:47-54.

4. Applegate RA, Trick LR, Meade DL, and Hartstein J: Radial keratotomy increases the effects of disability glare: initial results, Ann Ophthalmol 1987;19:293-297.

5. Arciniegas A, Amaya L, Velasquez G, et al: Corneal astigmatism induced by the combination of arc and radial keratotomies: experimental research in rabbits, J Refract Surg 1986;2:67-77.

6. Arrowsmith PN and Marks RG: Visual, refractive, and keratometric results of radial keratotomy: 1-year follow-up, Arch Ophthalmol 1984; 102:1612-1617.

7. Arrowsmith PN and Marks RG: Visual, refractive, and keratometric results of radial keratotomy: a 2-year follow-up, Arch Ophthalmol 1987; 105:76-80.

8. Arrowsmith PN and Marks RG: Visual, refractive and keratometric results of radial keratotomy: five-year follow-up. Arch Ophthalmol 1989; 107:506-511.

9. Arrowsmith PN, Deitz MR, Marks RG, et al: Radial keratotomy: ARK Study Group, Thorofare, NJ, 1984, Slack, Inc.

10. Asbell PA, Obstbaum S, and Justin N: Peripheral corneal endothelial evaluation post radial keratotomy in PERK patients, Ophthalmology 1984;91 (suppl 2):122.

11. Atkin A, Asbell P, Justin N, et al: Radial keratotomy and glare effects on contrast sensitivity, Doc Ophthalmol 1986;62:129-148.

12. Baldone JA and Franklin RM: Cataract following radial keratotomy, Ann Ophthalmol 1983;15:416-418.

13. Barker B and Swinger C: Complications of corneal refractive surgery. In Schwab IR, editor: Refractive keratoplasty, New York, 1987, Churchill-Livingstone, pp 227-272.

14. Barraquer J: Transient descemetocele following radial keratotomy, Refract Corneal Surg 1989;5:314.

15. Baum JL and Jones DB: Inteal therapy of suspected microbial corneal ulcers, Surv Ophthalmol 1979;24:97-116.

16. Beard C: Ptosis, ed 2, St Louis, 1976, The CV Mosby Co, p 67.

17. Beasley H and Fraunfelder FT: Retinal detachments and topical ocular miotics, Ophthalmology 1979;85:95-98.

18. Beatty RF, Robin JB, and Schanzlin DJ: Penetrating keratoplasty after radial keratotomy, J Refract Surg 1986;2:207-214.

19. Beatty RF and Smith RE: 30-year follow-up of posterior radial keratotomy, Am J Ophthalmol 1987;103: 330-331.

20. Beverman RW and Schimmelpfennig B: Sensory denervation of the rabbit cornea affects epithelial properties, Exp Neurol 1980;69:196.

21. Binder PS: Optical problems following refractive surgery, Ophthalmology 1986;93:739-745.

22. Binder PS: Presumed epithelial ingrowth following radial keratotomy, CLAO J 1986;12:247-250.

23. Binder PS, Able LR, Polack FM, et al: Keratoplasty wound separations, Am J Ophthalmol 1975;80:105-115.

24. Binder PS, Nayak SK, Deg JK, et al: An ultrastructural and histochemical study of long-term wound healing after radial keratotomy, Am J Ophthalmol 1987;103:432-440.

25. Binder PS, Waring GO, Arrowsmith PN, and Wang CL: Traumatic rupture of the cornea after radial keratotomy, Arch Ophthalmol 1988;106:1584-1590.

26. Bores L: Results of radial keratotomy after two years. In Schachar RA, Levy NS, and Schachar L, editors: Refractive modulation of the cornea, Denison, Tex, 1981, LAL Publishing, pp 123-131.

27. Bores LD: Radial keratotomy. I. A safe, effective way to correct a handicap, Surv Ophthalmol 1983;28:101-105.

28. Bores LD, Myers W, and Cowden J: Radial keratotomy: an analysis of the American experience, Ann Ophthalmol 1981;13:941-948.

29. Bourque LB, Cosand BB, Drews C, et al: Reported satisfaction, fluctuation of vision, and glare among patients one year after surgery in the Prospective Evaluation of Radial Keratotomy (PERK) study, Arch Ophthalmol 1986;104:356-363.

30. Bourque LB, Rubenstein R, Cosand B, et al: Psychosocial characteristics of candidates for the Prospective Evaluation of Radial Keratotomy (PERK) study, Arch Ophthalmol 1984;102: 1187-1192.

31. Brodsky ME, Bauerberg JM, and Sterzovsky A: Case report: probably fluorescein-induced uveitis following radial keratotomy, J Refract Surg 1987;3:28-29.

32. Busin M, Suarez H, Bieber S, and McDonald MD: Overcorrected visual acuity improved by antiglaucoma medication after radial keratotomy, Am J Ophthalmol 1985;101:374-375.

33. Busin M, Yau CW, Avini I, et al: The effect of changes in intraocular pressure on corneal curvature after radial keratotomy in the rabbit eye, Ophthalmology 1986;93:331-334.

34. Busin M, Yau CE, Yamaguchi T, et al: The effect of collagen cross-linkage inhibitors on rabbit corneas after radial keratotomy, Invest Ophthalmol Vis Sci 1986;27:1001-1005.

35. Calkins JL, Hochheimer BF, and Stark WJ: Corneal wound healing: holographic stress-test analysis, Invest Ophthalmol Vis Sci 1981;21:322-334.

36. Carlson KA and Goosey JD: Epikeratoplasty following overcorrected radial keratotomy, Invest Ophthalmol Vis Sci 1988;29:390.

37. Carroll RP and Lindstrom RL: Blepharoptosis after radial keratotomy, Am J Ophthalmol 1986;102:800

38. Chiba K, Oak SS, Tsubota K, et al: Morphometric analysis of corneal endothelium following radial keratotomy, J Cataract Refract Surg 1987;13:263-267.

39. Cogan DG, Donaldson DD, Kuwabara T, and Marshall D: Microcystic dystrophy of the corneal epithelium, Trans Am Ophthalmol Soc 1982;62:213-221.

40. Condon PI and Hill DW: The testing of experimental corneal wounds stitched with modern corneal scleral sutures: experimental corneal wound healing, Ophthalmol Res 1973;5:137-150.

41. Cottingham AJ, Berkeley RG, Nordan LT, et al: Bacterial corneal ulcers following keratorefractive surgery: a retrospective study of 14,163 procedures, read before the Ocular Microbiology and Immunology Group Meeting, San Francisco, September 28, 1986.

42. Cowden JW, Lynn MJ, Waring GO, and the PERK Study Group: Repeated radial keratotomy in the Prospective Evaluation of Radial Keratotomy study, Am J Ophthalmol 1987;103: 423-431.

43. Cross WD and Head WJ: Complications of radial keratotomy: an overview. In Sanders D, Hofmann RF, and Salz J, editors: Refractive corneal surgery, Thorofare, NJ, 1986, Slack, Inc, pp 347-399.

44. Darakjian NE and Marchese A: Assessment of corneal strength post radial keratotomy in rabbit eyes, Invest Ophthalmol Vis Sci 1982;22(suppl): 26.

45. Davis DB: Retrobulbar and facial nerve block? No; peribulbar? Yes? Ophthalmic Surg 1985;16:604.

46. Davis DB II and Mandel MR: Posterior peribulbar anesthesia: an alternative to retrobulbar anesthesia, Geriatr Ophthalmol 1987;3:27-34.

47. Davis RM, Miller RA, Lindstrom RL, et al: Corneal iron lines after radial keratotomy, J Refract Surg 1988;2:174-178.

48. Deg JK, Zavala EY, and Binder PS: Delayed corneal wound healing following radial keratotomy, Ophthalmology 1985;92:734-740.

49. Deitz MR and Sanders DR: Hyperopia in long-term follow-up of radial keratotomy, Ophthalmology 1985;92 (suppl 2):55.

50. Deitz MR and Sanders DR: Progressive hyperopia with long-term follow-up of radial keratotomy, Arch Ophthalmol 1985;103:782-784.

51. Deitz MR, Sanders DR, and Marks RG: Radial keratotomy: an overview of the Kansas City study, Ophthalmology 1984;91:467-478.

52. Deitz MR, Sanders DR, and Raanan MG: Progressive hyperopia in radial keratotomy: long-term follow-up of diamond knife and metal blade series, Ophthalmology 1986;93:1284-1289.

53. Deitz MR, Sanders DR, and Raanan MG: A consecutive series (1982-1985) of radial keratotomies performed with the diamond blade. II. Am J Ophthalmol 1987;103:417-422.

54. Dunn S, Jester JV, Arthur J, and Smith RE: Endothelial cell loss following radial keratotomy in a primate model, Arch Ophthalmol 1984;102: 1666-1670.

55. Edwards GA and Schaefer MK: Corneal flattening associated with daily wear soft contact lenses following radial keratotomy, J Refract Surg 1987;3:54-58.

56. Efron N, Holden BA, and Vannas A: Prostaglandin-inhibitor naproxen does not affect contact lens–induced changes in the human corneal endothelium, Am J Optom Physiol Optics 1984;61:741-744.

57. Ellis W: Radial keratotomy and astigmatism surgery, Irvine, Calif, 1986, Keith C. Terry and Associates, pp 117-130.

58. Evans DW and Ginsburg AP: Contrast sensitivity predicts age-related differences in highway sign discriminability, Hum Factors 1985;27:637-642.

59. Farley MK and Pettit TH: Traumatic wound dehiscence in penetrating keratoplasty, Am J Ophthalmol 1987;104:44-49.

60. Fiorentini A and Maffei L: Spatial contrast sensitivity of myopic subjects, Invest Ophthalmol Vis Sci 1976;16:437-443.

61. Forster RK: Endophthalmitis. In Duane TD, editor: Clinical ophthalmology, vol 4, Philadelphia, 1988, JB Lippincott Co, pp 1-24.

62. Forstot SL and Damiano RE: Trauma following radial keratotomy, Ophthalmology 1987;94:127.

63. Forstot SL, Damiano RE, and Duke D: Molding contact lenses for hyperopia following radial keratotomy (unpublished data).

64. Foulks GN: Refractive keratoplasty: keratomileusis, keratophakia, and epikeratophakia, Trans Pa Acad Ophthalmol Otolaryngol 1982;35:122-124.

65. Fox SA: Surgery for ptosis (blepharoptosis), New York, 1968, Grune & Stratton, p 23.

66. Franks JB and Binder PS: Keratotomy procedures for the correction of astigmatism, J Refract Surg 1985;1:11-17.

67. Franks S: Radial keratotomy undercorrections: a new approach, J Refract Surg 1986;2:171-173.

68. Friedman AH: Late traumatic wound rupture following successful partial penetrating keratoplasty, Am J Ophthalmol 1973;75:117-120.

69. Fritch CD: Post-RK patient presents retinal detachment after successful surgical treatment, Ophthalmol Times, Sept 1, 1987, p 18.

70. Fyodorov SN: Surgical correction of myopia and astigmatism. In Schachar RA, Levy NS, and Schachar L, editors: Keratorefraction, Denison, Tex, 1980, LAL Publishing, pp 141-172.

71. Fyodorov SN: Radial keratotomy. In Schachar RA, Levy NS, and Schachar L, editors: Refractive modulation of the cornea, Denison, Tex, 1981, LAL Publishing, pp 89-122.

72. Fyodorov SN and Durnev VV: Operation of dosaged dissection of corneal circular ligament in cases of myopia of mild degree, Ann Ophthalmol 1979;11:1885-1890.

73. Fyodorov SN and Durnev VV: Surgical correction of complicated myopic astigmatism by means of dissection of circular ligament of cornea, Ann Ophthalmol 1981;13:115-118.

74. Fyodorov SN, Sarkizova MB, and Kurasova TP: Corneal biomicroscopy following repeated radial keratotomy, Ann Ophthalmol 1983;15:403-407.

75. Garland MA: Monovision and related techniques in the management of presbyopia, CLAO J 1987;13:179-180.

76. Gasset AR and Dohlman CH: The tensile strength of corneal wounds, Arch Ophthalmol 1968;79:595-602.

77. Geggel HS: Delayed sterile keratitis following radial keratotomy requiring corneal transplantation for visual rehabilitation, Refract Corneal Surg 1990;6:55-58.

78. Gelender H, Flynn HW, and Mandelbaum SH: Bacterial endophthalmitis resulting from radial keratotomy, Am J Ophthalmol 1982;93:323-326.

79. Gelender H and Gelber EC: Cataract following radial keratotomy, Arch Ophthalmol 1983;101:1229-1231.

80. Gills JP: Trephination in combination with radial keratotomy for myopia. In Schachar RA, Levy NS, and Schachar L, editors: Radial keratotomy, Denison, Tex, 1980, LAL Publishing, pp 91-99.

81. Gills JP and Lloyd T: Peribulbar vs. retrobulbar anesthesia; a real difference? Ophthalmic Surg 1986;17:764 (letter).

82. Ginsburg AP: A new contrast sensitivity vision test chart, Am J Optom Physiol Opt 1984;61:403-407.

83. Ginsburg AP: Sine-wave gradings are more visually sensitive than disks or letters, J Opt Soc Am 1984;1:1301.

84. Ginsburg AP: The evaluation of contact lenses and refractive surgery using contrast sensitivity. In Dabezies OH, editor: Contact lenses: the CLAO guide to basic science and clinical practice, Update 2, 1987;6.1-56.17.

85. Ginsburg AP, Easterly J, and Evans DW: Contrast sensitivity predicts target detection field performance of pilots, Proceedings of the Human Factors Society 27th Annual Meeting, 1983;1:269-273.

86. Ginsburg AP, Evans DW, Cannon MR Jr, Owsley C, and Mulvanny P: Large-sample norms for contrast sensitivity, Am J Optom Physiol Opt 1984;61:80-84.

87. Ginsburg AP, Evans DW, Sekuler R, and Harp SA: Contrast sensitivity predicts pilots' performance in aircraft simulators, Am J Optom Physiol Opt 1982;59:105-109.

88. Ginsburg AP, Steinberg EB, Justin N, et al: Effects of radial keratotomy on contrast sensitivity in the Prospective Evaluation of Radial Keratotomy (PERK) study, Ophthalmology 1984; 91(suppl 2):121.

89. Ginsburg AP, Waring GO, Steinberg EB, et al: Contrast sensitivity under photopic conditions in the Prospective Evaluation of Radial Keratotomy (PERK) study, Refract Corneal Surg 1990;6:82-91.

90. Girard LJ, Rodriguez J, Nino N, and Wesson M: Delayed wound healing after radial keratotomy, Am J Ophthalmol 1985;99:485-486.

91. Girard LJ, Wesson ME, Vesequlinovic A, and Maghraby A: Case report: overcorrection of radial and arc keratotomies—two years postoperatively, J Refract Surg 1985;2:232.

92. Grady FJ: Experience with radial keratotomy, Ophthalmic Surg 1982;13: 395-399.

93. Grant MW: Toxicology of the eye, Springfield, Ill, 1974, Charles C Thomas Publishers, pp 136-139.

94. Grayson M: Disease of the cornea, St Louis, 1983, The CV Mosby Co, pp 241-244.

95. Guillon M, Schock SE, Holden BA, and Kotow M: Radial keratotomy: visual performance considerations, Arch Ophthalmol (in press).

96. Guth SK and McNelis JR: Threshold contrast as a function of target complexity, Am J Optom Physiol Opt 1969;46:98.

97. Harris DJ, Stulting RD, Waring GO, et al: Late bacterial and fungal keratitis following corneal transplantation, Ophthalmology 1987;94(suppl):75.

98. Havener WH: Ocular pharmacology, ed 5, St Louis, 1983, The CV Mosby Co, pp 77-79.

99. Hays JC, Rowsey JJ, and Balyeat HD: Effect of postoperative steroids on the refractive result of radial keratotomy, Invest Ophthalmol Vis Sci 1985; 26:150.

100. Hemenger RP, Tomlinson A, and Caroline PJ: Role of spherical aberration contrast sensitivity loss with radial keratotomy, Invest Ophthalmol Vis Sci 1989;30:1997-2001.

101. Hemenger RP, Tomlinson A, and McDonnell PJ: Optics of the post-RK cornea, Invest Ophthalmol Vis Sci 1990;31(suppl):29.

102. Hoffer KJ, Darin JJ, Pettit TH, et al: Three years experience with radial keratotomy: the UCLA study, Ophthalmology 1983;90:627-636.

103. Hofmann RF: The surgical correction of idiopathic astigmatism. In Sanders D, Hofmann RF, and Salz J, editors: Refractive corneal surgery, Thorofare, NJ, 1986, Slack, Inc, pp 20-32.

104. Hofmann RF: Reoperations after radial keratotomy and astigmatic keratotomy, J Refract Surg 1987;3:119-128.

105. Hofmann RF and Lindstrom RL: Sources of error in keratotomy knife incisions, J Refract Surg 1987;3:215-223.

106. Hofmann RF, Starling JC, and Hovland KR: Case report: retinal detachment after radial keratotomy surgery, J Refract Surg 1985;1:226-230.

107. Hofmann RF, Starling JC, and Masler W: Contact fitting after radial keratotomy: one year results, J Refract Surg 1986;2:155-162.

108. Holden BA, Sweeney DF, Vannas A, Kotow M, La Hood D, Grant T, Swarbrick H, and Efron N: Contact lens–induced endothelial polymegathism, Invest Ophthalmol Vis Sci 1985;suppl 26:275.

109. Holden BA, Sweeney DF, Vannas A, Nilsson KT, and Efron N: The effects of long-term extended wear of contact lenses on the human cornea, Invest Ophthalmol Vis Sci, 1984;suppl 25:192.

110. Holden BA, Vannas A, Nilsson K, Efron N, Sweeney D, Kotow M, La Hood D, and Guillon M: Epithelial and endothelial effects from the extended wear of contact lenses, Curr Eye Res 1985;4:739-742.

111. Holden BA, Williams L, and Zantos SG: The etiology of transient endothelial changes in the human cornea, Invest Ophthalmol Vis Sci 1985;26:1489-1501.

112. Holden BA, Sweeney DF, Vannas A, Nilsson KT, and Efron N: Effects of long-term extended contact lens wear on the human cornea, Invest Ophthalmol Vis Sci 1985;26:1489-1501.

113. Holden BA, Mertz GW, and McNally JJ: Corneal swelling response to contact lenses worn under extended wear conditions, Invest Ophthalmol Vis Sci 1983;24:218-226.

114. Holden BA and Zantos SG: The corneal endothelium and contact lenses, Int Contact Lens Clin 1978;5:10-14.

115. Holden BA and Zantos SG: Corneal endothelium: transient changes with atmospheric anoxia. In The cornea in health and disease, Proc VI Cong Europ Soc Ophthalmol, Royal Soc Med Series, London 1981;40:79-83.

116. Holladay LL: The fundamentals of glare and visibility, J Opt Soc Amer 1929;12:271-319.

117. Ingraham HJ, Guber D, and Green WR: Radial keratotomy: clinicopathologic case report, Arch Ophthalmol 1985;103:683-688.

118. Jaffe NS: Cataract surgery and its complications, ed 5, St Louis, 1990, The CV Mosby Co, pp 429-464.

119. Jester JV, Miyashiro JE, Rife L, and Smith RE: Radial keratotomy in primate eyes: pathologic studies, Invest Ophthalmol Vis Sci 1982;29(suppl):69.

120. Jester JV, Villasenor RA, and Miyashiro J: Epithelial inclusion cysts following radial keratotomy, Arch Ophthalmol 1983;101:611-615.

121. John ME and Schmitt TE: Traumatic hyphema after radial keratotomy, Ann Ophthalmol 1983;15:930-932.

122. Karlin J: Treatment of small undercorrections and overcorrections in radial keratotomy, Arch Ophthalmol 1986;104:177.

123. Karr DJ, Grutzmacher RD, and Reeh MJ: Radial keratotomy complicated by sterile keratitis and corneal perforation, Ophthalmology 1985;92:1244-1248.

124. Katz HR, Aizuss DH, and Mondino BJ: Inhibition of contact lens–induced corneal neovascularization in radial keratotomized rabbit eyes, Cornea 1984;3:65-72.

125. Katz HR, Duffin RM, Glasser DB, and Pettit TH: Complications of contact lens wear after radial keratotomy in an animal model, Am J Ophthalmol 1982;94:377-382.

126. Kaufman HE: Refractive surgery, Am J Ophthalmol 1987;103:355-357.

127. Keates RH, Watson SA, and Levy SN: Epikeratophakia following previous refractive keratoplasty surgery: two case reports, J Cataract Refract Surg 1986;12:536-540.

128. Kimble JA, Morris RE, Witherspoon CD, et al: Globe perforation from peribulbar injection, Arch Ophthalmol 1987;105:749.

129. Krasnov MM, Avetisov Se, Madashova NV, and Mamikonian VR: The effect of radial keratotomy on contrast sensitivity, Am J Ophthalmol 1988;105:651-654.

130. Kremer FB and Marks RG: Radial keratotomy: prospective evaluation of safety and efficacy, Ophthalmic Surg 1983;14:925-930.

131. Kremer FB and Steer RA: Stability of refraction following radial keratotomy over four years, J Refract Surg 1986;2:217-220.

132. Kwok LS: Endothelial oxygen levels during anterior corneal hypoxia, Aust J Optom 1985;68:58-62.

133. Larson BC, Kremer FB, Eller AW, and Bernardino VB: Quantitated trauma following radial keratotomy in rabbits, Ophthalmology 1983;90:660-667.

134. Lewicky A: Surgical technique and related complications. In Sanders D, Hofmann RF, and Salz J, editors: Refractive corneal surgery, Thorofare, NJ, 1986, Slack, Inc, pp 163-195.

135. Lewicky A and Salz J: Special report: radial keratotomy survey, J Refract Surg 1986;2:32-33.

136. Linberg JV, McDonald M, Safir A, and Googe JM: Ptosis following radial keratotomy: performed using a rigid eyelid speculum, Ophthalmology 1986;93:1509-1512.

137. Lindquist TD, Rubenstein JB, and Lindstrom RL: Correction of hyperopia following radial keratotomy: quantification in human cadaver eyes, Ophthalmic Surg 1987;18:432-437.

138. Luttrull JK, Jester JV, and Smith RE: The effect of radial keratotomy on ocular integrity in an animal model, Arch Ophthalmol 1982;100:319-320.

139. Lynn MJ, Waring GO, Arentsen J, et al: Prospective Evaluation of Radial Keratotomy (PERK) study: results four years after surgery, Invest Ophthalmol Vis Sci 1988;29:310.

140. MacRae SM, Matsuda M, and Rich LF: The effects of radial keratotomy on the corneal endothelium, Am J Ophthalmol 1985;100:538-542.

141. Maloney RK, Stark WJ, McCally RL, et al: The refractive change induced by radial keratotomy is not affected by intraocular pressure, Ophthalmology 1987;94(suppl):128.

142. Mandelbaum S, Waring GO, Forster RK, et al: Late development of ulcerative keratitis in radial keratotomy scars, Arch Ophthalmol 1986;104:1156-1160.

143. Manka RL and Gast TJ: Endophthalmitis following Ruiz procedure, Arch Ophthalmol 1990;108:21 (letter to the editor).

144. Markovits A: Extracapsular cataract extraction with posterior chamber intraocular lens implantation in a post radial keratotomy patient, Arch Ophthalmol 1986;104:329-331.

145. Marmer RH: Radial keratotomy complications, Ann Ophthalmol 1987;19:409-411.

146. Marmer RH: Ocular deviation induced by radial keratotomy, Ann Ophthalmol 1987;19:451-452.

147. Maurice DM: The biology of wound healing in the corneal stroma: Castroviejo lecture, Cornea 1987;6:162-168.

148. McClellan KA, Bernard PJ, et al: Suppurative keratitis: a late complication of radial keratotomy, J Cataract Refract Surg 1988;14:317-320.

149. McDonald MB: Epikeratophakia following radial keratotomy (personal oral communication, November 1989).

150. McDonald MB, Haik M, and Kaufman HE: Color vision and contrast sensitivity testing after radial keratotomy, Am J Ophthalmol 1987;103:468.

151. McDonnell PJ, Lean JS, and Schanzlin DJ: Globe rupture from blunt trauma after hexagonal keratotomy, Am J Ophthalmol 1987;103:241-242.

152. McDonnell PJ and Schanzlin DJ: Early changes in refractive error following radial keratotomy, Arch Ophthalmol 1988;106:212-214.

153. McKnight SJ, Fitz J, and Giangiacoma J: Corneal rupture following radial keratotomy in cats subjected to BB gun injury, Ophthalmic Surg 1988;19:165-167.

154. McMonnies CW and Zantos SG: Endothelial bedewing of the cornea in association with contact lens wear, Br J Ophthalmol 1979;63:478-481.

155. Menezo JL, Harto MA, and Cisneros AL: Light-induced maculopathy from the operating microscope in radial keratotomy, J Refract Surg 1988;4:179-182.

156. Milder B and Rubin M: The fine art of prescribing glasses without making a spectacle of yourself, Gainesville, Fla, 1978, Triad Scientific Publishers, pp 68-69.

157. Miller D and Miller R: Glare sensitivity in simulated radial keratotomy, Arch Ophthalmol 1981;99:1961-1962.

158. Moorhead LC, Carroll J, Constance G, et al: Effects of topical treatment with beta-aminopropionitrile after radial keratotomy in the rabbit, Arch Ophthalmol 1984;102:304-307.

159. Nelson JD, Williams P, Lindstrom RL, and Doughman DJ: Map-finger-dot changes in the corneal epithelial basement membrane following radial keratotomy, Ophthalmology 1985;92:199-205.

160. Neumann AC: Preliminary statistical analysis of radial keratotomy. In Schachar RA, Levy NS, and Schachar L, editors: Refractive modulation of the cornea, Denison, Tex, 1981, LAL Publishing, pp 277-284.

161. Neumann AC, Ochsner RH, and Fenzl RE: Radial keratotomy: a clinical and statistical analysis, Cornea 1983;2:47-55.

162. Neumann AC, Ochsner RH, and Fenzl RE: Radial keratotomy: a comprehensive evaluation, Doc Ophthalmol 1984;56:275-301.

163. Nordan LT and Havins WE: Undercorrected radial keratotomy treated with myopic keratomileusis, J Refract Surg 1985;1:56-58.

164. O'Day DM, Feman SS, and Elliott JH: Visual impairment following radial keratotomy: a cluster of cases, Ophthalmology 1986;93:319-326.

165. O'Neal MR, Polse KA, Holden BA, and Efron N: Time course of human cornea hydration recovery from induced edema—study of endothelial pump function, Invest Ophthalmol Vis Sci 1984;suppl 25:192.

166. Paris GL and Quickert MH: Disinsertion of the aponeurosis of the levator palpebrae superioris muscle after cataract extraction, Am J Ophthalmol 1976;81:337-340.

167. Pavan-Langston D: Viral diseases. In Smolin G and Thoft R, editors: The cornea, Boston, 1983, Little, Brown & Co, pp 178-195.

168. Peyman GA and Spigelman AV: Reduction of glare after radial keratotomy: an experimental study, Ophthalmic Surg 1981;12:727-730.

169. Poggio EC, Glynn RJ, Schein OD, Seddon JM, Shannon MJ, Scardino VA, and Kenyon KR: The incidence of ulcerative keratitis among users of daily-wear and extended-wear soft contact lenses, N Engl J Med 1989;321:779-783.

170. Polse KA, Holden BA, and Sweeney D: Corneal edema accompanying aphakic extended lens wear, Arch Ophthalmol 1983;101:1038-1041.

171. Powell K: Radial keratotomy: a continuing controversy, J Ophthalmol Nurs Tec 1986;4:6-13.

172. Raber IM, Arenson JJ, and Laibson PR: Traumatic wound dehiscence after penetrating keratoplasty, Arch Ophthalmol 1980;98:1407-1409.

173. Ramsay RC and Knobloch WH: Ocular perforation following retrobulbar anesthesia for retinal detachment surgery, Am J Ophthalmol 1978;86:61-64.

174. Reader AL and Salz JJ: Differences among ultrasonic pachymeters in measuring corneal thickness, J Refract Surg 1987;3:7-11.

175. Reed JW and Dohlman CH: Corneal cysts: a report of eight cases, Arch Ophthalmol 1971;86:648-652.

176. Richmond RD: Special report: radial keratotomy as seen through operated eyes, J Refract Surg 1987;3:22-27.

177. Robin JB, Beatty RF, Dunn S, et al: *Mycobacterium chelonei* keratitis after radial keratotomy, Am J Ophthalmol 1986;102:72-79.

178. Rowsey JJ and Balyeat HD: Preliminary results and complications of radial keratotomy, Am J Ophthalmol 1982;93:437-455.

179. Rowsey JJ and Balyeat HD: Radial keratotomy: preliminary report of complications, Ophthalmic Surg 1982;13:27-35.

180. Rowsey JJ, Balyeat HD, Monlux R, et al: Endothelial cell loss after radial keratotomy, Ophthalmology 1987;94 (suppl):97.

181. Rowsey JJ, Balyeat HD, Rabinovitch B, Burris TE, and Hays JC: Complications of radial keratotomy, Twenty-fifth International Congress of Ophthalmology, 1983.

182. Rylander HG, Welch AJ, and Fleming B: The effect of radial keratotomy in the rupture strength of pig eyes, Ophthalmic Surg 1983;14:744-749.

183. Salz JJ: Progressive endothelial cell loss following repeat radial keratotomy—a case report, Ophthalmic Surg 1982;13:997-999.

184. Salz JJ: Improving the results of radial keratotomy, J Refract Surg 1985;1:167-171.

185. Salz JJ: Multiple complications following radial keratotomy in an elderly patient: a case report, Ophthalmic Surg 1985;16:579-580.

186. Salz JJ: Four-incision radial keratotomy for low to moderate myopia and eight-incision radial keratotomy for high myopia. In Sanders DR, editor: Radial keratotomy: surgical technique, Thorofare, NJ, 1986, Slack, Inc, pp 3-34.

187. Salz JJ: How safe is radial keratotomy? J Refract Surg 1987;3:188-189.

188. Salz JJ, Villasenor RA, Elander R, et al: Four-incision radial keratotomy for low to moderate myopia, Ophthalmology 1985;92:73.

189. Sampson WG: Applied optical principles, Int Ophthalmol Clin 1971;11:81-102.

190. Sanders DR, editor: Radial keratotomy: surgical techniques, Thorofare, NJ, 1986, Slack, Inc.

191. Sanders DR, Deitz MR, and Gallagher D: Factors affecting predictability of radial keratotomy. In Sanders DR, Hofmann RF, and Salz JJ, editors: Refractive corneal surgery, Thorofare, NJ, 1986, Slack, Inc, pp 79-90.

192. Sanders DR, Hofmann RF, Salz JJ, editors: Refractive corneal surgery, Thorofare, NJ, 1986, Slack, Inc.

193. Santos CI: Herpes keratitis after radial keratotomy, Am J Ophthalmol 1982; 93:370 (letter).

194. Santos CI: Reply to letter to the editor (Porter J: Herpes keratitis after radial keratotomy), Am J Ophthalmol 1982;93:806-807.

195. Santos CI: Herpetic corneal ulcer following radial keratotomy, Ann Ophthalmol 1983;15:82-85.

196. Sawelson H and Marks RG: Two-year results of radial keratotomy, Arch Ophthalmol 1985;103:505-510.

197. Sawelson H and Marks RG: Three-year results of radial keratotomy, Arch Ophthalmol 1987;105:81-85.

198. Schachar RA: Understanding radial keratotomy, Ophthalmic Forum 1982;1:22-23.

199. Schachar RA: Indications, techniques, and complications of radial keratotomy, Int Ophthalmol Clin 1983;23: 119 128.

200. Schachar RA, Levy NS, and Schachar L: Refractive keratoplasty, Denison, Tex, 1983, LAL Publishing, pp 328-396.

201. Schanzlin DJ, Santos VR, Waring GO, et al: Diurnal change in refraction, corneal curvature, visual acuity, and intraocular pressure after radial keratotomy in the PERK study, Ophthalmology 1986;93:167-175.

202. Schein OD, Glynn RJ, Poggio EC, Seddon JM, Kenyon KR, and the Microbial Keratitis Study Group: The relative risk of ulcerative keratitis among users of daily-wear and extended-wear soft contact lenses: a case-control study, N Engl J Med 1989;321:773-778.

203. Shivitz IA and Arrowsmith PN: Delayed keratitis after radial keratotomy, Arch Ophthalmol 1986;104:1153-1155.

204. Shivitz IA and Arrowsmith PN: Corneal sensitivity following radial keratotomy, Ophthalmology 1987;94(suppl): 97.

205. Shivitz IA, Russell BM, and Arrowsmith PN: Contact lenses in the treatment of patients with overcorrected radial keratotomy, Ophthalmology 1987;94:899-903.

206. Shivitz IA, Russell BM, Arrowsmith PN, and Marks RG: Optical correction of postoperative radial keratotomy patients with contact lenses, CLAO J 1986;12:59-62.

207. Shultz R, Matsuto M, Yee R, et al: Corneal endothelial changes in type I and type II diabetes melitis, Am J Ophthalmol 1984;98:401-410.

208. Sigelman S and Friedenwald JS: Miotic and wound healing activities of the corneal epithelium: effect of sensory denervation, Arch Ophthalmol 1954;52:46.

209. Simmons KB and Linsalata RP: Ruptured globe following blunt trauma after radial keratotomy, Ophthalmology 1987;94:148.

210. Smith RE, Spence D, Dunn S, and Rife L: Assessment of chronic corneal endothelial changes in experimental radial keratotomy (primates), Invest Ophthalmol Vis Sci 1983;24:148.

211. Spigelman AV, Williams PA, Nichols BD, and Lindstrom RL: Four-incision radial keratotomy, J Cataract Refract Surg 1988;14:125-128.

212. Spivak L: Case report: radial keratotomy incisions remain intact despite facial trauma from plane crash, J Refract Surg 1987;3·59-60.

213. Stark WJ, Martin NF, and Maumenee EA: Radial keratotomy. II. A risky procedure of unproven long-term success, Surv Ophthalmol 1983;28:106-111.

214. Starling J and Hofmann R: A new surgical technique for the correction of hyperopia after radial keratotomy: an experimental model, J Refract Surg 1986;2:9-14.

215. Starling J and Hofmann R: Case report: anterior uveitis and transient hyperopia following radial keratotomy, J Refract Surg 1986;2:96-98.

216. Steinberg EB, Wilson LA, Waring GO, et al: Stellate iron lines in the corneal epithelium after radial keratotomy, Am J Ophthalmol 1984;98:416-421.

217. Stern GA, Weitzenkorn D, and Valenti J: Adherence of *Pseudomonas aeruginosa* to the mouse cornea: epithelial vs. stromal adherence, Arch Ophthalmol 1982;100:1956-1958.

218. Straatsma BR, Zeegan PD, Foos RY, et al: Lattice degeneration of the retina, Am J Ophthalmol 1974;77:619-649.

219. Sweeney DF, Holden BA, Vannas A, Efron N, Swarbrick H, Kotow M, and Chan-Ling T: The clinical significance of corneal endothelial polymegathism, Invest Ophthalmol Vis Sci 1985; (suppl) 26:53.

220. Swinger CA and Barker BA: Myopic keratomileusis following radial keratotomy, J Refract Surg 1985;1:53-55.

221. Theodore FH: Idiosyncratic reactions of the cornea from proparicaine, Eye Ear Nose Throat Monthly 1968;47: 286-291.

222. Topping TM, Stark WJ, Maumenee M, and Kenyon KR: Traumatic wound dehiscence following penetrating keratoplasty, Br J Ophthalmol 1982;66: 174-178.

223. Trick LR and Hartstein J: Investigation of contrast sensitivity following radial keratotomy, Ann Ophthalmol 1987; 19:251-254.

224. Vannas A, Holden B, Makitie J, Ruusuvaara P, and O'Donnell JJ: Specular microscopy and ultrastructure of endothelial blebs, Invest Ophthalmol Vis Sci 1979;suppl 18:143.

225. Vaughn ER: The four-cut radial keratotomy in low myopia, J Refract Surg 1984;2:164-169.

226. Villasenor RA, Salz J, Steel D, and Krasnow MA: Changes in corneal thickness during radial keratotomy, Ophthalmic Surg 1981;12:341-342.

227. Waring GO: Posterior collagenous layer of the cornea: ultrastructural classification of abnormal collagenous tissue posterior to Descemet's membrane in 30 cases, Arch Ophthalmol 1982;100:122-134.

228. Waring GO: The changing status of radial keratotomy for myopia, Part II. J Refract Surg 1985;1:119-137.

229. Waring GO: Short-term results of the Prospective Evaluation of Radial Keratotomy (PERK) study. In Sanders D, Hofmann RF, and Salz J, editors: Refractive corneal surgery, Thorofare, NJ, 1986, Slack, Inc, pp 313-346.

230. Waring GO, Lynn MJ, Culbertson W, et al: Three year results of the Prospective Evaluation of Radial Keratotomy (PERK) study, Ophthalmology 1987; 94:1339-1354.

231. Waring GO, Lynn MJ, Fielding B, et al: Results of the Prospective Evaluation of Radial Keratotomy (PERK) study 4 years after surgery for myopia, JAMA 1990;263:1083-1091.

232. Waring GO, Lynn MJ, Gelender H, et al: Results of the Prospective Evaluation of Radial Keratotomy (PERK) study one year after surgery, Ophthalmology 1985;92:177-198.

233. Waring GO, Moffitt SD, Gelender H, et al: Rationale for and design of the National Eye Institute Prospective Evaluation of Radial Keratotomy (PERK) study, Ophthalmology 1983;90:40-58.

234. Waring GO, Sperduto R, Moffitt SD, Bourque L, and the PERK Study Group: Changes in refraction, keratometry, and visual acuity during the first year after radial keratotomy in the PERK study, Invest Ophthalmol Vis Sci 1985;26(suppl):202.

235. Waring GO, Steinberg ED, and Wilson LA: Slit-lamp microscopic appearance of corneal wound healing after radial keratotomy, Am J Ophthalmol 1985;100:218-224.

236. Wilhelmus KR and Hamburg S: Bacterial keratitis following radial keratotomy, Cornea 1983;2:143-146.

237. Williams I and Holden BA: The bleb response of the endothelium decreases with extended wear of contact lenses, Clin Exp Optom 1986;69:90-92.

238. Wilson RP: Anesthesia. In Spaeth GL, editor: Ophthalmic surgery: principles and practice, Philadelphia, 1982, WB Saunders Co, pp 91-92.

239. Wyzinski P: Diurnal cycle of refraction after radial keratotomy, Ophthalmology 1987;94:120-124.

240. Wyzinski P: Why are refractive surgeons still wearing glasses? Ophthalmic Surg 1987;18:349-351.

241. Wyzinski P and O'Dell L: Subjective and objective findings after radial keratotomy, Ophthalmology 1989;86:108-111.

242. Yamaguchi T, Kanai A, Tanaka M, Ishii R, and Nakajima A: Bullous keratopathy after anterior-posterior keratotomy for myopia and myopic astigmatism, Am J Ophthalmol 1982;93:600-606.

243. Yamaguchi T, Kaufmann H, Fukushima A, et al: Histologic and electron microscopic assessment of endothelial damage produced by anterior radial keratotomy in the monkey cornea, Am J Ophthalmol 1981;92:313-327.

244. Yamaguchi T, Tamki K, Kaufman HE, et al: Histologic study of a pair of human corneas after anterior radial keratotomy, Am J Ophthalmol 1985; 100:281-292.

245. Zantos SG and Holden BA: Transient endothelial changes soon after wearing soft contact lenses, Am J Optom Physiol Optics 1977;54:856-858.

Stability of Refraction after Refractive Keratotomy

George O. Waring III
Michael J. Lynn
Michael H. Kutner

During the years of wound healing after refractive keratotomy, and perhaps for a long time afterwards, uncontrolled changes in corneal shape produce changes in refraction. Daily fluctuation of vision is at best an inconvenience and at worst a handicap. Long-term instability with a trend in the hyperopic direction can interfere with a successful result by hastening the onset of presbyopia. The question as to when refraction becomes stable after radial keratotomy is a compelling one for both patients and physicians.

In this chapter we examine the stability of the refraction and visual acuity from the time of surgery to approximately 5 years after refractive keratotomy. Since these changes occur primarily in the spherical component of the refraction, we discuss the changes in the spherical equivalent and not changes in astigmatism.

TERMINOLOGY OF STABILITY

We describe changes in refraction after radial keratotomy as an increase or decrease in the minus power. Decreasing minus power is a refractive change in the direction of a decrease in myopia or an increase in hyperopia. Increasing minus power is a refractive change in the direction of an increase in myopia or a decrease in hyperopia.

When describing a group of patients, refractive changes over time cannot ac-

BACKGROUND AND ACKNOWLEDGMENTS
This chapter was written at the PERK Statistical and Clinical Coordinating Centers, Emory University, based on information drawn from the published literature as cited. The information from the PERK study was previously published in the *American Journal of Ophthalmology* 1991;11:133-144.[39] The chapter was supported by National Institutes of Health grants EY03752 and EY03761. We acknowledge the assistance of our colleagues, Ellen Strahlman, Azhar Nizam, Brooke Fielding, and Ceretha Cartwright, and the staff of the Coordinating Centers, Portia Griffin, Brenda Henderson, Phyllis Newman, and Pamela O'Hagan. Drs. Michael Deitz and Donald Sanders provided unpublished data on long-term stability.

curately be referred to as increased/decreased myopia or increased/decreased hyperopia, since some patients are myopic whereas others are hyperopic. For example, it is inaccurate to call a change in refraction from −4.00 to −3.00 D "progressive hyperopia," just as it would be inaccurate to call a change from +2.00 to +1.00 D "progressive myopia." Therefore we are left with the awkward but accurate terms, "increase or decrease in minus power"; this is acceptable terminology because the goal of radial keratotomy is to decrease the minus power of the myopic refractive correction.

When Deitz and Sanders[8] first described a continued decrease in minus power in the years following radial keratotomy, they termed the phenomenon "progressive hyperopia." Although the term seems inaccurate, it does emphasize the major clinical consequence, which is a progression in the hyperopic direction, sometimes called a "hyperopic shift." It is certainly accurate to designate this as "a change in the hyperopic direction."

Probably the best way to conceptualize this is in terms of the surgery itself, an "increasing effect of radial keratotomy," since this term is accurate regardless of whether the patient is myopic or hyperopic. Some have called it a "continued effect" of the surgery, but strictly speaking the continuation of the initial reduction in myopia is the "continued effect" and the shift in the hyperopic direction represents an "increasing effect."

REFRACTIVE CHANGE IN UNOPERATED EYES OF PATIENTS WITH SIMPLE AND INTERMEDIATE MYOPIA

An evaluation of the refractive change after radial keratotomy requires some idea of the amount of change that occurs in unoperated myopic eyes (see Chapter 1, Myopia: A Brief Overview). Unfortunately, there are few studies in which a group of patients with myopic eyes have been followed longitudinally for a long time. Cohort studies that compare the refraction for myopic subjects of different ages to assess the change over time are not as sensitive an indicator of refractive changes as studies of individual eyes over time.

Most studies of myopic patients have been concerned with the age of onset and the progression of myopia. In a cohort study of persons 1 to 28 years of age, Lepard[17] found progression of myopia until age 25 years. Brown[6] performed atropine refractions at least 1 year apart on 1203 eyes for a total of 8820 comparative measurements from birth to age 51 years and concluded that the change in myopia was negligible after age 20 years.

A few studies have followed individual patients of different ages over time.[3,7,36] Bücklers[7] studied 120 eyes with refractive errors from approximately +5.00 to −20.00 D, which he followed for 20 to 70 years. His data indicate that stability of refraction typically occurs after age 20 and that significant reductions in myopia seldom occur.

Because the PERK study required that patients wait 1 year between surgery on the two eyes,[40] a group of patients with unoperated eyes (second eyes) having two measurements approximately 1 year apart (at the initial baseline visit and at 1 year after surgery on the first eye) were available for analysis. This gave an estimate of the refractive change over 1 year for eyes with simple and intermediate myopia between −2.00 and −8.00 D for patients 21 years or older.

To evaluate the change under as standardized conditions as possible, we included only eyes that were examined by the same clinical coordinator at both times and that did not wear a contact lens during the year between examinations; 156 eyes met these criteria[19] (Fig. 24-1). The change in refraction during this year was 0.25 D or less in 44% and 0.50 to 0.89 D in 56% of the eyes. None changed 1.00 D or more. Changes in the direction of increasing minus power were similar to changes in the direction of decreasing minus power, indicating a lack of a trend consistent with random variation.

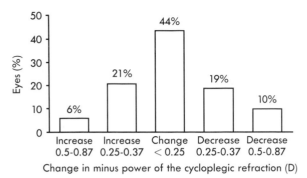

Figure 24-1
The change in refraction during a 1-year interval for 156 unoperated eyes with refraction of −2.00 to −8.00 D in the PERK study. Eyes did not wear a contact lens and were examined by the same individual using the same equipment. All eyes changed less than 1.00 D, and 84% changed by less than 0.50 D. A 1.00-diopter cutoff is reasonable for evaluating clinically meaningful refractive change after surgery.

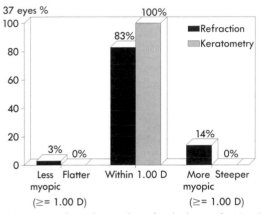

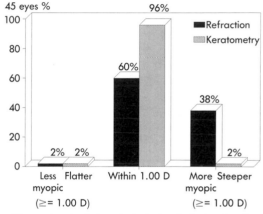

Figure 24-2
The change in spherical equivalent of the cycloplegic refraction and average central keratometric power between baseline and 5 years for the unoperated eyes of 37 non−contact lens wearers **(A)** and for 45 contact lens wearers **(B)** in the PERK study. In each case, not more than 3% of the eyes became less myopic or flatter by 1 D or more.

Based on these results, we chose 1.00 D as an indicator of a clinically meaningful change in refractive error over time in radial keratotomy patients.

There were 82 patients in the PERK study who did not have their second eye operated during the 5-year follow-up and for whom 5-year refractive data were available, so the stability of refraction in these individual eyes could be studied. The average age of these patients at the baseline examination was 35 years, and they were followed for an average of 5.3 years (range, 4.9 to 6.2 years). At baseline the mean spherical equivalent cycloplegic refractive error was −4.32 D (range, −7.62 to −2.00 D).

The baseline characteristics of patients who wore contact lenses and those who did not wear contact lenses on their unoperated eye were very similar. However, at the 5-year follow-up the cycloplegic refraction and central keratometric power results were different for contact lens wearers and non−contact lens wearers. Hence these results are broken down by contact lens wearing status.

For the 37 non−contact lens wearers at the 5-year follow-up, the mean change in refractive error was −0.22 D (statistically insignificant). The change was within 1.00 D for all but 5 patients (83%), and 14% became more myopic by 1.00 to 2.00 D. Three percent became less myopic by more than 1.00 D (Fig. 24-2, *A*). For the 45 contact lens wearers, the mean change in refractive error was −0.66 D (statistically significant). The change was within 1.00 D for 60% of

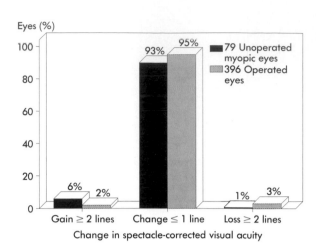

Figure 24-3
The change in spectacle-corrected visual acuity from baseline to 5 years after surgery for operated eyes in the PERK study was similar to the change in spectacle-corrected visual acuity in unoperated eyes. A change of two Snellen lines or more was considered significant.

patients; 38% became more myopic by 1.00 to 1.75 D, and 2% became less myopic by more than 1.00 D (Fig. 24-2, *B*).

The mean change in average central keratometric power for non−contact lens wearers was a decrease (that is, the corneas were flatter) of 0.02 D (statistically insignificant). The mean change for contact lens wearers was an increase of 0.15 D (statistically significant). For both groups the change was within 1.00 D for practically all patients.

The visual acuity results were very similar for contact lens wearers and non−contact lens wearers. Overall, the best spectacle-corrected visual acuity decreased by one Snellen line in 20% of patients (Fig. 24-3). Since there was no evidence of a pathologic process in these eyes, we interpreted this change of one Snellen line of best-corrected visual acuity as a normal biologic variation or a measurement error. In contrast, only 1% of the eyes had a loss of visual acuity of two or more lines. Therefore we recommend using the loss of two Snellen lines or more of best spectacle-corrected visual acuity as the cutoff point for meaningful change, since the loss of one line (three letters) is likely to occur as part of the standard measurement procedure.[26]

TIME INTERVALS FOR MEASUREMENT OF CHANGES IN REFRACTION

The following three periods occur during which we can conveniently study changes in refraction after radial keratotomy; we discuss each separately in this chapter:

1. The immediate postoperative and short-term adjustments after surgery, which span approximately 1 day to 3 months
2. Intermediate and long-term stability, beginning approximately 3 months after surgery and extending indefinitely
3. Morning to evening (diurnal) variation, which can persist for years after surgery

Selecting a cutoff point between short-term adjustment after surgery and intermediate to long-term follow-up is somewhat arbitrary. Using the PERK data, we observed extreme changes between the 2-week and the 3-month examination in most eyes and minimal changes between 3 and 6 months (Fig. 24-4). A retrospective study of 71 eyes of 44 consecutive patients 20 to 61 years of age who underwent a four-incision radial keratotomy was reported by Williams and colleagues.[42] Central keratotomy was carried out intraoperatively, at 1 day, and

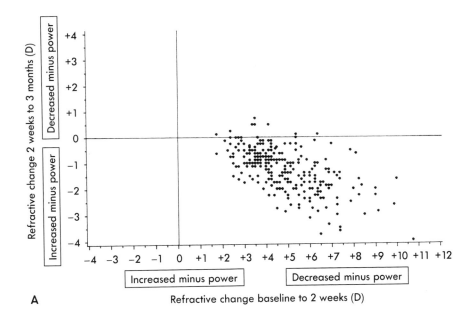

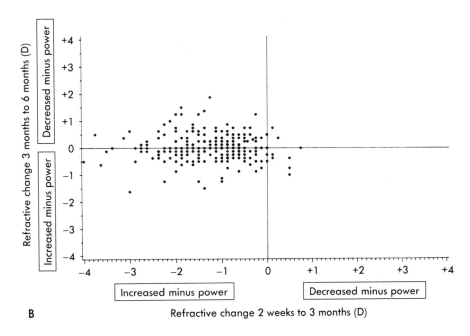

Figure 24-4

Scattergrams of change in refraction between baseline and 3 months for 341 eyes in the PERK study. **A,** Comparison of the refractive change between baseline and 2 weeks after surgery (x-axis) to that between 2 weeks and 3 months after surgery (y-axis) shows that all eyes had a reduction in myopia at 2 weeks after surgery. Most eyes lost some effect between 2 weeks and 3 months after surgery. Eyes that had a greater refractive change at 2 weeks tended to have a greater loss of effect between 2 weeks and 3 months (correlation, 0.4). **B,** The refractive change between 2 weeks and 3 months (x-axis) versus that between 3 months and 6 months (y-axis) after surgery. There was much less refractive change between 3 to 6 months, 50% of eyes changing by 0.25 D or less and only 5% of eyes changing by 1.00 D or more. The data points cluster around the "No Change" line between 3 to 6 months, indicating relative stability of refraction. (From Waring GO, Lynn MJ, Strahlman ER, et al: Am J Ophthalmol 1991;111:133-144.)

at 1, 3, 6, and 12 months after surgery. They found the keratometry measurements reasonably stable at 1 month after surgery when compared with 1 year (correlation coefficient equals 0.703), observing no statistically significant change in the keratometry readings taken at 1 and 3 months when compared with 6 and 12 months. Therefore somewhere between 1 and 3 months after surgery is a reasonable cutoff point to judge the overall short-term refractive result from radial keratotomy. Of course, significant changes in refraction in individual eyes may occur after that time.[4,12] Identifying this cutoff point has practical meaning for clinical studies of refractive keratotomy, since it suggests the time required for patient follow-up to measure the procedure's initial outcome. The literature on radial keratotomy, as well as on other refractive surgical procedures, has tended to report data 1 year after surgery as the first "definitive" representation of outcome, although many have reported results at 3 and 6 months after surgery. As seen in the following discussion, the large postoperative variations in refraction generally disappear in the first 3 months, suggesting that 3- to 6-month data on refractive keratotomy may be acceptable for reporting initial findings. This makes studies of refractive keratotomy easier to conduct, since to maintain a high follow-up rate is easier for 3 to 6 months than for 1 year.

Designating a cutoff time to mark intermediate-term versus long-term follow-up is also arbitrary. As of 1991, the longest published follow-up of radial keratotomy patients was approximately 5 years.[1,11,34,38a] The PERK study was funded for a 5-year follow-up; the results were published in 1991. Thus we have arbitrarily selected 5 years as a cutoff point for immediate-term follow-up and designated the years after that as long-term follow-up.

A 5-year cutoff point is also justified by histologic studies that have shown that an epithelial plug persists in human keratotomy wounds for approximately 4 to 5 years and generally is absent thereafter.[2] In addition, clinical observations of the corneal stroma adjacent to the wound show that the spicules and feathering that reflect stromal wound remodeling generally disappear by 4 to 5 years.[13,41]

1 DAY TO 3 MONTHS: POSTOPERATIVE ADJUSTMENT

As with any surgical procedure, the immediate postoperative period involves general recovery. We divide it into intervals of 1 day to 2 weeks and 2 weeks to 3 months (see Fig. 24-1).

1 day to 2 weeks: immediate postoperative course

Few published reports measure the changes that occur during the immediate postoperative period. In the PERK study,[39] all eyes became less myopic between surgery and 2 weeks (see Figs. 24-4 and 24-5). The average refractive change was a 4.83 D decrease in myopia. (The range was 1.75 to 10.75 D.)

During this time patients typically exhibit instability of refraction and visual acuity; thus physicians usually direct their efforts at explaining this to the patient rather than trying to assess the visual outcome of surgery. Many factors produce these large changes in refraction and visual acuity, including the amount of stromal edema, the depth of the incision, the extent of intraoperative epithelial abrasions, the amount of irrigation of the wounds, the amount of blood left in the wounds, the amount of time lids are kept closed after surgery, and the frequency of and vigor used in rubbing the eyes. As the epithelial plug fills the wounds, as the stromal edema subsides, and as the epithelial barrier function is reestablished, the variations in refraction, visual acuity, and glare gradually diminish. Laboratory models have demonstrated that corneal edema induces large changes in refraction immediately after surgery. For example, Parel and colleagues[28] showed that eyes flooded with balanced salt solution had the induction of more

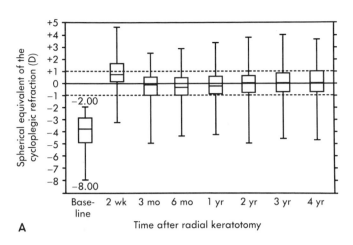
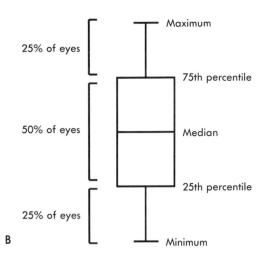

Figure 24-5
Refractive outcome for 341 eyes in the PERK study from 2 weeks to 4 years after surgery. **A,** Box and whisker plots showing the refractions at each of the follow-up visits for eyes in the PERK study. All eyes were at least 2 D myopic at baseline. Most eyes were overcorrected at 2 weeks after surgery, and there was a general loss of effect from 2 weeks to 3 months after surgery. At the 6-month to 4-year follow-up visits, there was a general trend on the average toward a continued effect of the surgery with a decrease in minus power. At least 50% of the eyes fell within 1 D of emmotropia. At 2, 3, and 4 years after surgery, the median value was a "perfect" plano; this observation emphasizes the fallacy of dealing solely with average values, since the range of residual error was from approximately −5.00 to +4.00 D. **B,** A schematic drawing showing the components of the box and whisker plot, which shows the distribution of refractions at each time interval.

than 10 D of astigmatism after transverse keratotomy and 5 D of flattening after radial keratotomy, but when the surfaces of the corneas were covered with dextran or silicon oil, no change greater than 1 D was recorded. Presumably the balanced salt solution produced marked swelling of the stroma within the wounds, causing greater wound gape and a greater change in curvature, whereas the dextran and silicone oil produced less stromal swelling and therefore essentially no measurable change in central corneal curvature.

Topical corticosteroids are used by some surgeons during this time to slow wound healing[14] (see Chapter 20, Corneal Wound Healing and Its Pharmacologic Modification after Refractive Keratotomy). Refractions during this time can give a general impression about the surgical results but cannot predict the outcome 6 to 12 months later.

Details of the refractive changes during the first 2 weeks after surgery are provided by two reports of ophthalmologists who had radial keratotomy. Wyzinski, who had preoperative myopia of −4.50 D, measured his refractive error every 3 to 5 days during the first 6 weeks after surgery.[43] He noted a transient hyperopia that was maximal (+2.75 D) at about 14 days after surgery (Fig. 24-6 and Table 24-1). One day after surgery the refractive error was +3.00 to +4.00 D, depending on the time of day. On the fourth day, the refractive error was +1.00 D; the hyperopia increased to +2.62 D on day 14 and then fell to approximately plano by 1 month where it remained until 6 months, when 1.00 D of hyperopia appeared.

Richmond[29] noted a rapid increase in minus power of 1.00 to 2.00 D between 1 and 2 weeks after surgery (Fig. 24-7) (see Chapter 25, The Patient Speaks: Testimonials after Refractive Keratotomy).

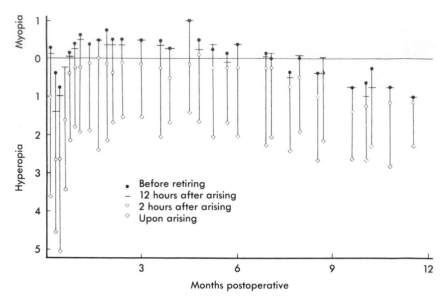

Figure 24-6

Stability of refraction after radial keratotomy in the right eye of ophthalmologist P. Wyzinski during the first year after radial keratotomy. The graph shows three major findings: (1) the general loss of effect in the first few weeks after surgery, (2) the persistent diurnal variation with the greatest change in the first 2 hours after arising, and (3) the gradual trend toward a continued effect of the surgery with a continued decrease in minus power over the first year. (From Wyzinski P and O'Dell LW: Ophthalmology 1987;94:120-124.)

Table 24-1

Self-Reported Diurnal Variation in Refractive Error (D) before and after Radial Keratotomy

Days before or after surgery	On arising (D)	Awake 2 hours (D)	Awake 12 hours (D)	Before retiring (D)
−3	−4.12	−4.25	−4.50	−4.62
−2	−3.87	−4.12	−4.25	−4.37
−1	−4.12	−4.25	−4.50	−4.50
Surgery				
1	+2.25	+3.25	+3.12	+3.87
4	+3.62	+1.00	−0.12	−0.37
7	+2.62	+1.75	−0.50	−0.12
11	+4.25	+2.75	+1.00	+0.62
14	+5.00	+2.62	+1.00	+0.75
17	+3.37	+1.75	+1.00	+0.75
24	+2.12	+0.37	0.00	−0.12
39	+1.87	+0.12	−0.37	−0.37
60	+2.12	+0.12	−0.37	−0.75

From Wyzinski P and O'Dell LW: Ophthalmology 1987;94:120-124.

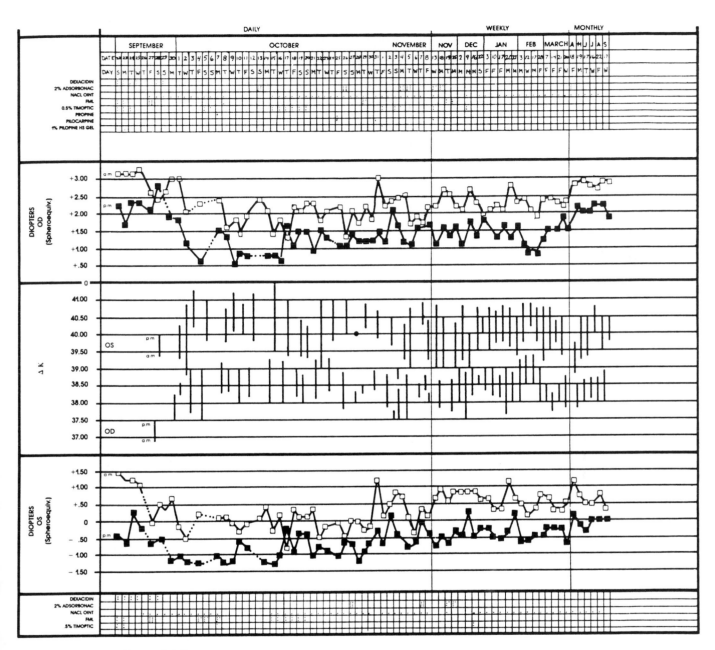

Figure 24-7

Stability of refraction in the right *(top)* and left *(bottom)* eyes of ophthalmologist R. Richmond during the first year after radial keratotomy. Charts at the top and bottom show medications used after surgery. The spherical equivalent of the refraction shows a persistent diurnal variation of 0.50 to 1.00 D in each eye during the first year. Changes in keratometric readings roughly parallel those of the refraction. During this shift, there is a slight trend toward a continued effect of the surgery with a decrease in minus power. (From Richmond RD: J Refract Surg 1987;3:22-27.)

2 weeks to 3 months: early postoperative course

As the early perturbations of corneal surgery subside, attention turns to evaluating how the patient's refraction has been affected by the surgery. In this early postoperative period most eyes experience a loss of the initial effect. As the early stromal edema gradually subsides, wound gaping diminishes and the central cornea steepens some (Fig. 24-8). Clinically this can be a time of great disappointment for a patient; some experience this as the "miracle that failed" because they had suddenly achieved nearly normal uncorrected acuity in the immediate preoperative period, only to have it fade with the return of some myopia. Ophthalmologists should advise patients in advance of these early swings and inform them to be cautious in interpreting the outcome immediately after surgery.

In the PERK study[39] most eyes lost some effect of surgery between 2 weeks and 3 months (see Fig. 24-5), with patients showing an average increase in mi-

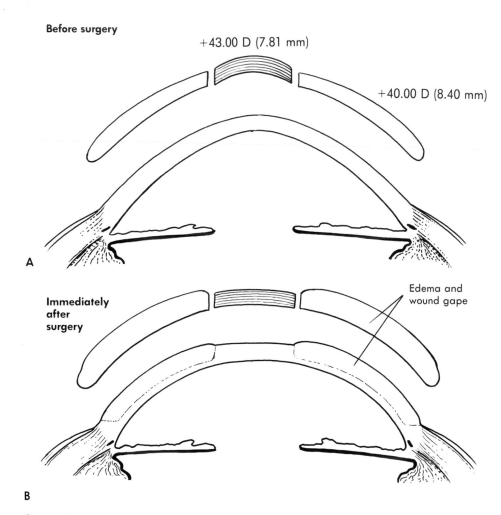

Figure 24-8

Drawings illustrate the changes in corneal curvature during the first few months after radial keratotomy. Each drawing consists of two components, an intact anterior ocular segment and a "detached cornea," that show the differential change in curvature of the unincised central zone and the incised paracentral and peripheral zones. **A,** Before surgery the central cornea is steeper than the paracentral cornea (positive asphericity). **B,** Immediately after surgery the stroma in the area of the incisions imbibes water and swells, enhancing the central flattening.

nus power of 1.25 D. Fifty-nine percent of eyes lost 1.00 D or more of effect, and 20% lost 2.00 D or more. Forty-one percent of eyes changed by less than 1.00 D, with most changing toward a loss of surgical effect.

Those eyes having the greatest initial effect of surgery at 2 weeks tended to have the largest regression of effect from 2 weeks to 3 months (correlation = 0.4). These may have been the eyes with the most stromal edema from the surgery.

Wyzinski and O'Dell[43] noted a 1.00 to 2.00 D decrease (depending on the time of day) in the amount of hyperopia between 2 weeks and 3 months after surgery (see Fig. 24-6 and Table 24-1). Richmond[29] reported that the regression had stopped by 2 weeks after surgery. Between 2 weeks and 3 months the refraction in Richmond's right eye fluctuated between +0.75 and +2.00 D, and his left eye had a gain in effect of approximately 1.00 D, the refraction changing from −1.25 to +0.25 D (see Fig. 24-7).

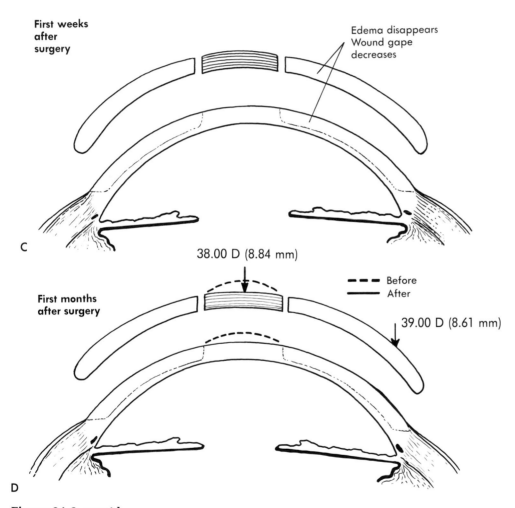

Figure 24-8, cont'd
C, During the first weeks after surgery the epithelium covers the wounds and the edema decreases, with a loss of some of the initial surgical effect. **D,** During the first few months after surgery scar formation determines the new shape of the cornea in which the central cornea is flatter than the paracentral cornea (negative asphericity). (Courtesy Jack Holladay, MD.)

Figure 24-9
The change in cycloplegic refraction between 2 weeks and 3 months in 126 eyes after radial keratotomy. Negative values indicate regression of effect; 59% of the eyes regressed by 1.00 D or more. (From McDonnell PJ and Schanzlin DJ: Arch Ophthalmol 1988;106:212-214.)

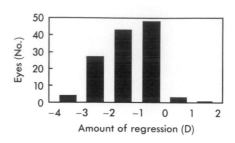

McDonnell and Schanzlin[23] reported early postoperative changes in 72 patients receiving radial keratotomy according to the PERK technique. Between 2 weeks and 3 months, a general regression of effect occurred: 38% of eyes became more myopic by less than 1.00 D, 34% by 1.00 to 1.87 D, and 25% by 2.00 to 3.50 D. Only four eyes (3%) had a decrease in myopia of 0.25 to 1.25 D (Fig. 24-9). The authors observed a correlation between the initial refractive error and the amount of regression between 2 weeks and 3 months (correlation, 0.41), a finding similar to that in the PERK study. The authors observed that eyes treated with topical steroids and patching after surgery had less regression of effect (mean, −0.31 D) than eyes with a similar preoperative refractive error and of similar age that had no steroids and were not patched (mean loss of effect, −1.57 D). The steroids may have retarded early stromal wound healing and contracture; the patching may have increased stromal edema and mechanically flattened the cornea. Whether these early differences in the two groups influence the intermediate-term and long-term outcomes is unknown.

3 MONTHS TO 5 YEARS: INTERMEDIATE TERM

The refraction is generally stable during 3 months to 5 years, although mild to moderate change occurs in some eyes. By 3 months (in fact, by approximately 4 to 6 weeks) the surgeon can determine reliably the intermediate-term outcome for the patient and discuss and plan surgery on the second eye. Surgeons who operate on both eyes simultaneously or within a week of each other obviate the advantage of modifying surgery on the second eye after identifying at 1 to 3 months those patients who have overresponded or underresponded to surgery or who have some other unexpected clinical course, such as satisfaction with a monocular correction.

Average change in refraction for all eyes

A simple way to characterize the change in refraction over time is to average the refraction in all eyes at each postoperative interval and to observe the change in this average refraction over time. Studying only the average change without considering variation among the eyes can be misleading, since the extent to which the refractive change for an individual patient differs from the mean cannot be determined. In addition, large changes in both the myopic and hyperopic directions will cancel each other out, making zero contribution to the average change.

One graphic method for describing an entire population is a box and whisker plot (see Fig. 24-5). This plot depicts the minimal and maximal values, the location of the central cluster of 50% of the eyes, and the median value.

Fig. 24-6 shows the refractions in the PERK study population at follow-up visits between baseline and 4 years after surgery. Before surgery, all refractions were −2.00 to −8.00 D. At all examinations from 3 months to 4 years, at least 50% of the eyes fell within 1.00 D of emmetropia. However, refractive errors varied widely, from approximately −5.00 to +4.00 D. Using the median value

Table 24-2

Studies of Refraction Stability after Radial Keratotomy

	PERK study[39]	Deitz and Sanders[8]	Deitz*	Arrowsmith and Marks[1]	Sawelson and Marks[34]	Neumann[25]
Population reported						
Number of eyes	435	225	916	156	198	118
Consecutive series	Yes	Yes	Yes	Yes	Yes	Yes
Knife blade	Diamond	Metal	Diamond	Metal	Metal	Metal
Eyes in analysis	341	165	149	122	103	118
Max follow-up (years)	4	4	4	5	5	5
Follow-up interval (years)	0.5 to 4	1 to 4	1 to 4	1 to 5	1.5 to 5	1 to 5
Refractive change (% of eyes)						
Decrease in minus power $\geq$1 D	23	31	19	22	17	26
Change <1 D	74	65	80	70	78	69
Increase in minus power $\geq$1 D	3	4	1	8	5	5

*Presented at the International Society of Refractive Keratoplasty, Oct. 6, 1988, Las Vegas, Nev.

only, which at 2, 3, and 4 years was approximately 0.00 D ("perfect emmetropia"), does not adequately summarize the refractive results.

Even though average values poorly represent the stability and change in refraction in the population, they can indicate a general trend. All intermediate-term studies have shown the average value moving in a hyperopic direction with an overall decrease in minus power. The following examples of average spherical equivalent refraction values illustrate the average trend toward hyperopia:

1. PERK study: 3 months, -0.23 D; 6 months, -0.33 D; 1 year, -0.18 D; 2 years, -0.03 D; 3 years, $+0.05$ D; 4 years, $+0.11$ D
2. Arrowsmith and Marks[1]: 1 year, -0.40 D; 2 years, -0.10 D; 4 years, $+0.30$ D; 5 years, $+0.30$ D
3. Sawelson and Marks[34]: 1.5 years, -0.8 D; 3 years, -0.5 D; 5 years, -0.5 D
4. Deitz (personal communication, October 6, 1988): *Metal blade series:* 3 to 12 months (214 eyes), $+0.01$ D; 12 to 24 months (142 eyes), $+0.11$ D; 24 to 48 months (134 eyes), $+0.35$ D; 48 to 72 months (65 eyes), $+0.44$ D; overall—12 to 72 months (66 eyes), $+1.1$ D. *Diamond knife series:* 3 to 12 months (519 eyes), $+0.17$ D; 12 to 24 months (157 eyes), $+0.32$ D; 24 to 48 months (54 eyes), $+0.25$ D; overall—12 to 72 months (17 eyes), $+0.97$ D

Change in refraction for individual eyes

A more meaningful description of average values for refractive change is to report the percentage of eyes that change less than 1.00 D; this also indicates the percentage having 1.00 D or more decrease in minus power (moving in a hyperopic direction) and the percentage having 1.00 D or more increase in minus power (moving in a myopic direction). This simple information should be included in every report of refractive keratotomy. Table 24-2 compares different studies of refraction stability.

Deitz and Sanders[8] first observed this unanticipated phenomenon after radial

Figure 24-10
The average spherical equivalent refraction at the beginning and end of various postoperative time intervals for eyes receiving radial keratotomy performed with metal or diamond blades. (From Deitz MR, Sanders DR, and Raanan MG: Ophthalmology 1986;93:1284-1289.)

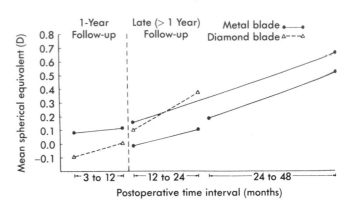

Figure 24-11
The change in the spherical equivalent of the cycloplegic refraction between 6 months and 4 years for 341 eyes in the PERK study. (From Waring GO, Lynn MJ, Strahlman ER, et al: Am J Ophthalmol 1991;111:133-144.)

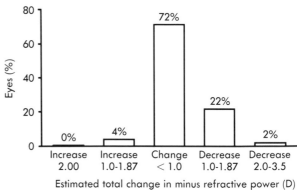

keratotomy—a continued effect of surgery. They reported that 31% of 225 eyes operated with a metal blade showed a decrease in minus power (a continued surgical effect) of 1.00 D or more between 1 and 3 to 4 years after surgery. A follow-up study[9] substantiated these findings (Fig. 24-10). All subsequent studies of stability have confirmed this finding, and as demonstrated in Table 24-2, the numbers from one report to another are remarkably consistent.

For example, in the PERK study, between 6 months and 4 years, 23% of the eyes showed 1.00 D or more decrease in minus power, whereas 74% changed less than 1.00 D (Fig. 24-11 and Table 24-2).

Deitz and Sanders[8] have presented longer-term follow-up data up to 8 years in selected eyes (Tables 24-2, 24-3, and 24-4), indicating that an increasing effect of the surgery may appear at 5 to 8 years postoperatively. The longest follow-up on radial keratotomy was done by Ivanova and Fyodorov,[15] who reported an average overall continued effect from surgery after 12 years.

When and if this increasing surgical effect stops is unknown. Based on histologic and slit-lamp microscopic studies, the suggestion that the unsutured corneal wounds might be healed by approximately 5 years offered hope that refraction would stabilize. The findings of Deitz and Sanders[8] and of Ivanova and Fyodorov[15] indicate that this is not true, which suggests that an increase in surgical effect might continue for many years in some individuals.

Table 24-3

Change in Refraction* During 8 Years after Refractive Keratotomy

Time (years)	Number of eyes	Average change (D)	Percentage of eyes changing <1 D	Percentage of eyes changing ≥1 D
Metal blade (289 eyes)				
1 to 2	142	0.11	88	9
1 to 4	188	0.46	69	28
1 to 6	66	1.10	36	61
1 to 8	15	1.80	13	87
Diamond blade (916 eyes)				
1 to 2	157	0.32	85	13
1 to 4	149	0.39	80	19
1 to 6	17	0.97	76	24

Deitz and Sanders series; presented at the International Society of Refractive Keratoplasty, Oct. 6, 1988, Las Vegas, Nev.
*Spherical equivalent of cycloplegic refraction.

Table 24-4

Individual Examples of Increasing Effect of Refractive Keratotomy

Patient and eye	Preoperative cycloplegic refraction	Postoperative cycloplegic refraction over years (D)					Change over longest interval (D)
		6 mo	1 to 2	3 to 4	5 to 6	7	
1 OD	−3.25	—	—	+2.50	+5.87	—	+3.37
OS	−3.50	—	+1.87	—	+3.50	—	+1.63
2 OD	−6.25	+3.00	+4.25	+4.75	—	+7.12	+4.12
3 OD	−6.37	—	+2.62	+3.75	+4.62	+5.62	+3.00
OS	−8.25	−0.12	+0.50	+1.50	+2.25	+3.37	+3.50
4 OS	−0.50	—	0.00	—	+4.50	—	+4.50

From Deitz MR: Personal communication, Oct. 6, 1988.

Stability of refraction in individual eyes in the PERK study

In clinical practice the patient and surgeon are concerned about the results and stability for an individual, not the overall outcome for a group. The stability of refraction in individual eyes should be the focus of long-term studies. The study of large numbers of eyes is difficult; for example, a graph of 400 time-course lines over many years would be difficult and confusing to interpret. Therefore some statistical summary of the change in refraction is needed. We describe the method used in the PERK study.[22]

Measures of change in refraction: trend and magnitude. We studied two aspects of the change in refractive error in individual eyes after radial keratotomy. The first aspect was a *trend* that indicated a persistent change in one direction, such as a continued effect of surgery. Such a trend may involve small changes between two examinations but may result in a large overall change. For example, an average decrease in minus power of 0.50 D between annual examinations would be considered reasonably stable. If this continues every year for 5 years, however, there would be a decrease in minus power of 2.50 D, a large trend.

The second aspect we considered was the *magnitude* of the change. The refraction in some eyes may not change consistently but may have large variations from one visit to another. For example, an eye with a refraction of −1.00 D at 1 year, a refraction of +0.50 D at 3 years, and a refraction of −1.50 D at 5 years shows an overall change of only 0.50 D from 1 to 5 years but clearly has experienced an unstable refraction.

We illustrate the trend and magnitude of refractive change in Fig. 24-12, which shows the refractive error at each of five follow-up examinations between 6 months and 4 years after surgery for an individual eye in the PERK study.

The trend in the refractive change (Fig. 24-12, *A*) is measured by computing

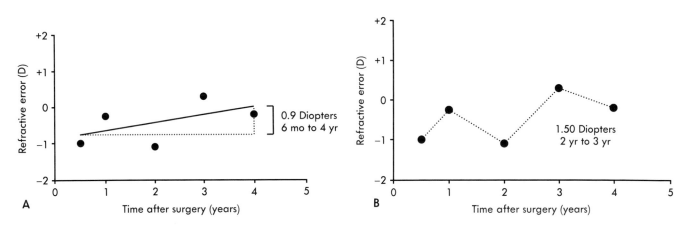

Figure 24-12
Illustrative example showing the refractions of a single patient between 6 months and 4 years after surgery. **A,** The regression line is used to evaluate the *trend* of the refractive change, 0.90 D between 6 months and 4 years. **B,** The *magnitude* of the refractive change is estimated by the largest change between any two visits, in this case, 1.50 D between the 2- and 3-year visits.

the regression line that relates the cycloplegic refraction at each of the five visits to the time after surgery. The slope of the regression line indicates if there is any trend toward a decrease or an increase in minus power. In this case a general trend is toward a decrease in minus power (a continued surgical effect), even though changes periodically occur in both directions. We can calculate an overall change that incorporates all the data points by multiplying the slope of the regression line by the time between the first and last examinations (from 6 months to 4 years after surgery). Rather than calculating the absolute change between 6 months and 4 years, this gives a better measure of the overall trend of the refractive error during the follow-up because it incorporates fluctuations in refraction during that time, not just the first and last points.

The magnitude of the refractive change (Fig. 24-12, *B*) is defined as the largest change in refraction between any two examinations, not necessarily successive ones. For example, the greatest change in this eye was 1.50 D between the 2- and 3-year examinations.

To categorize patients according to the overall stability of refraction, we used both the trend and the magnitude of change. We chose 1.00 D or more of change as a criterion for instability for both trend and magnitude.

Categories of refractive change in the PERK study. We classified eyes into four groups that characterized the stability of their refractive error (Table 24-5):
1. *Stable:* Less than 1.00 D change according to both criteria
2. *Fluctuating:* Less than 1.00 D change according to the regression criteria, but a maximum change between any two visits of 1.00 D or more
3. *Increasing effect:* 1.00 D or more change by both criteria in the hyperopic direction of decreased minus power
4. *Loss of effect:* 1.00 D or more change by both criteria in the myopic direction of increased minus power

Table 24-5

Categories of Refractive Stability 6 Months to 4 Years in the PERK Study According to Two Criteria

Refractive stability category	Change in the spherical equivalent cycloplegic refraction		Number of eyes (%)
	Overall change ≥1.00 D	Maximum interim change ≥1.00 D	
Stable	No	No	197 (58)
Fluctuating	No	Yes	49 (14)
Increasing effect in hyperopic direction	Yes	Yes	82 (24)
Loss of effect in myopic direction	Yes	Yes	13 (4)

Figure 24-13 shows the scattergram of the magnitude (the largest refractive change between any two visits) and the trend of refractive change (the estimated overall change from the regression line) for 341 eyes (one eye per patient, repeat surgery excluded) in the PERK study. The dotted lines indicate the 1.00 D cutoff points used in the definition of a stable refractive error and separate the population into four different categories of refractive change. The numbers on the graph are the percentages of eyes falling into the categories. The examples for each category are for one individual eye.

Stable. The 58% of eyes in the middle of the graph changed less than 1.00 D between any two visits and showed no evidence of a trend in the refractive change. The individual example *(C)* shows a flat line, which means no significant change was measured during 3½ years of follow-up (Fig. 24-13).

Fluctuation with no definite trend. This category is made up of the 14% of eyes in the two groups on either side of the stable box (Fig. 24-13). In these groups a change of 1.00 D or more occurred between two visits, but the overall change was not consistent enough to form a definite trend. In 10% of the eyes the change was a decrease in minus power, and in 4% the change was an increase in minus power. One graph of an individual eye *(B)* shows a change of 1.25 D between 2 and 4 years after surgery in the direction of a loss of surgical effect. However, because the refraction moved in both directions during this time, a consistent trend was not apparent. Similarly, the eye illustrated in Fig. 24-13, *E*, showed a change of 1.25 D between 2 and 3 years, but the overall trend was only +0.75 D between 6 months and 4 years.

In terms of overall stability this group is difficult to classify. Since no evidence of a consistent trend exists, a change of 1.00 D at some point during the follow-up may not be considered clinically meaningful. For example, the refraction may have been different at only one point. If one chooses to call this group stable and combines it with the group that was stable according to both criteria, a total of 72% of the eyes would be considered stable in the PERK study.

Unstable: decrease in minus power. Twenty-four percent of eyes had a change of 1.00 D or more in the direction of decreased minus power in both magnitude and trend measures, representing an increasing effect of the surgery in the hyperopic direction.

Most eyes showed a persistent trend in the direction of decreased minus power over the entire follow-up (Fig. 24-13, *D*). Some eyes showed a trend toward continued decrease in minus power over the early part of follow-up, then flattened off afterward so that they "became stable" in the last 1 or 2 years of follow-up.

Unstable: increase in minus power. The 4% of eyes in the lower left-hand box in Fig. 24-13 experienced an overall loss of surgical effect. The individual graph *(A)* shows a patient who steadily lost surgical effect, which amounted to slightly more than 1.00 D of increased minus power between 6 months and 4 years.

At one time some questioned whether the cornea had "memory" for its original shape and would therefore try to revert to its original curvature after keratotomy. This clearly has been shown to be false, since only a very small number of eyes show an increase in minus power after surgery and only rarely do eyes return to preoperative refractive error after modern refractive keratotomy.

Absolute change in refraction over time. The simplest way to determine the overall stability of refraction after surgery is to compare the values at some time after early stabilization (3 months, 6 months, 1 year) to values at a later time (5 years), which would indicate the number of eyes that change less than 1 D and more than 1 D in the hyperopic and myopic directions. This approach masks the fluctuation and instability that may occur during the follow-up interval, but accurately represents the overall change.

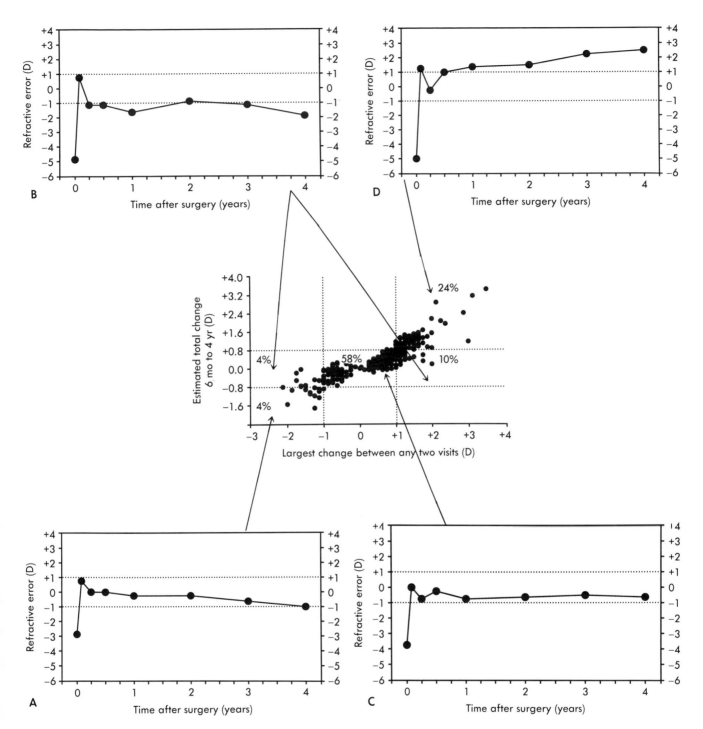

Figure 24-13

The categorization of eyes in the PERK study according to the two measures of stability: *trend* (estimated total change 6 months to 4 years) and *magnitude* (largest change between any two visits). The areas of the scattergram define the categories, as exemplified by the time course for one eye from each category. **A,** Loss of effect of surgery: 4% of eyes had an increase in minus power of 1.00 D or more according to both measures. **B,** Fluctuation: 14% of eyes did not have a definite trend but did have a change of 1.00 D or more during some follow-up interval. **C,** Stable course: 58% of eyes changed by less than 1.00 D on both measures. **D,** Continued effect of surgery: 24% of eyes had a decrease in minus power. Three patterns of change were noted in this group: 14% of eyes showed a persistent decrease in minus power during 6 months to 4 years **(D);** 4% of eyes showed a decrease in minus power in a fluctuating pattern (no example shown), and 6% of eyes showed an initial decrease in minus power that later became stable (no example shown). (From Waring GO, Lynn MJ, Strahlman ER, et al: Am J Ophthalmol 1991;111:133-144.)

Table 24-6

Percentage of Eyes in Each Interval of Refractive Error at 6 Months and 4 Years According to Refractive Stability Category in the PERK Study

Refractive stability category	Number of eyes	Refractive error at 6 months and 4 years*					
		< −1.00 D		±1.00 D		> +1.00 D	
		6 mo	4 yr	6 mo	4 yr	6 mo	4 yr
Stable	197	20%	15%	71%	74%	9%	11%
Fluctuating	49	29%	20%	55%	55%	16%	25%
Continued effect	82	29%	4%	56%	52%	15%	44%
Loss of effect	13	31%	61%	54%	31%	15%	8%
Total	341	24%	15%	65%	65%	11%	20%

From Waring GO, Lynn MJ, Strahlman ER, et al: Am J Ophthalmol 1991;111:133-144.
*For each stability category, the percentage of eyes in each refractive interval at 6 months and at 4 years after surgery.

In the PERK study the values for absolute change from 6 months to 4 years were almost identical to the values obtained by the more complex analysis involving both magnitude and trend. Thus, using the absolute change between two time points is a reasonable way to estimate stability of refraction after refractive keratotomy (see Fig. 24-11).

Effect of refractive instability on overcorrection and undercorrection. Although studies of the stability of refraction itself are interesting, the practical consequences of these relate primarily to the residual refractive error for individual patients. For example, a change in refraction in the hyperopic direction of 2 D would have a different effect on a person who started out undercorrected with a refraction of −2.00 D and then became emmetropic as opposed to an individual who started out emmetropic and then became +2.00 D hyperopic.

Table 24-6 indicates the changes in the number of eyes undercorrected and overcorrected between 6 months and 4 years in the PERK study. As expected, the eyes with the stable refraction changed little, whereas the eyes with a fluctuating refraction showed a slight trend toward increasing overcorrection. Marked changes were in those eyes with a continued effect of surgery; only 15% were overcorrected at 6 months, but 44% were overcorrected at 4 years. Similarly, the small number of eyes moving in a myopic direction showed an overall increase in undercorrections.

Table 24-7 shows the same information in a different way, demonstrating that approximately half of the eyes that were undercorrected at 6 months fell within ±1 D at 4 years and none became overcorrected. For these eyes, the continued effect of the surgery could be seen as an advantage. Interestingly, eyes with a refraction between −1.00 and +1.00 D at 6 months had an approximately 10% chance of moving into the undercorrected or overcorrected category.

Rate of change and duration of instability of refraction

It is difficult to calculate a meaningful rate of change for instability of refraction, since there is so much variation from one eye to another. However, overall, the number of eyes changing by 1 D or more over 4 years in the PERK study was reasonably uniform, increasing by approximately 5% per year. This does not mean that 5% per year are becoming overcorrected, but rather that 5% per year are changing by 1 D or more, most of them with a continuing decrease in minus power (Table 24-8).

Table 24-7

6-Month and 4-Year Comparison of the Number and Percentage of Eyes in Each Interval of Refractive Error in the PERK Study

Refraction at 6 months	Refraction at 4 years		
	Undercorrected (< −1.00 D)	−1.00 to +1.00 D	Overcorrected (> +1.00 D)
Undercorrected (<1.00 D)	45 (55%)	37 (45%)	0
−1.00 to +1.00 D	21 (10%)	166 (75%)	33 (15%)
Overcorrected (> +1.00 D)	4 (10%)	3 (8%)	32 (82%)
Total	70 (21%)	206 (60%)	65 (19%)

From Waring GO, Lynn MJ, Strahlman ER, et al: Am J Ophthalmol 1991;111:133-144.

Table 24-8

Percent of 341 Eyes with Increasing Effect of Surgery ≥1 D between Follow-up Visits after Radial Keratotomy

From	To				Approximate time intervals
	1 yr	2 yr	3 yr	4 yr	
6 mo	5.3	12.3	14.9	22.6	
1 yr		5.4	9.3	14.5	4 yr
2 yr			4.3	6.8	3 yr
3 yr				4.2	2 yr
					1 yr

How long this instability and overall trend toward hyperopia will last is unknown. Five studies have found it persisting up to 5 years (Table 24-2), with Deitz reporting it up to 8 years (Tables 24-3 and 24-4) and Ivanova and Fyodorov reporting it up to 12 years.[15] This uncertainty emphasizes the need for long-term follow-up of 10 to 20 years of a well-documented group of patients, such as those in the PERK study.

PRACTICAL ASPECTS OF REFRACTIVE INSTABILITY
Effect on daily living

The fact that only 58% of the patients' eyes in the PERK study were stable in all regards between 6 months and 4 years after surgery raises the specter of wild fluctuations in vision that might require multiple pairs of glasses every day and inexorable trends that may cause many patients to become hyperopic as they reach their forties. Some have speculated that rapid changes in refraction would be dangerous, particularly for individuals with military, aviation, or law-enforcement responsibilities. (Consider the pilot calling out from his jet fighter, "I can't see very well this morning.") Fortunately, these suspicions have *not* materialized because changes in refraction after 6 months occur slowly and are relatively small. Specifically, 98% of the eyes in the PERK study changed less than 2.00 D between 6 months and 4 years. The 82 eyes that showed an increasing effect of surgery had a mean change from 6 months to 4 years of 1.28 D, which averages 0.03 D per month. These changes do not seriously disrupt visual function from one day to another, and most individuals will be able to function without visual surprises or disability. Therefore patients, ophthalmologists, and employers can be reassured that the changes in refraction after refractive keratotomy are small and gradual.

Cumulative effect

The total number of patients who gradually become hypermetropic after radial keratotomy will increase (Table 24-8). This is well demonstrated by the 82 eyes that showed a continued effect of the surgery in the PERK study: only 15% were overcorrected at 1 D or more at 6 months, but 44% were overcorrected at 4 years after surgery. The longer the process lasts, the more overcorrections will occur.

Even a small cumulative effect can produce a meaningful clinical change. Consider a speculative example: a 25-year-old person who has radial keratotomy and achieves a perfect refractive outcome of emmetropia 6 months after surgery may demonstrate a continued effect of the surgery of 0.10 D annually; by age 55, the refraction will be +3.00 D and the person will require full-time refractive correction for both distance and near vision.

Early symptomatic presbyopia

The onset of symptomatic presbyopia is delayed in myopic individuals because most have a near point that is within arm's length, giving them the option of taking off their glasses for reading or of adjusting their contact lenses so that one eye is in focus at near while the other eye is in focus at distance (monovision). Most emmetropic and hypermetropic individuals must use plus lenses in the form of reading glasses or bifocals after approximately age 45 to achieve satisfactory near vision; the greater the hypermetropia, the earlier the need for near correction. A continued increase in the effect of radial keratotomy will cause early presbyopia in most individuals.

Most patients who have had radial keratotomy and become presbyopic in their early forties are happy to have exchanged the full-time use of their distance correction for part-time use of reading glasses. Those who become more than 1 D hypermetropic will likely need a correction for both distance and near vision, paradoxically thwarting the original goal for having surgery.

Effect on predictability of refractive keratotomy

Instability of refraction decreases the predictability of the outcome. In the PERK study 4 years after surgery, the 90% prediction interval for the refractive outcome was 4.12 D, approximately six times greater than that achieved by fitting glasses or contact lenses. The inability to identify before surgery who will exhibit an increasing effect of the surgery makes it more difficult to predict the outcome for an individual patient.

Intentional undercorrection

Most refractive keratotomy surgeons now aim for a final refractive error of −0.50 to −1.00 D rather than emmetropia. This has been accomplished by reducing the number of incisions from 16 to 8 to 4, by maintaining a diameter of the central clear zone of 3 mm or greater, by avoiding incisions of extreme depth (95% of corneal thickness or more), and by doing less extensive surgery on older individuals. Residual low myopia allows patients to retain good uncorrected visual acuity,[31] delays the onset of symptomatic presbyopia, and hedges against a continued increase in the effect of the surgery.

CHARACTERIZATION OF PATIENTS WITH UNSTABLE REFRACTION

Common sense might suggest that patients who have more surgery in the form of longer incisions (smaller-diameter clear zone), more incisions, and deeper incisions might be prone to more instability because a greater wound area must heal. Data from the PERK study[39] and Sawelson and Marks[34] support this concept, whereas the report of Deitz, Sanders, and Raanan[9] does not. In the PERK study,[39] among eyes that had less than 1.00 D of change between 6 months and 4 years, a higher percentage received a 4.0-mm clear zone, and therefore shorter incisions than the eyes showing an increasing surgical effect (Table 24-9). Sawelson and Marks[34] found a statistically significant larger decrease in minus power in eyes with greater myopia (-6.00 to -10.00 D) than those with less myopia (-1.50 to -5.88 D): 0.77 D in the former group and approximately 0.07 D in the latter (p < 0.006). The group with more preoperative myopia had smaller diameter clear zones and deeper incisions, but no analysis of specific surgical variables was reported.

Table 24-9

Diameter of Central Clear Zone According to Stability from 6 Months to 4 Years in the PERK Study

Category of stability	Number of eyes	Diameter of central clear zone*		
		4.0 mm	3.5 mm	3.0 mm
Stable	197	43%	35%	21%
Fluctuating	49	22%	33%	45%
Continued effect	82	20%	30%	50%
Loss of effect	13	38%	31%	31%

*For each stability category, the percentage of eyes in each clear-zone group. Note that stable category is significantly different from fluctuating and continued effect categories (p < 0.001).

None of these studies found a correlation between a change in refraction over time and the patient's age or sex, preoperative or intraocular pressure, preoperative keratometry, or central corneal thickness. Deitz, Sanders, and Raanan[9] did not find a correlation with the depth, number, length, or recutting of the incision.

Thus the surgeon knows that a certain percentage of patients will show a meaningful, progressive surgical effect but is unable to identify them. Therefore all patients must be warned of this potential long-lasting difficulty.

STABILITY OF REFRACTION AFTER REPEATED KERATOTOMY

The only published report addressing the question of stability after repeat radial keratotomy is from the PERK study. Of 62 eyes that had repeat procedures with eight additional incisions between the original eight incisions, patients representing 42 of these eyes made at least four visits at 3 months and 1, 2, 3, and 4 years. Changes in refraction from 3 months to 4 years were classified in the same way as for eyes with only one procedure, with these results—stable, 64%; fluctuating with no definite trend, 15%; unstable with a decrease of -1.00 D or more, 17%; and unstable with an increase of -1.00 D or more, 5%. This distribution of eyes was not statistically significantly different from that of eyes with one-time surgery ($p = 0.3$).[22]

Thus the number of incisions in the cornea, if they exceed eight, may or may not have a meaningful effect on the long-term stability. One might deduce that the length or depth of incisions would be more important.

STABILITY OF UNCORRECTED VISUAL ACUITY

Table 24-10 shows the change in uncorrected visual acuity for the categories of refractive stability. For eyes with a stable refraction, 76% had no change in visual acuity and the distribution of gain and loss was similar, suggesting normal biologic variation. Of eyes that showed a continued effect of surgery with a decrease in minus power, 31% gained two or more Snellen lines of visual acuity. This improvement in visual acuity occurred for undercorrected eyes whose refractive error moved closer to emmetropia; eyes that became more overcorrected did not have a change in uncorrected visual acuity, presumably because accommodation compensated for the increase in hyperopia. McDonnell and colleagues[22] have described diurnal variation in visual acuity in 26 eyes after radial keratotomy.

Table 24-10

Change in Uncorrected Visual Acuity According to Refractive Stability from 6 Months to 4 Years in the PERK Study

Category of stability	Number of eyes	Change in uncorrected visual acuity (Snellen lines)*		
		Loss ≥2	Change <1	Gain ≥2
Stable	197	9%	76%	15%
Fluctuating	49	16%	68%	16%
Continued effect	82	13%	56%	31%
Loss of effect	13	62%	38%	0%
Total	341	13%	68%	19%

*For each stability category, the percentage of eyes in each interval of change in uncorrected visual acuity.

CHANGES IN REFRACTION AND KERATOMETRIC POWER

To document that the changes in refraction were caused by changes in the curvature and power of the cornea, we correlated the change in the average central keratometric measurements with the change in the spherical equivalent cycloplegic refraction between 6 months and 4 years. The correlation between the two was -0.52 ($p = 0.001$), indicating a moderate association. We do not report the quantitative details of the keratotometric changes here.

MECHANISMS OF REFRACTIVE INSTABILITY

Both the inability to correlate patient and surgical variables with unstable refraction by regression analysis and the absence of biomechanical information about the material properties of the incised cornea leave the surgeon only one option in accounting for instability: speculation. It is not difficult to list a series of factors that might produce variations in refraction from morning to evening and over time, but identifying which of the following factors plays a role requires more extensive study[30]:

1. Depth, length, and number of incisions

2. Differential material properties of the corneal scar and the uncut corneal stroma
3. Wound healing: rate, strength, and individual variability
4. Individual variability in the properties of the cornea, especially age and ocular rigidity
5. External forces on the eye, such as eyelid pressure or rubbing the cornea
6. Corneal edema: postoperative and physiologic variation
7. Topical and systemic drugs
8. Partial pressure of oxygen and the effect of hyperbaric oxygen

MORNING-TO-EVENING (DIURNAL) VARIATION
Terminology

Changes in refraction and visual acuity that occur during a 24-hour period have a number of designations. In general, they assume a normal sleep-wake cycle, with sleeping during the nighttime hours. Changes that occur during the 24-hour period are called "variations" or "fluctuations." They are generally designated as "diurnal," indicating a morning-to-evening daily change. There are no published studies of changes in refraction during a 24-hour period for individuals with unusual sleep-wake cycles such as those who work night shifts. Also, there are no studies that correlate actual number of hours of sleep with refractive stability.

Diurnal variation in the PERK study

At 1 year and at 3.5 years after surgery, the PERK study measured the diurnal variation among a group of patients who complained of fluctuating vision at 2 months after surgery.[32,35] Patients were not randomly selected but were self-

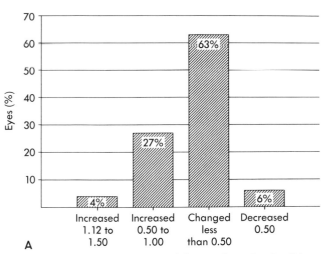

A

Change in minus power of the manifest refraction (D)
from morning to evening at 3½ years

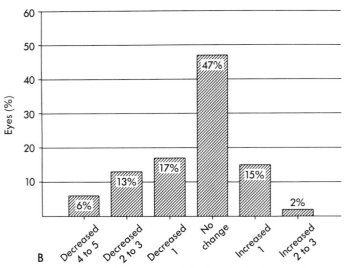

B

Change in uncorrected visual acuity (Snellen lines)
from morning to evening at 3½ years

Figure 24-14
The change in the manifest refraction (D) from morning to evening measured at 2 to 4 years after surgery in 52 eyes in the PERK study. Approximately one third of eyes show increased minus power of 0.50 to 1.50 D during the day. (From Santos VR, Waring GO, Lynn MJ, Schanzlin DJ, Cantillo N, Espinal M, Garbus J, Justin N, and Roszka-Duggan V: Ophthalmology 1988;95:1487-1493.)

Figure 24-15
The change in the uncorrected visual acuity (Snellen lines) from morning to evening measured at 2 to 4 years after surgery in 52 eyes in the PERK study. Approximately 20% of eyes lost two to five lines during the day. (From Santos VR, Waring GO, Lynn MJ, Schanzlin DJ, Cantillo N, Espinal M, Garbus J, Justin N, and Roszka-Duggan V: Ophthalmology 1988;95:1487-1493.)

Figure 24-16
The morning to evening change in refraction at 2 to 4 years after surgery compared with that at 1 year in 52 eyes shows four patterns of change: 46% had no measurable fluctuation; 17% had persistent fluctuation; 22% had an unstable refraction at 1 year, but appeared to have stabilized by 3.5 years later; the remaining 15% (7.5% and 7.5%) appeared stable at 1 year and subsequently had slightly greater changes. (From Santos VR, Waring GO, Lynn MJ, Schanzlin DJ, Cantillo N, Espinal M, Garbus J, Justin N, and Roszka-Duggan V: Ophthalmology 1988;95:1487-1493.)

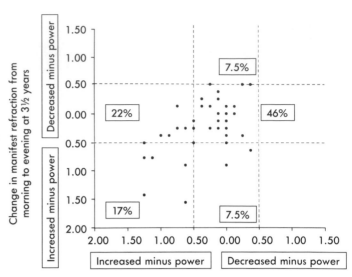

selected on the basis of their visual complaints and their willingness to participate in the study. It was not the intent to evaluate the incidence or magnitude of diurnal fluctuation in the total PERK population.

Of 52 eyes examined both morning and evening 3.5 years after surgery, 31% had an increase in the minus power of the manifest refraction of 0.50 to 1.50 D (Fig. 24-14), 19% had a decrease in uncorrected visual acuity by two to five Snellen lines (Fig. 24-15), and 29% showed central corneal steepening with a keratometer of 0.50 to 1.00 D. These data indicate that approximately one of four corneas had not stabilized, although 3.5 years had elapsed since surgery.

The diurnal variation in refraction was not consistent for all eyes studied at 1 and 3.5 years (Fig. 24-16). The morning-to-evening change was less at 3.5 years than at 1 year in 22%. Fifteen percent of eyes with no variation in manifest refractive error at 1 year changed 0.50 to 0.87 D at 3.5 years.

One of the drawbacks of the PERK study is that the full range of variation during the day was not determined because patients were examined a variable amount of time (usually one half to 2 hours) after waking; thus the study missed the larger changes of refraction and visual acuity that can occur immediately after waking and underestimated the total amount of fluctuation in some eyes.

MacRae and colleagues[20] studied diurnal variation in a group of patients, their study design differing in many respects from the PERK study. They studied a smaller number of patients (eight) at an earlier time postoperatively (1 to 2 weeks after surgery), keeping the eye taped shut between awakening and the time of measurements to capture the full range of diurnal change. Eyes were examined immediately after eyelid opening at 7:30 AM and again at 4:00 PM. The contralateral eye was used as a control. Refractive results showed that the treated eye was 1.48 ±0.24 D (mean ±SEM) more hyperopic in the morning than in the afternoon, whereas the unoperated control eyes had an insignificant change (0.16 ±0.06 D). Keratometric readings in the operated eye were significantly flatter (1.37 ±0.19 D) in the morning than in the afternoon as compared with the control eyes, which were only 0.11 ±0.09 D flatter. The major correlation with these changes was the corneal thickness, as measured by central ultrasonic pachometry; operated corneas were significantly thicker (5.7%) in the

Table 24-11

Comparison of Changes in Four Variables from Time of Eye Opening on Awakening (7:30 AM) to Afternoon (4 PM) after Radial Keratotomy (Mean ±SEM)*

Group (number of eyes)	Refraction (D)	Keratometry (D)	Corneal thickness (mm)	Intraocular pressure (mm Hg)
1. Radial keratotomy (n = 8)	−1.48 ±0.24†	1.37 ±0.19†	0.032 ±0.006†	0.50 ±0.53
2. Contralateral unoperated open eye (n = 8)	−0.16 ±0.06	0.11 ±0.09	0.004 ±0.003	0.50 ±0.84
3. Contralateral nonoperated eye closed until morning measurement (n = 4)	−0.22 ±0.16	0.06 ±0.12	0.009 ±0.003	0.25 ±0.48

Modified from MacRae S, Rich L, Phillips D, and Bedrosian R: Am J Ophthalmol 1989;107:262-267.
*Groups 2 and 3 do not differ significantly for any of the four variables.
†Group 1 differs from Groups 2 and 3 (p ≤ 0.01).

morning than in the afternoon, when compared with controls (1.7% thicker). There was no correlation with change in intraocular pressure (Table 24-11). The authors concluded that diurnal variations in corneal edema were the primary mechanism responsible for changes in refraction and keratometric measurements.

Diurnal variation reported by ophthalmologists

Two ophthalmologists who had radial keratotomy have measured changes in their refraction from morning to evening during the first year after surgery.

Wyzinski,[43] 38 years old, found that the greatest change in refractive error occurred in the first hour after awakening. Over the course of the day, the amount of change at 1 year was about a 2.00 D increase in myopia in each eye (see Fig. 24-6). Wyzinski noted that if the morning measurement had occurred about 2 hours after arising, the increase in myopia would not have been as extreme, about 0.75 D in each eye.

Richmond,[29] 51 years old, measured his refraction and keratometric power 90 minutes after awakening in the morning and at 4:30 PM. Over 2.5 years after surgery he measured significant variation in refraction of about 0.75 D consistently up to 2.5 years postoperatively; he estimated a total daily variation of 1.25 D from awakening to bedtime. His attempt to verify that changes in intraocular pressure were responsible for fluctuation by using glaucoma medications to reduce the overcorrection in one eye yielded a surprise—hyperopia increased (see Chapter 25, The Patient Speaks: Testimonials after Refractive Keratotomy).

Mechanism of diurnal variation

The forces that produce morning-to-evening variation in corneal shape—flattening during sleep and steepening during waking—have not been clearly defined. Candidates include corneal edema that occurs beneath the closed eyelid, early morning elevations in intraocular pressure, which amount to only a few millimeters of mercury, and mechanical pressure of the closed eyelids on the cornea.

During sleep the closed lids decrease the evaporation of the tears, which therefore become more dilute during sleep. This decreases the osmotic gradient of the tears across the epithelium, so that the normal human cornea thickens 4% to 8% during sleep.[20,21] On awakening the tonicity of the tears increases and corneal hydration decreases, measured as a decrease in corneal thickness. Most of these changes occur during the first 1 or 2 hours after awakening. These variations could account for the great changes in refraction noted by radial keratotomy patients 1 to 2 hours after awakening and may influence the daily fluctuation as well.

MacRae and colleagues[20] found a statistically significant correlation between decreasing corneal thickness and increasing minus power of the refraction and increasing corneal steepness on keratometric measurements. The greater diurnal change in corneal thickness and refraction in eyes that have had radial keratotomy may be caused by an exaggerated swelling of the cornea because the epithelial barrier is not as tight as in normal eyes or because the normal physiologic response can be exaggerated due to the decreased structural integrity produced by the incisions. Several reports support the concept that corneal thickness and corneal contour are related. In one report[37] an eye that developed an iridocyclitis after radial keratotomy showed a 12% increase in central corneal thickness (0.58 to 0.65 mm) associated with a marked change in refraction in the hyperopic direction (from -0.25 D to $+4.12$ D). Although the intraocular pressure was high initially, it fell and did not seem to be associated with the corneal flattening. As the uveitis subsided, the corneal thickness returned to normal and the refraction returned to the same level as that before the uveitis appeared. Contact lenses are well known to induce corneal edema, particularly soft contact lenses that span the corneal surface from limbus to limbus. Corneas may swell from 1% to 6%.[20] Edwards and Schaefer[10] reported 10 eyes that were left undercorrected after radial keratotomy and were fitted with soft contact lenses; these eyes changed refraction in the hyperopic direction, presumably because of the corneal edema induced by the hypoxia of the lenses, although a mechanical effect of the lenses cannot be ruled out. An example of this phenomenon is presented in Fig. 24-17.

Richmond[29] has demonstrated that lifting the lids off the globe produced steepening of the cornea, as measured by quantified keratographs. The continued pressure of the eyelid on the cornea during sleep may flatten the cornea, and the lids being open during the day may allow the cornea to steepen. Richmond has also suggested that high atmospheric pressure, low atmospheric humidity, and ocular convergence could produce a myopic shift.[30]

Practical aspects of daily fluctuation

The percentage of radial keratotomy patients who experience daily fluctuations in vision is unknown. Bourque et al.[5] administered a psychometric questionnaire to 355 patients in the PERK study before surgery and 1 year after surgery. This included four questions specifically referring to fluctuating vision in the operated eye, from which a fluctuation index was devised. "A lot of trouble" with fluctuating vision during the day was reported by 33.5% of patients; 42% indicated average trouble and the remaining 24.5% little or no trouble. The patients reported significantly more fluctuation in vision 1 year after radial keratotomy than they did before surgery, when only 12.1% patients reported great difficulty with fluctuation. Patients who had problems with fluctuating vision throughout the day were generally less satisfied with the results of surgery. Table 24-12 correlates the satisfaction index with fluctuation and glare indices.

Daily fluctuation of vision can persist for 5 years or more after refractive keratotomy, but its impact on each patient varies widely. Many patients have no fluctuation or state that the little they observe does not bother them. It is extremely rare for a patient to use different pairs of glasses during the day. Some

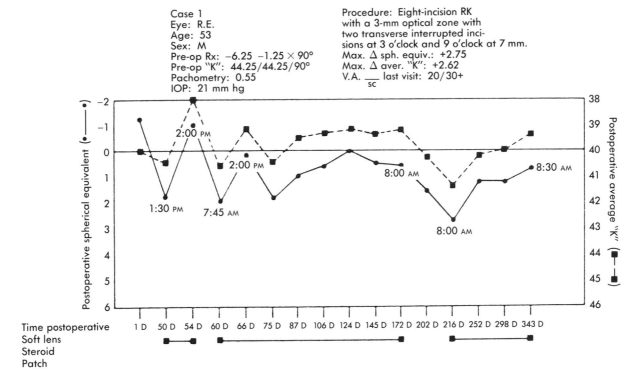

Case 1
Eye: R.E.
Age: 53
Sex: M
Pre-op Rx: −6.25 −1.25 × 90°
Pre-op "K": 44.25/44.25/90°
Pachometry: 0.55
IOP: 21 mm hg

Procedure: Eight-incision RK
with a 3-mm optical zone with
two transverse interrupted incisions at 3 o'clock and 9 o'clock at 7 mm.
Max. Δ sph. equiv.: +2.75
Max. Δ aver. "K": +2.62
V.A. $\frac{}{sc}$ last visit: 20/30+

Figure 24-17
Relationship of spherical equivalent refractive error and days after refractive keratotomy in a patient who wore soft contact lens intermittently. The 52-year-old man
had a preoperative refraction in his right eye of −6.25 − 1.25 × 90°. The intraocular
pressure was 21 mm Hg. He received an eight-incision radial keratotomy with a
3.0-mm diameter clear zone along with two transverse interrupted incisions at 3
o'clock and 9 o'clock at the 7-mm zone. At day 50 after surgery his refractive error
was −1.00 −1.50 × 100°. To correct the residual myopia, a daily wear lens, Sol-
Syntex CSI, 8.90, 14.80, −1.00 D was fitted. Four days later his refractive error was
+1.75 −1.50 × 125°. As the graph shows, when the contact lens was removed he
became more myopic, and when the contact lens was reinserted he moved toward
hyperopia, becoming essentially emmetropic. Diurnal variation from morning to
evening of approximately 1.00 D is present consistently during the approximate
1-year follow-up. (From Edwards GA and Schaefer KM: J Refract Surg 1987;3:54-
58.)

Table 24-12

**Correlation between the Satisfaction Index and Fluctuation Index
1 Year after Radial Keratotomy in the PERK Study***

		Satisfaction index, no. (%) of patients		
Fluctuation index	**No. of patients**	**Not satisfied (1.0 to 2.9)**	**Moderately satisfied (3.0 to 5.0)**	**Very satisfied (5.1 to 7.0)**
None (1.0 to 2.9)	87	3 (3.4)	15 (17.2)	69 (79.3)
Moderate (3.0 to 5.0)	149	11 (7.4)	71 (47.7)	67 (45.0)
Severe (5.1 to 7.0)	119	20 (16.8)	63 (52.9)	36 (30.3)
Total	355	34	149	172

From Bourque LB, Cosand BB, Drews C, Waring GO, Lynn M, and Cartwright C: Arch Ophthalmol
1986;104:356-363.
*p = 0.003; χ² test.

individuals, however, complain of the fluctuation, particularly when they become myopic in the evening and experience night myopia while driving or difficulty seeing television or screens in cinemas.

Longer-term follow-up should give more information about patients' experiences of and reaction to daily fluctuation. How long this will continue in affected patients is unknown.

STABILITY OF REFRACTION AFTER ASTIGMATIC KERATOTOMY

There are no published studies of changes in refraction or visual acuity from morning to evening or over an intermediate follow-up period in eyes that have had only astigmatic keratotomy. Most of these eyes have combined radial and transverse incisions; eyes with only isolated transverse incisions or trapezoidal patterns of incisions are few. Whether transverse incisions produce the same patterns of refractive instability as radial incisions is unknown.

UNFINISHED BUSINESS

The two major challenges concerning stability of refraction after refractive keratotomy are to identify before surgery those individuals who will have a continued increasing surgical effect and to determine how long this will last. Identifying patients before surgery will require more meticulous measurement of individual characteristics, particularly the topography and even the biomechanical properties of the cornea in vivo, for example, by holography. The persistent progression of surgical effect should sufficiently motivate researchers with established data bases to continue following patients over many years. This expensive, frustrating, time-consuming undertaking is the only way to determine the duration and severity of long-term instability. The PERK study has been funded by the National Eye Institute to perform examinations at 10 years (in 1993), which will help determine if stability has occurred by that time. Whether eyes with four incisions have more stable refractions than eyes with eight incisions is unknown.

Research in methods to speed corneal wound healing and stabilize the wounds involve biologically active substances. For example, inserting materials into the wound immediately after surgery has been proposed, as described in Chapter 20, Corneal Wound Healing and Its Pharmacologic Modification after Refractive Keratotomy. Filling the wound with substances such as a fibronectin gel impregnated with epidermal growth factor, proteoglycans, and collagen might keep the epithelial plug out of the wound and allow fibroblasts to invade the wound more quickly. This might speed wound healing and might even make a more stable wound, which could decrease long-term instability and possibly diurnal fluctuation. On the other hand, since the corneal scar will probably never have the material properties and tensile strength of the normal, nonincised cornea, some individuals may experience instability and fluctuation indefinitely.

REFERENCES

1. Arrowsmith PN and Marks RG: Visual, refractive and keratometric results of radial keratotomy: a five-year follow-up, Arch Ophthalmol 1989; 10:506-511.
2. Binder PS, Layak SK, Deg JK, Zavala EY, and Sugar J: An ultrastructural and histochemical study of long-term wound healing after radial keratotomy, Am J Ophthalmol 1987;103:432-440.
3. Blegvad O: Ueber die Progression der Myopic, Klin Montasbl Augenheilkd 1918;60:155.
4. Bores LD, Myers W, and Cowden J: Radial keratotomy: an analysis of the American experience, Ann Ophthalmol 1981;13:941-948.
5. Bourque LB, Cosand BB, Drews C, Waring GO, Lynn M, and Cartwright C: Prospective evaluation of radial keratotomy (PERK) study group: reported satisfaction, fluctuation of vision, and glare among patients 1 year after surgery in the Prospective Evaluation of Radial Keratotomy (PERK) study, Arch Ophthalmol 1986;104:356-363.
6. Brown EVL: Net average yearly changes in refraction of atropinized eyes from

birth to beyond middle life, Arch Ophthalmol 1938;19:719-734.

7. Bücklers M: Changes in refraction during life, Br J Ophthalmol 1953;37:587.

8. Deitz MR and Sanders DR: Progressive hyperopia with long-term follow-up of radial keratotomy, Arch Ophthalmol 1985;103:782-784.

9. Deitz MR, Sanders DR, and Raanan MG: Progressive hyperopia in radial keratotomy: long-term follow-up of diamond-knife and metal-blade series, Ophthalmology 1986;93:1284-1289.

10. Edwards GA and Schaefer KM: Corneal flattening associated with daily soft contact lenses following radial keratotomy, J Refract Surg 1987;3:54-58.

11. Fyodorov SN and Agranovsky AA: Long-term results of anterior radial keratotomy, J Ocular Therapy Surg 1982;1:217-223.

12. Fyodorov SN and Dunev VV: Operation of dosages dissection of corneal circular ligament in cases of myopia of mild degree, Ann Ophthalmol 1979;11:1885-1890.

13. Gemmill M and Waring GO: Slit-lamp microscopic observation of the healing of radial keratotomy wounds over a period of 5 years (unpublished data).

14. Hays JC, Rowsey JJ, and Balyeat HD: Effect of postoperative steroids on the refractive result of radial keratotomy, Invest Ophthalmol Vis Sci 1985; 26(suppl):150.

15. Ivanova P and Fydorov SN: Paper presented at Second International Cataract, Implant, Microsurgical and Refractive Keratoplasty Meeting, Nagoya, Japan, July 1-3, 1988.

16. Kiely P, Carney LG, and Smith G: Diurnal variations of corneal topography and thickness, Am J Optom Physiol Opt 1982;59:976.

17. Lepard CW: Comparative changes in the error of refraction between fixing and amblyopic eyes during growth and development, Am J Ophthalmol 1975;80:485-490.

18. Lipshitz I: Morning-to-evening changes in the PERK study, Ophthalmology 1989;96:926-927 (letter to the editor).

19. Lynn MJ, Waring GO, and PERK Study Group: Stability of refraction after radial keratotomy compared with unoperated eyes in the PERK study, Invest Ophthalmol Vis Sci (Suppl) 1987;28:223.

20. MacRae S, Rich L, Phillips D, and Bedrossian R: Diurnal variation in vision after radial keratotomy, Am J Ophthalmol 1989;107:262-267.

21. Maurice DM: The cornea and sclera. In Davison H, editor: The eye, vol 1b, ed 3, San Francisco, 1984, Academic Press, Inc, pp 1-158.

22. McDonnell PJ, McClusky DJ, and Garbus JJ: Corneal topography and fluctuating visual acuity after radial keratotomy, Ophthalmology 1989;96:665-670.

23. McDonnell PJ and Schanzlin DJ: Early changes in refractive error following radial keratotomy, Arch Ophthalmol 1988;106:212-214.

24. Mertz GW: Overnight swelling of the living human cornea, J Am Optom Assoc 1980;51:211.

25. Neumann AC: Personal written communication, Nov 1988.

26. Nizam A, Carter J, Lynn M, Waring G, Asbell P, Balyeat H, Cohen E, Culbertson W, Doughman D, Fecko P, McDonald M, Smith R, and the PERK Study Group: Changes in refractive error, keratometric power and best-corrected visual acuity for unoperated myopic eyes in the Prospective Evaluation of Radial Keratotomy (PERK) study, Invest Ophthalmol Vis Sci 1990; 31(suppl):30.

27. O'Day DM, Feman SS, and Elliot JH: Visual impairment follow radial keratotomy, Ophthalmology 1986;93:319-326.

28. Parel JM, Simon G, and Lowery J: The effect of wound hydration on central corneal curvature and laser and diamond knife keratotomy, Invest Ophthalmol Vis Sci 1990;31(suppl):479.

29. Richmond RD: Special report: radial keratotomy as seen through operated eyes, J Refract Surg 1987;3:22-27.

30. Richmond RD: Radial keratotomy as seen through operated eyes. Part II. J Refract Surg 1988;4:91-95.

31. Santos VR, Waring GO, Lynn MJ, Holladay JT, Sperduto RD, and the PERK Study Group: Relationship between refractive error and visual acuity in the Prospective Evaluation of Radial Keratotomy (PERK) study, Arch Ophthalmol 1987;105:86-92.

32. Santos VR, Waring GO, Lynn MJ, Schanzlin DJ, Cantillo N, Espinal M, Garbus J, Justin N, and Roszka-Duggan V: Morning to evening change in refraction, corneal curvature, and visual acuity 2 to 4 years after radial keratotomy in the PERK study, Ophthalmology 1988;95:1487-1493.

33. Sarver MD, Baggett DA, Harris MG, and Louie K: Corneal edema and hydrogel lenses and eye closure: effect of oxygen transmissibility, Am J Optom Physiol Opt 1981;58:386.

34. Sawelson H and Marks RG: Five-year results of radial keratotomy, Refract Corneal Surg 1989;5:8-20.

35. Schanzlin DJ, Santos VR, Waring GO, Lynn MJ, Bourque L, Cantillo N, Edwards M, Justin N, Reinig J, and Roszka-Duggan V: Diurnal change in refraction, corneal curvature, visual acuity, and intraocular pressure after radial keratotomy in the PERK study, Ophthalmology 1986;93:167-175.

36. Smith P: Introduction to a discussion on the diagnosis, prognosis and treatment of pernicious myopia, Ophthalmic Rev 1901;20:331.

37. Starling JC and Hofmann RF: Case report: anterior uveitis and transient hyperopia following radial keratotomy, J Refract Surg 1986;2:96-98.

38. Waring GO, Lynn MJ, Fielding B, Asbell PA, Balyeat HD, Cohen EA, Culbertson W, Doughman DJ, Fecko P, McDonald MB, Smith RE, Wilson LB, and the PERK Study Group: Results of the Prospective Evaluation of Radial Keratotomy (PERK) study 4 years after surgery for myopia, JAMA 1990;263:1083-1091.

38a. Waring GO, Lynn MJ, Nizam A, et al: Results of the Prospective Evaluation of Radial Keratotomy (PERK) study 5 years after surgery, Ophthalmology (in press).

39. Waring GO, Lynn MJ, Strahlman ER, et al: Stability of refraction during 4 years after radial keratotomy in the Prospective Evaluation of Radial Keratotomy study, Am J Ophthalmol 1991:111; 133-144.

40. Waring GO, Moffitt SD, Gelender H, Laibson PR, Lindstrom RL, Myers WD, Obstbaum SA, Rowsey JJ, Safir A, Schanzlin DJ, Bourque LB, and the PERK Study Group: Rationale for and design of the National Eye Institute Prospective Evaluation of Radial Keratotomy (PERK) study, Ophthalmology 1983;90:40-58.

41. Waring GO, Steinberg EB, and Wilson LA: Slit-lamp microscopic appearance of corneal wound healing after radial keratotomy, Am J Ophthalmol 1985; 100:218-224.

42. Williams PA, Chen V, Choi KY, Skelnik DL, and Lindstrom RL: The intraoperative and postoperative changes in K-readings following four-incision radial keratotomy, Invest Ophthalmol Vis Sci 1990;31(suppl):30.

43. Wyzinski P and O'Dell LW: Diurnal cycle of refraction after radial keratotomy, Ophthalmology 1987;94:120-124.

The Patient Speaks: Testimonials after Refractive Keratotomy

Mary C. Gemmill
George O. Waring III

Lost in the mass of statistics, tables, and graphs is the individual experience of each patient. We have attempted to capture the meaning and subjective aspects of refractive keratotomy by asking seven patients to relate concisely their experience with the surgery. We selected a full spectrum of stories, from fulfilled wishes to dashed dreams, including one that has been previously published—a candid assessment of refractive keratotomy by an ophthalmologist who underwent the procedure. The stories are not thorough case histories, but individual portrayals of the meaning of refractive keratotomy to these patients. To put the patients' comments in perspective, we have flanked their comments by a brief clinical history and our own editorial observations.

LIFELONG WISH COME TRUE
Clinical background

C.L.J. is a 36-year-old female registered nurse. Her preoperative refraction was −3.00 sphere in the right eye (20/15) and −2.75 sphere in the left eye (20/12). Her keratometry readings were 43.12 × 180°/43.87 × 82° in the right eye and 43.50 × 178°/43.75 × 80° in the left.

Her refractive keratotomy surgery was performed on the right eye in October 1982 in the PERK study. Eight single-pass centrifugal radial incisions were made with a 4.0-mm clear zone and the knife blade set at 100% of the thinnest para-

BACKGROUND AND ACKNOWLEDGMENTS
We asked each of the patients who contributed to this chapter to do so. The original contribution of each patient was moderately edited, but thereafter we have reproduced the patients' comments and observations with minimal editing. The observations are theirs, not necessarily ours. We thank each person for the time, effort, and content involved in his or her contribution. The contributions of Charles Snyder and Richard Richmond have been previously published, as acknowledged. Many of the patients were in the PERK study.

A Myope's View of Nearsightedness

I am a myope. To the best of my knowledge, I have always been a myope. At present I am O.S. −10.00, O.D. −8.25. This degree of correction enables me to review with a small amount of authority the world of the myopic patient.

When the myope removes his glasses the entire world is instantly covered by a great blanket of soft, merging colors, drifting mysteries, beautiful, muted. The myope looks at faces and to him they never smile, never frown; they are never ugly, never beautiful; for the myope sees all faces as pink, brown, or yellow balloons, moving in and out of a haze, opening slightly across the middle to speak to him. He is only vaguely aware of twisted bodies. Old age he cannot recognize. To him no room is ever badly decorated, no house ever in need of repairs or painting. The lawns he sees are smooth and green; crab grass does not exist. Streets are never shabby or dirty.

In brief, the unglassed myope looks at the world and sees no evil, no ugliness; all is soft, colorful, harmonious, indefinite. The myope often loves this world and, when pressures of the real world become too great for him, he may retreat from the definite into the indefinite by removing his glasses "to rest his eyes."

At an early age the myope learns he is different from his playmates. He does not mind too much, but his parents and teachers do, and one fine day he is fitted with his first pair of glasses. Now the world certainly looks different to him. He no longer stumbles over the cracks in the sidewalks and, wonder of wonders, he can read the blackboard in school. But little does he suspect that this is the first of endless pairs of glasses he will wear and that he will be a slave to his glasses until he dies.

The myope appreciates his glasses. He knows, oh so well, that he would be lost without them. Yet he resents them, for they are a badge of his physical inadequacy; they mark him as a weakling, as an incomplete human being. When he is young, the cost of examinations and new glasses are a drain on his small pocketbook; when he is older, each change in his prescription is a sign of his body's aging.

Consciously or unconsciously, every person who wears glasses wishes there was a simple, easy way he could eliminate them from his life. He wants something, anything, that will enable him to see the world as it really is. . . . .

Just as the obese of our population desire an effortless regime to relieve themselves of their excess poundage and to look slim and handsome, so the spectacle-wearers desire an easy path to good vision without glasses. It is inherent in human nature to want to be as nearly physically perfect as possible. Glasses—even though life is often impossible without them—are the mark of an incomplete or weak body. Provide any sort of hope, any program that gives even a glimmer of a promise that glasses are unnecessary, and the public will respond in droves.

From Snyder C: Bates, Huxley, and myself: a saga in visual reeducation. In Sloan AE: Refraction in children, Int Ophthalmol Clin 1962;2:921-934.

central intraoperative ultrasonic pachometry readings. Surgery on the left eye was done in November 1983 using eight incisions and a 4.0-mm clear zone.

In September 1987, her uncorrected visual acuity was 20/16 in the right eye, and 20/12 in the left eye. Her refraction was plano + 0.50 × 135°, right eye (20/16$^+$), and −0.25 sphere, left eye (20/12$^+$). Her keratometry readings in the right eye were 40.37 × 05°/40.87 at 95°, and in the left eye were 41.37 × 12°/42.00 × 106°. The patient gave this testimonial 5 years after her first surgery.

The patient speaks

"I began wearing glasses in the third grade and always hated them for cosmetic reasons. I started wearing contact lenses as a junior in high school and hated them because of all of the associated hassles of insertion, sensitivity, cleaning, etc. These hassles bothered me more than the cosmetic benefits, so that I would only wear contacts when cheerleading, going on dates, etc. (I was a real peer pressure victim.) I also at one time tried the orthokeratology contact lens procedure.

"I first heard of radial keratotomy when working as a registered nurse in Daytona Beach, Florida, around 1980. I attended a seminar regarding RK and decided I would do it. The only factor holding me back at the time was the cost. Insurance companies were not covering this procedure, so I decided to wait until I could afford it.

"A medical reporter told me about the PERK study, so I applied and was accepted. I had no reservations about the surgery and was eager to have it done. The actual procedure was minor surgery and caused me no anxiety. The discomfort postop for the first eye was the worse part. A year later when the second eye was done, I had prepared myself for the same severe pain. This time, however, the pain never came. This I attribute to the changed medications for pain—Dilaudid instead of Tylenol with codeine.

"The only negative aspect I have experienced occurs when driving at night. Headlights and traffic lights now have "points" related to the incision lines. There is a sensation of the lights being beyond normal brightness and this is sometimes disconcerting. This drawback is very minor compared to what I have gained. I would not give up my 20/20 vision because of it. Besides, when I wore contacts, I always experienced a "halo" effect at night with the same type lights.

"The benefits to me are well worth the surgery. First in importance is giving up the hassles involved with supportive vision care. Second is the freedom in such activities as swimming and other sports, and third is cosmesis. I really enjoy swimming and volleyball. Swimming is wonderful now. I don't have to deal with contacts or glasses and I can see. The surgery has also really helped in my work. I spend a lot of time at a computer terminal. My contact lenses would dry out and make it difficult to see. Not dealing with the hassles of contact lenses or glasses has given me much more time and freedom.

"I love telling people about my surgery and success. There are so many misconceptions about the procedure. I supply friends with materials from the PERK study and my own testimony. Since my procedure, two other people in my office have also had RK and one friend desires it in the near future.

"I am not fearful of what may happen to my eyes in the future. I truly do not believe anything horrible will happen 10 years from now. I'm confident technology will advance multifold over the years so that any possible problems will be dealt with. I'd rather enjoy my life right now to the fullest, and radial keratotomy has helped in a positive way.

"All my life I've made up a list of three wishes I'd love to have granted. They are always those 'impossible' things that are fun to dream about but could never come true. Well, *always* number one on my list was to have perfect vision. Thanks to RK, that wish is fulfilled and I can replace it with a new one. I'll never again believe that dreams can't come true!"

Editorial observation

She articulates clearly the motives that drive most patients to refractive surgery: ridding themselves of dependence on optical devices for normal, daily visual function—a motive much stronger than cosmesis alone. The persistent starburst pattern around lights at night occurs in the majority of patients, but is discounted by most as a minor nuisance, not dissimilar from what they experienced with dirty glasses or with contact lenses. Her exuberance cannot be taken lightly by the ophthalmic profession.

A 6-YEAR DELAY OF SECOND EYE SURGERY
Clinical background

W.H.S. is a 42-year-old businessman. His preoperative refraction was $-5.25 +0.25 \times 135°$, right eye, and $-6.00 +0.50 \times 50°$, left eye. His corrected visual acuity was 20/20 in each eye. His keratometry readings were $41.62 \times 90°/41.62 \times 180°$ in the right eye and were $41.37 \times 176°/41.87 \times 85°$ in the left eye.

Radial keratotomy was performed on his right eye on September 2, 1981, in the PERK study. Eight centrifugal radial incisions were made with a 3.0-mm diameter clear zone.

Six years postoperatively, in July 1987, the patient's uncorrected visual acuity in the right eye was $20/20^-$, and his refraction was $-1.00 +1.25 \times 175°$ (20/15). The refraction for the left eye was $-6.50 + 0.50 \times 20°$. His keratometry readings at this time were $37.75 \times 95°/38.37 \times 172°$, OD, and $41.87 \times 05°/41.87 \times 95°$, OS. Although the patient was more than 6 D anisometropic, he was most bothered by the "starburst" he describes in his testimonial and was never bothered by image disparity.

Surgery was performed on the left eye on July 13, 1987. Eight centrifugal radial incisions were made with the blade set at 110% of a paracentral corneal thickness, with a 3.0-mm diameter clear zone.

Three months postoperatively, the patient's uncorrected visual acuity in the left eye was 20/32. His refraction was $+0.50 +1.75 \times 05°$ $(20/20^-)$. His keratometry reading in the same eye was $36.25 \times 95°/37.12 \times 05°$. The patient gave this testimonial 6 years after his first eye surgery and 3 months after his second eye surgery.

The patient speaks

"When I first investigated radial keratotomy, I had an eye examination that I considered to be an extensive review of each eye. This examination established confidence in the surgeon and staff and made me anticipate good results. Even so, not knowing exactly what to expect created a certain level of anxiety while I was on the operating table. The operation was easier than I expected; there was no pain or discomfort. Listening to the doctors during the procedure also proved to be informative and relieving.

"The night after the operation passed with very little discomfort. The next 6 days were not as easy. I had soreness and problems rolling over while sleeping because of the increased discomfort.

"My vision as well as my mobility have been greatly improved by the operation. The first morning after surgery when I removed the patch, I saw the leaves on a tree without glasses for the first time. This was truly breathtaking, considering the fact that I was used to putting on my glasses to go to the bathroom.

"Not long after surgery, I noticed a starburst at night. This proved to be a greater problem than I expected, and was my primary reason for delaying surgery on the second eye. The starburst was a real concern to me. A starburst in one eye was difficult enough; both eyes seemed like an impossible problem.

"I was very satisfied with the improvement in vision in the right eye, and after several years, the starburst effect reduced greatly. Because of this, I decided to have my second eye surgery. I anticipated similar results or better ones than in my right eye.

"The anxiety level was greatly reduced during the second surgery. Those involved in the procedure seemed to be more at ease and the surgeon's method of inducing a relaxed state was also significantly improved over the first operation.

"Two days after surgery, I had an apparent reaction to the [gentamicin] drops. The eye burned every time I used the drops. It was also very sore and scratchy, as well as sensitive to light. The light sensitivity appeared to be greater than the first surgery. Double vision was present at all times, as well as the starburst effect at night.

"Now that 8 weeks have passed, I have no pain or soreness, the double vision has subsided, and my vision is very clear during the daylight hours. I still notice a considerable starburst at night.

"I have several recommendations I think may have helped my symptoms and postoperative problems:

1. I would have preferred to have the eye needing the greater correction have surgery first.
2. The postoperative eye drops did not give relief of soreness and scratchiness. I wonder if a topical pain medication could be used postoperatively. I would suggest this only if it would not harm the eye or affect healing.

3. Perhaps a perforated eye cover would prove helpful to decrease the starburst effect. I would need it only at night when driving."

Editorial observation

This patient's emphasis on postoperative pain, also echoed by C.L.J., emphasizes what a vivid aspect of the surgical procedure this can be, an aspect that is often downplayed by surgeons enthusiastic about the procedure. Topical gentamicin was used as the prophylactic antibiotic after surgery, and its toxic effect is articulated by this patient. Similarly, the starburst effect, which is often minimized by surgeons (as I did in my observations on the case of C.L.J.) caused this patient to delay surgery for 6 years, and yet apparently would not qualify as "disabling glare." Maybe we investigators are missing something in our assessment of glare.

HAPPY SWAP OF DISTANCE GLASSES FOR READING GLASSES
Clinical background

M.A.C. is a 42-year-old female secretary. Her preoperative refraction in the right eye was −3.00 sphere (20/20$^+$), and in the left was −3.50 +0.50 × 90° (20/20$^+$). Her preoperative keratometry readings were 45.62 × 170°/46.12 × 60°, right eye, and 46.12 × 180°/46.37 × 90°, left eye.

Her first refractive keratotomy was done as part of the PERK study on the right eye on April 1, 1982. Eight centrifugal radial incisions were made with a 4.0-mm diameter clear zone. The second (left) eye was done on May 18, 1983. Eight centrifugal radial incisions were made with a 4.0-mm diameter clear zone.

On April 13, 1987, five years after her first eye was operated, her uncorrected visual acuity was 20/20$^-$ in both eyes. Although able to read without correction, she had some blurring of print with each eye, the right eye being worse than the left. Her refraction in the right eye was −0.75 +1.75 × 180° (20/16) and in the left eye was −0.75 +1.25 × 10° (20/20). Her keratometry readings were 42.25 × 140°/42.37 × 60° in her right eye, and 42.50 × 94°/43.25 × 02° in her left eye.

On September 17, 1987, at 42 years of age, the patient returned for follow-up with symptoms of presbyopia. A repeat refraction was performed. The visual acuity of the right eye was 20/15 with −0.75 +0.50 × 180°. No change in the refraction was noted in the left eye. Reading glasses were prescribed. The following testimonial was given 5 years after the operation on her first eye.

The patient speaks

"At 8 years of age it became necessary for me to wear glasses full time, and for the next 30 years, I lived with the daily problems they caused.

"As a child, I was teased and left out of games. As I grew older, the teasing stopped, but I still could not participate in activities that required I remove my glasses, because I could not see without them. In addition to these problems, it seemed I was always looking through a layer of dust and dirt, no matter how often I cleaned the lenses.

"When I reached adulthood, I tried wearing contact lenses. During the period of about 10 years, I tried approximately 10 different pairs of lenses—all unsuccessfully. I finally gave up on them and resigned myself to the fact I would always have to wear glasses. I guess the thing I resented most was constantly being asked, 'Are you a school teacher?'

"During the spring of 1982, I heard about a new surgery called radial keratotomy that would correct myopia. I finally called Emory University School of Medicine when I was unable to get information through the media or by calling several doctors. I spoke with a secretary who informed me that I might qualify for a research program and told me how to apply.

"About 5 days later, I received a telephone call informing me, to my surprise, that I did qualify for their program. Two of the things required were a psychological test and an interview by the surgeon. Although radial keratotomy is now being done in private practice, I feel these two things should still be a major consideration in making the decision to have this elective surgery.

"In a matter of weeks, I had my left eye operated on. The only negative thing in connection with the surgery was the pain afterwards. It was like no pain I have ever experienced before or since. However, it did not last very long—only a few days. The most positive thing was that within 24 hours, I could look out my kitchen window and, with my right eye, actually count the leaves on the tree just outside. It took a few months for my vision to stabilize, but I didn't experience any real difficulty.

"Having had only one eye operated on left me with one good eye and one bad eye to contend with for the next year, when I could have my left eye operated on. To my good fortune, there was another 'miracle' in store for me. A new soft contact lens had been developed. I was able to get by for the next year wearing it in my right eye.

"By the time for surgery on my right eye, the research team had made some improvements involving procedures that made the surgery more comfortable. The pain afterwards was pretty much the same, but it seemed to me that my vision had stabilized much sooner.

"It has now been 5 years since my left eye surgery and 4 years since surgery on my right eye. I have to admit that the decision to go through with the surgery was a hard one to make, but after weighing the possibilities, I decided I had very little to lose if it didn't work and a lot to gain if it did.

"In the last few months I have experienced some difficulty from time to time doing close work and reading. It came as no surprise because I was told of the possibility this would happen. Had I not had the surgery I might not have had this problem for another 10 years, at the age most people experience this problem in the normal aging process. This means I will again have to depend on glasses. However, this does not alter my attitude toward the surgery because had I not decided to have the surgery I would be wearing glasses all of the time, not just for close work and reading.

"Yes, in spite of the pain involved and the fact that I must wear glasses for close work and reading, I would make the same decision again. I am thankful for the years I did not have to depend on glasses. (I haven't been asked once in the past 5 years if I am a school teacher!)

"Without people who are willing to weigh the possibilities and make positive decisions, there would be no research, and without research there would be no progress. By participating in this research program, I hope it may be possible for others, such as my son who has visual problems, to experience a miracle even greater than I have."

Editorial observation

Symptomatic presbyopia will come earlier for myopes like M.A.C., who end up with an approximately plano spherical equivalent correction. Her testimonial emphasizes two major points. First, she had been warned about the earlier onset of presbyopia and was therefore prepared to accept it when it arrived. Second, she articulates the most common point of view expressed by these individuals, "I hate my reading glasses, but not nearly as much as I hate my distance glasses. I would much rather wear reading glasses part of the time than have to wear distance glasses all the time."

The approximately 1.00 D increase in refractive astigmatism in each eye is not fully detected in the keratometric measurements and is an undesirable side effect of the surgery.

DECREASED VISUAL ACUITY BUT LESS DEPENDENCE ON GLASSES
Clinical background

P.A. is a 34-year-old man who is a major in the air force and is currently attending a local university for his doctorate; he was seen at the Emory Eye Center in consultation. His preoperative refraction in the right eye was −6.50 +1.50 × 122°, and in the left eye −5.00 sphere, which gave a visual acuity of 20/20 in each eye. The patient had three refractive keratotomy operations performed on each eye. The first surgery was in May 1983, the second in September 1983, and the third in September 1984. Both eyes were operated each time. No other clinical information was available.

In July 1987, his uncorrected visual acuity in the right eye was 20/40, and in the left eye 20/25. His cycloplegic refraction in the right eye was −0.50 +1.25 × 15° (20/30), and in the left eye −1.75 +2.00 × 115° (20/20). The patient had a 6 prism diopter exophoria at distance and near. Slit-lamp microscopy of the right cornea revealed 37 radial incision scars of 20% depth and four transverse incisions. The transverse incisions were located at 2:30, 5:30, 8:30, and 11:30. The left cornea had 19 radial incision scars of approximately 30% depth, with two transverse incisions at 3:00 and 9:00 of 80% depth. Keratography demonstrated severe irregular corneal astigmatism in each eye. Trial fitting with rigid gas-permeable contact lenses was recommended, but was not scheduled by the patient. Four years after his first procedure, the patient gave the following testimonial.

The patient speaks

"My major reason for considering radial keratotomy was because my work in the military requires frequent business trips. I was always concerned that I may lose my glasses and would not be able to see. I was just as worried about losing a contact lens down the drain.

"My surgeon is an ophthalmologist who has a special interest in radial keratotomy. In fact, he devotes his entire Friday to just radial keratotomy surgery. While he was very positive about the surgery, I felt well informed about possible side effects or complications. Two of the people in my office had surgery by the same physician and both had 20/15 uncorrected vision postoperatively.

"I expected radial keratotomy surgery to improve my vision appreciably, and it did. My vision improved greatly. I am very active in sports, including snow skiing and surfing. Before surgery, my vision was so bad that participation in sports was very difficult. My glasses interfered or did not fit properly because of perspiration. In some cases, like surfing, I couldn't wear them at all. I tried that once and lost a pair very quickly. Radial keratotomy has provided me with an additional degree of freedom. I am glad that I had the surgery.

"My dissatisfaction comes from the irregular healing that occurred, especially in my right eye. My corrected vision is not as crisp as it was before surgery. I am currently working on my PhD and am having difficulty reading the blackboard and acetate slides used in overhead projectors. My right eye is only 20/30 with glasses, and the difference in the acuity between my eyes brings out my exophoria. I did not have a problem with double vision in contact lenses.

"Overall, I am happy that I had the surgery. On business trips, I was always worried that I might lose my glasses or contact lenses. Now, I don't have that problem. I am even capable of driving without my glasses. I no longer feel dependent on my glasses; I use them only to enhance my vision.

"I did not realize there was a controversy among surgeons regarding the number of cuts and the time between surgeries. I understand that this may have contributed to the irregular healing. Had I known, I may have opted for a different surgical technique, but then again, hindsight is always 20/20."

Editorial observation

By 1990 standards, all would agree that excessive surgery was performed on P.A., with three operations in each eye, producing more than 30 incisions in one and approximately 20 in the other. Most ophthalmic surgeons would not do bilateral surgery at the same operation. This is a prescription for permanent irregular astigmatism, which he now experiences. This patient's statements illustrate the attitude that astounds most ophthalmologists: apparent satisfaction in spite of a loss of best-corrected visual acuity. This patient is no passive, ignorant dupe; he is a military man enrolled in a doctoral engineering program. His testimonial emphasizes the strong drive many patients have to rid themselves of dependence on glasses and contact lenses.

ASYMMETRIC RESULTS AND A RETURN TO CONTACT LENSES
Clinical background

M.V.F. is a 34-year-old female airline reservation agent. Her preoperative refraction in the right eye was −6.00 +0.75 × 45° and in the left eye −5.50 +0.25 × 45°. Best-corrected visual acuity was 20/20⁺ in both eyes. She had radial keratotomies performed on both eyes following the PERK protocol. In January 1983, eight centrifugal incisions were made in the right eye with a 3.0-mm diameter clear zone and the knife blade set at 100% of paracentral corneal thickness. In October 1984, eight centrifugal incisions were made in the left eye with the knife blade set at 110% depth and a 3.0-mm diameter clear zone.

On February 20, 1987, her uncorrected vision was 20/40 in the right eye and 20/80 in the left. The best-corrected visual acuity was 20/12 in the right eye with −1.25 +0.75 × 37°, and 20/16 in the left eye with −2.50 +0.50 × 114°. Keratography demonstrated no irregular astigmatism in either eye. The patient was unable to function without her glasses because of asymmetrical visual acuity. The patient gave the following testimonial 4 years after the first procedure.

The patient speaks

"In August 1982, I first considered radial keratotomy because I felt I was a danger to myself without my contact lenses or glasses. It seemed I was always running into walls or doors whenever I didn't wear correction. The main reason I elected to have my second eye operated was because I wanted to be a flight attendant. They require 20/100 vision without glasses. Little did I know at the time they would reject me because I had the surgery.

"I feel I was basically prepared for the surgery. I knew that cuts would be made on my cornea, but I was unaware of the marking and other testing that would be done before the cuts. I felt like I was under a mountain of sheets and was looking down a tunnel. The most frightening part of the surgery was when he was marking the incisions; it felt like my head would go through the table. I wished I could have been asleep instead of awake, or had watched a procedure before I had it. Of course, if I had watched, I probably wouldn't have had the surgery.

"I had no pain until after the anesthetic wore off, then I felt extreme pain for the next 24 hours. I found I could see television without my glasses the first night. I had severe nausea after both surgeries, especially when I rode an elevator. Returning for my follow-up appointment was very difficult. My eye was sore the day after surgery and was sensitive quite awhile afterward."

"Now that 4 years have passed, I found that my second eye did not turn out as well as the first. If I were to choose again I would not have had the surgery on my second eye. I am unable to read street signs and sometimes have double vision, especially when I wake up or am really tired. At night, when I look at lights, I notice a star effect, and I generally have more difficulty seeing at night.

"The only way to overcome the disparity in my vision is to wear glasses, which I really hate after being a successful contact lens wearer for eighteen years. I have difficulty with my routine activities. I enjoy clogging and if I wear glasses, they bounce all over my face. If I take them off, I have difficulty finding my way on and off stage. I also drive a motorcycle and have an extremely difficult time fitting my helmet over my glasses."

(Because of the patient's complaints about inability to be involved in recreational activities, she was fitted with hard contact lenses in March 1987. After wearing her contact lenses for 6 months, she wrote this letter.)

"Now that I have had time to adjust to hard contact lens once again, I can tell you how they are working out.

"I could tell from the first day that my vision was sharper and clearer, but the first time I was out at night, I was really surprised. The star effect was no longer there, my night blindness had decreased sharply, and I could read street signs easily. I still have trouble judging the distance of oncoming cars.

"We had a lot of trouble trying to get the contact lenses to fit, and they slide off the cornea more than any others. I have not attempted to wear them more than 16 hours like I did before because they are not as comfortable and I am more cautious.

"My decision about the surgery is the same as before. I would still have had the surgery, but probably on one eye only."

Editorial observation

M.V.F.'s anisometropic undercorrection has left her disappointed. Not only must she continue to wear correction during her avocational activities—the opposite of the goal she had set for herself by having the surgery—but she must also wear contact lenses uncomfortably and imperfectly for her best visual function. Presumably the contact lenses reduced some irregular astigmatism. Even at that she says she would have surgery again—albeit in only one eye. Her inability to become a flight attendant because of her surgery provides a good warning to surgeons and patients alike: check carefully the conditions for prospective employment before surgery.

HIGH EXPECTATIONS, POOR RESULTS, AND A LAWSUIT
Clinical background

D.L.K. is a 35-year-old minister who has been myopic since 2 years of age. An examination from 1971 indicated that his refraction in the right eye was −14.00 +3.00 × 160° (20/40) and in the left eye −13.00 +2.00 × 08° (20/25). His keratometry readings in 1971 were 43.50/44.62 × 161°, right eye, and 43.75/44.25 × 16°, left eye. In 1980 the patient had

16-incision radial keratotomy surgery on both eyes and a reoperation (additional incisions in the area of the first incisions) on each eye in 1981. No further details of the surgery were available.

In October 1984, he was seen in consultation at the Emory Eye Center. Visual acuity was 20/50 in the right eye with −12.25 +4.00 × 152°, and 20/80 with −13.00 +0.75 × 160° in the left eye. His keratometry readings were 37.50 × 75°/41.75 × 165° in the right eye and 41.00 × 10°/42.75 × 100° in the left. Keratoscopy revealed bilateral irregular astigmatism (see Chapter 18, Fig. 18-13). Endothelial cell count by specular photomicrography was 2000 cells/mm² in each eye.

Slit-lamp microscopy revealed 16 radial incisions with a 2.7-mm diameter clear zone in the right eye. Superficial vascularization was present in nine incisions. Several incisions were double. Examination of the left eye revealed 15 incisions with a clear zone diameter of 2.5 mm. Superficial vascularization was present in 11 incisions. All incisions were double. The incisions in both eyes were irregular, crossed each other, and did not end in a precise clear zone. The depth of the incisions was variable.

Fundus examination bilaterally revealed retinal pigment epithelial mottling in the posterior pole, myopic crescents around the optic discs, and posterior staphylomas.

As treatment for the irregular astigmatism, a trial fitting with rigid gas-permeable contact lenses was recommended, but never scheduled by the patient. Seven years after the first surgery the patient gave the following testimonial.

The patient speaks

"I first read about radial keratotomy in the *Palm Beach Post Times*. I still have the article 7 years later. It told the story of a postman who was legally blind and threw away his glasses after having surgery with this new technique. I contacted my local ophthalmologist to get more information. He was not personally familiar with RK, but gave me some ideas about the right questions to ask. Was I a suitable candidate, considering the size and curvature of my eye?

"The reason I had the surgery was that I was looking to see better without glasses in case of an emergency. I did not expect to decrease my visual acuity with glasses. I am also a minister. The most frequent complaint I heard was that people thought I was not looking at them. The glasses were so thick, they couldn't tell where I was looking. I wanted to try to improve that. I guess it was also vanity. I did know that I would have to wear glasses after surgery.

"When I considered radial keratotomy, I did not expect to go without my glasses. I was too myopic for that, but I expected to go without them if necessary. I wore very heavy glasses (like cataract glasses) and I still do.

"My expectations were pretty high. It was almost like being healed by a faith healer. You know how people get caught up in the moment with a faith healer; they feel better at first, and later realize that they are not much better than they were. I felt much better at first. The doctor was exuberant about the surgery and felt it was the greatest thing to come along, and I felt his exuberance.

"I was very apprehensive with the first set of surgeries. I had two. I was apprehensive about pain, but it didn't really hurt. It was pretty routine.

"Nine months after the surgery, I was really much better. My refraction had improved from about −14.00 to −7.00 and from −12.50 to −8.00. When I saw the doctor for a follow-up, he told me that astigmatism surgery would help. Also, at that time, there was no charge for the reoperation. It was covered by a blanket fee from the first surgery, so I went ahead. After the second pair of surgeries, the problems started. When I wasn't seeing clearly, the doctor told me it would take some time for the cornea to heal, and he felt it would continue to improve.

"I had 30 changes of glasses in 2 years. I moved back to my hometown and saw my old optometrist. When he looked at my eyes, he asked me, 'What the hell happened?' and 'Who did this?' He told me that he had seen several patients who had had RK, but none looked like me. This was the first time I considered filing a lawsuit. He referred me to an ophthalmologist who did an extensive workup and who then referred me to another ophthalmologist who specializes in RK. He also referred me to another RK specialist from a different school of thought. The latter two gentlemen had been known to not agree, but they agreed about the condition of my eyes.

"The reason I filed the lawsuit was because I was told by the surgeon that although my vision would not improve, I was also guaranteed that it wouldn't be worse. I am now 6 to 7 years postop, but my scars look like they are 1 year postop. I have been told that the scars cause irregular astigmatism, which makes my vision hard to correct. My prescription is now about −11.00 and −12.50, almost the same as preoperatively. My best visual acuity is 20/60 with both eyes. I am 20/60 with one and 20/70 to 20/80 with the other. I was 20/30 and 20/25 before my first surgery. I still have symptoms as if I just had the surgery; lights are distorted.

"After my first set of surgeries, I could tell my wife's shampoo from conditioner without my glasses. This only lasted 1 week, as the effects of the procedure regressed very quickly, but my vision was still 20/30 to 20/40 with glasses. After the second set of surgeries, my vision really got worse.

"My refraction has finally stabilized after 7 years. I have worn the same prescription for 2½ years. I still have fluctuation in my vision from morning to night, but I also have a symptom that seems to be uncharacteristic to other RK patients. I notice fluctuation in my vision from day to day. Some days, my vision is really good, then I'll have a bad day or two, followed by some average days.

"After more than 3½ years, the litigation is over. We won the lawsuit and were awarded $300,000 plus legal expenses. It is my understanding that our case set a precedent and was the first successful suit by a patient who has had radial keratotomy.

"Right now, I wouldn't touch RK with a 10-foot pole. If I were to start over, I would not have had the surgery at all. If I did have the surgery, I would go to someone experienced in the surgery, not some RK shop where the surgeon operates at 7 AM and 7 PM."

Editorial observation

This disastrous tale illustrates the catalytic relationship between a highly motivated patient and an enthusiastic physician. The patient's desire to reduce his need for spectacles—even with the full realization that he would not achieve normal, uncorrected acuity—and the surgeon's enthusiastic (but clearly unrealistic) promise to fulfill this desire fostered an adventure into surgery that resulted in the loss of the patient's ability to function as a minister, a loss so severe he sued the ophthalmologist. This scenario emphasizes the need for ophthalmologists to present candidly the strengths and weaknesses of refractive keratotomy and to insist that patients assess the probable outcome realistically, rather than enthusiastically wishing for miracles.

■ ■ ■

RADIAL KERATOTOMY AS SEEN THROUGH OPERATED EYES*

We conclude this chapter with excerpts from the previously published, extraordinarily candid experience of ophthalmologist Richard Richmond, MD, who had refractive keratotomy bilaterally. Not only does Dr. Richmond outline his motives for seeking radial keratotomy, but he meticulously relates his visual experiences over 2 years postoperatively, including a repeated operation for overcorrection. He concludes that his bilateral overcorrection should serve as an impetus to further research in refractive keratotomy to refine its predictability. We have edited the original contribution for clarity.

The patient speaks

"The desire to see unaided may transcend reason. As a 51-year-old ophthalmologist with a busy practice and everything to lose, I made a decision to have radial keratotomy (RK) done on my eyes. As with most others who consider radial keratotomy, the major stimulus for my decision was to rid myself of total dependence on glasses. In addition, I had already made the decision to become a radial keratotomy surgeon. I did not relish the task of having to explain to each RK candidate why I was wearing a moderately thick myopic correction, and yet was preparing to operate on them. So, on September 17, 1985, my left eye was operated upon and 2 days later, my dominant right eye was done.

"Before declaring me unwise for having my eyes done 2 days apart consider your need as an ophthalmologist for binocular vision. After radial keratotomy was performed OS, I had no satisfactory way to deal with 4.5 diopters (D) of anisometropia. Contact lenses and my eyes have always had a strong dislike for each other. My nondominant left eye was showing the expected overcorrection, of both sphere and cylinder, on the morning prior to my right eye surgery. I then made the decision to have my dominant right eye done, and there is a distinct advantage to healing only once.

Methods of examination

"Graphic representation of refractive and keratometric changes are illustrated in Fig. 25-1. Refractions were done by me using a B&L Green's refractor (minus cylinder). Final monocular endpoint was aided by the red-green test. Refractions were done 90 minutes after arising and at 4:30 PM. The early refraction time was chosen for convenience and did not represent the most hyperopic refractive error—greatest hyperopia was present upon awakening. The 4:30 PM time was within 0.25 D of greatest myopia during the full year of this study. Refractions were done without cycloplegia due to frequency of examinations, convenience, and expectation that at age 51, cycloplegia would show little difference from noncycloplegic refraction. Refractions were done at least 5 days per week during the first 2 months, weekly through 6 months, then monthly through 1 year.

"Keratometer (K) readings were done with a B&L

*Modified from Richmond RD: Radial keratotomy as seen through operated eyes, J Refract Surg 1987;3:22-27 and Richmond RD: Radial keratotomy as seen through operated eyes. Part II. J Refract Surg 1988;4:91-95.

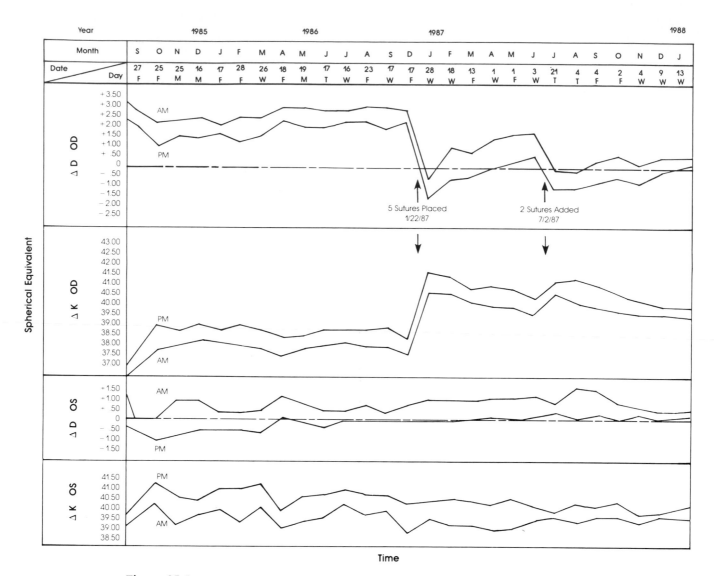

Figure 25-1

The patient's charting of his own refractions and keratometric readings over 3 years after bilateral radial keratotomy. The diurnal fluctuation with a flatter cornea and less minus power in the morning than in the evening has persisted for a 2½-year period. An additional loss of effect occurred in each eye during the first 6 weeks after surgery, and 3 months after surgery there have been fluctuations in refraction on the order of 0.50 to 1.00 D. Both eyes were overcorrected, but neither showed a marked tendency toward progressive, continued effect of the surgery during the period followed. For the markedly overcorrected right eye, wound revision was undertaken approximately 1 year after the initial surgery, resulting in a near emetropic refraction. (From Richmond RD: J Refract Surg 1988;4:91-95.)

keratometer, calibrated using a +42.50 steel ball. K readings were taken shortly after each refraction.

"Ocular pressure was measured by Goldman applanation tonometer calibrated as directed by the service manual.

"Pachometer measurements were done with a DGH 2000 pachometer with an angled probe.

Initial operations—both eyes

"My surgery was done under topical local anesthesia using 0.5% proparacaine, 0.5% tetracaine, and 1% unbuffered pontocaine. With these agents, surgery was painless. Ultrasonic pachometer measurements were taken with a DGH 2000 pachometer the day before surgery. Optical centers were marked using a Zeiss Opmi 6 microscope filament. The corneal reflex was marked at the opposite inferior edge, using monocular fixation. Incisions were made with an Xtal sapphire blade, Katena #K2-6505. Incisions were set at 100% of average pachometer measurements, plus 10 microns. Following calculations using a Bores-Fyodorov computer program, a 12-incision RL procedure was chosen OS. Incisions were performed from a 3.0 mm × 4.0 mm oval optical zone to the 6 mm optical zone. Blade length was extended to 100% of average measurements at 6 mm, plus 10 microns, and the incisions were extended to the limbal arcade. Peripheral redeepening was done from the 8 mm optical zone to the limbal arcade in all incisions. Six opposing L incisions, parallel to the 165° axis, were done first, followed by six radial incisions.

"Eight radial incisions were performed OD from 2.75 × 3.50 mm oval optical zone to the 6 mm optical zone. Blade length was then extended to 100% of average measurement at 6 mm, plus 10 microns. The incisions were then completed to the limbal arcade.

Repeated operations—right eye

"Revision of the [overcorrected] right eye by interrupted compression suture technique was initially done on January 22, 1987. Due to induced astigmatism and residual hyperopia, two additional sutures were placed on July 2, 1987.

"Anesthesia for the initial revision surgery was preceded by Brevital and followed by peribulbar injection using a 50-50 mixture of 2% lidocaine and 0.75% Marcaine with 1 cc of Wydase. The two additional sutures were placed using only topical 0.5% proparacaine.

"During the initial suturing, five incisions were opened by blunt dissection using a Sinsky hook and bluntly cleaned to remove epithelial plugs. When the additional two sutures were placed, the incisions were not opened. The incisions were closed using 10-0 Mersilene during the first operation; 11-0 Mersilene was used for the second operation. The knots were adjusted in slip knot configuration.

"On both occasions, sutures were placed perpendicular to the incision and extended 1 mm on either side of the incision at 75% of the stromal depth. All sutures were placed at the 7-mm optical zone. Sutures were tightened under keratometric control using a Terry keratometer capable of measuring 1.6 mm optical zone size. Fig. 25-2 illustrates the sequence of suture placement. There is no intent to remove the sutures.

"During [the suture revision] surgery, the first example of deceptive difficulty occurred, which shows this procedure is not simple. After incisions at 52°, 142°, 232°, and 322° had been opened and cleaned, and while sutures were being tightened, the incision at 187° opened spontaneously. A fifth suture was then necessary to close the gaping incision. Despite these sutures being tightened under keratometric control to a spherical reading of 43.00 D, postoperative astigmatism increased by 1.75 D (Table 25-1). This increase in astigmatism, and the presence of residual hyperopia, dictated addition of two sutures on July 2, 1987, instead of removing sutures to alter astigmatism.

"Again, when the two additional sutures were placed on July 2, 1987, the deceptive difficulty of this operation became more evident. Preoperative astigmatism showed the flattest corneal meridian to be 80°, with the nearest incision being at 97° (Fig. 25-2). A suture was placed perpendicular to the 97° incision at the 7-mm optical zone, and when tightened, vectored 4 D of astigmatism to 135°.

"The operating surgeon gave me the option of removing the suture or having a second suture placed. It took me about 10 seconds to decide to add a second suture. Hyperopic astigmatism still present after the original suturing gave uncorrected visual acuity no better than 20/50; meridional aniseikonia with correction was almost as uncomfortable, as was more symmetric aniseikonia following the original RK procedures.

"A second suture was then placed 90° from the vectored astigmatism, across the 52° incision. The sutures were again tightened under keratometric control to a reading of 42.25 D × 90° by 41.00 D × 180°. Sequential postoperative K and refraction measurements can be followed in Table 25-1.

"Postoperatively, I experienced the expected 2½ days of foreign body sensation prior to epithelial healing. Photophobia was not a serious problem for my brown eyes and relatively small pupils. Starbursts around lights cleared within 6 months OS, but a sig-

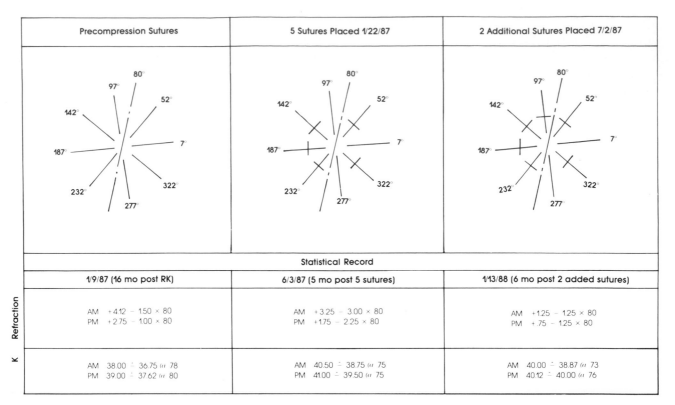

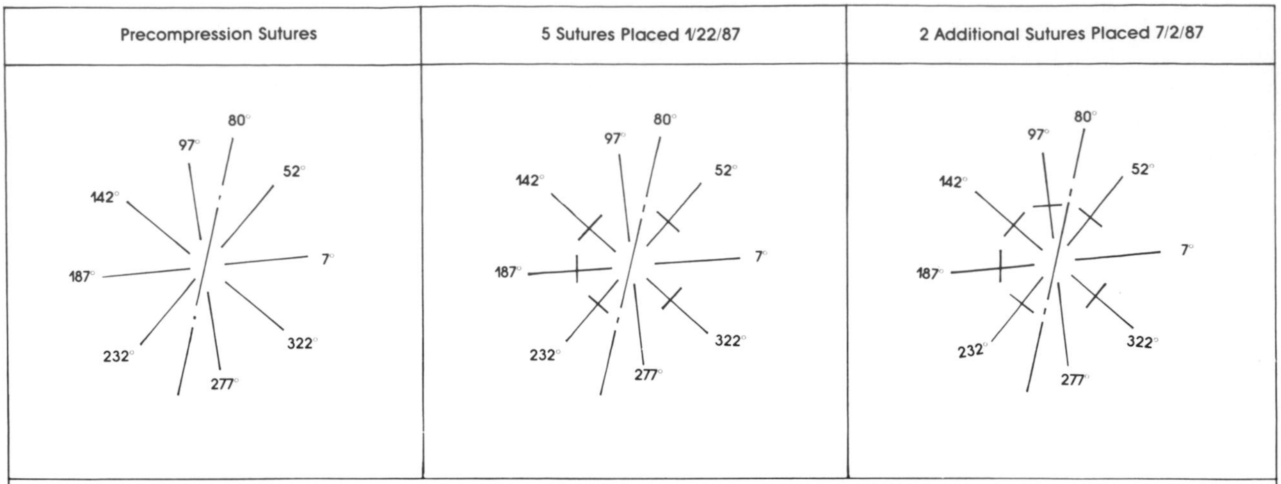
Precompression Sutures
5 Sutures Placed 1/22/87
2 Additional Sutures Placed 7/2/87
80°
97°
52°
142°
187°
7°
232°
322°
277°

	Statistical Record		
	1/9/87 (16 mo post RK)	6/3/87 (5 mo post 5 sutures)	1/13/88 (6 mo post 2 added sutures)
Refraction	AM +4.12 − 1.50 × 80 PM +2.75 − 1.00 × 80	AM +3.25 − 3.00 × 80 PM +1.75 − 2.25 × 80	AM +1.25 − 1.25 × 80 PM +.75 − 1.25 × 80
K	AM 38.00 / 36.75 @ 78 PM 39.00 / 37.62 @ 80	AM 40.50 / 38.75 @ 75 PM 41.00 / 39.50 @ 75	AM 40.00 / 38.87 @ 73 PM 40.12 / 40.00 @ 76

Figure 25-2
Illustrations and data resulting from placement of correcting compression sutures in the keratotomy wounds to reduce the overcorrection in the right eye. The three sketches show the original steep meridian at 80 degrees and the placement of sutures on two separate occasions. The statistical record shows the refraction and keratometric readings in the morning and the evening at specified times after surgery. (From Richmond RD: J Refract Surg 1987;3:22-29.)

nificant amount persisted until 7 months OD. Flare is present OU at one year, but I had some flare preoperatively that developed following hard contact lens wear in the late 1950s.

"Refraction data preoperatively, at 3 months, 6 months, and 1 year, are shown in Fig. 25-1. Preoperative spherical equivalent OD was −4.62 D; OS −4.37 D: only 0.25 D difference. Least myopia OD was −4.00 D and OS was −3.37 D: only 0.62 D difference. Astigmatism OD was −1.25 D, with 0.87 D being refractive and 0.37 D measurable by keratometer. Astigmatism was 1.75 D OS, with 1.25 D being refractive and 0.50 D measurable by keratometer. The data show fairly balanced refractive error, and yet, unbalanced surgery was chosen by Bores-Fyodorov computer program due to the difference in astigmatism of 1.25 D OD versus 1.75 D OS.

Postoperative course

"My postoperative course and medications used are shown in Fig. 25-1. Overcorrection was initially present OU. Rapid change of refraction was experienced, OU, for 2 weeks postoperatively. The right eye then settled into a band of overcorrection in which the spherical equivalent varied from +2.25 D in the morning to +1.00 D in the afternoon. The left eye moved from hyperopic to myopic after 2 weeks, then shifted back toward hyperopia in the morning and myopia in the afternoon 6 weeks postoperatively. This trend, with some decrease in fluctuation, is present at 1 year OS. Refractive changes OD are suggestive of progressive hyperopia from the fifth month through 1 year.

"Fluctuation of refractive error has been greater than 1 D (October 31, 1985; Fig. 25-1). Initial refraction done on this date was performed 15 minutes after arising. The diopter change from 7:30 AM to 8:50 PM was 1.62 D OD and 1.50 D OS. I estimate total dioptric change from awakening to bedtime to have been 2 D on that date. Diopter change 1 year postoperatively is still in the range of 0.75 D OU from the 90 minutes' refraction after awakening until the 4:30 PM refraction.

Table 25-1

Self-Collected Clinical Data Spanning 28 Months after Bilateral Radial Keratotomy

	Preoperative	3 months postoperative	6 months postoperative	1 year postoperative	5 mo postop initial suture revision, OD	2 weeks following addition of two sutures OD	1 yr postop original suture revision, OD; 28 mo postop RK, OU*
Refraction (D)							
OD Morning	−4.00 −1.25 × 97°	+3.00 −1.50 × 85°	+3.00 −1.50 × 80°	+3.50 −1.25 × 80°	+3.25 −3.00 × 80°	+1.50 −3.00 × 85°	+1.25 −1.25 × 80°
OD Afternoon	−4.12 −1.75 × 97°	+1.87 −1.00 × 85°	+2.25 −1.50 × 80°	+2.37 −1.00 × 75°	+1.75 −2.25 × 80°	+.25 −2.25 × 92°	+0.75 −1.25 × 80°
OS Morning	−3.37 −1.75 × 75°	+1.25 −0.75 × 145°	+0.75 −0.75 × 140°	+0.75 −0.75 × 150°	+1.50 −1.00 × 155°		+1.00 −0.75 × 155°
OS Afternoon	−3.50 −1.75 × 75°	+0.25 −0.50 × 145°	0 − 0.50 × 140°	+0.25 −0.50 × 150°	+.50 −0.75 × 155°		+0.62 −0.75 × 155°
Keratometry (D)							
OD Morning	44.62/44.25 × 97°	38.50/37.87 × 80°	38.25/37.12 × 78°	38.50/37.50 × 80°	40.50/38.75 × 75°	41.00/41.12 × 61°	40.00/38.87 × 73°
OD Afternoon	44.62/44.25 × 97°	39.25/38.75 × 80°	38.75/37.75 × 103°	39.37/38.37 × 81°	41.00/39.50 × 75°	41.25/41.00 × 61°	40.37/39.62 × 70°
OS Morning	44.50/44.00 × 75°	39.50/39.62 × 73°	39.62/39.75 × 78°	40.00/39.62 × 80°	39.25/39.50 × 81°		39.50/39.62 × 76°
OS Afternoon	44.50/44.00 × 75°	40.75/40.75 × 78°	40.50/40.25 × 78°	40.75/40.25 × 85°	40.12/40.00 × 76°		40.12/40.00 × 76°
IOP (applanation, mm Hg)							
OD	18	16	16	14			17
OS	19	16	15	15			16
Central pachometry (μm)							
OD	577	605		593			609
OS	592	607		584			588

*Measurements 36 months after the original surgery were unchanged from those at 28 months.

I estimate total dioptric change from awakening to bedtime still to be 1.25 D OU.

"How is it the eye with 12 radial incisions corrected nicely, while the eye with eight radial incisions overcorrected? One might speculate my right eye is an "overresponder," but I feel the results confirm the relative importance of optical zone size as the most critical predictability factor. One might also conclude that small optical zone sizes (2.75 mm) are as unpredictable when cut in one dimension of an oval optical zone as expected with a spherical optical zone.

"An equally important factor contributing to overcorrection OD is inaccuracy of optical center marking. I discovered early in my postoperative course that I could see reflected images of my corneal incisions, both with a direct ophthalmoscope and by backlighting a keratometer. The temporal inferior incision in the narrow dimension (2.75) may be as close as 1 mm to the optical center.

Fluctuation of refraction

"Corrected visual acuity at 2+ years following RK, OS, has remained 20/15. Fig. 25-1 and Fig. 24-7 in Chapter 24 provide graphic representation of dioptric and keratometric changes with time. Table 25-1 illustrates the comparison of refractive changes with time.

"The PERK study at 3 years reports 31% of eyes showing fluctuation of refractive error by at least 0.50 D from morning to night.[12] My left eye at nearly 2½ years is still fluctuating 0.75 D from 90 minutes after awakening to 4:30 PM. Greatest hyperopia is present in the morning. I estimate total daily changes to still be as much as 1.25 D. These numbers are not significantly different from those found 1 year postopera-

tively. Cylinder changes of 0.25 D occurred from morning to night.

"Keratometric changes are compatible with the dioptric changes, although they do not coincide exactly. The refractive trend is toward hyperopia, but rate of change is slow.

"Fluctuation of refraction error varies not only from morning to night but from day to day. Morning to afternoon cylinder changes of 0.50 D OD and 0.25 D OS are common, as is change of axis by 5° OU.

"Diurnal variation of intraocular pressure has been cited as a cause of visual fluctuation. My feeling is that within the normal physiologic range of intraocular pressure, other factors are more responsible for fluctuation. After reviewing my data and subjective refraction changes, I discovered on days I was in the office from 9:00 AM to 5:00 PM (Monday, Wednesday, Friday), fluctuations were significantly greater than on days I was in surgery ½ day (Tuesday, Thursday), or on weekends, during the first 6 months postoperatively. Changes of diurnal pressure would not account for the variations noted.

"I sought factors to explain the noted variations and concluded that three factors were important (Table 25-2):

1. Lid and orbital pressure. I discovered early in my postoperative course that "splinting" my eyes in a position of convergence (as with reading) resulted in a myopic shift after approximately 1 hour. At night, Bell's phenomenon places our eyes in a position of elevation and divergence, an opposite "splint" from that encountered during reading. Lid and orbital pressure are also changed frequently during exercise (Fig. 25-3).

Table 25-2

Factors That Subjectively Resulted in Refractive Fluctuation

Myopic shift	Hyperopic shift
1. Convergence—when performing reading or close work (probably combination of change of lid-orbital pressure and resolution of wound edema). Effect as much as 1 D during first 3 months postoperatively; effect minimal after 6 months. 2. Open lids	1. Sleep (probably combination of wound edema and physical alteration of K resulting from lid and orbital pressure). Effect as much as 2 D. 2. Exercise (probably combination of Valsalva, lid pressure changes, and wound edema). Effect no more than 0.5 D, but long-term cumulative effect unknown. Further research needed to determine if exercise is a factor in progressive hyperopia. 3. Low atmospheric pressure 4. High atmospheric humidity

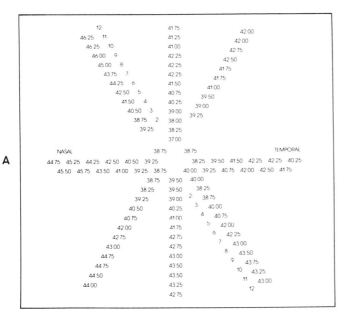
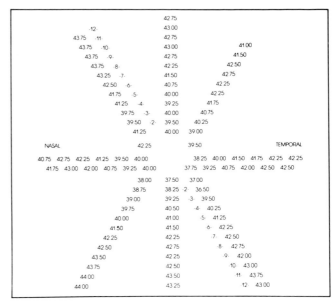

Figure 25-3
Faceplate from 12-ring Corneascope photograph gives corneal power readings
along eight hemimeridians in the right eye 4 months after surgery. **A,** Normal lid
pressure produces overall flattening of the cornea. **B,** With the lid lifted off the
globe, there is steepening of the superior cornea. Dr. Richmond suggests that the
pressure of the eyelid on the cornea flattens it and is one component that produces
diurnal fluctuation. (From Richmond RF: J Refract Surg 1987;3:22-29.)

2. Corneal wound edema. Prolonged lid closure, as during sleep, would certainly induce some wound edema. Subjectively, I also felt that exposure to weather conditions of wind, cold, or excessive heat caused corneal edema with resultant hyperopic shift.

3. Rapid changes of intraocular pressure. Exercise rapidly changes intraocular pressure as a result of the Valsalva maneuver. By applanation tonometer, we were able to demonstrate a change of intraocular pressure from 16 to 20 mm Hg with the Valsalva maneuver. The direction of refractive change resulting from the above factors is shown in Table 25-2.

"Although much of the evidence is circumstantial for the above factors causing refractive change, some concrete evidence can be presented in support of them. Figure 25-3 is the digital printout of corneoscope photographs of my corneas (courtesy of Dr. James Rowsey). The printouts demonstrate changes of corneal curvature with normal lid tone versus relief of lid pressure by elevating the lids manually.

"An example of increased hyperopia following excessive sleep can be seen on my postoperative chart (Fig. 25-1) on January 20, 1986. On the preceding two nights, prior to the measurement of January 20, I had slept 12 hours per night recovering from the first ISRK meeting in Las Vegas in January 1986.

"As suggested by others,[9] I tried glaucoma medications OD in an attempt to reduce the overcorrection. In my case, decreasing intraocular pressure probably resulted in increased lid pressure effect with increased hyperopia. Ocular pressure was lowered OD on those dates for periods extending up to 1 week. Ocular pressure was reduced from 19 mm Hg to 11 mm Hg. Instead of reducing hyperopia, each short-term trial of medication resulted in a hyperopic shift. Lowering of intraocular pressure also resulted in increased astigmatism by 0.5 D OD.

Suturing incisions for overcorrection

"The most disturbing consequence of the initial suturing was a two-line decrease in best-corrected Snellen visual acuity from 20/15 to 20/25. Addition of two sutures on July 2, 1987, did not cause a further reduction of best corrected visual acuity.

"Decreased visual acuity, accompanied by ghost images around Snellen letters, likely would be caused by lamellar distortion and irregular astigmatism. Visual acuity is showing some minor improvement with time. My experience is similar to reduced visual acuity following RK—vision improves under photopic conditions.

"Disturbingly, change of K resulting from the two sutures placed on July 2, 1987, did not cause an immediate change in refractive astigmatism (Table 25-1). One month was needed for astigmatism to decrease to an acceptable amount.

"Initial suturing done in association with incision opening caused an increase in refractive fluctuation for several months. It appeared that the sutures did very little to increase corneal rigidity.

"Despite the fact that incisions were not opened when the two additional sutures were placed on July 2, 1987, and yet refractive change was effected and astigmatism has remained relatively stable to the end of this study, I question the necessity of opening the incisions.

"The major question concerning interrupted compression suture surgery is: Will the effect be permanent, or will the sutures erode prior to healing, resulting in a loss of effect? Drs. Lindstrom and Lindquist feel the loss of effect stabilizes by 1 year (personal communication). But again the question must be asked: Will this be true of the slow healer? In my case, K readings flattened by 1 D from 1 through 5 months postoperatively following both surgery procedures (Fig. 25-1).

"Correction of secondary hyperopia by interrupted compression suture technique is deceptively difficult and should be undertaken only by those fully trained in corneal surgery.

"Keratometric control of interrupted compression suture surgery, as with RK, will only give "ball-park" control over the final outcome. Troutman[10] recently pointed out the poor correlation between K readings taken at the time of surgery versus those taken even one day later.

Hyperbaric oxygen treatment

(The following update is provided by the authors of this chapter.)

In attempt to reduce his overcorrection, based upon reports in the literature, Dr. Richmond came to Atlanta, Georgia, in September 1988 for hyperbaric oxygen treatments. Uncorrected visual acuity in the right eye was 20/50 (blur from 20/200 on) and in the left eye was 20/25 (blur from 20/50 on). His manifest refraction in the right eye was plano +1.25 × 180° for a visual acuity of 20/15 and in the left eye was +0.50 +0.50 × 60° for a visual acuity of 20/15. He received four 90-minute sessions of hyperbaric oxygen treatments at 2.4 atmospheres, but shortly after treatment, and at 6 months after treatment, his refraction, visual

acuity, and keratometric measurements remained unchanged. His endothelial cell density on wide field specular microscopy was 2766 cells/mm^2 in both eyes.

Conclusions

1. "An oval optical zone has not been effective,[4] up to 1 year postoperatively, in reducing astigmatism in my right eye. Most of my astigmatism preoperatively was refractive. Perhaps an oval optical zone would have been more effective with corneal astigmatism. The RL procedure was effective in reducing astigmatism OS.

2. Significant fluctuation of refraction is still present 1 year postoperatively. We are now being told by researchers that healing of the cornea may take 4 years.[1] Poor wound healing has been suspected to be the cause of progressive hyperopia. The operating surgeon stated that the incisions in my right eye "fell apart" during suture revision surgery, indicating at 16 months postoperatively that the incisions had healed poorly.

3. Short-term decrease of intraocular pressure did not reduce hyperopia; rather hyperopia increased, as did astigmatism.

4. Marking of optical centers using the corneal reflex of an operating microscope filament is not accurate enough when dealing with small optical zone sizes.

5. Overcorrection by RK should be avoided in a presbyopic patient. It is my impression the ideal correction for a presbyope is 0.5 D myopia, not emmetropia. It is necessary to approach presbyopes with caution because visual fluctuation will be more obvious to them. A progressive power bifocal is helpful to the presbyope in combatting visual fluctuation.

6. Personal habits of the patient may affect healing and the final result of RK. Sleep, exposure to the elements, exercise, and the position of the eyes at work may all be important.

7. Statistics concerning RK should be based on examination at the same time of day and the same day of the week. My direct experience with radial keratotomy indicates that although research has progressed at an astounding pace, we have just begun to refine this procedure. Developing quantitative methods to improve predictability should be our number 1 goal."

■ ■ ■

MEASUREMENT OF SUBJECTIVE SATISFACTION

This chapter has emphasized individual patient testimonials, illustrating a full spectrum of patients' responses. However, such an anecdotal approach is an unsatisfactory way to assess overall results of refractive keratotomy in a population. Two other approaches have been used to measure subjective satisfaction. The first involves simply asking patients to indicate how satisfied they are on a scale ranging from unsatisfied to very satisfied, and the other is to ask patients whether they would have the surgery again—a yes-or-no response. Numerous studies of radial keratotomy have incorporated this type of assessment in their results and have generally found patients to be highly satisfied with the operation. The studies of Neumann,[6] Cowden,[3] Salz,[8] Kim,[5] and Vaughan[11] all report on patient satisfaction and/or postoperative use of eye glasses or contact lenses.

A more systematic approach to measuring satisfaction is to use a psychometric instrument, that is, a questionnaire that is constructed to ask a variety of questions about satisfaction and to use the answers to construct a satisfaction index. Two such studies have been performed after refractive keratotomy, that by Bourque and colleagues[2] in the PERK study and that by Powers and colleagues.[7] The Bourque study started with 112 questions and repeatedly performed factor analysis to systematically reduce the number of questions needed to create a satisfaction index, ending up with 10 items. Powers and colleagues did not report the details of the questionnaire used. Both studies found a high level of patient satisfaction: Bourque, 48.5% very satisfied, 42.0% average satisfaction, and 9.6% dissatisfied; Powers and colleagues, 70.5% extremely satisfied, 13.6% somewhat satisfied, and 14.8% dissatisfied; 86.5% said they would undergo the surgery again.

DETERMINANTS OF SATISFACTION— REFRACTION AND VISUAL ACUITY

Bourque and colleagues[2] documented a high correlation between patient satisfaction and postoperative residual refractive error and the postoperative uncorrected visual acuity (Fig. 25-4). Overall, the smaller the residual refractive error and the better the uncorrected visual acuity, the higher the satisfaction index. In addition, in a multiple regression equation, uncorrected visual acuity and residual refractive error were the strongest predictors of patient satisfaction (Tables 25-3 and 25-4). These observations were supported by the study of Powers and colleagues[7], who found that the subjective appreciation in improvement in vision and in the quality of uncorrected vision were the two major determinants of patient satisfaction. Indeed, the improvement in vision and quality of uncorrected vision after surgery accounted for 73% of the variance in satisfaction.

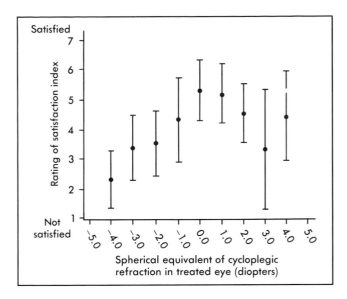

Figure 25-4
Regression analysis of reported satisfaction index and spherical equivalent of cycloplegic refraction shows curvilinear relationship between satisfaction and spherical equivalent of cycloplegic refraction. Persons whose vision was overcorrected or undercorrected were less satisfied with results of radial keratotomy. Larger standard deviation diagrammed around those whose vision was most severely overcorrected reflects small size of those two groups and extent to which problems with overcorrection increase with age. Eleven patients in the sample had a postoperative refractive error of +2.0 D or more. Of those 11, five were less than 35 years of age, two were between 35 and 44 years of age, and four were older than 45 years of age. (From Bourque LB et al: Arch Ophthalmol 1986; 104:356-363.)

These findings are extremely important for the ophthalmologist. The most important single reason patients give for seeking radial keratotomy is to have improved uncorrected visual acuity free from the bother of glasses and contact lenses. The most important factors determining postoperative satisfaction are the uncorrected visual acuity and residual refractive error. Thus both patients and ophthalmologists have the same major criteria for assessing the results of keratotomy. Some ophthalmologists have expressed the opinion that patients seek radial keratotomy only for improved appearance or improved function in their jobs; others think that patients are strongly affected by publicity or high expectations of their surgeon, so that they can be manipulated easily into an overly positive assessment of keratotomy surgery. The facts as presented in the studies of Bourque and Powers indicate otherwise. Patients judged the visual outcome as most important and did not seem too extensively influenced by other subjective or external influences.

Table 25-3

Correlation between the Satisfaction Index and the Uncorrected Visual Acuity 1 Year after Radial Keratotomy*

Uncorrected visual acuity	No. of patients	Satisfaction index, no. (%) of patients		
		Not satisfied (1.0-2.9)	Moderately satisfied (3.0-5.0)	Very satisfied (5.1-7.0)
20/40 or better	298	15 (5.0)	118 (39.6)	165 (55.4)
Worse than 20/40	57	19 (33.3)	31 (54.4)	7 (12.3)
Total	355	34	149	172

From Bourque LB, Cosand BB, Drews C, Waring GO, Lynn M, Cartwright C, and the PERK Study Group: Arch Ophthalmol 1986;104:356-363.
*$P < 0.001$, χ^2 test.

Table 25-4

Correlation between the Satisfaction Index and the Cycloplegic Refraction 1 Year after Radial Keratotomy*

Spherical equivalent of the cycloplegic refraction (D)	No. of patients	Satisfaction index, no. (%) of patients		
		Not satisfied (1.0-2.9)	Moderately satisfied (3.0-5.0)	Very satisfied (5.1-7.0)
−4.36 to −1.12	83	21 (25.3)	47 (56.6)	15 (18.1)
−1.00 to +1.00	232	11 (4.7)	82 (35.3)	139 (59.9)
+1.12 to +3.62	40	2 (5.0)	20 (50.0)	18 (45.0)
Total	355	34	149	172

From Bourque LB, Cosand BB, Drews C, Waring GO, Lynn M, Cartwright C, and the PERK Study Group: Arch Ophthalmol 1986;104:356-363.
*$P < 0.001$, χ^2 test.

Table 25-5

Correlation between the Satisfaction Index and Fluctuation Index 1 Year after Radial Keratotomy*

Fluctuation index	No. of patients	Satisfaction index, no. (%) of patients		
		Not satisfied (1.0-2.9)	Moderately satisfied (3.0-5.0)	Very satisfied (5.1-7.0)
No fluctuation (1.0 to 2.9)	87	3 (3.4)	16 (17.2)	69 (79.3)
Moderate fluctuation (3.0 to 5.0)	149	11 (7.4)	71 (47.7)	67 (45.0)
A lot of fluctuation (5.1 to 7.0)	119	20 (16.8)	63 (52.9)	36 (30.3)
Total	355	34	149	172

From Bourque LB, Cosand BB, Drews C, Waring GO, Lynn M, Cartwright C, and the PERK Study Group: Arch Ophthalmol 1986;104:356-363.
*$P < 0.0001$, χ^2 test.

DETERMINANTS OF SATISFACTION—SUBJECTIVE GLARE, FLUCTUATION IN VISION, AND PERSONAL APPEARANCE

Bourque and colleagues found a statistically significant correlation between the subjective satisfaction index and the subjective indices for fluctuating vision and glare 1 year after radial keratotomy (Tables 25-5 and 25-6). The association between fluctuating vision and satisfaction was much stronger than that between glare and satisfaction. Powers and colleagues evaluated more subjective factors. Although they found that the preoperative desire for a change in appearance, the willingness to pay more for the operation, and the amount of pain after the first eye influenced satisfaction, these factors did so much less than improvement in the amount and quality of uncorrected acuity. Interestingly, they found no relationship between the patient's satisfaction and the identity of the particular surgeon, the number of questions answered before surgery, or the changes in life-style, appearance, and self-esteem after surgery. Powers emphasized that "none of the predictors was related to life-style or what could be considered personality characteristics."

DETERMINANTS OF SATISFACTION—REGRESSION ANALYSIS

The regression analysis carried out by Bourque and colleagues (Table 25-7) and by Powers and colleagues (Table 25-8) emphasized two important factors. The first is that the visual acuity variable is the most important factor in determining patient satisfaction. The second is that the findings indicate the great variability for an individual person in judging the satisfactory outcome of keratotomy surgery. Bourque emphasized that only 46% of patient satisfaction could be explained by all the variables evaluated and that these factors cannot be very accurate in predicting the satisfaction for an individual patient. Although Powers's regression formula could explain approximately 80% of the patient satisfaction, it included only subjective factors.

Table 25-6

Correlation between the Satisfaction Index and the Glare Index 1 Year after Radial Keratotomy*

| | | Satisfaction index, no. (%) of patients | | |
| | | | | |
Glare index	No. of patients	Not satisfied (1.0-2.9)	Moderately satisfied (3.0-5.0)	Very satisfied (5.1-7.0)
No glare (1.0 to 2.9)	163	8 (4.9)	60 (36.8)	95 (58.3)
Moderate glare (3.0 to 5.0)	132	17 (12.9)	59 (44.7)	56 (42.4)
A lot of glare (5.1 to 7.0)	60	9 (15.0)	30 (50.0)	21 (35.0)
Total	355	34	149	172

From Bourque LB, Cosand BB, Drews C, Waring GO, Lynn M, Cartwright C, and the PERK Study Group: Arch Ophthalmol 1986;104:356-363.
*$P < 0.0001$, σ^2 test.
*P .003, σ^2 test.

Table 25-7

Regression of Satisfaction Index 1 Year after Radial Keratotomy on Refractive Error, Uncorrected Visual Acuity, Fluctuation of Vision, Glare, and Sex of Patient*

Independent variables	Unstandardized regression coefficient	Standard error	Standardized regression coefficient
Spherical equivalent of the cycloplegic refraction	.03	0.06	.03
Uncorrected visual acuity	.05	0.01	.47
Glare index (1, none; 7, a lot)	−.06	0.03	−.08
Fluctuation index (1, none; 7, a lot)	−.20	0.03	−.27
Sex (1, female; 0, male)	.43	0.11	.16
Refraction squared	−.10	0.04	−.20
Interaction of sex and acuity	−.02	0.01	−.10
Interaction of acuity and refraction squared	−.003	0.001	−.19

From Bourque LB, Cosand BB, Drews C, Waring GO, Lynn M, Cartwright C, and the PERK Study Group: Arch Ophthalmol 1986;104:356-363.

*Regression coefficients were significant at $P < .01$ for all variables except spherical equivalent of the cycloplegic refraction. The number of patients was 354, the Y intercept was 5.74, R^2 (the amount of variance in satisfaction explained by the equation) was 0.46, and the standard error was 0.997.

Table 25-8

Regression Analysis for Patient Satisfaction Postoperatively*

Variables	Results Beta†	P
In equation		
Improvement in vision due to operation	0.45	<0.00001
Quality of uncorrected vision postoperative	0.40	<0.00001
Preoperative desire for change in appearance	0.12	0.06
Willingness to pay more if insurance would not	0.16	0.02
Perceived pain following first operation	−0.14	0.03
Not in equation		
Importance of particular physician		
All questions answered prior to surgery		
Changes in life-style following surgery		
Changes in appearance due to surgery		
Level of self-esteem (SEI)		

Analysis of variance	df	MS	F
Regression	5	15.15	48.76+
Residual	59	.31	

From Powers MK, Meyerowitz BE, Arrowsmith PN, and Marks RG: Ophthalmology 1984;91:1193-1198.

df, Degrees of freedom.

*Multiple R = 0.90. $P < 0.00001$ for the overall regression, and N = 65 for this analysis because patients with missing values for any of the variables were not included.

†Beta values are standardized weighting coefficients for predicting patient satisfaction by each variable, after the presence of each other variable in the equation has been accounted for. The P values show the levels of significance of a *t* statistic computed for each Beta value by dividing Beta by its standard error. Although much of our data could be considered nonparametric in nature, we used Pearson correlation and multiple regression techniques in the analysis because of their robustness for non-normal data and, especially for regression, because of their predictive value. Spearman correlations were computed as well, and none of our conclusions would differ if those values had been used instead.

UNFINISHED BUSINESS

One of the most underestimated aspects of refractive corneal surgery is the patient's personal perspective. We need not only more research on the motivations of patients to have refractive surgery, but also more exacting assessment of the patient's subjective and functional response to the procedures. The customary clinical criteria of success (uncorrected visual acuity, residual refractive error, predictability of outcome, stability of results, and general safety) are not always the criteria by which patients judge the success or failure of a refractive surgical procedure. What are those criteria? How realistic are they? How well do they correlate with the customary clinical measures? Are the outcomes that are important to patients the ones that are important to ophthalmologists? To answer these and other questions, careful psychometric and psychologic information needs to be gathered on patients before and after surgery. The paucity of such studies speaks not only to their difficulty, but also to the limited perspective of ophthalmologists. There is a substantive need for the involvement of psychologists, sociologists, and public health workers in the assessment of refractive keratotomy.

REFERENCES

1. Binder P: Four-year postoperative evaluation of radial keratotomy, Arch Ophthalmol 1985;103:779-780.
2. Bourque LB, Cosand BB, Drews C, Waring GO, Lynn M, Cartwright C, and the PERK Study Group: Reported satisfaction, fluctuation of vision, and glare among patients one year after surgery in the PERK study, Arch Ophthalmol 1986;104:356-363.
3. Cowden JW: Radial keratotomy: a retrospective study of cases observed at the Kresge Eye Institute for six months, Arch Ophthalmol 1982;100:578-580.
4. Franks J and Binder P: Keratotomy procedures for the correction of astigmatism, J Refract Surg 1985;1:11-17.
5. Kim JH: A prospective clinical study of radial keratotomy in Koreans, Korean J Ophthalmol 1988;2:13-21.
6. Neumann AC, Osher RH, and Fenzl RE: Radial keratotomy: a clinical and statistical analysis, Cornea 1983;2:47-55.
7. Powers MK, Meyerowitz BE, Arrowsmith PN, Marks RG: Psychosocial findings in radial keratotomy patients two years after surgery, Ophthalmology 1984;91:1193-1198.
8. Salz JJ and Salz MS: Results of four- and eight-incision radial keratotomy for 6 to 11 diopters of myopia, J Refract Surg 1988;4:46-50.
9. Sanders DR, Hofmann RF, and Salz JJ: Refractive corneal surgery, ed 1, Thorofare, NJ, 1985, Slack, Inc, pp 297-298.
10. Troutman RC: Surgical keratometer in the management of astigmatism in keratoplasty, Ann Ophthalmol 1987;19:473-474.
11. Vaughan ER and Paschall WJ: A statistical analysis of radial keratotomy results, Ann Ophthalmol 1985;17:275-283.
12. Waring GO III, Lynn MJ, Gelender H, et al: Three-year results of the Perspective Evaluation of Radial Keratotomy (PERK) study, Ophthalmology 1987;97:1339-1354.

Summary of Factors That Affect the Outcome of Refractive Keratotomy

George O. Waring III

Throughout this book we consider factors that affect the outcome of refractive keratotomy surgery—subjective and objective, preoperative and postoperative, mechanical and biologic, surgeon and patient, controllable and uncontrollable. This mass of information may obscure the overall picture.

In this chapter I summarize the factors that affect the outcome of keratotomy to provide an overview of the complex interplay of some 50 variables that must be considered and (insofar as possible) controlled to achieve a successful outcome for the individual patient.

I define *outcome* in the broadest sense as the overall result of the surgery, both objective and subjective, for an indefinite time after the operation. I include the conditions of examination in the factors that affect the outcome because the methods we use to measure results may affect the results themselves.

Each of the variables affects the outcome to a different degree (small, medium, or large), but it is not now possible to create a formula that quantifies the sum total of these effects. Even those variables with a small influence are important. To illustrate, assume that each of these 50 variables makes a 1% difference in the outcome and that one surgeon handles each variable so that it increases the effect of the surgery, while another surgeon handles each variable so that it decreases the effect of the surgery. Theoretically, the first surgeon would have 50% more effect than average and the second surgeon 50% less effect than average—a difference between the two of 100%.

BACKGROUND AND ACKNOWLEDGMENTS
Although I have derived the information tabulated in this chapter from the published literature, the chapter represents my personal opinions, particularly when it comes to the quality of the assessment of the effect of each variable on the outcome and the surgeon's ability to control these effects. The accuracy or tolerance given for each variable is meant to reflect the average clinically encountered values and not necessarily numbers that have been validated as statistically significant. Documentation and references for these opinions are presented throughout this textbook, and it would be redundant to reference each topic and statement here.

Even though this unrealistic example exaggerates, it illustrates how easy it is to achieve variable and unpredictable results from refractive keratotomy. Fortunately, this kind of extreme variation does not exist; there is remarkable overall agreement about the outcome of surgery among surgeons using different techniques, as detailed in Chapter 21, Published Results of Refractive Keratotomy. Nevertheless, until there is more standardization and until surgeons gain more control over the variables discussed here, refractive keratotomy will still be considered an unpredictable procedure when compared with the fitting of glasses and contact lenses.

Factor	Approximate accuracy or tolerance	Estimated effect of factor on outcome (none, small, moderate, large)	Surgeon's ability to control the factor (none, poor, fair, good)	Methods used to control the factor
Surgical instruments				
1. Center mark	0.2 mm	Small	Good	Surgeon and patient fixate same object; mark center of pupil
2. Ultrasonic pachometry (1640 m/s)				
a. Single instrument	± 10 μm = $\pm 1.8\%$	Large	Poor	Select reliable company; calibrate instrument
b. Different instrument	10%	Moderate	Good	Use same instrument for all cases
3. Knife blade				
a. Tip and edge sharpness	Difficult to measure Visual inspection	Large	Fair	Buy good quality blade Inspect at 150 to 200$\times$ Meticulous cleaning and maintenance
b. Design (thickness, included angle, number of edges)	Varies	Moderate	None	Know characteristics of blade used
4. Micrometer on knife	± 1.0 to 10 μm	Large	Good	Calibrate on test micrometer
5. Knife footplates	Difficult to measure			
a. Design		Moderate	None	Select and use one style
b. Quality		Small	None	Check alignment, smoothness, contour at 150 to 200$\times$
6. Calibration gauge (ruler or ridge)				
a. Accuracy	10 to 100 μm	Small	None	Believe manufacturer or have independently calibrated
b. Parallax during setting	2% to 15%	Moderate	Fair	Practice to align blade and gauge properly

Factor		Approximate accuracy or tolerance	Estimated effect of factor on outcome (none, small, moderate, large)	Surgeon's ability to control the factor (none, poor, fair, good)	Methods used to control the factor
	c. Microscope with micrometer	±0.001 μm	None	None	Accurate alignment
7.	Circular zone markers				
	a. Accuracy	±0.2 mm	Moderate	None	Believe manufacturer or calibrate independently
	b. Bevel location	±0.2 mm	Moderate	None	Know whether it is inside or outside
	c. Alignment sight for centering	Difficult to measure	Small	Good	Use cross hairs or sight for centering

Surgical plan and technique

8.	Patient cooperation	Can disrupt procedure	Large	Good	Confidence in surgeon and staff Practical hypnotic suggestion Comfortable before and during surgery
9.	Anesthesia a. Topical	Difficult to measure	Large	Good	Cornea is anesthetized faster and deeper than conjunctiva
	b. Regional				Affects retropulsion of globe and intraocular pressure during surgery
10.	Drape and speculum	Difficult to measure	Small	Good	Keep speculum out of path of knife Avoid eyelid compression that may produce ptosis
11.	Fixation instrument	Difficult to measure	Moderate	Fair	Hold globe steadily during incisions Control intraocular pressure
12.	Incision markers				
	a. Radial markers	Unknown	Small	Good	
	b. Astigmatism markers	Unknown	Large	Fair	Identify anatomic landmarks for steep meridian or mark preoperatively
	c. Zone markers	Unknown	Large	Good	Use alignment sight for centering Check distance from center with calipers

Factor		Approximate accuracy or tolerance	Estimated effect of factor on outcome (none, small, moderate, large)	Surgeon's ability to control the factor (none, poor, fair, good)	Methods used to control the factor
Surgical plan and technique—cont'd					
13.	Predictability nomograms and programs	Variable	Large	Good	Use surgical technique from which program was derived Evolve personalized "surgeon factor" and modifications of program
	a. Data entered into program	Variable	Large	Good	Evaluate critically the variables requested by the program Calculate astigmatism surgery plan with refraction in minus cylinder form
	b. Relation of clear zone diameter, number of incisions and depth of incisions	Variable	Large	Fair	Easiest to keep depth constant and vary number of incisions and diameter of clear zone
14.	Diameter of clear zone	3 to 5 mm	Large	Good	Smaller diameter gives more effect
15.	Depth of incision (including perforation)	80% to 95% Effect not linear	Large	Fair	Deeper incision gives more effect Know knife and personal manual technique based on prior experience Draw cross section of each incision to establish personal "depth factor" Cornea usually thicker nasally and peripherally
	a. Paracentral part	±10%	Large	Fair	Gives relatively more effect
	b. Peripheral part	±15%	Moderate	Fair	Gives relatively less effect
	c. Deepening incisions	Difficult to measure	Small	Fair	Personal technique
16.	Radial incisions for myopia				
	a. Number of incisions	4 to 16 (most effect with initial four)	Moderate	Good	Use smallest number consistent with desired effect
	b. Spacing of radial incisions	Equal	Small	Good	Use radial markers or accurate visual inspection

Factor	Approximate accuracy or tolerance	Estimated effect of factor on outcome (none, small, moderate, large)	Surgeon's ability to control the factor (none, poor, fair, good)	Methods used to control the factor
Surgical plan and technique—cont'd				
c. Sequence of radial incisions	Varies	None known	Good	Cutting thicker nasal cornea first reduces chance of perforation early in case
17. Direction of radial incisions		Moderate	Good	Select direction that gives straightest incisions of most uniform depth
a. Centripetal, limbus to clear zone				Deeper, more uniform
b. Centrifugal, clear zone to limbus				Shallower, less uniform
18. Pattern of incisions for astigmatism	Multiple	Large	Good	
a. Transverse across steep meridian	More effect			See no. 19
b. Semiradial in steep meridian	Least effect			
c. Combined transverse and semiradial	Most effect			
19. Transverse incisions for astigmatism				
a. Length	1.0 to 5 mm (20° to 110°)	Large	Fair	Longer incision flattens steep meridian and steepens flat meridian more Mark length on cornea
b. Number	1 or 2 per semimeridian	Moderate	Good	3, 4, or 5 per semimeridian probably do not increase effect
c. Configuration	Straight or arc	Small	Fair	Arc cuts uniform tissue thickness but is harder to execute
d. Location	5 to 8 mm apart	Large	Good	Smaller zone gives more effect, but reduction of effect outside the 5- to 8-mm range Increased glare inside 5 mm
20. Sequence of incisions for astigmatism		Small	Good	
a. Transverse first				Transverse first produces less gaping and tissue movement during cutting

Factor	Approximate accuracy or tolerance	Estimated effect of factor on outcome (none, small, moderate, large)	Surgeon's ability to control the factor (none, poor, fair, good)	Methods used to control the factor
Surgical plan and technique—cont'd				
b. Radial first				Wound gape when transverse are made
21. Bias setting for length of blade	90% to 110% of pachometry reading	Large	Good	Know effect of knife and technique on depth of incision
22. Hydration of cornea	Varies	Small	Poor	
a. During surgery				Prevent thinning of cornea caused by leaving dry under microscope light Prevent thickening of cornea caused by epithelial abrasion and excess irrigating
b. At conclusion of surgery				Irrigation of wounds transiently increases effect of surgery
23. Intraocular pressure during surgery	10 to 100 mm Hg	Moderate	Fair	Try for consistency in force exerted by fixation instrument
24. Manual technique of incisions	Artistic	Large	Good	Consistent knife entry and seating of blade into tissue, rate of cutting, and indentation of cornea
25. Repeated operations	Less predictable than primary			
a. Additional incisions for uncorrection		Moderate	Fair	Additional incisions between previous ones or open and recut previous ones
b. Suturing incisions for overcorrection		Small	Poor	Effectiveness being studied
Patient factors				
26. Age	0.70 to 0.1 D per year based on age of 30 to 35 as zero	Moderate	Fair	Adjust baseline refraction by age factor before making surgical plan
27. Corneal curvature and topography	Effect unknown	Small	None	Effect of topographic shape of cornea on outcome needs further study

Factor	Approximate accuracy or tolerance	Estimated effect of factor on outcome (none, small, moderate, large)	Surgeon's ability to control the factor (none, poor, fair, good)	Methods used to control the factor
Patient factors—cont'd				
28. Intraocular pressure				Adjusting IOP by a few mm Hg using glaucoma medication has no desirable effect on outcome
a. Physiologic range	12 to 22 mm Hg	Small	Poor	No proven effect
b. Elevated	>22 mm Hg	Moderate	Poor	Flattens cornea
c. Lowered	<12 mm Hg	Small	Poor	Effect unknown
29. Corneal thickness	Central: 0.45 to 0.60 Peripheral: 0.60 to 0.75	Small	Good	Compensated for by blade length adjustment
30. Sex		None	None	No proven effect
31. Ocular rigidity	Increases with age	None	None	No proven effect Relationship between age effect and effect of increasing ocular rigidity is undefined
32. Corneal biomechanical properties	Variable among individuals	Moderate	None	No method available to measure stress, strain, or material properties of cornea in vivo
33. Corneal diameter	10.5 to 12.5 mm	None	None	No proven effect
34. Wound healing characteristics	Difficult to measure	Moderate	None	Major determinant for "overresponders," "underresponders," and "unpredictability"
35. Postoperative topical corticosteroids	Difficult to measure	Small	Poor	Retard wound healing Probably enhance effect short-term; effect on final outcome unknown
36. Glare	Difficult to measure	Small	Fair	Keep diameter of clear zone as large as possible
37. Contrast sensitivity	Normal range defined	Small	Fair	Minimal reduction with normal pupil diameter; more reduction with mydriasis
38. Amplitude of accommodation	Decreases with age	Moderate	Poor	Intentional undercorrection by 0.50 to 1.00 D delays onset of symptomatic presbyopia

Factor	Approximate accuracy or tolerance	Estimated effect of factor on outcome (none, small, moderate, large)	Surgeon's ability to control the factor (none, poor, fair, good)	Methods used to control the factor
Patient factors—cont'd				
39. Stability of refraction				
a. During first month after surgery	Loss of 0.1 to 1.5 D of effect	Small	None	Minimize corneal swelling during and after surgery
b. 6 mo to 5-6 yr	0 to 3 D; continued increase in effect in approximately 20% of patients	Small	None	Intentional undercorrection of −0.50 to −1.00 D can partially offset effect; decreases long-term predictability
c. Diurnal variation	0 to 1 D of corneal steepening; duration unknown	Small	None	None
40. Expectations and motivation	Variable from realistic to unrealistic for both patient and surgeon	Large	Good	Honest and realistic explanation of probable outcome, unpredictability, possible complications by surgeon to patient
41. Corrective lenses after surgery		Large	Fair	Whether the patient wears glasses or contact lenses after surgery depends on the residual refractive error and the patient's own preference
a. Distance	Needed by 20% to 50% of patients			
b. Near	Used by most emmetropic or hyperopic presbyopes 45 years of age and older			Intentional undercorrection delays onset of symptomatic presbyopia
Examination conditions				
42. Examiner	Variable skill and objectivity	Moderate	Good	Control bias by using independent examiner; ensure technical competence by training
43. Visual acuity testing	Variable conditions ± one Snellen line	Large	Good	Standardize testing conditions by using same clinical lane for all examinations on one patient; use high-contrast charts with known light conditions

Factor	Approximate accuracy or tolerance	Estimated effect of factor on outcome (none, small, moderate, large)	Surgeon's ability to control the factor (none, poor, fair, good)	Methods used to control the factor
Examination conditions—cont'd				
44. Refraction				
a. Cycloplegic	More accurate ±0.25 D	Large	Good	Prevents overestimating amount of myopia caused by uncontrolled accommodation
b. Manifest	More convenient ± 0.25 D	Moderate	Good	Reduces effect of multifocal cornea
45. Central keratometry	±0.12 D	Small	Good	Useful as long as measured area of cornea is regular and smooth
46. Corneal topography	±0.25 D	Small	Fair	Most useful in astigmatism surgery; increased asphericity after surgery may account for multifocal effect
47. Endothelial cell measurements	±10%	None	Fair	Most meaningful measurements made in area of incisions using morphometric analysis; perforations damage endothelium

UNFINISHED BUSINESS

Listing the factors that affect the outcome of refractive keratotomy is easy; controlling them is more difficult. The major factors on which more research needs to be done include methods of obtaining a uniformly deep incision, methods of measuring and controlling corneal wound healing, the effect of corneal curvature and topography on the outcome, preoperative biomechanical properties of individual corneas, and techniques of repeated surgery for undercorrection and overcorrection. Of course, the biggest challenge for the surgeon is to integrate all of these variables into a useful, predictable surgical procedure.

Corneal Biomechanics and Computer Modeling of Refractive Keratotomy

BACKGROUND AND ACKNOWLEDGMENTS

Refractive corneal surgery is essentially a problem in biomechanics—taking a single tissue (the cornea) and subjecting it to surgical incisions, excisions, and additions that alter its shape. If the cornea were made of plastic or some other well-defined homogeneous material, the ability to reshape it exactly predictably would be rather easy. However, the cornea is an inhomogeneous tissue, with different dimensions in different areas, that behaves in a nonlinear, viscoelastic fashion; it also undergoes wound healing postoperatively, so a proper biomechanical description of its behavior is an enormous challenge. The challenge has two practical aspects. First, a fundamental understanding of corneal biomechanics and its response to keratotomy can both explain and improve the effects of human surgery. Second, if the material properties of the cornea can be defined, computational mechanics can be used to create computer models of the cornea, which allow experimental surgery to be done mathematicaly on the computer rather than in the laboratory or the clinic—a much more efficient and cost-effective approach.

Because little has been published on corneal biomechanics, especially as applied to refractive keratotomy, a number of authors have prepared chapters for this book exploring the subject from many points of view. Since most ophthalmologists are not familiar with biomechanical and engineering concepts and terminology, Vito has written Biomechanics: a Primer for Corneal Surgeons (Chapter 27) to provide fundamental concepts and definitions that serve as a useful background for the other chapters. Seiler takes a mathematical approach to the overall effect of transverse keratotomy for astigmatism in a concise presentation of a biomechanical model (Chapter 33). To introduce the concept of a finite element model, Vito used commercially available software to model radial keratotomy and to depict the effects of different variables of that operation (Chapter 28). Hanna and colleagues present more complex original finite element models of radial keratotomy (Chapter 29) and transverse arcuate keratotomy (Chapter 34), reporting an increasingly sophisticated basis for computer similation of human surgery.

All of these chapters are written with the ophthalmologist in mind, and none has been prepared with the rigor that would be required of an engineer or physicist. Their purpose is to demonstrate to the ophthalmic profession the basic concepts and practical application of biomechanical and computer models of refractive keratotomy, in the hopes that further research in this area will be stimulated and that the development of computer modeling of human corneal surgery will become a practical reality in clinical practice.

Biomechanics: A Primer for Corneal Surgeons

Raymond P. Vito

The increased interest in refractive corneal surgery[7,15,20] has resulted in corneal surgeons becoming more aware of the importance of the mechanical factors that govern corneal shape before and after surgery. Therefore concepts such as stress, strain, and Hooke's law, long familiar to mechanical engineers, are finding their way into ophthalmic literature. Corneal surgeons are now being told by their engineering counterparts that these concepts are relevant to understanding the biomechanical basis for corneal shape and may even be useful in predicting the results of refractive surgery,[1,10,16] as demonstrated in Chapters 28, 29, 33, and 34.

Simply stated, mechanics is the study of the action of forces in promoting motion or equilibrium. Its importance to many engineering disciplines, including the design of buildings and machines, has resulted a long and interesting history[17,18] dating back to the early Greeks and Romans. Biomechanics is a subdiscipline of mechanical engineering that concerns the medical applications of mechanics. Biomechanical researchers have long been interested in the response of tissues, organs, organ systems, and whole organisms to the forces to which they are subjected in both normal (for example, in locomotion) and pathologic (for example, in locomotion using crutches or a wheelchair) situations. An excellent, though somewhat mathematical summary of modern biomechanics, especially the biomechanics of soft tissues, has been written by Fung.[6]

The eye is an organ that moves, or changes shape, when subjected to forces such as intraocular pressure, extraocular muscles, and supporting forces. It is

BACKGROUND AND ACKNOWLEDGMENTS
An ophthalmologist who spends a few minutes talking to a biomechanical engineer about the cornea realizes instantly the enormous gap in knowledge, language, and understanding that exists between the two professions. Ophthalmologists talk medicine; engineers talk math. Ophthalmologists manage patients; engineers manage materials. But bioengineers with expertise in tissue mechanics can help bridge this gap, as demonstrated in this essay on biomechanics by Dr. Vito, a professor of mechanical engineering at the Georgia Institute of Technology. This primer not only provides a useful background to help nonengineers better understand the chapters on finite element and bending moment modeling, but it also may whet their appetite to seek more information about the fascinating field of tissue biomechanics. I am indebted to Dr. Vito for the time and effort he has donated to his sister profession.

therefore not surprising that the eye has attracted the attention of biomechanical engineers. This attraction is not new. Many ideas from mechanics have been used in the study of tonometry.[22] Similarly, understanding corneal shape and its surgical alteration will require close collaboration between biomechanicians and corneal surgeons. An important element of such collaboration is communication, and it is in this spirit that this chapter is written—to present a nonmathematical introduction to biomechanics intended for corneal surgeons. The presentation relies on geometrical reasoning rather than mathematical formality and thus sacrifices mathematical rigor for clarity and simplicity. I hope this information facilitates productive collaboration between corneal surgeons and engineers on all aspects of biomechanics of the eye.

Certain basic ideas in mechanics are fundamental to understanding the subject. A discussion of these at an elementary level requiring some mathematics may be found in several texts.[2,8,14] A good text at the intermediate level is Fung.[5]

CONTINUUM

The concept of a continuum is fundamental. In a continuum, every element of volume, no matter how small, is assumed to contain many atoms and molecules. The individual atoms and molecules are "lost in the crowd," forces and motions at the atomic level are ignored, and only the behavior of the aggregate is examined.

Assuming that the cornea is a continuum does not mean that the existence of microstructure is ignored. For example, collagen fibrils are important force-carrying structures in ocular tissue. However, in biomechanical studies the individual protein molecules constituting the collagen need not be considered to obtain useful results.

Although some scientists study forces and motions at the atomic level, they tend to be physicists, not engineers.

HOMOGENEITY

Homogeneity simply means that any volume of a tissue looks like any other volume of that tissue. Structural metals like steel and aluminum are very close to being homogeneous, but most soft tissues, particularly those in the eye, are definitely not.

Many tissues are homogeneous over certain regions. For example, the corneoscleral connective tissue envelope of the eye can be considered homogeneous. The sclera may also be considered homogeneous, but the cornea has distinct layers—Bowman's layer, anterior and posterior stroma, and Descemet's membrane—each of which is not homogeneous in

terms of the type and orientation of collagen fibrils, the interfibrillar matrix, and the cellular content. This greatly complicates corneal biomechanics especially because nearly all studies make the simplifying assumption of homogeneity to get results. The basic idea is that assuming homogeneity is equivalent to considering some average microstructure. This kind of reasoning is common in soft tissue mechanics. It is used, for example, in studies of the mechanics of the arterial wall.[6]

DISPLACEMENT

The idea of displacement, here used synonymously with motion, is most easily explained using a coordinate system, such as the Cartesian system, and some ideas from mathematics. However, an example may be sufficient to get the idea across.

Suppose we can pinpoint the exact location of every point of the cornea, that is, every point of Bowman's layer, the stroma, and Descemet's membrane. Also suppose that we know the movement of every point of the cornea as it deforms in response to a particular surgery, for example, radial keratotomy. This movement is called the displacement field, and it represents the response of the cornea to forces acting on it as a result of surgery. The magnitude and direction of the movement of every point of the cornea is determined using a structural model as discussed in the following paragraphs.

For example, recall that when an airplane taxis down a runway, the wind and roughness of the runway cause the wings to displace. This motion is caused by the forces acting on the wings. It is highly predictable with the structural model used to design the airplane.

If we knew the displacement field resulting from a particular surgery, calculation of the correction in diopters would be straightforward. Clearly the prediction of displacement is an important goal of biomechanical modeling of the cornea.

STRESS
Definition

The precise definition of stress requires mathematics. However, a working definition can be given quite easily. Fig. 27-1 shows two arrows that represent forces. The length of an arrow is used to denote the magnitude (size) of the force, and the arrowhead denotes its sense (direction). In Fig. 27-2 these two forces, labeled F_1 and F_2, are shown acting on a surface, such as a part of the surface of the cornea, that has an area A. One force (F_1) acts parallel to the surface and one force (F_2) acts perpendicular to the surface. There is a stress associated with each force. With

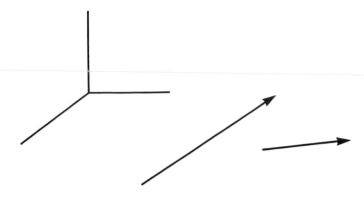

Figure 27-1
Two forces in space with arrows indicating direction and length indicating magnitude.

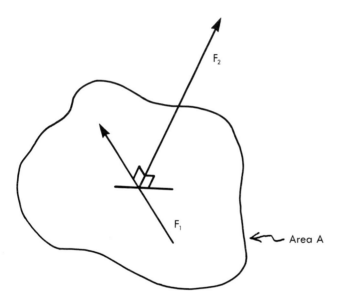

Figure 27-2
Forces F_1 and F_2 act parallel and perpendicular, respectively, to area A.

F_1, we associate the shear stress τ calculated from $\tau = F_1/A$, and with F_2 we associate the "normal" (perpendicular) stress σ calculated from $\sigma = F_2/A$.

The above definition, although adequate for our purposes, can be made exact if we can imagine the area A as being smaller than any number. Thus the precise definition of stress requires the notion of a limit. That is, area A is imagined to approach as mathematicians say, a point, or an area of zero size in the limit. The idea of limits is central to calculus.

Stress is a measure of force intensity. In the metric system, force is measured in dynes and area is measured in square centimeters. Thus both normal and

shear stresses have units of dynes per square centimeter (dynes/cm^2). In the familiar English system, the unit of stress is pounds per square inch (lb/in^2). For reference, 1 dyne/cm^2 = 1.4504 × 10^{-5} lb/in^2, 0.00101971 g/cm^2, or 7.5005 × 10^{-4} mm Hg.

Normal stresses whose force acts away from the surface on which they act are called tensile, or positive, stresses; normal stresses whose force acts toward the surface on which they act are called compressive, or negative, stresses. Shear stresses may also be positive or negative, but this depends on the directions of the stresses relative to a coordinate system.

As an example, consider the anterior and posterior surfaces of the cornea, on which both normal and shear stresses act (Fig. 27-3). There is a normal stress but no shear stress acting on the posterior surface, but on the anterior surface the action of the eyelid and the presence of the tear film result in both normal and shear stresses. The stress on the posterior surface of the cornea is known—it is compressive and equal to the intraocular pressure—but the stresses acting on the anterior surface are not known. On the anterior surface, the action of the eyelid results in normal and shear stresses that vary in magnitude both from point to point on the surface and in time because of the action of the eyelid. In addition, the shear stress acts in an unknown direction.

Stress in three dimensions

So far we have considered only a surface of area A. In reality the situation is more complicated. A very small volume of the ocular tissue may be considered as a cube having six sides, or for our purposes, three sides and the mirror images of these three sides each of which is a square (Fig. 27-4). On each of the three surfaces defined in this way, we can imagine a normal and a shear stress acting in much the same manner as on the surface of area A discussed above. Note that subscripts one to three are used to identify the planes on which the stress acts. In general, we do not know the direction of the shear stress; we know only that it acts in the plane of the surface. This ambiguity can be removed by replacing the single shear stress on any of the three surfaces by two *unique* shear stresses acting parallel to the sides of the surfaces and having an effect equivalent to the single shear stress that has an unknown direction. The proof of this requires an understanding of the rules for the adding forces and is therefore beyond the scope of this discussion. Fig. 27-5 is a graphic attempt to convince the reader of the reasonableness of this statement. It can be seen that the shear stress τ_1 forms the diagonal of a rectangle whose sides τ_{12} and τ_{13} represent two shear stresses equivalent to the given stress τ_1. Similarly, τ_2 is equiv-

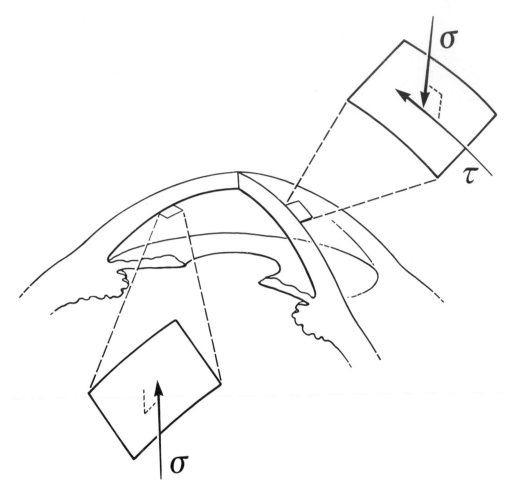

Figure 27-3
The posterior surface of the cornea is subjected to a normal stress σ, while on the anterior surface, both normal (σ) and shear (τ) stresses act.

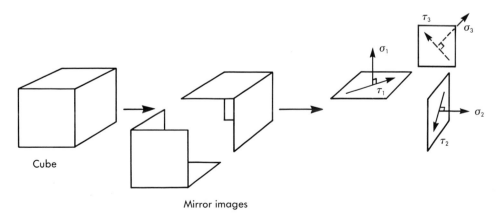

Cube

Mirror images

Figure 27-4
In three dimensions, the stresses act on areas that may be thought of as the faces of a cube. Different normal and shear stresses act on each face, and the subscripts 1 to 3 are used to distinguish them.

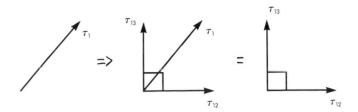

Figure 27-5
The given stress τ_1 is equivalent in its effect to the two orthogonal stresses τ_{12} and τ_{13} determined graphically. Shear stresses τ_2 and τ_3 can be similarly decomposed.

alent to τ_{23} and τ_{21}, and τ_3 is equivalent to τ_{31} and τ_{32}.

In summary, every very small cubic volume (point) of tissue generally has nine associated stresses—six shear stresses (τ_{12}, τ_{21}, τ_{13}, τ_{31}, τ_{23}, τ_{32}) and three normal stresses (σ_1, σ_2, σ_3). Each volume must be in equilibrium, that is, as each volume moves, the body deforms and the stresses change until there is a balance of force at which time no further motion can occur. An exception to this is the slow, creeping motion that occurs with constant stress and is exhibited by some tissues. For example, Nyquist[13] observed the elongation of weighted (loaded) corneal strips. Although such motions are usually small and occur over a limited period, they may be important in ocular biomechanics. For each volume to be in equilibrium, there are six relationships between the stresses. Considering these further requires mathematics, but we can say that the six relationships, referred to as the equilibrium equations, are not sufficient to determine the nine stresses. We must therefore either introduce additional ideas and equations or else consider problems where intuition tells us that some of the stresses are zero and equilibrium considerations may be used to determine the remaining stresses.

Fortunately in some problems of biomechanical interest, many of the stresses are zero or at least approximately zero. For example, on the surface of a normal cornea, the shear stresses, which are mostly a result of the action of the eyelid, are close to zero. However, refractive surgery can result in significant shear stress, at least in some regions, such as near radial keratotomy incisions.

Stress calculations

Stress is never measured directly. Typically, loads such as pressures and forces are measured and the stress is calculated using a mechanical model of varying complexity. Two particularly simple models are worth noting: the stress in a strip of tissue extended along its length and stresses in a thin-walled shell.

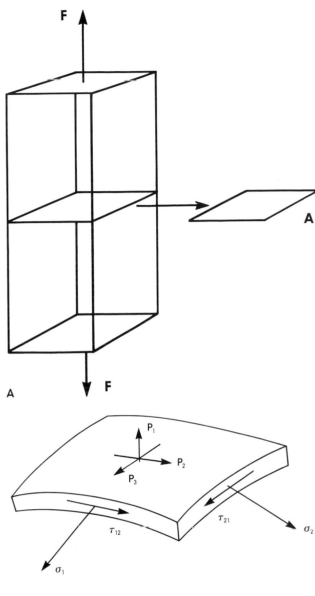

Figure 27-6
A, A representative "tension specimen" subjected to force *F* and having cross-sectional area *A*. **B,** An element of a thin shell is shown. The loads P_1, P_2, and P_3 and the stresses σ_1, σ_2, τ_{12}, and τ_{21} are shown.

A particularly simple state of stress exists when a strip of tissue having a uniform cross-sectional area A, often called a tension specimen, is extended by a force F acting lengthwise, as shown in Fig. 27-6, *A.* Every cross-sectional area A transverse to the length must support the force F, and it is reasonable to expect that the only stress acting in the tissue acts on the area A and is a uniform, normal stress of magnitude F/A. Actually this is only strictly true "far" from the ends where we expect the influence of the precise mechanism of applying F to be minimal. "Far" is usually interpreted by engineers to mean roughly 10 times the cross-sectional area divided by its perimeter. The extension of such a strip in the manner shown is an important experiment in biomechanics, and it will be discussed further in the following paragraphs.

As another example, the stresses σ_1, σ_2, τ_{12}, and τ_{21} in a shell structure that is very thin walled as compared to its radius may be calculated in terms of the loads P_1, P_2, and P_3 from equilibrium considerations only (Fig. 27-6, *B*). Since the shell is thin, the stresses may be assumed to be constant through the thickness and the shear stresses transverse to the thickness can be neglected. In general, partial differential equations must be solved. However, if the shell is spherical and subjected only to pressure, the shear stresses are zero and the result is the familiar Laplace's law: $\sigma_1 = \sigma_2 = P_1 R/2t$, where P_i is the pressure, R is the radius, and t is the thickness. Note that the calculation of the stress in terms of measurable quantities (pressure, radius, and thickness) is independent of the kind of material. The use of the Law of Laplace for corneal surgery, however, is debatable. The radius of the cornea is about 7 mm, and its thickness is about 0.5 mm, giving a radius/thickness ratio of 14. In engineering, the Law of Laplace is generally not used with radius/thickness ratios of 10 to 20. In any case, stress measurements derived using the Law of Laplace would be correct only in the central cornea "far" (several corneal thicknesses) from the effects of the bounding limbus. In the vicinity of the limbus, the stresses are more complex because the limbus is a material that is mechanically different from the cornea. This difference cannot be accounted for by the Law of Laplace.

In general, for ocular tissues a complex model, such as a "finite element" model,[21,25] must be used to determine the stresses from measured quantities. Although a discussion of these models is beyond the scope of this discussion, we note that the stresses determined in this way do depend on the material.

STRAIN
Definition

Strain is a geometrical concept. In its mathematical definition, it is intimately tied to the idea of displacement or motion that was discussed previously. There are also several possible definitions of strain, but we discuss only the simplest definition, the one most amenable to geometrical interpretation. As with stress, there are also two kinds of strain, extensional and shear; neither has any dimension. We consider each in turn.

The first strain is extensional strain. Suppose we can draw a very short line, OP, on the surface of the eye before any deformation occurs, as shown in Fig. 27-7. When we consider the application forces, such as intraocular pressure and muscle forces, to the eye, line OP deforms into line O'P' as shown in Fig. 27-7. The extensional strain, denoted by ϵ, is defined as the ratio of the lengths $\epsilon = (O'P' - OP)/OP$. Extensional strain is therefore the change in length divided by the original length of a very short line. In a similar way, we can define an extensional strain for any choice for the line OP drawn on any surface of the eye.

The second strain is shear strain, and it is denoted by γ. Consider the two very short lines, OP and OQ, drawn on the surface of the eye as shown in Fig. 27-8. The angle between lines OP and OQ is 90 degrees before any deformation occurs. When the loading, that is, intraocular pressure and other forces, is considered,

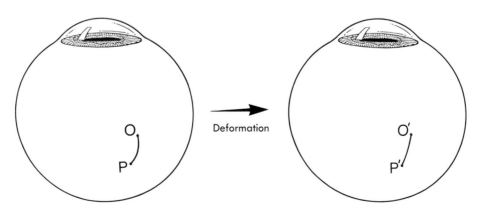

Figure 27-7
The line OP on the surface of the eye deforms into the line O'P' giving rise to the geometric interpretation of the extensional strain $\epsilon = (O'P' - OP)/OP$.

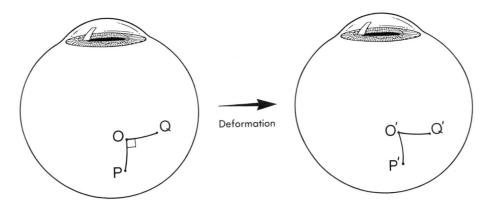

Figure 27-8
Lines OP and OQ are perpendicular lines on the surface of the eye that deform into lines O'P' and O'Q' giving rise to the geometric interpretation of shear strain γ. Shear strain γ is a measure of the distortion of right angles associated with a deformation.

the lines move so that the angle between them is no longer 90 degrees as shown in Fig. 27-8. The shear strain γ is defined as the change in right angles between two very short lines originally at right angles, that is, the difference between 90 degrees and the angle between lines O'Q' and O'P' of Fig. 27-8. By agreement, a positive shear strain means that the angle between the two very short lines decreases as in Fig. 27-8. Shear strain is therefore a measure of the distortion of the surface in the vicinity of the lines OP and OQ resulting from the deformation of the eye. For example, the shear strains in the cornea are normally quite small. However, surgery such as radial keratotomy can result in significant shear strains, especially in the vicinity of the incisions.

These working definitions of strain can be made exact if we let the lengths of the "short lines" discussed approach zero in the limit. Note that for all short lines emanating from a given point on a given surface there is an associated extensional strain, and for any two orthogonal lines emanating from the same point and on the same surface there is a shear strain. However, there are really only three unique strains, usually given as two extensional strains and one shear strain, associated with *all* lines emanating from a common point on a given surface. All the others may be calculated from the given three. The proof of this is beyond the scope of this discussion. However, intuitively we expect this to be true because a square drawn on the eye using four very short lines can deform only by having its sides extended and its right angles change as shown in Fig. 27-9. If the square is small enough, the magnitudes of the changes in all four right angles of the original square will be the same. Two right angles

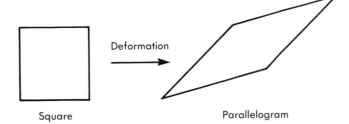

Figure 27-9
A small square shown deforming into a parallelogram. The sides extend giving rise to two extensional strains, while the right angles distort giving rise to a shear strain. These three strains determine the deformation.

become bigger and two become smaller, but all four angles change by about the same amount. This means that there is only one shear strain. Similarly, since the square is small, the extensions of the side opposite to any side of the originally square box will be almost the same as the side itself. In the limit these extensions will be the same. Therefore there are only two extensional strains, one associated with each of two adjacent sides of the original small square.

Strain in three dimensions

In the preceding discussion the short lines were drawn on a surface, but these ideas can be extended to three dimensions by considering a small cube in much the same manner as was done with stress. Such a cube of tissue can be generated using 12 lines—three lines emanating from each of the four vertices of the cube. Since the cube is small, we can consider each of the vertices to be essentially the same point. With the three lines emanating from a vertex, we can, using the

Figure 27-10
The cube deforms into a parallelepiped. A total of six strains, three extensional and three shear, is required to determine the deformation.

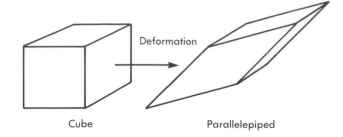

Cube   Parallelepiped

preceding ideas, associate three extensional strains, one for each line, and three shear strains, one for each unique pair of lines taken from the three. With a little imagination we can see that knowing these six strains defines the deformation of the small cube into a parallelopipid as shown in Fig. 27-10. An alternative way of coming up with the same conclusion is to make use of the arguments presented earlier. Recall that one shear and two extensional strains determine the deformation of a very small square as shown in Fig. 27-9. A very small cube can be generated from three squares and their mirror images as discussed earlier. Thus 3 sides × 3 strains per side = 9 strains. Accounting for sides common to more than one square reduces the number of extensional strains by three. The result is that the deformation of a very small cube is determined by six strains, three extensional strains and three shear strains, our previously reached conclusion.

Strain measurement

Strains in soft tissues must be measured without loading the tissue or else the measurement will be affected by the measurement technique. This almost always results in an optical technique, such as particle tracking, being used.[3,11,12] From the preceding discussions, tracking three closely spaced particles is sufficient to determine the average strain in the region of the particles. However, when the strains are relatively small as in the ocular tissue, this can be a difficult task.

As an example of a particularly simple state of strain, consider the strains in the long specimen, or tension specimen, of uniform cross section loaded along its length as shown in Fig. 27-11. The stresses in such a specimen were discussed previously. We do not expect any shear strains, and the most important strain will be an extensional strain along the length of the specimen. If we assume that the extensional strain is constant, its value may be computed $\epsilon = (L - L_0)/L_0$. Here ϵ is the extensional strain, L is the length of the specimen, and L_0 is the length before the application of the force F.

Finally we note that strain measurement is always made on an exterior surface. Strains at an interior

point are calculated using a mechanical model. There are optical techniques such as photoelasticity for measuring strains at interior points, but these use analog materials and are usually limited to engineering materials.

CONSTITUTIVE LAW

The previous discussion leads us to expect that there is a unique relationship between stress—intensity of force—and strain—a measure of deformation—for a specific tissue. This relationship is referred to as a constitutive law, or stress-strain law, and its determination is one of the major challenges in biomechanics. We also expect that measurements of stresses and strains in a particular tissue are required to establish the exact nature of the relationship between stress and strain.

Tension test

A complete discussion of constitutive laws for soft tissues is beyond the scope of this discussion. However, some insights may be obtained by considering the simple situation discussed previously: a specimen of undeformed length L_0 having uniform cross-sectional area A is loaded along its length by a force F causing the specimen length to change to L as depicted in Fig. 27-11. Using the arguments given before, we expect that the only stress will be a normal stress $\sigma = F/A$ and the most significant strain an extensional strain $\epsilon = (L - L_0)/L_0$ where L is the specimen length and L_0 is the unloaded length of the specimen.

Imagine the following experiment: the length L of the strip of cornea is gradually increased from L_0 while the force F is simultaneously measured. When F achieves a certain value, the process is reversed; the length is gradually decreased until the measured force reaches zero. There are several possible variations of the above description, but basically this is the simplest experiment we can perform. It is sometimes called a tension test. The results of a typical experiment (stress versus strain) are plotted in Figs. 27-12 to 27-14 for a few of the various kinds of material behavior.

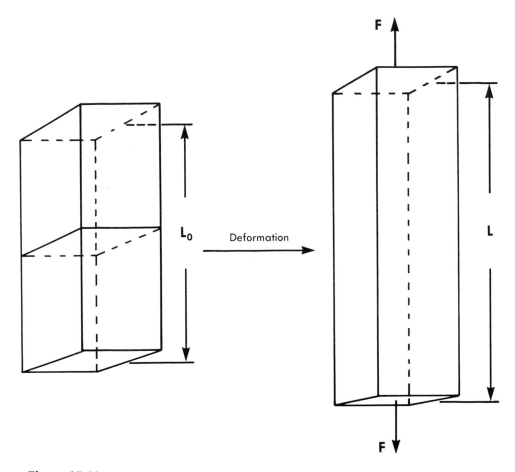

Figure 27-11
The tension specimen shown deforming from its original length L_0 to length L under the action of axial force F.

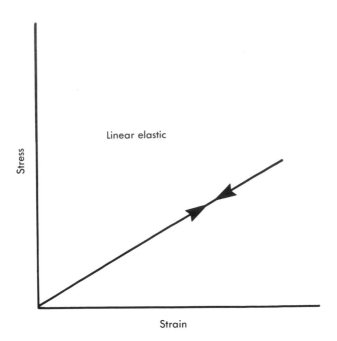

Figure 27-12
The stress-strain curve is a straight line representative of linear elastic material behavior.

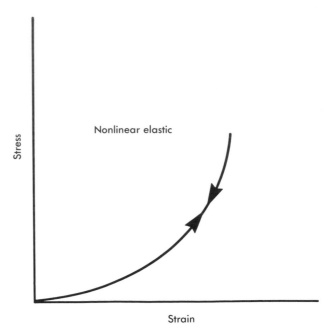

Figure 27-13
The stress-strain curve is not straight, but loading and unloading follow the same path—a result representative of nonlinear elastic material behavior.

Kinds of material behavior

Fig. 27-12 depicts linear elastic behavior: *linear* because the measured stresses and strains plot as a straight line and *elastic* because the strain resulting from loading (F increasing) is the same as for unloading (F decreasing). Fig. 27-13 therefore represents nonlinear elastic behavior; the stress and strain data do not plot as a straight line, but the loading and unloading curves are the same.

Fig. 27-14 represents a typical experimental result for a soft tissue, including the cornea. The curve is nonlinear and the loading and unloading curves are different, although they both appear to return to zero stress at zero strain. Since the only difference between loading and unloading is the time at which they occur, the resulting stress-strain curves must be time dependent. Materials that exhibit time-dependent stress-strain behavior are called viscoelastic. Materials that are viscoelastic are sometimes referred to as load history–dependent materials because the stress at any time depends on the stress history up to that time. Since the loading and unloading curves for soft tissues are nonlinear, these tissues exhibit what is called nonlinear viscoelastic behavior.

Other tests

When viscoelastic behavior is observed, other kinds of tests are often useful. We mention two such tests.

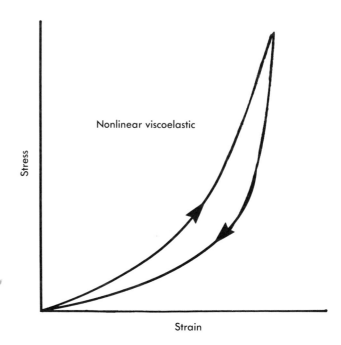

Figure 27-14
The stress-strain curve is not straight, and loading and unloading follow different paths—a result representative of nonlinear viscoelastic behavior. Such behavior is typical of soft tissues.

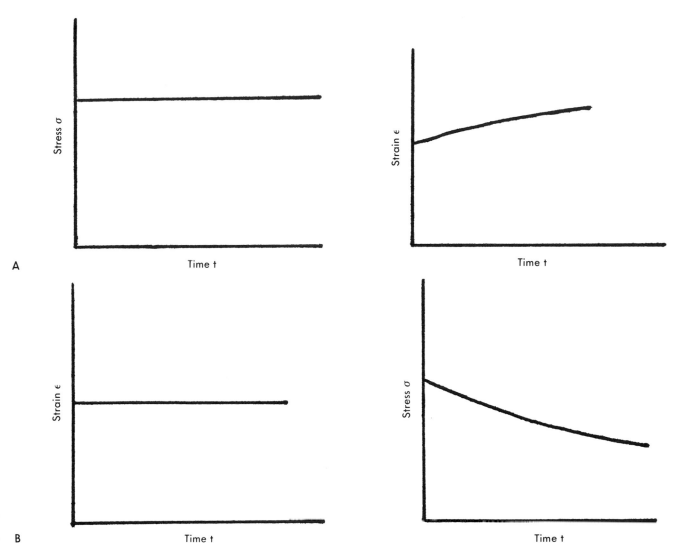

Figure 27-15
Creep **(A)** and relaxation **(B)** tests used to determine the magnitude of the viscous response for a viscoelastic material.

The first of these is a creep test in which the tension specimen described previously is subjected to a suddenly applied stress that is subsequently held constant in time. The resulting strain and its variation with time is one measure of the importance of viscous effects.

An analogous test is the relaxation test in which the specimen is subjected to a suddenly applied strain that is subsequently held constant over time. The resulting stress and its decay in time is yet another measure of viscous effects.

Fig. 27-15 illustrates creep and relaxation tests.

If the material is elastic, a creep test would result in a constant strain and a relaxation test in a constant stress. Thus these tests measure the deviation of the actual behavior of the material from elastic.

Hooke's law

For many linear elastic materials such as most structural metals the experiment described previously is sufficient to completely determine the six stress-strain relations, commonly referred to as Hooke's law, characterizing the material. Hooke's law depends on the Young's modulus, E, given in, for example: lb/in^2, and Poisson's ratio ν, which is nondimensional. Results for many soft tissues may be found in Yamada.[24] For the tensile test, Hooke's law takes on the particularly simple form $\sigma = E\epsilon$. Poisson's ratio is the negative of ratio of the strain transverse to the length of the tension specimen and the longitudinal strain. It is a measure of the transverse contraction in response to tensile loading.

Hooke's law is the simplest and most useful constitutive law. Engineers use it to design bridges, machines, and buildings successfully.

Many researchers have used Hooke's law as an approximation to the unknown constitutive law for ocular tissue, especially the cornea. In this approximation, E is about 5×10^5 dynes/cm^2 and ν is 0.49. This approach is not consistent with the experimental facts discussed previously and should be considered only as the crudest of approximations.

Soft tissues

For soft tissues, additional experiments are required and the stress-strain law is more complex. For example, the presence of viscoelasticity means that the stress-strain law for soft tissues should, unlike Hooke's law, depend on time.

There is a large and growing literature on the mechanics of soft tissues that is reviewed by Fung.[4,6] Some of the observations made on other tissues, such as arteries and skin, may be useful in research on ocular biomechanics. For example, the form of the stress-strain-time law for soft tissues has been extensively studied, and some of these results may be useful in interpreting the results of experiments using ocular tissue. However, the number of measurements of mechanical properties from experiments using ocular tissue that have been reported in the literature is limited.[9,19,23]

MATERIAL SYMMETRY

Intuition tells us that materials such as wood are stronger in one direction than in the other, whereas metals are equally strong in all directions. These differences reflect differences in microstructure and are important in the determination of a suitable stress-strain law. They are separate from the concept of homogeneity; both wood and most metals are homogeneous. Hooke's law holds for materials that behave mechanically the same in all directions. That is, no matter how one prepares the specimen used in a tension test, the experimental results will be the same. These kinds of materials are called isotropic. It is clear that wood is not isotropic. Wood has one strength along the grain and another perpendicular to it. It is referred to as an orthotropic material.

Few biologic tissues behave isotropically. For the cornea, each layer is not isotropic, although the entire structure may be nearly isotropic. Surgery such as radial keratotomy changes this, and mechanical models of the cornea must account for this.

BOUNDARY CONDITIONS

Everything is "connected" to everything else. The mechanical conditions that must be satisfied at the connections between a structure and its surroundings are called boundary conditions. For example, if we develop a mechanical model of the cornea, we must specify the mechanical constraints provided by the limbus at the boundary between the two.

It is clear that this is an important and difficult problem in the study of the whole eye. We understand qualitatively how the eye is supported, but our quantitative knowledge is limited. For example, the kinds of forces that the optic nerve, the extraocular muscles, the eyelids, and the orbital tissues exert on the eye, although important, are not well defined.

The importance of correctly accounting for conditions at the boundaries both in experimentation and in modeling cannot be overemphasized. For example, consider the simple extension experiment discussed earlier. Near the ends, the stresses depend on the exact nature of the application of the stretching force F and the strains depend on the kind of material. It is only away from the ends that the stress and strain are calculable from measured quantities using the formulas given previously. A similar situation holds in the so-called biaxial mechanical testing of planar tissue, such as the pleural membrane shown in Fig. 27-16.[11] It is only away from the points of application of the forces that the calculation of stress and measurement of the strain becomes relatively straightforward.

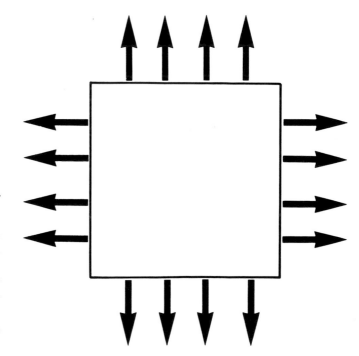

Figure 27-16
Biaxial mechanical testing of a planar sheet of tissue. Stresses and strains are uniform in the central region "far" from the application of the loads.

In experiments with a whole eye, we must correctly account for the supporting structures. This may be possible in vitro but the in vivo situation may only be qualitatively understood. Computation using a mechanical model of the eye may be useful here in simulating the possible boundary conditions and their effect on measurable quantities such as corneal curvature and intraocular pressure.

CONCLUSION

The mechanically significant ocular structures are generally considered to be the cornea, sclera, limbus, choroid, optic nerve, and the various muscles and tissues supporting the eye. Other structures, such as the retina, are probably not mechanically significant. However, the volume of published information on the mechanics of the eye is surprisingly small given the importance of the problem, and much more work must be done if the eye is to be modeled successfully in a clinically relevant way. This is the challenge to the surgeon and engineer.

One of the major challenges in any surgical procedure, particularly refractive surgery of the cornea, is to determine the exact surgical technique and variables that will produce a known predictable outcome. The ability to predict the outcome before surgery requires the creation of some type of model or predictive equation that can use preoperative variables to determine postoperative outcome.

The most common method used for determining surgical technique and variables in refractive surgery is a regression equation model that measures the postoperative results and conditions for a group of patients and then attempts to predict the outcome of a similar surgical technique on a similar group of subsequent patients with curve fitting and statistics. This approach has proved quite valuable, particularly in calculation of intraocular lens power during cataract surgery, as well as in predicting results of radial keratotomy, but the variability in regression modeling using current statistics does not provide a reliable means of predicting postoperative outcome. Since the regression model depicts the outcome for an overall group of patients, it is difficult to customize subsequent surgery for individual patients. Selecting patients for surgery depends almost entirely on previous clinical results with their wide standard deviation, making truly accurate patient selection difficult. Different regression models may identify different variables as important in determining postoperative results, thereby adding some confusion to the field.

A second approach to predicting the outcome of corneal surgery is to use mathematical, biomechanical models that assume the cornea is a structure that deforms in a predictable way according to accepted laws of physics when varying stresses are applied, as those from surgery. Such a model requires knowledge of the geometry of the cornea and supporting tissue, definition of the material properties of the cornea, and determination of the stresses and forces affecting the cornea, such as the intraocular pressure, pressure from the eyelids, and pressure from the orbital contents. Theoretically, such a model can be customized for individual corneas in individual patients by varying the geometry of that particular patient's cornea, the intraocular pressure, and (if measurements allow) the material properties of the cornea.

The practical outcome of mathematical models is the use of computer-generated surgery that will allow testing of a virtually unlimited number of operative techniques and variables for only the modest cost of computer time. This should improve the predictability of the outcome of surgery for individual patients and should allow development of new surgical techniques and strategies that will improve refractive surgery. Ultimately the techniques should allow computer simulation to select the best operation to achieve an exact outcome for an individual patient.

Currently the approach used by biomechanical engineers to model tissues is the finite-element model. Although such a model is mathematical and therefore described in terms of mathematical expressions that are beyond the scope of this chapter, we try to give here a simple definition of the process. A finite-element model conceptually breaks down a structure (the cornea) into a finite number of spatial pieces or elements. This can be conceptualized as taking apart a brick wall, the bricks being the individual elements constituting the wall. Usually the number of pieces, which are referred to as finite elements, is large. A model of the cornea might contain a minimum of 300 elements and a maximum of many more. Each element, or brick, has nodes at each corner and at the midpoint of each edge. These nodes are points at which the elements are attached to one another. The attachment is conceived of as a perfect coalescence— each finite element is compatible with the adjacent ones and deforms in synchrony with the adjacent elements. Within each of the elements, a simple displacement field or pattern based on polynomial interpolation is assumed and continuity of the element displacement fields is enforced at regions where the elements connect to each other.

Finally to use a finite element model, the geometry of the cornea, its material properties, and the stresses affecting it must be exactly defined. The veracity of using finite element model must be tested against real laboratory or clinical circumstances. Zienkiewicz[26] provides a detailed discussion of the model.

UNFINISHED BUSINESS

Biomedical engineering has emerged as a distinctive specialty within engineering, which has many subspecialties, among them the field of tissue mechanics. Similarly, ophthalmology is a distinctive specialty within medicine, which has many subspecialties, including refractive corneal surgery. The challenge ahead is to bring together the subspecialists in these related fields. More rapid and greater advances in refractive surgery will occur with the collaboration of biomechanical engineers, not only in understanding the structural behavior of cornea, but also in devising methods to simulate that behavior. Ophthalmologists interested in refractive surgery should seek out colleagues in the field of tissue mechanics and interest them in collaborative work. In fact, it is time to form a working group or society for ophthalmologists and engineers to share information. Periodic workshops, such as those held at the International Council on Eye Research and the National Eye Institute, are useful, but a group that meets regularly could refine and implement the seminal ideas propounded at these workshops on a more sustained basis. The Association for Research in Vision and Ophthalmology is an ideal setting for the assembly of such a group.

REFERENCES

1. Bryant MR, Velinshk SA, Plesha ME, and Clarke GP: Computer-sided surgical design in refractive keratotomy, CLAO J 1987;13:238-242.
2. Crandall S, Dahl N, and Lardner T: An introduction to the mechanics of solids, New York, 1972, McGraw-Hill, Inc.
3. Eliason J and Maurice D: Stress distribution across the in-vivo human cornea, Invest Ophthalmol Vis Sci 1981; 20(suppl):156.
4. Fung YC: Biorheology of soft tissue, Biorheology 1973;10:139-155.
5. Fung YC: The foundations of solid mechanics, Englewood Cliffs, NJ, 1965, Prentice-Hall.
6. Fung YC: The mechanics of living tissues, New York, 1981, Springer-Verlag.
7. Fyodorov SN: Surgical correction of myopia and astigmatism. In Schacher RA, Levy NS, and Schachar L, editors: Keratorefraction, Denison, Tex, 1980, LAL Publishing, pp 141-172.
8. Gere JM and Timoshenko S: Mechanics of materials, Pacific Grove, Calif, 1984, Brooks/Cole Publishing Co.
9. Graebel WP and vanAlphen GW: The elasticity of sclera and choroid of the human eye and its implications on scleral rigidity and accommodation, J Biomech Eng 1977;99:203-208.
10. Hanna KD, Jouve FE, Bercovie MH, and Waring GO: Computer simulation of lamellar keratectomy and laser myopic keratomileusis, J Refract Surg 1988; 4:222-231.
11. Humphrey J, Vawter D, and Vito RP: Quantification of strains during in plane bi-axial tests, J Biomech 1987;20:59-65.
12. Jue B and Maurice DM: The mechanical properties of the rabbit and human cornea, J Biomech 1986;19:10.
13. Nyquist GW: Rheology of the cornea: experimental techniques and results, Exp Eye Res 1968;7:183-188.
14. Popov E: Introduction to mechanics of solids, Englewood Cliffs, NJ, 1968, Prentice-Hall.
15. Sanders DR, Hofmann RF, and Salz JJ, editors: Refractive corneal surgery, 1986, Slack, Inc.
16. Schacher RA, Black RD, and Huang T: Linear small displacement mathematical model of radial keratotomy. In Schachar RA, Black TD, and Huang T, editors: Understanding radial keratotomy, Denison, Tex, 1981, LAL Publishing, pp 201-213.
17. Timoshenko S: History of strength of materials, New York, 1953, McGraw-Hill, Inc.
18. Truesdell C: Essays on the history of mechanics, New York, 1968, Springer-Verlag.
19. Vito RP, Kirschner S, Frazier J, Waring G, McCarey B, and Vawter D: The elastic and viscoelastic properties of human corneal strips, Proceedings of the Thirty-Fourth Annual Conference on Engineering in Medicine and Biology, Houston, Sept 1981.
20. Waring GO: Development and evaluation of refractive surgical procedures. Part I. J Refract Surg 1987;4:142-157.
21. Weaver W and Johnston PR: Finite elements for structural analysis, Englewood Cliffs, NJ, 1984, Prentice Hall.
22. Woo SL-Y, Kobayashi AS, Schlegel WA, and Lawrence C: Nonlinear material properties of intact cornea and sclera, Exp Eye Res 1972;14:29-39.
23. Wu W, Peters WH, and Hammer ME: Basic mechanical properties of retina in simple elongation, J Biomech Eng 1987;109:65-67.
24. Yamada H: Strength of biological materials, Baltimore, 1970, Williams & Wilkins.
25. Zienkiewicz OC: The finite element method, New York, 1977, McGraw-Hill, Inc.

A Finite Element Model of Radial Keratotomy Surgery

Raymond P. Vito

Jung-Woog Shin

The advent of refractive surgery has raised new questions for researchers in ophthalmology, questions that are inherently multidisciplinary and often do not fit within the usual confines of eye research. For example, radial keratotomy surgery alters the ability of the cornea to support the intraocular pressure to induce a change in corneal curvature. The shape of the cornea immediately after surgery is governed totally by mechanical factors, so the immediate surgical outcome ought to be predictable from a purely mechanical model. However, the relationship between the final change in shape of the cornea and the surgical and other parameters is not well understood[6,8] because wound healing and other biologic processes affect the outcome.

The cornea, like most soft tissues, is nonlinear, viscoelastic, nonhomogeneous, probably nonisotropic, and can exhibit large strains under physiologic loadings.[3] The whole eye is also geometrically complex. The only technique in biomechanics capable of systematically modeling this reality is the finite element method.[9,12] There is a growing literature on finite element−based models of the cornea and the eye.[1,4] The formulation of such a model, though difficult, is not beyond reach. The purpose of this chapter is to introduce the reader to the potential role of mechanical modeling in refractive corneal surgery. To this end, a finite element−based mechanical model of the cornea is used to simulate the

BACKGROUND AND ACKNOWLEDGMENTS

One simple approach to applying biomechanical principles to refractive keratotomy is to start with available information and tools. In this chapter, the authors, assisted by Alex Paine and Don Knasel, two very talented undergraduates who carried out many of the calculations, use their expertise as engineers at the Georgia Institute of Technology to select and apply "off-the-shelf" finite element model computer programs to the specific problems of radial keratotomy. The approach emphasizes the fundamentals of finite element modeling and serves as a valuable approach to the subject. I appreciate the time and effort contributed by these colleagues from a different discipline to our understanding of this subject.

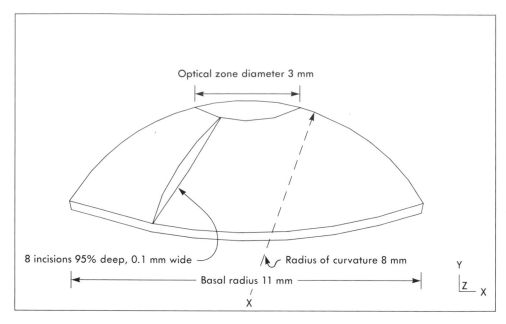

Figure 28-1
The baseline model was defined by data taken from a single operation on an individual human eye. The variables indicated were those actually used in the surgery.

immediate effect on corneal curvature of various choices for surgical and other parameters associated with radial keratotomy. The model assumes small strains and homogeneous, isotropic, nearly incompressible, linear elastic behavior. Though simple, the model shows good agreement with clinical observations and is indicative of the power and potential significance to refractive surgery of the finite element approach. Refinements of the model will be necessary to predict the acute response of the cornea to surgery more accurately.

DESCRIPTION OF THE FINITE ELEMENT MODEL
Software

The modeling uses a Computer Aided Design (CAD) software package called IDEAS (Integrated Designs, Engineering and Analysis System).* This program consists of various modules; in particular, a geometrical modeler, a finite element solver, and a post processor.

The geometric modeler accepts basic information defining the corneal shape. For example, Fig. 28-1 depicts the overall geometry of the "baseline" corneal model discussed below. To complete the generation of the finite element model, the user must select the kinds and sizes of the elements into which the structure is to be discretized, the material properties for each, the loading on each element, and the boundary conditions at the limbus. The resulting stresses, strains, and displacements are then determined using the finite element solver. The post processor reduces the results to graphic form (see Chapter 27, Biomechanics: A Primer for Corneal Surgeons).

Brick elements

The structure is discretized using so-called "brick" elements, with nodes at each corner (Fig. 28-2). These elements relate the three displacements and three

*Structural Dynamics Research Corporation, 2000 Eastman Dr., Milford, OH 45150.

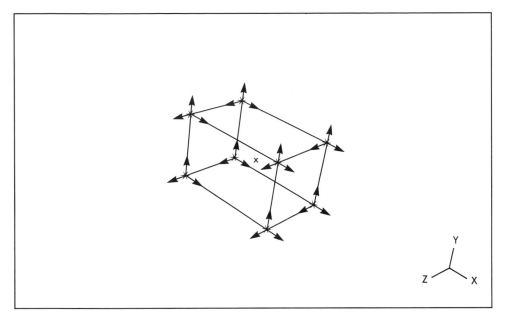

Figure 28-2

A single brick element shows the eight nodes at the vertices. Arrows are used to indicate loads or restraints on nodal deformation at boundaries.

rotations at each of the four nodes to loads applied to the element at the nodes. We used two bricks across the thickness of the cornea. The precise mathematical formulation of this finite element is beyond the scope of this discussion, and the interested reader is referred to Chapter 8 of *The Finite Element Method* by Zienkiewicz.[12]

Material properties of the cornea

In this model, the cornea is assumed to be a homogeneous, isotropic, incompressible, linear elastic material. Brief justifications for these simplifying assumptions follow.

Although the cornea has a lamellar, nonhomogeneous structure, we assume that microscopic observations, such as corneal curvature changes associated with the simulation of radial keratotomy surgery, can be accounted for by ignoring microscopic inhomogeneities. Accounting for differences in the mechanical properties of the layers of the cornea, such as Bowman's layer and Descemet's membrane,[5] requires a knowledge of both the mechanical properties of each layer and the nature of the mechanical interaction between them—information that is not available.

The presence of oriented collagen fibrils means that the individual layers of the cornea may not be isotropic. We are also aware that the corneal surface has an aspheric shape, steeper centrally and flatter peripherally. For simplicity, the cornea is assumed spherical in shape, indicating isotropic behavior.

To our knowledge there are no data on the compressibility of corneal tissue. However, its high water content (78%) means that the cornea, like most soft tissues, is nearly incompressible and, hence, Poisson's ratio was set to 0.49 in all our models.

The cornea is similar to other soft tissues in that it exhibits nonlinear viscoelastic behavior.[7] We expect, however, that the stress-strain relation is at least approximately linear in the range of intraocular pressures encountered in vivo

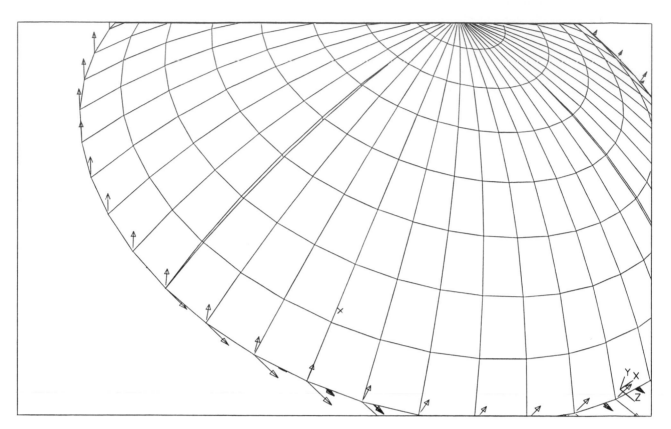

Figure 28-3
An incision is modeled as V shaped with 0.1-mm gap at its center and running from the limbus to the perimeter of the clear zone. Hidden lines are removed for clarity.

(12 to 22 mm Hg). We also expect that the viscous or time-dependent response is small when compared with the elastic or instantaneous response; hence, our focus is on the latter.

Strains in the cornea in vivo are a few percent, thus the borderline for ignoring nonlinear effects. For comparison, strains in the cornea are about 100 times larger than strains in engineering materials, such as steel, but only about one hundredth of the strains in other, more compliant soft tissues, such as arteries.

Values for the Young's modulus found in the literature[2,5,10,11] vary considerably. To choose an appropriate value, we simulated the results of an actual operation, using the patient data shown in Fig. 28-1. A Young's modulus of 5.5 MPa produced the same curvature change in our model as in the patient, and it is this value that is used in our baseline model discussed below.

Boundary conditions at the limbus

The exact simulation of the boundary conditions at the juncture of the cornea and limbus is difficult to construct because the mechanical properties of the limbus are unknown. In the finite element method, the specification of boundary conditions requires placement of restrictions on the translation and/or rotation at the various nodes located on the boundary. Since the limbus is much stiffer than the cornea and the resistance of the cornea to bending is not very great, the boundary nodes of the cornea are allowed to rotate freely about an axis tangent to the circles containing the boundary nodes. Any role played by the sclera is ignored.

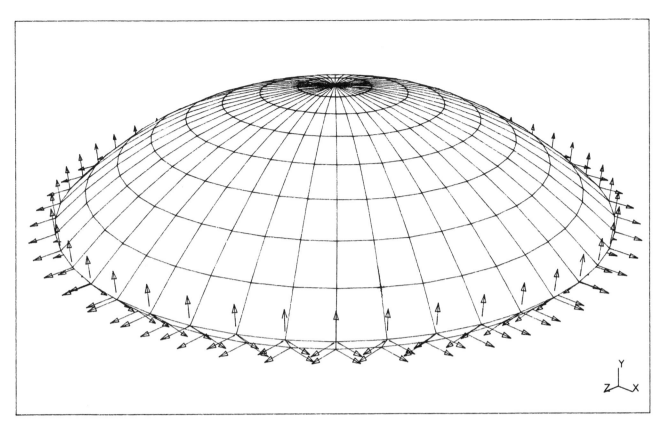

Figure 28-4
The baseline model of Figure 28-1 as discretized using brick elements. The arrows on the boundary with the limbus depict the boundary conditions described in the text. Hidden lines are removed for clarity.

Loading of the cornea

The cornea is loaded by the intraocular pressure on the posterior surface and by atmospheric pressure on the anterior surface. The loading produced on the anterior surface by the eyelids is ignored, as are other forces, such as the extraocular muscles and orbital tissues.

Radial incisions

The incisions run from the limbus to the perimeter of the clear zone. The clear zone is a circle of known diameter around the geometric center of the cornea. The incisions are V shaped and, on the anterior surface, are 0.1 mm wide at their center. Spline functions are used to locate the nodes on the anterior surface. Fig. 28-3 shows the geometry of an incision.

Calculation of anterior corneal curvature

The finite element model of the cornea deforms in response to the application of the intraocular pressure. However, in vivo the cornea is continuously subjected to the intraocular pressure and deforms in response to the surgical incisions. To simulate the effect of the incisions only, two models were constructed, one with and one without the incisions, but both subjected to the same intraocular pressure. Differences in the predicted deformation of these two models are the result of the incisions only and can be used to calculate a change in corneal curvature.

The deformed corneal anterior and posterior surfaces were usually close to being axis-symmetric (that is, differences in curvature from one meridian to another in a given surface were minimal). To calculate changes, we chose the meridian on the anterior surface of the cornea, which included the center line of an incision. Although shape information is known at many nodes along the meridian, three nodes suffice for the accurate determination of curvature: one node at the center of the clear zone and two 90 degrees apart on its periphery.

Baseline model

To determine the effect of various parameters, it was necessary to establish a baseline model. This model (Fig. 28-1) comes from an individual eye in the Pro-

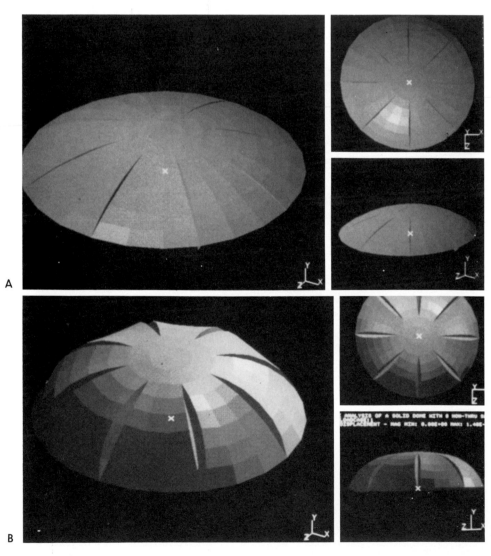

Figure 28-5
The baseline model of Figure 28-1 is shown both before **(A)** and after **(B)** the application of intraocular pressure. **A,** The sides of the radial incisions are approximated to each other without gaping, and the curvature remains normal. **B,** The incisions gape in the middle, producing central corneal flattening with paracentral corneal steepening. The graphic depiction of this central flattening is exaggerated for clarity.

spective Evaluation of Radial Keratotomy (PERK) study. The eye had eight incisions, 95% deep by slit-lamp microscopy and assumed to be 0.1 mm wide at their center. The central cornea measured 0.55 mm thick; the central radius of curvature was 8 mm; the clear zone was 3 mm in diameter; the horizontal corneal diameter was 11 mm. This patient had an approximately 8% decrease in the radius of curvature of the central cornea as measured by the keratometer at 20 mm Hg intraocular pressure. The Young's modulus, which simulates this curvature change, is 5.5 MPa, a value consistent with published data.

This baseline model, as discretized into brick elements, is shown in Fig. 28-4. Fig. 28-5 graphically shows the flattening predicted by the model in response to the application of the intraocular pressure.

Application and interpretation of the model

Our parameter study consisted of two parts. In the first, we investigated the effects of elastic modulus (Young's modulus, E), intraocular pressure, corneal thickness, incision depth, clear zone diameter, and number of incisions. Values for these parameters are as follows:

Parameter	Values
Elastic (Young's) modulus E (MPa)	1.0, 1.8, 2.4, 3.6, 4.8, 5.5, 6.0, 7.2
Intraocular pressure (mm Hg)	15, 20, 25
Corneal thickness (mm)	0.45, 0.55, 0.65
Incision depth (% of thickness)	55, 75, 95
Clear zone diameter (mm)	2.5, 3.0, 3.5, 4.0, 4.5
Number of radial incisions	4, 8, 16

In the second part of our study, we investigated the effects of surgical errors in the length, depth, and location of one of the eight incisions.

EFFECT OF VARIABLES ON CORNEAL CURVATURE
Effect of Young's elastic modulus

The effect of Young's modulus (E) on corneal curvature for two values of the intraocular pressure in the normal range is shown in Fig. 28-6. As E increased from 1 to 7.2 MPa, the change in the curvature of the central cornea decreased by approximately 35%.

The effect of changing the elastic modulus is not linear. When Young's modulus is low, from approximately 1 to 3 MPa, a small change in the elastic modulus is associated with a large change in the flattening of the cornea, whereas

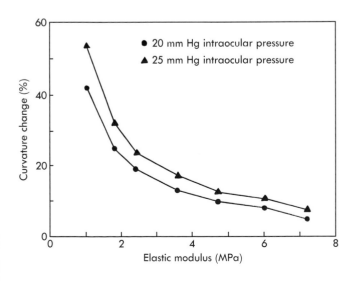

Figure 28-6
The effect of increases in Young's modulus on the amount of central corneal flattening. The calculations were carried out for two values of intraocular pressure. As Young's modulus increases from 1 to 7 MPa, the amount of change in corneal curvature decreases, indicating that the greater the elasticity of the cornea, the less change in curvature induced by radial keratotomy.

changes in the range of 3 to 7 MPa produced less change in curvature. These observations might be expected, in that a more elastic cornea would be likely to deform more easily and therefore show more central flattening, whereas a more rigid cornea might deform less easily.

These observations may have clinical meaning because it is likely the elastic modulus differs from one cornea to another and may decrease with age, so the same operation could be expected to have different effects in individuals. This may partially explain the greater effect of radial keratotomy with increasing age.

Effect of intraocular pressure

The effect of intraocular pressure, ranging from 15 to 25 mm Hg on corneal curvature, is linear (Fig. 28-7), with approximately a 4% greater change over this 10-mm Hg range. Thus, for a case with a total change after surgery of 5.00 D, raising the intraocular pressure from 15 to 25 mm Hg will add 0.20 D, not a clinically meaningful amount.

It is generally accepted that the intraocular pressure is the motive force that produces changes in the shape of the cornea after keratotomy. However, regression analyses of clinical series have not isolated intraocular pressure as a significant variable, probably because the effect of pressure in the normal range is small (as shown in our model) and because the effect of the other variables is so great. Thus, the intraocular pressure cannot emerge as significant. It is well documented, however, that elevated pressure outside the normal range, such as that induced by topical corticosteroids, can produce measurable increased flattening of the central cornea after keratotomy.

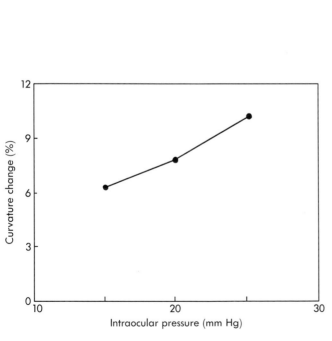

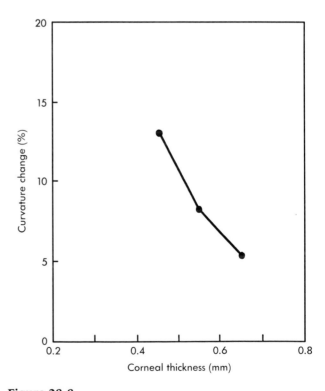

Figure 28-7
The effect of increasing intraocular pressure on the amount of central corneal flattening demonstrates that as the pressure increases from 15 to 25 mm Hg there is approximately a 4% increase in the amount of change in the central curvature. For an eye with a total of 5.00 D of change, this would represent about 0.25 D.

Figure 28-8
The effect of increasing corneal thickness on the amount of central corneal flattening demonstrates that for an incision of a given percentage depth, thicker corneas are somewhat stiffer and have less change in curvature than thinner corneas.

Effect of corneal thickness

The effect of corneal thickness is shown in Fig. 28-8 and is as expected: thin corneas flatten more.

Theoretically a 95% depth incision in a thinner cornea leaves less uncut tissue behind, which is more easily displaced, whereas in a thicker cornea, more uncut tissue is left behind, which is less easily displaced and therefore produces less central flattening of the cornea. A thicker cornea is simply stiffer.

However, regression analyses of clinical series have not isolated preoperative corneal thickness as an important variable, either because the incision depth is so variable as to mask the effect or because the thickness effect is "neutralized" by setting the knife blade length on the basis of the thickness reading itself.

Effect of incision depth

Fig. 28-9 shows that, as noted by the Dutch physician L.J. Lans in 1898, deeper incisions result in more corneal flattening. The effect is not linear. Incisions at 55% depth resulted in a 2% change, whereas incisions at 95% depth resulted in about an 8% change.

The fact that an incision must penetrate at least two thirds of the cornea to have a significant effect is of great clinical import, particularly when one realizes that a 5% difference in incision depth between 90% and 95% can make a significant difference in the amount of corneal flattening. Current manual techniques of radial keratotomy make it difficult to create an incision of uniform depth, but newer techniques, such as excimer laser linear keratectomy, might be able to achieve accurate and precise incision depth. Meanwhile, the surgeon using a diamond knife must exercise his or her best skill and judgment to cut deeply without perforating the cornea.

Effect of the clear zone diameter

As the diameter of the clear zone increases from 2.5 to 4.5 mm, the length of the incisions decreases and the amount of central corneal flattening decreases linearly by approximately 2% (Fig. 28-10).

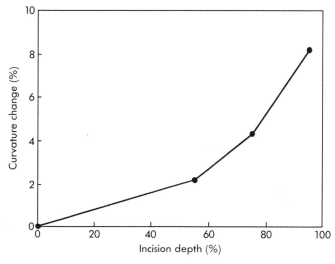

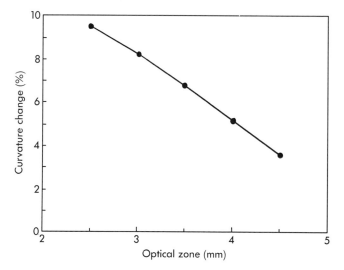

Figure 28-9
The effect of incision depth as a percentage of corneal thickness on the amount of central flattening indicates that incisions 60% or less deep have only a small effect; those 80% to 98% deep produce a much greater central corneal flattening. The relationship is not linear.

Figure 28-10
The relationship of increasing clear zone diameter to central corneal flattening is linear, showing that a larger diameter clear zone produces less central corneal flattening.

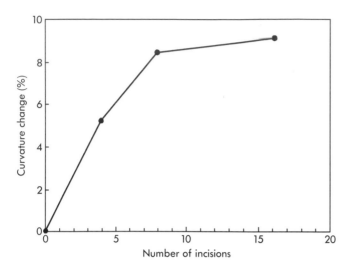

Figure 28-11
The relationship between the number of incisions and amount of central corneal flattening demonstrates that as the number of incisions increases from two to eight, there are relatively large increases in corneal flattening, whereas more than eight incisions produces little additional flattening. Thus the effect reaches a plateau at about eight incisions, and there is little to be gained in increasing this number.

Clinicians have known since the late 1970s that a larger diameter central clear zone produces shorter incisions and lesser effect, facts verified in this model. The effect is comparable to that of incision depth but is more easily controlled during the surgery. The fact this is a linear relationship means this variable can be controlled more easily during surgery.

Effect of number of incisions

It is well accepted that as the number of incisions increases beyond eight, the effect on corneal flattening decreases. This is borne out in our simulation (Fig. 28-11).

The fact that more than eight incisions contributes little to the amount of central flattening was demonstrated in early mathematical models, as well as in laboratory and clinical experience. Although some surgeons persist in using 16 and even 32 incisions, the majority are confining the number of incisions to eight or less, except in cases of attempted correction of higher amounts of myopia.

Effect of errors in incision length, depth, and offset

The following simulations were run:

1. One incision 7% longer than the others
2. One incision 7% shorter than the others
3. One incision offset by a 7.5-degree angle
4. One incision at 80% of depth and the rest at 95%

The clear zone in the first three of these models was irregular, and all four simulations resulted in some astigmatism. However, the differences in change in curvature, when compared with the baseline model, were less than 0.5%. The effect of combinations of errors was not investigated. Apparently, larger errors in more than one incision are required to give meaningful variation in results.

Effect of clear zone offset

In an attempt to simulate a "worst-case" scenario, the center of the clear zone was offset by 0.6 mm from the center of the cornea in a four-incision (95% depth) model (Fig. 28-12). All other parameters were as in the baseline model defined earlier. The effect on corneal curvature, as compared with a four-incision model with no offset, is shown in Fig. 28-13. There are significantly different curvature changes in the four meridians—0 degrees, 45 degrees, 90 degrees, and 135 degrees—creating irregular astigmatism.

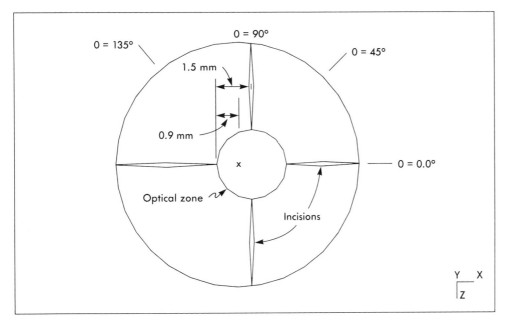

Figure 28-12
Drawing shows the central clear zone shifted by 0.6 mm to simulate the surgical error of poor centration with increasingly different lengths of the incisions.

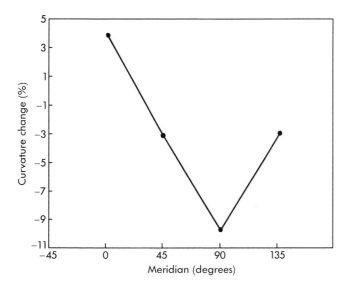

Figure 28-13
The effect of the eccentric placement of the clear zone illustrated in Figure 28-12 is the induction of astigmatism, with a much greater change in curvature at the 90-degree meridian than at the 180-degree (0-degree) meridian.

DIRECTIONS FOR REFINEMENT OF THE MODEL

Our model, though based on several simplifying assumptions, gives results that are in qualitative agreement with experimental and clinical observations. Although our model clearly demonstrates the potential benefit of finite element modeling to corneal surgeons, we are cautious when interpreting the results obtained using this or any model because the results are only as good as the assumptions made in the process of obtaining them.

We have emphasized the assumptions of our model concerning material behavior, geometric nonlinearities (that is, nonlinearities associated with large strains), and boundary conditions. Specifically, we assumed linear elastic, homogeneous, and isotropic material behavior, small strains (that is, linear, strain-displacement relations), and free rotation of the cornea at the limbus. It is likely that none of these assumptions truly applies. However, altering these assumptions requires experimental information that is, by and large, unavailable. For example, the stress-strain law characterizing the nonlinear mechanical properties of the cornea is not known. The variation of these properties through the different layers is also unknown. Consequently, one currently has considerable freedom in formulating a mechanical model for the cornea. We expect future efforts will be closely linked to experiments that measure the material properties of the human cornea directly.

Our model is of the cornea only. Other ocular structures, such as the sclera and the limbus, may be mechanically significant, although their effect on corneal shape is not well understood. In addition, little is known in a quantitative sense about how the eye is supported.

More realistic models of the cornea will require significant advances in computational mechanics. For example, a model assuming nonlinear elastic behavior requires the solution of thousands of simultaneous nonlinear algebraic equations. Techniques for accomplishing this task are an active area of research, and algorithms, when they work, require hours of computer time, even on the most powerful machines.

Finally, we suggest that finite element models can be helpful in both proposing and interpreting in vitro and in vivo experiments. They represent a unifying framework for communication among researchers interested in corneal surgery. Noteworthy is the graphic display of model results, especially corneal shape and curvature, often associated with finite element analysis. Graphic displays, such as Fig. 28-5, greatly facilitate the communication between surgeon and engineer. Continued development may give us finite element models that can design the surgery to fit individual patient needs.

UNFINISHED BUSINESS

As commercial software becomes increasingly available for finite element modeling, new programs and packages should be applied to refractive keratotomy. This will be particularly important if programs designed for biomechanical purposes become available and include anisotropic, nonlinear, and viscoelastic considerations.

REFERENCES

1. Bryant MR, Velinshk SA, Plesha ME, and Clarke GP: Computer-sided surgical design in refractive keratotomy, CLAO J 1987;13:238-242.
2. Eliason J and Maruice D: Stress distribution across the in vivo human cornea, Invest Ophthalmol Vis Sci 1981; 20(suppl):156.
3. Fung YC: The mechanics of living tissues, New York, 1981, Springer.
4. Hanna KD, Jouve FE, Bercovie MH, and Waring GO: Preliminary computer simulation of the effects of radial keratotomy, Arch Ophthalmol 1989; 107:911-918.
5. Jue B and Maurice DM: The mechanical properties of the rabbit and human cornea, J Biomech 1986;19:10.
6. Sanders DR, Hofmann RF, and Salz JJ, editors: Refractive corneal surgery, 1986, Slack, Inc.
7. Vito RP, Kirschner S, Frazier J, Waring G, McCarey B, and Vawter D: The elastic and viscoelastic properties of human corneal strips. Proceedings from the Thirty-Fourth Annual Conference on Engineering in Medicine and Biology, Houston, 1981, p 134.
8. Waring GO: Development and evaluation of refractive surgical procedures. Part 1. J Refract Surg 1987;4:142-157.
9. Weaver W and Johnston PR: Finite elements for structural analysis, Englewood Cliffs, NJ, 1984, Prentice Hall.
10. Woo SL-Y, Kobayashi AS, Schlegel WA, and Lawrence C: Nonlinear material properties of intact cornea and sclera, Exp Eye Res 1972;14:29-39.
11. Yamada H: Strength of biological materials, Baltimore, 1970, Williams & Wilkins.
12. Zienkiewicz OC: The finite element method, New York, 1977, McGraw-Hill, Inc.

Preliminary Computer Simulation of Radial Keratotomy

Khalil D. Hanna

Francois E. Jouve

The major unsolved problem for refractive keratotomy is the prediction of postoperative refraction for an individual eye.[19] The process of improving predictability focuses on three areas: (1) ensuring a reproducible surgical technique,[16,17,24] (2) determining the relevant variables that determine the outcome and establishing the values for each, and (3) using biologically active drugs to modulate wound healing and to control the results.

COMPUTER MODELING IN REFRACTIVE SURGERY

Two different approaches exist to make computational "models" of the cornea with computers. The first approach images corneal contours with keratography and projected slit beams through the cornea to measure corneal thickness and curvature. This information is digitized, and mathematical algorithms are used to create a geometric quantitative model of the cornea (see Chapter 3, Optics and Topography of Radial Keratotomy).

The second approach is biomechanical and uses either the imaged contours or an idealized geometry, but adds the constitutive equations that specify the me-

BACKGROUND AND ACKNOWLEDGMENTS

This chapter represents an interdisciplinary collaborative effort. Dr. Hanna, a practicing ophthalmologist, brings his background in mathematics to bear on the problems of computer simulation. Commencing in 1985, with the support of Dr. Herbert Budd at IBM-Europe and the IBM Science Centers in Paris, Dr. Hanna collaborated with mathematicians Francois Jouve, Philippe Ciarlet, and Michel Bercovier to develop a series of increasingly sophisticated and complex computational models of corneal surgery. The computational model of radial keratotomy presented in this chapter is somewhat simpler than the simulation of arcuate keratotomy presented in Chapter 34; for example, the radial keratotomy model is isotropic, the arcuate keratotomy model anisotropic. Nevertheless, it illustrates the process of doing surgery on a computer, which can obviate the expensive, time-consuming, and sometimes dangerous surgical experiments on animals and man. Work continues to develop more complex viscoelastic models, with collaboration with Professor Patrick Le Tallec at the Paris IX University. This chapter has been modified from work published separately in the *Archives of Ophthalmology* in 1989.[12]

chanical properties of the cornea and the eye. This approach predicts what will happen to the tissues when they are subjected to forces and external conditions such as surgery. These mathematical constructs are approximations based on assumptions about the mechanical properties of the cornea and other tissues in the eye. It is the approach we discuss in this chapter.

COMPUTER SIMULATION OF REFRACTIVE SURGERY

Computer simulation can be used to predict reactions of the eye to varying physiologic conditions, such as the internally applied force of intraocular pressure (IOP), externally applied forces of extraocular muscle tension and orbital pressure, or induced conditions such as keratotomy surgery. Computer simulation of the eye's mechanical behavior offers several advantages for the analysis of refractive corneal surgery; this is especially true for radial keratotomy, in which corneal curvature changes are produced by the mechanical effect of IOP. Computer simulation allows extensive and precise analysis, which is impossible in laboratory experiments and in living models. It can separate the instantaneous mechanical effects of surgery (the elastic, or time-independent, response) from the less immediate and longer term biologic and mechanical effects (the viscoelastic, or time-dependent, response). It allows assessment of interrelated variables that cannot be easily separated clinically, such as the effect of incision depth and length. Technically difficult or almost impossible surgical procedures can be simulated and evaluated.

To develop a mathematical model for the simulation of refractive corneal surgery, six components must be defined and employed:

1. Linear, nonlinear, or more complex viscoelastic mathematical laws that describe the behavior of the cornea
2. Mechanical constants and constitutive physical properties, such as Young's elastic modulus of the cornea
3. Boundary conditions
4. Computer programs that solve the equations and generate the data
5. Comprehensive interpretation of results
6. Computer programs that create a three-dimensional, geometric representation of the eye

Many mathematical and theoretical biomechanical models of the eye have been developed.[11] Most have been based on shell theory[23] or nonlinear membrane theory.[30] Some have defined the dynamics of the eye and tonometry.[7,15] Others have been applied to refractive surgery; these have varied from basic calculation to computer simulation of the cornea using linear or nonlinear laws to describe stress-strain behavior.[13,25-27] Computer simulation of the mechanical behavior of the eye using the finite element method and Hooke's law has been applied to highly myopic eyes and refractive surgery in two-dimensional models.[2] A sophisticated model that will simulate the response of the cornea to refractive surgery will have to include the anisotropic nature of the cornea, the viscoelastic response of the tissue, and the extraocular forces on the globe.

ASSUMPTIONS IN BIOMECHANICAL MODELS OF CORNEA AND SCLERA
Assumptions about constitutive properties

The assumptions about the values for the mechanical properties of the cornea and ocular tissues are derived from laboratory experiments, experience with other materials similar to the cornea, and measurements in living animals. The values derived from these sources may not be identical to the real ones present in the living tissues. For example, in trying to measure properties in living models, blood volume changes are important, both in the globe and in the orbit, and these are difficult to quantify in laboratory experiments and affect measurements of elasticity.[4,9] The values for Young's modulus are important but may be incorrect, since it is linked to linear laws. We used values on the order of 4860 kilopascals (kPa); unfortunately there are few reports that have measured the elastic coefficients of the cornea.

Assumptions about mechanical behavior

Various researchers attempted to characterize the stress-strain behavior of the cornea and the eye. Woo and colleagues[33] tried to determine the local, nonlinear elastic properties of the corneoscleral shell and concluded that viscoelastic and large deformation effects do not occur under physiologic conditions, an opinion not shared by everyone.[29] They expressed a different opinion and determined that the rheologic behavior of the eye is not elastic, but viscoelastic and quite complex. The most complex approach is to compute a nonlinear description of the viscoelastic model. However, Fung,[10] in his authoritative textbook, suggested that a linear viscoelastic model could be acceptable for finite deformations under physiologic conditions. We think that a nonlinear viscoelastic stress-strain relationship in tissues such as the cornea must be accounted for in a sophisticated model that can be used to predict the results of human surgery. However, the model becomes extremely complex when it is applied in three dimensions.

Few realistic computer simulations of radial keratotomy exist. The early ones[2,27] used linear laws for small displacement, assuming fixation of the cornea at the limbus.[27] More recent models are nonlinear.[13,32]

The advantage of the model we describe in this chapter lies in (1) the use of nonlinear mathematics, (2) the inclusion of the entire corneoscleral envelope, and (3) computation of the different stresses in a three-dimensional model. For most variables, our model is in general agreement with other models except for the correction related to the length of incisions. We have found that this length is an important variable.

Assumptions about distribution of physical properties in tissues

The simplest model assumes that the physical properties of a material are identical in all directions, the *isotropic* assumption. Therefore the application of stresses and the measure of the strain in any direction will result in the same elastic constants. This assumption is acceptable for homogeneous materials, such as metals or glass, but not for biologic materials, such as wood or connective tissue. For example, measurements on scleral samples have demonstrated an elastic modulus for radial stress across the thickness of the tissue that is more than 100 times less than the modulus for circumferential stress.[1] The anatomic structure of the cornea is obviously *anisotropic* because the cornea consists of multiple layers, and corneal stroma is lamellar, consisting of inextensible collagen fibrils enmeshed in a matrix of proteoglycans and other materials. The collagen fibrils are not intertwined and are regularly aligned in a parallel direction, so the stiffness of lamellae in the parallel direction is much higher than in the perpendicular direction. X-ray diffraction analysis has revealed the organization of collagen fibrils in the human stroma, which run in a superoinferior direction and a mediolateral direction in the central and paracentral cornea, and in a circumferential direction in the peripheral cornea.[22] Thus, the corneal stroma is anisotropic, requiring more complex mathematical models to account for its mechanical behavior. However, our model of radial keratotomy assumes isotropic behavior for ease of computation.

In terms of the cornea, even gross clinical experience demonstrates that Bowman's layer is stiff and inextensible, whereas Desccmet's membrane is flexible and more extensible. Jue and Maurice[14] have demonstrated that the behavior of the intact cornea seems to depend greatly on the behavior of the posterior stroma and Descemet's membrane.

All current models describe only an instantaneous change in the elastic response of the cornea at a single point in time; this is the instantaneous response for a given stress. This is an artificial assumption that does not take into account the time-dependent mechanical changes that occur. Also, it does not account for the effects of wound healing on the tissue. Realistic models will have to approximate these viscoelastic, time-dependent biologic conditions if they are to allow meaningful prediction of the surgical outcome.

Assumptions about extent of simulation and boundary conditions

One must define whether the model includes only the cornea, the corneoscleral envelope, all the tissues in the globe, or the entire orbital contents, including the forces of the extraocular muscles, orbital tissues, and eyelids. Our model simulates the cornea and the sclera fixated at the level of the optic nerve. All other current models assume a limbal fixation or a short distance beyond the limbus.

A NONLINEAR, FINITE ELEMENT MODEL OF RADIAL KERATOTOMY

We describe here a model of a moderately myopic eye based on the finite element method and the Mooney-Rivlin elastic, nonlinear law applied to almost incompressible materials.[6] We use this model to simulate radial keratotomy on a myopic eye.

Simulations of radial cuts on the cornea were performed according to an idealized surgical technique. The induced geometric and mechanical changes of the whole eye were evaluated. The effect of several variables, such as the number and length of the incisions, the radius of curvature, the IOP, and the corneal elasticity, also were determined.

This model cannot generate "real" clinical data, such as the change in refraction, because it describes only the instantaneous reactions of the eye to surgery, not the changes that occur with time, with reaction of the tissues, and with wound healing.

Numerical finite element method analysis

A finite element method (FEM) computer program was developed.[31,34] We used 27 nodes in a parametric curved, three-dimensional finite element for the mesh (Fig. 29-1). This is an optimal element for almost incompressible materials. All computations were carried out at the IBM Scientific Center in Paris on the IBM 4381 computer.

Geometric definition

To construct the model, we assumed perfect anteroposterior axial symmetry for the eye (Table 29-1). The spherical shape of the eyeball was accepted for both emmetropia and modest degrees of ametropia, whereas in severe myopia the shape of the eyeball was approximated to a prolate spheroid.[15,26,28] To allow representations of a slightly prolate shape of a moderately myopic eye (5 to 6 D) and the thickness variation of the sclera, we used two ellipses with a common axis to define the scleral boundaries. The accepted assumptions were that the sclera stretched mainly posteriorly and that the anteroposterior increase was three times the equatorial increase.[26] We assumed an axial length of 26.5 mm (range, 26.2 to 27.1 mm in myopia of 5.00 to 6.00 D). We assigned a value of

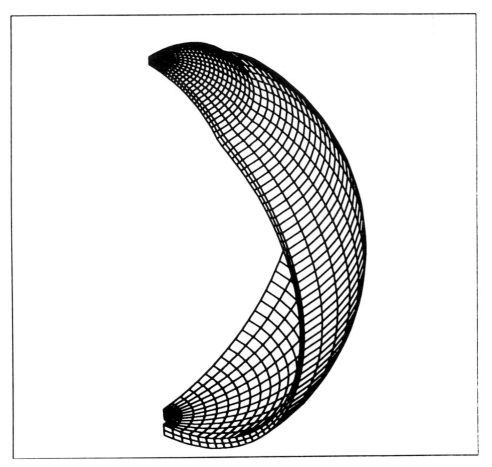

Figure 29-1

A computer-generated graphic three-dimensional quarter view model of a moderately myopic eye demonstrates the finite element mesh. Mathematically, the model includes only one element for thickness, even though the graphic depicts two elements.

Table 29-1

Values Used for Geometric Definition of the Eye in Mathematical Model

Measurement	Value
Axial length of eye	26.5 mm
Radius of curvature of corneal central zone	7.8 mm
Radius of curvature of posterior corneal surface	6.6 mm
Diameter of cornea	11.8 mm
Thickness of central cornea	0.5 mm
Thickness of peripheral cornea at 11 mm diameter	0.74 mm
Anterior corneal surface area	136.30 mm^2
Volume of cornea and sclera	916.36 mm^3
Internal volume of myopic eye	7433.56 mm^3

0.45 mm to thickness of the sclera at the equator and 0.825 mm at the limbus.

To define an idealized corneal profile, Lotmar's equation for the cornea was used[18]:

$$x = \frac{h^2}{2r_0}\left[1 + a\left(\frac{h}{r_0}\right)^2 + b\left(\frac{h}{r_0}\right)^4\right]$$

Where x is the profile of the cornea, r_0, the radius of curvature of the central cornea, h, the distance to the geometric axis, and a and b, the coefficients ($a = 5/28$, and $b = 1/12$). (Lotmar's equation is an approximation of Bonnet's profile, obtained by light diffused from talcum particles in the tear film.)[3]

An anterior radius of curvature of 7.8 mm for the 4-mm central zone and a 6.6 mm radius of the posterior surface were used in Lotmar's equation. Other variables included 11.8 mm for the corneal diameter, 0.74 mm for the corneal thickness at diameter 11 mm, and 0.5 mm thickness for the central cornea. The anterior corneal surface area was 136.30 mm². The volume of the cornea and sclera was 916.36 mm³, whereas the internal volume of this reference eye was 7433.56 mm³ (Fig. 29-1), 33.4% greater than that for the emmetropic eye.

Mathematical laws and definitions of coefficients

We made three assumptions about the cornea and sclera in this model: (1) the relationship between stress and strain is nonlinear; (2) the cornea and sclera are essentially incompressible[1,5]; and (3) the tissues are isotropic.

Nonlinearity. Woo and colleagues[33] and Vito and colleagues[31] have demonstrated the nonlinear stress-strain behavior of the corneoscleral envelope. Concerning the nonlinear relationship between stress and strain, we used the Mooney-Rivlin nonlinear law for almost incompressible materials:

$$W = \alpha I_1 + \beta I_2 + f\left[\det(\mathrm{Id} + 2\epsilon)\right]$$

This describes the strain energy at the level of the cornea and sclera, where W is the elastic potential or strain energy function, ϵ is the strain tensor at each point, I_1 and I_2 are the first main invariants of the strain tensor, and σ and β the coefficients of elasticity. The third term of the law is added to obtain incompressibility and zero stress when the displacement is equal to zero. Many functions of f are possible as long as the following relations are satisfied:

f is strictly convex and twice differentiable at the point 1
$f(1) = 0$
$f(x) \rightarrow +\infty$ when $x \rightarrow 0^+$
$f(x) \rightarrow +\infty$ when $x \rightarrow +\infty$
$f'(1) + \alpha + 2\beta = 0$

We took:

$$f(x) = \mathrm{pen}(x - 1) - (\mathrm{pen} + \alpha + 2\beta)\log(x)$$

where *pen* is a penalty coefficient for incompressibility, following Ciarlet.[6] Stress tensor Σ is then computed from the stored energy function as follows:

$$\epsilon = \begin{bmatrix} \epsilon_{11} & \epsilon_{12} & \epsilon_{13} \\ \epsilon_{21} & \epsilon_{22} & \epsilon_{23} \\ \epsilon_{31} & \epsilon_{32} & \epsilon_{33} \end{bmatrix} \qquad \Sigma = \begin{bmatrix} \sigma_{11} & \sigma_{12} & \sigma_{13} \\ \sigma_{21} & \sigma_{22} & \sigma_{23} \\ \sigma_{31} & \sigma_{32} & \sigma_{33} \end{bmatrix}$$

where ϵ and Σ are, respectively, the strain and stress tensor. We have the relationship:

$$\Sigma_{ij} = \frac{\partial W}{\partial \epsilon_{ij}}$$

Definition of elasticity coefficients. Young's modulus is a measure of the strength of a material and is expressed as the ratio of change in stress (σ = force per unit area) to the associated strain (ϵ = fractional change in length). We used data available in the literature for Young's elastic modulus, 4860 kPa for the cornea and 2000 kPa for the sclera. With these values, we derived the coefficients α and β from Lauvé constants by comparing both the Mooney-Rivlin law and Hooke's law for small displacement, which led to the relationship:

$$\alpha + \beta = \frac{\epsilon}{\sigma}$$

Incompressibility. The assumption that the cornea and sclera are essentially incompressible[1] is based on the volume of the tissue being reduced less than 0.001% under the force of an IOP of 15 mm Hg. Compressibility measurements have been performed on the sclera, which has been shown to be almost incompressible under physiologic loading.[1,5] The assumption is important, since the degree of compressibility of the cornea and sclera affects the stress distribution in the eye. If the eye wall were composed of a compressible material, the stress concentration would be relieved past the inner wall of the globe, whereas material that is nearly incompressible leads to more loading of the inner surface than the outer surface. Therefore the inner layers of the cornea bear more stress than the outer layers, contrary to experimental findings of McPhee and colleagues.[20]

Isotropia. Our third assumption, that the cornea and sclera are isotropic and exhibit the same physical properties in all directions, is incorrect because the collagenous structure of the cornea varies from anterior to posterior. However, anisotropic models require complex, extensive computation. Thus, for a first approximation, we assumed only different coefficients of elasticity for the cornea and sclera, but no differences across the thickness of either tissue. (See Chapter 34, Computer Simulation of Arcuate Keratotomy for Astigmatism, for an example of an anisotropic model.)

Idealized simulated surgical technique

To determine the effect of radial keratotomy with our model, we simulated surgery using several assumptions. The depth of the incisions used was nearly equal to the thickness of the cornea, including the peripheral increase in thickness. The incisions were made perpendicular to the anterior corneal surface. Perfect axial symmetry was present for the eye and for the distribution of incisions. The geometric and visual axes were superimposed, and no consideration was given to the physiologic angle between these two axes.

Optical calculations

We used Gullstrand's optical model of the eye to calculate the change in refractive power. We employed the elements in the Gullstrand model to compute the total refractive change for the eye, as well as simply computing the change in power in the cornea alone.[8]

SIMULATION OF BASELINE CONDITIONS IN LOW MYOPIA

Our model was based on the calculation of the different stresses in the cornea and sclera: the stress along a meridian (σ_1), the stress perpendicular to the surface (σ_2), and the stress tangent to the surface (hoop stress, σ_3) (Fig. 29-2). Shear stresses are $\Sigma_{r\theta}$, $\Sigma_{r\phi}$, and $\Sigma_{\theta\phi}$.

For initial computation, we describe stress changes very close to the edge of the simulated incision. We are not presenting the curves of these stresses between the incisions. (See Figs. 29-6 to 29-9 for what happens to the tissue only in the area adjacent to the incisions.)

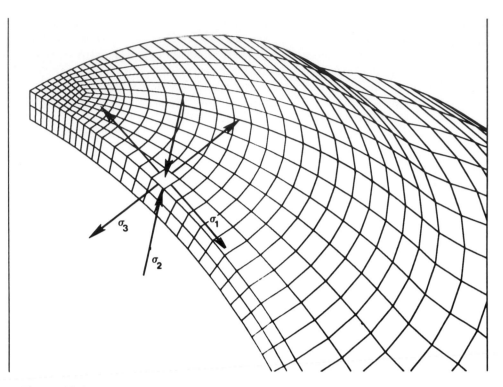

Figure 29-2

A computer-generated graphic model of the cornea demonstrates the direction of the three principal stresses: σ_1 = stress along a meridian, σ_2 = stress perpendicular to the surface, σ_3 = stress circumferentially around one zone.

Stress along a meridian (meridional stress, σ_1) (Fig. 29-3, *A*)

Stress along a single meridian from the center of the cornea to the equator is higher at the posterior surface, with a value in the center of the cornea of approximately 10 kPa. The amplitude increases slightly out to the 7 mm diameter point and then diminishes rapidly in the area of the limbus from approximately 10 to 15 mm, with a maximal amplitude at 12 mm where the junction occurs between the cornea and sclera. Here we find a negative value for the posterior layer, which arises from a change in curvature at the limbal zone. A small perturbation in this curve is also caused by the two different Young's moduli between the cornea and the sclera. Into the sclera, there is a new distribution of the meridional stress, with a continuous increase out to the equator from about 15 kPa and approximately the same values across the thickness of the tissue.

Stress perpendicular to surface (normal stress, σ_2) (Fig. 29-3, *B*)

This normal stress has a negative value and is also higher at the posterior surface. It equalizes near the limbus, shows an inversion across the limbus, and then becomes similar across the sclera and increases in absolute value toward the equator. This pattern generally is similar to that of the meridional stress, except it moves in a negative instead of a positive direction.

Stress around a circumference (circular or hoop stress, σ_3) (Fig. 29-3, *C*)

This stress is perpendicular to the meridional stress (σ_1) and is tangent to the surface, comprising the circular, circumferential, or hoop stress around the cor-

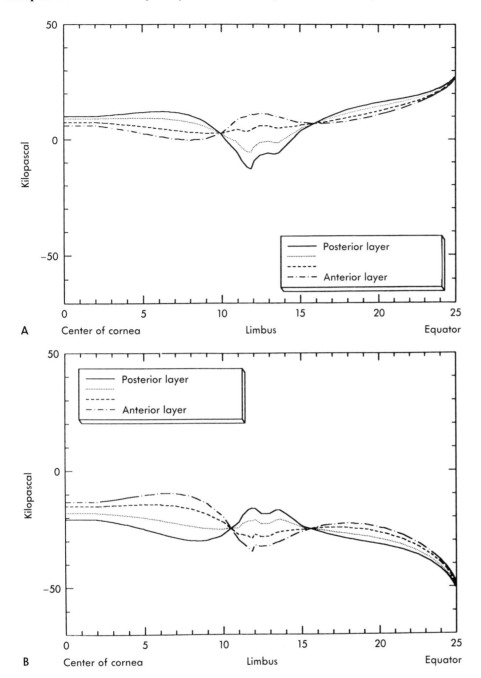

Figure 29-3

Distribution of three stresses in the normal cornea. **A,** Stress along a meridian (σ_1). Stress along a single meridian from the center of the cornea to the equator is higher at the posterior surface, with a value in the center of the cornea of approximately 10 kPa. The amplitude increases slightly out to the 7 mm diameter point and then diminishes rapidly in the area of the limbus with a maximum amplitude at 12 mm diameter at the junction between the cornea and sclera, where there is a negative value for the posterior layer, which arises from the change in curvature at the limbal zone. A small perturbation in this curve is also caused by the two different Young's moduli between the cornea and the sclera. **B,** Stress perpendicular to the surface (σ_2). This stress has a negative value and is also higher at the posterior surface, equalizing near the limbus, demonstrating an inversion in stress bearing across the limbus, becoming similar across the sclera, and increasing in absolute value toward the equator. This pattern is similar to that of the meridional stress, except it moves in a negative instead of positive direction.

Continued.

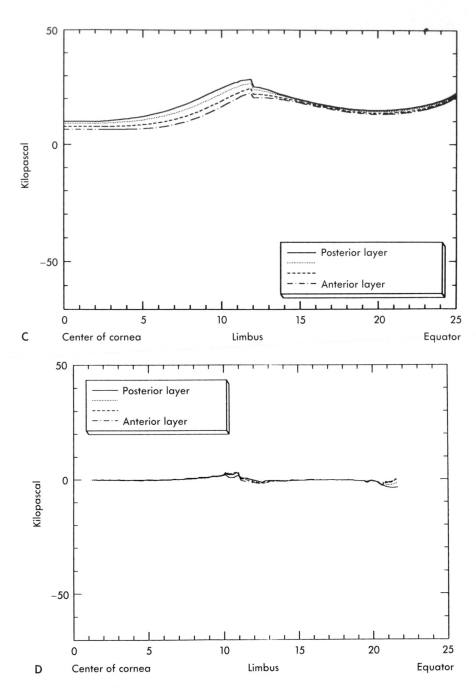

Figure 29-3, cont'd
C, Circumferential stress (hoop stress, σ_3) is perpendicular to the meridional stress (σ_1) and is tangent to the surface. At the center of the cornea it has the same value as the meridional stress, approximately 10 kPa, and increases in value by a small amount from the center to the periphery, the highest value being in the area of the limbus at 28 kPa for the posterior layer and 22 kPa for the anterior layer. The differences across the sclera are minimal out to the equator. **D,** Before surgery, there are three shear stresses: $\sigma\, r\, \theta$, $\sigma\, r\, \phi$, $\sigma\, \theta\, \phi$. This figure demonstrates that $\sigma\, \theta\, \phi$ is negligible except at the level of the limbus with a maximal value of 4 kPa.

nea. At the center of the cornea it has the same value as the meridional stress, approximately 10 kPa, and increases in value by a small amount from the center to the periphery. The highest value is in the area of the limbus, at 28 kPa for the posterior layer and 22 kPa for the anterior layer. The differences across the sclera are minimal out to the equator.

Stresses transverse to thickness (shear stresses) (Fig. 29-3, *D*)

The two shear stresses $\Sigma_{r\theta}$ and $\Sigma_{r\phi}$ are almost null because of the greater geometric axial symmetry (figures are not presented here). $\Sigma_{\theta\phi}$ is negligible except at the level of the limbus, with a maximal value of 4 kPa.

SIMULATION OF RADIAL INCISIONS

Using this model, we simulated the effect of radial incisions that extended from the edge of a specified central clear zone out to the diameter of 11 mm. During our initial simulations, we found that little change occurred out in the sclera from a diameter of 22 to 25 mm, that is, beyond approximately 5 mm from the limbus. Thus all our computations were done using one quarter of the eye, out to a diameter of 22 mm or less.

Preliminary simulation

We did a preliminary simulation using eight radial incisions at 99% depth, a 3-mm diameter clear zone, the endpoint of incisions at the 11 mm diameter, an IOP of 15 mm Hg, and a value for Young's modulus of 4860 kPa. The change in refractive power for the total eye was 3.00 D, much less than the expected clinical change. The value in the PERK study for this group was approximately 5.00 D. The reason for the discrepancy between the results from the model and the PERK study was the high value of Young's modulus. In addition, the model simulated only the instantaneous elastic change in the tissue, whereas the clinical circumstance included the entire viscoelastic alteration of the tissue over time, including wound healing.

Thus we modified Young's elastic modulus to consider individual difference. We progressively reduced the value for the elastic modulus until we reached approximately 6.00 D change in refraction at a Young's modulus of 2250 kPa, a value approximately half that given in the literature.[2] This is the number we used for Young's elastic modulus for all our subsequent simulations.

Change in corneal shape

The final model just described predicted: (1) a posterior displacement (flattening) of the central 6 mm diameter area of the cornea, (2) an anterior displacement (steepening) of the cornea and the sclera between diameters 6 and 11 mm, and (3) a slight but negligible anterior displacement between 11 and 22 mm (see Table 29-1 and Fig. 29-4, *A* and *B*).

The movement of the central cornea posteriorly (flattening) was very small and increased with greater IOP and more incisions (Tables 29-2 and 29-3).

Distribution of stress after radial incisions

This model took into account the response of the cornea under the influence of all stresses caused by IOP at one time. The model demonstrated that radial keratotomy changes the stress distribution in the cornea and the anterior part of the sclera back to about the 20 mm diameter point, but it does not affect the equatorial or posterior sclera. In general the stress levels were increased at the central clear zone of the cornea by about 300%, with most of this increase taken up by the posterior cornea. The stress is very high in the base of the incisions because only a thin layer of tissue remained to support all the forces.

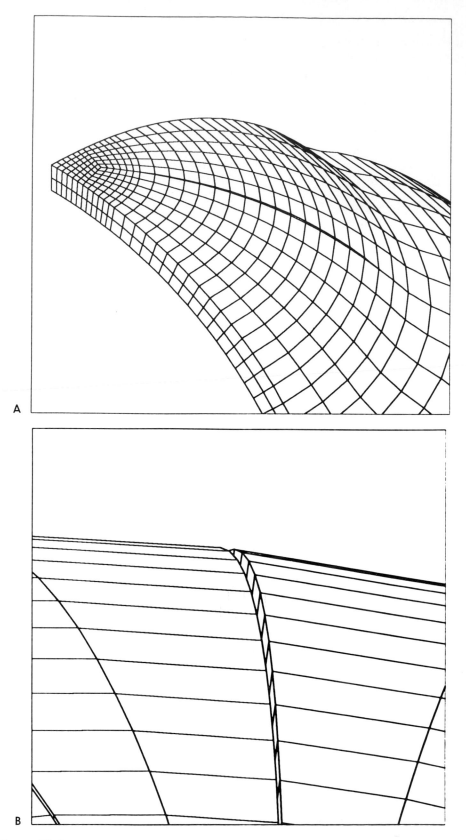

Figure 29-4
Pictorial representation of the effect of radial incisions in the cornea. **A,** The incision gapes open and the central cornea flattens. **B,** Magnified view of an incision.

Continued.

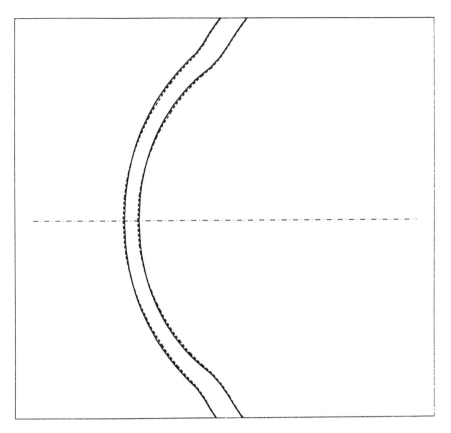

Figure 29-4, cont'd
C, Cross section shows the contour before *(dashed line)* and after *(solid line)* radial keratotomy with eight, 99% depth incisions. There is posterior displacement (flattening) of central cornea out to approximately 6 mm diameter and paracentral-peripheral anterior displacement (steepening) from 6 to 10 mm.

Table 29-2

Instantaneous Displacement of the Central Cornea Induced by Eight Radial Incisions That Extend from 3- to 11-mm Diameter Zones, 99% Depth, with an IOP of 15 mm Hg

Number of incisions	Posterior displacement (flattening) (μm)	Change in power (D)
2	8	2.50
4	15	4.50
8	24	6.10
12	29	6.90
24	34	7.50

Table 29-3

Instantaneous Displacement of the Central Cornea by Changes in IOP after Eight Radial Incisions That Extend from 3- to 11-mm Diameter Zones, 99% Depth

Intraocular pressure (mm Hg)	Posterior displacement (flattening) (μm)	Change in power (D)
10	17	4.40
13	21	5.40
15	24	6.10
17	27	6.80
20	30	7.80

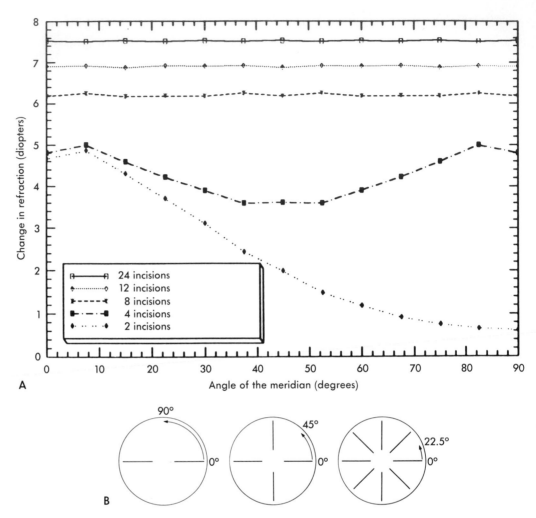

Figure 29-5
A, Effect of increasing the number of radial incisions from 2 to 24 on the power of the cornea from 0° to 90°. The effect of the incisions on the paracentral cornea is demonstrated. Two incisions at 180° flatten the horizontal meridian but have little effect at 90°. Four incisions at 180° and 90° flatten both of those meridians more than the area between them. Eight, 12, and 24 incisions flatten the entire circumference cornea equally. **B,** Drawings show the effect of increasing the number of incisions. Arrows indicate the decreasing difference between flatter and steeper areas of the cornea.

As might be expected, large focal changes in the stresses occurred at the paracentral and peripheral ends of the incisions, that is, the junctional zone between the intact and cut tissue. The major changes in these stresses occurred at 4.5 to 5.5 mm diameter and at 10 to 11 mm diameter, the areas close to the ends of the incisions. These stress changes at the edge of the incision explain the wound opening and the increase in surface area (Fig. 29-4, *C*). The zone limited by two incisions is under compressive forces, which explains the change in dioptric power from one point to another along a given diameter (Fig. 29-5, *A*). The meridian midway between two incisions is steep but disappears with an increase in number of incisions (Fig. 29-5, *B*).

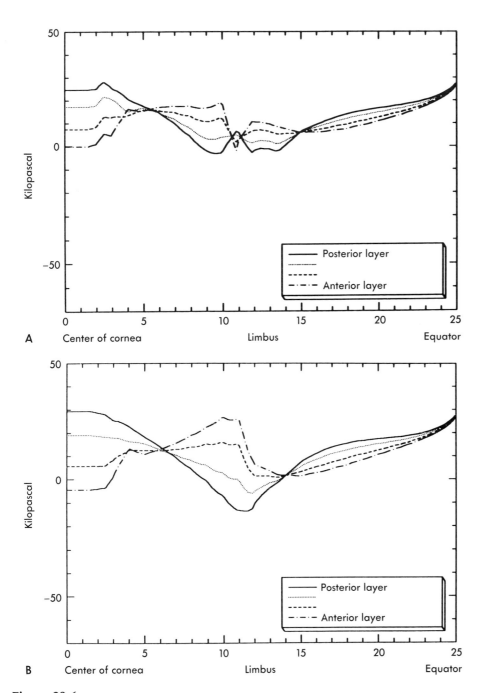

Figure 29-6

Graphic representation of distribution of meridional stress (σ_1) from 0 to 20 mm diameter after radial 99% deep incisions and 3.0 mm clear zone at an IOP of 15 mm Hg. **A,** With 8 incisions, the values (approximately 25 kPa) were greater in the posterior layers of the central region. All the values came together across the thickness of the cornea at approximately 15 kPa at a diameter of about 5.5 mm. Beyond this point, the anterior layers bore more stress than the posterior layers until another equalization point around 11 mm at the limbus. **B,** Increasing the number of incisions to 24 moved the equalization point out to about 7 mm diameter and produced a negative stress (a compressive force) along the posterior layers in the limbal area.

Stress along a meridian (σ_1). We evaluated the stress distributions from the center of the cornea at diameter 0 to approximately 20 mm diameter, along the edge of the incision. With eight incisions (Fig. 29-6, *A*), the values in the paracentral end were greater in the posterior layers by approximately 25 kPa at a diameter of 5.5 mm, but all the values came together at approximately 15 kPa across the thickness of the cornea. Beyond this point in the peripheral cornea, the anterior layers bore more stress than the posterior layers until another equalization point about 10 mm at the limbus. Increasing the number of incisions from 8 to 24 (Fig. 29-6, *B*) moved the equalization point out to about 7 mm diameter and produced a negative stress (a compressive force) along the posterior layers in the limbal area.

Stress perpendicular to the surface (σ_2). At the center of the cornea for eight incisions (Fig. 29-7, *A*), the amount of stress was much different between the anterior and the posterior layers. The stress became a positive extension stress for the anterior layers and remained a negative compression stress for the posterior layers. The posterior compression stress was two times greater than the stress before surgery. Here we did not find a point within the cornea where the stresses were the same across the thickness of the cornea; rather, this point occurred at the limbus, at the end of the incisions. When the number of incisions was increased to 24 (Fig. 29-7, *B*), even greater stress was supported by the posterior layers.

Circular, or hoop, stress (σ_3). In the center of the cornea for eight incisions, the values for the hoop stress were similar to those of the meridional stress. From the edge of the clear zone at 3 mm diameter, however, a great difference appeared in the stress between the anterior and posterior layers (a positive extension) and the stress along the anterior layers (a negative compression). The difference remained similar along the entire length of the incision, with the stresses coming together in a positive extension force of about 30 kPa near the limbus. An increase in the number of incisions to 24 (Fig. 29-8, *B*) caused the sudden stress change for the inner layers at the the 3-mm zone to disappear and induced a larger difference in stresses across the cornea out to the limbus.

Shear stresses. After eight incisions the three shear stresses were not affected at the center of the cornea. An important increase in these stresses occurred in the area outside the clear zone, particularly at the beginning and the ends of the incisions (Fig. 29-9).

Effect of number of incisions

Simulations were done using different numbers of incisions, keeping the clear zone diameter at 3 mm, the depth at 99%, and the IOP at 15 mm Hg. Figure 29-10 shows a rapid increase in the change of refraction from two to eight incisions and demonstrates that four incisions obtained two thirds of the effect of eight incisions. Using more than eight incisions produced only a small increase in the change in refraction, and with more than 10 incisions almost no change occurred. These results are in complete agreement with clinical observations and earlier calculations.[25-27]

To study the effect of different numbers of incisions further, we calculated the change in power along different meridians from 0° to 90° induced by varying the number of incisions (see Fig. 29-5). For two incisions placed at 0° and 180°, a change of 5.00 D occurred along the horizontal meridian, which dropped to almost no change in the vertical 90° meridian. When two more incisions were added in the vertical 90° and 270° meridians, a change of approximately 5.00 D occurred at both 0° and 90°, with a lesser change at about 45°. When 8, 12, and 24 incisions were placed, the change in curvature and refraction from 0° to 90° remained constant around the circumference of the cornea.

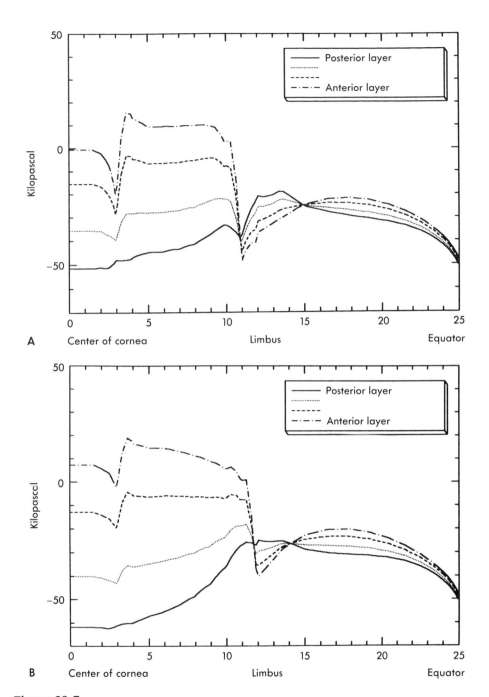

Figure 29-7

Model of distribution of stress perpendicular to the surface (σ_2) after radial 99% deep incisions and 3.0-mm diameter clear zone at an IOP of 15 mm Hg. **A,** With 8 incisions the amount of stress at the center of the cornea is much different between the anterior and the posterior layers. The stress becomes a positive extension stress for the anterior layers and remains a negative compression stress for the posterior layers, which is twice the stress before surgery. There is not a point within the cornea where the stresses are the same across the thickness of the cornea; rather, this point occurs at the limbus, at the end of the incisions. **B,** When the number of incisions is increased to 24, even greater stress is supported by the posterior layers.

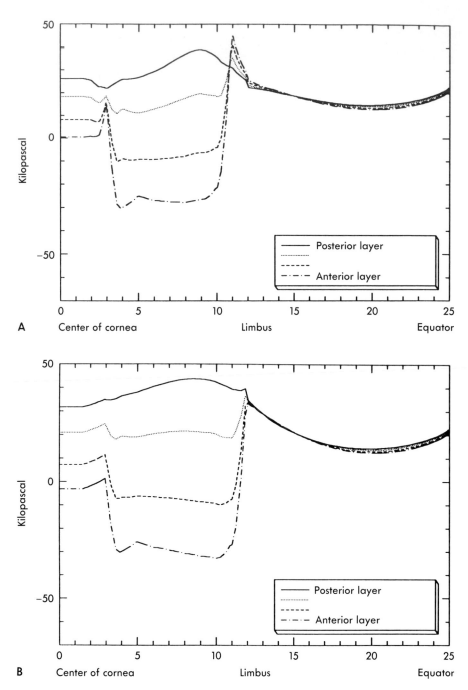

Figure 29-8

Model distribution of circular or hoop stress (σ_3) after radial 99% deep incisions and 3.0-mm diameter clear zone at an IOP of 15 mm Hg. **A,** For 8 incisions, the values for the hoop stress in the center of the cornea are similar to those of the meridional stress, but from the edge of the clear zone at 3 mm diameter, a large difference appears between the anterior and posterior layers, a difference of approximately 60 kPa. The stress along the posterior layers is one of positive extension, and the stress along the anterior layers is one of negative compression. The difference remains similar along the entire length of the incision, the stresses coming together in a positive extension force of about 30 kPa near the limbus. **B,** An increase in the number of incisions to 24 causes the disappearance of the sudden change for the inner layers at the 3-mm zone, and induces a larger difference in stresses across the cornea out to the limbus.

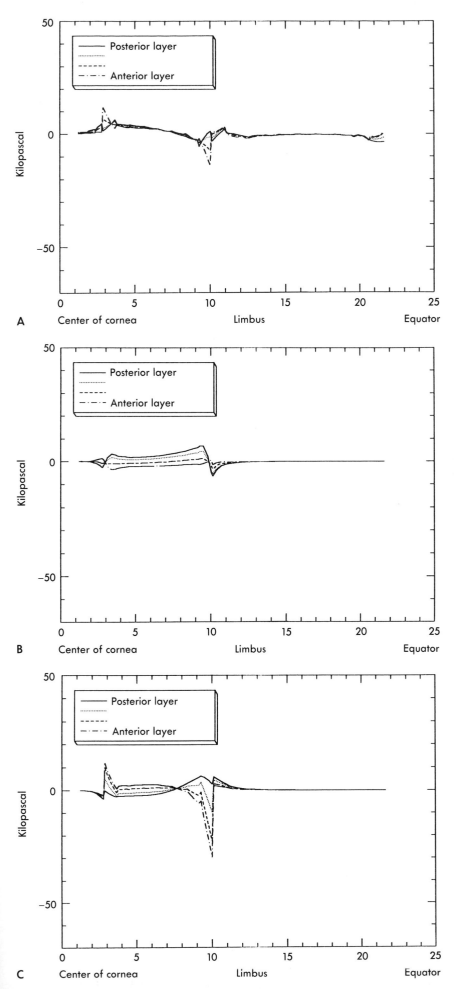

Figure 29-9
After eight incisions, the three shear stresses **(A, B,** and **C)** are not affected at the center of the cornea. There is a slight increase of these stresses in the area outside the clear zone, particularly at the beginning and end of the incisions.

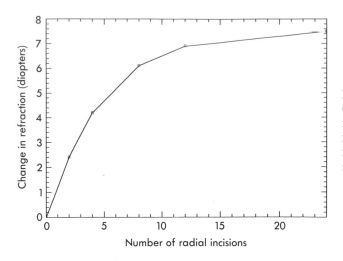

Figure 29-10
Graphic plot of the change in refraction with varying numbers of incisions, using a clear zone diameter of 3 mm, an incision depth of 99%, a length of incision of 4 mm, and an IOP of 15 mm Hg. More than 8 to 10 incisions increases the effect minimally.

Effect of intraocular pressure

As the IOP increased from 10 to 25 mm Hg, there was almost a linear correlation with the change in refraction (Fig. 29-11). A slightly greater change occurred when the IOP rose from 5 to 10 mm Hg than from 10 to 20 or from 20 to 25. Regression analysis showed that:

$$\text{Change in refraction} = 0.34 \times \text{IOP} + 1$$

Effect of length of incisions

The length of the incision was varied by changing the diameter of the clear zone and by changing the location of the peripheral end of the incision. To simulate the effect of the length of the incisions, we studied the effect of clear zones of 3, 4, and 5 mm in diameter and the effect of peripheral zones of 10 and 11 mm in diameter. In general, a change in the length of the incision of 0.5 mm produced a change of 1.00 D of correction. Interestingly, we did not find a significant change for incisions of equal length having different clear zones between 3 and 4 mm. For incisions extending from the clear zones of greater than 4 mm, however, there was always a decreased effect, no matter where the peripheral end in the cornea was located (Table 29-4).

Effect of depth of incisions

We did not study different depths of the incisions because our model had only one element (block) across the thickness of the cornea.

Effect of baseline corneal curvature

We varied the baseline radii of curvature of the cornea by increments of 0.3 mm, from 7.2 to 8.4 mm for the anterior surface and from 6.3 to 7.5 mm for the posterior surface, assuming a constant corneal thickness. We found the radius of curvature had a negligible effect on the amount of refractive change.

When we compared the change in the power of the cornea and the overall change in the refraction, we found that the refractive change was greater than the corneal power change by approximately 26%, with a fairly linear relationship.

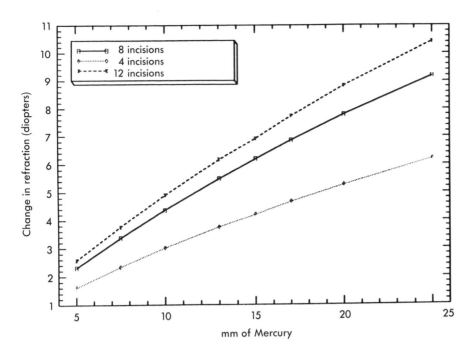

Figure 29-11
Increasing the IOP from 5 to 25 mm Hg produces a linear increase in the effect, more so for 8 and 12 incisions than for four.

Table 29-4			
Effect of Length of Radial Incisions			
Diameter of clear zone (mm)	Diameter of incision endpoint (mm)	Length of incision (mm)	Change in refractive power (D)
3	10	3.5	5.19
	11	4	6.18
4	10	3	4.20
	11	3.5	5.23
5	10	2.5	—
	11	3	3.96

Effect of Young's modulus

When we varied Young's modulus from 1000 to 5000 kPa in eyes with eight incisions, 99% deep, a 3-mm diameter clear zone, and a 15 mm Hg IOP (Fig. 29-12), we found that the lower the elastic modulus, the greater the correction. That is, we found less correction in a stiffer cornea, a finding that is mechanically correct but is at odds with clinical experience.

Multilayered model

To make a simple layered model, we did computations assuming three different moduli of elasticity across the thickness of the cornea. The central layer was kept at the previous value, and the elasticity was increased by 50% for the ante-

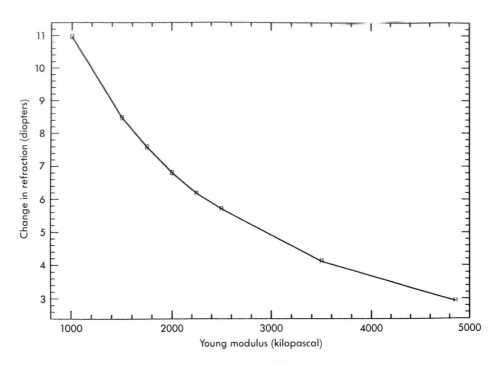

Figure 29-12
When Young's modulus increases from 1000 to 5000 kPa, the refraction change drops from 11.00 to 3.00 D.

rior layer and was decreased by 50% for the posterior layer. Using eight incisions, computations showed a greater change in refraction (4.8 D) with this layered model than with the isotropic model discussed earlier in this chapter.

SUMMARY OF CHANGES IN STRESS DISTRIBUTION

Our computerized mathematical model of the eye demonstrated that radial keratotomy changed the stress distribution in the cornea and in the anterior part of the sclera back to about the 20-mm diameter zone, but it did not affect the equatorial or posterior sclera. We studied only the changes in stress adjacent to the radial incisions.

In general the stress levels were increased at the central clear zone of the cornea by about 300%, with most of this increase taken up by the posterior cornea. The stress was very high in the base of the incisions. As might be expected, large, sudden changes in the stresses occurred at the paracentral and peripheral ends of the incisions, the junctional zone between the intact and cut tissue. The minimal increase in stress resulting when incisions were varied from eight to 24 explained the small amount of refractive change that occurred with more than eight incisions.

The elastic modulus seemed to be an important variable. We had to use a lower than expected value of 2250 kPa to achieve a simulated change in refraction of 6.00 D. We found that corneas with a lower modulus of elasticity underwent more changes.

COMPUTER SIMULATION AND CLINICAL OBSERVATIONS

Our computer simulation correlated well with many, but not all, known clinical observations and previous computer simulations. The number of incisions, up to about eight, increased the change in refraction, but using more than 10 incisions had little additional effect. IOP was an important factor and increased the amount of refractive change linearly, within the physiologic range. This is contrary to the results of regression analysis in clinical and laboratory studies.[21] It has been difficult to isolate the effect of IOP clinically.[28] The preoperative radius of curvature in the central cornea seems to have little effect on the outcome; this fact has been debated previously, with most investigators finding that the central corneal curvature is not an important variable.

The model demonstrated that the length of the incisions was clearly important, as shown clinically by the increased effect of a decrease in the clear zone diameter. However, we demonstrated that two incisions of the same length extending from the 3- to 10-mm diameter zones and from 4- to 11-mm diameter zones had the same effect, raising questions about the isolated role of the clear zone diameter itself. The PERK group found considerable overlap in the amount of effect from three different clear zones.[18]

We were not able to simulate the depth of the incisions because we have only one element across the thickness of the cornea in our model. All clinical and experimental evidence indicates that the deeper incisions produce a change in refraction, and Sato demonstrated clearly that incisions through the posterior cornea produce a greater change than incisions through the anterior cornea. We need more elements in the finite element mesh to simulate this.

Our prediction about the change in corneal power versus the change in the total refractive power, predicting approximately a 0.20 D greater change in refractive power than corneal power, corresponds to clinical observations.[29]

The strength of our model comes from the use of nonlinear mathematics, the inclusion of the entire corneoscleral envelope, and the computation of the three main different stresses. For most variables, our model is in general agreement with other models, except for the effect of the length of incisions, which we find to be an important variable. Improvements in the model are certainly needed to include the anisotropic nature of the cornea, to simulate the viscoelastic response of the tissue, and to include forces on the eye, such as extraocular ones. Such a challenge is formidable and will require collaboration between engineers, clinicians, basic scientists, and mathematicians, as well as enormous amounts of computer power.

UNFINISHED BUSINESS

Biomechanical and Computer Modeling

An accurate computer model of corneal surgery cannot be developed without knowing the material properties of the cornea: Young's modulus, Poisson's coefficient, and the like. Measurement of these properties depends on laboratory experiments using human donor corneas and eyes. Derivation of these properties from strip testing introduces many artifacts, and accurate measurements probably require experiments on whole eyes, using techniques such as video imaging of the surface or holographic imaging of corneal structure.

Although a computational model of the cornea itself would be very useful, simulation of the clinical response to corneal surgery in humans will require a model that involves both the whole eye and the external forces that impinge on the cornea, such as the extraocular muscles and the eyelids. This is a tall order, since our ability to measure such forces is limited; once such measurements are made, extensive computing power will be necessary to integrate them into a model that simulates the function of the living cornea. In addition, measurements of corneal viscoelasticity and wound healing will also be necessary to predict the outcome of surgery in a clinically meaningful way. Presently, no values for these phenomena are available.

In spite of these difficult obstacles, continued refinement of finite element modeling using the information available, with adjustment of variables based on clinical data, such as that achieved in the PERK study, will greatly foster the science of computational modeling of corneal surgery.

An essential ingredient in the success of this approach is establishment of interdisciplinary, well-funded groups of scientists that include corneal surgeons, biomechanical engineers, mathematicians, physicists, and physiologists. Few now exist.

REFERENCES

1. Battaglioli JL and Kamm RD: Measurement of the compressive properties of the scleral tissue, Invest Ophthalmol Vis Sci 1984;25:59-65.

2. Bercovier M, Hanna K, and Jouve F: An analysis of refractive surgery by the finite element method, Comput Mech 1986;4:143-148.

3. Boonet R and Cochet P: New method of topographical ophthalmometry, Am J Optom Physiol Opt 1962;39:227-251.

4. Brubaker RF, Ezekiel S, et al: The stress-strain behavior of the corneoscleral envelope of the eye, Exp Eye Res 1975;21:37-46.

5. Chuong CHJ and Fung YC: Compressibility and constitutive equation of arterial wall in radial compression experiments, J Biomech 1984;17:35-40.

6. Ciarlet PG: Elasticite tridimensionell, Paris, 1986, Masson.

7. Collins R and Van der Werff TJ: Mathematical model of the dynamics of the human eye, New York, 1980, Springer-Verlag New York, Inc.

8. Duke-Elder S and Abrams D: Ophthalmic optics and refraction. In Duke-Elder S, editor: System of ophthalmology, vol V, London, 1970, Kimpton.

9. Eisenlohr JR, Langham ME, and Maumenee ZE: Nanometric studies of the relationship in living and enucleated eyes of individual human subjects, Br J Ophthalmol 1962;46:536.

10. Fung YC: Mechanical properties of living tissues, New York, 1981, Springer-Verlag New York, Inc.

11. Green PR: Mechanical consideration in myopia, Am J Optom Physiol Opt 1980;57:902-914.

12. Hanna K, Jouve F, and Waring GO: Preliminary computer simulation of the effects of radial keratotomy, Arch Ophthalmol 1989;107:911-918.

13. Hofmann RF: The surgical correction of idiopathic astigmatism. In Saunders D et al, editors: Refractive corneal surgery, Thorofare, NJ, 1985, Slack, Inc, pp 250-258.

14. Jue B and Maurice DM: The mechanical properties of the rabbit and human cornea, J Biomech 1986;19:847-853.

15. Kobayashi AS: Mechanics and analysis of tonometry procedures by finite element modeling of the corneoscleral shell. In Ghista DN, editor: Biomechanics of medical devices, New York, 1981, Marcel Dekker, Inc.

16. Kramer SG, Yavitz EQ, and Sulonen J: Precision standardization of radial keratotomy, Ophthalmic Surg 1981;12:561-566.

17. Krueger RR and Trokel SL: Quantification of corneal ablation by UV laser light, Arch Ophthalmol 1985;1741-1742.

18. Lotmar W: Theoretical eye model with aspherics, J Opt Soc Am 1971;61:1522-1529.

19. Lynn MJ, Waring GO, Sperduto RD, and PERK Study Group: Factors affecting outcome and predictability of radial keratotomy, Arch Ophthalmol 1987;105:42-51.

20. MacPhee TJ, Bourne WM, and Brubacker RF: Location of the stress-bearing layers of the cornea, Invest Ophthalmol Vis Sci 1985;26:869-872.

21. Maloney RK: Effect of corneal hydration and intraocular pressure on keratometric power after experimental radial keratotomy, Ophthalmology 1990;97:927-933.

22. Meek KM, Blamires T, Elliott FG, et al: The organization of collagen fibrils in human corneal stroma, Curr Eye Res 1987;6:841-846.

23. Mow CC: A theoretical model of the cornea for use in studies of tonometry, Bull Math Biophysics 1968;30:437.

24. Pouliquen Y, Hanna K, and Saragoussi JJ: The Hanna radial microkeratome: presentation and first experiment, Dev Ophthalmol 1987;14:132-136.

25. Salz JJ, Rowsey JJ, Caroline P, et al: A study of optical zone size and incision redeepening in experimental radial keratotomy, Arch Ophthalmol 1985;103:590-594.

26. Salz J, Villasenor R, Elander R, et al: Four-incision radial keratotomy for low to moderate myopia, Ophthalmology 1986;93:727.

27. Schachar R, Black T, and Huang T: A physicist view of radial keratotomy with practical surgical implications. In Schachar R, Levy N, and Schachar L, editors: Keratorefraction, Denison, Tex, 1980, LAL Publishing, pp 195-200.

28. Southall JPC: Introduction of physiological optics, New York, 1961, Dover.

29. St. Helen R and McEwen WK: Rheology of the human sclera: an elastic behavior, Am J Ophthalmol 1961;52:539.

30. Taber LA: Large deformation mechanics of the enucleated eyeball, ASME J Biomech Eng 1984;16:229.

31. Vito RP, Kirschner S, Frazier J, et al: The elastic and viscoelastic properties of human corneal strips, proceedings of the Thirty-Fourth Annual Conference on Engineering in Medicine and Biology, Houston, Sept 21-23, 1981.

32. Waring GO, Lynn MJ, Culbertson W, et al: Three-year results of the Prospective Evaluation of Radial Keratotomy (PERK) study, Ophthalmology 1987;94:1339-1354.

33. Woo SL et al: Non-linear material properties of intact cornea and sclera, Exp Eye Res 1972;14:29-39.

34. Zienkiewicz OC and Cheung YC: The finite element method. In Structural and continuum mechanics, London, 1967, McGraw-Hill Book Co, p 193.

Keratotomy for Astigmatism

Optics and Topography of Corneal Astigmatism

George O. Waring III
Jack T. Holladay

DEFINITIONS OF ASTIGMATISM

In an eye with astigmatism, the refractive elements do not focus light to a point (Gk: *A* (privitive), without + *stigma,* point). This occurs because the refractive surfaces of the eye cannot form a clear image of an object at any distance. The major cause of astigmatism is usually the cornea, but astigmatism of the lens can occur also.

Corneal astigmatism may be regular or irregular as defined in Fig. 30-1. These designations generally refer to the astigmatism in the central optical zone of the cornea (depends on the pupil): if one considers the topography of the entire cornea, irregular astigmatism is always present because the refractive power changes from the center to the periphery by a few diopters, and the rate of change varies from one semimeridian to another. The box on p. 1061 defines some key terms used in describing astigmatism.

Regular astigmatism

In the astigmatic eye the refractive power is not the same in all meridians. When the astigmatism is regular, the maximal and minimal powers of the eye are 90° apart, or orthogonal. In with-the-rule astigmatism (so called because it occurs most commonly in young people), the refractive power of the eye is

BACKGROUND AND ACKNOWLEDGMENTS

The optics of astigmatism form the basis for surgical correction and are more complex than the optics of simple myopia. Chapter 3, Optics and Topography of Radial Keratotomy, summarizes the basic optical principles of myopia and methods of measuring corneal power. In this chapter we present similar information on astigmatism, without repeating the basic information presented in Chapter 3. Details of the optics of astigmatism are presented in standard textbooks.[6,11,12,19,21] We present here only basic information to help clarify the surgical correction of astigmatism. Robert Maloney, M.D., contributed the section on vector analysis of astigmatism. David Guyton, M.D., provided the information on the history of astigmatism. The other chapters in Section VII, Keratotomy for Astigmatism, present practical application of the information in this chapter. Portions of biomechanical computational models of transverse keratotomy have been used in this chapter. They are described in detail by YK Au and JJ Rowsey in GL Spaeth's text, *Current Therapy in Ophthalmic Surgery,* Philadelphia, 1989, BC Decker, pp. 47-53, by Seiler in Chapter 33, and by Hanna in Chapter 34.

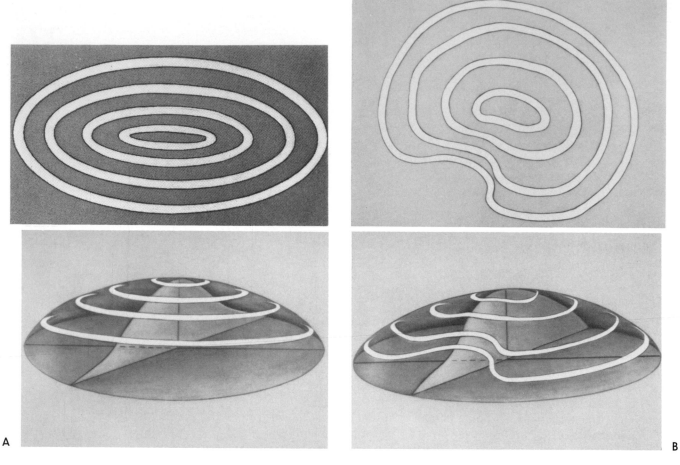

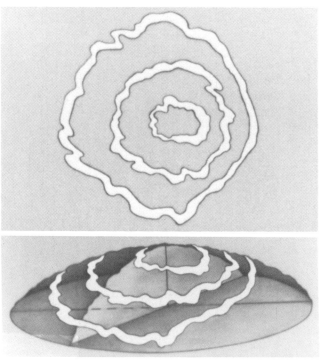

Figure 30-1

Drawings illustrate the topography of different types of corneal astigmatism. **A,** A cornea with regular astigmatism has a smooth surface. There is one steep meridian and one flat meridian, oriented orthogonally to each other. The reflected circular rings take on an oval, elliptical pattern, forming a toric surface. In this illustration the steep meridian is vertical and the flat meridian is horizontal (with-the-rule astigmatism). An example is naturally occurring astigmatism. **B,** A cornea with semimeridional irregular astigmatism has a smooth surface and radial asymmetry. In this example, the 7 o'clock semimeridian is focally steeper than other semimeridians, and the steep semimeridian is not orthogonal to the flat meridian. This circumstance can be caused by a tight suture after penetrating keratoplasty. **C,** A cornea with irregular astigmatism and a rough surface makes it difficult to identify the steep and flat meridians clearly, although this can be done if the mires are not too distorted. This circumstance can be produced by a rough epithelium in disorders such as epithelial basement membrane degeneration or Salzmann's nodular degeneration. (Courtesy R. Doyle Stulting.)

Definition of Terms Regarding Astigmatism

Because the language used in describing astigmatism is sometimes confusing, we include the following glossary of terms with simple definitions.

Refraction: Measurement of the spherocylindrical lens required to correct ametropia in an eye

Keratometry: Measurement of corneal curvature and power in steep and flat orthogonal meridians at points approximately 1.3 to 1.6 mm from the apex of the cornea

Keratoscopy: Clinical observation of the images of mires (usually concentric rings) reflected from the surface of the cornea

Keratography: Photographic or video recording of mires reflected from the corneal surface, also called photokeratography or videokeratography.

Meridian: A curved line on the surface of the cornea that passes through the center of the cornea and extends from two locations on the limbus 180° apart. Meridians are conventionally designated by angular notation using only the superior semimeridian, ranging from 0° to 180°. The steep meridian has the smallest radius of curvature and the greatest refractive power and corresponds to the shortest line that bisects an oval keratographic mire. The flat meridian has the largest radius of curvature and the least refractive power and corresponds to the longest line bisecting an oval keratographic mire.

Semimeridian: One half of a meridian that extends from the center of the cornea to a location on the limbus, usually designated by angular notation from 0° to 360° or by clock-hour notation from 1 o'clock to 12 o'clock (90°). The two semimeridians of a single meridian may have different radii of curvature.

Axis: The direction through a cylindrical lens that produces no refractive power. The axis of a cylindrical lens that corrects astigmatism is oriented along a corneal meridian designated from 0° to 180°. The axis of a plus cylinder is oriented along the steepest corneal meridian. It is incorrect to refer to the "steep axis" of the cornea, since the cornea has no axes, only meridians. Nevertheless, the term "axis of the cornea" is commonly used as shorthand for "the axis of the correcting plus cylinder is located along the steep meridian of the cornea."

Regular astigmatism: The deviation of the ocular refraction or corneal surface from a sphere, as measured by the correcting refractive cylinder or by the difference between the steep and flat keratometric measurements. Regular astigmatism can be corrected by a spherocylindrical lens.

Irregular astigmatism: Any astigmatism that cannot be corrected by a spherocylindrical lens; orientation of the steep and flat meridians at other than 90° to each other; or a diffusely rough corneal surface

Net change in astigmatism: The total astigmatic change between two refractions or two keratometric measurements, regardless of the change in the direction of the axis

Total induced astigmatism (vectorial change in astigmatism): The cylindrical component of the spherocylindrical lens that mimics the change in power of the cornea, as calculated by vector analysis; that is, the combined change of power and axis of the astigmatism

From Harris DJ, Waring GO, and Burk LL: Ophthalmology 1989;96:1597-1607.

greatest in the vertical meridian, where corneal curvature is the steepest, and the power is least in the horizontal meridian, where the corneal curvature is the flattest. In general, a range of 10° on either side of the 90° and 180° meridians is allowed for these designations. Any other astigmatism is considered oblique. In refractive keratotomy it is necessary to designate the exact meridian of the astigmatism, such as "the eye has 2.00 D of regular refractive astigmatism with the steep meridian at 100°." In regular astigmatism the corneal topography is uniformly nonspherical, usually designated as a toric surface, one on which elliptical curves can be described (see Fig. 30-1). The keratometry mires and keratoscopy rings are smooth, and each ring is shaped similarly to the other, allowing easy superimposition of the mires for measurement.

An astigmatic cornea is a spherocylindric lens that forms two focal lines, each parallel to a principal meridian and separated by a distance proportionate to the difference in power between the two meridians for a distant object. The three-dimensional surface formed by the resulting cone of limiting rays is known as the conoid of Sturm and the distance between the two principal focal lines as

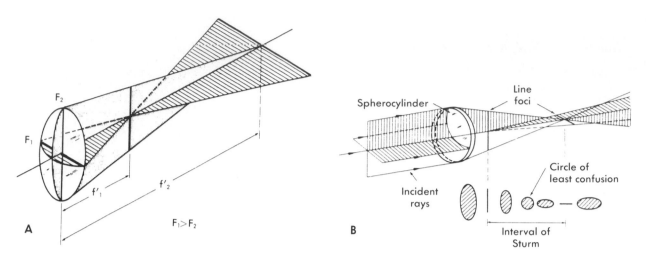

Figure 30-2
Optics of a spherocylindric lens: the conoid of Sturm. A spherocylindric (or toric) surface has one masimum and minimum meridianc called the principal meridians. **A,** The horizontal meridian (F_1) has the greatest curvature; hence the vertical focal line (f'_1) is focused first. **B,** There are two separated focal lines with series ellipsis and a circle that constitute the conoid of Sturm. The interval of Sturm is bounded by the two focal lines. At the dioptric mean is an image that is not elliptic, but round—the circle of least confusion that represents the best overall focal area for a correcting spherocylindric lens. What is seen depends on where the retina intersects it. In these illustrations the cornea has greater power in the horizontal meridian, against-the-rule astigmatism. (From Michaels DD: Visual optics and refraction: a clinical approach, ed 3, St Louis, 1985, The CV Mosby Co, p 48.)

the interval of Sturm (Fig. 30-2). The image on the retina is determined by where the conoid intersects the retina. If the conoid is located in front of the retina, compound myopic astigmatism is present; if the conoid overlaps the retina, mixed astigmatism is present; if the conoid is behind the retina, compound hyperopic astigmatism is present (Fig. 30-3). It is imperative that the refractive surgeon be able to visualize these different types of astigmatism as a basis for planning refractive surgical procedures. Without knowing the preoperative location of each of the focal lines with respect to the retina and without knowing the effect of the surgical techniques on the movement of both focal lines, the surgeon cannot properly plan and predict the refractive outcome.

Regular astigmatism may be corrected by a spherocylindric lens. The axis of the cylindrical component (the direction along which the cylinder has no refractive power) is oriented parallel to the focal line of the eye that is to be moved onto the retina. Thus the cylindrical lens collapses the conoid of Sturm: a plus cylinder lens will move the focal line from behind the retina anteriorly onto the retina, and a minus cylinder lens will move the focal line from in front of the retina posteriorly onto the retina. A rigid contact lens also can correct corneal astigmatism by creating a new spherical anterior optical surface on the eye, essentially masking the corneal astigmatism. Refractive surgery can correct regular astigmatism by making transverse incisions in the cornea perpendicular to the steep meridian, as described in Chapter 32, Atlas of Astigmatic Keratotomy.

Figures 30-4 to 30-6 summarize the basic optical concepts of regular corneal astigmatism and its correction. *Text continued on p. 1070.*

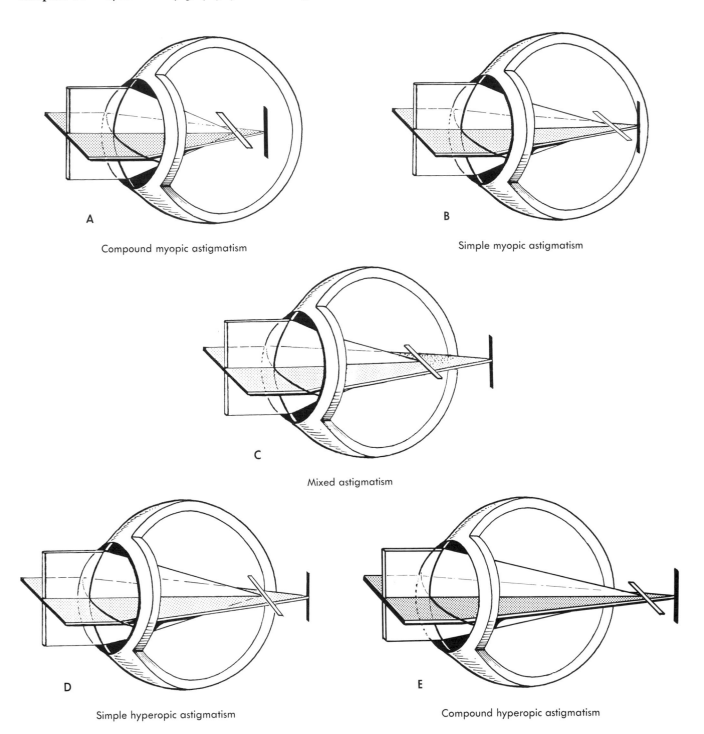

A Compound myopic astigmatism

B Simple myopic astigmatism

C Mixed astigmatism

D Simple hyperopic astigmatism

E Compound hyperopic astigmatism

Figure 30-3
Clinical types of regular astigmatic refractive errors. **A,** Compound myopic astigmatism in which both focal lines are located anterior to the retina. **B,** Simple myopic astigmatism in which only one focal line is located anterior to the retina. **C,** Mixed astigmatism in which one focal line is anterior to the retina, whereas the other is posterior to the retina. **D,** Simple hyperopic astigmatism in which one focal line is located posterior to the retina. **E,** Compound hyperopic astigmatism, in which both focal lines are located posterior to the retina. Clearly a different spherocylindrical lens and a different surgical procedure will be necessary to correct each of these astigmatic refractive errors.

FIGURE 30-4   BASIC CONCEPTS OF CORNEAL ASTIGMATISM

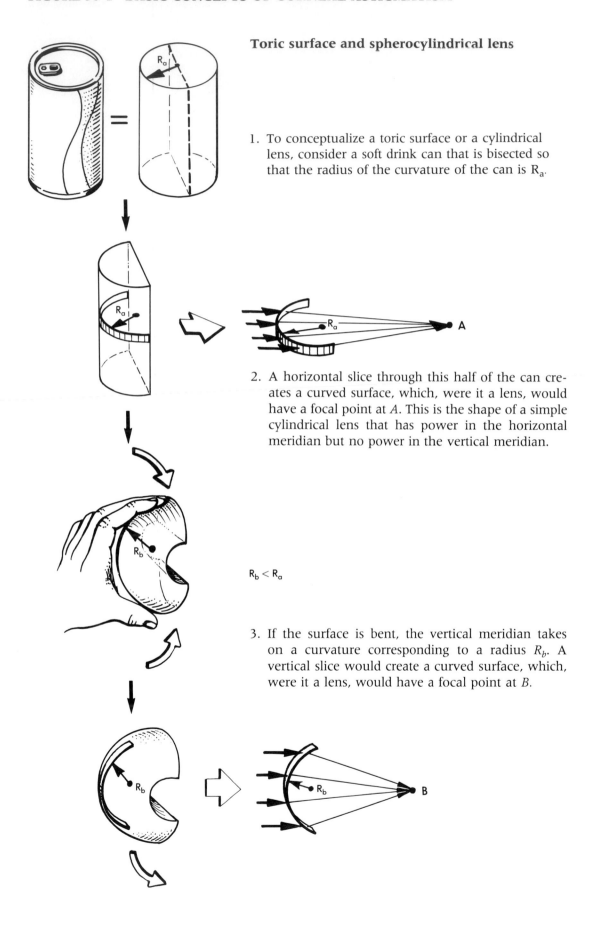

Toric surface and spherocylindrical lens

1. To conceptualize a toric surface or a cylindrical lens, consider a soft drink can that is bisected so that the radius of the curvature of the can is R_a.

2. A horizontal slice through this half of the can creates a curved surface, which, were it a lens, would have a focal point at *A*. This is the shape of a simple cylindrical lens that has power in the horizontal meridian but no power in the vertical meridian.

$R_b < R_a$

3. If the surface is bent, the vertical meridian takes on a curvature corresponding to a radius R_b. A vertical slice would create a curved surface, which, were it a lens, would have a focal point at *B*.

FIGURE 30-4, CONT'D

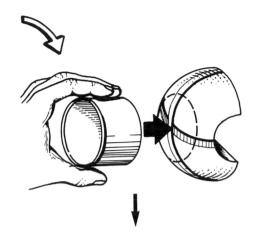

4. Taking a cookie cutter and carving out the center of this bent soft drink can give a toric surface. Considering it as a lens, the vertical meridian has the shorter radius of curvature (R_b) and therefore the greater refractive power (for example, 45 D), and the horizontal surface has the longer radius of curvature (R_a), so it has less refractive power (for example, 42 D).

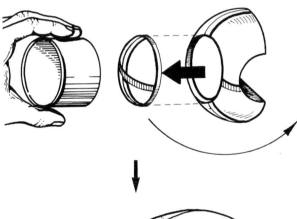

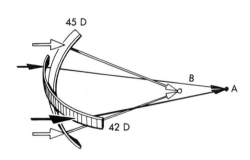

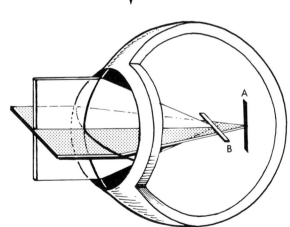

5. Converting this lens to a cornea can create compound myopic astigmatism, in which both focal lines fall in front of the retina. This is with-the-rule astigmatism because the focal line for the vertical meridian *(B)* lies anterior to the focal line for the horizontal meridian *(A)*. The interval between two focal lines is the conoid of Sturm.

Central keratometry

45.00 × 90°
42.00 × 180°

Refraction
Compound Myopic Astigmatism

−5.00 +3.00 × 90°
or
−2.00 −3.00 × 180°

FIGURE 30-5 SPHERICAL AND CYLINDRICAL LENSES AND THE POWER CROSS

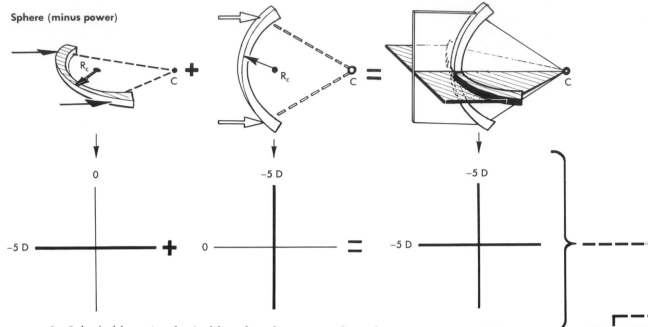

1. *Spherical lens.* A spherical lens has the same radius of curvature (R_c) and the same power in all meridians; it has a single focal point (C). Thus the horizontal and vertical components of the spherical lens are the same, so a power cross would have -5 D of refractive power in both the horizontal and the vertical meridians. We illustrate a minus power spherical lens here.

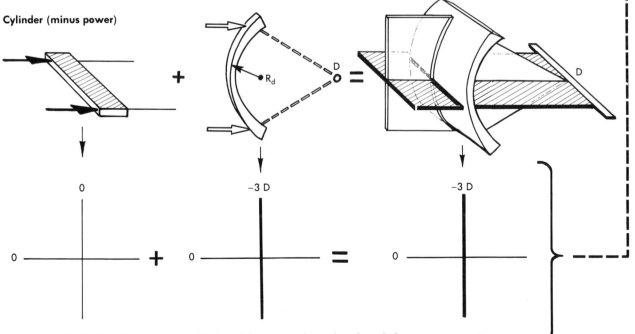

2. *Cylindrical lens.* A cylindrical lens, on the other hand, has no power in one meridian (the horizontal, in this case) and power in the orthogonal meridian (the vertical, in this case). In the vertical meridian the radius of curvature is R_d and the focal point is D. The power cross representing the minus power cylindrical lens has no power in the horizontal meridian and -3 D power in the vertical meridian.

FIGURE 30-5, CONT'D

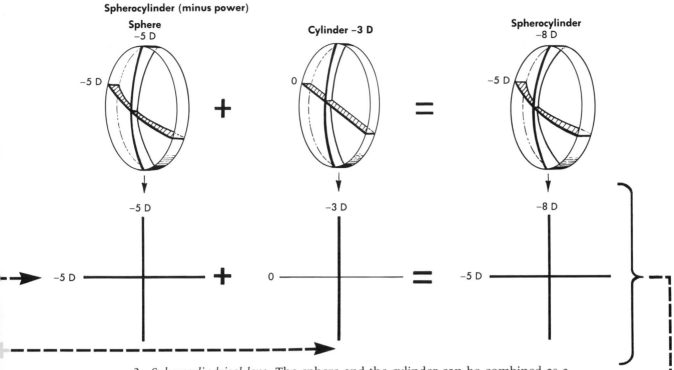

3. *Spherocylindrical lens.* The sphere and the cylinder can be combined as a minus power spherocylindrical lens that can correct the compound myopic astigmatism illustrated in Fig. 30-4. A −5.00 D sphere can be combined with a −3.00 D cylinder to produce a spherocylindrical lens with 8.00 D of minus power in the vertical meridian and 5.00 D of minus power in the horizontal meridian.

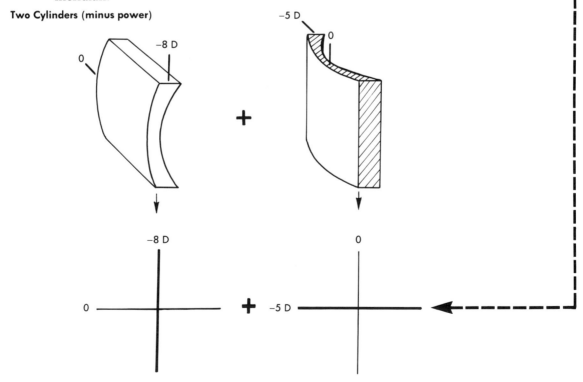

4. This spherocylindrical lens can be resolved into *two minus cylinders,* one with −8.00 D of power vertically and the other with −5.00 D of power horizontally.

FIGURE 30-6 CORRECTION OF COMPOUND MYOPIC ASTIGMATISM

Optical Correction of Compound Myopic Astigmatism

Original Refractive Error

−5.00 +3.00 × 90°
or
−2.00 −3.00 × 180°

Correct Spherical Error

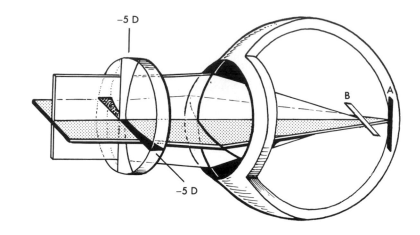

Residual Refractive Error

Plano +3.00 × 90°
or
+3.00 −3.00 × 180°

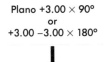

Correct Astigmatic Error

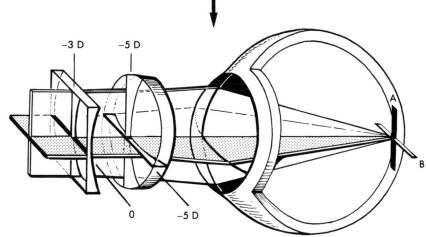

Residual Refractive Error

Plano

Final Correction

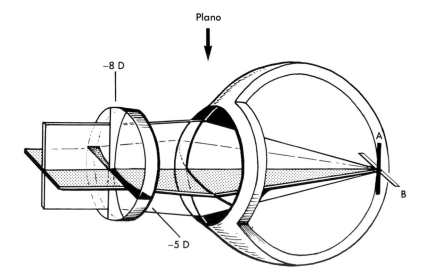

FIGURE 30-6, CONT'D

Surgical Correction of Compound Myopic Astigmatism

−5.00 +3.00 × 90°
or
−2.00 −3.00 × 180°

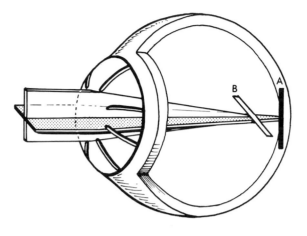

1. There are two ways to correct compound myopic astigmatism: *optical* and *surgical*. In each, the spherical component can be corrected first, followed by correction of the cylindrical (astigmatic) component.

2. *Optical correction* of the spherical error begins by using a −5.00 D sphere, which will place the focal line from the horizontal meridian *(A)* on the retina. This leaves a residual astigmatic refractive error.
   Surgical correction involves performing radial keratotomy to correct the −5.00 D of spherical refractive error.

Plano +3.00 × 90°
or
+3.00 −3.00 × 180°

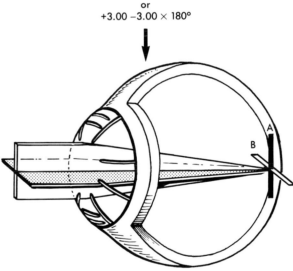

3. *Optical correction* of the astigmatism involves placing a cylindrical lens with −3.00 D of power acting in the vertical meridian and, with its axis in the horizontal meridian, placing the focal line from the vertical meridian *(B)* on the retina by collapsing the conoid of Sturm.
   Surgical correction of the residual astigmatic component requires making transverse incisions perpendicular to the vertical meridian. In surgical practice the transverse incisions are made first.

Plano

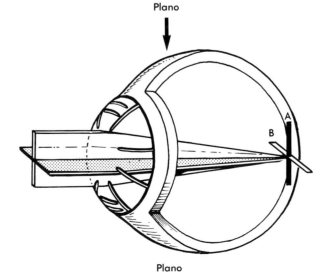

Plano

4. There is no residual refractive error now because the spherocylindrical lens and the corneal surgery have neutralized the refractive error of the eye.

Irregular astigmatism

Irregular astigmatism is any astigmatism that cannot be corrected with spherocylindrical spectacle lenses. Irregular astigmatism induces optical aberrations; some have specific designations, such as "coma" or "curvature of field," and others are simply called "irregular astigmatism." There are three general types of irregular astigmatism: semimeridional, oblique, and diffusely irregular.

Semimeridional irregular astigmatism occurs when the power changes irregularly along both sides of a given meridian, such as in keratoconus. Oblique astigmatism occurs when the steepest and flattest meridians are not perpendicular to each other, as occurs with a tight, compressive suture following cataract surgery or penetrating keratoplasty. Diffusely irregular astigmatism is the catch-all term used to describe anything else and can be caused by corneal scars, epithelial edema, filamentary keratopathy and the like.

Measuring irregular astigmatism is a difficult challenge for which there is currently no practical clinical solution. As emphasized in Chapter 3, Optics and Topography of Radial Keratotomy, keratometry measures an insufficient area of the corneal surface to accurately indicate its overall shape. Videokeratography provides a quantitative measure of the power of the cornea at many individual points, but the overall color-coded dioptric power map is interpreted qualitatively (Fig. 30-7). What is needed is an overall measure of the surface irregularity. One method of measuring surface irregularity was proposed by Dingeldein and colleagues[8] and refined by Wilson and Klyce.[25] Maloney and colleagues[17] have proposed an alternative method that uses mathematical algorithms to fit the measured corneal surface on the videokeratograph with the closest spherocylinder, and then subtracts the curvature of the spherocylinder from that of the actual corneal surface, the difference being the amount of irregular astigmatism Figure 30-8 illustrates this method and emphasizes that the color-coded dioptric power maps of cases of keratoconus cannot readily distinguish cases with less astigmatism and reasonably good spectacle-corrected visual acuity from those with more astigmatism and poor spectacle-corrected visual acuity. Nevertheless, color-coded videokeratography is the best current method of characterizing the overall shape of the cornea.

In the same way that the surgical correction of corneal astigmatism is more difficult than the correction of spherical refractive errors, the surgical correction of irregular astigmatism is more difficult than that of regular astigmatism. Of course, corneas with diffusely irregular surfaces, such as those with central corneal scars or with keratoconus, are not amenable to correction by keratotomy. Even though keratotomy can flatten the steep keratoconic cornea, it cannot do so predictably and irregular astigmatism will persist. Keratotomy is contraindicated in the management of keratoconus. However, there are corneas with reasonably smooth surfaces that have irregular astigmatism in the form of different curvatures along different semimeridians. This occurs commonly after penetrating keratoplasty, especially if there is a focal slippage of the wound. For example, a graft may have a spherical configuration while sutures are in place, but when the sutures are removed a focal anterior displacement of the donor may occur at 6 o'clock. Thus, along the 90° vertical meridian, the upper semimeridian (12 o'clock) would have a steeper curvature and the lower semimeridian (6 o'clock) would have a flatter curvature. This type of irregular astigmatism can be reduced by wound repair or by keratotomy (relaxing incisions), but keratography is necessary to define the location and extent of the irregular astigmatism; central keratometry is inadequate.

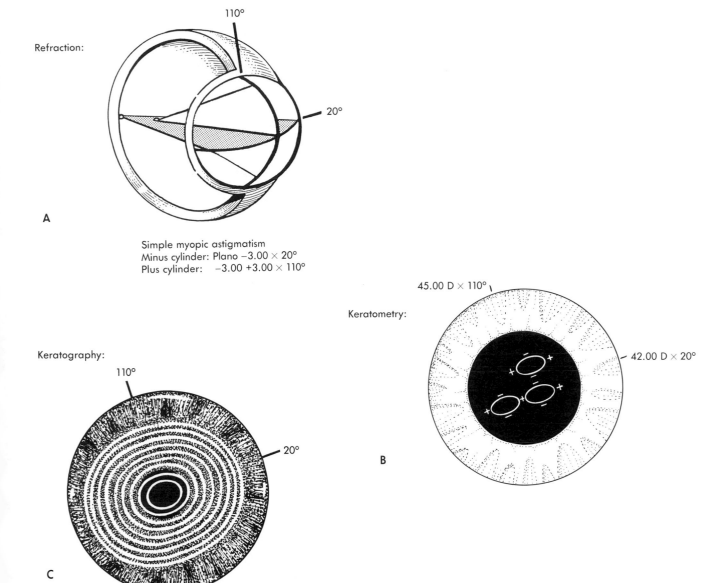

Refraction:

A

Simple myopic astigmatism
Minus cylinder: Plano −3.00 × 20°
Plus cylinder: −3.00 +3.00 × 110°

Keratometry:

45.00 D × 110°

42.00 D × 20°

B

Keratography:

110°

20°

C

Figure 30-7
Clinical methods of measuring corneal astigmatism. **A,** Simple myopic astigmatism is
illustrated with the steep meridian at 110° and the flat meridian at 20°. The refractive error can be written in minus or plus cylinder form. It should be written in minus cylinder form when planning astigmatic surgery. **B,** Keratometry mires show an
oval configuration with the steep meridian measuring 45 D and the flat meridian 42
D. **C,** Keratography mires also have an oval configuration, reflecting this regular corneal astigmatism. Computer programs can quantify the power at locations along
each ring and generate a power map of the corneal shape.

Figure 30-8
Topography of two corneas with keratoconus.

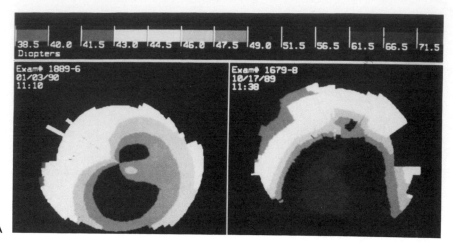

A, Gray scale dioptric maps. The cornea on the left has a distorted horizontal bowtie configuration characteristic of with-the-rule astigmatism; the manifest refraction has 2.5 D of astigmatism at the 60° axis. The cornea on the right has no clear meridian of astigmatism, but manifest refraction reveals 2.5 D of astigmatism at 60°. The best spectacle-corrected visual acuity of the eye on the left is 20/25. The eye on the right is steeper centrally, but has a more uniform central corneal power; however, its best spectacle-corrected visual acuity is only 20/60 (no apical scarring present).

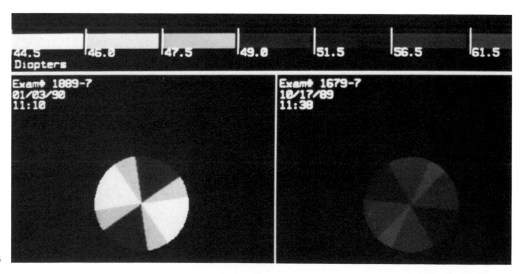

B, The best-fit spherocylinders of the corneas in **A**. The topographic astigmatism of the cornea on the left is +3.4 D × 6° and that of the cornea on the right is +3.6 D × 56°. The correlation with manifest astigmatism is good in both cases. The topographic measure detects astigmatism in the cornea on the right that is not apparent on inspection of the topographic map, but is clearly present by manifest refraction.

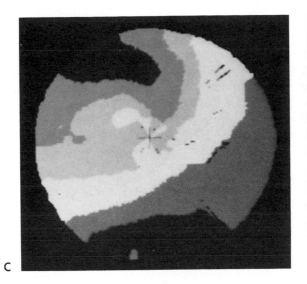
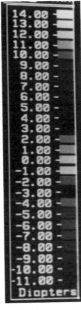
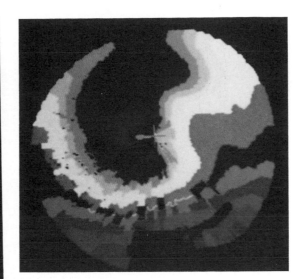

C

Figure 30-8, cont'd
C, Topographic irregularity of the corneas in **A.** Each map is obtained by subtracting, point by point, the color map of the best-fit spherocylinder from the color map of its cornea. These are maps of the local irregularities in each cornea; at each point the color value represents how much the cornea deviates from the best-fit spherocylinder at that point. The cornea on the left has deviations ranging from −3 D to +3 D. The cornea on the right is considerably more irregular, with deviations from −7 D to + 7 D. The topographic irregularity of the left and right corneas are 1.7 and 3.3 D, respectively, corresponding well to the visual acuities. (Courtesy Robert Maloney.)

HISTORY OF ASTIGMATISM

Historically the recognition of astigmatism grew out of the astute observations of scientists schooled in optics who had astigmatism themselves. They performed optical experiments on their own eyes to define the astigmatism and to devise optical corrections for it. This saga is detailed by Levine[16] and summarized by Bennett.[2]

Although Sir Isaac Newton was aware that light rays in different planes may be focused at different distances, it was Thomas Young who, while studying the mechanism of accommodation of the lens in 1800, described clinical astigmatism by refracting one of his own eyes, finding it to be about −4.00 D myopic in the vertical meridian and −5.75 D in the horizontal. Young further discovered that the same amount of astigmatism remained when his cornea was immersed in water, concluding that an obliquity of the crystalline lens caused the astigmatism. Young's observation is a good example of serendipitous discovery. A quarter of a century later, Sir George Biddell Airy measured the refraction of his own astigmatic eye and had a spherocylindrical lens especially made to correct it. He documented the changes in his own astigmatism for over 50 years and stimulated his colleagues at Cambridge University to develop an interest in the subject; thereafter, the Rev. Dr. Whewell coined the term "astigmatism" in approximately 1850, and Henry Goode devised a planocylindrical spectacle lens to correct not only his own astigmatism but also that of other gentlemen at Cambridge. Others interested in the subject deduced that the cornea was a probable cause for ocular astigmatism. The first thorough discussion of the subject was presented by Cornelius Donders[9] in 1864 in his book on optics. In the early twentieth century, Maurice Hans Eric Tscherning[24] described astigmatism and its correction. He also discussed in detail irregular astigmatism and emphasized "that there are in nearly all eyes optic differences between the different parts of the pupillary space," an observation that anticipated the current interest in the multifocal effects induced by refractive corneal surgery. Using a point source of light, Tscherning described his own astigmatic error very carefully in terms of the distorted images that he saw, illustrating not only the astigmatic aberration but also the spherical aberration. His drawings resemble those made by patients who see distorted images after refractive keratotomy.

CAUSES OF CORNEAL ASTIGMATISM

Corneal astigmatism has multiple causes (see the box below). The most common cause of regular astigmatism is naturally occurring, unassociated with corneal abnormalities.[3-5] This is sometimes called "congenital" astigmatism, a misnomer because it is not always present at birth and usually develops in the first years of life.

The cause of naturally occurring astigmatism is unknown. Investigators in the Finnish Twin Cohort Study[22] found no difference in the astigmatism between monozygotic and dizygotic twins, suggesting that genetic factors do not contribute to astigmatism and that environmental causes are the major influence. It is well known that higher amounts of astigmatism are associated with higher

---

Some Causes of Corneal Astigmatism with Selected Clinical Examples

I. Regular astigmatism

  A. Naturally occurring
    1. Acquired
    2. Inherited
  B. Postoperative—surgical procedure
    1. Circular corneal wound
      a. Penetrating keratoplasty
      b. Keratomileusis
      c. Epikeratoplasty
      d. Lamellar keratoplasty
      e. Intracorneal lens
    2. Linear corneal wound
      a. Cataract surgery
      b. Radial and transverse keratotomy
      c. Accidental corneal laceration
    3. No corneal wound: scleral buckle
  C. Postoperative—mechanisms
    1. Tight suture, tissue resection
      a. Tissue compression or removal
      b. Steeper meridian created
    2. Loose suture, wound separation, keratotomy
      a. Wound gape
      b. Flatter meridian created
    3. Asymmetric tissue distribution, wound volume, or healing from cataract or corneal surgery

II. Irregular astigmatism

  A. Irregular corneal surface
    1. Corneal edema
    2. Keratoconjunctivitis sicca
    3. Subepithelial scarring
  B. Central or paracentral corneal thinning
    1. Keratoconus
    2. Pellucid degeneration
  C. Marginal corneal thinning
    1. Terrien's degeneration
    2. Rheumatic keratopathy
    3. Mooren's ulcer
  D. Accidental corneal trauma
    1. Lacerations
    2. Chemical burns
  E. External pressure on cornea
    1. Contact lens warpage
    2. Eyelid mass
    3. Eye rubbing

III. Combined regular and irregular astigmatism

spherical ametropias. Fulton and colleagues[10] demonstrated a possible reason for this by observing that children with larger amounts of astigmatism in the early years of life developed higher amounts of increasing myopia, presumably because the uncorrected astigmatism during a period of visual immaturity blurred the retinal image and triggered the development of myopia, as occurs in occlusion experiments in animals (see Chapter 1, Myopia: A Brief Overview).

On the average, there is a small, gradual change in the predominant type of astigmatism with increasing age, from with-the-rule astigmatism in younger persons to against-the-rule astigmatism in older persons, fostering the speculation that the continual blinking of the eyelids may gradually flatten the vertical meridian of the cornea.

Astigmatism is a common finding in many corneal diseases, particularly those in which the cornea thins, such as in keratoconus, Terrien's marginal degeneration, and rheumatic keratopathy. Surgically induced corneal astigmatism may occur after any operation that affects the shape of the cornea, including cataract extraction, penetrating keratoplasty, pterygium excision, and scleral buckling. Severe irregular astigmatism may result from corneal trauma. Mild irregular astigmatism appears in ocular surface disorders such as corneal epithelial basement membrane degeneration and epithelial edema. Both regular and irregular astigmatism may occur after years of hard or soft contact lens wear.

Corneal astigmatism usually arises from the anterior surface of the cornea, since it is 10 times more optically powerful than the posterior surface. However, disorders such as posterior keratoconus can produce refractive astigmatism that would not be detected by keratometry or keratoscopy. The same is true for lenticular astigmatism.

PREVALENCE OF ASTIGMATISM

Table 30-1 summarizes some of the published studies of the prevalence of astigmatism in Western populations. The findings lead to three generalities:
1. There is considerable variability among different populations. For example, in Scandanavia less than 10% of eyes have astigmatism over 1.00 D, whereas in the United States approximately one third of eyes have astigmatism in that range.
2. If a cutoff of approximately 2.00 D is used as an indication for astigmatism surgery, then approximately 10% of the adult Western population might qualify.
3. Keratometric and refractive astigmatism may differ considerably in the same population.

MEASUREMENT OF ASTIGMATISM

Astigmatism is a vector quantity because it has both power and direction. Although it is common to state colloquially that an eye has "3.00 D of refractive astigmatism" or that a corneal transplant has "7.00 D of keratometric astigmatism," accurate communication requires more information such as designation of the steep or flat meridians or a description of the type of irregular astigmatism. Thus, after a penetrating keratoplasty, an accurate description of the astigmatism might be: "The transplant demonstrates 5.00 D of irregular astigmatism with the steep meridian at 120°, and the 11 o'clock semimeridian being much steeper than the 5 o'clock semimeridian."

There are three clinical methods used to measure astigmatism—refraction, keratometry, and keratography (see Fig. 30-7). In most cases the three measurements show general agreement but may differ quantitatively. Each method measures a different aspect of astigmatism and therefore can be expected to function differently in planning surgery for astigmatism. Surgeons use all three sources of information, appreciating the strengths and weaknesses of each.

Table 30-1

Amount of Naturally Occurring Astigmatism in Published Studies

	Buzard[*]	Shepherd[†]	Davison[‡]	Maloney[§]	Teikari[‖]
Year	1988	1989	1989	1989	1989
Method	Refraction	Keratometry	Keratometry	Keratometry	Refraction
Population	U.S.	U.S.	U.S.	U.S.	Finnish
Age range (yr)	40 to 100	Not reported	36 to 81	Not reported	30 to 31
Astigmatism (D)[¶]					
0	27.5	—	—	—	—
< 1.00	60.5	68	(≤ 1.50) 85	44	80.9
> 1.00	39.5	32	(≥ 1.50) 15	56	19.1
> 2.00	6.6	10	(1.67 to 3) 12	(1 to 2.50) 47	5.2
> 3.00	2.1	4	3	(≥ 2.50) 9	1.8
Number of eyes	756	458	40	4000 (approx)	228

[*]Buzard K, Shearing S, and Relyea R: Incidence of astigmatism in a cataract practice, Refract Surg 1988;4:173-178.
[†]Shepherd JR: Induced astigmatism in small incision cataract surgery, J Cataract Refract Surg 1989;15:85-88.
[‡]Davison JA: Transverse astigmatic keratotomy combined with phacoemulsification and intraocular lens implantation, J Cataract Refract Surg 1989;15:38-44.
[§]Maloney WF, Grindle L, Sanders D, and Pearcy D: Astigmatism control for the cataract surgeon: comprehensive review of surgically tailored astigmatism reduction (STAR), J Cataract Refract Surg 1989;15:45-54.
[‖]Teikari JM, and O'Donnell JJ: Astigmatism in 72 twin pairs, Cornea 1989;8:263-266.
[¶]Approximate percentage of eyes.

Astigmatism measurements as a guide to surgery

Refraction. The refraction measures the total amount of astigmatism in the pupillary zone of the optical system of the eye, as would be corrected by a spectacle lens. Therefore, if keratotomy surgery is to correct the astigmatism to the extent that spectacle lenses do, the refraction should be the basis for calculating astigmatism surgery.

Keratometry. Keratometry measures the radius of curvature between two points approximately 3 mm apart, assuming that the cornea is spherical. This works well for normal corneas, but for corneas that are aspheric or have irregular astigmatism (especially centrally), keratometry will not accurately represent the amount or direction of the astigmatism. Some surgeons reason that because they are operating on the cornea to correct astigmatism, it is the keratometric astigmatism, not the refractive astigmatism, that should be used as a basis for calculating their surgery. Given the inaccuracies of keratometry on an aspheric cornea and the desire to correct all of the patient's astigmatism, we think refraction is the optimal guide.

Keratography. A keratograph can depict the shape of the corneal surface qualitatively or quantitatively and theoretically would be the best basis for planning astigmatism surgery, because it can measure the entire surface subjected to surgery, with its various asymmetries. Currently there is little published information about how to use topography as a guide to astigmatism surgery, but as surgeons gain experience and publish their results, topographic analysis should become more useful. For example, after penetrating keratoplasty keratography can identify the extent of the steepest semimeridians, where the surgeon may place the longest or deepest arcuate relaxing incisions.

Corneal biomechanics. Currently there is no practical clinical way to measure the stress relationships within the cornea. This would be the most accurate basis for planning surgery because it is probably the stress within the cornea that keratotomy alters, with secondary changes in the surface curvature. For example, if holographic techniques were available to make a "stress map" that delineated the areas of greater and lesser stress within the cornea, then we might have a more accurate guide for locating and quantifying keratotomy surgery. Some surgeons presently use intraoperative keratometry and keratography to guide them in performing gradually graded incisions, the length and depth of which are increased until the oval mires are made round and then made slightly oval in the opposite direction. The theoretic basis for such an approach is that the stress patterns in corneas with similar keratometric or keratographic measurements may be quite different and require different amounts of surgery for correction.

Measurement of change in astigmatism

There are four ways to indicate the effect of surgery on astigmatism, whether it be measured by refraction, keratometry or keratography.

Net residual astigmatism. The final amount of refractive or keratometric astigmatism regardless of the axis is a commonly reported outcome of surgery. In a series of cases, the results can be reported as the number (percentage) of eyes with specific amounts of residual astigmatism in diopters (0 to 0.50; 0.62 to 1.00; 1.75 to 2.00; 2.25 to 3.00; 3.25 to 5.00; 5.25 to 10.00; 10.25 to 15.00; 15.25 and greater). Alternately the residual astigmatism can be reported as the mean, standard deviation, and range. Thus a study of residual astigmatism in a series of 100 penetrating keratoplasties might report (1) a mean refractive astigmatism 1 year after surgery of 3.25 ±1.50 D (range, 0 to 14 D), and (2) a distribution of astigmatism as 0 to 0.50 D in 2%, 0.75 to 1.00 D in 4%, 1.12 to 2.00 D in 10%, 2.12 to 3.00 D in 12%, 3.12 to 4.00 D in 22%, 4.12 to 5.00 D in 37%, 5.12 to 7.00 D in 10%, and 7.12 to 12.00 D in 3%.

The net residual astigmatism is a useful measure of clinical outcome, particularly in circumstances where preoperative astigmatism cannot be accurately measured, as is often the case with eyes requiring penetrating keratoplasty. Net residual astigmatism is probably the most important measurement in terms of optical function and patient satisfaction.

Net change in astigmatism. Net change in astigmatism is the total change of astigmatic power between two refractions or two keratometric measurements, regardless of the change in astigmatic axis. For example, a series of eyes with naturally occurring astigmatism might have a mean preoperative refractive astigmatism of 4.60 D ±1.25 D (range, 2.00 to 6.50 D) and a mean postoperative astigmatism of 1.25 D ±0.75 D (range, 0.25 to 4.50 D). This presents practical clinical information and allows an overall comparison of two different surgical techniques, but it does not take into account the surgical effectiveness of the techniques, because it ignores the change in axis.

Change in axis of astigmatism. Reporting the preoperative and postoperative axes of the correcting cylinder or steep keratometric meridian indicates how accurately a procedure corrects astigmatism in the desired meridian. For example, a surgical technique that produces a mean change in axis of the cylinder of 10° is preferable to one in which the mean change in axis is 30°.

Vectoral astigmatism. The most thorough way to describe the change in astigmatism induced by surgery is vectoral analysis, which indicates the change in both the power and the axis of the astigmatism. Serious study of astigmatic surgery must include vectoral analysis in the results.

Consider a hypothetic eye that preoperatively required +4.00 D of refractive cylinder correction at 90° and postoperatively required +1.00 D of cylinder correction at 180°. The net change in astigmatism was a 3.00 D reduction. However, the total change in astigmatism induced by the procedure was +5 D at 180°. This observation is fairly intuitive because +4 D at 180° were required to

---

Equations to Calculate Vectoral Change in Astigmatism

Preoperative plus cylinder D_1 diopters at axis A_1
Postoperative plus cylinder D_2 diopters at axis A_2

$$\text{Let } X = D_2 \cos 2A_2 - D_1 \cos 2A_1$$
$$Y = D_2 \sin 2A_2 - D_1 \sin 2A_1$$

The vector difference is: Magnitude $= \sqrt{x^2 + y^2}$

$$\text{If } X > 0 \text{ then axis} = \tfrac{1}{2} \tan^{-1} \frac{Y}{X}$$

$$\text{If } X < 0 \text{ then axis} = \tfrac{1}{2} \left(\tan^{-1} \frac{Y}{X} + 180 \right)$$

---

correct the preoperative astigmatism and an additional 1.00 D at 180° was required to neutralize the residual postoperative astigmatism. However, it is rare for the preoperative and postoperative astigmatic axes to be exactly 90° apart, and therefore this simple intuitive method of calculation does not usually work.

The accurate way to calculate the total change in astigmatism is to calculate the vectoral change. In this method, the preoperative and postoperative astigmatism are each represented by a vector. By subtracting the preoperative vector from the postoperative vector, the resultant vector represents the change in astigmatism induced by the procedure. Astigmatism is converted to a vector quantity by making a vector whose length is equal to the magnitude of the astigmatism in diopters and whose axis lies at twice the "steep axis" of the astigmatism. After subtraction of the preoperative vector from the postoperative vector, the resultant astigmatism has a magnitude equal to the length of the vector and an axis equal to half of the axis of the vector. For example, if the preoperative astigmatism is 1.00 D at 90°, then a vector is created 1.00 D in length at an angle of twice 90°, or 180°. If the postoperative astigmatism is 1.00 D at 45°, then the vector is created 1.00 D in length, oriented at 90°. The difference between these vectors can be calculated by either drawing the vectors or algebraically combining the coordinates of the endpoints, expressed in rectangular coordinates. The difference in this example is a vector 1.4 D in length oriented at 45°. Therefore the change in astigmatism induced by the procedure is 1.4 D of astigmatism at 22.5°.

In practice, calculating the change in astigmatism by vector subtraction is mathematically cumbersome because it requires an understanding of both trigonometry and vector algebra, as presented in the box above. The vector change in astigmatism can be calculated simply in the clinic by the following practical method. Express the preoperative and postoperative astigmatism in plus cylinder form. Place a plus cylinder trial lens with power equal to the postoperative cylinder in a lensometer and orient it in the postoperative axis. Place a minus cylinder trial lens with power equal to the preoperative astigmatism in the lensometer on top of the plus cylinder trial lens and orient it in the preoperative axis. Read this combination of lenses with the lensometer and record the magnitude and axis of this combination, which represents the vector difference between the preoperative and postoperative astigmatism; it is the change in astigmatism induced by the procedure.[15]

To illustrate the different methods of reporting the results of astigmatic surgery, we present the following fictitious case history.

A 28-year-old woman had naturally occurring astigmatism with a refraction of $+1.00 -3.00 \times 180°$ bilaterally. Her surgeon performed the "slicem" astigmatic keratotomy technique in the right eye and the "dicem" technique in the left, both operations being carried out in the 90° meridian. The refractive result in the right eye was plano $-1.00 \times 90°$ and the left was plano $-1.00 \times 30°$. The net residual corneal astigmatism was 1.00 D in each eye. The "slicem" technique did not alter the axis of astigmatism, which remained steep at 90°, but the "dicem" technique rotated the axis 60°. Vector analysis showed the total induced astigmatism by the "slicem" technique was 2.00 D and with "dicem" technique was 2.60 D.

Another simple way to determine the vectoral change in astigmatism after surgery is to use the table compiled by Hall and colleagues (Fig. 30-9).

The basic principles of vector analysis have been elaborated by Naylor[19a] and have been used in the study of astigmatic surgery by Neumann,[20] Merck,[18] Thornton and Sanders,[23] Agapitos,[1] and Jaffee and Clayman.[15]

CORRECTION OF ASTIGMATISM

Both optical and surgical methods can correct myopic astigmatism by correcting the spherical component and collapsing the conoid of Sturm to correct the astigmatic component. The differences between the optical and surgical techniques are emphasized in Fig. 30-10.

Details of the surgical correction of astigmatism are presented in Chapter 31, Keratotomy for Astigmatism.

In planning the correction of myopic astigmatism, the surgeon should aim for an undercorrection. Undercorrecting the sphere to leave the patient slightly myopic will keep the patient in the familiar visual territory of myopia, will delay the onset of symptomatic presbyopia, and will offset some of the continued increase in effect of radial keratotomy. Undercorrecting the cylinder to leave the patient with slight simple or compound myopic astigmatism will give presbyopic patients "pseudoaccommodation" of the type described in eyes with monofocal intraocular lenses. Huber[13,14] and Datiles and Gancayco[7] have observed that a low amount of compound myopic astigmatism, on the order of -2.00 D sphere and $+1.50$ D cylinder, is compatible with good distance visual acuity (20/40 or better) and good near visual acuity (Jaeger 3 or better). Datiles and Gancayco[7] theorize that this is based on the optics of the conoid of Sturm in which there are two distances at which an object is in focus along one meridian. The first distance corresponds to the first astigmatic meridian focal line and the second corresponds to the second astigmatic meridian focal line. Thus there is both a far point and a near point where things are relatively in focus, although there is a slight reduction in the visual acuity at each. If the pupil is between 1 and 2 mm in diameter, a pinhole effect with mild diffraction degradation occurs, further increasing the functional acuity. Whether the phakic presbyopic eye behaves like the pseudophakic eye in this regard requires further clinical study. Details of the optical correction of astigmatism are presented in standard textbooks.[2,18,19,21]

K_1	K_2	5	10	15	20	25	30	35	40	45	50	55	60	65	70	75	80	85
0.25	0.25	0.0	0.1	0.1	0.2	0.2	0.3	0.3	0.3	0.4	0.4	0.4	0.4	0.5	0.5	0.5	0.5	0.5
	0.50	0.3	0.3	0.3	0.3	0.4	0.4	0.5	0.5	0.6	0.6	0.6	0.7	0.7	0.7	0.7	0.7	0.7
	0.75	0.5	0.5	0.5	0.6	0.6	0.7	0.7	0.7	0.8	0.8	0.9	0.9	0.9	1.0	1.0	1.0	1.0
	1.00	0.8	0.8	0.8	0.8	0.9	0.9	0.9	1.0	1.0	1.1	1.1	1.1	1.2	1.2	1.2	1.2	1.2
	1.25	1.0	1.0	1.0	1.1	1.1	1.1	1.2	1.2	1.3	1.3	1.4	1.4	1.4	1.5	1.5	1.5	1.5
	1.50	1.3	1.3	1.3	1.3	1.4	1.4	1.4	1.5	1.5	1.6	1.6	1.6	1.7	1.7	1.7	1.7	1.7
	1.75	1.5	1.5	1.5	1.6	1.6	1.6	1.7	1.7	1.8	1.8	1.9	1.9	1.9	1.9	2.0	2.0	2.0
	2.00	1.8	1.8	1.8	1.8	1.8	1.9	1.9	2.0	2.0	2.1	2.1	2.1	2.2	2.2	2.2	2.2	2.2
	2.25	2.0	2.0	2.0	2.1	2.1	2.1	2.2	2.2	2.3	2.3	2.3	2.4	2.4	2.4	2.5	2.5	2.5
	2.50	2.3	2.3	2.3	2.3	2.3	2.4	2.4	2.5	2.5	2.6	2.6	2.6	2.7	2.7	2.7	2.7	2.7
	2.75	2.5	2.5	2.5	2.6	2.6	2.6	2.7	2.7	2.8	2.8	2.8	2.9	3.0	3.0	3.0	3.0	3.0
	3.00	2.8	2.8	2.8	2.8	2.8	2.9	2.9	3.0	3.0	3.1	3.1	3.1	3.2	3.2	3.2	3.2	3.2
	3.25	3.0	3.0	3.0	3.1	3.1	3.1	3.2	3.2	3.3	3.3	3.3	3.4	3.4	3.4	3.5	3.5	3.5
	3.50	3.3	3.3	3.3	3.3	3.3	3.4	3.4	3.5	3.5	3.6	3.6	3.6	3.7	3.7	3.7	3.7	3.7
	3.75	3.5	3.5	3.5	3.6	3.6	3.6	3.7	3.7	3.8	3.8	3.8	3.9	3.9	3.9	4.0	4.0	4.0
	4.00	3.8	3.8	3.8	3.8	3.8	3.9	3.9	4.0	4.0	4.1	4.1	4.1	4.2	4.2	4.2	4.2	4.2
	4.25	4.0	4.0	4.0	4.1	4.1	4.1	4.2	4.2	4.3	4.3	4.3	4.4	4.4	4.4	4.5	4.5	4.5
	4.50	4.3	4.3	4.3	4.3	4.3	4.4	4.4	4.5	4.5	4.6	4.6	4.6	4.7	4.7	4.7	4.7	4.7
	4.75	4.5	4.5	4.5	4.6	4.6	4.6	4.7	4.7	4.8	4.8	4.8	4.9	4.9	4.9	5.0	5.0	5.0
	5.00	4.8	4.8	4.8	4.8	4.8	4.9	4.9	5.0	5.0	5.0	5.1	5.1	5.2	5.2	5.2	5.2	5.2
	5.25	5.0	5.0	5.0	5.1	5.1	5.1	5.2	5.2	5.3	5.3	5.3	5.4	5.4	5.4	5.5	5.5	5.5
	5.50	5.3	5.3	5.3	5.3	5.3	5.4	5.4	5.5	5.5	5.5	5.6	5.6	5.7	5.7	5.7	5.7	5.7
	5.75	5.5	5.5	5.5	5.6	5.6	5.6	5.7	5.7	5.8	5.8	5.8	5.9	5.9	5.9	6.0	6.0	6.0
	6.00	5.8	5.8	5.8	5.8	5.8	5.9	5.9	6.0	6.0	6.0	6.1	6.1	6.2	6.2	6.2	6.2	6.2
	6.25	6.0	6.0	6.0	6.1	6.1	6.1	6.2	6.2	6.3	6.3	6.3	6.4	6.4	6.4	6.5	6.5	6.5
	6.50	6.3	6.3	6.3	6.3	6.3	6.4	6.4	6.5	6.5	6.5	6.6	6.6	6.7	6.7	6.7	6.7	6.7
	6.75	6.5	6.5	6.5	6.6	6.6	6.6	6.7	6.7	6.8	6.8	6.8	6.9	6.9	6.9	7.0	7.0	7.0
	7.00	6.8	6.8	6.8	6.8	6.8	6.9	6.9	7.0	7.0	7.0	7.1	7.1	7.2	7.2	7.2	7.2	7.2
	7.25	7.0	7.0	7.0	7.1	7.1	7.1	7.2	7.2	7.3	7.3	7.3	7.4	7.4	7.4	7.5	7.5	7.5
	7.50	7.3	7.3	7.3	7.3	7.3	7.4	7.4	7.5	7.5	7.5	7.6	7.6	7.7	7.7	7.7	7.7	7.7
	7.75	7.5	7.5	7.5	7.6	7.6	7.6	7.7	7.7	7.8	7.8	7.8	7.9	7.9	7.9	8.0	8.0	8.0
	8.00	7.8	7.8	7.8	7.8	7.8	7.9	7.9	8.0	8.0	8.0	8.1	8.1	8.2	8.2	8.2	8.2	8.2
	8.25	8.0	8.0	8.0	8.1	8.1	8.1	8.2	8.2	8.3	8.3	8.3	8.4	8.4	8.4	8.5	8.5	8.5
	8.50	8.3	8.3	8.3	8.3	8.3	8.4	8.4	8.5	8.5	8.5	8.6	8.6	8.7	8.7	8.7	8.7	8.7
	8.75	8.5	8.5	8.5	8.6	8.6	8.6	8.7	8.7	8.8	8.8	8.8	8.9	8.9	8.9	9.0	9.0	9.0
	9.00	8.8	8.8	8.8	8.8	8.8	8.9	8.9	9.0	9.0	9.0	9.1	9.1	9.2	9.2	9.2	9.2	9.2
	9.25	9.0	9.0	9.0	9.1	9.1	9.1	9.2	9.2	9.3	9.3	9.3	9.4	9.4	9.4	9.5	9.5	9.5
	9.50	9.3	9.3	9.3	9.3	9.3	9.4	9.4	9.5	9.5	9.5	9.6	9.6	9.7	9.7	9.7	9.7	9.7
	9.75	9.5	9.5	9.5	9.6	9.6	9.6	9.7	9.7	9.8	9.8	9.8	9.9	9.9	9.9	10.0	10.0	10.0
	10.00	9.8	9.8	9.8	9.8	9.8	9.9	9.9	10.0	10.0	10.0	10.1	10.1	10.2	10.2	10.2	10.2	10.2
0.50	0.50	0.1	0.2	0.3	0.3	0.4	0.5	0.6	0.6	0.7	0.8	0.8	0.9	0.9	0.9	1.0	1.0	1.0
	0.75	0.3	0.3	0.4	0.5	0.6	0.7	0.7	0.8	0.9	1.0	1.0	1.1	1.1	1.2	1.2	1.2	1.2
	1.00	0.5	0.6	0.6	0.7	0.8	0.9	1.0	1.0	1.1	1.2	1.3	1.3	1.4	1.4	1.5	1.5	1.5
	1.25	0.8	0.8	0.9	0.9	1.0	1.1	1.2	1.3	1.3	1.4	1.5	1.6	1.6	1.7	1.7	1.7	1.7
	1.50	1.0	1.0	1.1	1.2	1.2	1.3	1.4	1.5	1.6	1.7	1.7	1.8	1.9	1.9	1.9	2.0	2.0
	1.75	1.3	1.3	1.3	1.4	1.5	1.6	1.6	1.7	1.8	1.9	2.0	2.0	2.1	2.2	2.2	2.2	2.2
	2.00	1.5	1.5	1.6	1.6	1.7	1.8	1.9	2.0	2.1	2.1	2.2	2.3	2.4	2.4	2.4	2.5	2.5
	2.25	1.8	1.8	1.8	1.9	2.0	2.0	2.1	2.2	2.3	2.4	2.5	2.5	2.6	2.7	2.7	2.7	2.7
	2.50	2.0	2.0	2.1	2.1	2.2	2.3	2.4	2.5	2.5	2.6	2.7	2.8	2.8	2.9	2.9	3.0	3.0
	2.75	2.3	2.3	2.3	2.4	2.5	2.5	2.6	2.7	2.8	2.9	3.0	3.0	3.1	3.1	3.2	3.2	3.2
	3.00	2.5	2.5	2.6	2.6	2.7	2.8	2.9	3.0	3.0	3.1	3.2	3.3	3.3	3.4	3.4	3.5	3.5
	3.25	2.8	2.8	2.8	2.9	3.0	3.0	3.1	3.2	3.3	3.4	3.5	3.5	3.6	3.6	3.7	3.7	3.7
	3.50	3.0	3.0	3.1	3.1	3.2	3.3	3.4	3.4	3.5	3.6	3.7	3.8	3.8	3.9	3.9	4.0	4.0
	3.75	3.3	3.3	3.3	3.4	3.4	3.5	3.6	3.7	3.8	3.9	3.9	4.0	4.1	4.1	4.2	4.2	4.2
	4.00	3.5	3.5	3.6	3.6	3.7	3.8	3.9	3.9	4.0	4.1	4.2	4.3	4.3	4.4	4.4	4.5	4.5
	4.25	3.8	3.8	3.8	3.9	3.9	4.0	4.1	4.2	4.3	4.4	4.4	4.5	4.6	4.6	4.7	4.7	4.7
	4.50	4.0	4.0	4.1	4.1	4.2	4.3	4.4	4.4	4.5	4.6	4.7	4.8	4.8	4.9	4.9	5.0	5.0
	4.75	4.3	4.3	4.3	4.4	4.4	4.5	4.6	4.7	4.8	4.9	4.9	5.0	5.1	5.1	5.2	5.2	5.2
	5.00	4.5	4.5	4.6	4.6	4.7	4.8	4.9	4.9	5.0	5.1	5.2	5.3	5.3	5.4	5.4	5.5	5.5
	5.25	4.8	4.8	4.8	4.9	4.9	5.0	5.1	5.2	5.3	5.4	5.4	5.5	5.6	5.6	5.7	5.7	5.7
	5.50	5.0	5.0	5.1	5.1	5.2	5.3	5.3	5.4	5.5	5.6	5.7	5.8	5.8	5.9	5.9	6.0	6.0
	5.75	5.3	5.3	5.3	5.4	5.4	5.5	5.6	5.7	5.8	5.9	5.9	6.0	6.1	6.1	6.2	6.2	6.2
	6.00	5.5	5.5	5.6	5.6	5.7	5.8	5.8	5.9	6.0	6.1	6.2	6.3	6.3	6.4	6.4	6.5	6.5
	6.25	5.8	5.8	5.8	5.9	5.9	6.0	6.1	6.2	6.3	6.4	6.4	6.5	6.6	6.6	6.7	6.7	6.7
	6.50	6.0	6.0	6.1	6.1	6.2	6.3	6.3	6.4	6.5	6.6	6.7	6.8	6.8	6.9	6.9	7.0	7.0
	6.75	6.3	6.3	6.3	6.4	6.4	6.5	6.6	6.7	6.8	6.9	6.9	7.0	7.1	7.1	7.2	7.2	7.2
	7.00	6.5	6.5	6.6	6.6	6.7	6.8	6.8	6.9	7.0	7.1	7.2	7.3	7.3	7.4	7.4	7.5	7.5
	7.25	6.8	6.8	6.8	6.9	6.9	7.0	7.1	7.2	7.3	7.4	7.4	7.5	7.6	7.6	7.7	7.7	7.7
	7.50	7.0	7.0	7.1	7.1	7.2	7.3	7.3	7.4	7.5	7.6	7.7	7.8	7.8	7.9	7.9	8.0	8.0
	7.75	7.3	7.3	7.3	7.4	7.4	7.5	7.6	7.7	7.8	7.9	7.9	8.0	8.1	8.1	8.2	8.2	8.2
	8.00	7.5	7.5	7.6	7.6	7.7	7.8	7.8	7.9	8.0	8.1	8.2	8.3	8.3	8.4	8.4	8.5	8.5
	8.25	7.8	7.8	7.8	7.9	7.9	8.0	8.1	8.2	8.3	8.4	8.4	8.5	8.6	8.6	8.7	8.7	8.7
	8.50	8.0	8.0	8.1	8.1	8.2	8.3	8.3	8.4	8.5	8.6	8.7	8.8	8.8	8.9	8.9	9.0	9.0
	8.75	8.3	8.3	8.3	8.4	8.4	8.5	8.6	8.7	8.8	8.9	8.9	9.0	9.1	9.1	9.2	9.2	9.2
	9.00	8.5	8.5	8.6	8.6	8.7	8.8	8.8	8.9	9.0	9.1	9.2	9.3	9.3	9.4	9.4	9.5	9.5
	9.25	8.8	8.8	8.8	8.9	8.9	9.0	9.1	9.2	9.3	9.3	9.4	9.5	9.6	9.6	9.7	9.7	9.7
	9.50	9.0	9.0	9.1	9.1	9.2	9.3	9.3	9.4	9.5	9.6	9.7	9.8	9.8	9.9	9.9	10.0	10.0
	9.75	9.3	9.3	9.3	9.4	9.4	9.5	9.6	9.7	9.8	9.8	9.9	10.0	10.1	10.1	10.2	10.2	10.2
	10.00	9.5	9.5	9.6	9.6	9.7	9.8	9.8	9.9	10.0	10.1	10.2	10.3	10.3	10.4	10.4	10.5	10.5
0.75	0.75	0.1	0.3	0.4	0.5	0.6	0.8	0.9	1.0	1.1	1.1	1.2	1.3	1.4	1.4	1.4	1.5	1.5
	1.00	0.3	0.4	0.5	0.6	0.8	0.9	1.0	1.1	1.3	1.4	1.4	1.5	1.6	1.6	1.7	1.7	1.7
	1.25	0.5	0.6	0.7	0.8	1.0	1.1	1.2	1.3	1.5	1.6	1.7	1.8	1.8	1.9	1.9	2.0	2.0
	1.50	0.8	0.8	0.9	1.0	1.2	1.3	1.4	1.6	1.7	1.8	1.9	2.0	2.1	2.1	2.2	2.2	2.2
	1.75	1.0	1.1	1.2	1.3	1.4	1.5	1.7	1.8	1.9	2.0	2.1	2.2	2.3	2.4	2.4	2.5	2.5
	2.00	1.3	1.3	1.4	1.5	1.6	1.8	1.9	2.0	2.1	2.3	2.4	2.5	2.5	2.6	2.7	2.7	2.7
	2.25	1.5	1.6	1.6	1.7	1.9	2.0	2.1	2.2	2.4	2.5	2.6	2.7	2.8	2.9	2.9	3.0	3.0
	2.50	1.8	1.8	1.9	2.0	2.1	2.2	2.4	2.5	2.6	2.7	2.8	2.9	3.0	3.1	3.2	3.2	3.2
	2.75	2.0	2.1	2.1	2.2	2.3	2.5	2.6	2.7	2.9	3.0	3.1	3.2	3.3	3.4	3.4	3.5	3.5
	3.00	2.3	2.3	2.4	2.5	2.6	2.7	2.8	3.0	3.1	3.2	3.3	3.4	3.5	3.6	3.7	3.7	3.7
	3.25	2.5	2.6	2.6	2.7	2.8	2.9	3.1	3.2	3.3	3.5	3.6	3.7	3.8	3.9	3.9	4.0	4.0
	3.50	2.8	2.8	2.9	3.0	3.1	3.2	3.3	3.4	3.6	3.7	3.8	3.9	4.0	4.1	4.2	4.2	4.2
	3.75	3.0	3.1	3.1	3.2	3.3	3.4	3.6	3.7	3.8	3.9	4.1	4.2	4.3	4.4	4.4	4.5	4.5
	4.00	3.3	3.3	3.4	3.5	3.6	3.7	3.8	3.9	4.1	4.2	4.3	4.4	4.5	4.6	4.7	4.7	4.7
	4.25	3.5	3.6	3.6	3.7	3.8	3.9	4.1	4.2	4.3	4.4	4.6	4.7	4.8	4.8	4.9	5.0	5.0
	4.50	3.8	3.8	3.9	4.0	4.1	4.2	4.3	4.4	4.6	4.7	4.8	4.9	5.0	5.1	5.2	5.2	5.2
	4.75	4.0	4.1	4.1	4.2	4.3	4.4	4.5	4.7	4.8	4.9	5.1	5.2	5.3	5.3	5.4	5.5	5.5
	5.00	4.3	4.3	4.4	4.5	4.6	4.7	4.8	4.9	5.1	5.2	5.3	5.4	5.5	5.6	5.7	5.7	5.7
	5.25	4.5	4.6	4.6	4.7	4.8	4.9	5.0	5.2	5.3	5.4	5.6	5.7	5.8	5.8	5.9	6.0	6.0
	5.50	4.8	4.8	4.9	4.9	5.1	5.2	5.3	5.4	5.6	5.7	5.8	5.9	6.0	6.1	6.2	6.2	6.2
	5.75	5.0	5.1	5.1	5.2	5.3	5.4	5.5	5.7	5.8	5.9	6.0	6.2	6.3	6.3	6.4	6.5	6.5
	6.00	5.3	5.3	5.4	5.4	5.5	5.7	5.8	5.9	6.0	6.2	6.3	6.4	6.5	6.6	6.7	6.7	6.7
	6.25	5.5	5.6	5.6	5.7	5.8	5.9	6.0	6.2	6.3	6.4	6.5	6.7	6.8	6.8	6.9	7.0	7.0
	6.50	5.8	5.8	5.9	5.9	6.0	6.2	6.3	6.4	6.5	6.7	6.8	6.9	7.0	7.1	7.2	7.2	7.2
	6.75	6.0	6.1	6.1	6.2	6.3	6.4	6.5	6.7	6.8	6.9	7.0	7.2	7.3	7.3	7.4	7.5	7.5
	7.00	6.3	6.3	6.4	6.4	6.5	6.7	6.8	6.9	7.0	7.2	7.3	7.4	7.5	7.6	7.7	7.7	7.7
	7.25	6.5	6.6	6.6	6.7	6.8	6.9	7.0	7.2	7.3	7.4	7.5	7.7	7.8	7.8	7.9	8.0	8.0
	7.50	6.8	6.8	6.9	6.9	7.0	7.2	7.3	7.4	7.5	7.7	7.8	7.9	8.0	8.1	8.2	8.2	8.2
	7.75	7.0	7.0	7.1	7.2	7.3	7.4	7.5	7.7	7.8	7.9	8.0	8.2	8.3	8.3	8.4	8.5	8.5
	8.00	7.3	7.3	7.4	7.4	7.5	7.7	7.8	7.9	8.0	8.2	8.3	8.4	8.5	8.6	8.7	8.7	8.7
	8.25	7.5	7.5	7.6	7.7	7.8	7.9	8.0	8.2	8.3	8.4	8.5	8.6	8.8	8.8	8.9	9.0	9.0
	8.50	7.8	7.8	7.9	7.9	8.0	8.2	8.3	8.4	8.5	8.7	8.8	8.9	9.0	9.1	9.2	9.2	9.2
	8.75	8.0	8.0	8.1	8.2	8.3	8.4	8.5	8.7	8.8	8.9	9.0	9.1	9.2	9.3	9.4	9.5	9.5
	9.00	8.3	8.3	8.4	8.4	8.5	8.6	8.8	8.9	9.0	9.2	9.3	9.4	9.5	9.6	9.7	9.7	9.7
	9.25	8.5	8.5	8.6	8.7	8.8	8.9	9.0	9.1	9.3	9.4	9.5	9.6	9.7	9.8	9.9	10.0	10.0
	9.50	8.8	8.8	8.9	8.9	9.0	9.1	9.3	9.4	9.5	9.7	9.8	9.9	10.0	10.1	10.2	10.2	10.2
	9.75	9.0	9.0	9.1	9.2	9.3	9.4	9.5	9.6	9.8	9.9	10.0	10.1	10.2	10.3	10.4	10.5	10.5
	10.00	9.3	9.3	9.4	9.4	9.5	9.6	9.8	9.9	10.0	10.2	10.3	10.4	10.5	10.6	10.7	10.7	10.7
1.00	1.00	0.2	0.3	0.5	0.7	0.8	1.0	1.1	1.3	1.4	1.5	1.6	1.7	1.8	1.9	1.9	2.0	2.0
	1.25	0.3	0.5	0.6	0.8	1.0	1.1	1.3	1.5	1.6	1.7	1.8	2.0	2.0	2.1	2.2	2.2	2.2
	1.50	0.5	0.7	0.8	1.0	1.1	1.3	1.5	1.7	1.8	1.9	2.1	2.2	2.3	2.4	2.4	2.5	2.5
	1.75	0.8	0.9	1.0	1.2	1.3	1.5	1.7	1.9	2.0	2.2	2.3	2.4	2.5	2.6	2.7	2.7	2.7
	2.00	1.0	1.1	1.2	1.4	1.6	1.7	1.9	2.1	2.2	2.4	2.5	2.6	2.8	2.8	2.9	3.0	3.0
	2.25	1.3	1.4	1.5	1.6	1.8	2.0	2.1	2.3	2.5	2.6	2.8	2.9	3.0	3.1	3.2	3.2	3.2
	2.50	1.5	1.6	1.7	1.8	2.0	2.2	2.4	2.5	2.7	2.8	3.0	3.1	3.2	3.3	3.4	3.5	3.5
	2.75	1.8	1.8	1.9	2.1	2.2	2.4	2.6	2.8	2.9	3.1	3.2	3.4	3.5	3.6	3.7	3.7	3.7
	3.00	2.0	2.1	2.2	2.3	2.5	2.6	2.8	3.0	3.2	3.3	3.5	3.6	3.7	3.8	3.9	4.0	4.0
	3.25	2.3	2.3	2.4	2.6	2.7	2.9	3.1	3.2	3.4	3.6	3.7	3.8	4.0	4.1	4.1	4.2	4.2
	3.50	2.5	2.6	2.7	2.8	3.0	3.1	3.3	3.5	3.6	3.8	4.0	4.1	4.2	4.3	4.4	4.5	4.5
	3.75	2.8	2.8	2.9	3.1	3.2	3.4	3.5	3.7	3.9	4.0	4.2	4.3	4.5	4.6	4.6	4.7	4.7
	4.00	3.0	3.1	3.2	3.3	3.4	3.6	3.8	4.0	4.1	4.3	4.4	4.6	4.7	4.8	4.9	5.0	5.0
	4.25	3.3	3.3	3.4	3.5	3.7	3.8	4.0	4.2	4.4	4.5	4.7	4.8	5.0	5.1	5.1	5.2	5.2
	4.50	3.5	3.6	3.7	3.8	3.9	4.1	4.3	4.4	4.6	4.8	4.9	5.1	5.2	5.3	5.4	5.5	5.5
	4.75	3.8	3.8	3.9	4.0	4.2	4.3	4.5	4.7	4.9	5.0	5.2	5.3	5.4	5.6	5.6	5.7	5.7
	5.00	4.0	4.1	4.2	4.3	4.4	4.6	4.8	4.9	5.1	5.3	5.4	5.6	5.7	5.8	5.9	5.9	6.0
	5.25	4.3	4.3	4.4	4.5	4.7	4.8	5.0	5.2	5.3	5.5	5.7	5.8	5.9	6.1	6.1	6.2	6.2
	5.50	4.5	4.6	4.7	4.8	4.9	5.1	5.2	5.4	5.6	5.8	5.9	6.1	6.2	6.3	6.4	6.4	6.5
	5.75	4.8	4.8	4.9	5.0	5.2	5.3	5.5	5.7	5.8	6.0	6.2	6.3	6.4	6.5	6.6	6.7	6.7
	6.00	5.0	5.1	5.2	5.3	5.4	5.6	5.7	5.9	6.1	6.3	6.4	6.6	6.7	6.8	6.9	6.9	7.0
	6.25	5.3	5.3	5.4	5.5	5.7	5.8	6.0	6.2	6.3	6.5	6.7	6.8	6.9	7.0	7.1	7.2	7.2
	6.50	5.5	5.6	5.7	5.8	5.9	6.1	6.2	6.4	6.6	6.7	6.9	7.1	7.2	7.3	7.4	7.4	7.5
	6.75	5.8	5.8	5.9	6.0	6.2	6.3	6.5	6.6	6.8	7.0	7.2	7.3	7.4	7.5	7.6	7.7	7.7
	7.00	6.0	6.1	6.2	6.3	6.4	6.6	6.7	6.9	7.1	7.2	7.4	7.5	7.7	7.8	7.9	7.9	8.0
	7.25	6.3	6.3	6.4	6.5	6.7	6.8	7.0	7.1	7.3	7.5	7.6	7.8	7.9	8.0	8.1	8.2	8.2
	7.50	6.5	6.6	6.7	6.8	6.9	7.1	7.2	7.4	7.6	7.7	7.9	8.0	8.2	8.3	8.4	8.4	8.5
	7.75	6.8	6.8	6.9	7.0	7.1	7.3	7.5	7.6	7.8	8.0	8.1	8.3	8.4	8.5	8.6	8.7	8.7
	8.00	7.0	7.1	7.2	7.3	7.4	7.5	7.7	7.9	8.1	8.2	8.4	8.5	8.7	8.8	8.9	8.9	9.0
	8.25	7.3	7.3	7.4	7.5	7.6	7.8	8.0	8.1	8.3	8.5	8.6	8.8	8.9	9.0	9.1	9.2	9.2
	8.50	7.5	7.6	7.7	7.8	7.9	8.0	8.2	8.4	8.6	8.7	8.9	9.0	9.2	9.3	9.4	9.4	9.5
	8.75	7.8	7.8	7.9	8.0	8.1	8.3	8.5	8.6	8.8	9.0	9.1	9.3	9.4	9.5	9.6	9.7	9.7
	9.00	8.0	8.1	8.1	8.3	8.4	8.5	8.7	8.9	9.1	9.2	9.4	9.6	9.7	9.8	9.9	9.9	10.0
	9.25	8.2	8.3	8.4	8.5	8.6	8.8	9.0	9.1	9.3	9.5	9.6	9.8	9.9	10.0	10.1	10.2	10.2
	9.50	8.5	8.6	8.6	8.8	8.9	9.0	9.2	9.4	9.6	9.7	9.9	10.0	10.2	10.3	10.4	10.4	10.5
	9.75	8.8	8.8	8.9	9.0	9.1	9.3	9.5	9.6	9.8	10.0	10.1	10.3	10.4	10.5	10.6	10.7	10.7
	10.00	9.0	9.1	9.1	9.3	9.4	9.5	9.7	9.9	10.0	10.2	10.4	10.5	10.7	10.8	10.9	10.9	11.0
1.25	1.25	0.2	0.4	0.6	0.9	1.1	1.3	1.4	1.6	1.8	1.9	2.0	2.2	2.3	2.3	2.4	2.5	2.5
	1.50	0.3	0.5	0.8	1.0	1.2	1.4	1.6	1.8	2.0	2.1	2.3	2.4	2.5	2.6	2.7	2.7	2.7
	1.75	0.6	0.7	0.9	1.1	1.3	1.6	1.8	2.0	2.2	2.3	2.5	2.6	2.7	2.8	2.9	3.0	3.0
	2.00	0.8	0.9	1.1	1.3	1.5	1.8	2.0	2.2	2.4	2.5	2.7	2.8	3.0	3.1	3.1	3.2	3.2
	2.25	1.0	1.2	1.3	1.5	1.7	2.0	2.2	2.6	2.8	2.9	3.1	3.2	3.3	3.3	3.4	3.5	3.5
	2.50	1.3	1.4	1.5	1.7	1.9	2.2	2.4	2.6	2.8	3.0	3.2	3.3	3.4	3.5	3.6	3.7	3.7
	2.75	1.5	1.6	1.8	2.0	2.2	2.4	2.6	2.8	3.0	3.2	3.4	3.5	3.7	3.8	3.9	3.9	4.0
	3.00	1.8	1.9	2.0	2.2	2.4	2.6	2.8	3.0	3.3	3.4	3.6	3.8	3.9	4.0	4.1	4.2	4.2
	3.25	2.0	2.1	2.3	2.4	2.6	2.8	3.1	3.3	3.5	3.7	3.9	4.0	4.2	4.3	4.4	4.4	4.5
	3.50	2.3	2.4	2.5	2.7	2.9	3.1	3.3	3.5	3.7	3.9	4.1	4.3	4.4	4.5	4.6	4.7	4.7
	3.75	2.5	2.6	2.7	2.9	3.1	3.3	3.5	3.7	4.0	4.2	4.3	4.5	4.7	4.8	4.9	4.9	5.0
	4.00	2.8	2.9	3.0	3.1	3.3	3.5	3.8	4.0	4.2	4.4	4.6	4.8	4.9	5.0	5.1	5.2	5.2
	4.25	3.0	3.1	3.2	3.4	3.6	3.8	4.0	4.2	4.4	4.6	4.8	5.0	5.1	5.3	5.4	5.4	5.5
	4.50	3.3	3.4	3.5	3.6	3.8	4.0	4.2	4.5	4.7	4.9	5.1	5.2	5.4	5.5	5.6	5.7	5.7
	4.75	3.5	3.6	3.7	3.9	4.1	4.3	4.5	4.7	4.9	5.1	5.3	5.5	5.6	5.8	5.9	5.9	6.0
	5.00	3.8	3.8	4.0	4.1	4.3	4.5	4.7	4.9	5.2	5.4	5.6	5.7	5.9	6.0	6.1	6.2	6.2
	5.25	4.0	4.1	4.2	4.4	4.5	4.8	5.0	5.2	5.4	5.6	5.8	6.0	6.1	6.3	6.4	6.4	6.5
	5.50	4.3	4.3	4.5	4.6	4.8	5.0	5.2	5.4	5.6	5.8	6.0	6.2	6.4	6.5	6.6	6.7	6.7
	5.75	4.5	4.6	4.7	4.9	5.0	5.2	5.5	5.7	5.9	6.1	6.3	6.5	6.6	6.8	6.9	6.9	7.0
	6.00	4.8	4.8	5.0	5.1	5.3	5.5	5.7	5.9	6.1	6.3	6.5	6.7	6.9	7.0	7.1	7.2	7.2
	6.25	5.0	5.1	5.2	5.4	5.5	5.7	5.9	6.2	6.4	6.6	6.8	7.0	7.1	7.3	7.4	7.4	7.5
	6.50	5.3	5.3	5.5	5.6	5.8	6.0	6.2	6.4	6.6	6.8	7.0	7.2	7.4	7.5	7.6	7.7	7.7
	6.75	5.5	5.6	5.7	5.8	6.0	6.2	6.4	6.6	6.9	7.1	7.3	7.5	7.6	7.7	7.9	7.9	8.0
	7.00	5.8	5.8	6.0	6.1	6.3	6.5	6.7	6.9	7.1	7.3	7.5	7.7	7.9	8.0	8.1	8.2	8.2
	7.25	6.0	6.1	6.2	6.3	6.5	6.7	6.9	7.1	7.4	7.6	7.8	7.9	8.1	8.2	8.4	8.4	8.5
	7.50	6.3	6.3	6.4	6.6	6.8	7.0	7.2	7.4	7.6	7.8	8.0	8.2	8.4	8.5	8.6	8.7	8.7
	7.75	6.5	6.6	6.7	6.8	7.0	7.2	7.4	7.6	7.9	8.1	8.3	8.4	8.6	8.7	8.9	8.9	9.0
	8.00	6.8	6.8	6.9	7.1	7.3	7.5	7.7	7.9	8.1	8.3	8.5	8.7	8.9	9.0	9.1	9.2	9.2
	8.25	7.0	7.1	7.2	7.3	7.5	7.7	7.9	8.1	8.3	8.6	8.8	8.9	9.1	9.2	9.4	9.4	9.5
	8.50	7.3	7.3	7.4	7.6	7.8	7.9	8.2	8.4	8.6	8.8	9.0	9.2	9.4	9.5	9.6	9.7	9.7
	8.75	7.5	7.6	7.7	7.8	8.0	8.2	8.4	8.6	8.8	9.1	9.3	9.4	9.6	9.7	9.9	9.9	10.0
	9.00	7.8	7.8	7.9	8.1	8.3	8.4	8.7	8.9	9.1	9.3	9.5	9.7	9.9	10.0	10.1	10.2	10.2
	9.25	8.0	8.1	8.2	8.3	8.5	8.7	8.9	9.1	9.3	9.5	9.7	9.9	10.1	10.2	10.4	10.4	10.5
	9.50	8.3	8.3	8.4	8.6	8.7	8.9	9.1	9.4	9.6	9.8	10.0	10.2	10.3	10.5	10.6	10.7	10.7
	9.75	8.5	8.6	8.7	8.8	9.0	9.2	9.4	9.6	9.8	10.0	10.2	10.4	10.6	10.7	10.9	10.9	11.0
	10.00	8.8	8.8	8.9	9.1	9.2	9.4	9.6	9.9	10.1	10.3	10.5	10.7	10.8	11.0	11.1	11.2	11.2
1.50	1.50	0.3	0.5	0.8	1.0	1.3	1.5	1.7	1.9	2.1	2.3	2.5	2.6	2.7	2.8	2.9	3.0	3.0
	1.75	0.4	0.6	0.9	1.1	1.4	1.6	1.9	2.1	2.3	2.5	2.7	2.8	2.9	3.1	3.1	3.2	3.2
	2.00	0.6	0.8	1.0	1.3	1.5	1.8	2.0	2.3	2.5	2.7	2.9	3.0	3.2	3.3	3.4	3.4	3.5
	2.25	0.8	1.0	1.2	1.5	1.7	2.0	2.2	2.5	2.7	2.9	3.1	3.3	3.4	3.5	3.6	3.7	3.7
	2.50	1.1	1.2	1.4	1.7	1.9	2.2	2.4	2.7	2.9	3.1	3.3	3.5	3.6	3.8	3.9	3.9	4.0
	2.75	1.3	1.4	1.6	1.9	2.1	2.4	2.6	2.9	3.1	3.4	3.6	3.7	3.9	4.0	4.1	4.2	4.2
	3.00	1.5	1.7	1.9	2.1	2.3	2.6	2.9	3.1	3.4	3.6	3.8	4.0	4.1	4.3	4.4	4.4	4.5
	3.25	1.8	1.9	2.1	2.3	2.6	2.8	3.1	3.3	3.6	3.8	4.0	4.2	4.4	4.5	4.6	4.7	4.7
	3.50	2.0	2.2	2.3	2.5	2.8	3.0	3.3	3.6	3.8	4.0	4.3	4.4	4.6	4.7	4.9	4.9	5.0
	3.75	2.3	2.4	2.6	2.8	3.0	3.3	3.5	3.8	4.0	4.3	4.5	4.7	4.9	5.0	5.1	5.2	5.2
	4.00	2.5	2.6	2.8	3.0	3.2	3.5	3.8	4.0	4.3	4.5	4.7	4.9	5.1	5.2	5.4	5.4	5.5
	4.25	2.8	2.9	3.0	3.2	3.5	3.7	4.0	4.3	4.5	4.7	5.0	5.2	5.3	5.5	5.6	5.7	5.7
	4.50	3.0	3.1	3.3	3.5	3.7	4.0	4.2	4.5	4.7	5.0	5.2	5.4	5.6	5.7	5.8	5.9	6.0
	4.75	3.3	3.4	3.5	3.7	4.0	4.2	4.5	4.7	5.0	5.2	5.4	5.7	5.8	6.0	6.1	6.2	6.2
	5.00	3.5	3.6	3.8	4.0	4.2	4.4	4.7	5.0	5.2	5.5	5.7	5.9	6.1	6.2	6.3	6.4	6.5
	5.25	3.8	3.9	4.0	4.2	4.4	4.7	4.9	5.2	5.5	5.7	5.9	6.1	6.3	6.5	6.6	6.7	6.7
	5.50	4.0	4.1	4.3	4.5	4.7	4.9	5.2	5.4	5.7	5.9	6.2	6.4	6.6	6.7	6.8	6.9	7.0
	5.75	4.3	4.4	4.5	4.7	4.9	5.2	5.4	5.7	5.9	6.2	6.4	6.6	6.8	7.0	7.1	7.2	7.2
	6.00	4.5	4.6	4.8	4.9	5.2	5.4	5.7	5.9	6.2	6.4	6.7	6.9	7.1	7.2	7.3	7.4	7.5
	6.25	4.8	4.9	5.0	5.2	5.4	5.7	5.9	6.2	6.4	6.7	6.9	7.1	7.3	7.5	7.6	7.7	7.7
	6.50	5.0	5.1	5.3	5.4	5.7	5.9	6.2	6.4	6.7	6.9	7.2	7.4	7.6	7.7	7.8	7.9	8.0
	6.75	5.3	5.4	5.5	5.7	5.9	6.1	6.4	6.7	6.9	7.2	7.4	7.6	7.8	8.0	8.1	8.2	8.2
	7.00	5.5	5.6	5.8	5.9	6.1	6.4	6.6	6.9	7.2	7.4	7.6	7.9	8.0	8.2	8.3	8.4	8.5
	7.25	5.8	5.9	6.0	6.2	6.4	6.6	6.9	7.1	7.4	7.7	7.9	8.1	8.3	8.5	8.6	8.7	8.7
	7.50	6.0	6.1	6.2	6.4	6.6	6.9	7.1	7.4	7.6	7.9	8.1	8.4	8.5	8.7	8.8	8.9	9.0
	7.75	6.3	6.4	6.5	6.7	6.9	7.1	7.4	7.6	7.9	8.1	8.4	8.6	8.8	9.0	9.1	9.2	9.2
	8.00	6.5	6.6	6.7	6.9	7.1	7.4	7.6	7.9	8.1	8.4	8.6	8.8	9.0	9.2	9.3	9.4	9.5
	8.25	6.8	6.9	7.0	7.2	7.4	7.6	7.9	8.1	8.4	8.6	8.9	9.1	9.3	9.4	9.6	9.7	9.7
	8.50	7.0	7.1	7.2	7.4	7.6	7.9	8.1	8.4	8.6	8.9	9.1	9.3	9.5	9.7	9.8	9.9	10.0
	8.75	7.3	7.4	7.5	7.7	7.9	8.1	8.4	8.6	8.9	9.1	9.4	9.6	9.8	9.9	10.1	10.2	10.2
	9.00	7.5	7.6	7.7	7.9	8.1	8.4	8.6	8.9	9.1	9.4	9.6	9.8	10.0	10.2	10.3	10.4	10.5
	9.25	7.8	7.9	8.0	8.2	8.4	8.6	8.8	9.1	9.4	9.6	9.9	10.1	10.3	10.4	10.6	10.7	10.7
	9.50	8.0	8.1	8.2	8.4	8.6	8.8	9.1	9.4	9.6	9.9	10.1	10.3	10.5	10.7	10.8	10.9	11.0
	9.75	8.3	8.4	8.5	8.7	8.9	9.1	9.3	9.6	9.9	10.1	10.4	10.6	10.8	10.9	11.1	11.2	11.2
	10.00	8.5	8.6	8.7	8.9	9.1	9.3	9.6	9.9	10.1	10.4	10.6	10.8	11.0	11.2	11.3	11.4	11.5
1.75	1.75	0.3	0.6	0.9	1.2	1.5	1.8	2.0	2.2	2.5	2.7	2.9	3.0	3.2	3.3	3.4	3.4	3.5
	2.00	0.4	0.7	1.0	1.3	1.6	1.9	2.2	2.4	2.7	2.9	3.1	3.3	3.4	3.5	3.6	3.7	3.7
	2.25	0.6	0.9	1.1	1.4	1.8	2.0	2.3	2.6	2.9	3.1	3.3	3.5	3.6	3.8	3.9	3.9	4.0
	2.50	0.8	1.0	1.3	1.6	1.9	2.2	2.5	2.8	3.1	3.3	3.5	3.7	3.9	4.0	4.1	4.2	4.2
	2.75	1.1	1.3	1.5	1.8	2.1	2.4	2.7	3.0	3.3	3.5	3.7	3.9	4.1	4.2	4.4	4.4	4.5
	3.00	1.3	1.5	1.7	2.0	2.3	2.6	2.9	3.2	3.5	3.7	4.0	4.2	4.3	4.5	4.6	4.7	4.7
	3.25	1.6	1.7	1.9	2.2	2.5	2.8	3.1	3.4	3.7	3.9	4.2	4.4	4.6	4.7	4.8	4.9	5.0
	3.50	1.8	1.9	2.2	2.4	2.7	3.0	3.3	3.6	3.9	4.2	4.4	4.6	4.8	5.0	5.1	5.2	5.2
	3.75	2.0	2.2	2.4	2.7	2.9	3.3	3.6	3.9	4.1	4.4	4.6	4.9	5.1	5.2	5.3	5.4	5.5
	4.00	2.3	2.4	2.6	2.9	3.2	3.5	3.8	4.1	4.4	4.6	4.9	5.1	5.3	5.5	5.6	5.7	5.7
	4.25	2.5	2.7	2.9	3.1	3.4	3.7	4.0	4.3	4.6	4.9	5.1	5.3	5.5	5.7	5.8	5.9	6.0
	4.50	2.8	2.9	3.1	3.4	3.6	3.9	4.2	4.5	4.8	5.1	5.4	5.6	5.8	5.9	6.1	6.2	6.2
	4.75	3.0	3.2	3.4	3.6	3.9	4.2	4.5	4.8	5.1	5.3	5.6	5.8	6.0	6.2	6.3	6.4	6.5
	5.00	3.3	3.4	3.6	3.8	4.1	4.4	4.7	5.0	5.3	5.6	5.8	6.1	6.3	6.4	6.6	6.7	6.7
	5.25	3.5	3.7	3.8	4.1	4.3	4.6	4.9	5.2	5.5	5.8	6.1	6.3	6.5	6.7	6.8	6.9	7.0
	5.50	3.8	3.9	4.1	4.3	4.6	4.9	5.2	5.5	5.8	6.1	6.3	6.6	6.8	6.9	7.1	7.2	7.2
	5.75	4.0	4.1	4.3	4.6	4.8	5.1	5.4	5.7	6.0	6.3	6.6	6.8	7.0	7.2	7.3	7.4	7.5
	6.00	4.3	4.4	4.6	4.8	5.1	5.3	5.6	6.0	6.3	6.5	6.8	7.0	7.2	7.4	7.6	7.7	7.7
	6.25	4.5	4.6	4.8	5.0	5.3	5.6	5.9	6.2	6.5	6.8	7.0	7.3	7.5	7.7	7.8	7.9	8.0
	6.50	4.8	4.9	5.1	5.3	5.5	5.8	6.1	6.4	6.7	7.0	7.3	7.5	7.7	7.9	8.1	8.2	8.2
	6.75	5.0	5.1	5.3	5.5	5.8	6.1	6.4	6.7	7.0	7.3	7.5	7.8	8.0	8.2	8.3	8.4	8.5
	7.00	5.3	5.4	5.6	5.8	6.0	6.3	6.6	6.9	7.2	7.5	7.8	8.0	8.2	8.4	8.6	8.7	8.7
	7.25	5.5	5.6	5.8	6.0	6.3	6.6	6.9	7.2	7.5	7.7	8.0	8.3	8.5	8.7	8.8	8.9	9.0
	7.50	5.8	5.9	6.0	6.3	6.5	6.8	7.1	7.4	7.7	8.0	8.3	8.5	8.7	8.9	9.1	9.2	9.2
	7.75	6.0	6.1	6.3	6.5	6.8	7.0	7.3	7.6	7.9	8.2	8.5	8.8	9.0	9.2	9.3	9.4	9.5
	8.00	6.3	6.4	6.5	6.8	7.0	7.3	7.6	7.9	8.2	8.5	8.8	9.0	9.2	9.4	9.6	9.7	9.7
	8.25	6.5	6.6	6.8	7.0	7.3	7.5	7.8	8.1	8.4	8.7	9.0	9.3	9.5	9.7	9.8	9.9	10.0
	8.50	6.8	6.9	7.0	7.2	7.5	7.8	8.1	8.4	8.7	9.0	9.2	9.5	9.7	9.9	10.1	10.2	10.2
	8.75	7.0	7.1	7.3	7.5	7.7	8.0	8.3	8.6	8.9	9.2	9.5	9.7	10.0	10.2	10.3	10.4	10.5
	9.00	7.3	7.4	7.5	7.7	8.0	8.3	8.6	8.9	9.2	9.5	9.7	10.0	10.2	10.4	10.6	10.7	10.7
	9.25	7.5	7.6	7.8	8.0	8.2	8.5	8.8	9.1	9.4	9.7	10.0	10.2	10.5	10.7	10.8	10.9	11.0
	9.50	7.8	7.9	8.0	8.2	8.5	8.8	9.1	9.4	9.7	10.0	10.2	10.5	10.7	10.9	11.1	11.2	11.2
	9.75	8.0	8.1	8.3	8.5	8.7	9.0	9.3	9.6	9.9	10.2	10.5	10.7	11.0	11.1	11.3	11.4	11.5
	10.00	8.3	8.4	8.5	8.7	9.0	9.3	9.5	9.8	10.2	10.4	10.7	11.0	11.2	11.4	11.5	11.7	11.7
2.00	2.00	0.3	0.7	1.0	1.4	1.7	2.0	2.3	2.6	2.8	3.1	3.3	3.5	3.6	3.8	3.9	3.9	4.0
	2.25	0.4	0.8	1.1	1.5	1.8	2.1	2.4	2.7	3.0	3.3	3.5	3.7	3.9	4.0	4.1	4.2	4.2
	2.50	0.6	0.9	1.3	1.6	2.0	2.3	2.6	2.9	3.2	3.5	3.7	3.9	4.1	4.2	4.3	4.4	4.5
	2.75	0.9	1.1	1.4	1.8	2.1	2.5	2.8	3.1	3.4	3.7	3.9	4.1	4.3	4.5	4.6	4.7	4.7
	3.00	1.1	1.3	1.6	2.0	2.3	2.6	3.0	3.3	3.6	4.1	4.4	4.6	4.8	5.0	5.1	5.2	5.2
	3.25	1.3	1.5	1.8	2.1	2.5	2.8	3.2	3.5	3.8	4.1	4.4	4.6	4.8	5.0	5.1	5.2	5.2
	3.50	1.6	1.8	2.0	2.4	2.7	3.0	3.4	3.7	4.0	4.3	4.6	4.8	5.0	5.2	5.3	5.4	5.5
	3.75	1.8	2.0	2.3	2.6	2.9	3.3	3.6	3.9	4.3	4.5	4.8	5.1	5.3	5.4	5.6	5.7	5.7
	4.00	2.1	2.2	2.5	2.8	3.1	3.5	3.8	4.1	4.5	4.8	5.0	5.3	5.5	5.7	5.8	5.9	6.0
	4.25	2.3	2.5	2.7	3.0	3.3	3.7	4.0	4.4	4.7	5.0	5.3	5.5	5.7	5.9	6.1	6.2	6.2
	4.50	2.6	2.7	2.9	3.2	3.6	3.9	4.3	4.6	4.9	5.2	5.5	5.8	6.0	6.2	6.3	6.4	6.5
	4.75	2.8	3.0	3.2	3.5	3.8	4.1	4.5	4.8	5.2	5.5	5.7	6.0	6.2	6.4	6.6	6.7	6.7
	5.00	3.1	3.2	3.4	3.7	4.0	4.4	4.7	5.1	5.4	5.7	6.0	6.2	6.5	6.7	6.8	6.9	7.0
	5.25	3.3	3.4	3.7	3.9	4.3	4.6	4.9	5.3	5.6	5.9	6.2	6.5	6.7	6.9	7.1	7.2	7.2
	5.50	3.5	3.7	3.9	4.2	4.5	4.8	5.2	5.5	5.9	6.2	6.5	6.7	7.0	7.1	7.3	7.4	7.5
	5.75	3.8	3.9	4.1	4.4	4.7	5.1	5.4	5.8	6.1	6.4	6.7	7.0	7.2	7.4	7.5	7.7	7.7
	6.00	4.0	4.2	4.4	4.6	5.0	5.3	5.6	6.0	6.3	6.6	6.9	7.2	7.4	7.6	7.8	7.9	8.0
	6.25	4.3	4.4	4.6	4.9	5.2	5.5	5.9	6.2	6.6	6.9	7.2	7.5	7.7	7.9	8.0	8.2	8.2
	6.50	4.5	4.7	4.9	5.1	5.4	5.8	6.1	6.5	6.8	7.1	7.4	7.7	7.9	8.1	8.3	8.4	8.5
	6.75	4.8	4.9	5.1	5.4	5.7	6.0	6.4	6.7	7.0	7.4	7.7	7.9	8.2	8.4	8.5	8.7	8.7
	7.00	5.0	5.2	5.4	5.6	5.9	6.2	6.6	6.9	7.3	7.6	7.9	8.2	8.4	8.6	8.8	8.9	9.0
	7.25	5.3	5.4	5.6	5.9	6.2	6.5	6.8	7.2	7.5	7.8	8.2	8.4	8.7	8.9	9.0	9.2	9.2
	7.50	5.5	5.7	5.9	6.1	6.4	6.7	7.1	7.4	7.8	8.1	8.4	8.7	8.9	9.1	9.3	9.4	9.5
	7.75	5.8	5.9	6.1	6.3	6.6	7.0	7.3	7.7	8.0	8.3	8.6	8.9	9.2	9.4	9.5	9.7	9.7
	8.00	6.0	6.2	6.3	6.6	6.9	7.2	7.6	7.9	8.2	8.6	8.9	9.2	9.4	9.6	9.8	9.9	10.0
	8.25	6.3	6.4	6.6	6.8	7.1	7.5	7.8	8.1	8.5	8.8	9.1	9.4	9.7	9.9	10.0	10.2	10.2
	8.50	6.5	6.7	6.8	7.1	7.4	7.7	8.0	8.4	8.7	9.1	9.4	9.7	9.9	10.1	10.3	10.4	10.5
	8.75	6.8	6.9	7.1	7.3	7.6	7.9	8.3	8.6	9.0	9.3	9.6	9.9	10.2	10.4	10.5	10.7	10.7
	9.00	7.0	7.2	7.3	7.6	7.9	8.2	8.5	8.9	9.2	9.6	9.9	10.1	10.4	10.6	10.8	10.9	11.0
	9.25	7.3	7.4	7.6	7.8	8.1	8.4	8.8	9.1	9.5	9.8	10.1	10.4	10.6	10.9	11.0	11.2	11.2
	9.50	7.5	7.7	7.8	8.1	8.4	8.7	9.0	9.4	9.7	10.0	10.4	10.6	10.9	11.1	11.3	11.4	11.5
	9.75	7.8	7.9	8.1	8.3	8.6	8.9	9.3	9.6	10.0	10.3	10.6	10.9	11.1	11.4	11.5	11.6	11.7
	10.00	8.0	8.1	8.3	8.6	8.8	9.2	9.5	9.9	10.2	10.5	10.8	11.1	11.4	11.6	11.8	11.9	12.0
2.25	2.25	0.4	0.8	1.2	1.5	1.9	2.3	2.6	2.9	3.2	3.4	3.7	3.9	4.1	4.2	4.3	4.4	4.5
	2.50	0.5	0.9	1.3	1.6	2.0	2.4	2.7	3.1	3.4	3.6	3.9	4.1	4.3	4.5	4.6	4.7	4.7
	2.75	0.7	1.0	1.4	1.8	2.2	2.5	2.9	3.2	3.6	3.8	4.1	4.3	4.5	4.7	4.8	4.9	5.0
	3.00	0.9	1.2	1.5	1.9	2.3	2.7	3.1	3.4	3.8	4.1	4.3	4.6	4.8	4.9	5.1	5.2	5.2
	3.25	1.1	1.4	1.7	2.1	2.5	2.9	3.3	3.6	4.0	4.3	4.5	4.8	5.0	5.2	5.3	5.4	5.5
	3.50	1.3	1.6	1.9	2.3	2.7	3.1	3.5	3.8	4.2	4.5	4.8	5.0	5.2	5.4	5.6	5.7	5.7
	3.75	1.6	1.8	2.1	2.5	2.9	3.3	3.7	4.0	4.4	4.7	5.0	5.3	5.5	5.7	5.8	5.9	6.0
	4.00	1.8	2.0	2.3	2.7	3.1	3.5	3.9	4.2	4.6	4.9	5.2	5.5	5.7	5.9	6.1	6.2	6.2
	4.25	2.1	2.3	2.6	2.9	3.3	3.7	4.1	4.5	4.8	5.1	5.4	5.7	6.0	6.1	6.3	6.4	6.5
	4.50	2.3	2.5	2.8	3.1	3.5	3.9	4.3	4.7	5.0	5.4	5.7	6.0	6.2	6.4	6.5	6.7	6.7
	4.75	2.6	2.7	3.0	3.4	3.7	4.1	4.5	4.9	5.3	5.6	5.9	6.2	6.4	6.6	6.8	6.9	7.0
	5.00	2.8	3.0	3.3	3.6	3.9	4.3	4.7	5.1	5.5	5.8	6.1	6.4	6.7	6.9	7.0	7.2	7.2
	5.25	3.1	3.2	3.5	3.8	4.2	4.6	5.0	5.3	5.7	6.1	6.4	6.7	6.9	7.1	7.3	7.4	7.5
	5.50	3.3	3.5	3.7	4.0	4.4	4.8	5.2	5.6	5.9	6.3	6.6	6.9	7.2	7.4	7.5	7.7	7.7
	5.75	3.6	3.7	4.0	4.3	4.6	5.0	5.4	5.8	6.2	6.5	6.9	7.1	7.4	7.6	7.8	7.9	8.0
	6.00	3.8	4.0	4.2	4.5	4.9	5.3	5.6	6.0	6.4	6.8	7.1	7.4	7.6	7.9	8.0	8.2	8.2
	6.25	4.1	4.2	4.4	4.8	5.1	5.5	5.9	6.3	6.6	7.0	7.3	7.6	7.9	8.1	8.3	8.4	8.5
	6.50	4.3	4.5	4.7	5.0	5.3	5.7	6.1	6.5	6.9	7.2	7.6	7.9	8.1	8.3	8.5	8.6	8.7
	6.75	4.6	4.7	4.9	5.2	5.6	6.0	6.3	6.7	7.1	7.5	7.8	8.1	8.4	8.6	8.8	8.9	9.0
	7.00	4.8	4.9	5.2	5.5	5.8	6.2	6.6	7.0	7.4	7.7	8.1	8.4	8.6	8.8	9.0	9.1	9.2
	7.25	5.0	5.2	5.4	5.7	6.1	6.4	6.8	7.2	7.6	8.0	8.3	8.6	8.9	9.1	9.3	9.4	9.5
	7.50	5.3	5.4	5.7	6.0	6.3	6.7	7.1	7.4	7.8	8.2	8.5	8.8	9.1	9.3	9.5	9.6	9.7
	7.75	5.5	5.7	5.9	6.2	6.5	6.9	7.3	7.7	8.1	8.4	8.8	9.1	9.4	9.6	9.8	9.9	10.0
	8.00	5.8	5.9	6.2	6.4	6.8	7.1	7.5	7.9	8.3	8.7	9.0	9.3	9.6	9.8	10.0	10.1	10.2
	8.25	6.0	6.2	6.4	6.7	7.0	7.4	7.8	8.2	8.6	8.9	9.3	9.6	9.8	10.1	10.3	10.4	10.5
	8.50	6.3	6.4	6.6	6.9	7.3	7.6	8.0	8.4	8.8	9.2	9.5	9.8	10.1	10.3	10.3	10.6	10.7
	8.75	6.5	6.7	6.9	7.2	7.5	7.9	8.3	8.6	9.0	9.4	9.8	10.1	10.3	10.6	10.8	10.9	11.0
	9.00	6.8	6.9	7.1	7.4	7.7	8.1	8.5	8.9	9.3	9.6	10.0	10.3	10.6	10.8	11.0	11.1	11.2
	9.25	7.0	7.2	7.4	7.7	8.0	8.4	8.7	9.1	9.5	9.9	10.2	10.6	10.8	11.1	11.3	11.4	11.5
	9.50	7.3	7.4	7.6	7.9	8.2	8.6	9.0	9.4	9.8	10.1	10.5	10.8	11.1	11.3	11.5	11.6	11.7
	9.75	7.5	7.7	7.9	8.2	8.5	8.8	9.2	9.6	10.0	10.4	10.7	11.0	11.3	11.6	11.8	11.9	12.0
	10.00	7.8	7.9	8.1	8.4	8.7	9.1	9.5	9.9	10.3	10.6	11.0	11.3	11.6	11.8	12.0	12.1	12.2
2.50	2.50	0.4	0.9	1.3	1.7	2.1	2.5	2.9	3.2	3.5	3.8	4.1	4.3	4.5	4.7	4.8	4.9	5.0
	2.75	0.5	0.9	1.4	1.8	2.2	2.6	3.0	3.4	3.7	4.0	4.3	4.5	4.8	4.9	5.1	5.2	5.2
	3.00	0.7	1.1	1.5	1.9	2.4	2.8	3.2	3.6	3.9	4.2	4.5	4.8	5.0	5.2	5.3	5.4	5.5
	3.25	0.9	1.2	1.7	2.1	2.5	2.9	3.4	3.7	4.1	4.4	4.7	5.0	5.2	5.4	5.6	5.7	5.7
	3.50	1.1	1.4	1.8	2.3	2.7	3.1	3.5	3.9	4.3	4.6	4.9	5.2	5.5	5.6	5.8	5.9	6.0
	3.75	1.4	1.6	2.0	2.4	2.9	3.3	3.7	4.1	4.5	4.9	5.2	5.4	5.7	5.9	6.0	6.2	6.2
	4.00	1.6	1.9	2.2	2.6	3.1	3.5	3.9	4.3	4.7	5.1	5.4	5.7	5.9	6.1	6.3	6.4	6.5
	4.25	1.8	2.1	2.4	2.8	3.3	3.7	4.1	4.5	4.9	5.3	5.6	5.9	6.2	6.4	6.5	6.7	6.7
	4.50	2.1	2.3	2.6	3.0	3.5	3.9	4.3	4.8	5.1	5.5	5.8	6.1	6.4	6.6	6.8	6.9	7.0
	4.75	2.3	2.5	2.9	3.3	3.7	4.1	4.5	5.0	5.4	5.7	6.1	6.4	6.6	6.9	7.0	7.2	7.2
	5.00	2.6	2.8	3.1	3.5	3.9	4.3	4.8	5.2	5.6	6.0	6.3	6.6	6.9	7.1	7.3	7.4	7.5
	5.25	2.8	3.0	3.3	3.7	4.1	4.5	5.0	5.4	5.8	6.2	6.5	6.9	7.1	7.3	7.5	7.6	7.7
	5.50	3.1	3.3	3.6	3.9	4.3	4.8	5.2	5.6	6.0	6.4	6.8	7.1	7.4	7.6	7.8	7.9	8.0
	5.75	3.3	3.5	3.8	4.2	4.6	5.0	5.4	5.9	6.3	6.7	7.0	7.3	7.6	7.8	8.0	8.1	8.2
	6.00	3.6	3.7	4.0	4.4	4.8	5.2	5.7	6.1	6.5	6.9	7.2	7.6	7.8	8.1	8.3	8.4	8.5
	6.25	3.8	4.0	4.3	4.6	5.0	5.4	5.9	6.3	6.7	7.1	7.5	7.8	8.1	8.3	8.5	8.6	8.7
	6.50	4.1	4.2	4.5	4.9	5.3	5.7	6.1	6.5	7.0	7.4	7.7	8.0	8.3	8.6	8.8	8.9	9.0
	6.75	4.3	4.5	4.8	5.1	5.5	5.9	6.3	6.8	7.2	7.6	8.0	8.3	8.6	8.8	9.0	9.1	9.2
	7.00	4.6	4.7	5.0	5.3	5.7	6.1	6.6	7.0	7.4	7.8	8.2	8.5	8.8	9.1	9.2	9.4	9.5
	7.25	4.8	5.0	5.2	5.6	6.0	6.4	6.8	7.3	7.7	8.1	8.4	8.8	9.1	9.3	9.5	9.6	9.7
	7.50	5.1	5.2	5.5	5.8	6.2	6.6	7.0	7.5	7.9	8.3	8.7	9.0	9.3	9.6	9.7	9.9	10.0
	7.75	5.3	5.5	5.7	6.1	6.4	6.9	7.3	7.7	8.1	8.5	8.9	9.3	9.6	9.8	10.0	10.1	10.2
	8.00	5.6	5.7	6.0	6.3	6.7	7.1	7.5	8.0	8.4	8.8	9.2	9.5	9.8	10.0	10.2	10.4	10.5
	8.25	5.8	6.0	6.2	6.5	6.9	7.3	7.8	8.2	8.6	9.0	9.4	9.7	10.0	10.3	10.5	10.6	10.7
	8.50	6.1	6.2	6.5	6.8	7.2	7.6	8.0	8.4	8.9	9.3	9.6	10.0	10.3	10.5	10.7	10.9	11.0
	8.75	6.3	6.5	6.7	7.0	7.4	7.8	8.2	8.7	9.1	9.5	9.9	10.2	10.5	10.8	11.0	11.1	11.2
	9.00	6.6	6.7	6.9	7.3	7.6	8.0	8.5	8.9	9.3	9.8	10.1	10.5	10.8	11.0	11.2	11.4	11.5
	9.25	6.8	7.0	7.2	7.5	7.9	8.3	8.7	9.2	9.6	10.0	10.4	10.7	11.0	11.3	11.5	11.6	11.7
	9.50	7.1	7.2	7.4	7.8	8.1	8.5	9.0	9.4	9.8	10.2	10.6	11.0	11.3	11.5	11.7	11.9	12.0
	9.75	7.3	7.4	7.7	8.0	8.4	8.8	9.2	9.6	10.1	10.5	10.9	11.2	11.5	11.8	12.0	12.1	12.2
	10.00	7.6	7.7	7.9	8.2	8.6	9.0	9.4	9.9	10.3	10.7	11.1	11.5	11.8	12.0	12.2	12.4	12.5
2.75	2.75	0.5	1.0	1.4	1.9	2.3	2.8	3.2	3.5	3.9	4.2	4.5	4.8	5.0	5.2	5.3	5.4	5.5
	3.00	0.6	1.0	1.5	2.0	2.4	2.9	3.3	3.7	4.1	4.4	4.7	5.0	5.2	5.4	5.6	5.7	5.7
	3.25	0.7	1.2	1.6	2.1	2.6	3.0	3.5	3.9	4.3	4.6	4.9	5.2	5.4	5.6	5.8	5.9	6.0
	3.50	0.9	1.3	1.8	2.3	2.7	3.2	3.6	4.1	4.5	4.8	5.1	5.4	5.7	5.9	6.0	6.2	6.2
	3.75	1.1	1.5	1.9	2.4	2.9	3.4	3.8	4.2	4.7	5.0	5.4	5.7	5.9	6.1	6.3	6.4	6.5
	4.00	1.4	1.7	2.1	2.6	3.1	3.5	4.0	4.4	4.9	5.2	5.6	5.9	6.1	6.4	6.5	6.7	6.7
	4.25	1.6	1.9	2.3	2.8	3.3	3.7	4.2	4.6	5.1	5.4	5.8	6.1	6.4	6.6	6.8	6.9	7.0
	4.50	1.9	2.1	2.5	3.0	3.5	3.9	4.4	4.8	5.3	5.7	6.0	6.3	6.6	6.8	7.0	7.1	7.2
	4.75	2.1	2.4	2.7	3.2	3.7	4.1	4.6	5.1	5.5	5.9	6.2	6.6	6.8	7.1	7.3	7.4	7.5
	5.00	2.3	2.6	3.0	3.4	3.9	4.3	4.8	5.3	5.7	6.1	6.5	6.8	7.1	7.3	7.5	7.6	7.7
	5.25	2.6	2.8	3.2	3.6	4.1	4.5	5.0	5.5	5.9	6.3	6.7	7.0	7.3	7.6	7.8	7.9	8.0
	5.50	2.8	3.1	3.4	3.8	4.3	4.8	5.2	5.7	6.1	6.6	6.9	7.3	7.6	7.8	8.0	8.1	8.2
	5.75	3.1	3.3	3.6	4.0	4.5	5.0	5.5	5.9	6.4	6.8	7.2	7.5	7.8	8.1	8.2	8.4	8.5
	6.00	3.3	3.5	3.9	4.3	4.7	5.2	5.7	6.2	6.6	7.0	7.4	7.8	8.0	8.3	8.5	8.6	8.7
	6.25	3.6	3.8	4.1	4.5	5.0	5.4	5.9	6.4	6.8	7.3	7.6	8.0	8.3	8.5	8.7	8.9	9.0
	6.50	3.8	4.0	4.3	4.7	5.2	5.7	6.1	6.6	7.1	7.5	7.9	8.2	8.5	8.8	9.0	9.1	9.2
	6.75	4.1	4.3	4.6	5.0	5.4	5.9	6.4	6.8	7.3	7.7	8.1	8.5	8.8	9.0	9.2	9.4	9.5
	7.00	4.3	4.5	4.8	5.2	5.6	6.1	6.6	7.1	7.5	8.0	8.4	8.7	9.0	9.3	9.5	9.6	9.7
	7.25	4.6	4.8	5.1	5.4	5.9	6.3	6.8	7.3	7.8	8.2	8.6	8.9	9.3	9.5	9.7	9.9	10.0
	7.50	4.8	5.0	5.3	5.7	6.1	6.6	7.1	7.5	8.0	8.4	8.8	9.2	9.5	9.8	10.0	10.1	10.2
	7.75	5.1	5.3	5.5	5.9	6.3	6.8	7.3	7.8	8.2	8.7	9.1	9.4	9.7	10.0	10.2	10.4	10.5
	8.00	5.3	5.5	5.8	6.2	6.6	7.0	7.5	8.0	8.5	8.9	9.3	9.7	10.0	10.3	10.5	10.6	10.7
	8.25	5.6	5.7	6.0	6.4	6.8	7.3	7.8	8.2	8.7	9.1	9.5	9.9	10.2	10.5	10.7	10.9	11.0
	8.50	5.8	6.0	6.3	6.6	7.1	7.5	8.0	8.5	8.9	9.4	9.8	10.2	10.5	10.8	11.0	11.1	11.2
	8.75	6.1	6.2	6.5	6.9	7.3	7.8	8.2	8.7	9.2	9.6	10.0	10.4	10.7	11.0	11.2	11.4	11.5
	9.00	6.3	6.5	6.8	7.1	7.5	8.0	8.5	8.9	9.4	9.9	10.3	10.6	11.0	11.2	11.5	11.6	11.7
	9.25	6.6	6.7	7.0	7.4	7.8	8.2	8.7	9.2	9.7	10.1	10.5	10.9	11.2	11.5	11.7	11.9	12.0
	9.50	6.8	7.0	7.3	7.6	8.0	8.5	8.9	9.4	9.9	10.3	10.8	11.1	11.5	11.7	12.0	12.1	12.2
	9.75	7.1	7.2	7.5	7.8	8.3	8.7	9.2	9.7	10.1	10.6	11.0	11.4	11.7	12.0	12.2	12.4	12.5
	10.00	7.3	7.5	7.7	8.1	8.5	8.9	9.4	9.9	10.4	10.8	11.2	11.6	12.0	12.2	12.5	12.6	12.7
3.00	3.00	0.5	1.0	1.6	2.1	2.5	3.0	3.4	3.9	4.2	4.6	4.9	5.2	5.4	5.6	5.8	5.9	6.0
	3.25	0.6	1.1	1.6	2.2	2.7	3.1	3.6	4.0	4.4	4.8	5.1	5.4	5.7	5.9	6.0	6.2	6.2
	3.50	0.8	1.2	1.8	2.3	2.8	3.3	3.8	4.2	4.6	5.0	5.3	5.6	5.9	6.1	6.3	6.4	6.5
	3.75	1.0	1.4	1.9	2.4	2.9	3.4	3.9	4.4	4.8	5.2	5.5	5.9	6.1	6.3	6.5	6.6	6.7
	4.00	1.2	1.6	2.1	2.6	3.1	3.6	4.1	4.6	5.0	5.4	5.8	6.1	6.4	6.6	6.8	6.9	7.0
	4.25	1.4	1.8	2.2	2.7	3.3	3.8	4.3	4.8	5.2	5.6	6.0	6.3	6.6	6.8	7.0	7.1	7.2
	4.50	1.6	2.0	2.4	2.9	3.4	4.0	4.5	5.0	5.4	5.8	6.2	6.5	6.8	7.1	7.3	7.4	7.5
	4.75	1.9	2.2	2.6	3.1	3.6	4.2	4.7	5.2	5.6	6.0	6.4	6.8	7.1	7.3	7.5	7.6	7.7
	5.00	2.1	2.4	2.8	3.3	3.8	4.4	4.9	5.4	5.8	6.3	6.7	7.0	7.3	7.5	7.7	7.9	8.0
	5.25	2.4	2.6	3.0	3.5	4.0	4.6	5.1	5.6	6.0	6.5	6.9	7.2	7.5	7.8	8.0	8.1	8.2
	5.50	2.6	2.9	3.3	3.7	4.2	4.8	5.3	5.8	6.3	6.7	7.1	7.5	7.8	8.0	8.2	8.4	8.5
	5.75	2.8	3.1	3.5	4.0	4.5	5.0	5.5	6.0	6.5	6.9	7.3	7.7	8.0	8.3	8.5	8.6	8.7
	6.00	3.1	3.3	3.7	4.2	4.7	5.2	5.7	6.2	6.7	7.2	7.6	7.9	8.3	8.5	8.7	8.9	9.0
	6.25	3.3	3.6	3.9	4.4	4.9	5.4	5.9	6.4	6.9	7.4	7.8	8.2	8.5	8.8	9.0	9.1	9.2
	6.50	3.6	3.8	4.2	4.6	5.1	5.6	6.2	6.7	7.2	7.6	8.0	8.4	8.7	9.0	9.2	9.4	9.5
	6.75	3.8	4.1	4.4	4.9	5.3	5.9	6.4	6.9	7.4	7.8	8.3	8.6	9.0	9.3	9.5	9.6	9.7
	7.00	4.1	4.3	4.7	5.1	5.6	6.1	6.6	7.1	7.6	8.1	8.5	8.9	9.2	9.5	9.7	9.9	10.0
	7.25	4.3	4.5	4.9	5.3	5.8	6.3	6.8	7.3	7.8	8.3	8.7	9.1	9.5	9.7	10.0	10.1	10.2
	7.50	4.6	4.8	5.1	5.5	6.0	6.5	7.1	7.6	8.1	8.5	9.0	9.4	9.7	10.0	10.2	10.4	10.5
	7.75	4.8	5.0	5.4	5.8	6.3	6.8	7.3	7.8	8.3	8.8	9.2	9.6	9.9	10.2	10.5	10.6	10.7
	8.00	5.1	5.3	5.6	6.0	6.5	7.0	7.5	8.0	8.5	9.0	9.5	9.8	10.2	10.5	10.7	10.9	11.0
	8.25	5.3	5.5	5.8	6.3	6.7	7.2	7.8	8.3	8.8	9.3	9.7	10.1	10.4	10.7	11.0	11.1	11.2
	8.50	5.6	5.8	6.1	6.5	7.0	7.5	8.0	8.5	9.0	9.5	9.9	10.3	10.7	11.0	11.2	11.4	11.5
	8.75	5.8	6.0	6.3	6.7	7.2	7.7	8.2	8.7	9.3	9.7	10.2	10.6	10.9	11.2	11.4	11.6	11.7
	9.00	6.1	6.3	6.6	7.0	7.4	7.9	8.5	9.0	9.5	10.0	10.4	10.8	11.2	11.5	11.7	11.9	12.0
	9.25	6.3	6.5	6.8	7.2	7.7	8.2	8.7	9.2	9.7	10.2	10.7	11.1	11.4	11.7	11.9	12.1	12.2
	9.50	6.6	6.8	7.1	7.5	7.9	8.4	8.9	9.5	10.0	10.4	10.9	11.3	11.7	12.0	12.2	12.4	12.5
	9.75	6.8	7.0	7.3	7.7	8.2	8.6	9.2	9.7	10.2	10.7	11.1	11.5	11.9	12.2	12.4	12.6	12.7
	10.00	7.1	7.3	7.6	7.9	8.4	8.9	9.4	9.9	10.4	10.9	11.4	11.8	12.1	12.4	12.7	12.9	13.0
3.25	3.25	0.6	1.1	1.7	2.2	2.7	3.3	3.7	4.2	4.6	5.0	5.3	5.6	5.9	6.1	6.3	6.4	6.5
	3.50	0.6	1.2	1.8	2.3	2.9	3.4	3.9	4.3	4.8	5.2	5.5	5.8	6.1	6.3	6.5	6.6	6.7
	3.75	0.8	1.3	1.9	2.4	3.0	3.5	4.0	4.5	5.0	5.4	5.7	6.1	6.3	6.6	6.8	6.9	7.0
	4.00	1.0	1.5	2.0	2.6	3.1	3.7	4.2	4.7	5.2	5.6	6.0	6.3	6.6	6.8	7.0	7.1	7.2
	4.25	1.2	1.6	2.2	2.7	3.3	3.8	4.4	4.9	5.4	5.8	6.2	6.5	6.8	7.1	7.2	7.4	7.5
	4.50	1.4	1.8	2.3	2.9	3.5	4.0	4.6	5.1	5.6	6.0	6.4	6.7	7.0	7.3	7.5	7.6	7.7
	4.75	1.6	2.0	2.5	3.1	3.6	4.2	4.8	5.3	5.8	6.2	6.6	7.0	7.3	7.5	7.7	7.9	8.0

Figure 30-9

Tabular method of determining the vectoral change in astigmatism: (1) identify the lowest preoperative or postoperative keratometric or plus refractive cylinder power (D) in column K_1; (2) identify the highest preoperative or postoperative keratometric or plus refractive cylinder power (D) in column K_2; (3) identify the change in keratometric or refractive axis from K_1 to K_2 (degrees) along the top row; (4) find the number in the table at the intersection of these three values. It represents the vectoral change in astigmatism (D). (Courtesy Gary W. Hall, Michael Campion, and Robert R. McCulloch.)

Figure 30-9, cont'd
For legend see opposite page.

Minus Cylinder Correction
–5.00 –3.00 × 180°

Plus Cylinder Correction
–8.00 +3.00 × 90°

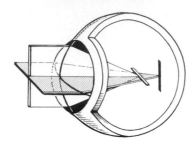
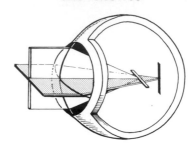

A, The refractive error can be written in minus cylinder or plus cylinder form.

Optical Correction of Sphere

–5.00 D sphere

–8.00 D sphere

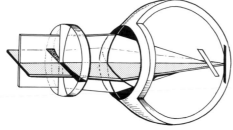
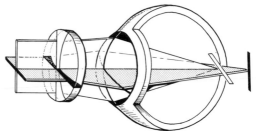

B, Optical correction commences with the correction of the sphere, which is
–5.00 D in the minus cylinder form and –8.00 D in the plus cylinder form.

Optical Correction of Astigmatism

–3.00 D × 180°

+3.00 D × 90°

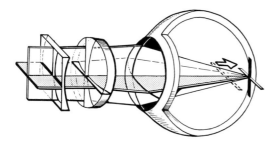
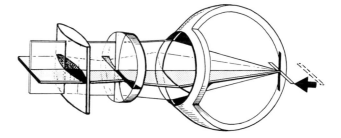

C, Optical correction of the astigmatism involves using a –3.00 D cylinder with
axis at 180° or a +3.00 D cylinder with axis at 90°; both collapse the conoid of
Sturm.

FIGURE 30-10, CONT'D

Surgical Correction of Sphere
Radial Keratotomy

Correct –5.00 D sphere

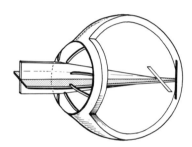

Correct –8.00 D sphere

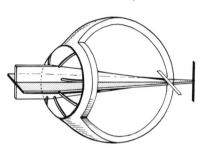

D, Surgical correction of the sphere by radial keratotomy corrects −5.00 D in the minus cylinder form and −8.00 D in the plus cylinder form.

Surgical Correction of Astigmatism
Transverse Keratotomy

Correct –3.00 D × 90°

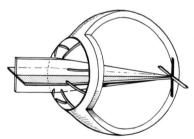

None

E, Because keratotomy can only flatten a meridian and because there are no surgical methods to reliably steepen a meridian, the residual 3.00 D of astigmatism can be corrected using only the minus cylinder refraction.

UNFINISHED BUSINESS

The biggest challenges facing the clinician concerning corneal astigmatism are to measure regular and irregular astigmatism accurately and to use these measurements as a guide to more accurate surgical and optical correction. This is particularly important for irregular astigmatism resulting from both disease and surgery. Even if accurate measures of overall corneal topography including measures of surface irregularity, were developed, the challenge remains to use these as a basis for planning surgery, whether it be astigmatic keratotomy, photorefractive keratectomy, or some future form of creating aspheric corneal surfaces.

There is a need to include vectoral analysis of astigmatism in reports of refractive surgery.

REFERENCES

1. Agapitos PJ, Lindstrom RL, Williams PA, and Sanders DR: Analysis of astigmatic keratotomy, J Cataract Refract Surg 1989;5:13-18.
2. Bennett AG and Rabbets RB: Clinical visual optics, London, 1984, Butterworth & Co, pp 92-93.
3. Binder PS: Reduction of postkeratoplasty astigmatism by selective suture removal, Dev Ophthalmol 1985;11:86-90.
4. Binder PS: The surgical correction of astigmatism. In Caldwell D, editor: Symposium on the cornea and refractive corneal surgery. Transactions of the New Orleans Academy of Ophthalmology, New York, 1987, Raven Press, pp 1-19.
5. Binder PS: The effect of suture removal on postkeratoplasty astigmatism, Am J Ophthalmol 1988;105:637-645.
6. Campbell CJ, Koester CJ, Rittler MC, et al: Physiological optics, Hagerstown, Md, 1974, Harper & Row.
7. Datiles MB and Gancayco T: Low myopia with low astigmatic correction gives cataract surgery patients good depth of focus, Ophthalmology 1990;97:922-926.
8. Dingeldein SA, Klyce SD, and Wilson SE: Quantitative descriptors of corneal shape derived from computer-assisted analysis of photokeratographs, Refract Corneal Surg 1989;5:372-378.
9. Donders FC: On the anomalies of accommodation and refraction of the eye, Boston, 1864, Milford House, pp 539-543 (Translated by WD Moore).
10. Fulton AB, Hanson RM, and Peterson RA: The relation of myopia and astigmatism in developing eyes, Ophthalmology 1982;89:298-302.
11. Guyton DL: Prescribing cylinders: the problem of distortion, Surv Ophthalmol 1977;22:177-188.
12. Holladay JT, et al: Optics, refraction and contact lenses. In the American Academy of Ophthalmology: basic clinical and science course, section II, San Francisco, 1986, The Academy.
13. Huber C: Myopic astigmatism, a substitute for accommodation in pseudophakia, Doc Ophthalmol 1981;52:123-178.
14. Huber C: Planned myopic astigmatism as a substitute for accommodation in pseudophakia, J Am Intraocular Implant Soc 1981;7:244-249.
15. Jaffe NS, Jaffe MS, and Jaffe GE: Cataract surgery and its complications, ed 5, St Louis, 1990, The CV Mosby Co, pp 109-127.
16. Levine JR: Clinical refraction in visual science, London, 1977, Butterworth & Co, pp 203-288.
17. Maloney RK, Bogan SJ, and Waring GO: Determination of corneal refractive properties from corneal topography (unpublished data).
18. Merck MP, Williams PA, Lindstrom RL: Trapezoidal keratotomy: a vector analysis, Ophthalmology 1986;93:719-726.
19. Michaels DD: Visual optics and refraction: a clinical approach, ed 3, St Louis, 1985, The CV Mosby Co.
19a. Naylor EJ: Astigmatic difference in refractive errors, Br J Ophthalmol 1968; 52:422-425.
20. Neumann AC, McCarty GR, Sanders DR, and Raanan MG: Refractive evaluation of astigmatic keratotomy procedures, J Cataract Refract Surg 1989;15: 25-31.
21. Rubin ML: Optics for clinicians, Gainesville, Fla, 1971, Triad Scientific Publishers.
22. Teikari JM and O'Donnell JJ: Astigmatism in 72 twin pairs, Cornea 1989; 8:263-266.
23. Thornton SP: Astigmatic keratotomy: a review of basic concepts with case reports, J Cataract Refract Surg 1990;16: 430-435.
24. Tscherning M: Physiologic optics, ed 3, Philadelphia, 1920, Keystone Publishing Co, pp 164-175 (Translated by C Welland).
25. Wilson SE and Klyce SD: Quantitative descriptors of corneal topography: a clinical study, Arch Ophthalmol 1991; 109:349-353.

Keratotomy for Astigmatism

Perry S. Binder
George O. Waring III

The surgical correction of astigmatism motivated the development of refractive keratotomy both for nineteenth century surgeons and for Sato and his colleagues in the early 1940s (See Chapter 5, Development of Refractive Keratotomy in the Nineteenth Century, and Chapter 6, Development of Radial Keratotomy in Japan, 1939-1960). The surgical correction of other spherical ametropias followed later. As of 1991 there was general consensus on the principles and practice of radial keratotomy for myopia, but development of keratotomy for astigmatism was in earlier stages; in addition, considerable difference in opinion existed about surgical techniques and patterns of astigmatic keratotomy.

Both Chapter 3, Optics and Topography of Radial Keratotomy, and Chapter 30, Optics and Topography of Corneal Astigmatism, outline basic concepts and principles, and we assume that the reader is familiar with this information. Chapter 32, Atlas of Astigmatic Keratotomy, spells out the specific details of surgical techniques now used in clinical practice. Many of the principles and precepts of keratotomy for astigmatism described in this chapter are also mentioned in a different context in Chapter 33, Biomechanics of Transverse Incisions of the Cornea, and Chapter 34, Computer Simulation of Arcuate Keratotomy for Astigmatism.

BACKGROUND AND ACKNOWLEDGMENTS

The information presented in this chapter is drawn from the published literature and our own experience. Dr. Binder's work comes from the Ophthalmology Research Laboratory, Sharp Cabrillo Hospital, La Jolla, California, and was sponsored in part by a grant from the National Vision Research Institute, San Diego, California, and National Eye Institute Grant No. EY0457-06. Individuals who have made specific contributions are cited throughout the text. The Prospective Evaluation of Astigmatic Keratotomy (PEAK) Study Group, which consisted of approximately 30 individuals who met biannually from 1987 to 1990, contributed much of the thinking of this chapter. We are particularly indebted to Drs. Richard Lindstrom, Peter Agapitos, Peter McDonnell, Alan Sugar, Stephen Klyce, and Marguerite McDonald for their contributions in the PEAK Study Group. Drs. Spencer Thornton and Albert Neumann provided considerable personal experience and counsel in addition to clinical data. Dr. Robert Maloney prepared the material on vector analysis. Dr. Osama Ibrahim provided research and personal material on trapezoidal keratotomy.

Some Causes of Corneal Astigmatism

I. Regular astigmatism
  A. Naturally occurring
    1. Acquired
    2. Inherited
  B. Postoperative—surgical procedure
    1. Circular corneal wound
      a. Penetrating keratoplasty
      b. Keratomileusis
      c. Epikeratoplasty
      d. Lamellar keratoplasty
      e. Intracorneal lens
    2. Linear corneal wound
      a. Cataract surgery
      b. Radial and transverse keratotomy
      c. Accidental corneal laceration
    3. No corneal wound
      a. Scleral buckle
      b. Extraocular muscle surgery
  C. Postoperative—mechanisms
    1. Tight suture, tissue resection
      a. Tissue compression or removal
      b. Steeper meridian created
    2. Loose suture, wound separation, keratotomy
      a. Wound gape
      b. Flatter meridian created
    3. Asymmetric tissue distribution, wound volume, or healing from cataract or corneal surgery

II. Irregular astigmatism—selected examples
  A. Irregular corneal surface
    1. Corneal edema
    2. Keratoconjunctivitis sicca
    3. Subepithelial scarring
    4. Others
  B. Central or paracentral corneal thinning
    1. Keratoconus
    2. Pellucid degeneration
    3. Others
  C. Marginal corneal thinning
    1. Terrien's degeneration
    2. Rheumatic keratopathy
    3. Mooren's ulcer
    4. Others
  D. Accidental corneal trauma
    1. Lacerations
    2. Chemical burns
  E. External pressure on cornea
    1. Contact lens warpage
    2. Eyelid mass
    3. Eye rubbing
    4. Others

III. Combined regular and irregular astigmatism
  A. Penetrating keratoplasty
  B. Lamellar refractive keratoplasty

In this chapter we summarize the published literature on keratotomy for naturally occurring and postoperative astigmatism, emphasizing general clinical principles, comparing different surgical techniques, presenting published results, and suggesting guidelines for planning astigmatic keratotomy.

Other authors have reviewed corneal surgery for astigmatism. Barner[13] surveyed the history of treating astigmatism surgically. Rowsey[143,144] emphasized basic principles of corneal curvature associated with corneal incisions and has applied some of these principles in a review of astigmatism surgery. Swinger[163] and Binder[22] have extensively reviewed different surgical techniques for managing postoperative astigmatism. Nordan[131,132] has spelled out his personal concepts underlying astigmatic keratotomy and corneal asphericity. Lindquist and colleagues[101] and Lindstrom[103] have described the overall principles of astigmatic keratotomy and recommended specific nomograms. Thornton[170,172] has discussed the concept of coupling and related his results for naturally occurring astigmatism. Much of the material these authors present on keratotomy for astigmatism has been incorporated into this chapter.

Some of the causes of corneal astigmatism are outlined in the box above. It is particularly important to separate these clinical categories when studying the results of keratotomy for astigmatism. The different categories and types of astigmatism should not be lumped together when reporting the results of surgery.

Methods of managing astigmatism are outlined in the box on p. 1087. The methods of keratotomy surgery are amplified in detail throughout this chapter.

Methods of Management of Astigmatism

I. Optical correction of astigmatism
  A. Spectacles[125]
  B. Contact lenses[47]
    1. Spheric or aspheric; rigid gas permeable (RGP) or soft
    2. Toric
    3. Piggyback RGP and soft[156]
    4. Concentric RGP in soft carrier
    5. Soft with spectacle overcorrection[47]
    6. Orthokeratology*[16]
II. Surgical correction of astigmatism
  A. Intraoperative manipulation of suture and wound
    1. Wound placement, configuration, approximation
    2. Suture location, length, tension
  B. Postoperative suture adjustment
    1. Selective removal of interrupted sutures
    2. Distribution of tension on running sutures
    3. Addition of sutures
    4. Removal of all sutures
  C. Postoperative wound revision (limbal, corneal)
    1. Open, realign, and resuture

  2. Relaxing incision in wound, with or without compression sutures
  3. Wedge resection
  4. Combination with keratotomy
  D. Transverse keratotomy
    1. Straight or arcuate incision (relaxing incision)
    2. Combined transverse and radial incisions
    3. Combined transverse and semiradial incisions (trapezoidal)
    4. Simultaneous transverse incisions and cataract surgery
  E. Repeat penetrating keratoplasty
  F. Radial and arcuate thermal stromal collagen shrinkage (thermokeratoplasty)
    1. Hot wire in stroma
    2. Intrastromal holmium YAG laser
  G. Partial thickness corneal trephination and suturing
  H. Lamellar astigmatic refractive keratoplasty*
    1. Toric keratomileusis
    2. Toric epikeratoplasty
    3. Toric intracorneal lens
  I. Photorefractive keratectomy
    1. Transverse keratectomy
    2. Astigmatic laser surface area ablation

*Techniques not currently in clinical use.

SELECTION OF PATIENTS

Patients who are candidates for astigmatic keratotomy are those who cannot achieve an acceptable level of visual function with spectacles or contact lenses or who do not want to depend on these optical devices. The principles of patient selection are enunciated in Section III, Patient Selection and Planning for Refractive Keratotomy, and are not repeated here.

PRINCIPLES OF ASTIGMATIC KERATOTOMY

The basic principles of astigmatic keratotomy apply to all types of astigmatism; specific subtleties in each group require special attention, as described subsequently.

1. Keratotomy for astigmatism is placed in the steep corneal meridian, which is the meridian that is parallel to the plus cylinder refraction axis, that has the greatest power on central keratometry, and that crosses the short direction of the ellipse seen on keratography (Fig. 31-1).
2. Planning for astigmatic keratotomy is done on the basis of the minus cylinder refraction, which helps the surgeon conceptualize the focal lines of the conoid of Sturm within the vitreous and move them back toward the retina by flattening the cornea; this also allows consideration of the effect of keratotomy on the spherical component of the refraction (Fig. 31-2).
3. Transverse incisions across the steep meridian will flatten that meridian and steepen the unincised meridian 90° away—the coupling effect. In general, the longer the transverse incision, the greater the steepening 90° away, until an arc length of 100° to 120° is reached (Fig. 31-3).

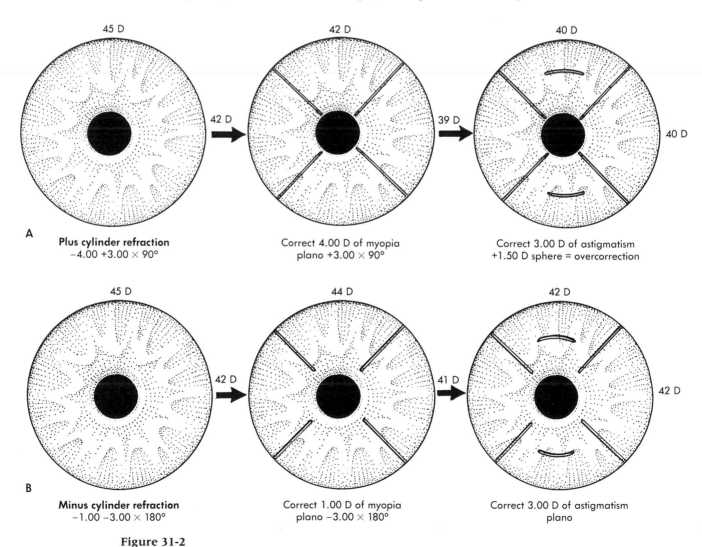

Figure 31-1

Analogy of the surgical correction of astigmatism. Consider an astigmatic cornea to be like a football, with a steep meridian perpendicular to the laces and a flat meridian parallel to the laces. To convert the football to a basketball, the surgeon can "tighten the tip" by doing a wedge resection or applying tight sutures, or "loosen the laces" by doing a transverse keratotomy. (Courtesy Dr. James Gills.)

A

45 D

42 D

Plus cylinder refraction
−4.00 +3.00 × 90°

42 D

39 D

Correct 4.00 D of myopia
plano +3.00 × 90°

40 D

40 D

Correct 3.00 D of astigmatism
+1.50 D sphere = overcorrection

B

45 D

42 D

Minus cylinder refraction
−1.00 −3.00 × 180°

44 D

41 D

Correct 1.00 D of myopia
plano −3.00 × 180°

42 D

42 D

Correct 3.00 D of astigmatism
plano

Figure 31-2

Demonstration of the advantage for calculating astigmatism surgery based on the minus cylinder refraction. **A,** If the calculations are done on the basis of the plus cylinder refraction, residual hyperopia occurs with no reasonable surgical way to correct it. **B,** If the calculations are done on the basis of the minus cylinder refraction, both focal lines of the conoid of Sturm can be moved from the vitreous to the retina with an emmetropic result.

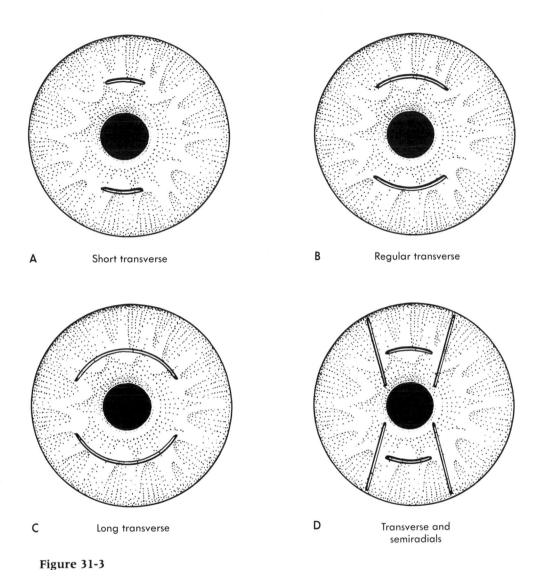

A   Short transverse   B   Regular transverse

C   Long transverse   D   Transverse and
                                  semiradials

Figure 31-3
Relationship of the length of transverse incisions to the flattening/steepening ratio (coupling phenomenon). **A,** Short incisions flatten the incised meridian more than they steepen the unincised orthogonal meridian; the flattening/steepening ratio is greater than 1. **B,** Medium length incisions produce an equal amount of flattening of the incised meridian and steepening of the unincised meridian; the flattening/steepening ratio is 1. **C,** Long incisions flatten both the incised and the unincised meridians, the incised meridian more than the unincised; the flattening/steepening ratio is greater than 1. **D,** Combined transverse and semiradial incisions (trapezoidal, Ruiz) produce much more flattening in the incised meridian than in the orthogonal unincised meridian; the flattening/steepening ratio is greater than 1 but becomes smaller as the transverse incisions become longer. There is great variability in the coupling ratio for all techniques.

4. Semiradial incisions flatten both the parallel operated meridian and the meridian 90° away (Fig. 31-3).

5. In general, transverse incisions closer to the center of the cornea (that is, a smaller diameter clear "optical" zone) produce greater change in astigmatism.

6. More than two pairs of transverse incisions across the same meridian do not significantly increase the amount of change in astigmatism.

7. The depth of a transverse incision should not exceed approximately 80% of the corneal thickness to prevent excessive uplift of the central edge of the incision.

8. As emphasized throughout this book, reports of astigmatic keratotomy should present not only average results, but also standard deviations, ranges, percentage of eyes with specific amounts of residual astigmatism, scattergrams, and vectoral analysis—all designed to depict the clinical reality of the results and the relative variability and predictability of the outcome. A mere recitation of data is insufficient. Analytic interpretation, clarifying discussion, and graphic summaries are all necessary to make sense out of a subject as complex as astigmatic keratotomy.

CLASSIFICATION OF ASTIGMATIC KERATOTOMY

In this section we discuss the different patterns of keratotomy for astigmatism. In subsequent sections we discuss the variables that affect the outcome and the laboratory and clinical studies that have been reported.

The box below lists the techniques of keratotomy for astigmatism. Figure 31-4 presents a simplified pictorial classification of the techniques.

Classification of Keratotomy Techniques for Correction of Astigmatism

I. Transverse incisions perpendicular to the steep meridian (T-cuts, tangential incisions)
   A. Isolated (bare) transverse incisions (Bates, Lans, Sato)
      1. Patterns
         a. Straight or arcuate
         b. Single or multiple
         c. Symmetric or asymmetric
      2. Clinical indications—type of astigmatism
         a. Naturally occurring
         b. After cataract surgery
         c. Combined with small incision cataract surgery
   B. Arcuate keratotomy after penetrating keratoplasty (relaxing incisions) (Troutman, Krachmer)
      1. In wound
      2. In donor
      3. With or without compression sutures in flat meridian
II. Combined transverse and radial incisions
   A. Transverse incisions between radials, one or two pair (Lans, Thornton)

   B. Nonintersecting, interrupted incisions
      1. Interrupted transverse incisions
         a. Jump-T (one or two pair)
         b. Jump staggered T (Hofmann)
      2. Interrupted radial incisions (jump radial) (Mallinger, Nordan)
      3. Transverse incisions across end of short radial incisions (end-T) (Arrowsmith)
III. Grouped incisions parallel to steep meridian*
   A. Parallel radial incisions (L, RL, Fyodorov)*
   B. Fan-shaped semiradial incisions (Binder, Azar)*
IV. Variable length radial incisions (oval clear zone with longer incisions in steep meridian, R procedure) (Sato, Fyodorov)*
V. Deep circular keratotomy with sutures (trephination) (Krumeich)
VI. Delimiting keratotomy after accidental corneal trauma
   A. Incision central and parallel to corneal scar
   B. Incision perpendicular to steep meridian
VII. Scleral incisions or excisions (Barraquer)*

*Techniques not currently in use.

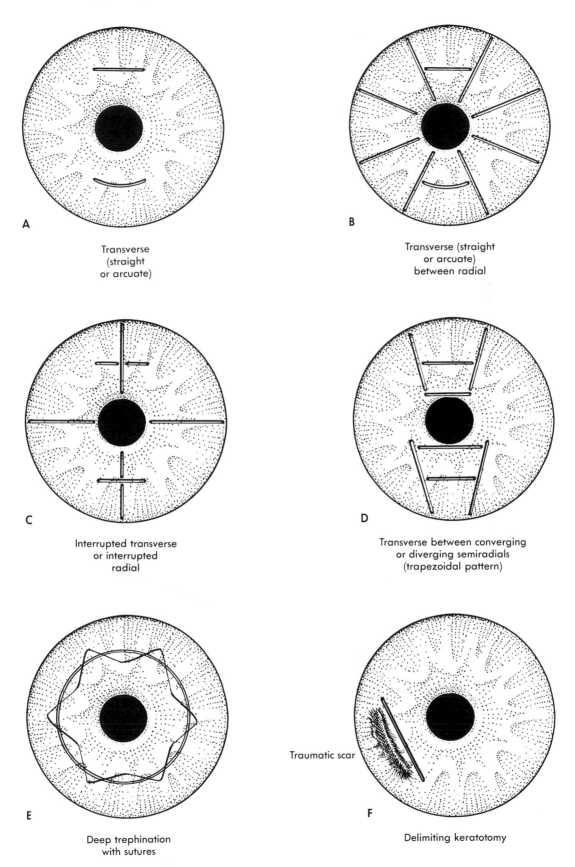

A

Transverse
(straight
or arcuate)

B

Transverse (straight
or arcuate)
between radial

C

Interrupted transverse
or interrupted
radial

D

Transverse between converging
or diverging semiradials
(trapezoidal pattern)

E

Deep trephination
with sutures

F

Traumatic scar

Delimiting keratotomy

Figure 31-4
A-F, Classification of keratotomy for astigmatism into six general patterns that are in
clinical use in 1991.

Transverse incisions perpendicular to the steep meridian

Transverse incisions perpendicular to the steep meridian have been the cornerstone for the surgical correction of astigmatism for almost a century, since they were first described by Bates and Lans, studied by Sato, and "rediscovered" by American surgeons after a brief detour with the use of grouped radial incisions and oval optical zones (see Section II, Development of Refractive Keratotomy). The incisions are made perpendicular to the steep meridian and are properly called "transverse incisions," indicating that they cut across the steep meridian. They also have been called "tangential incisions," because they are made tangent to a circular zone, and, colloquially, "T-cuts."

A transverse incision may be straight or arcuate, both being transverse to the steep meridian (Fig. 31-5).

Transverse incisions alone are commonly used to treat naturally occurring astigmatism, astigmatism after penetrating keratoplasty (relaxing incisions), and astigmatism associated with cataract surgery. The number of incisions ranges from one in a single semimeridian to four (one pair in each semimeridian).

Figure 31-6 illustrates different patterns of isolated transverse incisions. A single incision is usually made superiorly beneath the upper lid. One pair of incisions is used most commonly. The basis for asymmetric incisions is questionable and will require a detailed analysis of corneal topography to see if asymmetric incisions can correct semimeridional astigmatism. Incisions in the limbus or sclera have less effect on the central cornea than those made within the cornea itself; their clinical use is questionable.

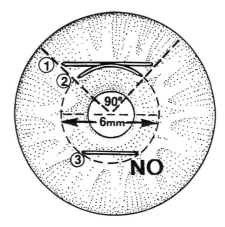

Figure 31-5

Two types of transverse incisions reduce astigmatism: straight linear transverse incisions and arcuate linear transverse incisions. The location is defined in terms of the circular zone (clear zone, optical zone); the zone mark is described in terms of its diameter (6 mm); and the location of the incision is described in terms of the zone radius (3 mm from the center). *1,* The straight transverse incision is made tangential to the circular zone mark and is measured in millimeters. *2,* The arcuate transverse incision is made along the circular zone mark and is measured in degrees. *3,* Transverse incisions are not placed across the chord of the delimiting circular zone.

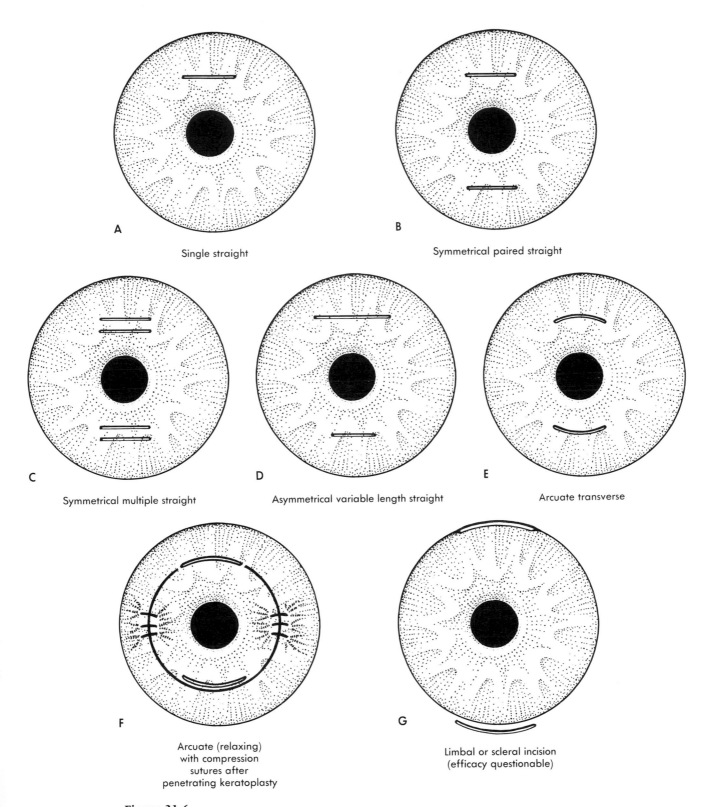

A — Single straight

B — Symmetrical paired straight

C — Symmetrical multiple straight

D — Asymmetrical variable length straight

E — Arcuate transverse

F — Arcuate (relaxing) with compression sutures after penetrating keratoplasty

G — Limbal or scleral incision (efficacy questionable)

Figure 31-6
A-E, Patterns of isolated straight or arcuate transverse ("T") incisions made perpendicular to the steep meridian (90°). **F,** The pattern includes arcuate relaxing incisions for astigmatism after penetrating keratoplasty. **G,** Limbal or scleral incisions are less effective.

Combined transverse and radial or semiradial incisions

Three basic combined patterns are currently in use (Fig. 31-7; see Fig. 31-9):

1. Transverse incisions between radial incisions
2. Transverse incisions between semiradial incisions (trapezoidal, Ruiz)
3. Interrupted transverse incisions (jump-T, flags) or interrupted radial incisions (jump radial)

Each of these three patterns has a complex set of interactions, particularly when considering the coupling phenomenon—flattening of the incised meridian and the steepening of the unincised meridian 90° away.

Further comparative studies are necessary to decide which of these patterns (Fig. 31-7) is preferable and to identify the differences and subtleties that affect the outcome. Placing the transverse incisions between radial incisions probably has overall less effect on astigmatism than interrupting either the transverse or the radial, where both are placed in the steep meridian.

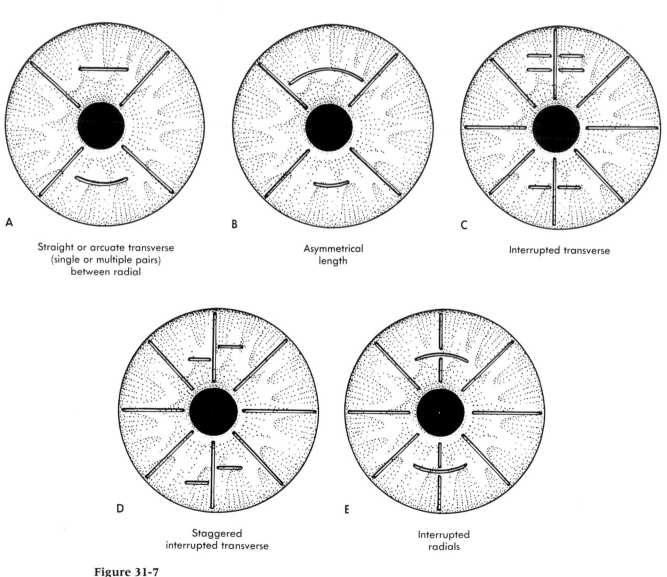

A Straight or arcuate transverse (single or multiple pairs) between radial

B Asymmetrical length

C Interrupted transverse

D Staggered interrupted transverse

E Interrupted radials

Figure 31-7
Combined radial incisions and transverse ("T") incisions in the steep meridian (90°) to reduce astigmatism. There are three general categories. **A-E,** Nonintersecting incisions are used most commonly.

Continued.

Intersecting incisions. During the development of astigmatic keratotomy, Sato, Fyodorov, and American surgeons used intersecting transverse and radial incisions in a variety of patterns. Unfortunately, it took many years and hundreds of damaged corneas for surgeons to realize that intersecting incisions create excessive wound gape, with persistence of a large epithelial plug, anterior displacement of the corners of the wounds, delayed wound healing, accentuated scarring, and a mechanically unstable cornea. Fenzl[58] introduced the concept of the flag incisions, with intersection only on one side of the radial wound, to reduce these problems, which can also be treated by opening and suturing the wounds to achieve more rapid wound healing and a better surface contour.

Hofmann[76] demonstrated that intersecting transverse and radial or semiradial incisions tended to produce an unstable cornea, with a gradual progression of effect over 9 months (Fig. 31-8). On this basis he abandoned intersecting the incisions and recommended a minimum of 0.2 mm between the end of a transverse incision and a radial incision.

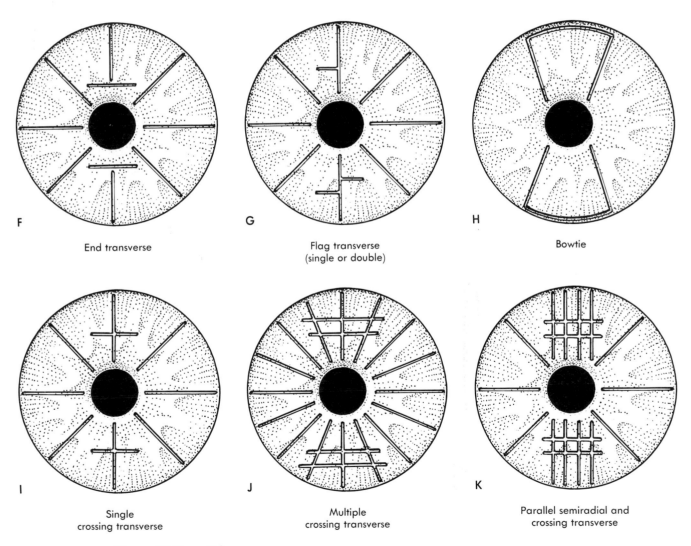

F — End transverse

G — Flag transverse
(single or double)

H — Bowtie

I — Single
crossing transverse

J — Multiple
crossing transverse

K — Parallel semiradial and
crossing transverse

Figure 31-7 cont'd
F-H, These three patterns of incisions are used rarely. **I-K,** Crossing incisions are not in clinical use.

Figure 31-8

Instability of refraction after three types of intersecting incisions (x-axis): intersecting radial and single transverse, intersecting radial and double transverse, and intersecting trapezoidal (Ruiz). The unstable continued effect of the surgery is shown at 3, 6, and 9 months in terms of the mean increase in the net vector-corrected refractive astigmatism (y-axis). This is one reason that crossing incisions are no longer used. (From Hofmann RF: The surgical correction of idiopathic astigmatism. In Sanders DR, Hofmann RF, and Salz JJ, editors: Refractive corneal surgery, Thorofare, NJ, 1986, Slack, Inc.)

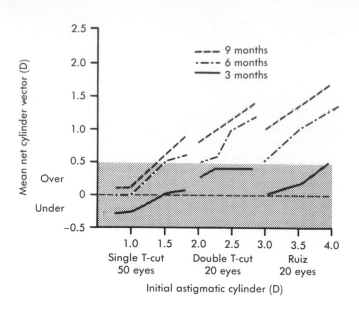

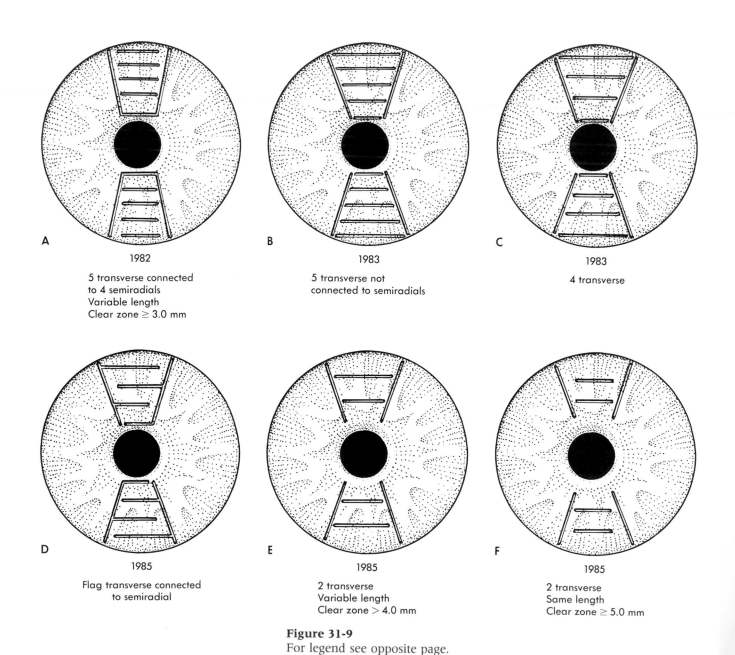

A 1982

5 transverse connected
to 4 semiradials
Variable length
Clear zone ≥ 3.0 mm

B 1983

5 transverse not
connected to semiradials

C 1983

4 transverse

D 1985

Flag transverse connected
to semiradial

E 1985

2 transverse
Variable length
Clear zone > 4.0 mm

F 1985

2 transverse
Same length
Clear zone ≥ 5.0 mm

Figure 31-9
For legend see opposite page.

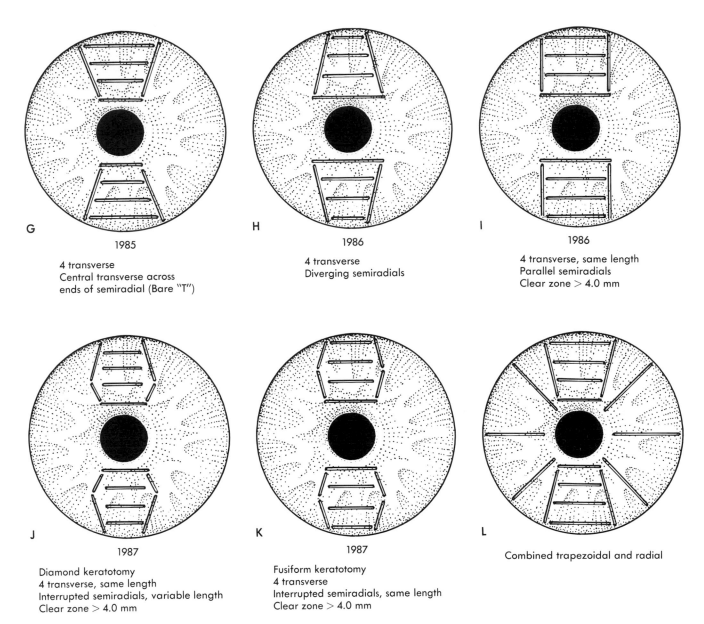

G 1985

4 transverse
Central transverse across
ends of semiradial (Bare "T")

H 1986

4 transverse
Diverging semiradials

I 1986

4 transverse, same length
Parallel semiradials
Clear zone > 4.0 mm

J 1987

Diamond keratotomy
4 transverse, same length
Interrupted semiradials, variable length
Clear zone > 4.0 mm

K 1987

Fusiform keratotomy
4 transverse
Interrupted semiradials, same length
Clear zone > 4.0 mm

L

Combined trapezoidal and radial

Figure 31-9
Development of trapezoidal keratotomy. **A,** The original procedure described in 1982 by Ruiz called for five pairs of transverse incisions, the inner incisions connecting to the semiradial incisions. **B,** The first modification of the procedure consisted of not connecting the transverse and semiradial incisions. **C,** The number of transverse incisions was reduced from five pairs to four pairs. **D,** The transverse incisions touched the semiradial incisions to form "flag" incisions. **E,** The number of transverse incisions was decreased to two pairs. **F,** Shortening the semiradial incisions and more peripheral placement of the transverse incisions to decrease glare. **G,** The innermost transverse incisions were placed across the ends of the semiradial incisions for greater effect. **H,** Diverging semiradial incisions created greater steepening of the orthogonal unincised meridian. **I,** The use of parallel "corridor" incisions in an attempt to stabilize the effect of the surgery. **J** and **K,** Diamond and fusiform keratotomies with short transverse incisions flatten the incised meridian with minimal change in the unincised meridian. **L,** Combined trapezoidal and radial keratotomy for compound myopic astigmatism. (Modified from Ruiz LA: The astigmatic keratotomies (Ruiz procedures). In Boyd B, editor: Highlights of ophthalmology, vol 2, Refractive surgery with the masters, Coral Gables, Fla, 1987, Highlights of Ophthalmology.)

The uplift of tissue from intersecting incisions is used to advantage in the bow tie pattern of Tate, in which a peripheral arcuate keratotomy is connected to two semiradial keratotomies. This produces an intentional uplift of the cornea peripherally to flatten the incised meridian. Most surgeons avoid intersection of corneal incisions.

Trapezoidal keratotomy. Trapezoidal keratotomy has evolved through a number of patterns (Fig. 31-9). Ruiz initially performed a large number of cases with intersecting transverse and semiradial incisions, but this technique was abandoned when other surgeons found it created the wound healing problems described above. Nordan[131] advocated making the incisions 90% deep instead of the original 80% made by Ruiz. Fenzl[58] modified the procedure by disconnecting the transverse and semiradial incisions, and Ellis[56] suggested joining one end of the transverse incision to the semiradial incision, creating a series of "flag" incisions. The next development was to enlarge the diameter of the clear zone to reduce glare, and, on the basis of the laboratory experiments of Lindquist and colleagues[96,97,102] to reduce the number of transverse incisions from five pairs to approximately two pairs. Thereafter the central transverse incision was placed across the ends of the semiradial incisions for greater effect and to allow adjustment of the length of the transverse incisions to modulate the coupling ratio.[145] The overall pattern has been again modified by Ruiz: for simple myopic astigmatism, a diamond or fusiform pattern with short transverse incisions; for compound myopic astigmatism, converging semiradial incisions; and for mixed astigmatism or hyperopic astigmatism, an inverted pattern of diverging semiradial incisions with longer paracentral incisions. One optic theory for these patterns is discussed in the next section. No comparative clinical studies of these patterns have been published. Presently, tapezoidal incisions are limited to a few selected cases.

Grouped radial incisions and oval clear zone

Modification of the pattern of the radial incisions themselves has not proven effective in the management of astigmatism (Fig. 31-10). The concept of making multiple parallel semiradial incisions or a group of fan-shaped radial incisions along the steeper meridian to cause greater flattening is theoretically appealing but not clinically effective.[62] Similarly the idea of making longer incisions in the steeper meridian (oval "optical zone")[63] does not produce enough differential flattening of the cornea to meaningfully decrease astigmatism. These methods have been abandoned.

Circular and delimiting keratotomy

Making a deep partial thickness circular trephination and then suturing the cornea in place has been described by Krumeich[91] in an attempt to let the natural forces of the cornea produce a rounded shape and eliminate astigmatism.

Creating a single linear delimiting keratotomy just inside a traumatic scar may separate the distorting effect of the scar from the central cornea, allowing the central cornea to round up and decrease astigmatism.[143,144]

Scleral surgery

Surgery outside the limbus to alter astigmatism, in the form of sclerotomies to flatten the cornea or scleral resections to steepen the cornea, is minimally effective because the limbus acts as a mechanical boundary for the cornea and greatly reduces the effect of remote scleral surgery on the central cornea. There is little published literature on these techniques except for Arciniegas and Amaya's[3] scleral fold, resection, and imbrication in rabbits and Barraquer's[14] scleral resection.

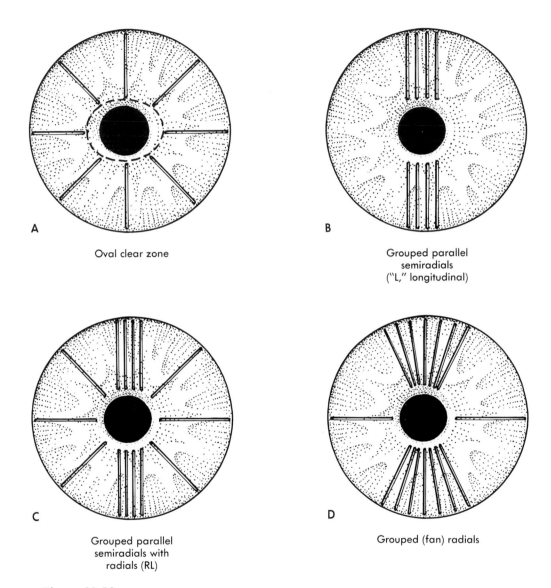

A — Oval clear zone

B — Grouped parallel
semiradials
("L," longitudinal)

C — Grouped parallel
semiradials with
radials (RL)

D — Grouped (fan) radials

Figure 31-10
A-D, Patterns of radial incisions grouped in the steep meridian are not now in clinical use.

COMPARATIVE STUDIES OF TECHNIQUES OF ASTIGMATIC KERATOTOMY
Evaluation of astigmatic keratotomy

The creativity of ophthalmic surgeons in designing patterns of keratotomy for astigmatism has been as varied as the multitude of designs of intraocular lenses for cataract surgery. One of the difficulties in interpreting the published literature is that some papers describe a combination of procedures used for a combination of etiologies, making it impossible to determine the effectiveness of a given technique for a given indication. For example, Agapitos and colleagues[1] described six different astigmatic keratotomy procedures for three different indications, making it difficult to determine the results of each technique in each disorder.

The challenge of quantitatively evaluating surgical techniques is made more difficult by their informal promulgation in a series of cases without laboratory evaluation or careful clinical analysis. Indeed, much of astigmatic surgery has developed in the confusing stages of trial-and-error refinement and informal case series (see Chapter 4, Development and Classification of Refractive Surgical Procedures). Many of the early patterns of keratotomy—including the parallel "L" and intersecting "TL" techniques of Fyodorov, the intersecting trapezoidal incisions of Ruiz, the oval optical zone, and the intersecting flag techniques—were once touted as the accepted norm for astigmatic correction and have now been abandoned because of complications or ineffectiveness.[76,130] This kind of sporadic clinical application of untested procedures should make ophthalmologists critical when they hear that a new technique "works well in the hands" of another surgeon. Originators of such techniques must responsibly compile and publish their experimental and clinical results. For example, Ruiz has promulgated many variations of trapezoidal keratotomy but has never published a clinical series.[145] Conversely, some surgeons publish a detailed analysis of results without describing the surgical technique.[51]

We summarize here the laboratory and clinical studies that have compared multiple techniques.

In 1980 Fyodorov[63] presented the first clinical results of the changes in refraction produced by parallel radial incisions with or without intersecting transverse keratotomy. None of the five patterns is now in use. Franks and Binder[62] used enucleated human eye bank and canine eyes with keratometric readings to evaluate six different patterns. However, the intraocular pressure was not controlled during the experiments, and different methods of measuring the knife depth and corneal thickness were used. They concluded that parallel semiradial, fan-shaped radial, and oval "optical zone" patterns were quantitatively and qualitatively unacceptable. Trapezoidal incisions were most effective but produced variable results.

Chi-Wang and associates[36] used rabbits to compare six different patterns of keratotomy. Keratometric measurements were taken 2 weeks to 4 months after surgery. All eyes received a standard eight-incision radial keratotomy. Those that had additional double parallel incisions in the steep meridian and/or an oval "optical" zone did not show a greater increase in astigmatism than the standard radial keratotomy with the circular optical zone; these patterns were deemed ineffective. Transverse incisions across one or two of the radial incisions induced 1 to 2 D of astigmatism and were deemed the more effective technique. Neumann (personal communication, International Society of Refractive Keratoplasty meeting, Las Vegas, October 7, 1988) compared four different techniques of astigmatic keratotomy in humans using vector analysis. He concluded that the parallel semiradial incisions *(L)* and the combined radial and parallel semiradial *(RL)* incisions were neither effective nor predictable. The eyes with combined radial and transverse incisions (staggered flags, interrupted transverse, modified trapezoidal) had a more effective and predictable reduction in astigmatism, as described in a subsequently published article,[128] which we discuss in a later section.

Agapitos and colleagues[1] compared six different techniques of astigmatic keratotomy in eyes with naturally occurring, postcataract and postpenetrating keratoplasty astigmatism. The details are reported in subsequent sections. They concluded that oval "optical" zones are ineffective (correcting less than 1.00 D of astigmatism), that trapezoidal keratotomy produced the largest corrections (mean of 8.00 to 13.00 D), that the intersecting trapezoidal pattern was unacceptable, that transverse or transverse and radial incisions corrected small to moderate amounts of astigmatism (mean of 3.00 to 6.00 D), that arcuate relaxing incisions after penetrating keratoplasty with compression sutures gave the most consistent and predictable effect, and that all techniques produced results that were highly variable and poorly predictable.

Arciniegas[4,5] performed a series of theoretic biomechanical calculations and laboratory studies in rabbits combining radial, arcuate, and circular incisions. He abandoned intersecting incisions. The rabbit model proved to be unstable, but the theoretic calculations are instructive. Arciniegas reasoned that the combination of paired radial incisions in each of the primary orthogonal meridians and arcuate incisions across the intervening quadrants would produce greater flattening of the entire cornea than that achieved by radial incisions alone, and he demonstrated in rabbits the creation of approximately 18 D of myopia with this technique; this pattern has not been reported in humans.

THE COUPLING EFFECT: RELATIONSHIP BETWEEN INCISED AND UNINCISED MERIDIANS

Both Lans in the late 1890s and Sato in the 1940s demonstrated experimentally that a transverse incision flattens the meridian it incises and steepens the unincised meridian 90° away (See Chapter 5, Development of Refractive Keratotomy in the Nineteenth Century, and Chapter 6, Development of Radial Keratotomy in Japan, 1939-1960).

Minus cylinder refraction

Planning for astigmatic keratotomy should be done on the basis of the minus cylinder refraction, since this allows the use of astigmatic and radial keratotomies to correct both the astigmatism and myopia (see Fig. 31-3). For example, in compound myopic astigmatism, the minus cylinder form of the refraction allows both of the astigmatic focal lines that define the conoid of Sturm to be moved from their location in the vitreous cavity posteriorly to the retina by first correcting the spherical component and then by collapsing the conoid during the correction of the astigmatic component, just as one does during a minus cylinder refraction (Fig. 31-11) (see Chapter 30, Optics and Topography of Corneal Astigmatism). If the plus cylinder form of the refraction is used, correction of the spherical myopic refractive error will leave the astigmatic focal line located behind the retina, requiring a steepening of the cornea to move it forward, something that cannot be achieved readily by keratotomy surgery. The magnitude of the spherical refractive error is always less in the minus cylinder form, which also helps to prevent overcorrection.[21] Minus cylinder parallels flat meridian.

Definition of coupling effect

The term "coupling effect" refers to the changes in curvature that occur in the incised meridian and in the orthogonal unincised meridian 90° away. The basic concept derives from Gauss' law of total curvature, which states that if a flexible and extensible surface (such as a hula hoop or basketball) is bent in one meridian, the total curvature of the surface remains constant because the second orthogonal meridian moves an equal amount in the opposite direction. This idea derives from the premise that the circumference, or perimeter, of the corneal surface remains constant.[124,170] Thus when a transverse incision induces flattening in the 90° meridian, there should be an equal compensatory steepening in the 180° meridian. This is known as the flattening/steepening ratio, or coupling ratio. If the amount of flattening and steepening are the same, there would be no change in the spherical equivalent refraction.

This relationship changes if radial or semiradial incisions are added because these incisions increase the circumference of the surface, so the requirement of Gauss' law is not fulfilled and there is not an equal compensatory steepening in the orthogonal unincised meridian because the circumference of the cornea can become larger. That is, radial or semiradial incisions flatten the entire cornea and that flattening offsets the steepening that would be induced by the transverse incisions, so the flattening/steepening, or coupling, ratio becomes larger. Conceptually, the surgeon can think of the radial or semiradial incisions as blocking the effect of the transverse incisions on the unincised orthogonal meridian.[76,97]

In expressing the coupling ratio, it seems most logical to place the major effect, the flattening from the transverse incision, as the numerator and express the coupling ratio as the following:

$$\text{Coupling ratio} = \frac{\text{Flattening of incised meridian}}{\text{Steepening of unincised meridian}} = \frac{\text{Flattening}}{\text{Steepening}} = \frac{F}{S}$$

Some authors, such as Ruiz and Nordan,[131,145] have expressed the coupling ratio as steepening/flattening. Readers must be cautious in reading reports of changes in the coupling ratio to know how the ratio is being expressed.

Effect of coupling ratio on astigmatic surgery

What is the practical effect of the coupling ratio on refractive keratotomy? Surgery done on an eye with a refraction of −3.00 −2.00 × 180° has the goal of flattening the steep meridian at 90° to eliminate the 2 D of astigmatism and to flatten the entire cornea to eliminate the 3 D of spherical myopia. Correction of the astigmatism can be done by transverse incisions across the 90° meridian, but these will steepen the orthogonal 180° meridian. Therefore there are two components to the amount of myopia that must be corrected, the underlying 3 D of the spherical component and the approximately 1 D of steepening induced by the transverse incisions. Thus radial incisions must be used to correct both of these components and calculations for the radial incisions are done on the basis of the spherical equivalent refraction (−4.00 D), not the spherical component of the spectacle refraction (−3.00 D), since the spherical equivalent can take into account both the original myopia and the steepening induced by the transverse incisions. Of course, the exact surgical procedure depends on the surgeon's individual nomogram.

Factors that affect the coupling ratio

If the cornea were an ideal shell that followed Gauss' law, clinical calculations for astigmatic surgery would be easier. But as a biologic tissue, the cornea exhibits a time-dependent viscoelastic response that includes wound healing. Therefore there is considerable variability in the response of corneas among individuals, and fixed flattening/steepening ratios cannot be established. In addition, surgeons do not create identical incisions, so surgical variability will also effect the flattening/steepening ratio.

The major factor that affects the coupling ratio is the length of the incision (see Fig. 31-3). Short incisions (1.0 to 1.5 mm, 20°) tend to flatten the incised meridian more than steepening the unincised meridian, with a coupling ratio of 1.5 to 2. Intermediate length incisions (2 to 5 mm long, 30° to 90°) tend to create a coupling ratio of 1.0. Longer incisions (5 to 6 mm, 90° to 100°) tend to induce more steepening in the unincised meridian than flattening in the incised meridian with a coupling ratio less than 1.0. Incisions 6 mm or longer (110° or more) tend to flatten both meridians (Table 31-1). Of course, these generalities will be affected by the distance of the incisions from the central cornea (zone diameter).

These facts can be used to modulate the overall refractive effect of the transverse incisions; for eyes with compound myopic astigmatism, shorter incisions (20° to 40°) are used to prevent inducing more myopia, whereas in eyes with mixed or hyperopic astigmatism, longer (40° to 90°) incisions are used to induce more steepening that will partially reduce the hyperopic component of the refraction (see Fig. 31-52).

Table 31-1

Change in Corneal Power (D) Produced by Arcuate Transverse Incisions at 7.5-mm Zone in Human Donor Eyes

	Single incision			Symmetric paired incisions		
Arc length of incision	Incised meridian (D)	Unincised meridian 90° away (D)	Total astigmatic change (D)	Incised meridian (D)	Unincised meridian 90° away (D)	Total astigmatic change (D)
30°	−0.33	+0.25	0.58	−1.08	−0.30	0.78
60°	−2.58	+1.59	4.17	−3.15	+1.49	4.64
90°	−2.95	+2.98	5.93	−9.07	+4.90	13.97

From Lundergan MK and Rowsey JJ: Ophthalmology 1985;92:1226-1236.
− indicates flattening; + indicates steepening.

The addition of radial or semiradial incisions to transverse incisions greatly reduces the amount of steepening in the unincised meridian. A demonstration of how radial incisions decrease the coupling ratio was made by Tchah[151] and colleagues, who studied the bow tie configuration of keratotomy in a stepwise manner in eye bank eyes (Fig. 31-11). They demonstrated that short 2-mm radial incisions made from a 10-mm zone into an 8-mm zone made little change in the central corneal curvature. The addition of connected arcuate keratotomies along the 10-mm zone induced a moderate amount of flattening in the incised meridian with slight steepening in the unincised meridian. Extensions of the radial incisions for 1 mm centrally enhanced the flattening effect in the incised meridian and essentially eliminated the steepening effect 90° away. These dynamics are similar to those achieved by trapezoidal keratotomy and by combined transverse incisions between radial incisions, but the effect of the transverse incisions is taken to an extreme by connecting them to the radial incisions, which creates a flap of cornea that elevates and probably slides forward slightly, essentially uncoupling the effect of the arcuate incisions from the unincised meridian.

Whether the coupling effect is different for straight transverse and arcuate transverse incisions with the same chord length is unknown.

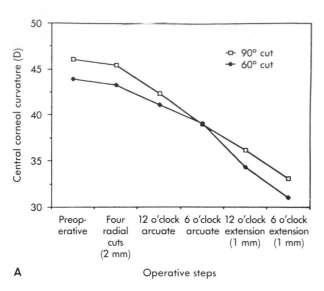

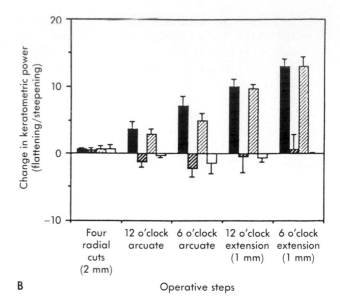

Figure 31-11

Cumulative effect of the components of bowtie keratotomy demonstrated in human eye bank eyes. The components were added sequentially in the following order: (1) four 2-mm long radial cuts from the 8- to 10-mm zone, (2) a 60° or 90° long arcuate keratotomy connected to the radial incisions at the 10-mm zone, first at 12 o'clock and then at 6 o'clock, and (3) 1-mm extensions of the radial incisions centrally, first at 12 o'clock and then at 6 o'clock. **A,** The central corneal curvature at the incised 90° meridian decreases with each operative step. The initial 2-mm long radial incisions induced little change. The peripheral connecting arcuate keratotomies induced the most change. The central extensions of the radial incisions produced additional change. **B,** The cumulative change in keratometric power is depicted at both the 90° and 180° meridians after each step in the operation. Almost all of the change is in the 90° meridian. *Solid bar,* Change in power at 90° meridian for 90° incision; *heavy hatched bar,* change in power at 180° meridian for 90° incision; *hatched bar,* change in power at 90° meridian for 60° incision; *open bar,* change in power 180° meridian for 60° incision. (From Tchah H, Hofmann R, Duffey R, et al: J Refract Surg 1988;5:183-190.)

Reports of coupling ratios

Although simple fixed coupling ratios have been proposed, such as 1:1 for a 3 mm transverse incision and 6:1 for trapezoidal keratotomy with 2 mm long transverse incisions,[131] fixed coupling ratios do not correspond to clinical reality, even though they are useful guidelines. The variability of the coupling ratio in trapezoidal keratotomy was illustrated by Buzard,[32] who observed no difference in the coupling ratio between 1.5 mm long and 5.0 mm long transverse incisions when the semiradial incisions were parallel, but also noticed a large difference when the semiradial incisions were converging, such that the 1.5 mm long incisions produced a flattening to steepening ratio of 0.71. Table 31-2 summarizes the coupling ratios from various published reports.

Using the model of a standard limbal incision after extracapsular surgery, Binder[26] measured the ratio of the change in the flat and steep corneal meridia before and after surgery. Sixty-six percent of the eyes had a coupling ratio of 0 to 2, suggesting that the two principal meridia were linked or coupled. Binder[25] performed a similar analysis, following suture removal in eyes after penetrating keratoplasty, and reached similar conclusions. Both studies were performed without calculation of vectoral astigmatism.

Table 31-2

Astigmatic Keratotomy: Ratio of Flattening of Incised Meridian to Steepening of Unincised Meridian 90° Away (Coupling Ratio) Reported in the Literature

Author (year)	Subject and type of astigmatism	Pattern of keratotomy (length, zone diameter)	Flattening/ steepening ratio Mean	Range
Merlin[124] (1987)	Human, naturally occurring	Paired arcuate transverse (100° and 160°)	1	Not reported
Duffey[55] (1988)	Eye bank eyes	Paired arcuate transverse (45° to 120°, 5- to 9-mm zone)	1.5	0.8 to 2.6
Lundergan[107] (1985)	Eye bank eyes	Paired arcuate transverse (30° to 90°, 7.5-mm zone)	2	1.9 to 2.1
Hofmann[76a] (1987)	Human, naturally occurring	Paired straight interrupted transverse with radial (jump T) (6- to 7-mm zone, 4-mm length)	—	—
Ibrahim[77] (1990)	Human, naturally occurring	Paired trapezoidal with four transverse (1.5 to 5 mm long, 3- to 5-mm zone)	6	2.5 to 6
Merck[122] (1986)	Human, after keratoplasty and cataract	Paired trapezoidal with four transverse (2.5 to 3 mm long, 3- to 5-mm zone)	1.75	1 to 7.5

The practical clinical question of how to use the coupling ratio most advantageously requires further study, with documentation of the effect of different lengths, locations, and patterns of incisions on the coupling ratio and the overall refractive effect. We think the coupling concept is useful, but it cannot be applied rigorously in all cases. Studies of various procedures can further define the coupling ratio for many cases,[25,26] but surgeons must be aware that different coupling ratios can produce unwanted postoperative spherical errors.

VARIABLES THAT DETERMINE THE EFFECT OF TRANSVERSE INCISIONS

Table 31-3 presents the variables that determine the effect of transverse keratotomy.

Configuration

Transverse incisions can be made either straight or arcuate. Arcuate incisions have several advantages: (1) they are concentric to the center mark; (2) they cut through cornea of approximately equal thickness; (3) they can be made parallel to penetrating keratoplasty wounds; and (4) intuitively, they seem more physiologic. Two disadvantages of arcuate incisions are that they are more difficult to make with a diamond knife, and they are measured in degrees not millimeters. When the incisions are short (2 mm or less), it probably makes little difference which configuration is used. However, the arcuate pattern is preferable when longer incisions are made. No published studies have compared the effectiveness of arcuate versus straight incisions. Arcuate incisions theoretically have a greater effect than straight incisions with the same chord length because the entire length of the incision is equidistant from the center of the cornea, whereas the ends of a straight incision are farther from the center, where they may have less effect, and because the incision itself is longer (see Table 31-4).

Table 31-3

Variables That Determine the Effect of Transverse Keratotomy

Incision variables	Effect	Options	Commonly used
Configuration	Arcuate incisions produce more effect than straight ones at lengths approximately 30° or more.	Straight or arcuate	Both
Length	Longer incisions give slightly more flattening in incised meridian and much more steepening in unincised orthogonal meridian up to 120° length.	1 to 5 mm or 10° to 120°	1.5 to 4 mm 20° to 100°
Location (zone diameter)	Incisions closer to the center give greater effect between 5 to 8 mm.	3 to 9 mm	6 to 8 mm (sweet spot)
Number	One pair induces most of the change.	Single to two pairs	Single to two pairs
Depth	Deeper incisions produce more effect; very deep incisions give uplift of central edge.	60% to 99%	75% to 85%
Direction	Vertical blade gives more uniform depth.	Push vertical blade (back-cutting); pull angled blade (front-cutting)	Vertical blade (back-cutting)
Sequence	Avoid fishmouth of previous incisions.	Transverse first or radial first	Transverse first (for jump-radial, radial first)

Length

Straight incisions are measured in millimeters and arcuate incisions in degrees (Fig. 31-12 and Table 31-4). The length of transverse incisions between radial incisions can be estimated in "segment widths"; one segment width for an eight-incision radial keratotomy is 40°, allowing space for nonintersection. The segment width will vary depending on the distance from the center of the procedure.

In general, longer incisions produce more flattening of the incised meridian, at least for incisions from 30° to approximately 120° in length (Table 31-5). For example, in an eye bank eye model of arcuate incisions, Duffey and colleagues[47]

Table 31-4

Arc Length (Degrees and Millimeters) and Chord Length (Millimeters) of Transverse Corneal Incisions

Angular length (degrees)	Chord length (mm) Zone diameter (mm)				Segment width for eight radial incisions	Arc length (mm) Zone diameter (mm)			
	5	6	7	8		5	6	7	8
22°	0.95	1.14	1.34	1.53	½	1.92	2.30	2.69	3.07
30°	1.29	1.55	1.81	2.07	⅔	2.62	3.14	3.67	4.19
45°	1.91	2.30	2.68	3.06	1	3.93	4.71	5.50	6.28
60°	2.50	3.00	3.50	4.00	1½	5.24	6.28	7.33	8.38
90°	3.54	4.24	4.95	5.66	2	7.85	9.42	11.00	12.57
120°	4.33	5.20	6.06	6.93	3	10.47	12.57	14.66	16.76

Courtesy of Robert Maloney, MD.

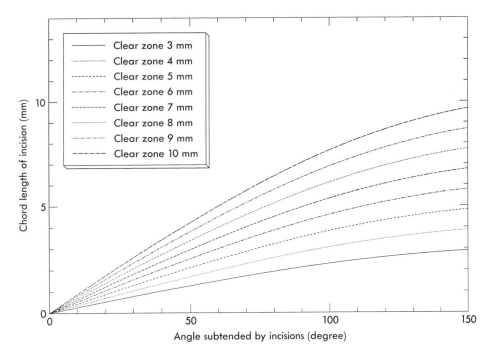

Figure 31-12

Relationship between angular length of arcuate transverse incision and chord length of straight transverse incision. (Courtesy Khalil Hanna.)

showed that there was an increased flattening in the incised meridian of approximately 2.00 D for every 30° lengthening of the incisions (Table 31-6). Similarly, in a study of 60 eyes with straight transverse incisions placed between eight radial incisions, Thornton and Sanders[157] demonstrated statistically significant increases in the amount of surgically corrected astigmatism as the incisions became longer; there was an increase of approximately 0.50 D as incision length increased from 22° to 30° and approximately 0.50 D as incision length increased from approximately 30° to 45° (Table 31-6). However, there was considerable scatter, with a range of about 1.5 D for each incision length (Fig. 31-13).

Table 31-5

Straight Transverse Incisions between Radial Incisions: Effect of Transverse Incision Length on Vectoral Change in Naturally Occurring Astigmatism (D)*

Length of one pair or two pairs of transverse incisions	Number of eyes	Surgically induced astigmatism (D) mean (SEM)†
½ segment (20°)	30	1.02 (0.09)
⅔ segment (30°)	13	1.48 (0.14)
1 segment (40°)	17	2.09 (0.12)

Modified from Thornton SP and Sanders DR: J Cataract Refract Surg 1987;13:27-31.
*Eight radial incisions, T incisions, at 6- to 8-mm diameter zone, blade length 95% of corneal thickness.
†The mean surgically induced astigmatism changes are significantly different from each other for all three lengths of incisions; LSD test 1-way ANOVA, overall $p < 0.001$.

Table 31-6

Effect of Paired Arcuate Transverse Keratotomy of Different Lengths Placed at Different Zone Diameters on Corneal Curvature in Human Donor Eyes

Incision length	45°				60°				90°				120°			
Clear zone diameter (mm)	F	S	F/S	ΔK	F	S	F/S	ΔK	F	S	F/S	ΔK	F	S	F/S	ΔK
5	2.70	1.85	1.46	4.55 ± 1.66	5.95	4.25	1.40	10.20 ± 3.14	8.50	7.95	1.07	16.45 ± 3.85	9.85	12.20	0.81	22.05 ± 3.55
6	3.25	2.15	1.51	5.40 ± 2.85	5.40	4.80	1.13	10.20 ± 4.60	8.75	8.60	1.02	17.35 ± 3.83	10.20	8.45	1.21	18.65 ± 6.88
7	2.10	0.80	2.63	2.90 ± 0.84	4.15	2.30	1.80	6.45 ± 1.37	7.25	3.70	1.96	10.95 ± 2.32	7.75	4.30	1.80	12.05 ± 3.15
8	1.85	1.15	1.61	3.00 ± 0.81	3.55	2.20	1.61	5.75 ± 1.27	5.70	3.30	1.73	9.00 ± 1.96	7.45	4.45	1.67	11.80 ± 1.66
9	1.40	1.25	1.12	2.65 ± 1.07	2.15	1.90	1.13	4.05 ± 1.02	4.90	4.10	1.20	9.00 ± 1.72	6.30	4.35	1.45	10.65 ± 1.91

Average corneal flattening, steepening, and induced astigmatism (D)*

Modified from Duffey RJ, Vivanit NJ, Hungwon T, et al: Arch Ophthalmol 1988;106:1130-1135.

*F, Diopters of corneal flattening in meridian of incision; S, diopters of corneal steepening 90° away from incised meridian; F/S, coupling ratio (overall F/S, 1.47 ± 0.41; ΔK, diopters of surgically induced astigmatic change (average ±SD).

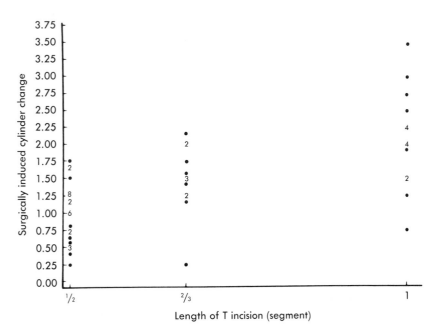

Figure 31-13
Relationship of the length of straight transverse incisions placed between radial incisions (x-axis) and the vectoral surgically induced change in astigmatism (y-axis) in 60 eyes with naturally occurring astigmatism. Longer incisions induced more change in astigmatism, but there was a wide variation for each length. Single dot represents one eye. Numbers represent multiple eyes. Incision length expressed as fraction of 45°, which is one segment between eight radial incisions. (From Thornton SP: J Cataract Refract Surg 1987;13:30.)

However, the change is not always computed so simply. For example, Ibrahim and colleagues[77] reported a series of trapezoidal keratotomies, observing that an increase in the length of the transverse incisions from 1.5 to 2.5 mm increased the flattening of the primary incised meridian, but an increase in length from 2.5 to 5.0 mm had little effect on flattening the primary meridian, although it induced more steepening of the secondary meridian (Table 31-7). Ruiz[145] has suggested that longer incisions in trapezoidal keratotomy produce greater steepening in the unincised meridian 90° away.

A somewhat paradoxic effect occurs as transverse incisions become longer than 120° because they induce a flattening of the unincised meridian 90° away, thereby inducing a change in the spherical equivalent refraction in the hyperopic direction.[124,170] In a sense the effect of these long incisions has "wrapped around" the circumference of the cornea and the incisions have become transverse relaxing incisions in the secondary meridian, which is now actually under the influence of the incision. Thus incisions placed at the 6- to 7-mm diameter zone should have a length less than 100° (approximately 5 mm). Merlin[124] has documented these effects in humans, emphasizing that incisions longer than 120° decrease the amount of change in astigmatism when compared with incisions shorter than 120° (Tables 31-8 to 31-10).

Table 31-7

Change in Refractive Astigmatism (D) (Mean ± SD) with Different Lengths of Transverse Incisions in Nonintersecting Trapezoidal Keratotomy for Naturally Occurring Astigmatism

	1.5 mm	2.5 mm	5.0 mm
Length of transverse incisions	1.5 mm	2.5 mm	5.0 mm
No. of eyes (total = 64)	37	19	8
Surgically corrected astigmatism (D)	3.2 ±1.2	4.5 ±1.9	4.2 ±1.5
Flattening of primary meridian (D)	3.2 ±1.5	3.9 ±1.8	2.9 ±1.3
Steepening of secondary meridian (D)	0.5 ±0.4	0.7 ±0.3	1.2 ±0.3
Flattening to steepening ratio	6:1	5:1	2.5:1

Modified from Ibrahim O, Husein JA, El-Sahn MF, El-Nawawy S, Kassem A, and Waring GO: Arch Ophthalmol, in press.

Table 31-8

Relationship between Angular Length of Arcuate Transverse Incisions and Change in Spherical Equivalent Refractive Error in Naturally Occurring Astigmatism

	100°	120°	140°	160°
Angular length of incision	100°	120°	140°	160°
Change in spherical equivalent (D)	0	+0.33	+1.06	+1.67
Number of eyes	45	104	40	16

Modified from Merlin U: J Refract Surg 1987;3:92-97.

Table 31-9

Change in Astigmatism (D) Produced by One Pair of Transverse Arcuate Incisions in 205 Eyes with Naturally Occurring Astigmatism

Zone diameter (mm)	Angular length of incisions (degrees)			
	100° incision (n) (SD)	120° (n) (SD)	140° (n) (SD)	160° (n) (SD)
5		5.10 (6) (0.60)		
R		4.00-5.75		
5.5	4.10 (3) (0.82)	4.40 (12) (0.85)	3.75 (2) (0.70)	
R	3.37-5.00	3.00-5.75	3.25-4.25	
6	3.25 (25) (0.66)	4.10 (55) (0.83)	3.20 (18) (0.91)	2.40 (10) (0.98)
R	2.00-4.25	2.50-5.50	1.75-5.00	1.5-3.75
6.5	2.80 (15) (0.46)	3.60 (20) (0.73)	2.75 (15) (0.84)	1.75 (6) (0.96)
R	1.50-3.50	2.50-4.75	1.50-4.50	0.75-3.25
7	2.10 (2) (0.53)	2.90 (11) (0.77)	2.40 (5) (0.80)	− (0)
	1.75-2.50	1.75-4.00	1.25-3.25	
Total no. of eyes	45	104	40	16

From Merlin LL: J Refract Surg 1987; 3:92-97.

n, Number of eyes; *SD*, standard deviation; *R*, range. The incisions were always performed leaving 0.02 mm of uncut tissue in the posterior cornea.

Table 31-10

Effect of Length of Transverse Keratotomy on Corneal Curvature

	Length of incision		Effect on corneal curvature	
Category	Arcuate (angular, degrees)	Straight (chord, mm)	Incised meridian	Unincised meridian 90° away
Short	≤20°	≤1.5	Flatten	Steepen, mild
Medium	25 to 110°	2 to 5	Flatten	Steepen, moderate
Long	≥120°	>5	Flatten	Flatten

Distance of incision from center of cornea—zone diameter

There are two designations for the location of transverse incisions. The most commonly used is the diameter of the circular zone (optical zone, clear zone) along which the incision is made; a straight incision is tangential to the zone mark. A second designation is the distance from the center point of the surgery, that is, the radius of the circular zone. Sometimes these designations are confused: "The present studies suggest that tangential corneal incisions 5 mm from the optical center have the greatest effect on alteration of corneal topography."[92] The authors probably meant tangential incisions at a 5-mm diameter zone, which would be 2.5 mm from the optical center as they indicated in the remainder of the paper.

In general, the closer a transverse incision is to the center of the cornea, the greater the flattening effect is in the incised meridian, as demonstrated by Duffey and colleagues[47] in eye bank eye experiments (Fig. 31-14; see Table 31-2), by

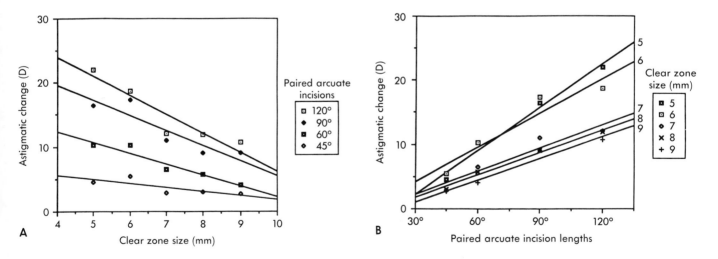

Figure 31-14

Relationship of zone diameter, incision length, and change in average central keratometric power for paired arcuate transverse keratotomies in human donor eyes. Superimposed regression lines demonstrate the linear relationship of the sum of corneal flattening and steepening (change in average central keratometry). **A,** Larger diameter zones produced greater changes in astigmatism, the amount of change increasing as the incisions became longer, mostly because of increased steepening in the unincised orthogonal meridian. **B,** Incisions made at the 5- to 6-mm zones created more change than those made in the 7- to 9-mm zones, when the incisions were 45° to 120° long. (From Duffey RJ: Arch Ophthalmol 1988; 106:1130.)

Merlin[124] in a clinical series of isolated arcuate keratotomies (Tables 31-9 and 31-11), and by Hofmann's clinical series[76] using interrupted transverse incisions with radial keratotomy (Fig. 31-15).

The relationship of corneal flattening to zone diameter is probably not linear because there seems to be a "sweet spot" between diameters of 5 and 8 mm where a maximum effect occurs, the effect decreasing somewhat at very small diameters of 3 to 4 mm and at large diameters of 8 to 12 mm. The concept of a "sweet spot" is based on the work of Lavery and Lindstrom,[87] who demonstrated in eye bank eyes that paired isolated transverse incisions 2.5 mm long placed at the 5- to 7-mm zone flattened the incised meridian effectively, whereas those placed at the 3-mm and 4-mm zones actually steepened the incised merid-

Table 31-11

Relationship between Diameter of Clear Zone and Change in Astigmatism with 120° Arcuate Incisions in Eyes with Naturally Occurring Astigmatism

Diameter of clear zone (mm)	Mean change in astigmatism (D)	No. of eyes
5	5.10	6
5.5	4.40	12
6	4.10	55
6.5	3.60	20
7	2.90	11

Modified from Merlin U: J Refract Surg 1987;3:92-97.

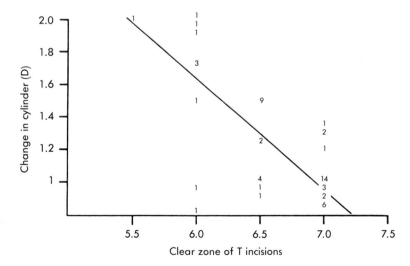

Figure 31-15
Effect of zone diameter for straight transverse incisions on the change in refractive astigmatism in human eyes. The smaller the diameter of the zone the greater the change in astigmatism, although there was considerable variability for each diameter. Scattergram represents results of 56 eyes with interrupted paired transverse incisions in conjunction with radial incisions. (From Hofmann RF: The surgical correction of idiopathic astigmatism. In Sanders DR, Hofmann RF, and Salz JJ, editors: Refractive corneal surgery, Thorofare, NJ, 1986, Slack, Inc.)

ian; those placed at the 8-mm and 9-mm zones showed minimal effect with little difference between each other. These findings are supported by other laboratory and clinical research[96,168] (Table 31-12).

Tripoli and colleagues[174] have used keratography to define the change in corneal topography after arcuate keratotomy in human eye bank eyes (Fig. 31-16). They also concluded that maximal flattening occurred with a 5- to 7-mm diameter zone and that only a small effect occurred at the 3-mm zone and a negligi-

Table 31-12

Change in Keratometric Power (D) Induced by One Pair of Straight Transverse Incisions 2.5 mm Long at Different Zone Diameters in Human Donor Eyes

Zone diameter (mm)	Mean change in power in incised meridian (D) (SD, range)	Mean change in power in unincised meridian (D) 90° away (SD, range)	Net change in corneal power (D)
3	+1.25 steeper (±0.73, +0.75 to +2.50)	+3.45 steeper (±1.14, +2.25 to +5.00)	2.20
4	+0.80 steeper ±1.19, −1.00 to +2.25)	+3.90 steeper (±0.72, +3.25 to +5.20)	3.10
5	−1.45 D flatter (±0.67, 0.75 to −2.50)	+2.20 steeper (±0.76, +1.50 to +3.25)	3.65
6	−0.50 flatter (±0.95, 0 to −2.25)	+1.80 steeper (±0.57, +1.25 to +2.50)	2.50

Modified from Lavery GW and Lindstrom RL: J Refract Surg 1985;1:18-24.

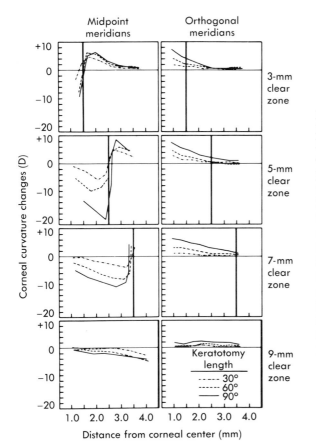

Figure 31-16
Keratographic analysis of paired arcuate keratotomy in human eye bank eyes. The left column demonstrates the changes in power in the incised meridian (the "midpoint meridian"). Vertical line shows location of incision. The right column shows the changes along the unincised orthogonal meridian 90° away. The x-axis shows the distance along the keratograph rings from the center of the cornea for both meridians. The y-axis shows the change in corneal curvature. Incisions were placed at four different diameter zones: 3, 5, 7, and 9 mm. The length of the keratotomies were 30°, 60°, and 90° as demonstrated by the three different lines within each box. The figure shows the complex interplay among the length, location, and meridional effect. (From Tripoli NK, Cohen KL, and Holman RE: J Refract Surg 1987;3:129-136.)

ble effect at the 9-mm zone. They also showed that incision length has a variable effect at different zones. At the 5- to 7-mm zone, the 90° long incision had considerably more effect than a 30° long incision. In the 3-mm and 9-mm zone groups, the length of the incisions did not make much difference. In all zone groups, there was steepening of the unincised orthogonal meridian 90° away with flattening/steepening ratios varying from 1.0 to 2.0 (Fig. 31-16).

There is little information about the effect of transverse incisions made at a 3- or 4-mm diameter zone because of the danger that such small zones will induce irregular astigmatism and glare. Lavery and colleagues[96,97] found an unexpected "steepening" of the incised meridian by using a 3-mm diameter zone, possibly because the keratometer mires were actually reading outside of the incision where the cornea becomes slightly steeper. This is possible with a 3-mm and even a 4-mm zone, as was subsequently suggested by the same research group.[55] It does not make sense for the cornea to steepen on the inside of the two transverse incisions, even at 3 mm and 4 mm. Tripoli and colleagues[174] have shown a high flattening to steepening ratio with 3-mm and 4-mm diameter zones.

There is also little information about the effect of incisions at the 9- to 11-mm zones. Merlin[123] found variable results with paralimbal keratotomies caused by regression over time because of the increased fibrosis and occasional neovascularization that reached these incisions.

Trapezoidal keratotomy has two clear "optical" zones. The one most commonly referred to is that delimiting the length of the semiradial incisions, as discussed below. Although no studies have systematically analyzed the effect of transverse incisions at different zone diameters as part of trapezoidal keratotomy, it is reasonable to assume that the transverse incisions in trapezoidal keratotomy will have more effect when placed closer to the center of the cornea, as occurs in isolated transverse incisions. Such a study would involve making the semiradial incisions and then making the first pair of transverse incisions at specifically different diameter zones, such as one set at 4 mm diameter in one series of eyes, at 5 mm in diameter in a second series of eyes, and so forth. Once a single pair of incisions is in place, it is not possible to determine the isolated effect of another pair of incisions placed at a different zone diameter; such a study could measure the cumulative effect of these incisions[102] (Table 31-12).

There are no published studies of varying the effect of the zone diameter of arcuate relaxing incisions after penetrating keratoplasty because most incisions are made either in the keratoplasty wound or just inside the wound, with a diameter of approximately 7 mm to 8.5 mm.

Number of transverse incisions

The first transverse incision across a semimeridian produces almost all of the change that will occur in that semimeridian, no matter where it is placed. The addition of a second parallel incision may enhance the effect slightly. The addition of third and fourth incisions across that semimeridian will produce little additional change in curvature. For example, Terry and Rowsey[168] demonstrated in eye bank eyes a flattening of the incised meridian of 2.00 D with the first pair of straight transverse incisions, an additional flattening of 0.5 D with the second pair, and less than 0.5 D with the third and fourth pairs (Table 31-13). Lindquist and colleagues[102] have reported similar findings (Table 31-14). Some surgeons prefer to use more than one pair of incisions, particularly in trapezoidal keratotomy, because they contend it smooths out the contours of the cornea and makes less of an acute inflection point at the edge of the single incision.

No clinical studies have quantified the change in curvature produced by progressively increasing the number of incisions, which would require meticulous intraoperative keratometry.

Table 31-13

Effect of Increasing the Number of Paired Transverse Incisions in the Vertical Meridian on Induced Astigmatism (D) in Human Donor Eyes

Data from photokeratographs indicate change in astigmatism (D) in vertical and horizontal meridians

Number of incisions	Ring 3: central change (D) (range)		Ring 9: peripheral change (D) (range)	
	Vertical	Horizontal	Vertical	Horizontal
0 to 2	−2.05 (−4.66 to +2.19)	+3.05 (+0.76 to +5.29)	+0.64 (0.03 to +1.13)	+0.25 (−0.68 to 11.51)
2 to 4	−0.54 (−1.48 to 11.15)	−0.09 (−3.38 to +2.20)	+0.24 (−10.09 to +1.30)	+0.30 (−0.36 t +0.89)
4 to 6	−0.33 (−1.79 to +0.62)	−0.15 (−1.12 to +2.46)	−0.23 (−1.56 to +1.45)	+0.27 (−1.39 to +2.12)
6 to 8	+0.14 (−1.31 to +4.06)	−0.10 (−2.07 to +0.95)	−0.52 (−1.74 to +0.55)	−0.23 (−1.50 to +0.86)
8 → added four semiradial incisions	−6.71 (−12.61 to −4.18)	−1.48 (−8.22 to +1.90)	+0.52 (−1.27 to +2.17)	−0.66 (−2.55 to +0.27)

Modified from Terry MA and Rowsey JJ: Arch Ophthalmol 1986;104:1611-1616.
Minus sign indicates flattening; plus sign indicates steepening.

Table 31-14

Change in Keratometric Astigmatism (D) with Sequential Addition of Incisions in Trapezoidal Keratotomy Performed in the 180° Meridian in Five Human Donor Eyes

	Eye bank eye number					
	1	2	3	4	5	All five eyes mean ±SD
Semiradial incisions alone						
At 90° (unincised)	−3.50	−3.00	−4.25	−4.75	−4.00	−3.90 ±0.68
At 180° (incised)	−4.75	−4.25	−5.75	−5.75	−6.00	−5.30 ±0.76
Cumulative effect at 90° (unincised meridian) from addition of transverse incisions at different zones						
At 5 mm	+9.25	+9.25	+10.75	+9.00	+10.00	+9.65 ±0.72
At 7 mm	+8.50	+7.50	+9.00	+8.75	+8.00	+8.35 ±0.62
At 3 mm	+8.00	+5.75	+3.75	+6.76	+8.75	+6.60 ±1.97
At 9 mm	+6.25	+7.75	+8.25	+5.75	+10.75	+7.75 ±1.97

Modified from Lindquist TD, Rubenstein JB, Rice SW, Williams PA, and Lindstrom RL: Arch Ophthalmol 1986;104:1534-1539.
Minus sign indicates flattening; plus sign indicates steepening.

Depth of transverse incision

As in radial keratotomy, deeper transverse incisions produce greater corneal flattening. To demonstrate this in humans, Seiler and colleagues[151] used argon fluoride 193-nm excimer laser ultraviolet radiation to make arcuate transverse excisions for the correction of astigmatism. They demonstrated an exponential relationship between the depth of the incision and the change in astigmatism (Fig. 31-17). This emphasizes the difficulty of controlling the exact effect of the incision depth, since a small difference in the depth between 80% and 98% of corneal thickness will create a large effect in the astigmatism. Ruiz[145] has stated

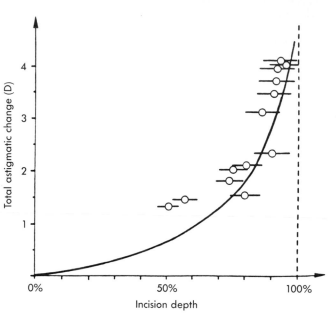

Figure 31-17

Effect of incision depth on total astigmatic change using arcuate transverse excisions made with a 193-mm argon fluoride excimer laser through a contact lens mask in eyes with naturally occurring astigmatism. The excision depths for each eye are represented by the data points and were determined from slit-lamp photographs with a measurement error of ±8%. The curved line is the calculated theoretical curve. The clinical values show a greater change in astigmatism than expected from the theoretical curve. The curve emphasizes the extreme importance of incisions greater than 80% depth, where a small change in the depth produces a relatively large change in astigmatism. (From Seiler T, Bende T, Wollensak J, and Trokel S: Am J Ophthalmol 1988; 105:117-124.)

Table 31-15

Effect of Single Arcuate Transverse Keratotomy 90° Long Made from 12:00 to 3:00 at a 7.5-mm Zone on the Change in Corneal Power (D) along Different Semimeridians (Designated in Clock Hours) in Human Donor Eyes

Keratoscope ring number	Mean change in corneal power (D) (range)			
Semimeridian (clock hour)	*12:00*	*2:30*	*3:00*	*4:30*
9	+3.22 (+2.15 to +7.24)	−1.83 (−1.44 to −2.23)	+2.19 (+1.41 to +3.12)	−0.50 (−2.74 to +2.06)
7	+3.29 (+2.05 to +5.40)	−1.89 (−3.51 to +0.01)	+2.14 (+0.44 to +3.15)	+0.68 (−0.85 to +2.08)
3	+1.39 (+0.61 to +2.74)	−3.76 (−1.05 to −7.50)	+1.55 (−0.44 to +3.53)	+2.58 (+2.32 to +2.95)
Semimeridian (clock hour)	*6:00*	*7:30*	*9:00*	*10:30*
3	−1.17 (−2.70 to +0.63)	−2.14 (−0.74 to −4.35)	+0.03 (−0.78 to +1.03)	+3.38 (+2.11 to +4.90)
7	−0.39 (−1.30 to +0.57)	−0.77 (−0.07 to −1.88)	−0.63 (−1.67 to +0.81)	+2.69 (+0.86 to +6.11)
9	+0.43 (−0.88 to +1.07)	−0.55 (−2.25 to +0.77)	−0.61 (−1.86 to +1.07)	+1.96 (−0.06 to +5.25)

Modified from Lundergan MK and Rowsey JJ: Ophthalmology 1985;92:1226-1236.
*Diopters of change for three eyes.
Plus sign indicates steepening; minus sign indicates flattening.

that incision depths greater than 90% commonly lead to overcorrections and that incision depths shallower than 70% commonly lead to undercorrection. He prefers incision depths of 80%. Binder and colleagues[49] have demonstrated that the incision depth of astigmatic cuts tends to be shallower than the radial cuts using the same blade length.

A single transverse incision intersects only the *semi*meridian in which it is made, but it flattens both the semimeridian that it intersects and the semimeridian 180° away. The amount of flattening in the incised semimeridian is greater than that in the unincised semimeridian, as demonstrated by Lundergan and Rowsey[107] (Table 31-15).

The change in topography is somewhat different after transverse incisions than after radial incisions. A transverse incision causes an uplift and flattening of

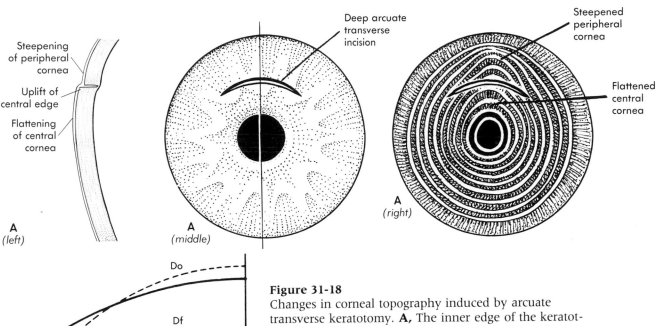

Figure 31-18
Changes in corneal topography induced by arcuate transverse keratotomy. **A,** The inner edge of the keratotomy incision elevates and the region central to it flattens (*left* and *middle*), creating pear-shaped mires on the keratograph (*right*). The outer edge of the incision compensates by becoming slightly steeper. **B,** Combined theoretical drawing of the geometry of corneal curvature before *(Do)* and after *(Dc)* arcuate transverse keratotomy. The center of the cornea is on the right of the figure, and the limbus is on the left of the figure. Before surgery the cornea *(Do, dotted line)* is flatter peripherally and steeper centrally. After surgery *(Dc, solid line)* the cornea is steeper peripherally and flatter centrally. The other notations on the drawing form the mathematical basis for the determination of the diameter of the clear zone, the length of the incisions, and the resultant change in corneal power and curvature. (From Arciniegas A and Amaya LE: J Refract Surg 1988;4:51-59.)

the central edge of the incision, while the peripheral edge of the incision remains in place and may steepen slightly (Fig. 31-18). The deeper and longer the incision, the greater the amount of central uplift. This phenomenon has been demonstrated with keratography by Lundergan and Rowsey,[107] Terry and Rowsey,[168] and Tripoli and Cohen[174] and is illustrated in Fig. 31-19. This uplift or "cliff" created by the transverse incision has a number of undesirable consequences: (1) it causes more distance between the two edges of the incision, which delays wound healing; (2) it creates irregular astigmatism that can produce glare and visual distortion in the pupillary zone; and (3) it can create an overcorrection with excessive flattening in the incised meridian.

Arciniegas[4,5] used a theoretic bioengineering approach to mathematically describe the changes in curvature induced by arcuate incisions, emphasizing that the central portion of the cornea flattened and the peripheral portion of the cornea steepened (see Fig. 31-18). This uplift phenomenon described is similar to

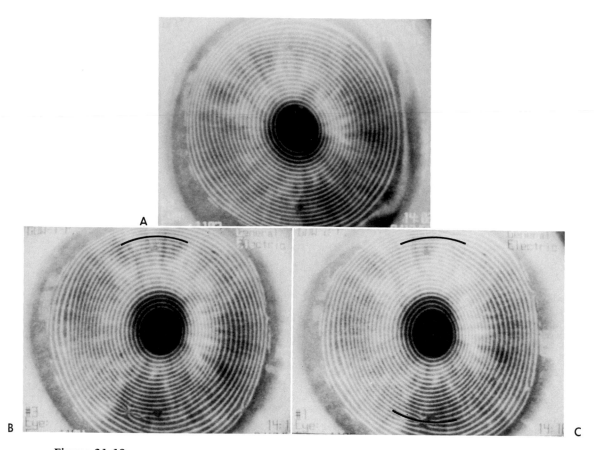

Figure 31-19
Effect of progressive lengthening of arcuate keratotomy in human eye bank eyes. Eyes were presoaked in solution containing dextran to obtain a normal corneal thickness. The epithelium was removed. The eyes were mounted in an artificial orbit where an intraocular pressure of 22 mm Hg was maintained throughout the procedure. Incisions were made along a 7-mm diameter zone mark with vertical-bladed diamond knife set to achieve an incision depth of 80% to 90% of corneal thickness. The Corneal Modeling System was used to obtain the videokeratographs. **A,** Preoperative keratograph demonstrates essentially round mires. **B,** A single 45° incision across 12 o'clock produces flattening in the 90° meridian. **C,** A second 45° incision across the 6 o'clock semimeridian produces further flattening of vertical meridian.

anterior slippage of a penetrating keratoplasty wound or a cataract wound.

The transverse keratotomy must be controlled to prevent excessive uplift by making the incision no deeper than approximately 80% of the local corneal thickness and no longer than approximately 90° (5 mm), unless the surgeon is intentionally trying to induce steepening of the unincised meridian 90° away. To correct large amounts of astigmatism we think it is better to move the incision closer to the center of the cornea than to make it excessively long or deep.

Variables that affect radial or semiradial incisions

Configuration. The configuration of the radial incisions has been described in the foregoing section on the classification of keratotomy for astigmatism. The variety of configurations of semiradial incisions bespeaks lack of standardization (see Figs. 31-7 and 31-9).

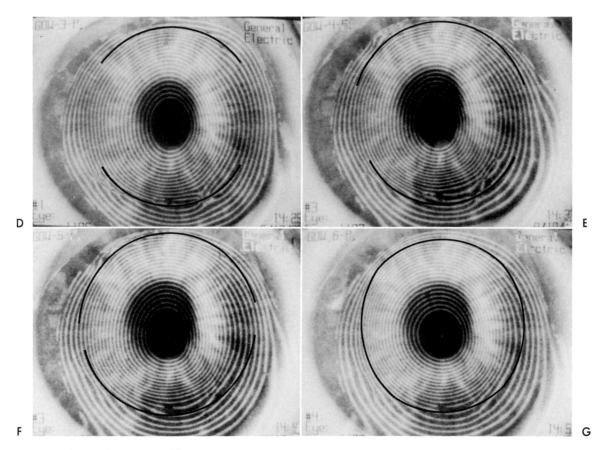

Figure 31-19, cont'd
D, Extension of both incisions to a length of 90° creates even more flattening with an increase in the ovality of the central mires. **E,** Extension of both incisions to 135° produces little change in vertical flattening but shows a slight increased steepening horizontally. **F,** Extension of the incisions to 165° produces little change. **G,** Connection of the incisions to create a 360° circular keratotomy restores the mires to a more round configuration. (Keratographs courtesy of Quishi Ren.)

Clear zone diameter. The flattening of the entire cornea is greater when the diameter of the clear zone is smaller, as with radial keratotomy. This has been demonstrated in trapezoidal keratotomy in numerous laboratory and clinical studies (Figs. 31-20 and 31-21 and Table 31-16).

Length. The length of the semiradial and radial incisions is determined by the diameter of the clear zone and the proximity of the incision to the limbus. The longer the incision, the greater the effect.

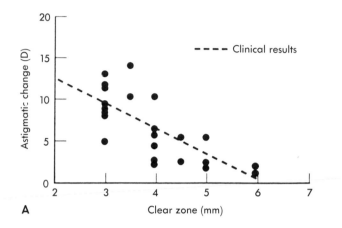

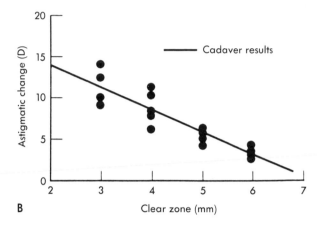

A

B

Figure 31-20

Relationship of clear zone diameter for semiradial incisions in nonintersecting trapezoidal keratotomy and change in astigmatism. Smaller clear zones created a greater change in keratometric astigmatism. **A,** Data from clinical series of eyes after penetrating keratoplasty or cataract extraction. **B,** Data from laboratory studies of human donor eyes. The linear regression line is parallel for both groups, but the clinical results are proportionately lower than the laboratory results. An exact ratio between clinical and laboratory results cannot be made for individual eyes. (From Merck MP: Ophthalmology 1986;93:719-726.)

Figure 31-21

Relationship between clear zone diameter for semiradial incisions in intersecting trapezoidal keratotomy and the change in astigmatism in human donor eyes. Smaller diameter zones created a greater change in keratometric astigmatism ($y = 21.7872 - 3.7588x$; $R = 0.49$). (From Agapitos PJ, Lindstrom RL, Williams PA, and Sanders DR: J Cataract Refract Surg 1989;15:13-18.)

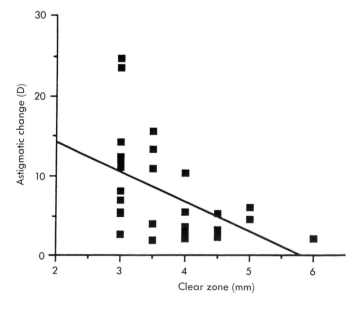

Table 31-16

Effect of Clear Zone Diameter for Semiradial Incisions in Trapezoidal Keratotomy for Naturally Occurring Astigmatism

Clear zone diameter (mm)	Number of eyes	Mean change in astigmatism (D) (range)
3.00	6	4.63 (3.50 to 6.50)
3.50	4	3.31 (2.00 to 4.50)
3.75	2	1.37 (1.00 to 1.75)
4.00	10	3.14 (0.50 to 7.25)
4.50	3	0.67 (0.00 to 1.50)
5.00	3	0.75 (0.50 to 1.00)

Modified from Villaseñor RA and Stimac GR: J Refract Surg 1988;4:125-131.

Depth. The semiradial and radial incisions may be made 90% to 95% deep, based on the nomogram used, because there is not a problem with the uplift of the edges of the incision as there is with a transverse incision.

Effect of other variables on transverse keratotomy

The roles of patient variables such as age, sex, preoperative intraocular pressure, central keratometric power, corneal topography, corneal diameter, ocular rigidity, and the like have not been studied as thoroughly in astigmatic keratotomy as they have been in radial keratotomy (see Chapter 13, Predictability of Refractive Keratotomy). There is no reason to think that the effect of age should be different for transverse keratotomy than for radial keratotomy, where greater age produces greater effect for the same surgery.

CLINICAL RESULTS OF KERATOTOMY FOR NATURALLY OCCURRING ASTIGMATISM
Isolated transverse keratotomy

A few human series have been reported using isolated transverse keratotomy. Most have combined transverse and radial keratotomies for the treatment of compound myopic astigmatism; see Fig. 31-2.

Merlin[124] used arcuate transverse keratotomies to correct naturally occurring astigmatism in 205 eyes, reporting the results 6 months or more after surgery, as presented in Tables 31-8 and 31-9. He described the change in astigmatism in these eyes but did not give the outcome in terms of residual astigmatism.

Seiler and colleagues[151] used a 193-nm argon fluoride excimer laser and a contact lens mask to create straight transverse excisions (not incisions) in 13 eyes (see Fig. 31-17 and Chapter 19, Laser Corneal Surgery). The excisions were placed tangential to a 6-mm diameter zone mark and were 4.5 mm long and 150 μm wide. The preoperative astigmatism ranged from 0.75 to 6.5 D (mean, 3.70 D). The change in astigmatism ranged from 1.32 to 4.16 D. Residual astigmatism varied from 0.01 to 4.60 D. Postoperatively, four eyes had 1.00 D or less astigmatism, and eight eyes had 2.50 D or less. In 10 of the 13 eyes, there was less flattening in the meridian of surgery than in the meridian 90° away; the flattening/steepening ratio varied from 0.08 to 1.30. Four eyes had approximately equal flattening and steepening; seven eyes had two to twelve times as much steepening as flattening; and one eye had half as much steepening as flattening.

Case 1: Staged Isolated Transverse Keratotomies

A 47-year-old with an uncorrected visual acuity in the right eye of 20/80 had a refraction of OD: +1.50 −3.75 × 10° and central keratometric readings of OD: 43.75 × 174°/47.12 × 84°. Transverse keratotomy was performed using a 5-mm zone and a 3-mm straight incision placed across the superior semimeridian at approximately 85% depth. Three months after surgery the uncorrected visual acuity was 20/50 with a manifest refraction of +0.25 −2.00 × 135° and keratometric readings of 44.75 × 158°/ 47.50 × 68°. At that time an additional transverse keratotomy was placed across the inferior semimeridian at the 5-mm zone, 2.5 mm long and 85% deep. Four months after the second operation the uncorrected visual acuity was 20/30, the manifest refraction was +0.75 −1.25 × 160°, and the keratometric readings were 44.00 × 162°/46.75 × 72°. The spherical equivalent refraction remained unchanged, being approximately plano before and after surgery.

Comment: This case illustrates several aspects of isolated transverse incisions. The expression of the refraction in the minus cylinder form obviously indicates that the surgeon would operate only to correct the astigmatism while preventing the creation of more hyperopia. By staging the procedure the surgeon achieves a more predictable and satisfactory outcome. If both incisions were made simultaneously at the same 3-mm length, overcorrection may have occurred. The spherical equivalent was unchanged after the second incision. The mean corneal power of 45.35 D was essentially unchanged. A coupling ratio of 1:1 most likely occurred. The flat meridian steepened from 43.75 D to 44.00 D, and the steep meridian flattened from 47.12 D to 46.75 D. These apparently small central changes reduced the refractive astigmatism from 3.75 D to 1.25 D, suggesting that topographic changes outside the area measured by keratometry produced the refractive results.

This result is different from that described by Merlin with arcuate diamond knife keratotomy and may be related to the effect of a keratectomy (tissue removal), as opposed to a keratotomy (tissue severing).

Shepherd[153] reported 395 transverse keratotomy procedures using from one to ten incisions, but the results were combined with operations using other techniques, so the effect of the transverse incisions alone could not be determined.

Agapitos[1] used isolated transverse incisions to correct astigmatism in three eyes with naturally occurring astigmatism, but combined his results with those after cataract and penetrating keratoplasty surgery. However, for all 10 eyes the mean preoperative keratometric cylinder was 5.3 D (range, 1.50 to 11.00 D), and the mean change in keratometric astigmatism was 6.3 ±5.7 D. The shift in astigmatic axis was less than 30° for all eyes. The change in spherical equivalent refraction was a mean of +1.13 D, indicating an overall steepening of the cornea.

Combined transverse and radial nonintersecting incisions

The pattern of astigmatic keratotomy used most frequently for naturally occurring astigmatism is combined transverse and radial incisions (Fig. 31-22).

Transverse incisions between radial incisions. Thornton has described and refined the use of straight transverse incisions made between radial incisions for the correction of compound myopic astigmatism[169,172] (Fig. 31-23). He reported the results of 60 eyes with 1.00 to 2.25 D of preoperative refractive astigmatism out of 106 consecutive procedures. He made eight incisions for myopia and one straight transverse incision at an 8-mm zone across each side of the steep meridian. The length of the transverse incision was graduated as a fraction of the 45°

Case 2: Transverse Incisions between Radial Incisions with Variable Effect

A 25-year-old patient had an uncorrected visual acuity in the right eye of 20/800 with a refraction of −6.50 −1.00 × 175° and keratometry measurements of 45.75 × 175°/47.50 × 85°. Surgery consisted of six radial incisions with a 3-mm diameter clear zone and the placement of four pairs of transverse incisions superiorly and inferiorly along the steep meridian, the transverse incisions being 2.5 mm long at axis 85°. One year after surgery the visual acuity without correction was 20/70, and the manifest refraction was −1.75 −1.25 × 75°, with keratometric measurements of 43.37 × 180°/45.00 × 90°. The net amount of astigmatism was approximately the same before and after surgery, although the vectoral amount had changed approximately 2 D because of the axis shift of almost 100°.

In the left eye, the uncorrected visual acuity was 20/400. The manifest refraction was −6.50 −2.00 × 75° with keratometric readings of 45.75 × 75°/47.87 × 85°. Surgery consisted of eight radial incisions with a 3-mm diameter clear zone and the placement of two transverse incisions, 3 mm long, at the 5-mm zone mark. Six months after surgery the uncorrected visual acuity was 20/60 and the manifest refraction was −1.00 −2.00 × 170° with keratometric readings of 41.75 × 180°/44.00 × 90°. In this eye, there was also no change in the net amount of astigmatism, 2 D being present before and after surgery, in the same meridian.

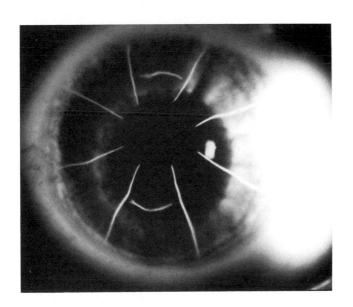

Figure 31-22
Slit-lamp photograph in scleratic scatter demonstrates combined arcuate transverse keratotomy and eight-incision radial keratotomy. A 34-year-old woman had a preoperative refraction of −4.00 −2.50 × 180°. She had eight centripetal incisions using a 3-mm diameter clear zone and two arcuate transverse incisions 40° long at the 6-mm zone. The incisions are irregular. Six months after surgery her uncorrected visual acuity was 20/25, and her refraction was −0.50 −0.50 × 180°.

distance between two adjacent radial incisions (one "segment length") using a previously published nomogram.[169] The results were reported at 3 months after surgery using vectoral analysis.

The preoperative mean astigmatism was 1.5 D ±3.1 D (range, 1.00 to 2.25 D), a narrower range than that reported in the series by Neumann.[128] The mean postoperative refractive cylinder was 0.40 D ±0.61 D. The mean decrease in astigmatism was 1.10 D. The effectiveness of this technique was emphasized by the fact that none of the eyes had less than 1.00 D of astigmatism preoperatively, but postoperatively 85% of the eyes had less than 1.00 D of astigmatism (Table 31-17), and by the fact that only one eye had an increase in refractive astigma-

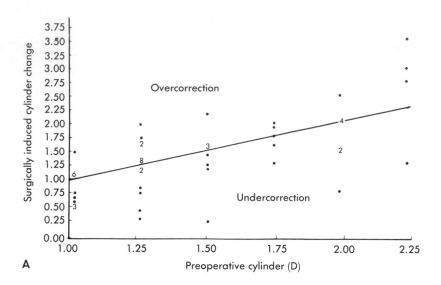

A

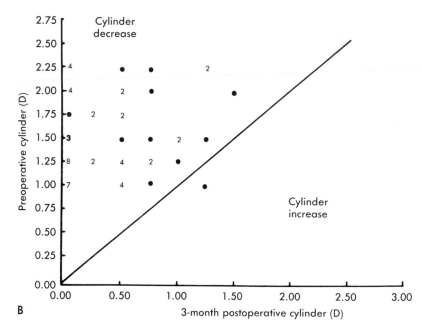

B

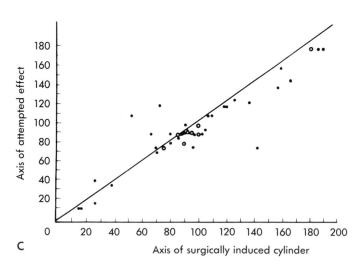

C

Figure 31-23

Scattergrams demonstrating the results of straight transverse incisions between radial incisions in 60 eyes with naturally occurring astigmatism. **A,** The amount of refractive astigmatism decreased in all but one eye. **B,** The surgically induced vectoral astigmatism along the axis perpendicular to the transverse incision indicated a clustering around the desired result, but a spread of approximately 1.50 D. A dot represents one eye. Numbers represent number of eyes at each point. **C,** Comparison of the refractive axis of attempted astigmatic effect to the axis of surgically induced vectoral cylinder. Oblique line indicates the line of equality between the two; few eyes deviated more than 20° from the attempted axis. Dots represent one eye, open circles represent two eyes, triangles represent three eyes, and asterisks at (90°, 90°) data point represent 10 eyes. (From Thornton SP: J Cataract Refract Surg 1987;13:29.)

Table 31-17

Results of Transverse Keratotomy between Radial Incisions for Naturally Occurring Astigmatism

Refractive cylinder (D)	Preoperative			Postoperative		
	Number of eyes	%	Cum %*	Number of eyes	%	Cum %*
0.00 - 0.25	0	0	0	31	52.0	52
0.50 - 0.75	0	0	0	20	33.0	85
1.00 - 1.25	31	52	52	7	12.0	97
1.50 - 1.75	13	22	74	1	1.7	99
2.00 - 2.25	16	26	100	0	0	99
3.00 - 3.75	—	—	—	1	1.7	100

Modified from Thornton SP and Sanders DR: J Cataract Refract Surg 1987;13:27-31.
* Cumulative percentage of all eyes operated.

Case 3: Successful Combined Transverse and Radial Incisions

A 31-year-old patient had a history of amblyopia in the right eye with an uncorrected visual acuity of 20/400, a spectacle-corrected visual acuity of 20/40, and a refraction of −2.50 −4.00 × 14°. Central keratotomy readings were 40.50 × 15°/43.87 × 105°. Keratotomy surgery consisted of six radial incisions with a 3-mm diameter clear zone and two straight transverse incisions 3 mm long at the 5-mm zone between the radials across the steep meridian. Depth was approximately 90%. Eight months after surgery the refraction was plano −0.75 × 55° with corrected visual acuity of 20/30. Keratometry measurements were 38.75 × 57°/39.75 × 147°. Uncorrected visual acuity was 20/40. This case illustrates a less commonly used technique of combined radial and astigmatic keratotomy with the transverse incision placed closer to the center (at the 5-mm zone) to achieve a greater effect. The spherical equivalent refraction was reduced 4.12 D, and the refractive astigmatism was reduced 3.67 D.

---

tism (Fig. 31-23). However, the vectoral results indicated a wide spread in the outcome, indicating a range of vectoral astigmatic correction of approximately 1.50 D. The effect of the surgery was concentrated in the intended corneal meridian, the axis of the surgically induced astigmatism being quite close to that of the attempted effect.

Based on this experience, Thornton devised an updated guide to astigmatism surgery (see Tables 31-41 and 31-42). Differences from the technique described in the published paper include making the pair of incisions at a 7-mm zone instead of an 8-mm zone and using two pairs of incisions placed at the 6- and 8-mm zones if the astigmatism is 2.50 D or more. He now prefers arcuate instead of straight incisions (personal written communication, June 1991).

Interrupted transverse or radial incisions. Neumann and colleagues[128] compared three types of combined radial and transverse keratotomy, with all incisions made in the steep meridian. The three techniques were used sequentially in three different series of eyes with different follow-up times. The first series used radial and intersecting staggered transverse incisions (mean follow-up, 8.1 months); the second series used radial and nonintersecting interrupted transverse incisions ("jump-T") (mean follow-up, 5.2 months); the third series used transverse and nonintersecting interrupted radials (mean follow-up, 3.0 months). Both refractive and vectoral astigmatic results were presented (Fig. 31-24 and Tables 31-18 to 31-20). Preoperatively, all eyes had between 0.50

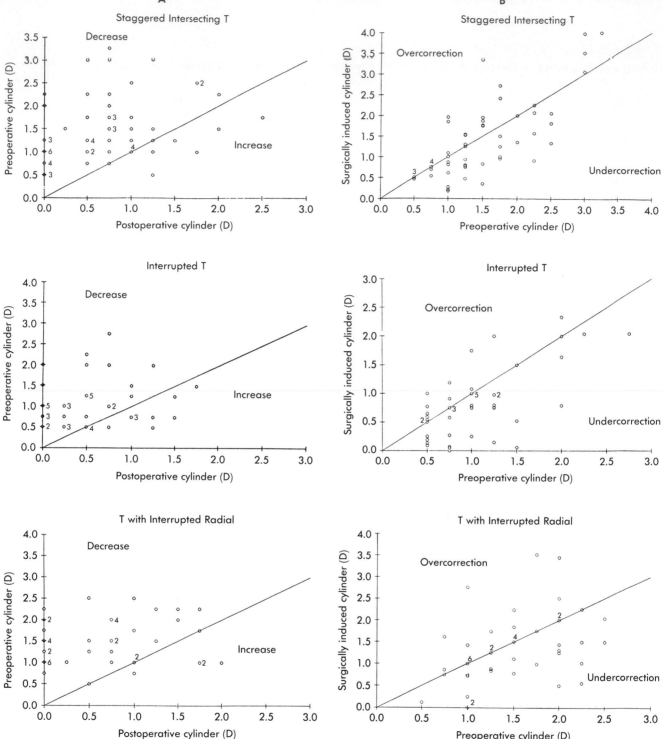

Figure 31-24

Results of combined transverse and radial keratotomy in three different patterns: staggered intersecting transverse, interrupted transverse, and interrupted radials in eyes with naturally occurring astigmatism. Column **A,** Scatterplots of the refractive astigmatism compare preoperative and postoperative refractive cylinders for each of the three techniques. Column **B,** Scatterplots compare the surgically induced vectoral astigmatism in the meridian perpendicular to the incision with the preoperative refractive astigmatism. Multiple eyes are indicated with numbers. All three techniques decreased refractive astigmatism, but there was a wide scatter in the results. (From Neumann AC, McCarty GR, Sanders DR, and Raanan MG: J Cataract Refract Surg 1989;15:78-84.)

Table 31-18

Comparison of Three Patterns of Combined Transverse (T) and Radial Keratotomy for Naturally Occurring Astigmatism Showing Preoperative and Postoperative Refractive Cylinder (D) and the Number (Percentage) of Eyes

Refractive astigmatism (D)	Staggered touching T		Interrupted T		T with interrupted radial	
	Preoperative	Postoperative	Preoperative	Postoperative	Preoperative	Postoperative
< 0.5	0	19 (31.7)	0	19 (40.4)	0	18 (38.3)
0.5 to 0.99	10 (16.6)	23 (38.3)	21 (44.7)	17 (36.2)	18 (38.3)	13 (27.7)
1.0 to 1.49	24 (40.0)	12 (20.0)	17 (36.2)	8 (17.0)	11 (23.4)	8 (17.0)
1.5 to 1.99	13 (21.7)	3 (5.0)	3 (6.4)	3 (6.4)	12 (25.5)	7 (14.9)
2.0 to 2.99	9 (15.0)	3 (5.0)	6 (12.8)	0	2 (4.3)	1 (2.1)
3.0 to 3.99	4 (6.7)	0	0	0	0	0

Modified from Neumann AC, McCarty GR, Sanders DR, and Raanan MG: J Cataract Refract Surg 1989;15:25-31.

Table 31-19

Comparison of Three Patterns of Combined Transverse (T) and Radial Keratotomy for Naturally Occurring Astigmatism

	Pattern		
	Staggered touching T	Interrupted T	T with interrupted radial
Number of eyes	60	47	47
Mean age (yr)	35.5	34.4	32.6
Follow-up (mo.)			
mean (range)	8.1 (2 to 16)	5.2 (1 to 14)	3.0 (1 to 9)
Preoperative refractive cylinder	1.44	1.05	1.47
Mean (SD)	0.68	0.53	0.52
Range	0.5 to 3.25	0.5 to 2.75	0.5 to 2.5
Eyes with postoperative refractive cylinder < 1 D	70%	77%	66%
Surgically induced vectoral cylinder	1.39	0.84	1.33
Mean	0.88	0.59	0.76
Range	0.19 to 3.99	0 to 2.33	0 to 3.5
Eyes with surgically induced cylinder ≤ 0.5 D in attempted axis	63%	72%	60%
Percentage correction	96.4	82.3	93.1
Mean	37.9	46.9	51.9
Range	18 to 222	0 to 200	0 to 275
Eyes with deviation of surgically induced axis from attempted axis < 20°	78%	77%	89%

Modified from Neumann AC, McCarty GR, Sanders DR, and Raanan MG: J Cataract Refract Surg 1989;15:25-31.

Table 31-20

Deviation of the Surgically Induced Vectoral Refractive Cylinder Axis from the Axis of Attempted Effect (the Steep Meridian Perpendicular to the Transverse [T] Incision) for Three Combined Techniques

Amount of axis deviation	Staggered touching T	Interrupted T	T with interrupted radial
< 10°	58%	64%	72%
< 20°	78%	77%	89%
≥ 30°	13%	23%	11%

Modified from Neumann AC, McCarty GR, Sanders DR, and Raanan MG: J Cataract Refract Surg 1989;15:25-31.

and 3.75 D of refractive astigmatism. All transverse incisions were straight, placed at the 6-mm zone, and were calculated so that the total transverse incision length in millimeters was equal to the preoperative astigmatism in diopters. The length of the blade was 100% of the central corneal thickness. A basic premise of this paper is that better control of astigmatism can be achieved when both the radial and transverse incisions are centered over the steep corneal meridian.

All three techniques effectively reduced astigmatism, correcting more than 80% of the preexisting astigmatism, although a few eyes showed 0.50 to 1.00 D increase in astigmatism (Fig. 31-24). In terms of the surgically induced vectoral change in the desired preoperative meridian, the percentage of correction of astigmatism was generally similar: intersecting transverse incisions, 96.4% ±37.9% (range, 18% to 222%; interrupted transverse incisions 83.3% ±46.9% (range, 0% to 200%); and interrupted radial incisions, 93.1% ±51.9% (range, 0% to 275%). Thus there was generally poor predictability, with the range of correction spanning over 200% and the standard deviations being approximately half of the mean values for all three techniques. In addition, it was difficult to reduce the postoperative refractive astigmatism to less than 1.00 D, the percentage of eyes having more than 1 D of residual astigmatism being 70%, 77%, and 66% for the three groups. There was good correlation between the meridian of surgery and the refractive axis of the surgically induced cylinder, approximately 80% of the eyes deviating by less than 20% from the desired axis. No statistical analyses were reported for comparing the three groups.

The authors[128] abandoned the staggered, intersecting transverse incisions because of increased scarring at the junctions and because the other procedures seemed to be slightly more effective. They preferred the transverse incisions with interrupted radial incisions because they achieved a somewhat higher amount of correction, had the best correlation between the desired and achieved vectoral axis of correction, and avoided intersection of incisions.

Hofmann[76] reported a prospective study of 104 eyes using staggered, intersecting transverse and radial incisions in eyes with 1.00 to 3.25 D of refractive astigmatism and a follow-up of at least 1 year. The average preoperative refractive astigmatism was 1.95 D, and the average postoperative refractive astigmatism was 0.47 D. However, 83% of the eyes had 1.25 D or more of residual astigmatism. Hofmann also reported a series of 56 eyes with interrupted transverse incisions, 90% deep, placed across the steep meridian at zone diameters of 5.5, 6.0, 6.5, and 7.0 mm, with 0.2 mm between the end of the transverse incision and the radial incision. Each incision was 2 mm long for a total transverse

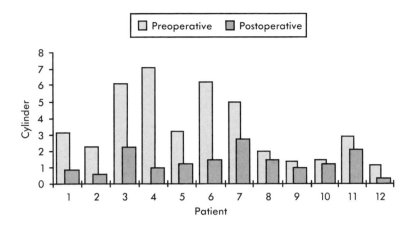

Figure 31-25
Bar graph demonstrates refractive cylinder before and after bowtie keratotomy in 12 eyes with different types of astigmatism. Seven of the 12 eyes demonstrated a clinically meaningful decrease in astigmatism. (From Tate GW: International Society of Refractive Keratoplasty, Las Vegas, October 7, 1988.)

incision length of 4 mm in each semimeridian. Fifty-nine percent of the eyes achieved a reduction of 1 D or less of astigmatism, so the overall effectiveness was less than desired.

Agapitos and colleagues[1] reported 20 eyes that had combined transverse and radial incisions, 10 with the transverse between the radials, eight with interrupted transverse incisions, and two with flag transverse incisions. The average follow-up was 7.7 months. The average preoperative keratometric astigmatism was 2.50 D, and the average change in keratometric astigmatism was 2.90 D. The change in spherical equivalent refraction was +2.27 D, indicating an overall flattening of the cornea.

Bow tie keratotomy. Tate described a clinical series of the bow tie technique. The operation consisted of a standard 4-incision radial keratotomy with the incisions 90° apart. A peripheral arcuate incision was made across the steep meridian at the 10- to 12-mm diameter zone, which connected two of the radial incisions. The clear zone of the radial incisions ranged from 4 to 6 mm. For seven primary and six secondary procedures with an average follow-up of approximately 100 days, the overall change in spherical equivalent refraction was a flattening of approximately 1.50 to 2.50 D. Seven of the 12 eyes showed a clinically meaningful decrease in refractive astigmatism of between 1 and 6 D, whereas five eyes showed a minimal decrease in refractive astigmatism (Fig. 31-25).

Trapezoidal keratotomy—nonintersecting incisions. Trapezoidal keratotomy in its classical form—a pair of semiradial incisions converging centrally with two to four transverse incisions between them—is one of the most thoroughly studied astigmatic keratotomy procedures, although the many frequent modifications bespeak the inherent problems with the procedure and may reflect why the operation has lost popularity (see Fig. 31-9).

Ibrahim and colleagues[77] reported the results of nonintersecting trapezoidal keratotomy in 64 eyes of 45 consecutive patients with naturally occurring astigmatism (Fig. 31-26). Preoperative refractive astigmatism ranged from 2.25 to 7.00 D (mean, 3.8 D ±1.16 D); 62.5% of the eyes were between 3.00 and 5.00 D. The diameter of the central clear zone for the radial incisions ranged from 3 to 5 mm and was proportionate to the amount of preoperative refractive astig-

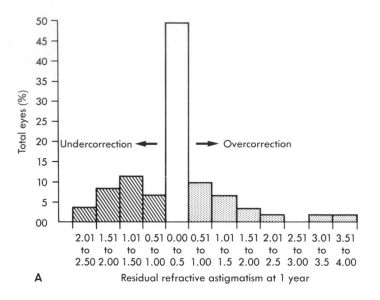

A

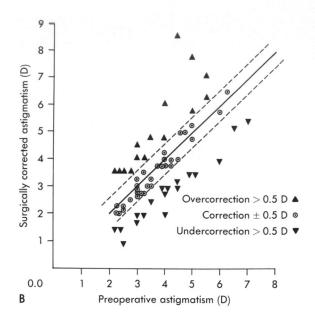

B

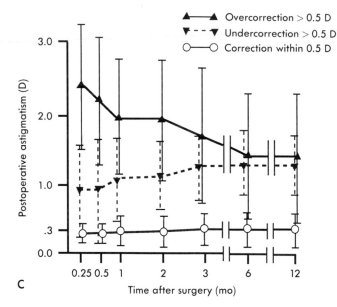

C

Figure 31-26

Results of nonintersecting trapezoidal keratotomy in 64 eyes with naturally occurring astigmatism. **A,** Bar graph of astigmatism after surgery demonstrates that 64% of eyes had residual astigmatism of 1.00 D or less. **B,** Scattergram compares the preoperative astigmatism to the surgically induced vectoral astigmatism. Dotted lines represent a correction of ±1.50 D. **C,** Changes in surgically induced vectoral astigmatism during 1 year after surgery. In general, eyes corrected to within ± 0.50 D or undercorrected showed a stable postoperative course, but overcorrected eyes showed a gradual loss of effect up to about 6 months. Symbols represent mean values; error bars represent standard deviation. (From Ibrahim O, Hussein HA, Kassem A, et al: Arch Ophthalmol, in press.)

matism. The length of the transverse incisions depended on the spherical component of the minus cylinder refraction: myopic = 1.5 mm long; plano to +2.00 D = 2.5 mm long, greater than +2.00 D = 5.0 mm long. The mean preoperative refractive astigmatism was 3.18 D ±1.16 D (range, 2.25 to 7.00 D). One year after surgery the mean surgically corrected vectoral astigmatism was 3.70 D ±1.50 D (range, 0.75 to 8.50 D), and the mean residual refractive astigmatism was 0.85 D ±0.72 D (range, 0.25 to 4.00 D); 64% of the eyes had 1 D or less of refractive astigmatism. The scatter of the results and the similar distribution of undercorrections and overcorrections indicate the lack of predictability of the procedure (Table 31-21).

Ibrahim and colleagues[77] observed that a smaller diameter clear zone for the semiradial incisions enhanced the effect, roughly on the order of 1.00 D for each 0.50 mm length. Eyes with clear zone diameters of 3.0 to 4.0 mm for the semi-radial incisions showed a flattening to steepening ratio of approximately 6,

Table 31-21

Comparison between Preoperative and Postoperative Refractive Astigmatism at 1 Year after Nonintersecting Trapezoidal Keratotomy for Naturally Occurring Astigmatism

Astigmatism (D)	Preoperative			1 Year postoperative		
	No. of eyes	Percent of total eyes	Cumulative percent	No. of eyes	Percent of total eyes	Cumulative percent
0.00 to 0.50				31	48.4	48.4
0.51 to 1.0				10	15.6	64.0
1.01 to 1.5				11	17.2	81.2
1.51 to 2.0				7	11.0	92.2
2.01 to 3.0	11	17.2	17.2	3	4.7	96.9
3.01 to 4.0	23	35.9	53.1	2	3.1	100.0
4.01 to 5.0	17	26.5	79.6			
5.01 to 6.0	8	12.5	92.1			
6.01 to 7.0	4	6.3	98.4			
7.01 to 8.0	1	1.6	100.0			
Total	64	100.0		64	100.0	

Modified from Ibrahim O, Hussein JA, El-Sahn MF, El-Nawawy S, Kassem A, and Waring GO: Arch Ophthalmol, in press.

Case 4: Trapezoidal Keratotomies with Nonintersecting Incisions and Variable Results

A 44-year-old patient had a refractive error in the right eye of plano $-2.75 \times 180°$, a corrected visual acuity of 20/25, and keratometric readings of $44.00 \times 4°/47.12 \times 94°$. Surgery consisted of a nonintersecting trapezoidal keratotomy with a 3-mm diameter clear zone for the semiradial incisions with two pairs of 3 mm long transverse incisions placed at the 5- and 7-mm zones at 90°. Five months after surgery, visual acuity without correction was 20/70. The manifest refraction was $+0.50 -2.50 \times 130°$ with keratometric readings of $40.12 \times 115°/43.50 \times 25°$. This result was unsatisfactory, showing almost no change in astigmatism.

In the left eye the preoperative refractive error was $-0.75 -4.00 \times 165°$, the corrected visual acuity 20/25, and the keratometric readings $43.00 \times 170°/47.62 \times 80°$. Surgery consisted of a nonintersecting trapezoidal keratotomy with a 3-mm diameter clear zone for the semiradial incisions and with two pairs of 3 mm long transverse incisions placed at the 5- and 7-mm clear zones at 75°, the same procedure performed in the right eye. However, in this case the outcome was better, because 2 months after surgery the refraction was $+0.50 -0.75 \times 135°$ with keratometry readings of $41.50 \times 170°/41.87 \times 80°$. This case emphasizes the variability that can be seen in trapezoidal keratotomy.

---

whereas eyes with a 5-mm zone showed a flattening to steepening ratio of approximately 4. The length of the transverse incisions of 1.5 mm, 2.5 mm, and 5.0 mm showed that the 5-mm incisions produced approximately twice as much steepening of the unincised meridian, so the flattening to steepening ratio was 2.5 for the 5-mm incisions, whereas it was approximately 5 for the 1.5- and 2.5-mm incisions (see Table 31-7). They observed that two pairs of incisions achieved as much result (mean, 2.4 D) as three pairs or four pairs when the clear zone diameter of the semiradial incisions was 5.0 mm. With the smaller clear zone of 4.0 mm for the semiradial incisions, two pairs of incisions achieved a mean correction of 2.0 D, whereas three and four pairs achieved a mean correction of 3.2 D. In general, two pairs of incisions were preferred.

The authors analyzed the stability of results during 1 year after surgery, observing that eyes with a residual astigmatism of ±0.50 D or eyes that were undercorrected showed a generally stable course, whereas eyes that were overcorrected showed a gradual decay of refraction over the first 6 months (see Fig. 34-26).

Lara[95] reported the results of 15 out of 32 eyes that had nonintersecting trapezoidal keratotomy based on the nomogram of Nordan.[130] The mean preoperative refractive astigmatism was 3.85 D (range, 2.5 to 7.0 D), and postoperatively it was 1.13 D (range, 0.00 to 3.00 D).

Trapezoidal keratotomy—intersecting incisions. A number of articles have been published regarding the now abandoned technique of intersecting the innermost transverse incision with the two semiradial incisions. An initial study of 17 eyes by Lavery and Lindstrom[96] was updated by Merck and colleagues[122] using vectoral analysis. Twenty-three eyes were operated, 14 after penetrating keratoplasty, eight after cataract extraction, and one with naturally occurring astigmatism. The clear zone diameter for the semiradial incisions ranged from 3 to 6 mm and the achieved incision depth was approximately 80%. Four pairs of transverse incisions were made, the inner pair intersecting the tips of the semiradial incisions. Preoperative keratometric astigmatism ranged from 3.13 to 13.00 D. The mean follow-up was 5 months. The surgically induced vectoral astigmatism varied from 1.28 to 14.21 D. Frequently, due to a shift in the axis of surgically induced change, the change in keratometric astigmatism was not the same as the reduction of the refractive astigmatism; therefore in many cases a residual astigmatic error was created in a meridian that was significantly different from that of the preoperative astigmatism. The authors found that approximately one third of the eyes obtained a reduction of astigmatism in the intended meridian, whereas the other two thirds either had an inadequate reduction in the amount of astigmatism or sustained a surgically induced change in the astigmatic axis. This lack of predictability of refractive effect in a specified meridian was the chief problem with the technique.

The group of eyes reported by Lavery[96] and then by Merck[122] was included in a subsequent report of 30 eyes with interesecting trapezoidal keratotomy by Agapitos and collagues.[1] The mean preoperative keratometric astigmatism was 8.3 D (range, 3.00 to 23.30 D), and the mean change in keratometric astigmatism was 8.0 D ±6.0 D. The large standard deviation indicated the wide scatter in the results. Although there was a reasonably good correlation between the axis attempted and the axis achieved, 30% of the eyes had a deviation of 10° to 30° from the intended axis of correction.

Villasenor and Stimac[185] reported the results of trapezoidal keratotomy in 35 consecutive eyes with naturally occurring astigmatism after keratoplasty, cataract extraction, and keratomileusis. Fifteen of the eyes had intersecting radial and transverse incisions and the remainder were nonintersecting. The largest group—the 29 eyes with naturally occurring astigmatism—had a mean preoperative astigmatism of 4.61 D ±1.05 D and a mean postoperative astigmatism of 2.16 D ±1.86 D, with the mean change in astigmatic axis of 24° ±27°. A residual astigmatism of 1.00 D or less was present in 31% of the eyes, and 55% had a residual astigmatism of 2.00 D or less. The results were worse for the five eyes with astigmatism after penetrating keratoplasty. The authors concluded that trapezoidal keratotomy produced less than satisfactory results with lack of predictability. They also found an unacceptably high complication rate including macroperforations, vascularization of the wounds, and late wound separation. The overall perforation rate was 23%. The authors concluded, "The risk-benefit ratio does not warrant the use of trapezoidal keratotomy in its present forms."[185]

Trapezoidal keratotomy—general observations. Although trapezoidal keratotomy can effect a large vectoral change in astigmatism, the residual refractive
astigmatism may remain large because of a difference in the original astigmatic
axis and the surgically induced axis.[77,122,185] Most eyes change their spherical
equivalent refraction in the hyperopic direction, indicating an overall flattening
after the procedure, but there can be great variation in the flattening/steepening
ratio. Most observers[105,131,145] agree that an optimal incision depth is approximately 80% to 85%. The amount of corneal flattening is roughly proportionate
to the diameter of the clear zone for the semiradial incisions, and there is a general tendency to keep the zone diameter at 4 mm or larger to prevent irregular
astigmatism and glare.[131,185] In general, the length of the transverse incisions
does not greatly affect the amount of flattening in the incised meridian, but the
longer the incision, the greater the steepening in the orthogonal unincised meridian up to a length of about 5 mm, as discussed previously. Opinions differ on
the optimal number of transverse incisions; most surgeons use one or two pairs.
The innermost transverse incisions are usually made central to the ends of the
semiradial incisions, which increases their effect and allows lengthening in a reoperation.

Grouped radial incisions

Grouped radial incisions (see Fig. 31-10) are no longer in clinical use, simply
because they correct only small amounts of astigmatism and are generally ineffective.

In 1980 Fyodorov[63] presented clinical results of different patterns of astigmatic keratotomy procedures. Seven cases of parallel semiradial incisions (L procedure) achieved a mean correction of 1.68 D; 16 cases combining the parallel
semiradial incisions with radial incisions (RL procedure) achieved a mean correction of 1.15 D. In 1981 Fyodorov and Durnev[64] described 16 eyes with combined radial incisions and parallel semiradial incisions (RL procedure), stating
that eight of the 16 cases had no astigmatism postoperatively. Neumann (personal communication, International Society of Refractive Keratoplasty Meeting,
Las Vegas, Nevada, October 7, 1988) reported 56 eyes that received parallel
semiradial incisions (L procedure) or combined radial incisions and parallel
semiradial (RL) incisions. He concluded that these techniques were not effective
or predictable because there was only a 57% reduction in the preoperative astigmatism and 30% of the eyes exhibited a change in refractive astigmatic axis of
30° or more. Grady[69] performed parallel semiradial incisions (L procedure) on
33 eyes with 1.75 to 3.00 D of astigmatism, achieving an uncorrected visual acuity of 20/20 or better in 27 of the eyes. No refractive results were reported.

Shepard[153] reported the results of 279 parallel semiradial procedures (L) using between one and 16 parallel incisions, but there was no way to determine
the results of this technique because they were combined with those of other
techniques in the report. Zelman[191] reported the use of parallel semiradial incisions in the steep meridian combined with radial incisions (RL), but reported no
data.

The laboratory results of Franks and colleagues[62] and Yau and colleagues[190]
also have concluded that group radial and semiradial incisions are not effective.

Oval clear zone

The oval clear zone also has been found to be ineffective and is no longer
used, although the logic of making longer incisions in the steep meridian was
appealing. Fyodorov[63] described 10 eyes with an oval clear zone with an average correction of 0.58 D. Fyodorov and Durnev[64] reported five more oval clear

zone cases with a mean correction of 1.60 D. Grady[69] and Hofmann[76] considered oval clear zones to be ineffective. Agapitos and colleagues[1] reported five eyes treated with radial incisions and an oval clear zone; the average preoperative keratometric astigmatism was 1.30 D, and the average change induced was 0.90 D. The overall spherical equivalent change was +2.27 D, indicating the overall flattening effect.

Deep circular trephination

Krumeich[92] has described making a simple circular trephination 90% deep in the cornea with antitorque suturing of the incision for the correction of astigmatism. The principle of the operation is Gauss' law; a deep circular incision releases the stress within the central cornea so that an island of "stress-free" tissue is created in which Gauss' law of coupling does the work—the steep meridian flattens, the flat meridian steepens, and the central cornea becomes spherical. The diameter of the incision is usually 7 mm. Krumeich employs the guided trephine system with a Barraquer-style suction ring on the cornea, which does not raise the intraocular pressure. A calibrated trephine is attached to the suction ring and remains perpendicular to the surface. If necessary, sutures are removed or transverse incisions are added to correct more than 4 D of residual astigmatism. The technique depends on the ability to make a trephination 90% deep without perforating the cornea, on the adequate placement of sutures so as not to induce astigmatism, on the assumption of uniform circumferential wound healing, and on the realization that the astigmatism may change when the sutures are removed.[23]

Krumeich[92] reported 14 eyes selected from a larger number and followed for at least 1 year. The causes of astigmatism included postoperative and posttraumatic cases. Preoperatively, the mean astigmatism was 5.66 D (range, 3.0 to 9.0 D). At 12 months after surgery with sutures in place, the mean astigmatism was 1.33 D, with 28% of eyes having 1.00 D or less of residual astigmatism and 93% of eyes (all but one) having 2.00 D or less.

The technique takes advantage of improved instrumentation and warrants further study to verify Krumeich's results. Final astigmatism with all sutures removed should be reported, along with the change in the spherical equivalent refraction.

Scleral surgery for astigmatism

Jose Barraquer[15] has used wedge resection of the limbus to steepen the flat meridian in naturally occurring astigmatism. No data have been published using this technique.

Incisions made outside the limbus have less effect on the central cornea than those made inside the limbus. Therefore scleral incisions are not used for the correction of naturally occurring or postkeratoplasty astigmatism, but they do play a role in the generation of astigmatism after cataract surgery, as discussed in a subsequent section.

ASTIGMATISM AFTER CATARACT SURGERY

The evolution of techniques of cataract extraction over the last 250 years, since Daviel established the method of extracting a cataractous lens through an incision in the cornea, has included a mind-boggling variety of incision and suture techniques, many designed to reduce postoperative astigmatism. Interestingly, all this experience and information may be heading for the archives of history if small-incision, sutureless cataract surgery becomes the standard of practice. Until that time, however, surgeons must continue to attempt to control the factors that affect astigmatism after cataract surgery (Table 31-22).

Table 31-22

Effect of Cataract Incision Variables on Postoperative Astigmatism

Variable	Options	Effect on astigmatism in meridian of incision
Incision		
Location (zone diameter)		Smaller zone results in more astigmatism.
	Scleral (14 to 15 mm)	Least
	Limbal (12 to 13 mm)	Intermediate
	Corneal (10 to 11 mm)	Most
Surgical technique and incision (chord) length		
	Phacoemulsification plus foldable intraocular lens (3 to 4 mm)	Least
	Phacoemulsification plus rigid intraocular lens (5 to 7 mm)	Least
	Extracapsular cataract extraction (10 to 11 mm)	Intermediate
	Intracapsular cataract extraction (12 mm)	Most
Incision depth and configuration	One plane; anterior or posterior bevel	Deeper incision results in more astigmatism.
	Two plane or three plane; anterior flap of variable depth	Thicker anterior flap results in more astigmatism.
	Scleral pocket	More distance from limbus may reduce astigmatism.
Suture		
Material		More elasticity results in less wound compression and astigmatism at same suture tension.
	Polypropylene (Prolene)	
	Nylon	Least
	Polyester (Mersilene)	Intermediate
	Stainless steel	
	Silk	Most
Diameter		Larger diameter results in more compression for same suture material and tension.
	11-0	Least
	10-0	Intermediate
	9-0	Most
Volume of tissue in each suture bite		More volume results in more steepening.
	Small—short and shallow bite	Least
	Large—long and deep bite	Most
Number of suture bites		More sutures result in more steepening.
Compression of tissue = suture tension		More tension results in more steepening.
	Edges separated	Flatten the operated meridian
	Edges approximated	No change in the operated meridian
	Edges compressed	Steepen the operated meridian
Pattern	Interrupted	Astigmatism depends on suture location, bite size, and tension.
	X	
	Single	
	Continuous	
	Double continuous	
	Parallel to wound (vertical mattress)	

Development of techniques to control astigmatism

Interest in reducing astigmatism after cataract surgery is only approximately 20 years old, commencing in the late 1960s with the advent of monofilament nylon sutures placed after the cataract was extracted. Earlier studies glossed over the problem of postcataract astigmatism. For example, the standard European and American textbook of ocular surgery by Arruga[8] published in 1952 details an enormous variety of cataract incision and suture techniques, but dismisses astigmatism in one sentence as a minimal postoperative problem. Similarly the manual on cataract surgery published by the American Academy of Ophthalmology and Otolaryngology in 1967[141] gives details of cataract incision and suture techniques, but never mentions astigmatism. The major concern of cataract surgeons before the era of microsurgery was to obtain a good anatomic closure of the cataract wound. However, astigmatism after cataract surgery was not completely ignored. In fact, almost a century ago, Snellen noticed the occurrence of astigmatism with-the-rule following cataract surgery and suggested making an incision perpendicular to the meridian of greatest refractive power to decrease the postoperative astigmatism (see Chapter 5, Development of Refractive Keratotomy in the Nineteenth Century). In 1936 Groenholm and Kangasniemi[70] found that increasing the number of silk sutures would decrease the amount of against-the-rule astigmatism. Studies of the change in astigmatism over time after surgery were also reported, such as that by Floyd in 1951,[60] who observed that with-the-rule astigmatism occurring soon after cataract surgery would change to against-the-rule astigmatism in more than half of the eyes when only one to two silk sutures were used.[52]

In the late 1960s and early 1970s Troutman[175] used his experience with the operating microscope and monofilament nylon suture to emphasize the importance of astigmatism after cataract and corneal surgery, observing that absorbable sutures produced more against-the-rule astigmatism than did monofilament sutures because of early postoperative wound stretch. He also emphasized the importance of correcting preexisting astigmatism by the use of a limbal wedge resection in the flat meridian as part of the cataract incision. Jaffe and Clayman[79,80] made major contributions in the early 1970s by emphasizing the different effects of wound and suture patterns on astigmatism after cataract surgery and by emphasizing the need for vectoral analysis. The trend toward shorter, more posteriorly placed incisions in the 1980s has reduced postoperative astigmatism; most studies report less than 3 D in over 90% of eyes.

A detailed discussion of the pathogenesis of astigmatism after cataract surgery and the multitude of methods proposed to control it is beyond the scope of this book. In this chapter we concentrate on current surgical techniques, present the similarities between the cataract surgery incision and transverse keratotomy for astigmatism, and emphasize the use of transverse keratotomy to correct astigmatism during and after cataract surgery.

Cataract surgery as refractive surgery

Modern cataract surgery is a form of refractive surgery from two points of view:

1. Intraocular lens implantation attempts to correct spherical refractive errors, both at distance and, with the advent of multifocal intraocular lenses, at near. There is even recurrent interest in implantation of intraocular lenses in phakic eyes to correct myopia.[12,39,125a,150a] Discussion of intraocular lens implantation is beyond the scope of this book.
2. Cataract surgeons attempt to minimize postoperative astigmatism both by reducing preexisting astigmatism and by preventing the induction of astigmatism from the surgical procedure. In most cases the surgeon attempts no

alteration in astigmatism in eyes with minimal preoperative astigmatism. However, in eyes that have 1.50 D or more of astigmatism before surgery, the surgeon may modify the cataract incision or do intraoperative transverse keratotomy to reduce the preexisting astigmatism.[22,159]

Effect of cataract wound on astigmatism

The incision made for cataract surgery can be considered a type of transverse arcuate or straight keratotomy, even though it is often made in the limbus or the sclera.[117] Therefore its effect follows the basic principles of transverse keratotomy (Table 31-22).

The variables that affect transverse astigmatic keratotomy also affect cataract incisions, with the additional effect of the sutures.

Location of incision—zone diameter. The smaller the clear zone ("optical zone") diameter the greater the effect of a transverse keratotomy. The same principle applies to cataract incisions. Those placed within the cornea or the anterior limbus will have more effect on corneal astigmatism than those placed in the posterior limbus or in the sclera. Of course, the cataract incisions placed at zones of 11 to 14 mm in diameter will have much less effect on the central corneal curvature than a transverse astigmatic keratotomy placed in the 5- to 8-mm diameter zones.

Hanna and colleagues[72] devised a finite element computer model with anisotropic, nonlinear assumptions to demonstrate that an incision placed in the cornea induces more radial deformation than one placed in the sclera, which produces almost no corneal deformation (see Chapter 34).

Many surgeons have concluded that a posteriorly placed scleral wound will induce less astigmatism.[57,67,113,173] An early study that demonstrated the effect of the location of the cataract incision was carried out by Jaffe,[80] demonstrating less astigmatism in eyes where a markedly beveled scleral incision was made (Table 31-23). Shepherd[155] described 99 eyes with a 4-mm scleral incision made 2 mm posterior to the limbus and closed with a single suture. The mean induced astigmatism 3 months after surgery was 0.22 D ±0.47 D. At 1 month the induced astigmatism was 1.00 D or less in 98% of the eyes. The change in astigmatism from 1 to 3 months was 1.00 D or less in 100% of the eyes. This demonstrated considerable wound stability in the short term.

Table 31-23

Effect of Three Types of Limbal Incisions on Astigmatism after Cataract Extraction

	Anterior limbal incision	Posterior limbal incision	Beveled scleral incision
Number of eyes	138	248	276
Average postoperative astigmatism (D)	2.69	1.56	0.77
Percentage of eyes with no astigmatism	2	21	42
Percentage of eyes with astigmatism with-the-rule	3	8	22
Percentage of eyes with astigmatism against-the-rule	95	71	36

Modified from Jaffe NS, Jaffe MS, and Jaffe GF: Cataract surgery and its complications, St Louis, 1990, CV Mosby Co, pp 109-127.

Table 31-24

Astigmatism Induced by Three Different Posterior Limbal Cataract Incision Lengths at 3 Months after Surgery

Surgical technique and style	Number of eyes (percent examined at 3 mo)	Incision chord length (mm)	Suture pattern (10-0 nylon)	Preoperative refractive astigmatism (D) (mean, SD, range)	Net change in refractive astigmatism (D) (mean, SD, range)	Vectoral change in refractive astigmatism (D) (mean, SD, range)
Phacoemulsification and silicone IOL	67 (75%)	3 to 4	Interrupted	0.8 ±0.16 (0 to 3.25)	0.14 (0.97) (−2.0 to +3.5)	1.29 (0.96) (0 to 3.25)
Phacoemulsification and PMMA IOL	56 (89%)	6	Interrupted	0.78 ±0.05 (0 to 2.50)	0.21 (0.86) (−1.0 to +3.0)	1.06 (1.09) (1 to 7.42)
Extracapsular cataract extraction	59 (92%)	10	Running	0.82 ±0.73 (0 to 2.75)	1.43 (1.41)* (−1.5 to +7.0)	2.27 (1.28)* (0.5 to 7.0)

Modified from Neumann AC, McCarty GR, Sanders DR, and Raanan MG: J Cataract Refract Surg 1989;15:78-84.
*Significantly different; $p = 0.0001$.

The location of the cataract incision should center on either the steep meridian in with-the-rule astigmatism or the flat meridian in against-the-rule astigmatism. This will give a better opportunity for using wound modifications to alter the astigmatism because the axis of astigmatism does not shift markedly during such a procedure.[112]

Incision length. Longer incisions have a greater tendency to alter corneal curvature. Therefore, if the surgeon wishes to leave the curvature unchanged, a 3- to 4-mm incision, as used with phacoemulsification and a foldable intraocular lens, will be of greater advantage. In the future, cataract surgery may be done through smaller puncture wounds, further decreasing the induced astigmatism. On the other hand, attempts to change corneal curvature will require a 6- to 10-mm long incision, as is commonly used in extracapsular cataract extraction with implantation of an unfolded intraocular lens.

Armeniades and colleagues[7] used a finite element model to demonstrate that a 12-mm scleral incision induced up to seven times as much radial deformation on the cornea as did a 3-mm long incision. They concluded that the length of the incision was more important than the location of the incision or the configuration of the incision in determining corneal deformation and astigmatism after cataract surgery.

Numerous studies have compared longer wounds placed closer to the cornea with shorter wounds placed in the sclera.[173] Neumann and colleagues[129] compared three different incision lengths: a 3- to 4-mm incision used with a foldable IOL, a 6-mm chord length incision used with phacoemulsification, and a 10-mm chord length used with extracapsular cataract extraction (Table 31-24). The two shorter phacoemulsification incisions induced less astigmatism at 3 months and at 6 months than the longer incision. The cases were not done concurrently and did not represent consecutive series of eyes; different suturing techniques were used, so the results must be interpreted cautiously. Nevertheless, the differences were statistically significantly different and clinically meaningful. The authors concluded that the small-incision phacoemulsification produced earlier visual rehabilitation with better uncorrected and corrected visual acuity. Lindstrom and Destro[104] compared retrospectively a series of eyes that had a 6- to 7-mm chord length incision for phacoemulsification with a series of eyes that had a 10- to 11-mm chord length incision for extracapsular cataract extraction, both incisions being placed 1.5 to 2 mm posterior to the limbus. Intraoperative keratometry

Table 31-25

Eyes with Different Length Cataract Incisions Achieving Each Level of Keratometric Astigmatism at 6 to 10 Weeks Postoperatively (Incision Placed 1.5 to 2.0 mm behind the Limbus)

		Postoperative astigmatism (D)			
Surgical technique	Number of eyes	< 1 N (%)	1 to 2 N (%)	2 to 3 N (%)	>3 N (%)
Phacoemulsification with 6- to 7-mm incision	120	78 (65)*	31 (26)	5 (4)	6 (5)*
Extracapsular cataract extraction with 10- to 11-mm incision	80	22 (27)*	34 (43)	5 (6)	19 (24)*

Modified from Lindstrom RL and Destro MA: Am Intraocular Implant Soc J 1985;11:469-473.
*$p < 0.05$.

was used selectively in both groups. They found less postoperative astigmatism in the group with the shorter incision (Table 31-25).

Incision depth and configuration. All incisions for cataract surgery are 100% deep (full thickness). As with astigmatic keratotomy, the deeper the incision, the greater the potential change in curvature. Therefore a two-plane or three-plane incision that has a shallow superficial flap theoretically may create less astigmatism than a three-plane incision with a thick superficial flap, assuming all other variables are equal. The variety of configurations for cataract incisions makes this a truly artistic aspect of the surgery.

Suture materials and patterns. An unsutured or loosely sutured limbal or corneal cataract incision induces flattening of the vertical meridian. Many suture variables affect the amount of astigmatism after surgery (Table 31-22). Suture-less cataract surgery uses 3 to 5 mm long scleral tunnels that enter the anterior chamber through a clear cornea. If these techniques are widely adapted, suture problems may become obsolete.

A suture acts like a wedge resection: it functionally "removes" tissue from the meridian by compressing it. This has the effect of flattening the cornea in the region of the suture and steepening the central cornea. The greater the volume of tissue and the greater the compression, the greater the induced central steepening[183] (Figs. 31-27 and 31-28). Thus a longer suture bite, a deeper bite, and a more tightly tied bite will steepen the cornea in that meridian.[159,160] Conversely, short, shallow, loosely tied bites will flatten the meridian. The pattern of suture placement is probably less important than the volume of the bite and the amount of tissue compression in determining postoperative astigmatism. To produce no change in astigmatism, suture bites should be short and tied to a tension that coapts the wound edges with sufficient compression to allow for the natural decay in wound edema and suture elasticity.

More elastic, smaller-diameter sutures conform more easily to the contours of the wound, stretching to accommodate wound edema and contracting when the edema disappears and the wound remodels. Larger, stiffer sutures tend to compress the wound more when it is swollen, steepening the sutured meridian, and tend to loosen as the wound contracts, flattening that meridian. The most commonly used suture material is nylon because it strikes the best balance between too much and too little elasticity. However, nylon biodegrades and loses its strength over a few years after surgery, compressing less tissue, so against-the-rule astigmatism may occur.

Figure 31-27

Three theories used to explain the effect of a limbal corneal suture on central corneal curvature. **A,** Before suture *(ab)* is tied, the cornea has a radius of r1. **B,** The suture might pull the tissue taut, flattening the cornea centrally, but keratometric measurement demonstrates that the cornea steepens centrally. **C,** The circle theory suggests that the circumference of the cornea is reduced, creating a smaller radius of curvature *(r2)* and a steeper cornea, but the predicted amount of steepening is far less than the amount measured clinically or experimentally. **D,** The tissue compression theory suggests that the suture compresses the tissue focally, depressing the cornea and steepening it centrally. This theory explains clinical and experimental observations.

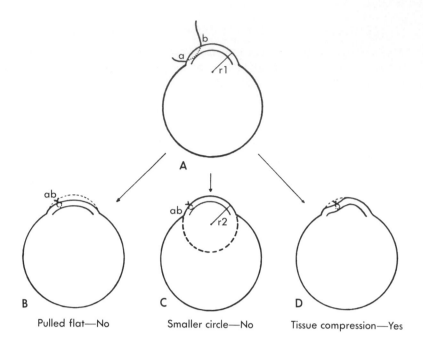

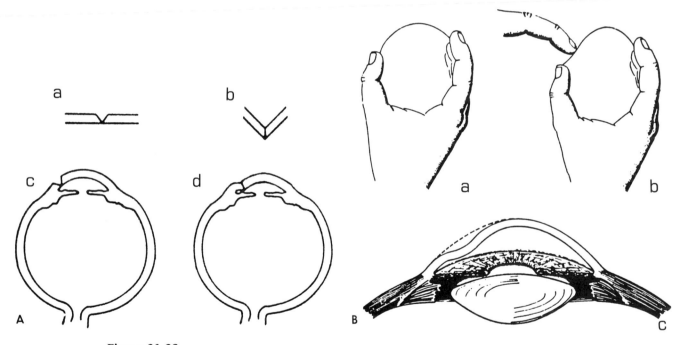

Figure 31-28

Illustration of how a tight limbal suture produces flattening in the area of the suture and steepening in the central cornea. **A,** A wedge is removed from a piece of wood *(a)* and from the corneascleral limbus *(c)*. When the two sides are approximated by glue *(b)* or sutures *(d)*, the area around the wedge resection is depressed, and the area remote from the wedge is steepened. **B,** Demonstration of this phenomenon with a calling card. A card is arched between the thumb and first two fingers *(a)*. The forefinger depresses the area near the end of the arched card, causing a steepening of the central part of the card *(b)*. This is the phenomenon that occurs with depression of peripheral cornea where sutures compress the tissue, steepening the central cornea *(c)*. (From van Rij G and Waring GO: Am J Ophthalmol 1984;98:773-783.)

Examples of studies of suture material are those conducted by Wishart and colleagues,[188] who demonstrated that 8-0 virgin silk suture produced an earlier and larger shift in the against-the-rule direction than 10-0 monofilament nylon. Masket[114] compared the change in astigmatism associated with 10-0 nylon, 9-0 nylon, and 10-0 polyester (Mersilene) sutures for the closure of a 6.5-mm long scleral pocket incision under tonometric and operating keratometric control. During the first 2 weeks after surgery, the eyes closed with 10-0 nylon exhibited less with-the-rule cylinder than the other two groups, presumably because the greater elasticity adapted to the postoperative wound edema. At 6 weeks and 4 months after surgery, there was no difference in the mean astigmatism in the three groups. Stainer and colleagues[161] found no difference between interrupted and double-running 10-0 nylon suture, but demonstrated a decay in astigmatism to against-the-rule using absorbable 8-0 polyglactin suture.

Cravy[45] performed studies of consecutive series of different types of limbal and pocket incisions using 10-0 nylon, 9-0 nylon, 10-0 polypropylene (Prolene), and 10-0 polyester (Mersilene). He found that the nylon sutures demonstrated clinically significant hydrolysis beginning at 5 months for the 10-0 diameter and at 12 months for the 9-0 diameter, producing changes in the against-the-rule direction. The elasticity of the polypropylene suture produced more against-the-rule astigmatism than desired (see Table 31-32). The author favored the stiffer, nonbiodegradable, less elastic polyester (Mersilene) suture. None of the suture-incision combinations displayed ideal behavior: early stabilization, little or no change from the first visit to the end of follow-up, and negligible shift to against-the-rule astigmatism. In contrast, Drews[54] found no difference in induced astigmatism between 10-0 nylon and 11-0 polyester over 6 months, with a mean decay of approximately 2 D.

The effects of different suture patterns on postoperative astigmatism have been studied and described by numerous authors, and a thorough discussion is beyond the scope of this chapter.[144,145] One of the most extensive studies, conducted by Jaffe and Clayman,[79,80] compared 11 different suturing techniques, varying the type, placement, and pattern of sutures. They concluded that techniques producing wound compression (long, deep bites, tightly tied) increased with-the-rule astigmatism. Running sutures steepened the cornea near the end of the incisions. Few data have been published about astigmatism after a single mattress suture closure of a scleral tunnel incision.

Intraoperative keratoscopy and keratometry

Attempts to control astigmatism during cataract surgery require some method of intraoperative measurement, either qualitative or quantitative. These methods are reviewed in detail in Chapter 3, Optics and Topography of Radial Keratotomy. A pertinent summary is presented here.

To correlate intraoperative keratometric measurements with postoperative ones, the intraocular pressure must be brought to a normal level during the intraoperative measurements by inflating the eye with a balanced salt solution until the pressure is approximatey 20 mm Hg. Some studies of intraoperative keratoscopy and keratometry have not controlled intraocular pressure, and therefore it is not surprising that intraoperative and postoperative measurements correlated poorly. Some surgeons simply inflate the globe until it "feels normal." The best approach is to measure the intraocular pressure using an instrument such as the Astigmatism Control Enforcer (ACE), which contains a Barraquer-style applanation tonometer. If the intraocular pressure is low, it is easier to tie sutures too tightly and compress more tissue, which will induce more steepening in the meridian of the suture when the postoperative pressure rises to normal values. Conversely, if the intraocular pressure is too high during the tying of sutures, it

Sources of Error in the Use of a Quantitative Keratometer during Surgery

Eyelid speculum distortion of cornea
Intraocular pressure too low or too high
Keratometer out of calibration
Keratometer and corneal surface not parallel
Operating microscope tilted off axis
Rectus muscle sutures distorting cornea
Parallax induced by monocular or binocular fixation
Variable magnification during readings
Rough epithelial surface with irregular mires
Erroneous reading from fluid meniscus
Inexperienced user

Modified from Samples JR and Binder PS: Ophthalmology 1984;91:280-284.

will be more difficult to close the wound and less tissue will be compressed within the suture, resulting in flattening of that meridian when the pressure lowers postoperatively. Masket[115] found that meticulous attention to measurement of intraocular pressure before tying cataract sutures produced a better correlation between astigmatism at the end of surgery and 1 day postoperatively; the mean difference was 0.36 D when the pressure was controlled, and 0.74 D when it was not.

Numerous qualitative keratoscopes have been designed, including simple metal (Flieringa) rings and plastic (Barrett) rings, comparators (Hyde, Karikoff), hand-held, Placido-type instruments that project concentric rings on the cornea (ACE, Medical Workshop, Maloney), and qualitative surgical keratoscopes mounted on the operating microscope (Troutman, Cravy).[179,191] Simcoe[157] suggested placing a contact lens with a flat back curvature of 20 to 30 D on the cornea to produce an area of central touch that depicts the corneal astigmatism. Herman and colleagues[75] inject an air bubble into the anterior chamber, using its ovality to determine the amount of corneal astigmatism.

Quantitative surgical keratometers have been designed by Terry,[167] Smirmaul, and the NIDEK Corp. Samples and Binder[149] compared keratometric readings before, at the start of, and at the end of surgery with the Terry keratometer and the morning after surgery with the Bausch & Lomb keratometer. Preoperative readings differed from those taken at the start of surgery by more than 1.00 D in 37% of 27 eyes, possibly because ocular massage had taken place and decreased the intraocular pressure. At the end of surgery, readings differed by more than 2 D from the postoperative readings obtained the morning after surgery. The authors concluded that numerous factors must be controlled to obtain accurate correlations between intraoperative and postoperative measurements (see box above).

There is little doubt that adjustment of sutures using intraoperative keratometry can reduce the amount of astigmatism in the first few weeks after surgery, possibly up to 2 or 3 months, although there is no prospective randomized trial to establish this fact. The restrospective studies of Colvard and colleagues[40,41] and of Lindstrom and Destro[104] demonstrated that at 6 weeks after surgery there was a substantial decrease in the amount of astigmatism present in eyes that had had intraoperative Terry keratometry with adjustment of sutures compared with eyes that did not have adjustment of sutures (Table 31-26). Kratz and colleagues[40,41,89] described similar findings (Table 31-27). However, Perl and col-

Table 31-26

Effect of Intraoperative Terry Keratometry on Keratometric Astigmatism (D) 6 to 10 Weeks after Cataract Surgery Using a Scleral Pocket Incision

Surgical technique	Intraoperative keratometer	Number of eyes	Mean postoperative astigmatism (D) (range)	Percentage of eyes with postoperative astigmatism (D)				Percentage of eyes requiring cutting of sutures
				< 1.00	1–2	2–3	> 3.00	
Phacoemulsi-fication, 6.5- to 7.0-mm incision, running suture	Terry	80	1.03* (0 to 4.50)	71	23	3	3	—
	None	40	1.62* (0 to 8.00)	53	32	5	10	—
Extracapsular cataract extraction, 11.0-mm incision, interrupted and running suture	Terry	50	1.60* (0 to 4.00)	38	43	5	14	—
	None	30	3.00* (1.00 to 7.00)	8	42	8	42	—
Both techniques combined	Terry	130	—	60*	28	4	8*	1.6*
	None	70	—	35*	35	7	23*	30.0*

Modified from Lindstrom RL and Destro MA: Am Intraocular Implant Suc J 1985; 11:469-473.
*Significantly different; *p* is less than .05.

Table 31-27

Effect of Intraoperative Terry Keratometry on Astigmatism 6 weeks after Cataract Extraction

Time	Astigmatism (D)	No keratometry (n = 100 eyes) (%)	Intraoperative Terry keratometry (n = 200 eyes) (%)
Preoperative	0 to 1	68	69
	1 to 2	22	20
	2 to 3	7	8
	> 3	3	3
Postoperative (6 weeks)	0 to 1	28	66
	1 to 2	30	25
	2 to 3	13	5
	> 3	29	4

Modified from Kratz RP and Johnson SH: Int Ophthalmol Clin 1983;23:87-99.

leagues[126] found in a series of eyes with an 11-mm long wound with planned extracapsular cataract extraction that although the intraoperative measurements with the Terry keratometer reduced the number of eyes with large amounts of postoperative astigmatism, it did not decrease the average amount of astigmatism.

Few studies have reported the amount of astigmatism more than 6 months after cataract surgery with and without intraoperative keratometry in eyes that had no suture adjustment postoperatively, so it is impossible to tell whether intraoperative keratometry affects the "final" amount of astigmatism after cataract surgery.

Intraoperative adjustment of cataract wound to modify astigmatism

Maloney[110-112] has described techniques of intraoperative wound and suture adjustment and intraoperative transverse keratotomy to reduce preexisting astigmatism and to prevent an increase in astigmatism after surgery (Fig. 31-29). These techniques were only moderately successful (Table 31-28 and Fig. 31-30)

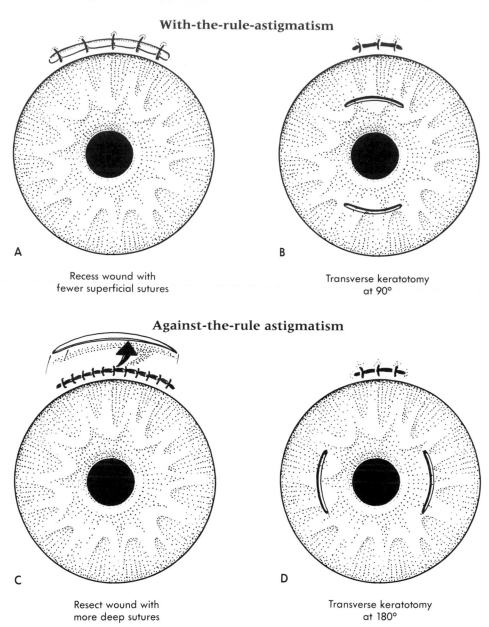

With-the-rule-astigmatism

A — Recess wound with fewer superficial sutures

B — Transverse keratotomy at 90°

Against-the-rule astigmatism

C — Resect wound with more deep sutures

D — Transverse keratotomy at 180°

Figure 31-29
Techniques to attempt to correct corneal astigmatism during cataract surgery. **A** and **B,** To correct preoperative astigmatism with the rule, the goal is to flatten the vertical 90° meridian. Theoretically this can be achieved by recessing the limbal or scleral wound to flatten the meridian **(A)** or by placing transverse keratotomies across the 90° meridian in association with a small scleral pocket incision **(B). C,** For preoperative against-the-rule astigmatism, tightening or resecting the limbal wound will steepen the vertical meridian. **D,** Transverse keratotomy at 180° will flatten the horizontal meridian and steepen the vertical meridian in association with a small scleral pocket incision.

in eyes with less than 1.00 D of preoperative astigmatism; only 62% had less than 1.00 D after surgery. Of eyes with 1 to 1.9 D of astigmatism preoperatively, 42% had less than 1 D postoperatively, and of eyes with 2 to 4.5 D preoperatively, only 30% had less than 1 D of astigmatism postoperatively. However, intraoperative wound modification was able to reduce approximately 75% of the preexisting astigmatism in these latter two groups of eyes.

Jensen[82] and Azar[11] have advocated resecting a strip of sclera from the posterior edge of the wound and resuturing it to steepen the vertical meridian and correct against-the-rule astigmatism.

Table 31-28

Results of Intraoperative Adjustment of Cataract Wound to Reduce Preexisting Astigmatism

Preoperative refractive astigmatism (D)	Number of eyes	Follow-up (mo) mean (range)	Preoperative astigmatism (D) mean (range)	Postoperative astigmatism (D) mean (range)	Percentage of eyes with < 1.00 D postoperative astigmatism	Percentage of eyes with ≥ 2.00 D postoperative astigmatism
< 1	47	7.4 (3 to 68)	0.4 (0 to .9)	0.84 (0 to 3.50)	62	4
1 to 1.9	67	7.8 (3 to 32)	1.3 (1.0 to 1.87)	1.1 (0 to 3.75)	42	10
2 to 4.5	27	10.9 (2 to 68)	2.68 (2.12 to 4.50)	1.46 (0 to 3.37)	30	37

Modified from Maloney WF, Sanders DR, and Pearcy DE: J Cataract Refract Surg 1990;16:297-304.

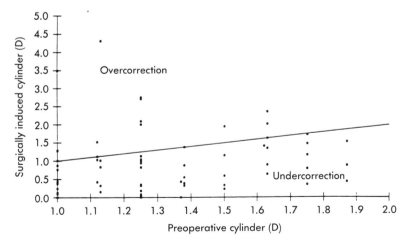

Figure 31-30

Scatterplot demonstrates the effect of modification of a 6.0- to 7.5-mm long cataract wound to reduce preoperative astigmatism in 67 eyes with 1.0 to 1.9 D of naturally occurring astigmatism. X-axis indicates the amount of preoperative cylinder, and y-axis indicates the surgically induced vectoral change in cylinder. Results show general undercorrection with considerable variability. (From Maloney WF: J Cataract Refract Surg 1990;16:297-304.)

Transverse keratotomy during cataract surgery

Instead of modifying the cataract incision, some surgeons attempt to reduce preexisting astigmatism by using transverse keratotomy at the same time as cataract surgery. This approach has been reported by numerous authors* (Table 31-29). All published reports (Table 31-30) have used phacoemulsification and a 4- to 6-mm long, sclerally placed cataract incision and have emphasized the following generalities:

1. There was considerable variability in the response of individual eyes (Fig. 31-31).
2. Transverse keratotomy should be made before the cataract incision because the eye is in an undisturbed state; doing it after the cataract extraction is more difficult because of the influence of the cataract wound and the variable intraocular pressure.
3. Because transverse incisions change the spherical equivalent refraction minimally (they flatten the incised meridian and steepen the unincised meridian approximately the same amounts), the calculation of the spherical intraocular lens power was not affected in most eyes, although it was affected in a few.[134]
4. Transverse keratotomy has a more predictable effect if the cataract incision is short and sclerally placed, such as a 4-mm pocket incision.
5. The interplay between a superior transverse keratotomy incision across the 90° meridian and the parallel limbal-scleral cataract incision has not been well defined. A tight suture in the cataract wound can pull open the transverse keratotomy and increase its effect.[48,71]

*References 34, 40, 51, 63, 100, 121, 140, 141.

Table 31-29

Reports of Combined Straight Transverse Keratotomy and Phacoemulsification Cataract Surgery

Author	Keratotomy before or after cataract extraction	Length (mm) and location of cataract wound	Intra-operative kerato-metry	Transverse incisions (diamond knife)			Number of eyes	Mean follow-up, mo (range)
				Number of pairs	Length (mm)	Zone diameter (mm)		
Maloney[112]	Before	6 to 7.5 Scleral	Yes	1, 2	3	7, 8	151	4 (1 to 20)
Shepherd[154]	Before	4 Scleral	No	1	1 mm/D (1 to 4)	7	48	Not reported (2 to 14)
Osher[134]	After	6 Scleral	No	1	3	7 to 10	75	Not reported
Davison[48]	Before	Not reported Scleral	Yes	1, 2	3.5	7, 8	40	5.5 (2 to 16)
Hall[71]	Before	6 Scleral	No	2	3	5.5, 6, 7	61	3 (not reported)

Modified from Maloney WF, Sanders DR, and Pearcy DE: J Cataract Refract Surg 1990;16:297-304.
For results, please see the following: Table 31-30 and Fig. 31-31 (Maloney), Fig. 31-32 (Shepherd), Fig. 31-33 (Davison), and Table 31-31 (Hall).

6. All surgeons used straight transverse keratotomies, but some authors[48] acknowledged that an arcuate keratotomy might be more physiologic.
7. Most surgeons used a 7-mm diameter zone for placement of a 3-mm long transverse keratotomy depending on the circumstances for an individual eye. Incision depth varied, but it is likely that the achieved incision depth (which was not reported in any of the articles) was on the order of 80%, based on the described knife settings.
8. The major complications were unpredictability of the outcome and shifts in the axis of astigmatism. Corneal perforations were rare, but lacerations of Descemet's membrane have occurred, requiring suturing and complicating subsequent phacoemulsification.[48]

The individual surgical plans varied widely. The most complex was that of Maloney,[111,112] who utilized intraoperative keratoscopy. He placed the first set of paired incisions at the 7-mm zone, followed by a second set of paired incisions at the 8-mm zone (making the incisions 0.5 mm apart), followed by short semiradial incisions flanking the transverse ones until the ovality of the keratoscopy mires was neutralized. If residual astigmatism was still present, cataract wound modifications were made (see Fig. 31-31). He reported a high correlation between the axis of the attempted effect of the incisions and the axis of the surgically induced vectoral cylinder ($r^2 = 0.96$) (Table 31-30). Nordan supplemented the transverse incisions with a peripheral, perpendicular radial one in the steep meridian.

Shepherd[154,155] emphasized that a reduction of astigmatism in most eyes was an advantage, even if all astigmatism was not eliminated (Fig. 31-32). He cautioned that a 4-mm long scleral incision induced 1.00 D or more of astigmatism

Table 31-30

Effect of Transverse Keratotomies and a 6-mm Long Scleral Incision to Reduce Preexisting Astigmatism during Phacoemulsification Cataract Surgery

Pairs of transverse incisions	Preoperative refractive astigmatism (D)	Number of eyes	Follow-up (mo) mean (range)	Preoperative astigmatism (D) mean (range)	Postoperative astigmatism (D) mean (range)	Percentage of eyes with < 1.00 D postoperative astigmatism	Percentage of eyes with ≥ 2.00 D postoperative astigmatism
One	1 to 1.9	27	2.6 (1 to 6)	1.55 (1.13 to 1.87)	0.90 (0 to 2.75)	56	11
	2 to 4.5	16	3.7 (1 to 12)	2.79 (2.0 to 7.1)	1.98 (0.14 to 4.02)	44	25
Two	1 to 1.9	41	4.4 (1 to 16)	1.54 (1.1 to 1.87)	0.73 (0 to 3.12)	71	10
	2 to 4.5	66	5.3 (1 to 20)	2.85 (2 to 6.63)	1.24 (0 to 4.0)	42	23

Modified from Maloney WF, Sanders DR, and Pearcy DE: J Cataract Refract Surg 1990;16:297-304.

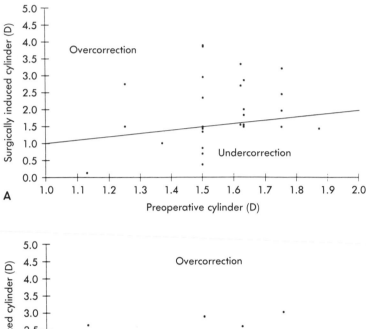

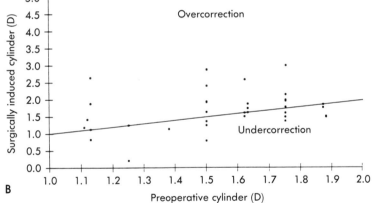

Figure 31-31
Effect of combined cataract surgery with a 6-mm long scleral incision and 3-mm long transverse keratotomies for eyes with a preoperative naturally occurring astigmatism of 1.0 to 1.9 D. Y-axis indicates surgically induced vectoral astigmatism in the attempted meridian of correction. **A,** Results for a single pair of transverse keratotomies at the 7-mm zone in 27 eyes. **B,** Results of two pairs of transverse keratotomies at 7-mm and 8-mm in 41 eyes. Points cluster around the line of desired correction, but there is considerable variability in the results. (From Maloney WF: J Cataract Refract Surg 1990;16:297-304.)

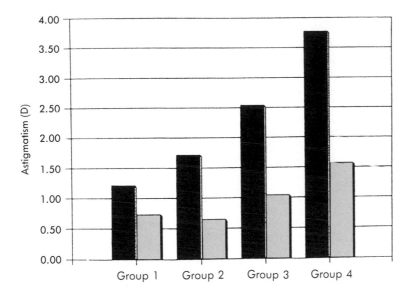

Figure 31-32

Effect of combined cataract surgery with a 4-mm scleral pocket incision and one pair of transverse keratotomy incisions on preoperative naturally occurring astigmatism. Incisions were placed at the 7-mm zone. X-axis indicates four groups of preoperative astigmatism. Black bar depicts average preoperative keratometric astigmatism. Gray bar depicts average postoperative keratometric astigmatism. All groups showed a mean reduction in astigmatism. (From Shepherd JR: J Cataract Refract Surg 1989;15:55-57.)

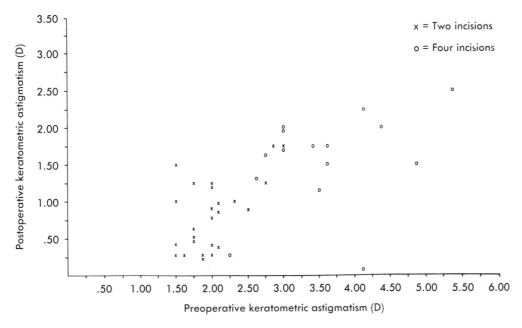

Figure 31-33

Scattergram depicts the net preoperative and postoperative keratometric astigmatism in 40 eyes with naturally occurring astigmatism that received combined cataract surgery and one or two pairs of 3.5-mm long transverse keratotomy incisions at the 7.0-mm zone. All eyes but one had a reduction in astigmatism, but there was considerable variability in the results. (From Davison JA: J Cataract Refract Surg 1989;15:38-44.)

Table 31-31

Effect of One Pair of Straight Transverse Keratotomies and a 6-mm Long Scleral Incision Done During Cataract Surgery on Keratometric Astigmatism

Preoperative astigmatism (D)	Number of eyes	Transverse keratotomy zone diameter (mm)	Average (SD) preoperative astigmatism (D)	Average (SD) postoperative astigmatism (D)	Percentage of eyes with residual astigmatism < 1 D		Average surgically induced vectorial astigmatism (D)	
					Pre-operative	Post-operative	Total	Transverse keratotomy only
< 1.00 (control)	105	None	0.53 ±0.43	0.82 ±0.63	100	Not reported	0.78 ±0.57	Not reported
1.00 to 2.00	30	7.0	1.24 ±0.33	0.74 ±0.56	6	63	1.57 ±0.76	2.04 ± 0.74
2.12 to 3.00	19	6.0	2.36 ±0.44	0.91 ±0.81	0	52	2.59 ±0.93	2.85 ± 0.90
> 3.00	12	5.5	3.62 ±0.63	1.76 ±1.00	0	25	3.49 ±1.60	3.52 ± 2.10

From Hall GW, Campion M, Sorenson CM, and Monthofer S: Personal communication, Jan. 17, 1990.

in 6% of eyes and that this could greatly affect the results of the transverse keratotomies. He suggested limiting transverse keratotomies to eyes with 1.50 D or more of preexisting astigmatism.

Davison[48] pointed out that a shallow knife setting avoids large corneal perforations and that tight cataract wound sutures can induce with-the-rule astigmatism despite transverse keratotomies across the vertical meridian. He reported an average preoperative astigmatism of 2.5 D and an average postoperative astigmatism of 1.1 D (Fig. 31-33). The results of Hall and colleagues[71] are presented in Table 31-31.

Because the cataract wound can change corneal shape, the use of transverse keratotomy intraoperatively may be less predictable than if it were used postoperatively, as discussed in a subsequent section.

Natural course of astigmatism after cataract surgery

The natural course of corneal curvature following cataract surgery has been well studied.* Most authors report that eyes with nylon sutures, particularly those sutures placed across limbal incisions, demonstrated a gradual flattening in the 90° meridian, usually in a two-phase response. The first phase occurs during 2 to 3 months after surgery, which presumably reflects the decreased suture tension from decreased edema and remodeling of the wound. The second phase lasts up to 3 or 4 years, presumably reflecting the biodegradation of the nylon suture and some stretching of the incision scar.

Cutting tight sutures postoperatively. One method of decreasing excessive with-the-rule astigmatism in the early postoperative period is to cut the suture(s) that create the excessive tension and excessive wound compression in the steep meridian[90] (Fig. 31-34). Sutures can be cut with a knife blade or with an argon laser.[28,146] Colvard and colleagues[40] cut interrupted sutures so that the amount of astigmatism in eyes operated without surgical keratometry was similar to that in eyes in which intraoperative keratometry was used.

Numerous reports describe the effect of different types of sutures on the natural course of astigmatism after cataract surgery: interrupted 7-0 chromic gut,[79] interrupted 9-0 silk,[68] interrupted 8-0 silk,[188] interrupted polyglactin,[158] running 10-0 nylon,[158,188] interrupted 10-0 nylon,[62,158] and combined interrupted

*References 44, 45, 68, 91, 139, 159-161.

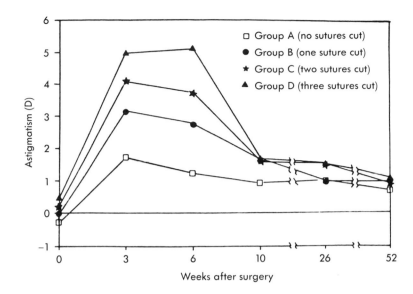

Figure 31-34
Effect of cutting interrupted 10-0 nylon sutures in a limbal cataract wound on postoperative keratometric astigmatism in 75 eyes. The number of sutures cut was determined by the amount of with-the-rule astigmatism 6 weeks after surgery. Cutting a larger number of sutures produced a greater decrease in astigmatism, which rcmained generally stable thereafter. (From Kronish JW and Forster RK: Arch Ophthalmol 1987;105:1650-1655.)

10-0 and 9-0 nylon.[81] Most of these studies are of historical interest because the sutures or suture combinations or incision lengths and placements are not now in use.

Changes in astigmatism from nylon sutures. Four studies using modern techniques have reported instability of astigmatism over approximately 4 years after extracapsular cataract surgery using an approximately 10-mm chord length limbal incision closed with 10-0 nylon sutures: Axt[10] in 1987 (503 eyes), Richards and colleagues[140] in 1988 (229 eyes), Cravy[45] in 1989 (41 eyes), and Parker and Clorfeine[135] in 1989 (66 eyes). The results of the four studies are remarkably similar. From approximately 3 months to 3 to 4 years after surgery, the change in astigmatism averagcd approximately 1.50 D with a general shift in the against-the-rule direction. Eyes that had minimal astigmatism or already had against-the-rule astigmatism at 3 months changed less than eyes that had with-the-rule astigmatism, showing a more rapid and steady rate of "decay" in the against-the-rule direction (Fig. 31-35). In general, this shift in astigmatism was unrelated to the preoperative astigmatism, the number of sutures used, the number of sutures cut to reduce astigmatism in the early postoperative period, and the age of the patient.

These findings have led to a search for methods to stabilize astigmatism in the early postoperative period. One approach is to use sutures that are neither absorbable nor biodegradable; for example, Cravy[45] preferred polyester (Mersilene) in the study described in the previous section on suture material (Table 31-32). Another approach has been to use a smaller incision, assuming that it influences corneal astigmatism less and that suture biodegradation and wound slippage therefore will produce less drift of astigmatism in the against-the-rule direction. An informal study by Shepherd[155] with only a 3-month follow-up supported this concept (Fig. 31-36), but long-term studies of the stability of astigmatism associated with small incisions are still needed.

Surgical management of astigmatism after cataract surgery

There are few studies of the surgical correction of astigmatism after cataract extraction. In fact, there is considerable difference of opinion among surgeons about whether induced against-the-rule astigmatism from wound slippage after cataract surgery should be managed surgically by wound revision or by astigmatic keratotomy (Fig. 31-37). Of course, if the cataract wound dehiscence

Figure 31-35
Four studies depict the change in astigmatism after extracapsular cataract extraction using a 10- to 11-mm chord length incision closed with 10-0 nylon suture.

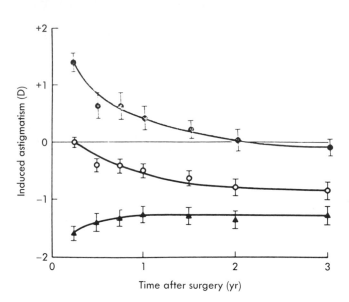

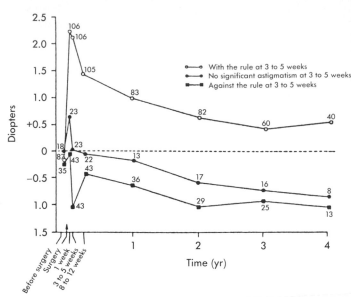

A, Study of Parker and Clorfeine of 66 eyes shows evolution of induced corneal astigmatism plotted for three groups of eyes defined by the amount of induced astigmatism present 3 months after posterior limbal incision. Group 1 *(open circles)* began with 0.50 D or less; group 2 *(triangles)* began with greater than 0.50 D against-the-rule astigmatism; group 3 *(closed circles)* began with greater than 0.50 D with-the-rule astigmatism. Lines represent exponential regression fits. Decay toward with-the-rule astigmatism was greatest for group 3. (From Parker WT and Clorfeine GS: Arch Ophthalmol 1989;107:353-357.)

B, Study of Richards and colleagues divided cases into three groups based on amount of astigmatism at 3 to 5 weeks after posterior limbal incision. The preoperative astigmatism for the three groups was similar, but the postoperative change was different. The with-the-rule astigmatism group decayed more rapidly and to a greater amount in the against-the-rule direction than the other two groups. Positive y-axis values denote with-the-rule-astigmatism; negative y-axis values denote against-the-rule astigmatism. Numbers indicate eyes evaluated at each time point. (From Richards SC, Brodstein RS, Richards WL, et al: J Cataract Refract Surg 1988;14:270-276.)

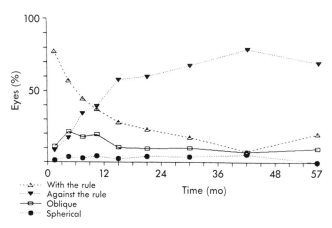

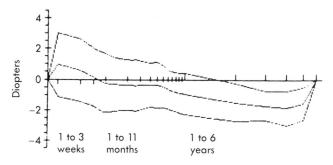

C, Study of Axt of 503 eyes shows the percentage of eyes (y-axis) with different types of astigmatism during the postoperative period. Sceral wound was made 1mm posterior to limbus. As the number of eyes showing against-the-rule astigmatism increased, the number of eyes showing with-the-rule astigmatism decreased. Eyes with oblique astigmatism or spherical measurements remained relatively constant. (From Axt JC: J Cataract Refract Surg 1987;13:381-388.)

D, Study of Cravy of 41 eyes (reduced to 22 eyes followed for 6 years) demonstrates the change in astigmatism. Limbal incision varied from 60° to 140° long. On the y-axis positive values indicate with-the-rule vectoral astigmatism and negative values against-the-rule vectoral astigmatism. The x-axis shows the logarithm of time as labeled. The central line represents the mean and the upper and lower lines the standard deviation. There is a continued trend toward against-the-rule astigmatism throughout the 6 years of follow-up. (From Cravy TV: J Cataract Refract Surg 1989;15:61-69.)

Table 31-32

Comparison of the Effect of Different Types of Sutures on the Change in Astigmatism after Extracapsular Cataract Extraction with a 60° to 140° Long Wound

	Time		Change in astigmatism toward against-the-rule			
Suture	Time to zero astigmatism (mo)	Time to initial stability (mo)	Onset of hydrolysis (mo)	Decay to stability (mo)	Total decay (D)	Total against-the-rule (D)
Limbal incision						
10-0 nylon	0.75	1	5	1.15	2.80	1.85
9-0 nylon	8	4	12	1.77	3.32	1.35
10-0 Prolene	3	12	—	2.29	2.42	0.91
10-0 Mersilene	2.5	2.5	—	2.00	2.79	0.65
Scleral incision						
9-0 nylon	6	12	12	2.49	2.95	1.07
10-0 Prolene	2.25	12	—	3.75	3.75	1.43
10-0 Mersilene	5	6	—	2.69	3.03	0.59

Modified from Cravy TV: J Cataract Refract Surg 1989;15:61-69.

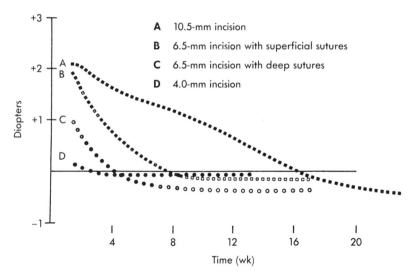

Figure 31-36
A theoretical summary graph of the general changes in astigmatism after cataract surgery using incisions of different lengths closed with nylon suture. The shorter scleral tunnel incision may demonstrate a more stable postoperative course than longer scleral or limbal incisions. (From Shepherd JR: J Cataract Refract Surg 1989-15:55-57.)

poses a structural threat to the eye, such as a large filtering bleb, a fistula with epithelial ingrowth, chronic hypotony, or iris incarceration with an ectopic pupil and symptomatic glare, then an anatomic wound repair is essential. However, if the structural integrity of the globe is acceptable, then the challenge becomes one of refractive rehabilitation with the reduction of spherical and astigmatic anisometropia and their associated diplopia and asthenopia. Two journals published consultation sections in 1989-1990[116,171] that presented problem cases of patients with refractions of approximately +2.00 −6.00 × 90° after cataract surgery. Among those offering opinions about how to reduce the astigmatism, 11 surgeons elected to use isolated pairs of astigmatic keratotomies across the 180° meridian; three surgeons suggested combined transverse and radial keratotomies; six surgeons recommended opening and resuturing the wound; four surgeons preferred wound repair with resection of tissue; and one surgeon advocated a relaxing scleral flap in the 180° meridian (Fig. 31-38).

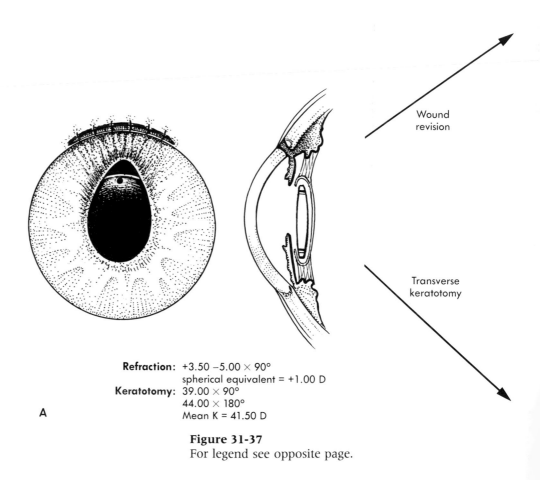

Wound revision

Transverse keratotomy

Refraction: +3.50 −5.00 × 90°
spherical equivalent = +1.00 D
Keratotomy: 39.00 × 90°
44.00 × 180°
Mean K = 41.50 D

A

Figure 31-37
For legend see opposite page.

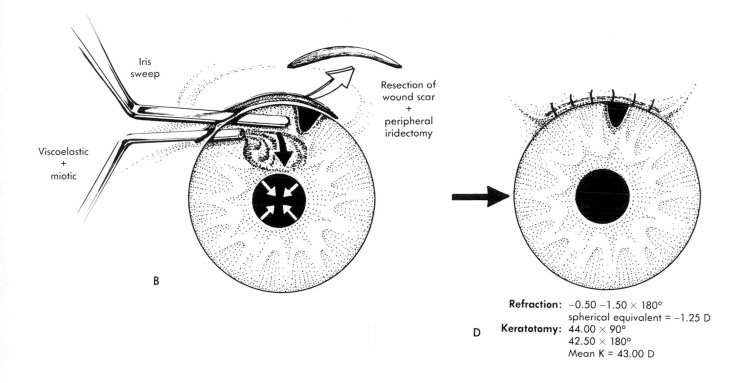

Iris
sweep

Resection of
wound scar
+
peripheral
iridectomy

Viscoelastic
+
miotic

B

D   **Refraction:** −0.50 −1.50 × 180°
spherical equivalent = −1.25 D
Keratotomy: 44.00 × 90°
42.50 × 180°
Mean K = 43.00 D

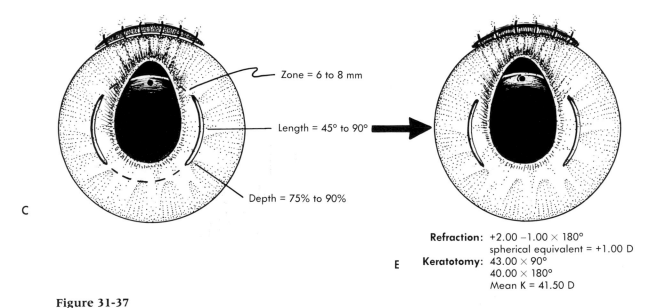

Zone = 6 to 8 mm

Length = 45° to 90°

Depth = 75% to 90%

C

E   **Refraction:** +2.00 −1.00 × 180°
spherical equivalent = +1.00 D
Keratotomy: 43.00 × 90°
40.00 × 180°
Mean K = 41.50 D

Figure 31-37
Two alternatives to the surgical management of residual astigmatism after cataract
extraction. **A** (*opposite page*), Wound dehiscence with iris incarceration has induced
5 D of astigmatism against the rule. *Left,* Alternatives to correction include wound
revision, repositing of the iris, resection of the wound scar, and resuturing **(B)** or
arcuate transverse keratotomy across the steep 180° meridian **(C).** *Right,* The anatomic outcome of the two techniques is different **(D** and **E),** although each greatly
reduces the postoperative astigmatism.

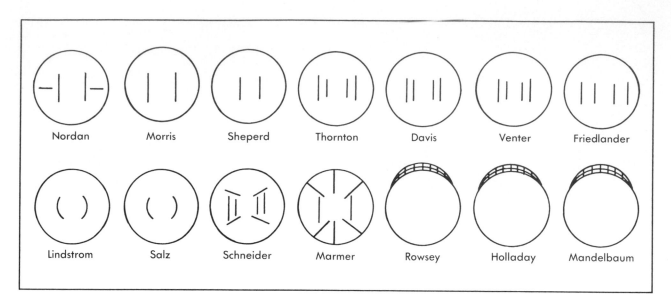

Figure 31-38

Variations in opinion among refractive surgeons concerning the correction of astigmatism after cataract surgery in 1990. Each surgeon proposed the illustrated surgical technique as management for the following case:

> A 65-year-old man had cataract surgery with IOL implantation in the right eye 2 years ago. The refraction is -0.50 $-0.75 \times 90°$, with a visual acuity of 20/20. The left eye had cataract surgery 1 year ago with a posterior chamber IOL, and the refraction is now $+2.00$ $-5.50 \times 90°$ with a visual acuity of 20/25. His keratometry readings are OD, 42.00/43.00 $\times$ 180° and OS 39.25/45.50 $\times$ 180°. Slit-lamp biomicroscope examination shows the limbal wound to be well healed and shows no wound defect. The vision in the left eye corrects to 20/30. The patient complains of glare, eye fatigue, poor depth perception, and headaches. (From Thornton SP: Refract Corneal Surg 1990;6:131-136.)

Astigmatic keratotomy after cataract surgery. Making transverse astigmatic keratotomies after cataract surgery, with or without accompanying radial or semiradial incisions, follows the principles discussed earlier in this chapter. In general, many eyes with against-the-rule astigmatism will have a hyperopic spherical equivalent refraction associated with overall flat keratometry readings as a result of the flattening in the vertical meridian from the wound slippage. Thus longer transverse keratotomies (60° to 90°) made across the steep horizontal meridian will have the coupling effect of steepening the flat vertical meridian at 90°, reducing the hyperopic spherical equivalent refraction. Unfortunately the coupling ratios are not constant, as Merck and colleagues[122] showed in eight cases of trapezoidal keratotomy for postcataract astigmatism, where the flattening to steepening ratio varied from 1.12 to 7.50. In a study of more than 300 eyes, Binder[26] found 66% of eyes to have a flattening to steepening ratio of about 1, but 18% of the eyes had unpredictable and excessive ratios (as much as 10 to 1).

The advantage of astigmatic keratotomy over wound revision is surgical simplicity: surgery can be done outside the operating room; the eye is not entered; the procedure is less involved; recovery time is more rapid; morbidity is less; and wound revision can be done at a later date if necessary. The primary disadvantage is the lack of predictability, particularly in view of the preexisting surgery, which will alter the expected effect and curvature ratios. The anatomic defect itself—the wound slippage or dehiscence—is not repaired.

Case 5: Successful Arcuate Transverse Keratotomy for Astigmatism after Cataract Surgery

A 73-year-old man had an extracapsular cataract extraction with intraocular lens implantation using a 10-mm chord length limbal incision. Postoperatively he developed a wound slip and astigmatism against-the-rule, which produced occasional monocular diplopia and an oblique orientation of lights and objects. The refraction was $-4.50 + 5.25 \times 20°$, with a corrected visual acuity of 20/25. Central keratometric power was $40.50 \times 105°/47.25 \times 15°$. The cornea was clear and compact. A multiflex style anterior chamber intraocular lens was in good position with slight haze of the posterior capsule. Videokeratography demonstrated a symmetrical bowtie pattern with the steep meridian at 15°.

Two arcuate transverse keratotomy incisions were made in the cornea with a vertical-bladed diamond knife along a 7-mm zone, each incision 50° long and 80% of the corneal thickness. Four months after surgery his manifest refraction was $-1.25 + 0.75 \times 105°$, 20/40. Central keratometric measurements were $42.87 \times 12°/43.25 \times 101°$. The approximate preoperative spherical equivalent refraction of -2.00 D is similar to the postoperative spherical equivalent refraction of -1.12 D.

Agapitos and colleagues[1] reported trapezoidal keratotomies in eight eyes with against-the-rule astigmatism after cataract surgery with highly variable results, including large shifts in preoperative and postoperative astigmatic axis and variable final outcomes that ranged from little residual astigmatism to no effect.

Since the majority of patients are over 60 years of age, the effect of the keratotomies may be greater than that usually expected, so it is wise to aim for an undercorrection by placing the incisions farther from the center and making them more shallow, doing a reoperation if needed later.

Astigmatism after cataract surgery also may result from a tilt of the intraocular lens that exceeds 20°[75,138] or from an oversized rigid anterior chamber lens that mechanically distorts the corneal cornea.[147]

ASTIGMATISM AFTER PENETRATING KERATOPLASTY

Improvements in corneal transplantation such as the operating microscope, monofilament nylon sutures and ultrasharp needles, intermediate term donor storage in nutrient media, better education of ophthalmologists in the signs and management of allograft reaction, improved case selection, immunosuppressive agents such as cyclosporin, and tissue matching techniques have combined to produce clear, structurally intact grafts in approximately 85% of eyes at 1 year after surgery. Therefore the major concern of corneal surgeons has gradually moved to the refractive aspects of penetrating keratoplasty—minimizing astigmatism and reducing spherical refractive errors, especially with concomitant intraocular lens implantation. Penetrating keratoplasty, like cataract surgery, is now as much a refractive surgical procedure as it is a therapeutic one.

Causes of astigmatism after penetrating keratoplasty

The exact factors that cause astigmatism after penetrating keratoplasty are not known, although discussion and speculation have filled many chapters and textbooks. Astigmatism results from a combination of factors, many of which are listed in the box on p. 1158 and have been discussed by many authors,[16,35,133,177] including a review by Binder.[27]

The average astigmatism after penetrating keratoplasty is 3 to 4 D using current techniques (Table 31-33), but the range extends from 0 to 20 D, making

Factors That Affect Astigmatism after Penetrating Keratoplasty

I. General surgical factors

  A. Pressure of eyelid speculum
  B. Distortion from scleral ring
  C. Distortion from traction sutures

II. Donor cornea

  A. Asymmetric shape and edge contour
    1. Method of removing donor button
    2. Punch block curvature
    3. Donor trephine blade quality
    4. Donor trephine technique
      a. Manual
      b. Mechanical
      c. Suction
      d. Punch
      e. Cut down
  B. Preexisting astigmatism

III. Host cornea

  A. Asymmetric trephine opening
  B. Eccentric trephine opening
  C. Irregular or asymmetric edge contour
  D. Host corneal astigmatism
  E. Host trephine blade quality
  F. Trephine style and technique
    1. Manual
    2. Mechanical
    3. Suction
    4. Obturator

IV. Sutures

  A. Needle and suture size
  B. Variation in bite size
  C. Variation in suture tension
  D. Variation in distribution and direction of bites
  E. Variation in depth of bites
  F. Wound slippage or decompression after suture removal

V. Wound configuration and healing

  A. Mismatch of donor and host configurations
  B. Mismatch of donor and host thicknesses
  C. Poor approximation of donor and host surfaces (Bowman's layer and Descemet's membrane)
  D. Variable wound volume
  E. Iris incarceration
  F. Wound fistula
  G. Keratolysis (melting) of donor or host
  H. Progressive host disease

astigmatism one of the major complications and challenges of corneal transplantation. Four major factors influence the amount of astigmatism after penetrating keratoplasty:

1. Host disease
2. Configuration of the donor and host keratoplasty wounds
3. Sutures
4. Wound healing

Discussion of these factors involves essentially the entire field of penetrating keratoplasty and therefore is beyond the scope of this chapter. However, we can make a few generalities.

Host disease. The preoperative distortion in many corneas undergoing keratoplasty makes the accurate measurement of corneal curvature difficult. There are few published studies of the relationship between preoperative and postoperative keratometry. Binder and colleagues[23] demonstrated no correlation between preoperative host astigmatism and postoperative graft astigmatism (Table 31-34). The small amount of astigmatism present in most corneas before surgery contributes minimally to the postoperative astigmatism. However, in corneas that have large amounts of astigmatism before surgery—such as keratoconus, corneal trauma with dense peripheral corneal scars, and marginal thinning dis-

Table 31-33

Astigmatism after Penetrating Keratoplasty

First author	Year	Number of eyes (suture technique)	Average astigmatism (D) at 1 year
Donor diameter greater than recipient—sutures retained			
Binder	1986	148 (interrupted running)	2.9
Binder	1988	188 (interrupted running)	3.5
Burke	1988	24 (interrupted running)	2.25 (4 mo)
McNeill	1989	289 (single running)	2.87 (6 mo)
Musch	1989	53 (double running)	4.0
Pradera	1989	44 (interrupted running)	2.50
Donor diameter greater than recipient—sutures removed			
Troutman	1972	75	4.4 to 5.1
Foulks	1979	32	3.5
Perl	1981	47	6.4
Perlman	1981	?	4.5 to 5.8
Bourne	1981	33	4.1
Davison	1981	33	4.1
Heidemann	1985	86	5.2
Insler	1987	31	3.9
Binder	1986	55	4.3
Donor diameter same as recipient—sutures removed			
Boruchoff	1975	42	4.6
Anseth	1967	50	4.2
Foulks	1979	32	5.7
Perl	1981	36	4.2
Perlman	1981	?	4.5 to 5.8

Modified from Binder PS: Controlled reduction of postkeratoplasty astigmatism. In Brightbill FS, editor: Corneal surgery, St Louis, 1986, CV Mosby Co, pp 333-343.

Table 31-34

Effect of Preoperative Corneal Astigmatism on Astigmatism after Penetrating Keratoplasty

Amount of preoperative keratometric astigmatism (D)	No. of eyes*	Mean astigmatism (D)	
		Before suture removal	After suture removal
< 3	68	3.73	3.34
3 to 5	21	3.01	2.52
> 5	19	3.70	3.03

Modified from Binder PS: Am J Ophthalmol 1988;105:637-645.
*Preoperative keratometry was not obtainable on all eyes.

orders—the shape of the host cornea can affect the shape of the graft. For example, when trephining a keratoconus cornea using an instrument with an obturator, the central cone is flattened and distorted, which may create an incision that is not completely circular. Hatch[74] has proposed using thermal surface cautery to flatten the cone immediately before trephination. Fig. 31-39 illustrates how a host scar can induce astigmatism in penetrating keratoplasty.

Configuration of donor and host incisions. Ever since circular grafts replaced square grafts, the surgeon's goal has been to create an incision as radially symmetric as possible for both the donor button and the host opening, on the assumption that more uniform tissues around the entire circumference will create more uniform wound healing and less astigmatism. Thus most surgeons have tried to place a perfectly circular donor button with smooth edges into a per-

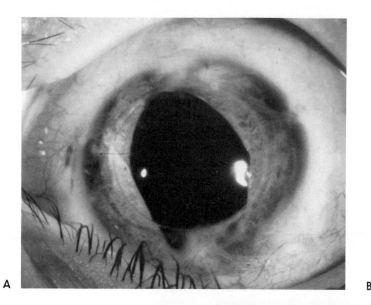

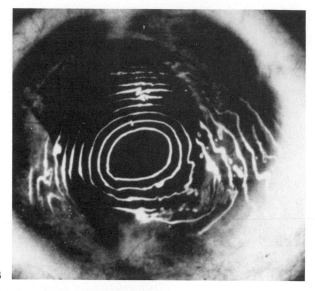

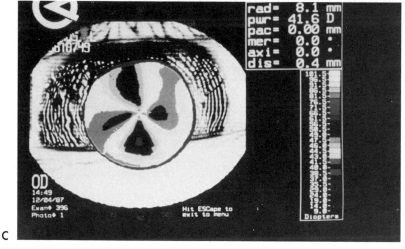

Figure 31-39

Effect of preoperative scarring and astigmatism on astigmatism after penetrating keratoplasty. A 15-year-old boy suffered a full-thickness corneal laceration while surfing. The laceration was repaired, primarily resulting in a dense vascularized corneal scar that extended from 6 o'clock to 12 o'clock. **A,** A penetrating keratoplasty was performed with technical success, but the residual scarring at the superior and inferior limbus produced high postoperative astigmatism. At 9 months after penetrating keratoplasty the graft is clear and compact and the dense scar *(arrows)* is seen in the 6 o'clock and 12 o'clock host cornea and limbus. **B,** Photokeratograph shows horizontally oval mires that corresponded to central keratometric readings of 39.75 × 10°/50.75 × 110°. **C,** Videokeratograph (gray scale) demonstrates the typical bowtie pattern that shows 9 D of astigmatism.

fectly circular host opening with smooth edges, minimizing the disparity in shape between the two. However, many variables alter this ideal goal. Distortion of the donor and host during trephination can create irregular wounds. Extensive clinical, laboratory, and technical research continues to improve donor and host trephination systems.[92,133,165,184] Troutman and colleagues[180] attempted to orient the donor button so it fit into the host opening more readily in eyes with keratoconus in an attempt to distribute the tissue appropriately and diminish postoperative astigmatism. The approach was ineffective.

Not all surgeons think a round wound is best, as illustrated by the research of Lang and colleagues,[94] who used an excimer laser to create an oval host wound and an oval donor that they think improve the fit between the two tissues. Other surgeons create a shelf on the posterior aspect of the host wound, which they think better supports the graft, preventing prolapse of the graft into the anterior chamber and sealing the posterior wound. It is virtually impossible, however, to manually create a uniform, radially symmetric posterior shelf.

Disparate diameters of the donor and the host incisions, either oversizing the donor[137] or undersizing the donor as in keratoconus,[66] also may affect postoperative astigmatism.

Techniques of trephination of the donor and host incisions continue to improve with the development of mechanical suction trephines that employ the following principles:

1. Accurate centering mechanism
2. Adaptability to donor and host corneas of different curvatures
3. Ability to select depth of trephination
4. Uniform support inside and outside the blade on the surface of the cornea during cutting
5. Perpendicular alignment to the cornea throughout trephination
6. Absence of distortion of tissue during cutting
7. Visualization of the blade during the incision with recognition of entry into the anterior chamber
8. Control of intraocular pressure during trephination
9. Avoidance of damage to donor endothelium and host intraocular structures

The suction mechanical trephine systems designed by Hanna[187] and by Krumeich[91] and the point-cutting trephine systems, such as those designed by Crock[46] and Lieberman,[98a] embody many of these principles.

The studies of Cohen, Tripoli, and colleagues[37,38] in cats have demonstrated the complexity of trying to correlate corneal incision shape and wound morphology with postoperative astigmatism. These researchers could not demonstrate a distinct correlation between postkeratoplasty astigmatism and the ovality of the donor and host incisions or the cross-sectional morphology of the wound. However, they showed that a thicker corneal epithelium within the wound (indicating the amount of anterior wound separation) correlated with more astigmatism. Basing their study on the histopathology of human eyes, Lange and colleagues[93] postulated that the alignment of the anterior surface was more important than the alignment of the posterior surface in reducing astigmatism. Every corneal surgeon has cases in which there is minimal astigmatism with considerable irregularity of the healed wound, including visible overlap and underlap of the anterior and posterior edges, as well as varying thickness of the wound on slit-lamp microscopy. Thus the factors that determine the final amount of astigmatism after all sutures are removed remain complex and to some degree beyond the surgeon's control.

Suture pattern, technique, and adjustment. The wide variety of suture patterns and techniques that have been used for penetrating keratoplasty reflects the fact that none predictably eliminates postoperative astigmatism without postoperative adjustment.[21,133] The ideal suture technique has the following goals:

1. Uniform distribution of sutures 360° with similar size and configuration of suture bites
2. Uniform moderate tension on each suture bite without excess tissue compression
3. Deep suture bites for full wound apposition
4. Absence of long, deep, tightly tied sutures that increase corneal curvature and astigmatism in that semimeridian

Intraoperative keratoscopy and keratometry (as described in the previous section on cataract surgery) can be used to adjust the sutures at the conclusion of keratoplasty, decreasing the amount of astigmatism immediately after surgery. Nevertheless, the relatively high average amount of postoperative astigmatism with sutures still in place is a testimony to the limitations of manual suture placement and to the need for postoperative suture adjustment. Even if the sutures can be adjusted to minimize astigmatism, they probably cannot set the wound in a configuration so that when the sutures are removed, there is no change in astigmatism. The underlying wound configuration still exerts an important force on the corneal shape. Whether postoperative suture adjustment can reduce the final amount of astigmatism that remains after all sutures have been removed is unknown.

Considerations of astigmatism after penetrating keratoplasty can be divided into two time periods: (1) the months to years during which sutures are in place, and (2) the time after sutures are removed. As long as sutures are in place, they are probably the major factor that determines the shape of the donor cornea, so suture manipulation after penetrating keratoplasty can reduce astigmatism. Once all sutures are removed, the configuration and biomechanical stress of the wound as influenced by the shape of the donor and host corneas and by wound healing determine the amount of astigmatism; therefore surgical modification by keratotomy or keratectomy is presently the preferred method for reducing astigmatism. Other techniques, such as holmium-YAG laser intrastromal thermokeratoplasty, are under consideration.

Because large amounts of astigmatism can be present after removal of all sutures and because modern techniques of keratoplasty allow early visual rehabilitation, techniques of postoperative adjustment of sutures have developed to reduce astigmatism and to allow prescription of spectacles or contact lenses within the first few months after surgery (Fig. 31-40).

Sutures produce astigmatism after keratoplasty by the same mechanisms described for cataract surgery. The goal of suture adjustment is to decrease the suture tension in the steep meridian and increase the suture tension in the flat meridian, equalizing the corneal curvature 360°. This can be done by identifying and removing tight interrupted sutures[18,19,23]—as initially described by Cottingham,[43] popularized by Binder and colleagues,* and refined by Waring and colleagues[29,30,73,86]—or by moving a portion of the running suture from the flat meridian, where tension is presumably less, to the steep meridian, where the tension is presumably more, as proposed by Atkins and Roper-Hall,[9] McNeill and Wessels,[121] and others.[100,181,189] The basic principles for suture adjustment are based on the following facts:

1. The axis of the plus refractive cylinder indicates the steep corneal meridian.

*References 19, 23, 29, 30, 73, 86, 159-161.

2. The steep keratometric meridian may have a different axis and power than that found by refraction.
3. The astigmatism is not radially symmetric. Along any steep meridian one half of that meridian may have an acceptable curvature and the other half may be responsible for the astigmatism. Thus keratography is an enormous aid in identifying the semimeridians with the tight sutures.

Keratography helps identify the tight suture; focally indented rings on the keratograph indicate a greater amount of astigmatism and portend a greater change after the removal of the indenting tight suture (Tables 31-35 and 31-36 and Figs. 31-40 and 31-41; see also Stainer and colleagues[161]). Once the surgeon has identified the tight suture, then, using topical anesthesia at the slit-lamp microscope, he or she can cut it and remove it with a tying forceps, jerking the suture briskly to accelerate the exit of the knot from the tissue. We use a bent, disposable 22-gauge hypodermic needle that acts as a sterile pic to lift the suture from beneath the epithelium, that cuts the suture with the sharp edge, and that is inexpensive. The suture ends should retract immediately when cut; if the ends remain approximated, the suture probably was not tight enough to induce astigmatism, and the surgeon should search for another tighter suture. Adjustment of a running suture requires not only identifying the steep and flat meridians, but also using a Tennant-style fine-tipped, blunt, smooth-edged tying forceps to lift the suture and pull it from the flat meridian around to the steep meridian. The amount of tension pulled up on each loop, the cumulative amount of slack taken up over the total number of loops, and the exact redistribution of the slack all will influence the results of the running adjustment.[121]

Postoperative suture adjustment can decrease the astigmatism present in the months after surgery and can promote rapid visual rehabilitation. For example, Binder[19] performed selective suture removal in 143 eyes, reducing an initial average keratometric astigmatism of 7.6 D at 1 month to a final average astigmatism of 2.9 D at 12 months.

Pradera and colleagues[138] studied 44 eyes after penetrating keratoplasty and intraocular lens implantation or exchange, in which the mean astigmatism present at the first postoperative refraction was 5.11 $\pm$2.48 D; by selectively removing an average of 2.5 $\pm$2 sutures per eye, the mean astigmatism was reduced to 2.5 $\pm$1.5 D, 55% of the eyes having 3 D or less and 90% of the eyes having 4 D or less (Fig. 31-42). Similarly, Burk and colleagues[29] reported 24 consecutive eyes with an initial postoperative astigmatism of 5.8 D; removal of an average of two sutures per eye achieved a mean astigmatism of 2.25 D at 4 months, with 67% of the eyes showing 3 D or less of astigmatism.

Musch and colleagues[127] performed a prospective randomized trial comparing a double-running suture, with removal of the 10-0 nylon, at approximately 3 months postoperatively with a combined 12-bite running and interrupted suture technique, with selective removal of the interrupted sutures. Differences in the two groups were not apparent until 1 year after surgery, when the median astigmatism in 53 eyes in the selective removal group was 2.50 D, compared with 4.00 D in three eyes in the double-running suture group. It is possible that more frequent suture adjustments earlier in the postoperative course could have shown an earlier difference in the two techniques.

Therefore selective suture removal can reduce the average astigmatism to less than 3 D within the first few months after surgery, a considerable improvement over that achieved with no suture adjustment.

Results for adjusting a single-running suture have been reported by McNeill and colleagues,[121] who showed that for 289 eyes the mean astigmatism was 2.87 D at 6 months, as compared with a nonadjusted control group of 83 eyes, in which the mean astigmatism was 4.80 D (Fig. 31-43). In a small pilot study

Figure 31-40
After penetrating keratoplasty photokeratographs and drawings demonstrate patterns
of astigmatism induced by the keratoplasty wound and sutures. These patterns can
serve as a guide to postoperative suture adjustment for the reduction of astigmatism.
(From Harris DJ, Waring GO, and Burk LL: Ophthalmology 1989;96:1597-1607.)

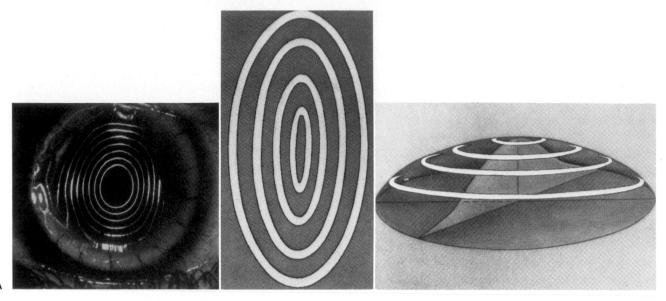

A, Symmetrically oval keratographic mires. *Left,* Clinical example shows the steep
meridian at approximately 175° and the flat meridian at approximately 85°. A single
steep semimeridian cannot be identified. *Middle and right,* Schematic representations
of oval mires and a corneal contour that is flat in one meridian and steep 90° away.

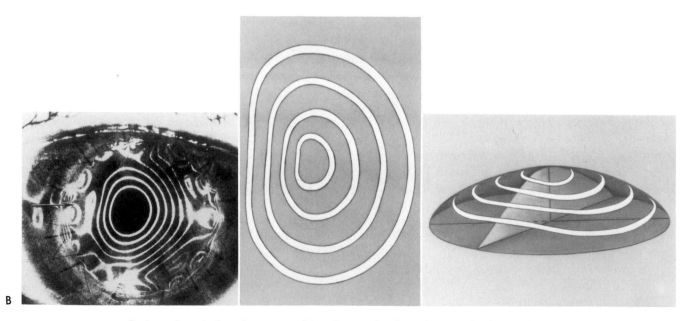

B, D-shaped oval photokeratographic mires. *Left,* Clinical example shows the steep
meridian at 165°. The 9:30 semimeridian is steeper than the 3:30 semi-meridian;
therefore the 9:30 suture *(arrow)* should be removed. *Middle and right,* Schematic
representation of D-shaped mires and corneal contour.   *Continued.*

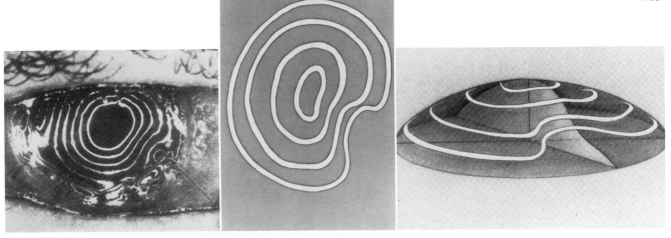

C, Focally indented photokeratographic mires. *Left,* Clinical example shows a focal indentation of the mires at the 330° semimeridian at 4:00, locating the tightest suture *(arrow). Middle and right,* Focally indented mires and corneal contour.

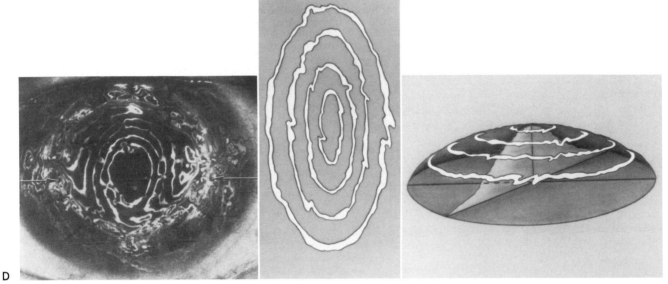

D, Mildly disrupted photokeratographic mires. *Left,* Clinical example shows a rough epithelial surface that precludes accurate manifest refraction and keratometry, but the photokeratograph clearly demonstrates astigmatism with its steep meridian at approximately 180°. Therefore either the 3:00 or the 9:00 suture could be considered for removal. *Middle and right,* Mildly disrupted mires and corneal contour.

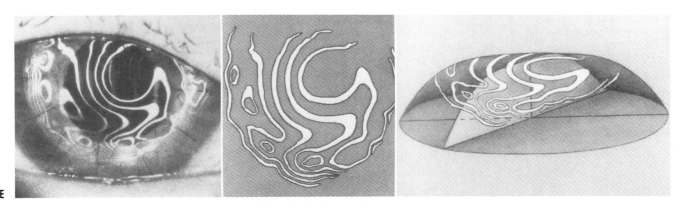

E, Incomplete photokeratographic mires. *Left,* Clinical example shows incomplete photokeratographic mires. Keratometry was not possible, and interpretation of the photokeratograph was difficult; however, manifest refraction revealed minimal astigmatism, and no sutures were removed. *Middle and right,* Incomplete mires and "barrel-top" corneal contour, that is, centrally flat and peripherally steep.

Table 31-35

Effect of Keratographic Pattern on Change in Penetrating Keratoplasty Astigmatism after Removal of One Interrupted Suture*

Pattern of keratographic mires (no. of eyes)	Net reduction in keratometric astigmatism (D)	Amount of vectoral induced astigmatism (D)	Axis of induced astigmatism†
Symmetric oval (9)	0.44 ±1.69	3.60 ±2.43	0° ±10°
D-shaped (14)	2.07 ±2.48	4.81 ±1.84	−10° ±18°
Focal indentation (6)	6.60 ±2.54	7.65 ±1.95	−4° ±3°

Modified from Harris DJ, Waring GO, and Burk LL: Ophthalmology 1989;96:1597-1607.
*Keratometric measurements taken immediately before and at least 2 weeks after single suture removal. Values presented are mean ±SD.
†The difference between the actual axis of the induced astigmatism as calculated by vector analysis and the location of the removed suture.

Table 31-36

Change in Corneal Astigmatism after Removal of One Interrupted Suture under Keratographic Guidance in 29 Eyes

Direction of change in astigmatism	Amount of change in astigmatism (D)*	Pattern of photokeratograph mires		
		Oval	D-shaped	Indented
Decrease	8.00 to 10.00	0	0	2
	6.00 to 7.87	0	1	1
	4.00 to 5.87	0	3	2
	2.00 to 3.87	2	3	1
	1.00 to 1.87	1	3	0
No change	0.87 to 0.87	4	1	0
Increase	1.00 to 1.87	1	1	0
	2.00 to 2.50	1	1	0

Modified from Harris DJ, Waring GO, and Burk LL: Ophthalmology 1989;96:1597-1607.
*Keratometric measurements taken immediately before and at least 2 weeks after removal of one interrupted suture.

of eight eyes, Lin and colleagues[100] showed a mean astigmatism after adjustment of the running suture of 1.7 D, all eyes having less than 2.6 D at 4 months, in contrast to a group of 10 eyes with a double-running suture, from which one of the sutures had been removed, that showed a mean astigmatism of 5.4 D.

The ideal method of postoperative suture adjustment has not been identified. Adjustment of a single-running suture is more flexible because it can be done repeatedly in any direction, whereas the selective removal of interrupted sutures allows only for flattening of the steep meridian unless interrupted sutures are again added to steepen the flat meridian. Wood[189] has advocated opening the anterior portion of the wound at the time of the adjustment of running sutures. This is done with the blunt tip of a tying forceps or a blunt intraocular lens hook and is designed to destabilize the wound in the same way that a relaxing incision within the wound does so that the change in tension on the suture can create a change in the wound configuration and presumedly reestablish the wound in a configuration that will induce less astigmatism. No data are published on this technique. Prospective randomized trials are the best way to evaluate these techniques.

Disadvantages of suture adjustment include the need for more frequent postoperative visits with increased manipulation of the eye and frequent breaks in the healed epithelium. Problems may result from sutures left in place indefi-

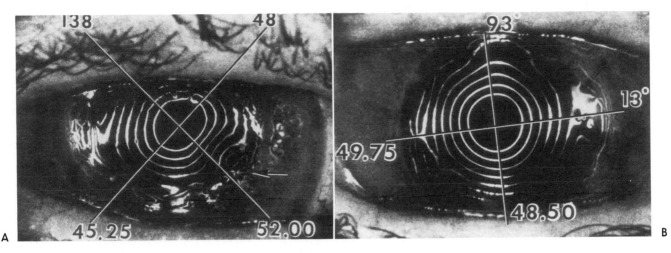

Figure 31-41
Selective removal of tight interrupted sutures to reduce astigmatism after penetrating keratoplasty. **A,** Photokeratograph shows focally indented mires with 6.75 D of keratometric astigmatism. Arrow indicates suture chosen for removal at 4 o'clock. **B,** At three weeks after removal of one tight suture there was a 5.50 D net reduction in astigmatism producing reasonably round keratograph mires and a residual keratometric astigmatism of 1.25 D. (From Harris DJ, Waring GO, and Burk LL: Ophthalmology 1989;96:1596-1607.)

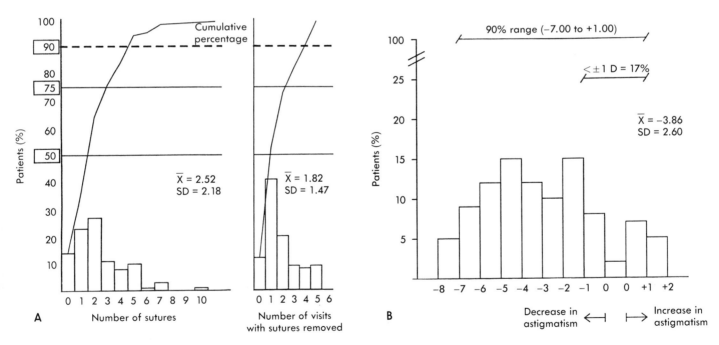

Figure 31-42
Results of selected interrupted suture removal in 44 eyes with penetrating keratoplasty and intraocular lens insertion. **A,** Graphs illustrate the total number of selected interrupted sutures that required removal *(left)* and the total number of clinical visits during which the sutures were removed *(right)* to achieve visual rehabilitation. Over 90% of the eyes achieved acceptable visual function with the removal of four sutures during four suture removal visits. **B,** Change in refractive astigmatism during the time of selective removal of interrupted sutures indicates that 95% of the 44 eyes showed a decrease in astigmatism or a net change of less than 1 D. Ninety percent of the eyes had a change in astigmatism ranging from a decrease of 7 D to an increase of 1 D. (From Pradera I, Ibrahim O, and Waring GO: Refract Corneal Surg 1989;5: 231-239.)

Figure 31-43
Effect of postoperative adjustment of running 10-0 nylon suture in penetrating keratoplasty. The eyes with suture adjustment *(black bars)* showed a large and persistent decrease in astigmatism compared with the nonadjusted control groups *(gray bars).* (From McNeill JI and Wessels IF: Refract Corneal Surg 1989;5:216-223.)

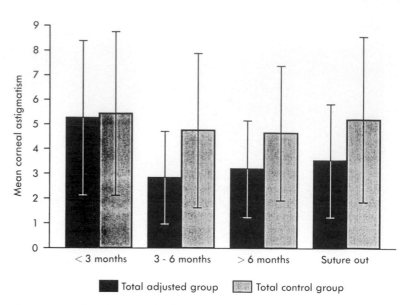

nitely, such as late suture breakage with discomfort, the stimulation of microbial keratitis or allograft reaction, and changes in refraction.

Corneal wound healing. The fourth major factor that determines astigmatism after penetrating keratoplasty is corneal wound healing as modified by corticosteroids. Presumedly the shape of the corneal graft is determined by the symmetry of wound healing, contracture, vascularization, slippage, and the like. Each of these aspects varies greatly from one eye to another and at different locations around a keratoplasty wound. Presently there is no clinically useful method of accurately controlling corneal wound healing, although topical corticosteroids can decrease fibroplasia and vascularization.

Changes in astigmatism after removal of all sutures

Large changes in shape of the donor cornea, refraction, and astigmatism can occur any time that sutures are removed, whether in the early postoperative period during intentional adjustment or years after surgery when the suture breaks spontaneously or is removed voluntarily. For example, Mader and colleagues[109] studied the removal of a single-running suture from 130 eyes between 1 and 6 years after penetrating keratoplasty, observing a range of change in keratometric astigmatism from an increase of 11 D to a decrease of 18 D. The average vectoral change was 6.5 ±4.3 D (range, 0.59 to 19.8 D). In general, eyes that had a small amount of astigmatism with the sutures in place demonstrated an increase of astigmatism when the sutures were removed, whereas eyes that had a large amount of astigmatism with the sutures in place demonstrated a decrease. In spite of these trends, the authors concluded that it was impossible to predict the direction or amount of change in astigmatism induced by late suture removal in an individual eye (Fig. 31-44).

Binder[19] showed similar findings in a series of 143 eyes, demonstrating that after suture removal, 34% had an increase in astigmatism of 1 D or more and 45% had a decrease in astigmatism of 1 D or more. He[19] and Mader[109] also showed that eyes with a large amount of astigmatism tended to show a decrease after suture removal, whereas eyes with a small amount of astigmatism tended to show an increase. Similar findings were reported by Musch and colleagues,[126] who reported that 41% of 131 eyes showed more than 2 D of astigmatic change after removing a 10-0 running nylon suture, and 19% showed more than 2 D of astigmatic change after removing an 11-0 nylon suture, the distribution of increases and decreases being similar. Burk and colleagues[30] reported similar findings.

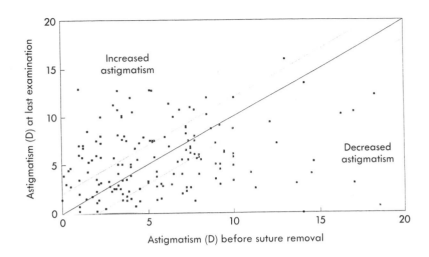

Figure 31-44
Scattergram shows the change in keratometric astigmatism occurring after removal of all sutures in 135 eyes with penetrating keratoplasty. All eyes were between 1 and 6 years after surgery. X-axis shows astigmatism before suture removal, and Y-axis shows astigmatism after suture removal. Increases and decreases occurred after suture removal; there was no way to predict the change in astigmatism for an individual eye. (From Mader TH, Yuan R, Lynn MJ, et al: Invest Ophthalmol Vis Sci 1990;31(suppl):574.)

Recently Binder[26] reported on corneal shape after removal of 11-0 nylon sutures in 300 eyes that were followed for more than 40 months after surgery. Sutures were removed at an average of 22 months postoperatively. In 199 eyes that had keratometry readings available immediately *before* suture removal, the mean astigmatism was 3.83 D. About 50% of the eyes had less than 3 D of astigmatism. A decrease in astigmatism of 1 D or more (up to 7D) occurred in 52 eyes, and an increase of 1 D or more (up to 8 D) occurred in 84 eyes.

Because all previous studies of the effect of 10-0 suture removal demonstrated unpredictable changes after suture removal and because large shifts are possible even with removal of 11-0 nylon sutures, we can be certain that removal of a previously adjusted nylon suture also will produce significant changes. Although the short-term follow-up published by McNeill suggested that the adjusted topography remained after the removal of the 10-0 suture, long-term studies will most likely show changes similar to those found by previously published studies. It is difficult to imagine that removal of an adjusted 10-0 nylon suture will produce results different from those of nonadjusted continuous sutures or following selective suture removal.*

Nonkeratotomy surgery for astigmatism after penetrating keratoplasty

Patients with unacceptable astigmatism after penetrating keratoplasty and suture removal are candidates for surgery, usually transverse keratotomy. Surgical modification of astigmatism after penetrating keratoplasty has developed over the past two decades through the following stages:

1. Repair of wound slippage or dehiscence
2. Wedge resection in the flat meridian (Troutman)
3. Arcuate keratotomy in the steep meridian (Troutman, Krachmer)
4. Arcuate keratotomy in the steep meridian with placement of compression sutures in the flat meridian (Troutman)
5. Trapezoidal keratotomy (Ruiz, Lindstrom)
6. Graduated, "tailored" relaxing keratotomy with intraoperative keratoscopy or sequential surgery

The fundamental decision for the surgeon is whether to flatten the steep meridian or to steepen the flat meridian.

*References 19, 23, 29, 30, 73, 86, 160, 161.

Wound revision. The first consideration in wound revision is the configuration of the wound, such as anterior displacement of the graft or obvious wound gaping, both visible with slit-lamp microscopy. Keratography identifies the area of anterior slippage of the graft as a flatter zone producing pear-shaped mires that point to the area of displacement. Buzard[31] has proposed that "microdehiscences" may produce focal flattening in the keratoscopy mires without visible displacement of the graft, especially when a running suture may have unequal distribution of tension. To steepen this flat area, Buzard proposes opening the wound, removing any epithelial plug, freshening the edges, and suturing the wound back together with moderately tight sutures that temporarily overcorrect and steepen that meridian.[87,143] Alternatively, one or two long, deep interrupted sutures may be placed across the focal flat area and tied to compress the wound and steepen that semimeridian. The sutures can be added with the preexisting sutures in place without disruption of the keratoplasty wound.[31,142] Limberg and colleagues[99] described a similar procedure, using an operating keratoscope to place one or two 9-0 nylon sutures across the flat meridian, tightening the sutures to reverse the oval mires. In the first weeks after surgery, the overcorrection gradually decayed, and subsequently the procedure was not as effective as desired. In 10 eyes followed for 9 to 12 months, an average preoperative keratometric astigmatism of 9.9 D was decreased to 5.1 D. Seven of the ten eyes had more than 3 D of residual astigmatism (range, 3.4 to 8.0), and the procedure corrected only approximately 41% of the astigmatism.

Wedge resection. A more complex method of steepening the flat meridian is to perform a wedge resection from the host at the wound in one flat semimeridian (avoid a pair of wedge resections),* to flatten the steep meridian and to steepen the flat meridian. A wedge of tissue is created with a freehand knife by making a vertical incision in the wound adjacent to the donor tissue and a beveled incision in the host. The length is approximately 90°, and the width is roughly proportionate to the amount of astigmatism to be corrected, at a rate of 0.1 mm per diopter, although the results are highly variable and not nearly this quantifiable. Six to eight interrupted radial 10-0 nylon sutures are used to close the wound after paracentesis lowers the intraocular pressure.

There is less published information about the results of wedge resections than of other procedures. The sutures are tightened to overcorrect the astigmatism by an amount approximately equal to that present preoperatively; the overcorrection can be reduced gradually by selective suture removal. It can take many months to stabilize the refraction. The flat meridian steepens, and the steep meridian flattens.

In general, a wedge resection is difficult to perform: the wound is often ragged[182]; the early postoperative course is fraught with induced irregular astigmatism; the recovery period is long; and the predictability of the procedure is poor. Van Rij[182] described the postoperative course of an eye that had 12 D of induced astigmatism after wedge resection, which gradually decayed along with suture removal to 2 D at 19 months after surgery. Nevertheless, wedge resection offers an alternative to repeat penetrating keratoplasty in eyes with high astigmatism. The surgeon would consider a wedge resection in an eye with a flat corneal curvature, where as a relaxing incision is indicated for an eye with a steep corneal curvature.

Secondary limbal surgery after corneal transplantation. Following keratoplasty, cataracts may form or an aphakic eye may become contact lens intolerant. In such situations a limbal wound will be made. Using the techniques described in the cataract astigmatism section, the surgeon may attempt to reduce postkeratoplasty astigmatism by proper placement of the wound in relation to

---

*References 14, 88, 106, 175, 176, 178.

Case 6: Cataract Surgery after Penetrating Keratoplasty

A 68-year-old woman had undergone a penetrating keratoplasty on July 1, 1978. Her keratometry readings were $46.12 \times 90°/43.12 \times 180°$. A left extracapsular cataract extraction and posterior chamber intraocular lens implant was performed in 1983, 60 months after her corneal transplant, using eight interrupted Vicryl sutures to induce some flattening of the vertical meridian and correct her keratoplasty astigmatism. When the patient was last examined in July 1985, her keratometry readings were $46.62 \times 90°/43.12 \times 180°$, or approximately 3.5 D of with-the-rule astigmatism. This case example points out the difficulties in using limbal manipulation at cataract surgery to affect preexisting astigmatism after a corneal transplant.

---

the steep meridian and by using suture techniques to reduce astigmatism. In a series of 32 postkeratoplasty eyes undergoing cataract or IOL surgery, Binder[24] used these approaches to reduce preexisting astigmatism. Although astigmatism was reduced in a few eyes, the mean astigmatism remained unchanged. Binder concluded that limbal surgical manipulation was unable to modify the shape of the graft, probably because the keratoplasty wound functioned as a new "limbus" that blocked the transmission of the changes induced by the cataract wound.

Another approach to correcting postkeratoplasty astigmatism is to perform a limbal wedge resection at the time of secondary intraocular lens implantation.[65,82] The technique has the advantage of accomplishing two refractive corrections at one time—correction of aphakia and astigmatism—but suffers from the same problems and unpredictabilities that wedge resection in the keratoplasty wound does. Geggel[65] reported 13 such procedures, 11 of which showed reduction of astigmatism of an average of 3.1 ± 1.77 D (range, 0.50 to 6.25 D). There was approximately as much steepening of the wedge resection meridian as there was a flattening of the unoperated meridian 90° away.

Transverse relaxing keratotomy for astigmatism after penetrating keratoplasty

Table 31-37 summarizes the published results of different techniques of relaxing transverse keratotomy after penetrating keratoplasty. A review of these data indicates the following generalities:

1. Astigmatism is reduced in the vast majority of eyes, indicating that the procedure has general clinical utility (Fig. 31-45).
2. The amount of reduction varies greatly from one eye to another, even using the same technique, indicating that the outcome is unpredictable for individual eyes (Fig. 31-46).
3. Surgical techniques vary from one study to another, including variations in the location, length, depth, number, and pattern of incisions, and the use of compression sutures. Some surgeons use graded sequential keratotomy and intraoperative keratometric monitoring. This emphasizes the considerable art underlying the procedure and the lack of consensus on the most effective techniques (Fig. 31-47).
4. The surgery is done either at the slit-lamp microscope or in the operating room, usually under topical anesthesia, depending on the complexity of the technique.
5. Although the use of compression sutures is said to enhance the results, no prospective randomized trial comparing relaxing incisions with and without compression sutures has been done.

6. The lowest amounts of residual astigmatism were achieved by graded sequential keratotomy with intraoperative monitoring as reported by Troutman,[179] Forstot,[61] Arffa,[6] and Salmeron,[148] suggesting that a fixed surgical nomogram is inadequate for the varieties of astigmatism after penetrating keratoplasty. This approach also has been advocated by McDonald and colleagues[119,120] and by Duffey and colleagues.[55]

7. The resultant spherical equivalent refraction (a result of the flattening to steepening ratio) remained roughly unchanged from preoperative values or became hyperopic, indicating more flattening than steepening. There is great variability.

8. Serious complications are rare; perforation of the cornea that sometimes requires suturing is the most frequent. However, severe problems can occur, including cystoid macular edema,[34] the vitreous wick syndrome,[158] traumatic dehiscence with endophthalmitis and loss of all vision (personal observation). The risk of the procedure cannot be minimized by the surgeon or the patient.

9. Trapezoidal keratotomy has the disadvantage of intersecting semiradial incisions with the previous keratoplasty wound,[49,50] but if the wound is well healed, gaping may not occur. The cautions about trapezoidal keratotomy discussed in the previous section apply to its use after penetrating keratoplasty. Its major advantage is to minimize steepening in the unincised meridian.

   Buzard[32] reported a series of 13 eyes using two techniques of trapezoidal keratotomy for astigmatism after penetrating keratoplasty. Five eyes were treated with converging semiradial incisions and eight eyes were treated with parallel ("corridor") semiradial incisions. All eyes had four pairs of transverse incisions. The mean follow-up was 23 months (range, 9 to 55). None of the incisions were connected. The average preoperative astigmatism was 7.03 ±2.64 D, and the average reduction of refractive cylinder was 6.12 ±3.50 D. Eight of the 13 eyes had less than 3.00 D of refractive astigmatism after surgery. The authors concluded that the effect of the surgery remained confined around the meridian of surgery, but that the overall predictability was less than desired (Fig. 31-48).

   Agapitos and colleagues[1] reported seven eyes with nonintersecting trapezoidal keratotomy, one after cataract surgery and six after penetrating keratoplasty. The mean follow-up was 2.6 months. The mean preoperative refractive astigmatism was 9.4 D (range, 2.50 to 20.00 D). The mean change in keratometric astigmatism was 13.4 ±9.2 D. The authors concluded that the overall results in the group with nonintersecting trapezoidal incisions were more predictable than those in a previous group with intersecting trapezoidal incisions.

10. Incisions are made in the donor or in the wound. None of the reports placed relaxing incisions outside the keratoplasty wound in the host cornea because the keratoplasty wound in effect forms a new "limbus," a barrier that minimizes the effect of incisions made in the host, just as with limbal cataract surgery.

11. There are no detailed studies of the stability of refraction after relaxing incisions. However, there are reports of prolonged individual fluctuation of vision and refraction.[105] *Text continued on p. 1182.*

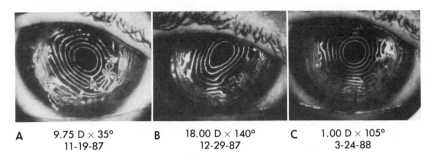

A   9.75 D × 35°   **B**   18.00 D × 140°   **C**   1.00 D × 105°
         11-19-87   12-29-87   3-24-88

Figure 31-45
Example of arcuate transverse relaxing keratotomy and compression sutures to treat high astigmatism after penetrating keratoplasty. **A,** With all sutures removed from the graft, 9.75 D of astigmatism remain. **B,** After one pair of arcuate keratotomy incisions placed 0.5 mm inside the keratoplasty wound in the 35° meridian and the placement of compression sutures in the 145° meridian, a large overcorrection was achieved. **C,** Three months after the removal of the compression sutures, only 1 D of astigmatism remained.

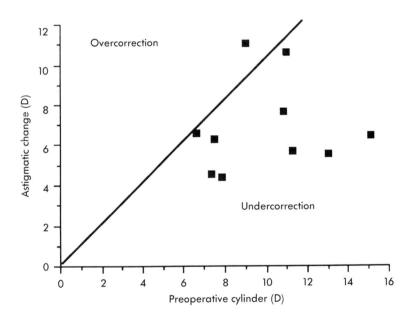

Figure 31-46
Results of arcuate relaxing keratotomy with compression sutures still in place for the treatment of astigmatism after penetrating keratoplasty. Change in keratometric astigmatism shows an overall undercorrection. The mean change in astigmatism was 6.90 ±2.00 D. The change in the spherical equivalent refraction was −1.50 D, indicating overall flattening of the cornea. (From Agapitos PJ, Lindstrom RL, Williams PA, et al: J Cataract Refract Surg 1989;5:13-18.)

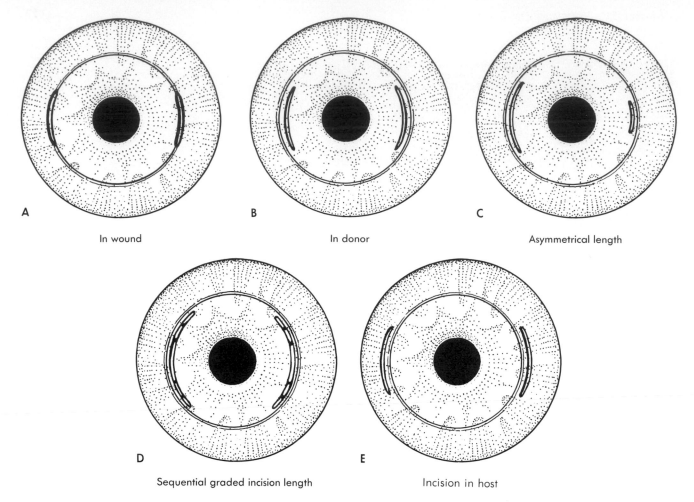

A In wound

B In donor

C Asymmetrical length

D Sequential graded incision length

E Incision in host

Figure 31-47
Placement and patterns of arcuate transverse keratotomy to reduce astigmatism after penetrating keratoplasty. **A,** Incisions placed in the wound ("classic" technique). **B,** Incisions placed in the donor avoid uncertainties of variable thickness of the wound and allow a smaller diameter clear zone for greater effect. **C,** Incisions of asymmetrical length based on corneal topography are under investigation. **D,** A titrated approach in which incisions are lengthened or deepened or in which repeated operations are done to enhance the original incisions may be preferred because it allows incision adjustment to fit the corneal response. **E,** Incisions in the host cornea are ineffective because the keratoplasty wound forms a new "limbus," blocking the effect of the relaxing incisions on the central cornea.

Figure 31-48
Results of trapezoidal keratotomy in 13 eyes after penetrating keratoplasty, comparing astigmatism before *(solid bar)* and after *(dotted bar)* keratotomy surgery. The age of each patient is indicated on the x-axis, and the vectoral change in astigmatism on the y-axis. Although all eyes had a decrease in astigmatism and six had a residual astigmatism of 3 D or less, the variability in results indicated the unpredictability of this technique (From Buzard KA, Haight D, and Troutman D: J Refract Surg 1987;3:40-45.)

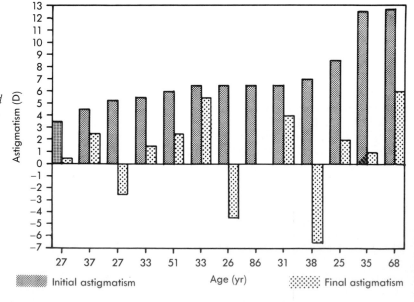

Table 31-37

Results of Relaxing Transverse Keratotomy Techniques for Reduction of Astigmatism after Penetrating Keratoplasty

First author, year	Pattern of incisions	Number of eyes	Reason for surgery
Isolated relaxing transverse keratotomy			
Krachmer, 1980	Paired arcuate	16	High postkeratoplasty astigmatism; glasses and contact lenses discussed or tried
Sugar, 1983	Paired arcuate	17	Astigmatism > 8.5 D
Agapitos, 1989	Transverse cuts alone	5	
Price, 1987	Paired arcuate	37	Postkeratoplasty astigmatism with functional vision <6/60
Relaxing transverse keratotomy and compression sutures			
Mandel, 1987	Paired arcuate—six compression sutures. Sutures removed if > 3D cylinder at 3 months. Sutures retained in 85%	19	High astigmatism and unable to wear glasses or contact lenses
McCartney, 1987	Paired arcuate. Incisions in host in four eyes. Compression sutures. No. eyes with retained sutures not specified	11	Functionally disabling astigmatism for > 6 months after surgery
Agapitos, 1989	Paired arcuate compression sutures. No. eyes with retained sutures not specified	10	Postcataract. Postkeratoplasty
Price, 1987	Paired arcuate—four compression sutures. No. eyes with retained sutures not specified	8	Postkeratoplasty astigmatism with functional vision < 6/60
Lustbader, 1990	Paired arcuate—six compression sutures. No. eyes with retained sutures not specified	10	Not reported
Trapezoidal keratotomy			
Lavery, 1985	Intersecting trapezoidal	9	High, regular astigmatism
Buzard, 1987	Intersecting rectangular, nonintersecting trapezoidal	13	High astigmatism
Agapitos, 1989	Intersecting trapezoidal	20	
	Nonintersecting trapezoidal	6	
Graded incremental transverse keratotomy			
Troutman, 1980	Cut down, one or two incisions	4	Significant astigmatism
Arffa, 1988	One or two straight incisions ± semiradial incisions depending on intraoperative keratotomy (goal = 25% to 30% overcorrection)	6	Poor vision with spectacles and contact lens intolerance
Forstot, 1988	Paired arcuate, subsequent wound spreading, deepening, lengthening	7	Unsatisfactory spectacle correction and poor contact lens fit
Salmeron, 1989	Relaxing incisions following penetrating keratoplasty; 90° arcuate relaxing keratotomies and intraoperative keratometric controls	9	Keratoconus patients with high degree of postkeratoplasty astigmatism

Prepared by Stephen Bogan, MD.

Continued.

Table 31-37—cont'd

Results of Relaxing Transverse Keratotomy Techniques for Reduction of Astigmatism after Penetrating Keratoplasty

First author	Knife	Slit-lamp (SL) or operating room (OR)	Anesthesia	Depth (%)	Length	Location
Isolated relaxing transverse keratotomy						
Krachmer	Metal	SL	Topical	50%	60°	In wound 180° apart
Sugar	Metal	SL	Not reported	66%	90°	In wound 180° apart
Agapitos	Diamond	OR	Topical	Not reported	Not reported	Not reported
Price	Not reported	Not reported	Not reported	75%	60° to 90°	In wound Paired incisions
Relaxing transverse keratotomy and compression sutures						
Mandel	Metal	Minor OR	Topical	60%	60°	In wound 180° apart
McCartney	Diamond	OR	Retrobulbar	70%	60° to 90°	0.5 mm central to wound 180° apart
Agapitos	Diamond	OR	Topical	Not reported	Not reported	Graft-host interface
Price	Not reported	Not reported	Not reported	75%	60° to 90°	In wound Paired incisions
Lustbader	Diamond	Not reported	Topical	75%	90°	0.5 mm central
Trapezoidal keratotomy						
Lavery	Not reported	OR	Topical	90%	T = 2.5 to 3 mm	Ruiz nomogram Clear zone = 3 to 6 mm
Buzard	Diamond	Not reported	Retrobulbar General	80%	1.5, 5	Ruiz computer program Does not intersect post-keratoplasty wound
Agapitos	Diamond	OR	Topical	Not reported	Not reported	3- or 5-mm clear zone (four or five pairs of transverse incisions)
	Diamond	OR	Topical	Not reported	Not reported	3- or 5-mm clear zone nonintersecting semiradial incisions
Graded incremental transverse keratotomy						
Troutman	Metal	SL	Topical	33%	60° to 80°	In wound 100° apart
Arffa	Diamond	OR	Topical	100%	3 mm linear	5-mm clear zone None in wound
Forstot	Metal	SL	Topical	60%	60° to 90°	In wound 180° apart
Salmeron	Not reported	OR	Not reported	Not reported	90°	Not reported

Table 31-37—cont'd

Results of Relaxing Transverse Keratotomy Techniques for Reduction of Astigmatism after Penetrating Keratoplasty

First author	Pachometry	Spectacle refraction	Photokeratoscopy
Isolated relaxing transverse keratotomy			
Krachmer	No	Not reported	No
Sugar	No	Not reported	No
Agapitos	No	Yes	No
Price	No	Yes	No
Relaxing transverse keratotomy and compression sutures			
Mandel	No	Yes	Yes (safety pin)
McCartney	No	Not reported	No
Agapitos	No	Yes	No
Price	No	Yes	No
Lustbader	No	Not reported	No
Trapezoidal keratotomy			
Lavery	Yes	No	No
Buzard	No	Not reported	No
Agapitos	Not reported	Yes	No
	Not reported	Yes	No
Graded incremental transverse keratotomy			
Troutman	No	Not reported	No
Arffa	Yes	Yes	Yes
Forstot	No	Yes	Yes
Salmeron	Not reported	Yes	Not reported

Continued.

Table 31-37—cont'd

Results of Relaxing Transverse Keratotomy Techniques for Reduction of Astigmatism after Penetrating Keratoplasty

First author	Evaluation		
	Keratometry		
	Preoperative	Intraoperative	Postoperative
Isolated relaxing transverse keratotomy			
Krachmer	Yes	Yes	Yes
Sugar	Yes	Yes	No
Agapitos	Yes	Not reported	Yes
Price	Yes	Not reported	Not reported
Relaxing transverse keratotomy and compression sutures			
Mandel	Yes	Yes	Yes
McCartney	Yes	Yes	Yes
Agapitos	Yes	Not reported	Yes
Price	Yes	Not reported	Not reported
Lustbader	Not reported	No	Yes
Trapezoidal keratotomy			
Lavery	Yes	No	Yes
Buzard	Yes	No	Yes
Agapitos	Yes	No	Yes
Graded incremental transverse keratotomy			
Troutman	Yes	Yes	Yes
Arffa	Yes	Yes	Yes
Forstot	Yes	Yes	No
Salmeron	Yes	Yes	Yes

Table 31-37—cont'd

Results of Relaxing Transverse Keratotomy Techniques for Reduction of Astigmatism after Penetrating Keratoplasty

First author	Undercorrected/ overcorrected	Follow-up (months)	Results Preoperative cylinder (mean ± SD, range)	Postoperative cylinder (mean ± SD, range)	Change in cylinder (mean ± SD, range)
Isolated relaxing transverse keratotomy					
Krachmer	Not reported	8.25 (3 to 31)	10.0 (7.00 to 14.25)	5.75 (1.50 to 11.37)	4.25 (2.00 to 7.75)
Sugar	12/2	7.5 to 23 months	12.47 ± 3.11 (8.50 to 18.00)	4.95 ± 2.00 (2.00 to 8.50)	7.5 ± 3.13 (2.5 to 11.5)
Agapitos	Not reported	3.4	5.30 (1.50 to 11.00)	Not reported	Not reported
Price	Not reported	Not reported	Not reported	Not reported	4.49 ± 6.22
Relaxing transverse keratotomy and compression sutures					
Mandel	8/4	Not reported (6 to 9)	9.73 (4.50 to 14.50)	3.17 (0 to 7.00)	6.56 (1.00 to 11.00)
McCartney	6/2	13.5 (6 to 21)	11.68 ± 3.75 (6.50 to 19.00)	3.91 (2.00 to 9.00)	7.59 ± 3.03 (4.50 to 13.00)
Agapitos	10/5	4.5	9.96 (6.60 to 15.10)	Not reported	Not reported
Price	Not reported	Not reported	Not reported	Not reported	5.80 ± 7.23
Lustbader	Not reported	6 to 12	14.25 (7 to 25)	7.42 (5 to 13)	Not reported
Trapezoidal keratotomy					
Lavery	Not reported	Not reported	(5.50 to 12.75)	(1.50 to 5.50)	(1.75 to 10.00)
Buzard	5/3	Not reported	7.03	2.94	4.09
Agapitos	10/5	14	8.30 (3.00 to 23.30)	Not reported	Not reported
	0/2	2.6	9.40 (2.5 to 20.00)	Not reported	Not reported
Graded incremental transverse keratotomy					
Troutman	2/1	<4	11.2 (7.00 to 13.25)	2.8 (2.00 to 3.00)	8.4 (5.00 to 10.25)
Arffa	1/1	15.7 (8 to 23)	9.63 ± 3.54 (4.00 to 14.00)	2.17 ± 2.23 (0.25 to 5.50)	7.46
Forstot	Not reported	12.5 (4 to 19)	9.96 (7.25 to 19.50)	1.8 (0.12 to 2.75)	8.3 (4.75 to 12.13)
Salmeron	Not reported	14 (2 to 29)	6.34 D ± 0.89 D	3.19 D ± 1.05 D	3.1 D

Continued.

Table 31-37—cont'd

Results of Relaxing Transverse Keratotomy Techniques for Reduction of Astigmatism after Penetrating Keratoplasty

First author	Vector-corrected change in cylinder (mean ± range)	Change in spherical equivalent refraction	Percentage of absolute reduction in cylinder	Percentage of effect in cylinder (corrected for change in axis)
Isolated relaxing transverse keratotomy				
Krachmer	Not reported	−0.42 (4.25 to −6.00)	47%	77%
Sugar	Not reported	+1.69 ±2.29 (5.5 to −0.43)	60%	76%
Agapitos	6.3 ±5.70	+1.13	116%	Not reported
Price	Not reported	−2.01 ±3.20	Not reported	Not reported
Relaxing transverse keratotomy and compression sutures				
Mandel	8.40 (1.13 to 14.26)	−0.54 (2.50 to −7.50)	67%	86%
McCartney	Not reported	+0.52 (3.00 to −1.75)	68%	Not reported
Agapitos	6.9 to 2.00	−1.50	71%	Not reported
Price	Not reported	−4.1 ±5.97	Not reported	Not reported
Lustbader	Not reported	Not reported	48%	Not reported
Trapezoidal keratotomy				
Lavery	Not reported	Not reported	Not reported	Not reported
Buzard	Not reported	Not reported	56%	Not reported
Agapitos	8.0 ±6.00	−0.39	93%	Not reported
	3.4 ±5.70	+2.40	137%	Not reported
Graded incremental transverse keratotomy				
Troutman	9.35 (5.04 to 15.92)	About 2:1 (flattening to steepening)	75%	84%
Arffa	10.23 (5.73 to 16.44)	−0.86	77%	106%
Forstot	Not reported	Not reported	83.3%	Not reported
Salmeron	Not reported	Not reported	Not reported	Not reported

Table 31-37—cont'd

Results of Relaxing Transverse Keratotomy Techniques for Reduction of Astigmatism after Penetrating Keratoplasty

First author	Complications	Author's observations
Isolated relaxing transverse keratotomy		
Krachmer	Two perforations requiring sutures	Incisions should be < 50% depth
		Relaxing incisions method of choice, then wedge resection
		Incisions in the wound are risky because of unpredictable thickness
Sugar	One perforation	Amount of preoperative cylinder may correlate with effect of
	One wound dehiscence	relaxing incision
		Repeat incisions performed in 4 patients because of insufficient gape of superficial incision
Agapitos	None reported	—
Price	Eight perforations	Compression sutures more reliable than wedge resection
	One rejection	No benefit to reopening wound when compression sutures used
Relaxing transverse keratotomy and compression sutures		
Mandel	Three perforations	Time after keratoplasty and amount of preoperative cylinder
	One allograft reaction	may affect outcome
		Decreased incidence of wound dehiscence with incisions in donor
McCartney	One stitch abscess	—
Agapitos	None reported	Significant undercorrections
		Most predictable of astigmatic keratotomy procedures
Price	Eight perforations	Compression sutures more reliable than wedge resection
	One rejection	No benefit to reopening wound when compression sutures used
Lustbader	None	Titrated removal of six sutures useful; overcorrection essential initially
Trapezoidal keratotomy		
Lavery	Wound leak, choroidal effusion	Variable effect
	Diplopia, monocular	Some large overcorrections
Buzard	Microperforation	Variable decrease in cylinder or different optical zones
		No decrease in endothelial cells
		Flattening/steepening variable
		Steepening greater than flattening if transverse incision is >5 mm
Agapitos	None reported	Increasing effect with smaller optical zones
		No significant difference with intersecting group for vector-corrected changes in cylinder when just keratoplasties are compared
Graded incremental transverse keratotomy		
Troutman	One wound dehiscence requiring sutures	Incisions should be 50% depth or less to prevent dehiscence
Arffa	Two perforations	Semiradial incisions should be omitted because of risk of perforation and poor wound healing
	Two allograft reactions	
		Graded technique preferable
Forstot	None reported	Graded approach decreases risk of complications
		No sutures means less rehabilitation time
Salmeron	None reported	Spherical equivalent not affected by relaxing incisions until after 6 months postoperatively

Corneal topography and astigmatism after penetrating keratoplasty

As emphasized in Chapter 3, Optics and Topography of Radial Keratotomy, the topography of the cornea after surgery is often radially asymmetric, and this is especially true for corneas after penetrating keratoplasty.[33] Ibrahim and colleagues[78] used computer-assisted videokeratography to classify the topography of 45 eyes after penetrating keratoplasty and suture removal. Their classification is depicted in Fig. 31-49, and the correlations with astigmatism are listed in Table 31-38.

Table 31-38

Qualitative Classification of Corneal Topography after Penetrating Keratoplasty with Sutures Removed in 45 Eyes and Correlation with Postoperative Astigmatism (D)

Qualitative pattern	Number of eyes (% of total)	Refractive astigmatism		Keratometric astigmatism	
		Mean	SD	Mean	SD
Prolate	14 (31)	5.1	2.4	6.3	3.5
Oblate	14 (31)	6.2	2.6	6.9	2.5
Mixed	8 (17)	7.0	2.0	7.2	3.2
Asymmetric	3 (8)	3.8	1.3	4.8	2.1
Steep/flat	6 (13)	2.9	2.0	2.8	1.7

Modified from Ibrahim OS, Tripoli NK, Coggins JM, Bogan S, Cohen KL, and Waring GO: Arch Ophthalmol (unpublished data).

The complex topography of penetrating keratoplasty can produce a greater disparity among refraction, keratometry, and keratography. For example, Judge and colleagues[85] observed a much greater disparity between refractive and keratometric astigmatism in eyes with sutures in place than in eyes with sutures removed. In 65 eyes retaining a running 10-0 nylon suture, the average keratometric astigmatism was 5.43 D, whereas the average refractive astigmatism was 2.95 D; however, in 50 eyes with all sutures removed, the average keratometric astigmatism was 4.27 D and the average refractive astigmatism was 3.70 D, not statistically significantly different. This disparity probably results from the increased irregular astigmatism, distortion, and asphericity induced by the sutures. The disparity between astigmatism measured by refraction and keratometry cannot be overstated. The difference was pointed out by Sampson[150] in 1975 to be dependent on the spherical component of the refraction. Because refractive astigmatism is usually less than keratometric astigmatism, reports of postkeratoplasty refractive astigmatism cannot be compared directly with reports using keratometric astigmatism.

Whether keratographic power maps can provide a guide for the placement and length of keratotomy to correct astigmatism, as they can for selective suture adjustment, is unknown. If the keratography shows an asymmetric distribution of power along a single meridian, asymmetric relaxing incisions might be appropriate. For example, in an eye with a refraction of $-5.00 +10.00 \times 90°$ and keratometry readings of $45.00 \times 180°/55.00 \times 90°$, relaxing keratotomies would be made across the vertical steep 90° meridian. If the keratograph demonstrated that the 12 o'clock semimeridian had an average power of 60 D and the inferior 6 o'clock semimeridian had an average power of 50 D, and if the map of power distribution showed an area of steepening superiorly that was twice as large as the area of steepening inferiorly, it might be appropriate to make the superior relaxing keratotomy closer to the center, longer, or deeper than the inferior one (see Fig. 31-46).

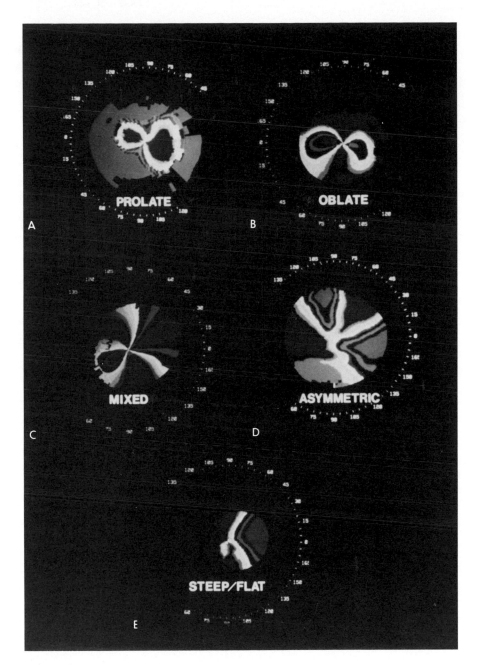

Figure 31-49

Qualitative classification of corneal topography after penetrating keratoplasty with sutures removed. Videokeratography was done with the Corneal Modeling System. The pattern categories are described according to the appearance of the normalized, color-coded corneal power maps. (From Ibrahim O, Tripoli NK, Coggins JM, Bogan S, Cohen KL, and Waring GO: unpublished data.)

A, *Prolate.* The cornea had regular astigmatism featured as a symmetric, red bowtie pattern. Along the semimeridians of the bowtie, color gradations showed steep central regions becoming flatter toward the periphery. **B,** *Oblate.* The cornea had regular astigmatism features as a symmetric, blue bowtie pattern. Along the semimeridians of the bowtie, color gradations showed flat central regions becoming steeper toward the periphery. **C,** *Mixed prolate and oblate.* The cornea had regular astigmatism with at least one of the four principal semimeridians depicted as a half red bowtie as seen in the prolate pattern and another principal semimeridian depicted as a half blue bowtie as seen in the oblate pattern. The half bowties could be approximately 90° or 180° from one another. **D,** *Asymmetric.* The principal semimeridians could be depicted by any of the previous patterns (red or blue, partial or complete), but the two steep semimeridians were not aligned into a single meridian. **E,** *Steep/flat.* The cornea was steeper on one side and became progressively flatter toward the other side.

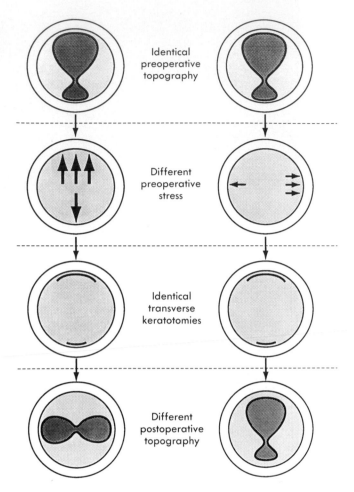

Identical
preoperative
topography

Different
preoperative
stress

Identical
transverse
keratotomies

Different
postoperative
topography

Figure 31-50
Illustration depicts the theoretical effect of corneal stress
distribution in penetrating keratoplasties on the response
to arcuate transverse keratotomy. Two corneas with
similar corneal topography might have different stress
distributions, so identical relaxing keratotomies would
have different topographic outcomes. (Courtesy Steve
Bogan.)

Dresner and colleagues[53] used keratography on human donor eyes to suggest
that transverse incisions should be made at the inflection point along a semimeridian where the change in curvature was the greatest. Their laboratory model
demonstrated twice as much astigmatism correction when incisions were placed
at the inflection point as when they were placed central to or peripheral to that
point. McClusky and colleagues[118] used videokeratography as a guide to placing
transverse incisions in the steep meridians in 10 eyes. They observed that this
flattened the steep meridian without overcorrection or shift of cylinder axis, or
appreciably steepening the unincised meridian 90° away. Prospective randomized trials using variable length incisions based on keratography compared with
the standard placement of symmetric incisions are needed to see if this more
complex modality can lead to more accurate correction of astigmatism.

Clinical reports of relaxing keratotomy after penetrating keratoplasty have
shown large variability in the results (see Table 31-37). We think that even if

topography were used as a guide to tailor the incisions for an individual eye, the results might still be highly variable, since the distribution of stress within the graft and host cornea is not known. For example, Fig. 31-50 illustrates a hypothetic situation in which two eyes have similar corneal topography after penetrating keratoplasty, but there is a different distribution of corneal stress in each. If identical relaxing transverse keratotomies were performed on the basis of the pattern of the keratographs, the two eyes may have completely different outcomes because the large amount of stress in the first eye might produce a large wound gape with a greater change in shape, whereas the small amount of stress in the second eye would produce less change in shape. If the distribution of stress in the cornea could be measured and combined with topographic measurements, the accuracy and predictability of transverse relaxing keratotomy might improve. Of course variability in individual wound healing limits the predictability.

These limitations have led a number of surgeons to advocate intraoperative keratoscopy or keratometry as a basis for determining the length and depth of incisions, titrating the incisions on an individual basis by lengthening and deepening the incisions enough to reverse the shape of the mires and then later using repeated "touch up" procedures to lengthen or deepen the incisions as needed until a stable reduction of astigmatism is achieved. At the time of this writing, no prospective comparison of preoperative versus intraoperative measurements as a basis for relaxing keratotomy has been published.

Repeat penetrating keratoplasty for high astigmatism. Only rarely does the corneal surgeon encounter a clear penetrating keratoplasty with high astigmatism that cannot be reduced by relaxing incisions in a patient who is intolerant of contact lenses. In this circumstance, a repeat corneal transplant can be performed to reduce the astigmatism. No studies of such cases have been conducted to determine whether the astigmatism can be reduced.

Preoperative planning

Table 31-39 and Fig. 31-47 present patterns of transverse arcuate relaxing keratotomy for correcting astigmatism after penetrating keratoplasty.[186] In the absence of published standards, we recommend the following guidelines:

1. Incisions made in the donor approximately 0.5 mm central to the keratoplasty wound will probably decrease the number of microperforations and will provide a more uniform tissue in which to make graded incisions. They may be more effective in altering the curvature of the donor cornea because they are placed at a smaller diameter clear zone.
2. Intraoperative keratoscopy or keratometry or a graded sequential surgical technique may help to customize the procedure to the response of the individual eye.
3. The use of compression sutures will enhance the effect by producing a temporary overcorrection but will prolong the rehabilitation because of the need for sequential selective removal.
4. The factors that affect transverse keratotomy in general (location, zone diameter, length, and depth) have been discussed in a previous section and also apply after penetrating keratoplasty. In general, incisions should not be longer than 90°, deeper than 80%, or more central than a 6- to 7-mm zone.
5. The change in the mean curvature of the cornea and the spherical equivalent refraction must be planned in advance to reduce postoperative problems with anisometropia, contact lens fitting, and correlation between corneal curvature and intraocular lens power. If the present mean corneal curvature is acceptable, then relaxing keratotomies alone may be suffi-

cient. If the cornea is excessively flat, however, a wedge resection or wound revision with the addition of compression sutures might be preferable to produce overall steepening. If the cornea is excessively steep, an arcuate keratotomy longer than 100° might be planned to create overall flattening. Unfortunately, current techniques are not predictible enough to allow the surgeon to accurately determine the final refractive error.

Table 31-39

Surgical Protocols for Correction of Astigmatism after Penetrating Keratoplasty Recommended by Krachmer

Amount of corneal astigmatism (D)	Surgical technique
0 to 4	Observation or relaxing incisions
4 to 8.5	Relaxing incisions only*
8.5 to 16	Relaxing incisions with compression sutures
16 to 20	Wedge resection, double wedge resection, or repeat penetrating keratoplasty†
> 20	Repeat penetrating keratoplasty

Modified from Vrabec MP, Florakis GJ, and Krachmer JH: Int Ophthalmol Clin 1988;28:145-149.

*If relaxing incisions have been tried 4 to 6 weeks before and failed, or if perforation occurs during the relaxing incision procedure and requires sutures in the wound, then relaxing incisions with compression sutures are used.

†A wedge resection greater than 1.5 mm can lead to irregular astigmatism.

ASTIGMATISM AFTER LAMELLAR REFRACTIVE SURGERY

The most bothersome type of astigmatism after lamellar refractive surgery (keratomileusis, keratomileusis in situ, epikeratoplasty, intracorneal lenses, keratophakia) is irregular astigmatism that distorts the optical zone.[132] A small or decentered optical zone that will place the transition curves over the pupil will create optical aberrations. Other possible causes of irregular astigmatism include an irregular microkeratome cut, irregular absorption of the cryoprotectant, irregular approximation of the corneal tissue to the base of the cryolathe, irregular expansion during the freezing process, asymmetric cutting with the cryolathe, and asymmetric suturing and healing of the lenticule to the bed.[164] Prevention is achieved by having a large optical zone with smooth surface contours centered over the pupil. Management includes gas-permeable contact lenses and repeated surgery.

Regular astigmatism also occurs after lamellar refractive surgery, but little is published about its surgical management. Swinger and colleagues[164] described postoperative keratometric astigmatism after suture removal in 49 eyes with keratophakia performed at the time of cataract surgery and reported a mean of

2.38 ±1.87 D (range, 0 to 8 D) of astigmatism, which was a considerable increase over the less than 1 D that was present preoperatively. In 13 other eyes with secondary keratophakia, minimal astigmatism was induced. Most of the astigmatism was against-the-rule.

Barraquer[15] described a series of 100 eyes that received myopic keratomileusis, with an induced average astigmatism of 2.39 D in eyes that had more than 2 D of preoperative average astigmatism and an induced average astigmatism of 1.33 D in eyes with less than 2 D of preoperative astigmatism. He described making linear transverse incisions through the lenticule in the bed across the steep meridian to reduce astigmatism.[15]

Numerous clinical reports of aphakic and myopic epikeratoplasty have described the spherical equivalent refraction, but few have discussed the problem of astigmatism. In a nationwide study of adult aphakic keratoplasty in 310 eyes with more than 1-month follow-up, the mean keratometric astigmatism was 2.7 ±2.6 D.[119] In a previous study of aphakic epikeratoplasty 29 eyes were reported to have 2.2 ±0.29 D of keratometric astigmatism at 1 year.[120] These results suggest that regular astigmatism after epikeratoplasty is not as big a problem as it is after penetrating keratoplasty. Since the donor lenticule has minimally strong attachments to the underlying Bowman's layer, the edge of the epikeratoplasty wound can be broken and lifted and a gentle lamellar dissection done to release tension in the steep meridian. Often, an extensive dehiscence of the wound is necessary to accomplish flattening of the steep meridian. Alternatively, arcuate keratotomy can be performed. No publications have described the results of such surgery.

ASTIGMATISM AFTER REFRACTIVE KERATOTOMY

Radial keratotomy alone can induce astigmatism, presumably because of asymmetry in the configuration or wound healing of the incisions. Lynn and colleagues[108] described 435 eyes that underwent an eight-incision radial keratotomy in the PERK study. Maximal preoperative astigmatism was 1.50 D. Fourteen percent of the eyes had an increase in astigmatism of 1 D, and 2% of the eyes had a decrease in astigmatism of this amount. The mean absolute change in astigmatism was 3.50 D, and the mean vectorial induced astigmatism was 0.78 D (range, 0 to 4.31 D). Eyes with smaller diameter clear zones had induction of significantly more astigmatism.

Surgical management of astigmatism after refractive keratotomy follows the basic principles of transverse keratotomy. The variation, however, is that there are incisions already in the eye that may not be oriented symmetrically around the steep meridian; therefore transverse keratotomy must be done in an interrupted pattern, centering the transverse incision on the postoperative steep meridian but making the incision asymmetric, "jumping" over the preexisting radial incisions. There are no published studies of results of this technique.

As discussed in Chapter 18, Repeated Surgery for Residual Myopia and Hyperopia after Refractive Corneal Surgery, refractive keratotomy can be considered a staged procedure, particularly in terms of correcting astigmatism, so that radial keratotomy is done initially to correct the myopia and to allow for any changes in astigmatism that are induced by that procedure, followed if necessary by transverse keratotomy to reduce the astigmatism.

PREOPERATIVE PLANNING FOR ASTIGMATISM SURGERY

We suggest the following steps as a guide to planning astigmatic keratotomy for the correction of naturally occurring astigmatism and astigmatism after cataract surgery, penetrating keratoplasty, and previous refractive keratotomy. Because there are so many different patterns of astigmatic keratotomy and because the art and skill of an individual surgeon have a major effect on the results, numerous different approaches, techniques, patterns, and nomograms have been published and can be effective. Thus the surgeon must understand the principles of keratotomy and then adopt one or two techniques with which he or she can become facile.

1. Ensure proper patient selection by establishing the ineffectiveness of optical correction, the reasonable stability of the astigmatism, the anatomic acceptability of the cornea for keratotomy surgery, and the patient's realistic understanding of the advantages and disadvantages (particularly the unpredictability) of astigmatic keratotomy.
2. Examine the cycloplegic refraction in two forms.
   a. Plus cylinder form to identify the steep meridian
   b. Minus cylinder form as a basis for calculating the amount of astigmatism surgery (see Fig. 31-2)
3. Compare the central keratometric power and axis measurements with those of the refraction and attempt to account for any disparity. The amount of keratometric astigmatism may be influenced by irregular topography and does not take into account astigmatism induced by the lens. When disparity exists, refraction, not keratometry, is the basis for calculating the amount of surgery needed to produce an optimal functional correction; however, controversy surrounds the refraction versus keratometry issue. If the eye is pseudophakic, a search for a tilt or decentration of the IOL may help explain some of the astigmatism; the IOL may need repositioning before keratotomy surgery.
4. Examine the corneal topography on keratographs, particularly in complex postoperative cases, to see if the steep topographic meridian correlates with the keratometric and refractive findings, if there is asymmetry along the steep meridian, and if there is irregular topography that might affect the outcome (see Fig. 31-49).

Table 31-40

Guide to Effect of Patterns of Transverse and Semiradial Incisions on Different Types of Astigmatism*

Type of astigmatism	Desired effect of surgery on focal lines in conoid of Sturm	Effect of length of transverse incision	Effect of semiradial or radial incisions
Compound myopic	Move both posteriorly	Short—move steep meridian posterior	Move all meridians posterior
Simple myopic	Move steep meridian posteriorly	Short—move steep meridian posterior	None
Mixed	Move steep meridian posteriorly and move flat meridian anteriorly	Long—incision may produce desired effect	None
Simple hyperopic	Move flat meridian anteriorly	Intrastromal thermokeratoplasty with hot probe or Ho:YAG laser (under evaluation)	
Compound hyperopic	Move both meridians anteriorly		

*Assume a depth of 80% of corneal thickness and a zone diameter of 7 mm.

5. Decide how much flattening of the steep meridian is desired and determine the desirable change in power in the unincised meridian 90° away (the flattening/steepening ratio) (see Fig. 31-3). Calculate the spherical equivalent refraction and decide whether it should remain the same, become more myopic, or become more hyperopic. Select an overall goal for refractive change in the cornea and the technique to achieve it, as indicated in Table 31-40.

   a. Compound myopic astigmatism: flatten both meridians.
   b. Simple myopic astigmatism: flatten the steep meridian and leave the other meridian unchanged.
   c. Mixed astigmatism: flatten the steep meridian and steepen the flat meridian.
   d. Simple and compound hyperopic astigmatism: flatten the steep meridian and steepen the flat meridian more.

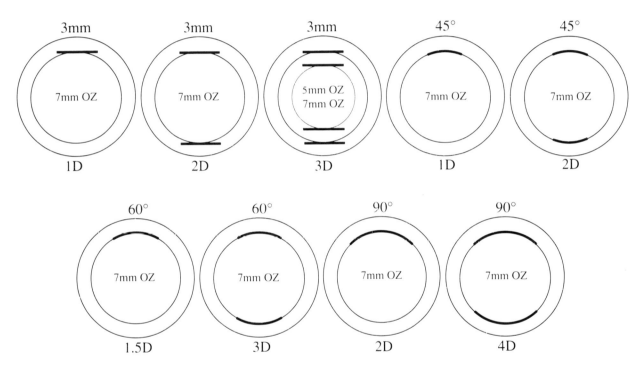

Figure 31-51

Lindstrom nomogram for astigmatic keratotomy. Modifiers of the Lindstrom nomogram include the following:

1. Zone: 7 mm for arcuate keratotomy, 7 mm and 5 mm for straight keratotomy
2. Knife setting: 100% of thinnest paracentral pachometry at zone mark in the meridian of astigmatism
3. Over/under age 30: Increase or decrease efficacy 2% per year:
   Age 20 = 80% of age 30
   Age 55 = 150% of age 30
   Age 80 = 200% of age 30
4. Although mild overall corneal flattening may occur, assume a coupling of ratio of 1:1
5. The procedure may be combined with a four-incision or eight-incision radial keratotomy, although radial and transverse incisions should not touch.
6. Assume a range of effect of ±2.00 Di when planning surgery. (From Lindstrom RL: Refract Corneal Surg 1990;6:437-454.)

6. Select the surgical technique that meets the following criteria (see Fig. 34-1 to 34-7, and 34-9).
   a. Accomplishes the stated refractive goals
   b. Is familiar to the surgeon with his/her technical capabilities
   c. Has reasonably well-established guidelines based on the clinical results of other investigators (unless a new technique is being explored)
   d. Has the potential for reoperation to adjust the outcome if necessary
7. For the technique selected, consult nomograms to determine the surgical variables for the desired amount of correction (Fig. 31-51 and Tables 31-41 and 31-42).
   a. Published nomograms
   b. Computer programs
   c. Personal nomogram
   d. Intraoperative monitoring with keratoscopy or keratometry
   e. Staged surgery with successive operations (When in doubt, perform the myopia surgery first and then the astigmatic correction later, if needed.)
8. Select the specific variables for the eye (see Table 31-4).
   a. Location of transverse incisions; zone diameter or distance from center of the pupil
   b. Orientation of transverse incisions with respect to the steep meridian using a reticle on the slit-lamp microscope (Identify the steep meridian by anatomic landmarks on the iris, limbus, or conjunctiva as drawn on the clinical record or as seen on a keratograph or as marked on the cornea directly at the slit-lamp microscope.)
   c. Number of transverse incisions (number of pairs)
   d. Length of each transverse incision in terms of degrees of arc or millimeters of length
   e. Depth of incision with length of the knife blade set on the basis of ultrasonic pachometry in the location of the incision
   f. For radial or semiradial incisions, select the number and location of incisions, the clear zone diameter, and the knife blade length
9. Create a simple planning sheet for the operating room that contains most of the above information, including a labeled sketch of the proposed operation. The sketch should be mounted with the 12 o'clock location downward (the same view the surgeon has through the microscope) to facilitate simple copying of the pattern from the drawing onto the patient's cornea.
10. Check ahead of time that the necessary equipment is available for surgery, particularly the knife intended for use and the appropriate astigmatism markers.
11. Execute the operation as detailed in Chapter 32, Atlas of Astigmatic Keratotomy.

Table 31-43 presents a series of examples with proposed preoperative plans by different surgeons, based on published cases. This compilation emphasizes the variety of approaches to the management of a specific astigmatic refractive error. Because we cannot determine which technique is superior, each surgeon must understand the principles and master a particular technique using his or her own personal fudge factors to achieve the optimal result.

Table 31-41

Nomogram of Thornton for Correction of Astigmatism by Paired Straight or Transverse Incisions with or without Radial Incisions

Change in astigmatism	Straight Length of one pair of straight transverse incisions at 7-mm zone*	Arcuate Chord length of one pair of arcuate transverse incisions at 7-mm zone *
0.50 D	1.3 mm	1.2 mm
0.75 D	1.5 mm	1.3 mm
1.00 D	1.7 mm	1.5 mm
1.25 D	1.8 mm	1.7 mm
1.50 D	2.1 mm	1.9 mm
1.75 D	2.3 mm	2.1 mm
2.00 D	2.5 mm	2.3 mm
2.25 D	2.7 mm	2.5 mm

Change in astigmatism	Length of two pairs of straight transverse incisions		Chord length of two pairs of arcuate transverse incisions	
	6-mm zone	8-mm zone	6-mm zone	8-mm zone
2.00 D	1.3 mm	1.7 mm	1.2 mm	1.5 mm
2.25 D	1.5 mm	2.0 mm	1.4 mm	1.8 mm
2.50 D	1.7 mm	2.3 mm	1.6 mm	2.0 mm
2.75 D	1.9 mm	2.6 mm	1.8 mm	2.3 mm
3.00 D	2.1 mm	2.9 mm	2.0 mm	2.6 mm
3.25 D	2.3 mm	3.2 mm	2.2 mm	2.9 mm
3.50 D	2.5 mm	3.4 mm	2.4 mm	3.1 mm
3.75 D	2.7 mm	3.6 mm	2.6 mm	3.3 mm

Modified from Thornton SP: Personal communication, June 4, 1991.
1. For every year below age 30, add 1% to the astigmatic error; for every year above age 30, subtract 1/2%.
2. For every 1.0 mm Hg pressure below 15, add 2% to the astigmatic error; for every 1.0 mm Hg above 15, subtract 2%.
3. Length of knife blade is 95% to 98% of corneal thickness.
*See Table 31-4 for lengths in millimeters and degrees and segment width.

Table 31-42

Binder's Guide to Astigmatic Keratotomy for Naturally Occurring Myopic Astigmatism

Myopia (D)	Astigmatism (D)				
	0 to 1	1 to 2	2 to 3	3 to 4	> 4
0 to 1	No surgery	"T" 3.0-mm zone	Two "T" 2.5 mm long	Trap with one "T" 2.5 mm long	Trap with two "T" 2.5 mm long
1 to 4	4 to 8 radial incisions 3- to 4-mm zone	"T" 3.0-mm zone	Two "T" 3.0 mm	2.5 mm long	2.5 mm long
4 to 6	4 to 8 radial incisions 3- to 4-mm zone	"T" 3.0-mm zone	Two, 2.5 to 3.0 mm	2.5 mm long	2.5 mm long
> 6	4 to 16 radial incisions 3- to 4-mm zone	"T" 3.0-mm zone	Two 2.0 to 3.0 mm	2.5 mm long	2.5 mm long

"T", Transverse incision placed at 5.0-mm or 5.0- and 7.0-mm zone.
Trap, Trapezoidal keratotomy.

Table 31-43

Examples of Surgical Plans to Reduce Various Astigmatic Refractive Errors in a 30-Year-Old Patient

Case 1

+2.00 −6.00 × 90°

Nordan	*Binder*	*Hofmann*
5.0-mm "T"	Two, 3.0-mm "T"	Four, RK at 4.0-mm zone
3.75-mm zone	5.0-mm zone	TK at 4.0-mm zone
		Eight "T," 4.0-mm each

Case 2

−2.00 −1.50 × 180°

Nordan	*Binder*	*Hofmann*
Eight, RK	Four, RK	Eight, RK
4.0-mm zone	3.5-mm zone	4.25-mm zone
Jump T, 1.5 mm each	Two, "T" at 5.0-mm zone	Two, flag at 7.0-mm zone
7.0-mm zone	3.0 mm long	½ segment

Case 3

−2.00 −6.00 × 180°

Nordan	*Binder*
Six, RK with"redeepening" 3.0-mm zone	Six, RK at 3.00-mm zone
TK at 3.5-mm zone	TK at 5- and 7-mm zones
Eight, "T," 1.5-mm each	Four, T, = 2.5 mm each

Case 4

−2.00 −3.00 × 180°

Nordan	*Binder*
Six, RK with "redeepening" 3.0-mm zone	Six, RK at 3.00-mm zone
TK at 3.5-mm zone	TK at 5- and 7-mm zones
Eight, T, 1.5 mm each	Four, T, 2.5 mm each

Case 5

−2.00 −3.00 × 180°

Nordan	*Binder*	*Hofmann*
Two, RK at 3.25-mm zone	Four, RK at 3.0-mm zone	Six, RK at 3.5-mm zone
Six, partial RK at 3.25-mm zone	TK at 5- and 7-mm zones	TK at 4.75-mm zone and greater
Double jump radial T 7.0-mm zone	2.5 mm long	Eight, 2.0 mm long

Case 6

pl −6.00 × 180°

Lindstrom	*Nordan*	*Binder*
TK at 4.0-mm zone	RK at 3.25-mm zone	TK at 5- and 7-mm zones
Four, T, 2.5 mm each	Eight, T, 2.5 mm each	Four, T, 3.0 mm each

Case 7

+1.00 −2.00 × 180°

Lindstrom	*Nordan*	*Binder*	*Hofmann*
Two, T at 5.0-mm zone	One, T at 7.0-mm zone	Two, T at 5-mm zone	Four, T at 5.5-mm zone
3.0 mm long	2.0 mm long	3.0 mm long	4.0 mm long

"T", Transverse incision; *RK*, radial keratotomy; *TK*, transverse keratotomy.

COMPLICATIONS

The complications of keratotomy are discussed in detail in Chapter 23, Complications of Refractive Keratotomy. The major complications in the earlier development of astigmatic keratotomy were caused by intersection of transverse and radial incisions, but these techniques are not now in use.[49,50,83,162] Complications such as undercorrections, overcorrections, and corneal perforations* are inherent in the current techniques.

*References 87, 88, 98, 107, 158, 179.

UNFINISHED BUSINESS

Measuring the topography of astigmatic corneas is becoming increasingly sophisticated with videokeratography, which has emphasized the radially asymmetric asphericity of such corneas and has accentuated their irregular astigmatism. Whether topographic power maps can improve the outcome of keratotomy surgery remains to be proved. Theoretically, asymmetric incisions would be appropriate for asymmetric astigmatism, but careful studies are needed to compare these techniques to standard symmetric surgery.

Preoperative nomograms based on past experience and published data are certainly useful in selecting the location, length, and depth of the transverse incisions. These should be compared with intraoperative monitoring using keratometry or keratoscopy to titrate the response to the surgery. Development of methods to measure the stress patterns within the living cornea and to relate these patterns to the change induced by keratotomy would probably improve the results of keratotomy surgery. There is no currently available technology that can make such measurements in a clinically meaningful way, but holography may be useful in the future.

There is a need for improved clinical trials of different patterns and techniques of astigmatic keratotomy. Surgical cases should be grouped homogeneously (naturally occurring astigmatism separated from postcataract, postpenetrating keratoplasty disorders), as should different surgical techniques so that specific comparative analyses can be made. Consecutive case series with high rates of follow-up should be performed to define the limits of different types of refractive keratotomy. Prospective randomized trials could compare preoperative nomograms with intraoperative monitoring or relaxing incisions with and without compression sutures. In naturally occurring astigmatism, specific preoperative nomograms comparing different techniques of radial keratotomy should be randomized using the right and left eyes of the same individual. For example, comparison of transverse keratotomy between radial incisions versus interrupted radials versus interrupted transverse incisions would help to define the strengths and weaknesses of each technique.

Long-term data should be collected on series of eyes with good follow-up to identify the stability of refraction after astigmatic keratotomy and to see if there is a continued increase in the effect of the surgery as it occurs after eight-incision radial keratotomy.

REFERENCES

1. Agapitos PJ, Lindstrom RL, Williams PA, and Sanders DR: Analysis of astigmatic keratotomy, J Cataract Refract Surg 1989;5:13-18.
2. Alpar JJ: Modification of the Kratz incision with a scleral marking and a temporary silk suture for astigmatic control, Am Intraocular Implant Soc J 1985;11:491-493.
3. Arciniegas A and Amaya LE: Experimental modification of the corneal curvature by means of scleral surgery, Ann Ophthalmol 1984;16:1155-1166.
4. Arciniegas A and Amaya LE: Combined semiradial and arcuate keratotomy for correction of ametropia: a theoretical bioengineering approach, Refract Surg 1988;4:51-59.
5. Arciniegas A, Amaya LE, Velasquez G, and Hernandez L: Corneal astigmatism induced by the combination of arc and radial keratotomies: experimental research in rabbits, J Refract Surg 1986;2:68-77.
6. Arffa RC: Results of graded relaxing incision technique for postkeratoplasty astigmatism, Ophthalmic Surg 1988; 19:624-628.
7. Armeniades CD, Boriek A, and Knolle GE: Effect of incision length, location, and shape on local corneoscleral deformation during cataract surgery, J Cataract Refract Surg 1990;16:83-87.
8. Arruga H: Ocular surgery, New York, 1952, McGraw-Hill.
9. Atkins AD and Roper-Hall MJ: Control of postoperative astigmatism, Br J Ophthalmol 1985;69:348-351.
10. Axt JC: Longitudinal study of postoperative astigmatism, J Cataract Refract Surg 1987;13:381-388.
11. Azar RF: Corneal tuck for postcataract astigmatism. In Binder PS, editor: Refractive corneal surgery: the correction of astigmatism, Int Ophthalmol Clin 1983;23:101-110.
12. Baikoff G and Joly P: Comparison of minus power anterior chamber intraocular lenses and myopic epikeratoplasty in phakic eyes, Refract Corneal Surg 1990:6:252-260.
13. Barner SS: Surgical treatment of corneal astigmatism, Ophthalmic Surg 1976;7:43-48.
14. Barraquer J: Results of the crescentic resection for the correction of congenital astigmatism and astigmatism secondary to keratoplasty, Arch Soc Am Ophthalmol Optom 1982;16:211-220.
15. Barraquer JI:: Cirugia refractiva de la cornea, Bogota, Colombia, 1989, Instituto Barraquer de America, pp 454, 480, 764-765.
16. Barraquer J and Rutlan J: Microsurgery of the cornea: an atlas and textbook, Barcelona, 1984, Scriba.
17. Binder PS: An evaluation of orthokeratology, 1980;87:729-744.
18. Binder PS: Reduction of postkeratoplasty astigmatism by selective suture removal, Dev Ophthalmol 1985; 11:86-90.
19. Binder PS: Selective suture removal can reduce postkeratoplasty astigmatism, Ophthalmology 1985;92:1412-1416.
20. Binder PS: Controlled reduction of postkeratoplasty astigmatism. In Brightbill PS, editor: Corneal surgery: theory, technique and tissue, St Louis, 1986, The CV Mosby Co, pp 326-332.
21. Binder PS: Optical complications following refractive surgery, Ophthalmology 1986;93:739-745.
22. Binder PS: The surgical correction of astigmatism. In Caldwell D, editor: Symposium on the cornea and refractive corneal surgery, Transactions of the New Orleans Academy of Ophthalmology, New York, 1987, Raven Press, pp 1-19.
23. Binder PS: The effect of suture removal on postkeratoplasty astigmatism, Am J Ophthalmol 1988; 105: 637-645.
24. Binder PS: Intraocular lens implantation after penetrating keratoplasty, Refract Corneal Surg 1989;5:224-230.
25. Binder PS: The effect of suture removal post penetrating keratoplasty on the principal corneal meridia, Switzerland, SS Karger (in press).
26. Binder PS: The relationship between the corneal meridia—the coupling phenomenon, J Cataract Refract Surg (in press).
27. Binder PS: The theoretical and practical factors that determine corneal transplant topography: their effect on astigmatism and refractive errors (submitted for publication).
28. Brown NP, Sparow JM: Control of astigmatism in cataract surgery, Br J Ophthalmol 1988;72:487-493.
29. Burk LL, Waring GO, and Harris DJ: Simultaneous and sequential selective suture removal to reduce astigmatism after penetrating keratoplasty, Refract Corneal Surg 1990;6:179-187.
30. Burk LL, Waring GO, Radjee B, and Stulting RD: The effect of selective suture removal on astigmatism following penetrating keratoplasty, Ophthalmic Surg 1988;19:849-854.
31. Buzard KA: Repair of the "microdehiscence" to correct postkeratoplasty astigmatism, Ophthalmic Surg 1989; 20:876-882.
32. Buzard K, Haight D, and Troutman D: Ruiz procedure for postkeratoplasty astigmatism, J Refract Surg 1987; 3:40-45.
33. Camp JJ, Maguire LJ, Cameron BM, and Robb RA: A computer model for the evaluation of corneal topography on optical performance, Am J Ophthalmol 1990;109:379-386.
34. Carter J, Baron BA, and McDonald MB: Cystoid macular edema following corneal relaxing incisions, Arch Ophthalmol 1987;105:70-72.
35. Casey TA and Mayer DJ: Corneal grafting, Philadelphia, 1984, WB Saunders Co.
36. Chi-Wang Y, Busin M, McDonald MB, et al: The effect of different radial keratotomy patterns on astigmatism in rabbits, J Refract Surg 1985;1:201-205.
37. Cohen KL, Tripoli NK, and Moecker RJ: Prospective analysis of photokeratoscopy for arcuate keratotomy to reduce postkeratoplasty astigmatism, Refract Corneal Surg 1989;5:388-393.
38. Cohen KL, Tripoli NK, and Proia AD: Cat keratoplasty wound healing and corneal astigmatism, Invest Ophthalmol Vis Sci 1989;30(suppl):339.
39. Colin J, Mimaini F, Robinet A, Conrad H, and Mader P: The surgical treatment of high myopia: comparison of epikeratoplasty, keratomileusis and minus power anterior chamber lenses, Refract Corneal Surg 1990;6:245-251.
40. Colvard DM, Kratz RP, Mazocco TR, et al: The Terry surgical keratometer: a 12-month follow-up report, Am Intraocular Implant Soc J 1981;7:348-350.
41. Colvard DM, Mazzoco TR, Kratz RP, et al. Clinical evaluation of the Terry surgical keratometer, Am Intraocular Implant Soc J 1987;6:249-251.
42. Cory CC: Prevention and treatment of postimplantation astigmatism, J Cataract Refract Surg 1989;15:58-60.
43. Cottingham AJ: New techniques for preventing high astigmatism in keratoplasty, In Boyd BE, editor: Highlights of ophthalmology: silver anniversary, Panama, 1979, Highlights of Ophthalmology, Publisher, pp 1182-1189.
44. Cravy TV: The surgical correction of postoperative astigmatism by wound revision, Am Intraocular Implant Soc J 1980;6:160-163.
45. Cravy TV: Long-term corneal astigmatism related to selected elastic, monofilament, nonabsorbable sutures, J Cataract Refract Surg 1989;15:61-69.

46. Crock GW, Pericic L, Chapman-Smith JS, et al: A new system of microsurgery for human and experimental corneal grafting, Br J Ophthalmol 1978; 62:74-80.

47. Dabezies OH Jr and Holladay JT: Measurement of corneal curvature: keratometer (ophthalmometer) in contact lenses. In Dabezies OH Jr, editor: The CLAO guide to basic science and clinical practice, Philadelphia 1984, Grune & Stratton, Inc.

48. Davison JA: Transverse astigmatic keratotomy combined with phacoemulsification and intraocular lens implantation, J Cataract Refract Surg 1989;15:38-44.

49. Deg JK and Binder PS: Wound healing after astigmatic keratotomy procedures in human eyes, Ophthalmology 1987;94:1290-1298.

50. Deg JK, Zavala EY, and Binder PS: Delayed corneal wound healing following radial keratotomy, Ophthalmology 1985;92:734-740.

51. Deitz MR, Sanders DR, and Raanan MG: A consecutive series (1982-1985) of radial keratotomies performed with the diamond blade, Am J Ophthalmol 1987;103:417-422.

52. Devoe AG: Discussion of Troutman RC: microsurgical control of corneal astigmatism in cataract and keratoplasty, Trans Am Acad Ophthalmol Otolaryngol 1973;77:572.

53. Dresner NS, Novak I, Hugg J, and Schanzlin JJ: Topographic guidance in the placement of relaxing incisions, Invest Ophthalmol Vis Sci 1988; 30(suppl):340.

54. Drews RC: Astigmatism shift after extracapsular surgery: Mersilene versus nylon, Ophthalmic Surg 1989;20:695-696.

55. Duffey RJ, Vivanti NJ, Hungwon T, Hofmann RF, and Lindstrom RL: Paired arcuate keratotomy: a surgical approach to mixed and myopic astigmatism, Arch Ophthalmol 1988; 103:477-488.

56. Ellis W: Radial keratotomy and astigmatism surgery, ed 2, Irvine, Calif, 1986, Keith C. Terry & Associates.

57. Ernest PH: Trapezoidal wound construction, Curr Concepts Ophthalmic Surg 1984;7:9-11.

58. Fenzl RE: Control of astigmatism using corneal incisions. In Sanders D and Hofmann RF, editors: Refractive surgery: a text of radial keratotomy, Thorofare, NJ, 1985, Slack, Inc, pp 153-165.

59. Flaharty PM and Siepser SB: Surgically induced astigmatism in human cadaver eyes, J Cataract Refract Surg 1989;15:19-24.

60. Floyd G: Changes in the corneal curvature following cataract extraction, Am J Ophthalmol 1951;34:1525-1533.

61. Forstot SL: Modified relaxing incision technique for postkeratoplasty astigmatism, Cornea 1988;7:133-137.

62. Franks JB and Binder PS: Keratotomy procedures for the correction of astigmatism, J Refract Surg 1985;1:11-17.

63. Fyodorov SN: Surgical correction of myopia and astigmatism. In Schachar RA, Levy NS, and Schachar L, editors: Keratorefraction, Denison, Tex, 1980, LAL Publishing, pp 141-172.

64. Fyodorov SN and Durnev VV: Surgical correction of complicated myopic astigmatism by means of dissection of circular ligament of cornea, Ann Ophthalmol 1981;13:115-118.

65. Geggel HS: Limbal wedge resection at the time of intraocular lens surgery for reducing postkeratoplasty astigmatism, Ophthalmic Surg 1990;21:102-108.

66. Girard LJ, Eguez I, Esnaola N, Barnett L, and Maghraby A: Effect of penetrating keratoplasty using grafts of various sizes on keratoconic myopia and astigmatism, J Cataract Refract Surg 1988;14:541-547.

67. Girard LJ, Rodriguez J, and Mailman ML: Reducing surgically induced astigmatism by using a scleral tunnel, Am J Ophthalmol 1984;97:450-456.

68. Gorn RA: Surgically induced corneal astigmatism and its spontaneous regression, Ophthalmic Surg 1985;16:152-164.

69. Grady FJ: Radial keratotomy for astigmatism, Ann Ophthalmol 1984;16:942-944.

70. Groenholm V and Kangasniemi M: Uber Hornhautnaht Beim Starschnit un den Postoperativen Astigmatismus, Acta Ophthalmol 1936;14:158-167.

71. Hall GW, Campion M, Sorenson CM, and Monthofer S: Reduction of corneal astigmatism at cataract surgery, J Cataract Refract Surg (in press).

72. Hanna KD, Jouve FE, and Waring GO: Computer simulation of arcuate and radial incisions involving the corneoscleral limbus, Eye 1989;3:227-239.

73. Harris DJ, Waring GO, and Burk LL: Keratography as a guide to selective suture removal for the reduction of astigmatism after penetrating keratoplasty, Ophthalmology 1989;96:1596-1607.

74. Hatch JL: Thermal wedge with penetrating keratoplasty to reduce high corneal cylinder, Am J Ophthalmol 1980;90:137-141.

75. Herman WK, Harris WS, and Kogan I: Intraoperative air bubble keratometry to control postoperative astigmatism, Am Intraocular Implant Soc J 1982;8:373-375.

76. Hofmann RF: The surgical correction of idiopathic astigmatism. In Sanders DR, Hofmann RF, and Salz JJ, editors: Refractive corneal surgery, Thorofare, NJ, 1986, Slack, Inc, pp 241-290.

77. Ibrahim O, Hussein HA, Kassem A, El-Shan MF, and El-Nawawy S: Trapezoidal keratotomy for the correction of naturally occurring astigmatism, Arch Ophthalmol (in press).

78. Ibrahim O, Tripoli NK, Coggins JM, Bogan S, Cohen KL, and Waring GO: Corneal topography after clear penetrating keratoplasty: qualitative and quantitative topography classification, Arch Ophthalmol (unpublished data).

79. Jaffe NS and Clayman HM: The pathophysiology of corneal astigmatism after cataract extraction, Trans Am Acad Ophthalmol Otolaryngol 1975;79:615-630.

80. Jaffe NS, Jaffe MS, and Jaffe GE: Cataract surgery and its complications, ed 5, St Louis, 1990, The CV Mosby Co, pp 109-127.

81. Jampel HD, Thompson JR, Baker CC, et al: A computerized analysis of astigmatism after cataract surgery, Ophthalmic Surg 1986;17:786-790.

82. Jensen RP and Jensen AC: Surgical correction of astigmatism by microwedge resection of the limbus, Ophthalmology 1978;85:1288-1298.

83. Jester JV, Villasenor RA, and Miyashiro J: Epithelial inclusion cysts following radial keratotomy, Arch Ophthalmol 1983;101:611-615.

84. Jolson AS and Seidel FJ: Postoperative astigmatism induced by intraocular lens tilt, Am Intraocular Implant Soc J 1985;10:213-216.

85. Judge D, Gordon L, Vanderzwagg R, and Wood TO: Refractive versus keratometric astigmatism postkeratoplasty, Refract Corneal Surg 1990;6:174-178.

86. Kozarsky AM and Waring GO: Postkeratoscopy in the management of astigmatism following keratoplasty, Dev Ophthalmol 1985;11:91-98.

87. Krachmer JH and Ching ST: Relaxing corneal incisions for postkeratoplasty astigmatism. In Binder PS, editor: Refractive corneal surgery: the correction of astigmatism, Int Ophthalmol Clin 1983;4:153-161.

88. Krachmer JH and Fenzl RL: Surgical correction of high postkeratoplasty astigmatism: relaxing incisions versus wedge resection, Arch Ophthalmol 1980;98:1400-1402.

89. Kratz RP and Johnson SH: Clinical results of the surgical keratometer, Int Ophthalmol Clin 1983;23:87-99.

90. Kronish JW and Forster RK: Control of astigmatism following cataract extraction by selective suture cutting, Arch Ophthalmol 1987;105:1650-1655.

91. Krumeich JH: Circular keratotomy for the correction of astigmatism, Refract Corneal Surg (in press).

92. Krumeich JH, Binder PS, and Knull EA: The theoretical effect of trephine tilt on postkeratoplasty astigmatism, CLAO J 1988;4:213-219.

93. Lang GK, Green WR, and Maumenee AE: Clinicopathologic studies of keratoplasty eyes obtained postmortem, Am J Ophthalmol 1986;101:28-40.

94. Lang GK, Maxeiner R, and Naumann GOH: Corneal outline: morphometric evaluation for noncircular keratoplasty, Invest Ophthalmol Vis Sci 1990;31(suppl):575.

95. Lara RT: Personal experience in the surgical correction of astigmatism, Ocular Surg 1987;3:15-17.

96. Lavery GW and Lindstrom RL: Clinical results of trapezoidal astigmatic keratotomy, J Refract Surg 1985;1:70-74.

97. Lavery GW and Lindstrom RL: Trapezoidal astigmatic keratotomy in human cadaver eyes, J Refract Surg 1985;1:18-24.

98. Lavery GW, Lindstrom RL, Hoffer LA, et al: The surgical management of corneal astigmatism after penetrating keratoplasty, Ophthalmic Surg 1985;16:165-169.

98a. Lieberman DM: A new corneal trephine, Am J Ophthalmol 1976;81:684-685.

99. Limberg MB, Dingeldein SA, Green MT, Klyce SD, Insler MS, and Kaufman HE: Corneal compression sutures for the reduction of astigmatism after penetrating keratoplasty, Am J Ophthalmol 1989;108:36-42.

100. Lin DTC, Wilson S, Reidy JJ, Klyce SD, McDonald MB, Kaufmann HE, and McNeill JI: An adjustable single-running suture technique to reduce postkeratoplasty astigmatism: a preliminary report, Ophthalmology 1990;97:934-938.

101. Lindquist TD, Rubenstein JB, Hofmann RF, and Lindstrom RL: Astigmatic keratotomy. In Sanders DR, editor: Radial keratotomy surgical techniques, Thorofare, NJ, 1986, Slack, Inc, pp 115-130.

102. Lindquist TD, Rubenstein JB, Rice SW, et al: Trapezoidal astigmatic keratotomy: quantification in human cadaver eyes, Arch Ophthalmol 1986; 104:1534-1539.

103. Lindstrom RL: Surgical correction of astigmatism: a clinician's perspective, Refract Corneal Surg 1990;6:437-454.

104. Lindstrom RL and Destro MA: Effect of incision size and Terry keratometer usage on postoperative astigmatism, Am Intraocular Implant Soc J 1985;11:469-473.

105. Lindstrom RL and Lindquist TD: Surgical correction of postoperative astigmatism, Cornea 1988;7:138-148.

106. Lugo M, Donnefeld ED, and Aronson JJ: Corneal wedge resection for high astigmatism following penetrating keratoplasty, Ophthalmic Surg 1987; 18:650-653.

107. Lundergan MK and Rowsey JJ: Relaxing incisions: corneal topography, Ophthalmology 1985;92:1226-1236.

108. Lynn MJ, Waring GO, Culbertson W, and the PERK Study Group: Change in astigmatism after radial keratotomy in the Prospective Evaluation of Radial Keratotomy (PERK) study, Invest Ophthalmol Vis Sci 1990;31(suppl): 300.

109. Mader TH, Yuan R, Lynn MJ, Stulting RD, Wilson LA, and Waring GO: Change in the keratometric astigmatism following suture removal more than 1 year after penetrating keratoplasty, Invest Ophthalmol Vis Sci 1990;31(suppl):574.

110. Maloney WF and Grindle L: Textbook of phacoemulsification, Lasenda Farbrook, Calif, 1988, Lasenda Publishers, pp 85-111.

111. Maloney WF, Grindle L, Sanders D, and Pearcy D: Astigmatism control for the cataract surgeon: a comprehensive review of surgically tailored reduction (STAR), J Cataract Refract Surg 1989;15:45-54.

112. Maloney WF, Sanders DR, and Pearcy DE: Astigmatic keratotomy to correct preexisting astigmatism in cataract patients, J Cataract Refract Surg 1990;16:297-304.

113. Masket S: Astigmatic analysis of the scleral pocket incision and closure technique for cataract surgery, CLAO J 1985;11:206-209.

114. Masket S: Comparison of suture materials for closure of the scleral pocket incision, J Cataract Refract Surg 1988;14:548-551.

115. Masket S: Correlation between intraoperative and early postoperative keratometry, J Cataract Refract Surg 1988;14:277-280.

116. Masket S: Consultations, J Cataract Refract Surg 1989;15:109-113.

117. Masket S: Keratorefractive aspects of the scleral pocket incision and closure method for cataract surgery, J Cataract Refract Surg 1989;15:70-77.

118. McClusky DA, Garbus J, and McDonnell PJ: Computer-assisted corneal topographic analysis in preoperative planning of surgery for astigmatism, Invest Ophthalmol Vis Sci 1989; 30(suppl):189.

119. McDonald MB, Kaufman HE, Aquavella JV, Durrie DS, et al: The nationwide study of epikeratophakia for aphakia in adults, Am J Ophthalmol 1987;103:358-365.

120. McDonald MB, Klyce SB, Safir A, Friedlander MH, Kaufman HE, and Granet N: Epikeratophakia: the surgical correction of aphakia: update 1982, Ophthalmology 1983;90:668-672.

121. McNeill JI and Wessels IF: Adjustment of single continuous suture to control astigmatism after penetrating keratoplasty, Refract Corneal Surg 1989;5: 216-223.

122. Merck MP, Williams PA, and Lindstrom RL: Trapezoidal keratotomy: a vector analysis, Ophthalmology 1986; 93:719-726.

123. Merlin U: Cheratotomie paralimbari nell' astigmatismo indicazione limiti, Contatologia Medicae Chirurgia Refrattiva 1986;2:215-220.

124. Merlin U: Curved keratotomy procedure for congenital astigmatism, J Refract Surg 1987;3:92-97.

125. Milder B and Rubin ML: The fine art of prescribing glasses without making a spectacle of yourself, Gainesville, Fla, 1978, Triad Scientific Publishers.

125a. Mimouni F, Colin J, Koffi V, and Bonnet P: Damage to the corneal endothelium from anterior chamber intraocular lenses in phakic myopic eyes, Refract Corneal Surg (in press).

126. Musch DC, Meyer RF, and Sugar A: The effect of removing running sutures on astigmatism after penetrating keratoplasty, Arch Ophthalmol 1988; 106:488-492.

127. Musch DC, Meyer RF, and Sugar A: Corneal astigmatism after penetrating keratoplasty, Ophthalmology 1989;96: 698-703.

128. Neumann AC, McCarty GR, Sanders DR, and Raanan MG: Refractive evaluation of astigmatic keratotomy procedures, J Cataract Refract Surg 1989;15:25-31.

129. Neumann AC, McCarty GR, Sanders DR, and Raanan MG: Small incisions to control astigmatism during cataract surgery, J Cataract Refract Surg 1989;15:78-84.

130. Nordan LT: Current status of refractive surgery, San Diego, 1983, CL Printing.

131. Nordan LT: Quantifiable astigmatism correction: concepts and suggestions, J Cataract Refract Surg 1986;12:507-518.

132. Nordan LT and Grene BR: The importance of corneal asphericity and irregular astigmatism in refractive surgery, Refract Corneal Surg 1990;6:200-204.

133. Olson RJ: Corneal transplantation techniques. In Kaufman HE et al, editors: The cornea, New York, 1988, Churchill Livingstone, pp 743-787.

134. Osher RH: Paired transverse relaxing keratotomy: a combined technique for reducing astigmatism, J Cataract Refract Surg 1989;15:32-37.

135. Parker WT and Clorfeine GS: Long-term evolution of astigmatism following planned extracapsular cataract extraction, Arch Ophthalmol 1989;107: 353-357.

136. Perl T, Binder PS, and Earl K: Postcataract astigmatism with and without the use of the Tery keratometer, Ophthalmology 1984;91:489-493.

137. Perl T, Charlton KH, and Binder PS: Disparate diameter grafting: astigmatism, intraocular pressure, and visual acuity, Ophthalmology 1981;88:774-781.

138. Pradera I, Ibrahim O, and Waring GO: Refractive results of successful penetrating keratoplasty: intraocular lens implantation with selective suture removal, Refract Corneal Surg 1989; 5:231-239.

139. Reading VM: Astigmatism following cataract surgery, Br J Ophthalmol 1984;68:97-104.

140. Richards SC, Brodstein RS, Richards WL, Olson RJ, et al: Long-term course of surgically induced astigmatism, J Cataract Refract Surg 1988;14:270-276.

141. Roper KL: The cataract operation: a study of details, Rochester, Minn, 1967, Custom Printing.

142. Roper-Hall MJ and Atkins AD: Control of astigmatism after surgery and trauma, a new technique, Br J Ophthalmol 1985;69:352-356.

143. Rowsey JJ: Ten caveats in keratorefractive surgery, Ophthalmology 1983; 90:148-155.

144. Rowsey JJ: Current concepts in astigmatism surgery, J Refract Surg 1986;2:85-94.

145. Ruiz LA: The astigmatic keratotomies (Ruiz procedures). In Boyd B, editor: Highlights of ophthalmology, vol 2, refractive surgery with the masters, Coral Gables, Fla, 1987, Highlights of Ophthalmology, pp 162-193.

146. Sachdev MS, Kumar H, Dada VK, Mehta MR, and Jain AK: Argon laser suturotomy: a technique for the correction of surgically induced astigmatism, Ophthalmic Surg 1990;21:277-281.

147. Saleh-Eddin A and Hakim A: Corneal astigmatism induced for oversized rigid anterior chamber implants, Am Intraocular Implant Soc J 1985;11: 474-479.

148. Salmeron B, McDonald M, Naguchi B, Hogan C, and Kaufman HE: 90° arcuate relaxing incisions, using intraoperative keratometric control, for astigmatism after penetrating keratoplasty for keratoconus, Invest Ophthalmol Vis Sci 1989;30(suppl):339.

149. Samples JR and Binder PS: The value of the Terry keratometer in predicting postoperative astigmatism, Ophthalmology 1984;91:280-284.

150. Sampson WG: Applied optical principles: keratometry, Trans Am Acad Ophthalmol Otolaryngol 1979;86: 347-351.

150a. Saragoussi JJ, Cotinat J, Renard G, et al: Damage to the corneal endothelium by minus power anterior chamber intraocular lenses, Refract Corneal Surg (in press).

151. Seiler T, Bende T, Wollensak J, and Trokel S: Excimer laser keratectomy for the correction of astigmatism, Am J Ophthalmol 1988;105:117-124.

152. Sevak JG, Kreuzer RO, and Hildebrand T: Intraocular lenses, tilt and astigmatism, Ophthalmic Res 1985; 17:54-59.

153. Shepard DD: Radial keratotomy: analysis of efficacy and predictability in 1058 consecutive cases, Part I. Efficacy, J Cataract Refract Surg 1986; 12:632-643.

154. Shepherd JR: Correction of preexisting astigmatism at the time of small-incision cataract surgery, J Cataract Refract Surg 1989;15:55-57.

155. Shepherd JR: Induced astigmatism in small-incision cataract surgery, J Cataract Refract Surg 1989;15:85-88.

156. Shivitz IA, Arrowsmith PN, and Russell BM: Contact lenses in the treatment of patients with overcorrected radial keratotomy, Ophthalmology 1987;94:899-903.

157. Simcoe WC: Two simple intraoperative measuring techniques: keratometry by contact lens and intraocular lens power verification, Am Intraocular Implant Soc J 1982;8:165-169.

158. Stainer GA and Binder PS: Vitreous wick syndrome following a corneal relaxing incision, Ophthalmic Surg 1981;12:567-570.

159. Stainer GA, Binder PS, and Parker WT: Modulation of postcataract astigmatism by suturing techniques. In Binder PS, editor: Refractive corneal surgery: the correction of astigmatism, Boston, 1983, Little, Brown & Co, pp 57-68.

160. Stainer GA, Binder PS, Parker WT, et al: The natural and modified course of postcataract astigmatism, Ophthalmic Surg 1982;13:822-828.

161. Stainer GA, Perl T, and Binder PS: Controlled reduction of postkeratoplasty astigmatism, Ophthalmology 1982;89:668-676.

162. Stainer GA, Shaw EL, Binder PS, et al: Histopathology of a case of radial keratotomy, Arch Ophthalmol 1982; 100:1473-1477.

163. Swinger CA: Postoperative astigmatism, Surv Ophthalmol 1987;31:219-248.

164. Swinger CA, Troutman RC, and Forman JS: Keratophakia: postoperative astigmatism, Cornea 1987;6:202-206.

165. Tanne E: Corneal trephines and cutting blocks. In Brightbill SS, editor: Corneal surgery: theory, technique and tissue, St Louis, 1986, The CV Mosby Co, pp 258-264.

166. Tchah H, Hofmann R, Duffey R, Vivanti J, and Lindstrom R: Delimited peripheral arcuate keratotomy for astigmatism: "bowtie" configuration, J Refract Surg 1988;5:183-190.

167. Terry CM: Surgical keratometry and optics of cornea alteration. In Schachar RA, Levy NS, and Schachar L, editors: Keratorefraction, Denison, Tex, 1980, LAL Publishing, pp 15-25.

168. Terry MA and Rowsey JJ: Dynamic shifts in corneal topography during the modified Ruiz procedure for astigmatism, Arch Ophthalmol 1986;104: 1611-1616.

169. Thornton SP: Thornton guide for radial keratotomy incisions and optical zone size, J Refract Surg 1985;1:28-31.

170. Thornton SP: Astigmatic keratotomy: a review of basic concepts with case reports, J Cataract Refract Surg 1990; 16:430-435.

171. Thornton SP: Consultations: correction of astigmatism after cataract surgery, Refract Corneal Surg 1990;6: 131-136.

172. Thornton SP and Sanders DR: Graded nonintersecting transverse incisions for correction of idiopathic astigmatism, J Cataract Refract Surg 1987;13:27-31.

173. Thrasher BH and Boerner CF: Control of astigmatism by wound placement, Am Intraocular Implant Soc J 1984;10:176-179.

174. Tripoli NK, Cohen KL, and Holman RE: Corneal topographic response to circumferential keratotomies, J Refract Surg 1987;3:129-136.

175. Troutman RC: Microsurgical control of corneal astigmatism in cataract and keratoplasty, Trans Am Acad Ophthalmol Otolaryngol 1973;77:563-572.

176. Troutman RC: Corneal wedge resection for correction of astigmatism. In Troutman RC: Microsurgery of the anterior segment of the eye, vol 2, St Louis, 1977, The CV Mosby Co, pp 263-286.

177. Troutman RC: Microsurgery of the anterior segment of the eye, St Louis, 1977, The CV Mosby Co.

178. Troutman RC: Corneal wedge resections and relaxing incisions for postkeratoplasty astigmatism, Int Ophthalmol Clin 1983;23:161-168.

179. Troutman RC and Swinger CA: Relaxing incision for control of postoperative astigmatism following keratoplasty, Ophthalmic Surg 1980;11:117-120.

180. Troutman RC, Swinger CA, and Belmont S: Selective positioning of the donor cornea in penetrating keratoplasty for keratoconus: postoperative astigmatism, Ann Ophthalmol 1984; 3:135-139.

181. Van Meter WS, Gussler JR, Steinemann TL, and Wood TO: Control of astigmatism following keratoplasty with an adjusted single continuous suture compared to combined running/interrupted suturing, Invest Ophthalmol Vis Sci 1990;31(suppl):302.

182. van Rij G and Vijsvinkel G: Correction of postkeratoplasty astigmatism by razor blade and V-shaped knife wedge resection, Ophthalmic Surg 1983;14: 406-410.

183. van Rij G and Waring GO: Changes in corneal curvature induced by sutures and incisions, Am J Ophthalmol 1984;98:773-783.

184. van Rij G and Waring GO: Configuration of corneal trephine opening using five different trephines in human donor eyes, Arch Ophthalmol 1988; 106:1228-1233.

185. Villasenor R and Stimac GR: Clinical results and complications of trapezoidal keratotomy, J Refract Surg 1988; 4:125-131.

186. Vrabec MP, Florakis GJ, and Krachmer JH: Corrective surgery for astigmatism, Int Ophthalmol Clin 1988;28: 145-149.

187. Waring GO and Hanna KD: The Hanna suction punch block and trephine system for penetrating keratoplasty, Arch Ophthalmol 1989;107: 536-539.

188. Wishart MS, Wishart PK, and Gregor ZJ: Corneal astigmatism following cataract extraction, Br J Ophthalmol 1986;70:825-830.

189. Wood TO, Nabors G, Van Meter WS, and Zwagg RV: Wound revision for postkeratoplasty astigmatism, Invest Ophthalmol Vis Sci 1990;31(suppl): 575.

190. Yau CW, Busin M, McDonald M, and Kaufman HE: The effect of different radial keratotomy patterns on astigmatism in rabbits, Refract Surg 1985; 1:201-205.

191. Zelman J: Controlling astigmatism with radial keratotomy. In Schachar RA, Levy NS, and Schachar L, editors: Refractive keratoplasty, Denison, Tex, 1983, LAL Publishing, pp 284-286.

Atlas of Astigmatic Keratotomy

George O. Waring III
Perry S. Binder

Our goal in this chapter is to present a practical surgical approach to astigmatic keratotomy with techniques in use in the early 1990s. The optics and principles of astigmatism and astigmatic keratotomy are discussed in Chapter 30. Chapter 31 discusses the types of astigmatic keratotomy, the variables that influence the results, and the results achieved in published reports. This chapter presupposes basic knowledge of the material in Chapters 30 and 31, although we repeat some of the information here for continuity and so that the surgical atlas can be read as a unit.

As emphasized throughout this book, refractive keratotomy is an art, and individual instruments, surgical techniques, nomograms, and experience are extremely important in determining the actual techniques used during surgery. Thus this atlas presents the overall schematic principles and some details of surgical technique, but it does not pretend to substitute for personal clinical experience.

Many of the general principles of astigmatic keratotomy have already been presented in Chapter 17, Atlas of Surgical Techniques of Radial Keratotomy, and such principles are not repeated here.

We omit techniques not currently in use, such as intersecting incisions or grouped radial incisions. The techniques represented here reflect our own experience and bias, and we have not tried to be encyclopedic in representing all techniques currently in use.

BACKGROUND AND ACKNOWLEDGMENTS

This surgical atlas derives from the cumulative personal and published experience of numerous surgeons, as detailed in other chapters of Section VII, Keratotomy for Astigmatism. In this atlas we have specifically avoided using eponyms and acknowledging priority for description of specific techniques because the atlas is focused on the execution of the techniques themselves. Some eponyms are used where they serve to enhance communication. Our debt to those who derived and fostered these techniques is acknowledged in Section II, Development of Refractive Keratotomy, and the other chapters in Section VII, Keratotomy for Astigmatism. We reaffirm these acknowledgments here. We express special appreciation to the following individuals: Drs. Norman Jaffe, Jay Krachmer, Richard Lindstrom, William Maloney, Albert Neumann, Luis Ruiz, Donald Sanders, Spencer Thornton, and Richard Troutman, who have contributed repeatedly and substantively to our knowledge of astigmatic keratotomy.

PLATE 32-1:   Transverse Keratotomy and the Steep Corneal Meridian
(Figs. 32-1 to 32-3)

FIGURE 32-1   FOUR METHODS OF MEASURING AND REPRESENTING ASTIGMATISM

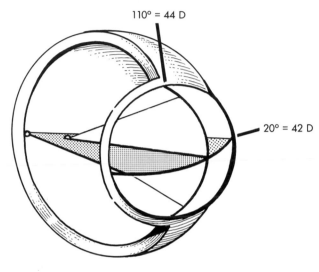

A   Refraction:
  Minus cylinder: −3.00 −2.00 × 20°
  Plus cylinder: −5.00 +2.00 × 110°

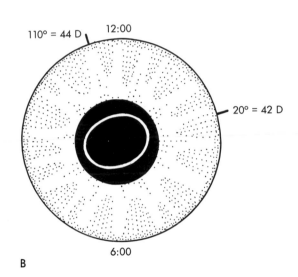

B

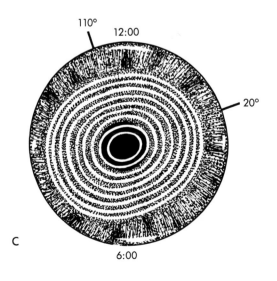

C

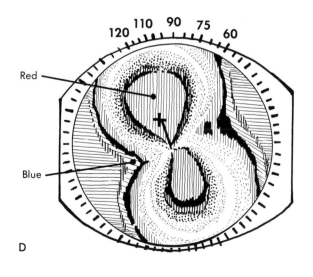

D

Four methods of measuring and representing astigmatism. A, Optics: Drawing demonstrates steep meridian at 110°, creating simple myopic astigmatism. Both the minus cylinder and the plus cylinder forms of refraction have a spherical equivalent of −4.00 D. The minus cylinder form is used to plan astigmatism surgery. **B,** Keratometry: Mire is oval, the narrowest section of the oval is oriented along the steepest meridian (44 D) at 110°. The widest section of the oval is oriented along the flattest (42 D) meridian at 20°. **C,** Qualitative keratography: Concentric oval mires are closer to each other along the 110° steep meridian. **D,** Quantitative videokeratography: Power map shows steep 110° meridian in the classical "bow tie" or "hourglass" configuration that results from the smaller surface area in the center of the cornea compared with the larger surface area in the peripheral cornea.

Throughout this atlas this specific orientation is used, with the steep meridian at 110° and the flat meridian at 20°. The purpose of this is to alter the customary 90° and 180° orientation to challenge the reader's thinking and to emphasize the importance of orienting the entire surgical procedure around the steep meridian.

FIGURE 32-2   EFFECT OF ASTIGMATIC KERATOTOMY

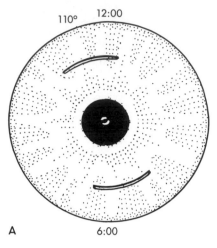

A   6:00

Transverse—straight or arcuate

Refractive effect
Flattens incised meridian, steepens unincised meridian, spherical equivalent unchanged

Clinical indication
Low (1.5 to 4 D) or mixed astigmatism

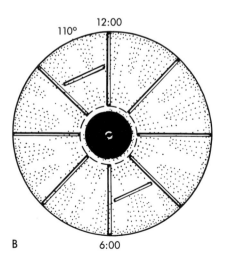

B   6:00

Transverse between radials

Refractive effect
Flattens all meridians, incised meridian flattened more

Clinical indication
Compound myopic astigmatism

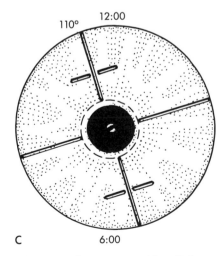

C   6:00

Interrupted transverse with radials

Refractive effect
Flattens all meridians, incised meridian flattened more

Clinical indication
Compound myopic astigmatism or repeated astigmatic keratotomy after previous radial keratotomy

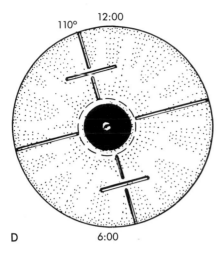

D

6:00

Transverse with interrupted radials

Refractive effect
Flattens all meridians, incised meridian flattened more

Clinical indication
Compound myopic astigmatism; repeated radial keratotomy after previous astigmatic keratotomy

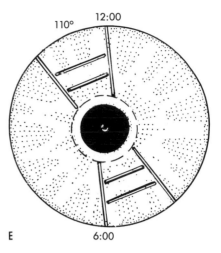

E

6:00

Transverse and semi-radial (trapezoidal, Ruiz)

Refractive effect
Flattens incised meridian, unincised meridian steepens slightly, spherical equivalent more hyperopic

Clinical indication
High compound myopic astigmatism

FIGURE 32-3   ORIENTATION OF INCISIONS

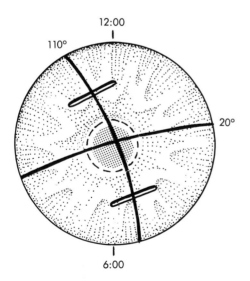

Orientation of incisions. Transverse incisions are oriented perpendicular to the steep 110° meridian to reduce the refractive power in that meridian. Throughout this atlas we use this representation of two straight transverse incisions oriented perpendicular to the 110° meridian, either from the frontal view as seen at the slit-lamp microscope (Figs. 32-1 to 32-14) or from the surgeon's point of view as seen through the operating microscope (Figs. 32-16 to 32-41). Drawings from the surgeon's view have a conjunctival vessel and an iris nevus drawn as anatomic orientation for the steep meridian. Many surgeons use arcuate incisions instead of straight incisions, but that pattern is not illustrated in most of this atlas.

PLATE 32-2:   Variables Used for Planning Astigmatic Keratotomy
(Figs. 32-4 to 32-14)

FIGURE 32-4   LOCATION OF TRANSVERSE INCISIONS

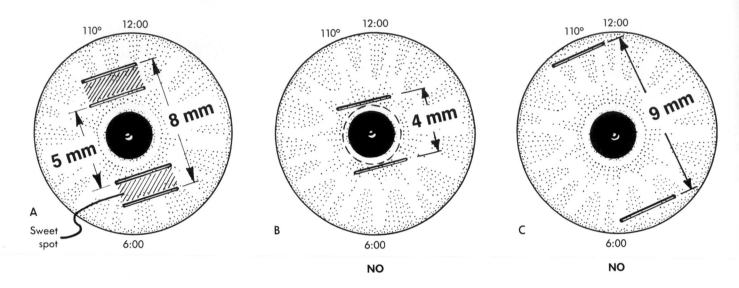

Location of transverse incisions. A, The incisions are centered around the steep meridian and generally extend equidistant from that meridian. The incisions are placed between the 5-mm diameter zone (2.5 mm from the center of the pupil) and the 8-mm zone (4 mm from the center of the pupil). Incisions closer to the center of the pupil create a greater flattening effect. **B,** Transverse incisions placed inside the 5-mm zone may greatly increase glare. **C,** Transverse incisions placed outside the 8-mm zone do not effectively flatten the cornea.

FIGURE 32-5   INTERSECTING INCISIONS

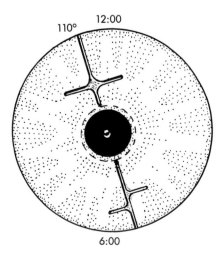

Intersecting—NO

Intersecting incisions. Intersecting incisions will create gaping of the cornea, increased scarring, and sometimes elevated corneal flaps. Incisions should not intersect.

FIGURE 32-6   NUMBER OF TRANSVERSE INCISIONS

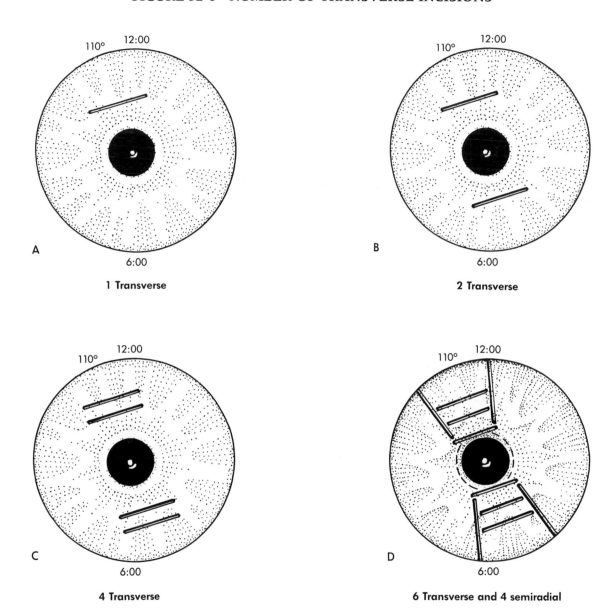

A — **1 Transverse**

B — **2 Transverse**

C — **4 Transverse**

D — **6 Transverse and 4 semiradial**

Number of transverse incisions. The greater the number of transverse incisions the greater the decrease in astigmatism, up to approximately four incisions (two pairs). **A,** One superior incision can be used to correct minor amounts of astigmatism and to prevent the possible glare that might come from a transverse incision placed inferiorly. Superior incisions seem to gape less and heal faster. **B,** Symmetric placement of two transverse incisions is used most commonly. **C,** The main reason for using four or six incisions is to create a smooth transition zone for the flattened meridian. The fifth and sixth incisions add little to the overall flattening. **D,** In general, six incisions (three pairs) are used in combination with semiradial incisions. The most central transverse incision is often placed across the end of the semiradials to enhance its effect.

FIGURE 32-7   CONFIGURATION OF TRANSVERSE INCISIONS

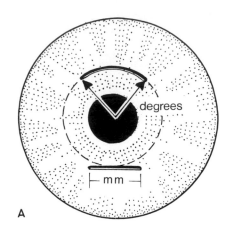

A

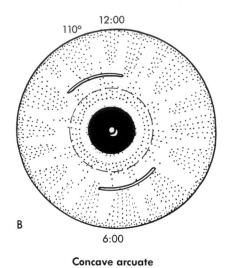

B

Concave arcuate

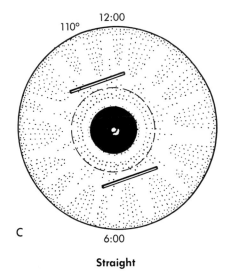

C

Straight

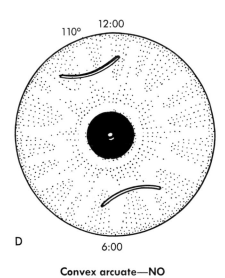

D

Convex arcuate—NO

Configuration of transverse incisions. A, Concave arcuate incisions and straight incisions are used clinically. **B,** Arcuate incision placed along the circumference of the zone mark. **C,** Straight incision tangential to the zone mark. **D,** Convex arcuate incisions have less effect and should not be used. Arcuate incisions have numerous theoretic advantages: (1) the entire incision is equidistant from the center of the pupil; (2) they cut cornea of approximately the same thickness; (3) their length is measured in degrees as is the axis of astigmatism; and (4) they have a theoretic biomechanical advantage. They are, however, more difficult to make uniformly than straight incisions. Straight incisions have been used successfully on numerous cases.

FIGURE 32-8   LENGTH OF TRANSVERSE INCISIONS

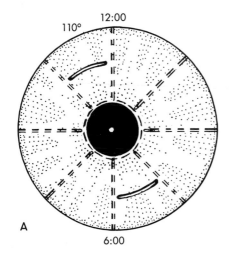

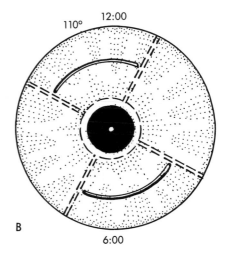

Segment width		Angular length		Straight length
1/2	≅	20°	≅	1.34 mm
2/3	≅	30°	≅	1.81 mm
Full	≅	45°	≅	2.68 mm

Segment width		Arc length		Straight width
1/2	≅	45°	≅	2.68 mm
2/3	≅	60°	≅	3.50 mm
Full	≅	85°	≅	4.95 mm

Length of transverse incisions. Transverse incisions vary in length from approximately 15° to approximately 100°. The longer the incision the greater the flattening of the incised meridian and the greater the steepening of the orthogonal unincised meridian up to approximately 120°. The length of the incisions is often defined and delimited by preexisting radial incisions or by the topography of a corneal transplant. **A,** With eight radial incisions, the surgeon can grade the length of the transverse incision in fractions of the space between the radials, in degrees, or in millimeters. **B,** The same is true with four radials. (See Table 31-8 for additional relative angular, arc, and chord lengths.)

FIGURE 32-9   VARIABLE LENGTH INCISIONS

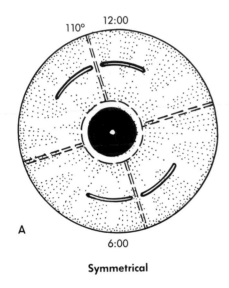

A

Symmetrical

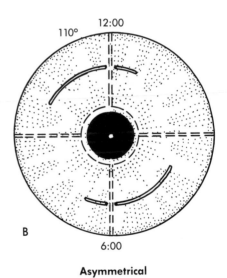

B

Asymmetrical

Variable length incisions. When desired in a primary operation or necessary in a repeated operation, the length of the interrupted transverse incision can be varied as symmetric **(A)** or asymmetric **(B)**.

FIGURE 32-10   COUPLING EFFECT

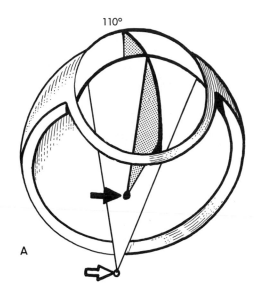

Mixed astigmatism

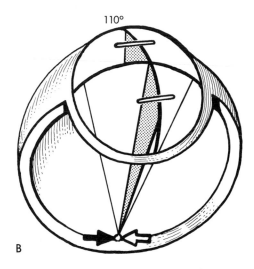

Shorter incision = proper correction

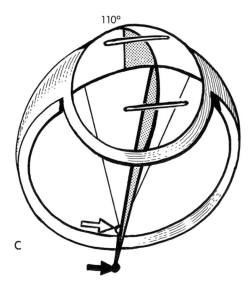

Long incision = overcorrection

Coupling effect. A, Optical diagram of mixed astigmatism. **B,** A shorter (2- to 3-mm) incision flattens the incised meridian and steepens the orthogonal unincised meridian approximately an equal amount. **C,** A longer (4- to 5-mm) incision can create astigmatism by producing excess flattening in the incised meridian and excess steepening in the unincised meridian. Longer incisions will create a change in the refraction away from myopia and toward hyperopia.

FIGURE 32-11   ASYMMETRIC INCISIONS

Asymmetric incisions. Asymmetric transverse incisions theoretically can be used to correct astigmatism that has a steeper semimeridian and a flatter semimeridian, as occurs commonly after penetrating keratoplasty. The longer incision would be used on the side of the steeper semimeridian. There is little published information on this technique.

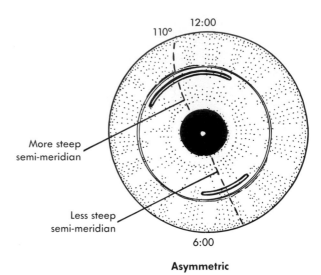

Asymmetric

FIGURE 32-12   DEPTH OF TRANSVERSE INCISIONS

Depth of transverse incisions. The depth of transverse incisions should be shallower than that of radial incisions: 80% to 85% of the measured corneal thickness—especially for longer arcuate incisions, which tend to an uplifted central edge. To achieve this depth, the surgeon must control numerous factors: (1) where the corneal thickness measurements are taken (central, paracentral, or over the area of the intended incision), (2) how the length of the knife blade is calculated as a percentage of the measured corneal thickness (for example, 95% of the thickness in the location where the incision will be made), (3) the configuration and sharpness of the knife blade, (4) calibration of the blade extension, and (5) the manual technique of executing the incision.

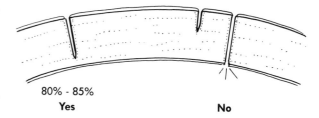

FIGURE 32-13   DIRECTION OF TRANSVERSE INCISIONS

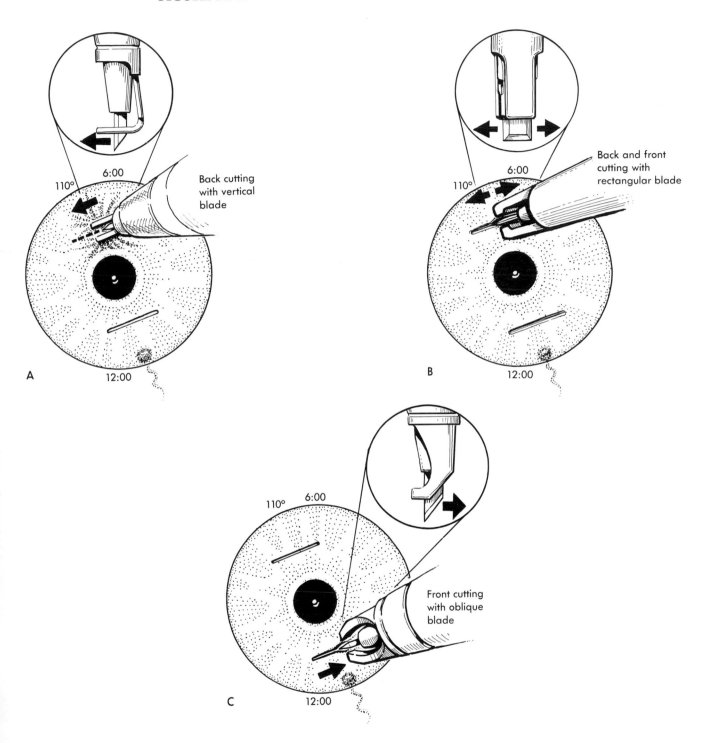

Direction of transverse incisions. A, The preferred direction for transverse incisions is to push a vertical blade along the straight or arcuate incision mark. The main advantage of this technique is the visibility of the cutting edge of the blade, which allows a more exact starting and stopping point at each end of the incision. **B,** Alternatively a rectangular diamond blade can be used with the same technique, which may have the advantage of squaring off each end of the incision better but cannot readily make an arcuate incision. **C,** Pulling an angled blade along the mark can produce an acceptable incision, but it is more difficult to see the blade at the end of the incision and to square off the ends of the incision.

FIGURE 32-14   SEQUENCE OF COMBINED TRANSVERSE
AND RADIAL INCISIONS

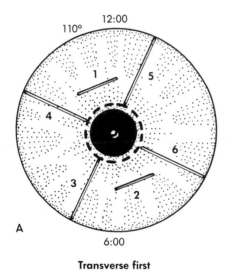

Transverse first

A

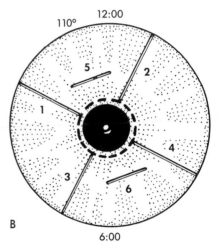

Radial first—No

B

Sequence of combined transverse and radial incisions. A, Making the transverse incisions first is easier because the tissue is more stable and the placement of the transverse incisions with respect to the steep meridian can be delineated with greater care. Placement of the radial incisions can then be made to avoid intersecting the transverse incisions. **B,** Placing the radial incisions first may appear simpler because the transverse incisions can then be spaced between the radials, but there are two drawbacks: (1) the wedge of tissue between the radial incisions becomes somewhat mobile during the transverse incisions (particularly when eight incisions are used), making it more difficult to create an incision with vertical ends and of uniform depth; and (2) if the radial incisions are not placed in the correct position, the transverse incisions may not be centered exactly on the steep meridian.

FIGURE 32-15   SURGICAL PLAN IN THE OPERATING ROOM

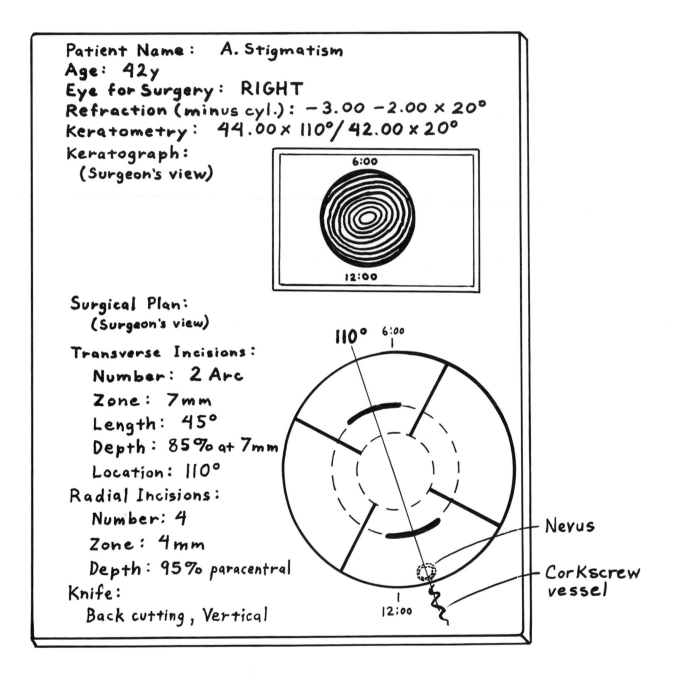

Patient Name: A. Stigmatism
Age: 42y
Eye for Surgery: RIGHT
Refraction (minus cyl.): −3.00 −2.00 × 20°
Keratometry: 44.00 × 110°/ 42.00 × 20°
Keratograph:
  (Surgeon's view)

6:00

12:00

Surgical Plan:
  (Surgeon's view)

Transverse Incisions:
  Number: 2 Arc
  Zone: 7mm
  Length: 45°
  Depth: 85% at 7mm
  Location: 110°
Radial Incisions:
  Number: 4
  Zone: 4mm
  Depth: 95% paracentral
Knife:
  Back cutting, Vertical

110° 6:00

12:00

Nevus

Corkscrew vessel

Surgical plan in the operating room. It is absolutely necessary for astigmatism surgery that the surgeon post the plan for the incisions in an easily visible location, for example, hanging from the microscope or on an IV pole. The amount of information presented varies from surgeon to surgeon, but the minimal information includes the name of the patient, the eye for surgery, and a drawing of the incision pattern from the surgeon's view (12 o'clock facing downward). The methods relating to positioning, preparing, and draping the patient for astigmatic keratotomy are the same as those depicted in Chapter 17, Atlas of Surgical Techniques of Radial Keratotomy.

FIGURE 32-16　IDENTIFICATION OF ANATOMIC LANDMARKS

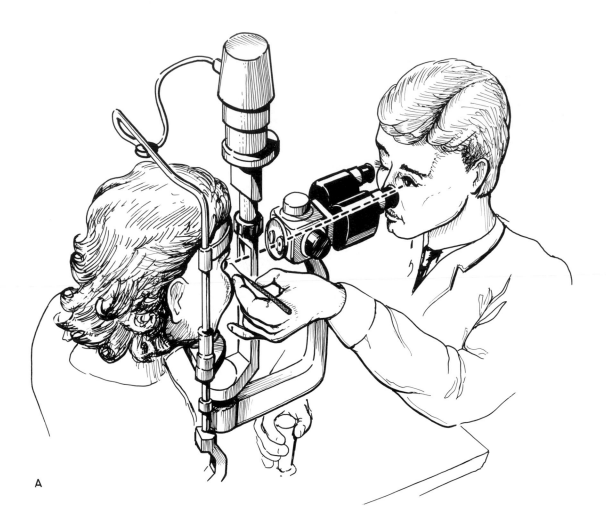

A

Identification of anatomic landmarks. A, Before surgery the surgeon should examine the patient with a slit-lamp microscope and identify anatomic landmarks that will make it easy to locate the position of the steep meridian during surgery. Some surgeons mark the steep meridian with a sharp needle at the slit-lamp microscope immediately before surgery. A protractor reticle in the eyepiece can help identify the anatomic location of the steep meridian. This gives the advantage of familiar orientation, good patient cooperation, normal position of the globe as determined by the extraocular muscles, and a chance to double-check the location of the anatomic landmarks with respect to the measured steep meridian.

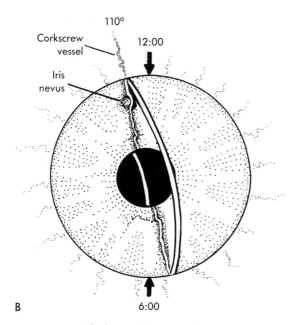

B

Slit-lamp microscope view

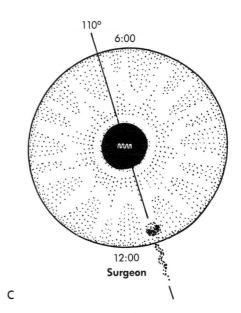

C

Surgeon's view through the operating microscope

B, For example, the steep meridian (110°) can be identified by an iris nevus or a limbal vessel with a specific configuration; this can be drawn on the chart and the steep meridian identified. **C,** During surgery the surgeon's view through the operating microscope is upside down from the frontal view seen with a slit-lamp microscope (as depicted in Figs. 32-1 to 32-14), so the location of the landmarks will be rotated 180°. The surgeon's view is used in all subsequent illustrations in this atlas (Figs. 32-16 to 32-42).

FIGURE 32-17   MARKING THE CENTER OF THE PUPIL

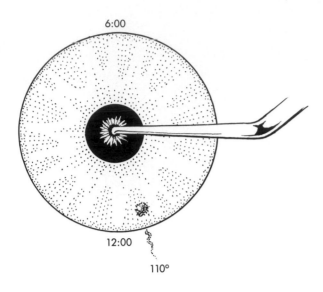

Marking the center of the pupil. The incisions are centered around a mark made in the center of the pupil with a blunt instrument, such as an intraocular lens hook, as discussed in Chapter 16, Centering Corneal Surgical Procedures.

FIGURE 32-18   MARKING THE CENTRAL CLEAR ZONE

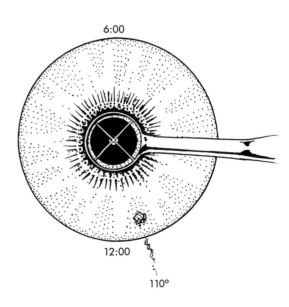

Marking the central clear zone. The surgeon centers a clear zone marker around the center of the pupil and indents the corneal epithelium without rotating the instrument to delineate the end of the radial incisions.

FIGURE 32-19　MARKING THE STEEP MERIDIAN

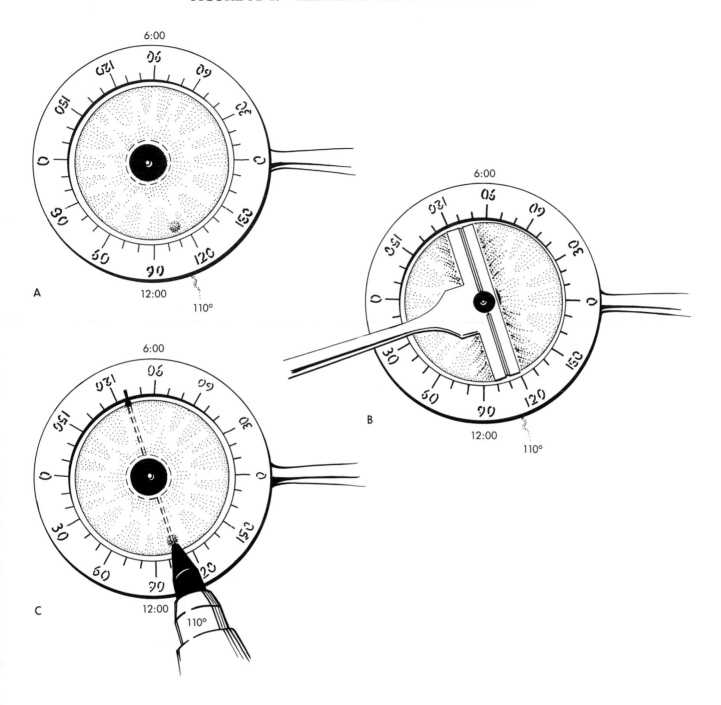

Marking the steep meridian. A, The surgeon orients a circular protractor (Mendez) around the limbus so that the previously determined landmarks are aligned with the measured steep meridian. In this case, the iris nevus and the conjunctival vessel are aligned with the steep 110° meridian. Some protractors have teeth on the back to help secure them to the limbus, and the surgeon must be careful to avoid abrading the corneal surface with the teeth. Some have a large enough outer diameter that they must be wedged beneath the eyelids and eyelid speculum. A rotating handle and dial on some instruments allows the surgeon to place the dial in the desired location on the cornea and rotate the handle to any desired, comfortable position. A swivel handle can be pivoted from one side to the other, making it easier to use for right and left eyes. **B,** A linear marker with a straight, prominent ridge (Bores marker) is aligned with the steep corneal meridian and pressed into the cornea to mark epithelium. **C,** A sterile methylene blue surgical marking pen can also be used to mark the orientation of the steep meridian by placing a blue dot at the limbus.

**FIGURE 32-20   MARKING THE LOCATION OF TRANSVERSE
                 INCISIONS**

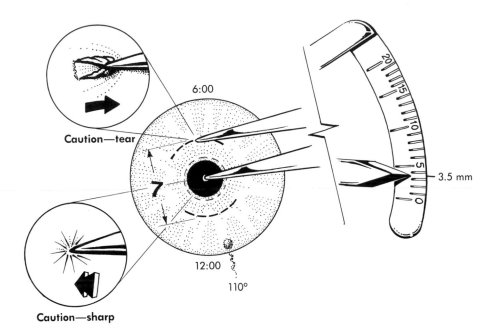

Marking the location of transverse incisions. Marking the transverse incisions
consists of locating the incision along the steep meridian at a predetermined distance from the center of the pupil and straddling the meridian equidistantly. After
that, the length of the incision is marked. A Castroviejo or other type of caliper is
an easy, inexpensive instrument to mark the incision. The diameter of the zone (7
mm in this example) for the incisions is determined, and half that diameter (the
radius) is dialed on the caliper (3.5 mm in this example). The tips of the caliper are
often sharp and must be applied gently to the corneal surface or blunted with a
file. One tip is placed on the mark in the center of the pupil and the other tip used
to outline the location of the transverse incision with a series of small dots. Sweeping the tip across the corneal surface will produce an epithelial abrasion.

FIGURE 32-21   CIRCULAR ZONE MARKER

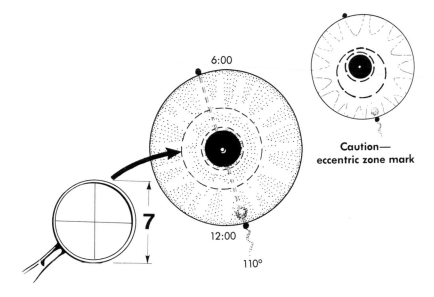

Caution—
eccentric zone mark

Circular zone marker. A circular zone marker with an alignment sight can be used to delimit the zone, but it is sometimes difficult to make this mark exactly concentric with the central clear zone mark. The surgeon can ensure the zone marks are concentric by using markers with two or three circular ridges.

FIGURE 32-22   INCISION MARKERS

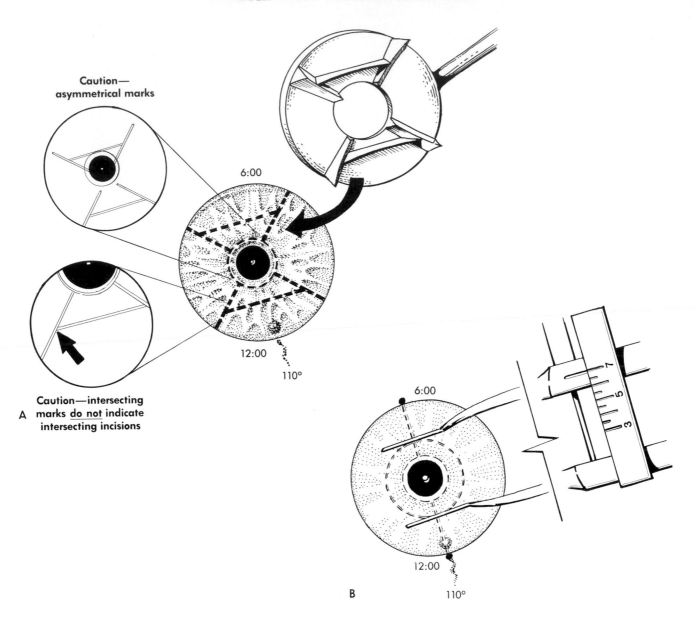

Incision markers. A variety of incision markers are available to the surgeon for locating the transverse incisions. **A,** Combined radial and transverse markers (Hoopes) have the advantage of making all marks at once but the disadvantage that, if the marks are made in the wrong location the first time, a second set of marks must be made, creating confusion. A full set of these markers must be available so that the desired number of radial marks is combined with the desired zone diameter of the transverse marks (for example, four and eight radials combined with transverse incisions at 6, 7, and 8 mm transverse, for a total of six markers). Paired parallel transverse markers (not illustrated) are available; some have notches in the middle for straddling the radial marks. The proper alignment of the central clear zone mark, the radial marks, and the transverse marks with three different markers is sometimes difficult. **B,** A caliper designed to make two parallel marks on the cornea (Ruiz) allows adjustability in a single instrument, but still poses the problem of ensuring that the marks are equidistant from the center. This can be resolved by making a circular zone mark first and then making the two parallel marks on either side with the caliper.

FIGURE 32-23 MARKING THE LENGTH OF THE INCISIONS

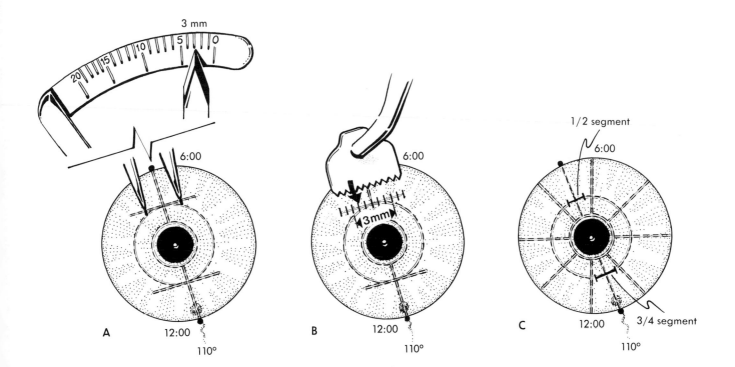

Marking the length of the incisions. A, A caliper (Castroviejo) can be set for the length of the incision (3 mm in this example) and used to mark either end of the transverse incision straddling the steep meridian. **B,** A calibrated marking ruler (Thornton) can be coated with methylene blue and used to make a series of calibrated marks along the location of the transverse incision. **C,** The length of the incision can be established by visual inspection, as a fraction of the distance between the radial marks (Thornton). Although this has the advantage of simplicity, it makes accurate determination of the length of the incision difficult. The angular length of an arcuate incision is marked with the circular protractor in place, placing marks the required distance on either side of the steep meridian (see Fig. 32-19, *C*).

FIGURE 32-24   FIXATION OF THE GLOBE DURING INCISIONS

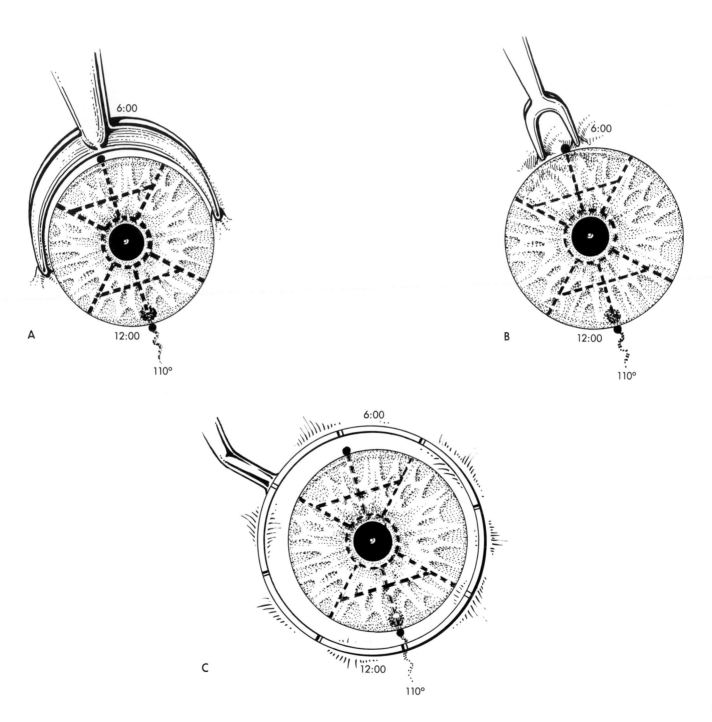

Fixation of the globe during incisions. The surgeon fixates the globe in a manner similar to that for radial keratotomy, but since the incisions are made in a variety of directions, wide two-point fixation such as that with spanning forceps (Kremer, Arrowsmith) **(A)** or with a compression ring (Thornton) **(C)** is preferable. Single-point fixation and narrow double-point fixation (Bores) **(B)** are less stable for transverse keratotomy.

FIGURE 32-25   SEQUENCE OF INCISIONS

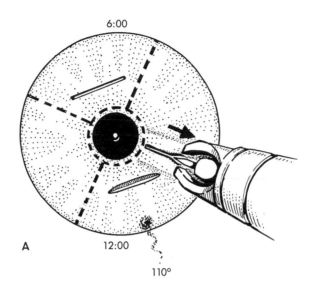

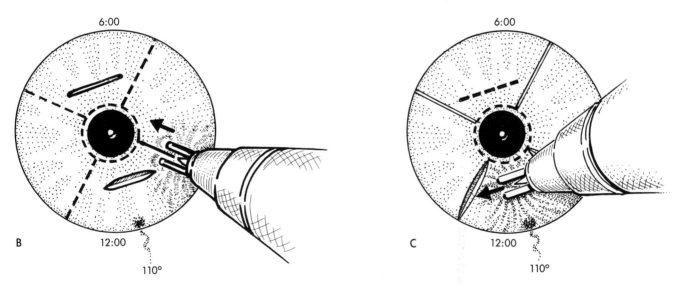

Sequence of incisions. The transverse incisions are made first followed by the radial incisions. The radial incisions may be made centrifugally **(A)** or centripetally **(B). C,** Making the transverse incisions after the radial incisions is more difficult because the tissue between the radial incisions is less stable.

FIGURE 32-26 EXECUTING A STRAIGHT TRANSVERSE INCISION

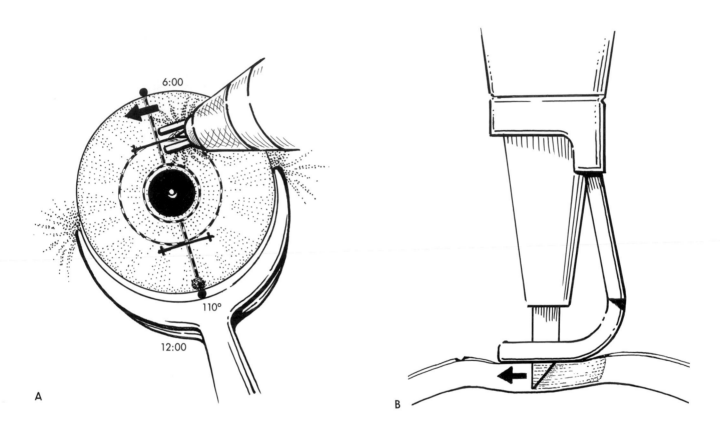

Executing a straight transverse incision. The corneal surface is lightly moistened with a balanced salt solution and the epithelial marks dried for visibility. The manual technique of making a transverse incision is similar to that for making a centripetal (limbus to clear zone, Russian technique) radial incision, except that the knife is held in a constant perpendicular orientation across one plane of the cornea, so the handle does not need to be tilted during the procedure. The surgeon plunges the blade into the cornea at one end of the transverse mark, holds it or bounces it for a count of three, and pushes the knife forward smoothly and steadily to the other end of the mark **(A)**, maintaining a slight indentation of the cornea during the incision **(B).** Because the back edge of the knife is bevelled, the initial end of the incision will not be vertical. Turning the knife in the other direction and squaring up the initial end of the incision can ensure verticality. A blade with both edges sharp will make the initial end closer to vertical. A rectangular knife will make both ends vertical. Note the depth on the drawing is 90% to 95%, but the preferred depth for transverse incisions is 80% to 85%.

FIGURE 32-27   EXECUTING AN ARCUATE TRANSVERSE INCISION

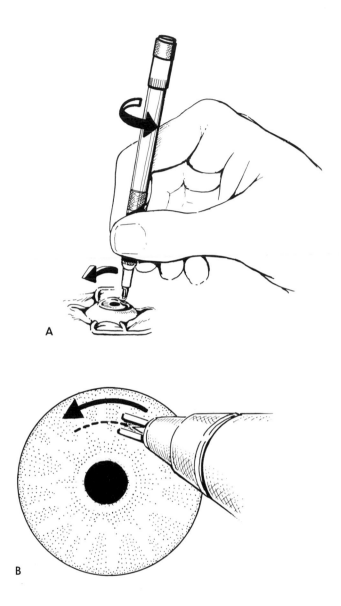

Executing an arcuate transverse incision. It is more difficult to make a curved arcuate incision than a straight incision. To make the arcuate incision, the knife must not only be pushed in the back-cutting direction, but must also be rotated between the fingers so that the blade follows the path of the arc **(A).** This is not done by swinging the arm or the wrist in a curved position, but rather by rotating the knife between the fingers along the arcuate path **(B).** The longer the incision is, the more latitude there is to follow a gentle arc. Short arcuate incisions are more difficult to make smoothly.

FIGURE 32-28   INTERSECTING INCISIONS

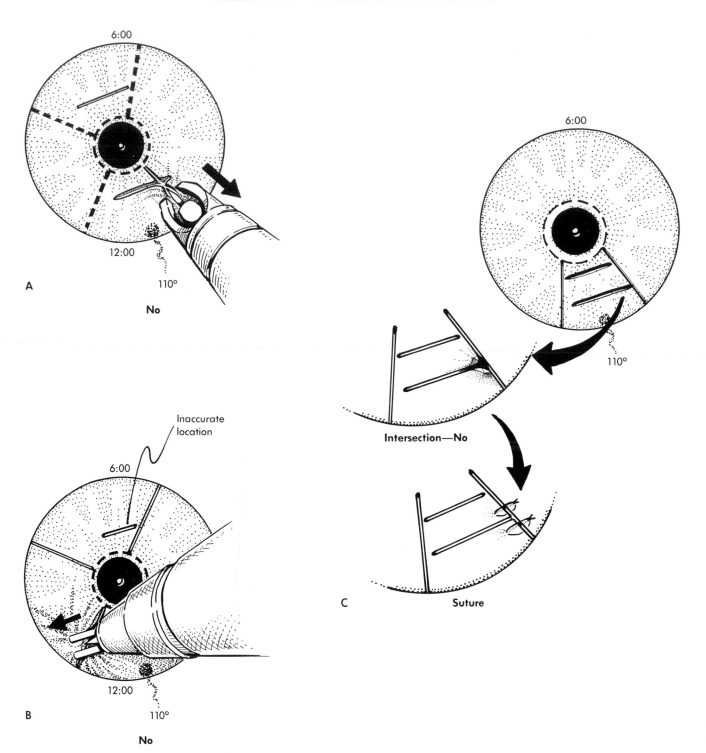

Intersecting incisions. The surgeon should avoid intersecting incisions **(A, B,** and **C).** This includes intersecting incisions made during previous surgery, although healed wounds will not gape open like freshly made ones. If an incision is intersected, it is prudent to place a short superficial interrupted 10-0 nylon suture, tied moderately firmly with the knot buried in the tissue, to prevent wound gaping **(C).**

PLATE 32-5: Trapezoidal Keratotomy (Figs. 32-29 to 32-33)

FIGURE 32-29   MARKING OF SEMIRADIAL INCISIONS

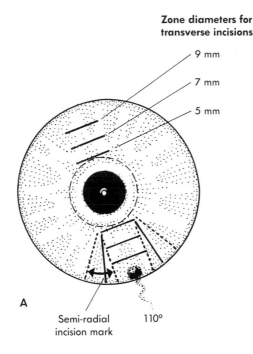

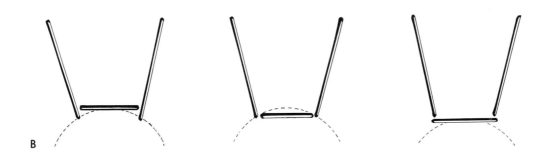

Marking of semiradial incisions. A, In general, the semiradial incisions are placed along imaginary lines outside the ends of the transverse incisions. Many patterns have been described (parallel, converging, semiradial, diverging semiradial, diamond, and fusiform). **B,** Alignment of the innermost transverse incision with the ends of the semiradial incisions varies among surgeons. It may be placed within the semiradials *(left)*, just between the tips of the semiradials *(middle)*, and across the tips of the semiradials *(right)*, which is probably the preferred alignment.

FIGURE 32-30   MARKING TRAPEZOIDAL INCISIONS

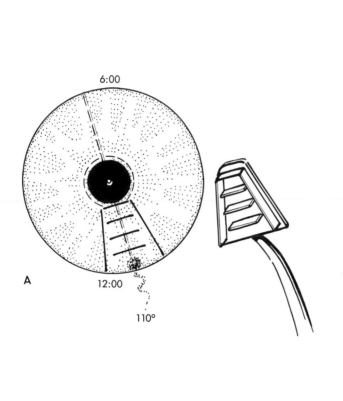

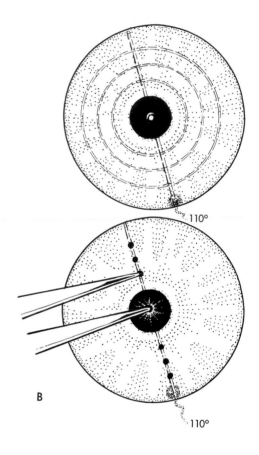

Marking trapezoidal incisions. A, A variety of markers can imprint the pattern of the transverse and semiradial incisions on the cornea. Most do not adjust for variable length of the transverse incisions. **B,** Marking location of the transverse incisions can be done either using circular zone markers (some companies manufacture multiple circular zone markers on a single marking instrument) or using a caliper to measure the desired distance along the steep meridian from the center mark or a parallel mark caliper (Ruiz, see Fig. 32-22, *B*).

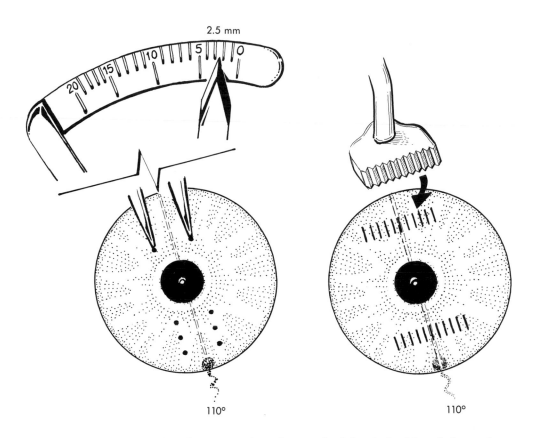

C, The callipers can then be reset and used to marked the desired length for each incision, or a marking ruler (Thornton) can be used.

FIGURE 32-31 SEQUENCE OF INCISIONS IN TRAPEZOIDAL KERATOTOMY

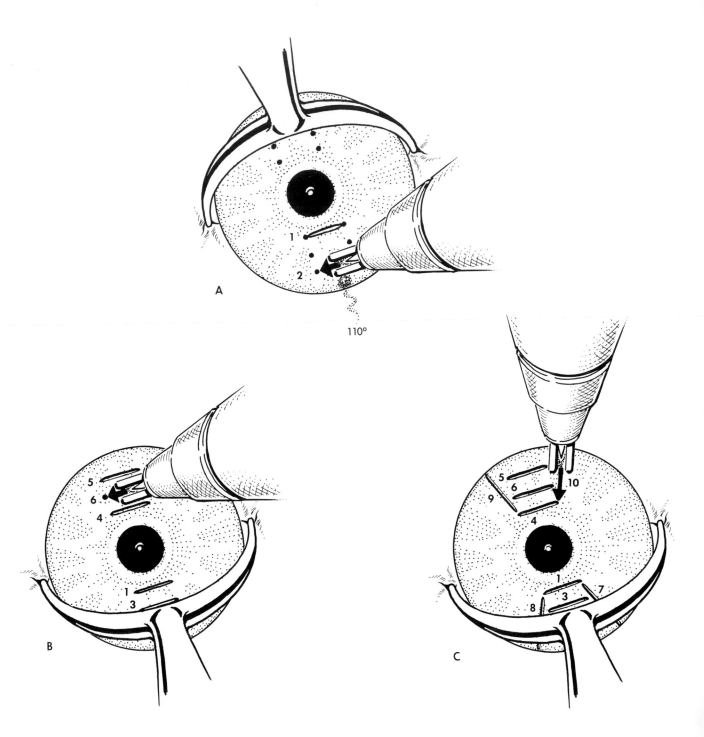

Sequence of incisions in trapezoidal keratotomy. A, The transverse incisions are made first. The innermost *(1)* and outermost *(2)* incisions are placed initially followed by the complementary pair *(3 and 4)*. **B,** The third pair *(3 and 6)* is placed between the initial pairs *(1 and 2, 4 and 5)*. **C,** The surgeon makes the semiradial incisions last, cutting centripetally and being careful not to intersect the transverse incisions.

FIGURE 32-32 ALIGNMENT OF SEMIRADIAL INCISIONS

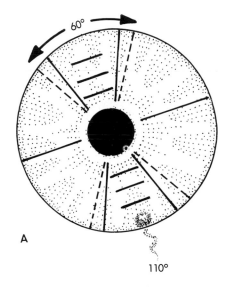

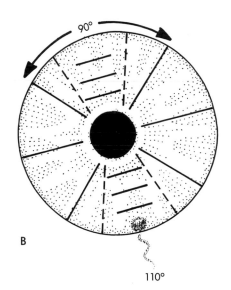

Alignment of semiradial trapezoidal incisions. A, The closer the radial incisions are brought to the trapezoidal pattern, the greater the flattening in the steep meridian and the less the steepening in the orthogonal meridian. This would be preferred for an eye with a refractive error of −3.00 −5.00 × 180°. **B,** If the radial incisions are placed farther away from the trapezoidal pattern, there is less flattening of the steep meridian and more flattening of the orthogonal meridian. This would be preferred for an eye with a refractive error of −5.00 −3.00 × 180°.

**FIGURE 32-33   TECHNICAL ERRORS IN TRAPEZOIDAL
KERATOTOMY**

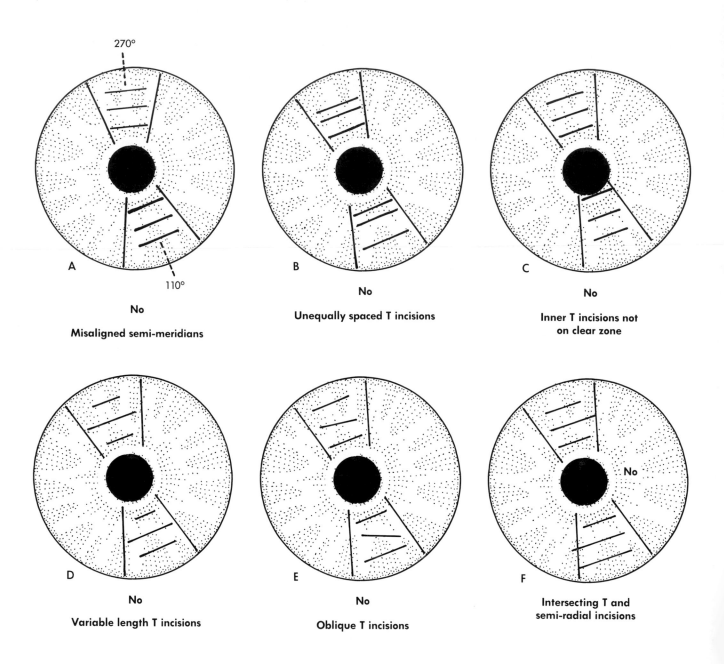

A

No

Misaligned semi-meridians

B

No

Unequally spaced T incisions

C

No

**Inner T incisions not
on clear zone**

D

No

Variable length T incisions

E

No

Oblique T incisions

F

No

**Intersecting T and
semi-radial incisions**

Technical errors in trapezoidal keratotomy. A, Misaligned semimeridians. **B,**
Unequal spacing of the transverse *(T)* incisions. **C,** Placement of the transverse incisions off of the zone marks. **D,** Variable length transverse *(T)* incisions. **E,** Variable
direction transverse *(T)* incisions. **F,** Intersection of transverse *(T)* and semiradial
incisions.

PLATE 32-6: Astigmatism after Cataract Surgery
(Figs. 32-34 and 32-35)

FIGURE 32-34   AGAINST-THE-RULE ASTIGMATISM

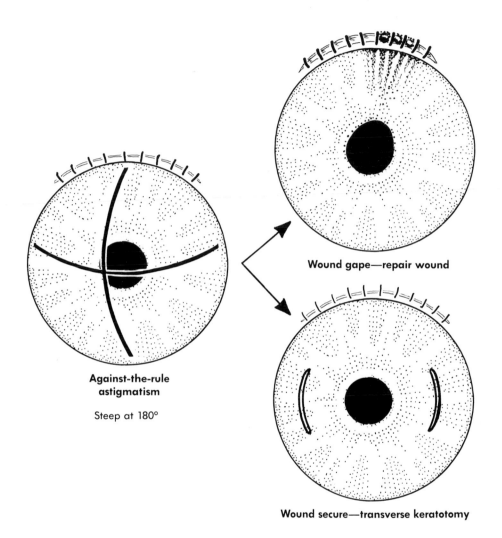

Against-the-rule astigmatism

Steep at 180°

Wound gape—repair wound

Wound secure—transverse keratotomy

Against-the-rule astigmatism. There are two causes for against-the-rule astigmatism after cataract extraction. The first is a wound gape, sometimes accompanied by iris incarceration, which may require opening the surgical wound. The second circumstance is where the surgical wound shows no visible wound disruption, and transverse incisions in the steep horizontal meridian are an appropriate method of management. The technique of performing these transverse incisions is the same as that described earlier in this atlas for naturally occurring astigmatism (see Chapter 31, Keratotomy for Astigmatism).

FIGURE 32-35   LOCATION OF ARCUATE RELAXING INCISION
AFTER PENETRATING KERATOPLASTY

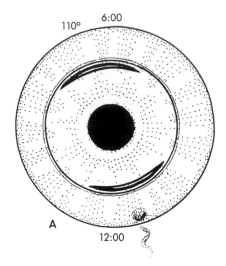

Donor—Yes

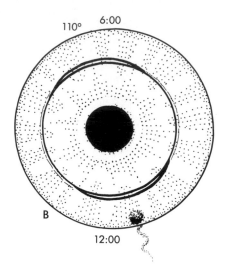

In wound—symmetrical

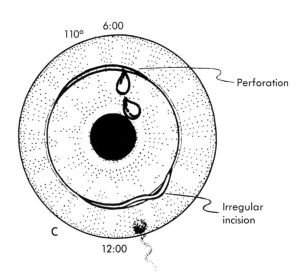

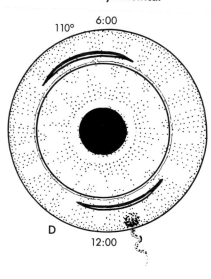

In host—No

Location of arcuate relaxing incision after penetrating keratoplasty. A,
Making the incisions in the donor cornea 0.5 mm inside the keratoplasty wound
cuts into tissue of relatively uniform thickness, decreasing the chance of perforation,
allows creation of a new cleaner scar than that achieved by recutting the old wound,
and probably allows a more predictable mechanical effect from the incision on the
shape of the donor. **B** and **C,** Incisions commonly have been made in the wound
and can effectively alter the shape of the donor, but because it is difficult to trace the
course of the wound exactly, because the wound may have posterior gaping that
predisposes to corneal perforation, and because the biomechanical properties of the
wound are not uniform, this may be a more precarious location for the incisions. **D,**
Relaxing incisions placed in the host are ineffective because the corneal transplant
scars form an effective blockade for the transmission of the effect of the incisions, so
the shape of the donor is not substantially altered.

**FIGURE 32-36   FIVE METHODS TO IDENTIFY THE STEEP
MERIDIAN IN A CORNEAL TRANSPLANT**

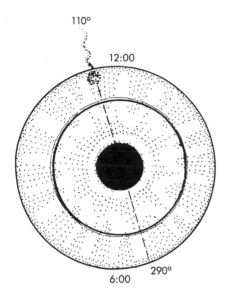

A   Refraction
   −5.00 + 8.00 × 110°

B   Keratometry
   55.00 × 100°
   46.00 × 10°

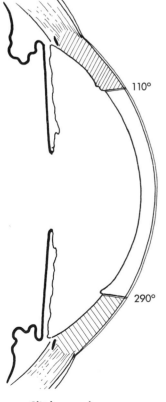

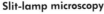
E   **Slit-lamp microscopy**

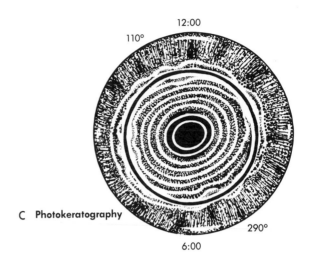
C   Photokeratography

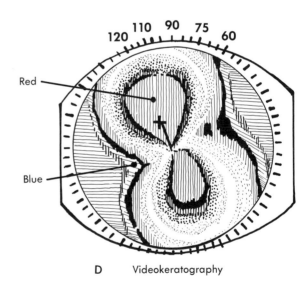
D   Videokeratography

Five methods to identify the steep meridian in a corneal transplant.
A, *Refraction,* in which the axis of the plus cylinder lies on the steep meridian, and
B, *Keratometry,* in which the meridian with the greatest power can be identified; **C,**
Qualitative keratography, in which the ovality and configuration of the mires indicate the steeper and flatter semimeridians; **D,** *Quantitative computer-assisted videokeratography,* which can depict semimeridional variations as color-coded power
maps; **E,** *Slit-lamp microscopy* in which the surgeon sometimes can identify the area
of corneal steepening by visual inspection. The steep meridian identified by these
five methods is not always in the same direction because each method measures a
slightly different area of the cornea, but all measurements should be within approximately 20° of each other. Keratography and slit-lamp microscopy have the
advantage of identifying differences along the semimeridians, such as the illustrated
circumstance in which the 110° semimeridian at approximately 11 o'clock is
steeper than the 290° semimeridian at approximately 5 o'clock.

FIGURE 32-37   MARKING THE LOCATION OF THE INCISION

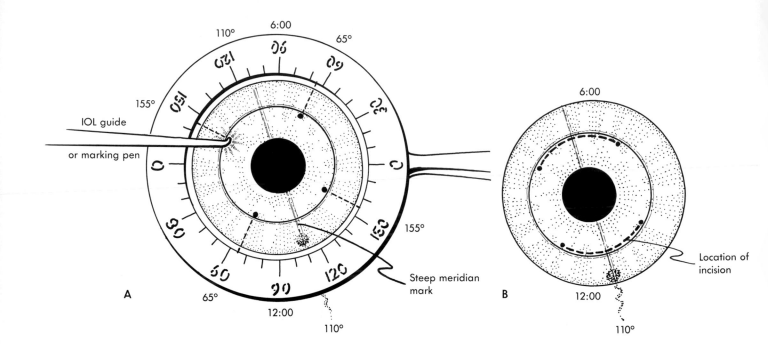

Marking the location of the incision. A, Four steps are involved: (1) identification of landmarks as recorded from the slit-lamp examination, in this case a nevus and corkscrew vessel in the steep 110° semimeridian; (2) placing the circular protractor in the correct 90° to 180° orientation; (3) marking the steep meridian with the linear astigmatism marker or marking pen; and (4) marking the length of the incision (commonly 90°) with an intraocular lens hook or a marking pen. **B,** The penetrating keratoplasty wound serves as a guide for the configuration of the arcuate transverse incision, and therefore an arcuate incision marker is not necessary.

FIGURE 32-38   INTRAOPERATIVE ULTRASONIC PACHOMETRY

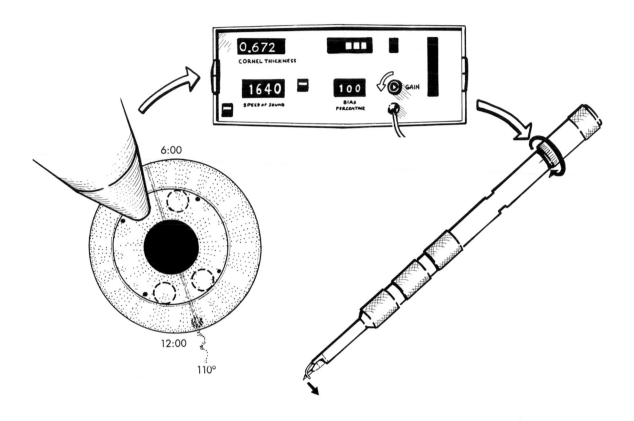

Intraoperative ultrasonic pachometry. If a fixed depth of the wound is part of the surgical plan, measurement of corneal thickness in the area of the incisions is carried out and recorded. The length of the knife blade is determined by the surgeon's nomogram, experience, and instruments.

FIGURE 32-39   MAKING THE INCISION

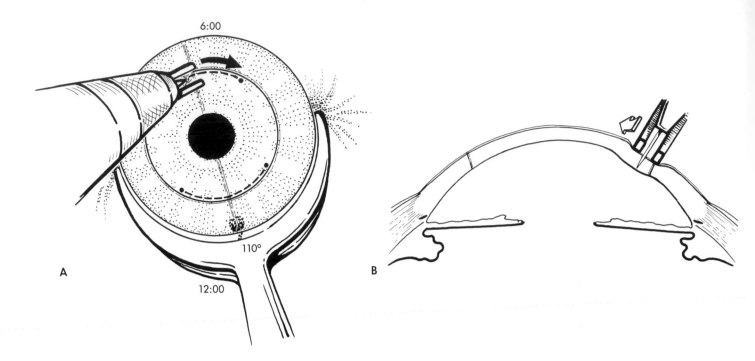

Making the incision. A, The surgeon can see the cutting edge of a vertical back-cutting blade easier; this is the knife preferred for these incisions. **B,** The incision is made by rotating the knife between the fingers to follow the arc, with moderate indentation of the cornea (see Fig. 32-26).

FIGURE 32-40   DEPTH OF RELAXING INCISION

Depth of relaxing incision. As with other types of keratotomy, the flattening of the steep meridian is affected by the depth of the incision. When incisions become very deep, more than 80%, the inner edge of the cut tissue tends to displace anteriorly, and this gaping can cause overcorrection and slow wound healing.

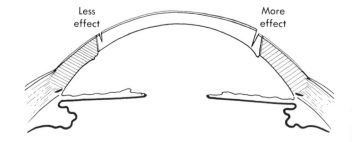

FIGURE 32-41 COMPRESSION SUTURES

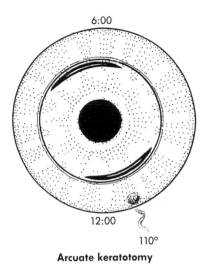

Arcuate keratotomy

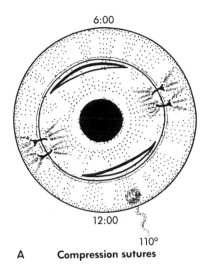

A   Compression sutures

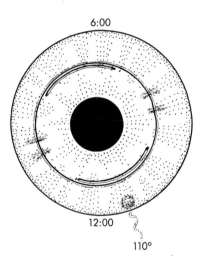

B   Compression sutures removed

Compression sutures. A, Compression sutures placed in the flat meridian and tied moderately tightly will pull open the arcuate relaxing incisions. Tighter sutures produce more gaping. **B,** The sutures can be removed either selectively to titrate the effect or all at once to achieve a final effect. If sutures are to be left in place indefinitely to try to control the final amount of astigmatism, it might be preferable to use a nonabsorbable suture such as polyester (Mersilene), although it lacks the elasticity to conform to changes in wound volume.

FIGURE 32-42   INTRAOPERATIVE TITRATION OF INCISION
LENGTH AND DEPTH

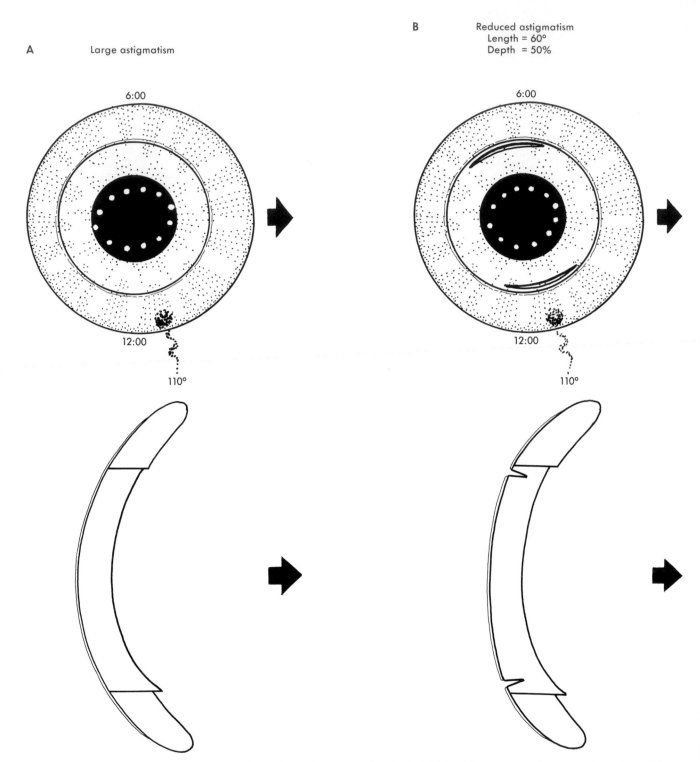

A   Large astigmatism

B   Reduced astigmatism
Length = 60°
Depth = 50%

6:00

12:00

110°

6:00

12:00

110°

Intraoperative titration of incision length and depth. The surgeon can use intraoperative keratometry or keratoscopy to monitor the effects of the transverse incisions as they are made. **A,** The steep meridian is at 110° as shown by the oval qualitative keratoscopy mires. The cross section shows variable approximation of the donor and host posterior wound.

B, The initial incisions are made approximately 60° long at a depth of approximately 50% of the corneal thickness. It is not necessary to use ultrasonic pachometry to measure this depth because this is an initial approximation; the knife blade can be set arbitrarily at an extension of approximately 300 μm. After the incisions are made just inside the keratoplasty wound, the keratoscopy mires are still slightly oval, indicating residual astigmatism in the steep 110° meridian.

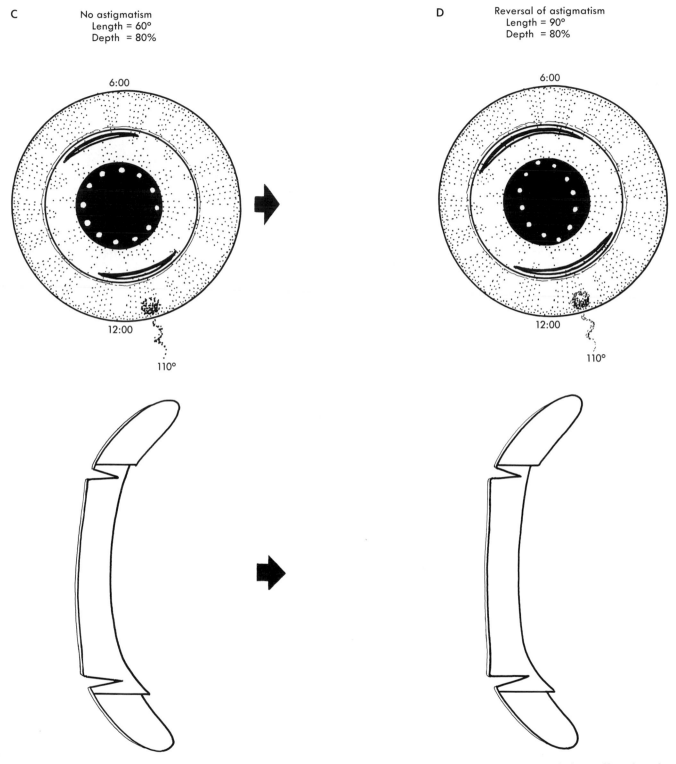

C
No astigmatism
Length = 60°
Depth = 80%

D
Reversal of astigmatism
Length = 90°
Depth = 80%

6:00

12:00

110°

6:00

12:00

110°

C, The knife blade is advanced approximately 100 μm and the depth increased to approximately 80% of the corneal thickness, resulting in round keratoscopy mires and the disappearance of astigmatism. The amount of deepening of the incisions is dictated by the shape of the keratoscopy mires. Two or three deepenings may be necessary to effect the desired change.

D, Since some overcorrection is needed to offset the effect of wound healing, the incisions are extended a small amount at each end until the keratoscopy mires become oval with the flat direction in the 110° meridian. The amount of lengthening of the incisions is determined intraoperatively by the shape of the keratoscopy mires. An alternative approach is to stage the surgical instruments over a series of procedures, lengthening or deepening the incisions as needed.

UNFINISHED BUSINESS

The results of astigmatic keratotomy are less predictable than those of radial keratotomy, emphasizing the need for better preoperative planning and intraoperative execution. Improved methods of identifying the steep meridian would help the surgeon orient the incisions more accurately. Methods of titrating the surgery should be studied in more detail, with more careful intraoperative monitoring and the use of prospective randomized trials to compare different techniques. Improved markers for astigmatic surgery might decrease some of the inaccuracy. More experience with newer knife blade and footplate designs, such as the Thornton rectangular blade, will demonstrate whether these improve the results of astigmatic keratotomy. Reports of surgical techniques of astigmatic keratotomy should be detailed, particularly those techniques using intraoperative keratoscopy and keratometry, so that they can be replicated and the results interpreted more accurately.

Biomechanics of Transverse Incisions of the Cornea

Theo Seiler

The main elements of astigmatism surgery of the cornea are straight or arcuate transverse incisions. I present here a biomechanical theory that explains the flattening of the cornea in the meridian perpendicular to the incisions and the steepening 90 degrees away.

GENERAL CONCEPTS

Because of the incisions, the stress in the deeper, nonincised corneal layers increases up to 20-fold, depending on the incision's depth. This greater stress results in increased strain on the nonlinear viscoelastic cornea, leading to a greater curvature radius and consequent flattening of the incised meridian. Quantitative calculations of astigmatic changes, as demonstrated in this chapter, show a strong dependence on incision depth. According to Poisson's ratio, a contraction of the unincised meridian explains the steepening effect. Unfortunately, the value of Poisson's ratio has not been determined for the cornea; however, in making an analogy to other biologic materials, an approximate value between 0.3 and 0.7, probably 0.5, is suggested.

The factors involved in experimentally and clinically corrected astigmatism are in agreement with biomechanical theory. Geometric parameters, such as incision zone diameter and incision length, are theoretically studied and compared with clinical data in this chapter.

BIOMECHANICAL COMPUTATIONS

In a simple approach, the cornea behaves as a viscoelastic spheric shell. Because of intraocular pressure (IOP) in the normal eye, corneal tissue is pre-

BACKGROUND AND ACKNOWLEDGMENTS
Theo Seiler has both a Ph.D. in physics and an M.D. degree and is thus able to integrate both biomechanical and physiological processes to increase our understanding of the effects of transverse keratotomy. In addition to his clinical responsibilities as professor of ophthalmology at the Charlottenburg Clinic in Berlin, Seiler maintains an active research laboratory affiliated with the Freie University, where he works not only on corneal biomechanics, but also on laser corneal surgery and magnetic resonance imaging.

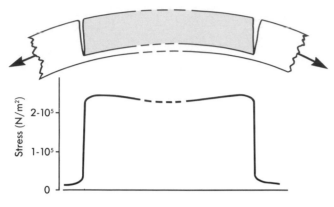

Figure 33-1
Stress distribution inside the incised cornea. The stress of the posterior layers increases in the area between the incisions because the tension is borne only by the unincised layers of the cornea.

Table 33-1

Standard Geometric Values for the Human Cornea

Corneal measurement	Value (mean ± SD)
Thickness	
Central	0.52 ±0.04 mm
Peripheral	0.65 mm
Anterior diameter	
Horizontal	11.7 ±0.25 mm
Vertical	10.5 ±0.25 mm
Central curvature radius	
Anterior	7.86 ±0.26 mm
Posterior	6.5 to 6.8 mm

stretched to a linear strain of 0.8%.[3] For an inflated spheric shell with an approximate internal pressure of p_i, inner radius of R_i, and an outer radii R_e, where $R_i < r < R_e$, the circumferential stress (σ_c) has the following distribution[19]:

$$\sigma_c = p_i \cdot [2 + (R_e/r)^3]/[2 \cdot (1 - (R_e/R_i)^3] \quad (1)$$

When approximating to an infinitesimal thickness, $h = R_e - R_i << R_i R_e = R$, this formula reduces to the well-known Laplace's law:

$$\sigma_c = p_i \cdot R/2h \quad (2)$$

With the standard values of the cornea (Table 33-1), formula *1* yields for the circumferential stresses,

$$\sigma_{c,i} = 12.840 \text{ N/m and } \sigma_{c,e} = 11840 \text{ N/m} \quad (3)$$

at the posterior and anterior surfaces of the cornea, respectively. As this holds only for a spheric approximation, the inner radius of corneal curvature ($R_i = 6.65$ mm) was used, whereas for R_e only the central thickness of the cornea (0.52 mm) was added to R_i.

When performing transverse incisions into the cornea at a depth of x%, the stress originating from IOP is unchanged. Because the tissue between the incisions is mechanically decoupled from the limbus, only the untouched deeper layers bear the stress. Therefore the stress in these remaining layers of the thickness increases (Fig. 33-1):

$$h = 0.52 \text{ mm} \cdot (100 - x)/100$$

This assumption may be justified by the observation that the cornea has a very low shear modulus. Maurice[8] points out that the stroma has little resistance to shear forces, in contrast to the sclera. This low shear modulus can be explained by the structure of the stro-

mal lamellae that run parallel to the corneal surface and are minimally interwoven. Therefore the anterior and posterior surfaces of the cornea may slide quite freely relative to one another. Table 33-2 lists the stress at the posterior corneal surface as a function of incision depth. The values are obtained by using the first formula in this section.

The increased stress leads to increased strain on the nonincised layers. To calculate the strain ϵ(x%), the elastic properties of the cornea must be considered. Biologic tissues show a nonlinear elasticity, including the effect of stress-induced stiffening, which implies that constant increments of stress produce successively smaller increments of strain; the material resists further stretching more forcefully as it is stressed. A formula describing this behavior was suggested by Kenedi, Gibson, and Daly[4]:

$$\epsilon = \alpha^{-1} \ln (\alpha/A + 1) \quad (4)$$

Nash, Greene, and Foster[9] showed that this equation holds true for the cornea for stresses up to more than 200,000 N/m^2. For determination of the constants A and α (exponential stiffening constant), the authors used strips of swollen corneas but claimed that at least α does not depend on stromal swelling. Thus their value for α can be accepted:

$$\alpha = 59.12 \pm 3.47$$

In contrast to α, the constant A must be applied to the standard in vivo situation. Using data of Jue and Maurice[3] yields the following value for A:

$$A = 21224 \text{ N/m}^2$$

With these assumptions, the resulting strain ϵ(x%) can be calculated from formula *4*.

Table 33-2

Stress (σ) at Posterior Corneal Surface as a Function of Incision Depth

Incision depth (% of corneal thickness)	Stress (N/m²)
0	$\sigma(0) = 12.835$
50	$\sigma(50) = 25.596$
75	$\sigma(75) = 51.181$
90	$\sigma(90) = 128.958$
95	$\sigma(95) = 255.715$

Table 33-4

Flattening of Corneal Anterior Surface in Diopters as a Function of Incision Depth

Incision depth (% of corneal thickness)	Flattening (D)
0	$P(0) = 0$
50	$P(50) = -0.51$
75	$P(75) = -1.16$
90	$P(90) = -1.93$
95	$P(95) = -2.64$

Table 33-3

Total Strain (ε) of Posterior Corneal Surface as a Function of Incision Depth

Incision depth (% of corneal thickness)	Strain (%)
0	$\epsilon(0) = 0.8$
50	$\epsilon(50) = 2.72$
75	$\epsilon(75) = 4.26$
90	$\epsilon(90) = 6.78$
95	$\epsilon(95) = 8.96$

Another effect complicates the biomechanical processes within the incised cornea. Besides the nonlinear elasticity, previous studies of corneal mechanics describe rheologic or viscoelastic properties in the plane of the surfaces.[9,11] Under a constantly applied stress, a continuous stretching of the cornea occurs, sometimes termed *creep*. This viscoelastic extension is reported to vary from twice to three times the instantaneous (elastic) strain. However, shear spectrometry shows evidence that the viscous component varies from three to six times the elastic component.[15] Thus we will assume the viscoelastic strain to be twice the elastic (immediate) strain, a rather conservative estimate. Using these data, the final strain on the expanded cornea in the meridian perpendicular to the incision can be calculated and correlated with the incision depth (Table 33-3).

The expansion of a spheric shell produces an increase in its radius of curvature:

$$\epsilon = \Delta L/L = \Delta R/R \qquad (5)$$

From the strains listed in Table 33-3, we can calculate the flattening of the posterior surface of the cornea directly. We chose the approximation for the posterior surface because in refractive keratotomy the posterior

cornea remains unincised. The anterior radius of curvature is determined by addition of the standard difference, $R_e - R_i = 1.21$ mm; this holds at least for the central part of the cornea. Table 33-4 demonstrates the refractive changes induced by the described flattening of the anterior surface. The strong dependence on incision depth, especially at greater depths, is obvious.

As already mentioned, besides the flattening of the cornea in one direction, there is some steepening in the unincised meridian 90° away. This effect can be explained by the so-called transverse contraction. Although the longitudinal incised dimension increases in a uniaxial tensile stress situation, the transverse unincised dimensions decrease. Therefore, transverse strains are associated with the longitudinal strain but are negative to signify contraction. Poisson's ratio is a

$$\text{Poisson's ratio} = \frac{\text{transverse strain}}{\text{longitudinal strain}}$$

constant for elastic and some viscoelastic materials. To our knowledge, Poisson's ratio for the cornea (surface parallel) has not yet been determined. In similar tissues, such as vessel walls, Poisson's ratio has values of 0.25 to 0.75.[12] If we assume the cornea to be almost incompressible, as has been proved for the sclera, values of approximately 0.5 can be expected. As already demonstrated, after transverse incisions the cornea undergoes an extension that leads to flattening in the incised meridian. With a Poisson's ratio of 0.5, a contraction in the unincised meridian 90° away must occur and amounts to 50% of the extension (Fig. 33-2). Consequently the curvature in this meridian increases and there is a steepening of about 45% of the flattening. Thus the total astigmatic correction is 1.45 times the amount caused by the flattening listed in Table 33-4. The overall astigmatism change correlated to the incision depth is shown in Fig. 33-3.

So far the geometric dimensions of the incisions and their influence on the refractive change have not

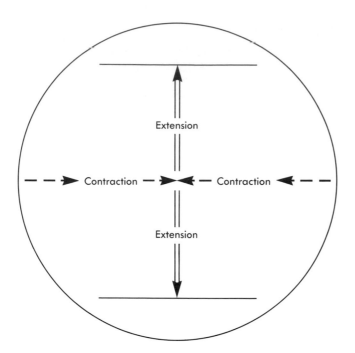

Figure 33-2

Mechanical processes induced by transverse incisions. Although extension produces flattening in the meridian perpendicular to the incisions, this effect is associated with transverse contraction leading to steepening 90° away from the incised meridian.

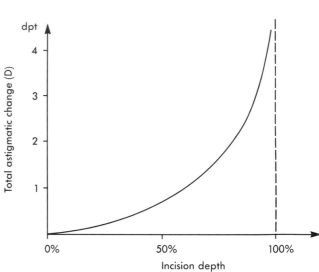

Figure 33-3

Total astigmatism change as a function of incision depth. The values are calculated for straight incisions 5 mm long and a zone diameter of 6 mm. In the region of interest (incision depths greater than 90%) the curve is very steep and small variations in incision depth greatly affect changes in refractive outcome.

Figure 33-4

Flattening effect in central cornea by incisions of different length and location. Larger diameter zones result in a decrease of refractive change, but for identical angular lengths *(0)* nearly identical refractive changes are achieved. The calculations were carried out for incision depths of 95% local corneal thickness.

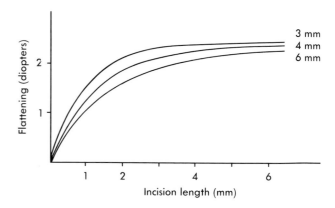

been considered. Undoubtedly the effect depends on the total amount of incised corneal lamellae. To calculate the changes at the central cornea, we will assume that the lamellae cross the center more or less radially. Each of these lamellae bears a stress, which in a physical view is a vector; this means the stress includes a component in the alpha-direction. Setting the alpha-direction as the symmetry meridian of the incisions (of the length 2 γ), the total stress $\sigma(x\%)$ in the alpha-direction can be calculated by integration:

$$\sigma(x\%) = 2\,\sigma_0 + 2\,(\sigma_1 - \sigma_0)\cdot\sin\gamma \qquad (5)$$

where σ_0 is the stress in the nonincised area, σ_1 is the stress in the incised area, and γ is the angular length of incisions.

Using the previously described formulas, the resulting strain and refractive change can be calculated. Fig. 33-4 demonstrates the flattening effect for several combinations of zone diameter and lengths of straight incisions (incision depth = 95%).

COMPARISON OF BIOMECHANICAL THEORY AND PUBLISHED STUDIES

Clinical and experimental studies have gathered data on transverse corneal incisions (see Chapter 31, Keratotomy for Astigmatism).

Fenzl[1] reported clinical experience with transverse incisions 4 to 5 mm long and with a 5-mm zone, as made by Fyodorov. Astigmatism corrections of 3.26 ± 0.35 D were obtained, but the incision depth was not stated. In comparison with other studies, this standard deviation is extremely small.

Nordan[10] reported 85% as the optimal depth of incisions when he applied transverse cuts to corneas astigmatic up to 3.5 D.

Lundergan and Rowsey[7] performed systematic experiments on eye bank eyes with swollen corneas. They made circular incisions of 30° to 90° length and a zone of 7.5 mm. With 60° incisions they found flattening of −3.15 D and steepening of +1.50 D, with variabilities of about ±2.00 D. The incision depth varied from 66% to 90%. When 30° incisions were made, the corneal flattening was −1.08 D with a negligible steepening 90° away. The effect increased greatly when 90° cuts were made; the authors observed flattening of −9.10 D and steepening of +4.90 D. The obtained astigmatism corrections in these swollen human donor corneas correspond well with those expected by our biomechanical theory, except for very long incisions of 90°. At 90° the effects are higher than predicted, but even then the flattening/steepening ratio is 2:1, close to our theoretic value of 2.3:1.

Terry and Rowsey[17] made 2.5 mm transverse incisions 8 mm apart in unswollen corneas. The depth of the cuts was 75% to 99% of local corneal thickness. Flattening in the meridian perpendicular to the incisions was −2.00 D, but steepening was greater than 3.00 D. Although the flattening effect agrees closely with theory, the amount of steepening is quite different.

In all these reports, astigmatism correction varied greatly, and no correlation between incision depths and refractive change was established. On the other hand, Jester et al.[2] demonstrated that incision depth was the parameter most significant for refractive outcome in radial incisions. However, this strong dependence on incision depth may be the reason for the extreme spread and therefore unreliable changes in refraction. As seen in Fig. 33-3, a difference in incision depth, such as 95% versus 90%, leads to astigmatism changes of 3.8 D versus 2.8 D, an increase of more than 35%. From these data we therefore must conclude that to obtain more reliable results, we need to find ways to adjust incision depth better, such as excimer laser keratectomy[16] (see Chapter 19, Laser Corneal Surgery).

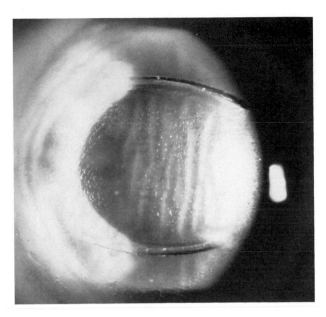

Figure 33-5
Folds in the deeper layers of the stroma after transverse excisions (IOP = 50 mm Hg). When increasing the IOP the posterior corneal folds can be seen clearly.

Lindquist and colleagues[6] discuss the influence of the geometric dimensions of transverse cuts on refractive outcome. The authors state that zone diameter is not as important as it is in radial keratotomy. A maximal effect is achieved when the transverse incisions are placed coincident with a 5-mm zone mark. Thornton[18] suggests that using shorter incisions with a smaller diameter zone gives the same astigmatism change as using longer transverse incisions placed at a larger diameter zone. This corresponds exactly with our theory, as shown in Fig. 33-4.

Clinical experience points out that refractive outcome is influenced by the patient's age.[6] With identical procedures, the change in astigmatism in an eye of an 80-year-old person is twice that of a 30-year-old person. This may be explained by variations in the elastic parameters of the cornea, but a convincing analysis of the effect of age on the elastic constants is unfortunately not yet available.

A fundamental premise of the biomechanical model presented here is the thinning of the stress-bearing layers by incisions, which leads to an extension of the unincised layers of corneal stroma. To verify this assumption, Fig. 33-5 shows data on an enucleated eye with two transverse excisions (depth, 85%). When pressure is increased to 50 mm Hg, the posterior surface folds may resemble a rubber foil that is stretched in one direction. The folds occur only in the deeper, unincised layers of the stroma and Descemet's membrane.

LIMITATIONS OF THE BIOMECHANICAL MODEL

The theoretical model presented here has its limitations. First, the theory suffers from a lack of knowledge on biomechanical constants of the cornea, such as Poisson's ratio and the linear or viscoelastic properties. Second, the model starts from a more or less isotropic radial distribution of the stromal lamellae. This might be correct for the center of the cornea but is definitely incorrect in the periphery.

Nevertheless, the theory in its present state can provide understanding of the parameters that govern biomechanical processes during astigmatism surgery.

REFERENCES

1. Fenzl RE: Control of astigmatism using corneal incisions. In Sanders D and Hofmann R, editors: Refractive surgery: a text of radial keratotomy, Thorofare, NJ, 1985, Slack, Inc, pp 151-165.
2. Jester J, Venet T, Lee J, et al: A statistical analysis of radial keratotomy in human cadaver eyes, Am J Ophthalmol 1981;92:172-177.
3. Jue B and Maurice D: The mechanical properties of the rabbit and human cornea, J Biomech 1986;19:1-7.
4. Kenedi R, Gibson T, and Daly G: Structure and function of connective and skeletal tissue. In Fung Y: Biomechanics, New York, 1981, Springer-Verlag New York, Inc, p 226.
5. Lans LJ: Experimentelle Untersuchungen über Entstehung von Astigmatismus durch nicht-perforierende Corneawunden, A von Graefes Arch Ophthalmol 1898;45:117-152.
6. Lindquist T, Rubenstein J, and Lindström R: Keratotomy for corneal astigmatism, Semin Ophthalmol 1986;1:246-253.
7. Lundergan M and Rowsey J: Relaxing incisions: corneal topography, Ophthalmology 1985;92:1226-1236.
8. Maurice D: The cornea and sclera. In Davson H, editor: The eye, Orlando, Fla, 1984, Academic Press, Inc, pp 1-158.
9. Nash J, Greene P, and Foster S: Comparison of mechanical properties of keratoconus and normal corneas, Exp Eye Res 1982;35:413-423.
10. Nordan L: Quantifiable astigmatism correcting: concepts and suggestions, J Cataract Refract Surg 1986;12:507-518.
11. Nyquist G: Rheology of the cornea: experimental techniques and results, Exp Eye Res 1968;7:183-188.
12. Patel D and Voishnov R: Basic hemodynamics, Baltimore, 1980, University Park Press, p 208.
13. Rowsey J: Current concepts in astigmatism surgery, J Refract Surg 1986;2:85-94.
14. Schiötz H: Ein Fall von hochgradigem Hornhautastigmatismus, Arch für Augenheilk 1885;15:178-181.
15. Seiler T: Laserchirurgie der Kornea, Habilitationsschrift, 1987, Freie Universität Berlin.
16. Seiler T, Bende T, Wollensak J, and Trokel S: Excimer laser keratectomy for correction of astigmatism, Am J Ophthalmol 1988;105:117-124.
17. Terry M and Rowsey J: Dynamic shifts in corneal topography during modified Ruiz procedure for astigmatism, Arch Ophthalmol 1986;104:1611-1616.
18. Thornton SP and Sanders DR: Graded nonintersecting transverse incisions for correction of idiopathic astigmatism, J Cataract Refract Surg 1987;13:27-31.
19. Timoshenko S: Theory of elasticity, New York, 1934, McGraw-Hill, pp 323-326.

Computer Simulation of Arcuate Keratotomy for Astigmatism

Khalil D. Hanna
Francois E. Jouve
George O. Waring III
Philippe G. Ciarlet

STAGES IN DEVELOPMENT OF MATHEMATIC MODELS OF KERATOTOMY

The development of new surgical techniques in general, and of refractive corneal surgery in particular, involves numerous attempts to isolate the effect of individual factors on the surgical outcome. Methods include laboratory evaluation in enucleated human or animal eyes, experiments in living animals, and experimental investigation in humans. Computer simulation of refractive keratotomy allows the surgeon to alter variables of the technique and to isolate the effect of specific factors independent of other factors, something that cannot easily be done in any of the currently available experimental models.

In its current state of development, computer simulation is applicable only to assess the instantaneous change immediately after the incisions are made (the elastic change independent of time). It does not purport to simulate fully the clinical situation of keratotomy surgery, which also involves viscoelastic re-

BACKGROUND AND ACKNOWLEDGMENTS
The collaborative effort among ophthalmologists and mathematicians that yields sophisticated models is well illustrated by this chapter. We have mentioned the background and other collaborators in this work in our acknowledgments in Chapter 29. The anisotropic model presented in this chapter is the most sophisticated model of corneal surgery to be published as of 1991. The model is based now on the ultrastructure of the cornea and is being generalized to model the entire globe. Some of the fundamental definitions in the model are presented in Chapter 29, Preliminary Computer Simulation of Radial Keratotomy, and are not repeated here.

sponses (as can be represented by human cadaver eye experiments), and wound healing responses as would affect the outcome of surgery in living animals or humans.

Our computer model has developed through numerous phases. The initial two-dimensional computer model of superficial keratectomy assumed that the corneoscleral shell obeyed Hooke's law, which states that the stress tensor is a linear function of the strain tensor. This early model also assumed that the corneoscleral shell was isotropic, that is, that the mechanical properties were identical in all directions.[10] The second step in development was to create a three-dimensional nonlinear model that still assumed the tissue to be isotropic, but acknowledged the fact that the response of biologic tissues is truly nonlinear. This was applied to radial keratotomy[12] in Chapter 29, Preliminary Computer Simulation of Radial Keratotomy.

The third model assumes tissues are nonlinearly elastic and anisotropic. We published a first approximation of this model in describing the effect of limbal incisions.[11] In this chapter we take the anisotropic assumption further. "Transversal isotropia" takes into account the fibrillar structure of the cornea and sclera but assumes that the collagen fibrils are arrayed in lamellae parallel to the surface in both tissues. We are aware that the superficial cornea and the sclera do not have such an ideal structure, and therefore this assumption is still an approximation.

Our finite element computer model gives reasonably accurate information about the relative effects of different surgical variables but only approximates information about the absolute refractive effect in diopters. Therefore the absolute refractive values presented in the text cannot be directly applied to clinical surgery.

The effect of paired arcuate incisions for the correction of astigmatism was described in eye bank eyes[5,15,27] and in living human eyes.[17] These papers are discussed in Chapter 31, Keratotomy for Astigmatism. All these studies address the effect of the length of the incisions, the distance of the incisions from the centering point, and the number of incisions. There are no specific data on variable depth of the incisions or variables such as age, intraocular pressure, and preexisting corneal curvature.

DESCRIPTION OF THE MATHEMATIC MODEL
Assumptions concerning geometry and properties of the eye

The theoretic reference eye was assumed to have naturally occurring corneal astigmatism. The model was designed as symmetric around an anteroposterior plane, not around a single anteroposterior axis as in our previous simulations.[10,12] The simulations were done on a quarter of the eye; to simulate the effect of a single arcuate incision, we used half of the eye because of the asymmetric circumstance created by the single incision. The generally aspheric shape of the cornea and the variation in the thickness of both the cornea and the sclera were considered, as described in detail in previous publications.[8,12,26] We assumed a normal axial length of 23.4 mm and an intraocular pressure of 15 mm Hg (2 kiloPascal).

We made three assumptions about the cornea and sclera: (1) three-dimensional, nonlinear elasticity equations were used to describe the stress-strain relationship accurately; (2) the cornea and sclera were essentially incompressible; and (3) the cornea and sclera were anisotropic. These assumptions were supported in part by publications of other authors.[2,19] We have discussed nonlinear elasticity and incompressibility in a previous publication.[12] We discuss here in more detail the anisotropic behavior of the cornea and sclera.

Anisotropy of the cornea and sclera

An anisotropic tissue is one in which the tissue has an oriented structure, so it exhibits a different amplitude of mechanical response to forces applied from different directions. The anisotropic behavior of the cornea arises from its lamellar and fibrillar structure (see Chapter 2, Corneal Anatomy and Physiology as Applied to Refractive Keratotomy). Nyquist[19] has evaluated the mechanical behavior of the pig's cornea and found that the tissue is anisotropic and behaves as if the fibrils were randomly arrayed parallel to the surface. This indicates that transverse isotropy can be used to describe the behavior of the cornea. However, no published studies have quantified the anisotropic behavior of the human cornea. Battaglioli and Kamm[2] demonstrated in the sclera that the elastic modulus for perpendicular compressive stress was 100 times less than the elastic modulus for circumferential tangential stress.

The tissue we are modeling is the stroma itself (and by extension the sclera), and we do not include in the computations the anisotropic effects of Bowman's layer and Descemet's membrane; that will require a future development.

To compute realistic elastic moduli for an anisotropic model, we used the technique of homogenization mathematically applied to elasticity,[3,6,22,23] taking into account the fibrillar structure of the corneal stroma and of the sclera. An outline of the mathematic approach used in homogenization appears in Appendix A at the end of this chapter. The purpose of homogenization in elasticity allows us to describe macroscopically stress-strain relationships of materials whose microscopic structure is periodic. These techniques are widely used in mechanical engineering for the study of composite materials, such as reinforced concrete and tires. However, there are limitations to using computations of homogenization to describe the corneal stroma because these mathematic techniques in homogenization have been developed only for systems of linear elasticity; when describing tissues, we must apply them to nonlinear elastic behavior.

Macroscopic model of stromal lamellae

The mechanical properties of collagenous tissue, specifically of a collagen lamella, depend on the diameter of the collagen fibrils that constitute the lamella, on their spatial orientation, on their mechanical properties, and on the amount of intrafibrillar proteoglycan ground substance. The hydration of both the collagen fibrils and the ground substance affects the mechanical behavior of the lamella. X-ray diffraction measurements made on wet rat tail tendon (which is composed primarily of collagen type I and ground substance) showed that 55% of the volume of the fiber is occupied by collagen molecules and the remaining 45% by water.[18] Such information is available for fixated human corneal stroma but not for stroma in its normal hydrated state. To compute the elastic coefficients of a stromal lamella, the lamella can be considered as composed of a large number of fibrils of uniform diameter, cylindric shape, and oriented parallel to the long axis of the lamella itself. The collagen fibrils are interspersed among the ground substance, and the spacing of the fibrils is assumed to be uniform, an approximating assumption, even though transmission electron-microscopy demonstrates that the collagen fibrils are not exactly spaced in a perfect lattice.

The collagen fibrils are assumed to have a linear elastic response to small stress with the Young's modulus of $E = 10^{10}$ dynes/cm^2, that is, 10^9 Pascals (Pa).[7] Three coefficients, two Poisson's ratios for the collagen fibrils and ground substance and Young's modulus for ground substance, were defined by computation because no data from measurements are available in the literature. They were adjusted so that the final coefficients for the cornea after mathematic ho-

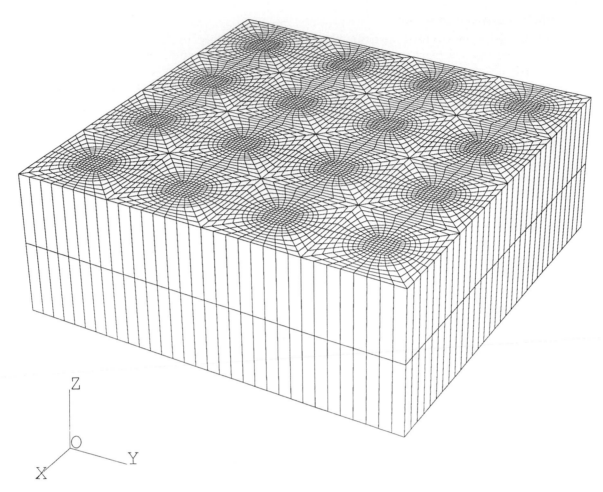

Figure 34-1
Graphic representation of the finite element model of a corneal lamella. The model consists of multiple central zones surrounded by squares. Each central zone represents a collagen fibril in a square that represents the ground substance. The fibrils are assumed to run from one side of a lamella to the other. They are divided into elements along their length. This figure demonstrates two elements along the longitudinal aspect of each fibril; that is, it represents a simple section perpendicular to one lamella.

mogenization match the experimental results of Battaglioli and Kamm,[2] who measured Young's modulus and Poisson's ratio of the sclera in the direction perpendicular to the surfaces. They found values for Young's modulus in the perpendicular direction between 2.69×10^4 Pa and 4.12×10^4 Pa, and for Poisson's ratio between 0.46 and 0.50. We assumed the following values:

υ Poisson's ratio for the collagen fibrils = 0.40

υ Poisson's ratio for ground substance = 0.45

Young's modulus for ground substance = E = 1×10^4 Pa

Although these coefficients were determined by homogenization in linear elasticity, we will use them in this model for computations to simulate the effect of surgery in the framework of nonlinear elasticity.

The finite element method was used to simulate corneal lamellae (Fig 34-1).

We based this on transmission electron micrographs of normal human corneal stroma. We estimated the relative contribution of the collagen fibrils and the ground substance. We found that the fibrils filled approximately 35% of the total volume. We gave an average fibril diameter of 25 nm and an average space between the center of two fibrils of 48 nm, and we assumed that corneal shrinkage induced by fixation was 20%,[20] identical in both collagen fibrils and the ground substance (even though it may be different in reality).

Transversely isotropic model of cornea and sclera

We assumed that the corneal stroma and the sclera were composed of many lamellae that ran parallel to the surface and were randomly arrayed in many directions. We are aware that the sclera does not have the same lamellar structure as the cornea, but we did not make any mathematic distinction between the two for these computations. The difference in mechanical properties of the cornea parallel to the surface as compared with those perpendicular to the surface can be more easily appreciated if one visualizes taking cylindric trephinations out of the cornea, one perpendicular to the surface and one parallel to the surface. Pulling on the cylinder taken perpendicular to the surface will separate the lamellae and give a different set of mechanical properties than pulling on the cylinder taken parallel to the surface, which is almost nondistensible.

We applied the homogenization method of Dumontet to the cornea as a stratified periodic structure (Appendices B and C), and found a value of Young's modulus of $E_1 = 1.1 \times 10^7$ Pa in the direction parallel to the corneal surface. This was not in the approximate range of that reported in the literature, which is between 2.0×10^6 and 5.5×10^6 Pa. But Nyquist[19] found Young's modulus in the direction parallel to the corneal surface as $E_1 = 4.86 \times 10^6$ Pa after stabilization of the experimental process (that is, after integration of long-time viscoelastic effect) and $E_1 = 1.65 \times 10^7$ Pa for the instantaneous Young's modulus. Our value of 1.1×10^7 Pa is in the range of his experimental values.

We estimated coefficients not reported in literature, including Poisson's ratio for collagen fibrils and the ground substance and Young's modulus perpendicular to the surface and for the ground substance using computational analysis. In the direction perpendicular to the surface, we computed Young's modulus as $E_2 = 3.9 \times 10^4$ Pa. Battaglioli and Kamm measured E_2 in the range between 2.69×10^4 Pa and 4.12×10^4 Pa. Values of Poisson's ratio were different in the two directions. Perpendicular to the surface the value was 0.47, and parallel to the surface the value was 0.26.

The respective values of E_1 and E_2 indicated that the cornea is more resistant to deformation parallel to the surface than perpendicular to the surface, where the lamellae can separate to some degree. Poisson's ratios are more complex. Roughly, Poisson's ratio specifies the reaction of the material in a direction when stretched in the direction perpendicular to that being measured. It is a two-dimensional effect, whereas Young's modulus is a one-dimensional effect.

The shear modulus was also computed and found to be 6.4×10^3 Pa.

Finite element computer program

A computer program was developed that used a finite element method (FEM) to discretize the equations of the three-dimensional nonlinear elasticity. Curved elements with 27 nodes were used in the finite element mesh. This curved element is more accurate because of the geometry of the cornea and sclera.

Mesh that covered half of the eye consisted of about 800 elements and 8500 nodes. Two elements were used across the thickness, and more elements were attributed to the 2-mm central zone for accuracy. Newton's method was used to solve the discretized nonlinear equations. Convergence was reached in about 10 iterations. Each iteration involved approximately 22,500 equations and took approximately 150 minutes of central processing unit (CPU) time on an IBM 4381 computer; the disk memory needed to store intermediate results was 150 megabytes of temporary storage. These programs require a supercomputer for practical analysis.

To generate the mesh, we developed several original programs that were more adapted to our needs than the existing programs. Once the three-dimensional mesh of a perfectly axisymmetric eye was obtained, a distortion was generated in the stress-free mesh to create 6.00 D of astigmatism along the vertical 90° meridian when the intraocular pressure was applied as the single force. We ignored other forces, such as the extraocular muscles and eyelids.

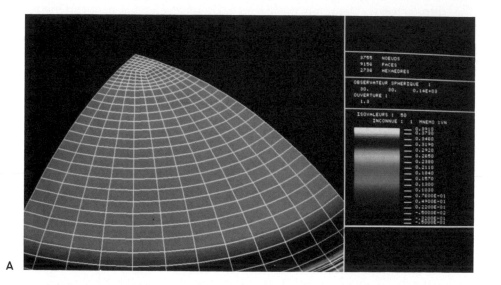

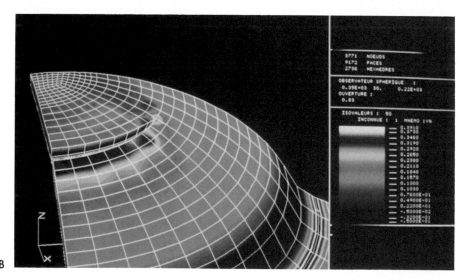

Figure 34-2
Color-coded maps (represented here as various shades of black, white, and gray) of the effect of arcuate transverse keratotomy on stress distribution in the superficial cornea using finite element modeling. White and red indicate more stress, yellow and green indicate moderate stress, and blue represents less stress (dark blue represents negative values of stress). The colors correspond to stress values measured in megapascals. Hoop stress is shown in **A** and **B. A,** There is nearly uniform hoop stress before surgery in the central and paracentral cornea (light blue). Hoop stress at the limbus (dark blue) has a compressive effect. **B,** After arcuate keratotomy, there is more hoop stress on either side of the incision, with the greatest concentration on the outer edge of the incision. Meridional stress is shown in **C** and **D.**

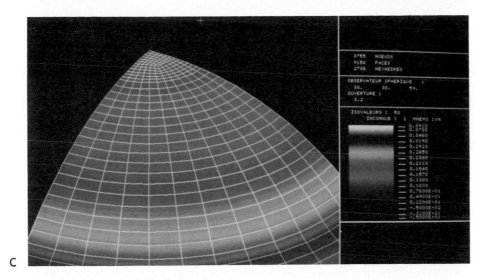

C

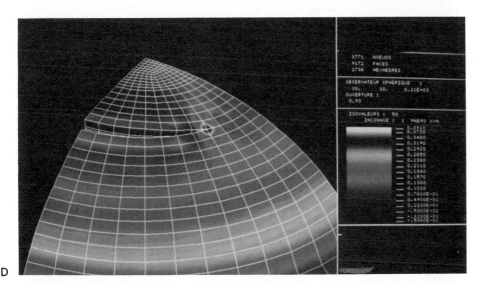

D

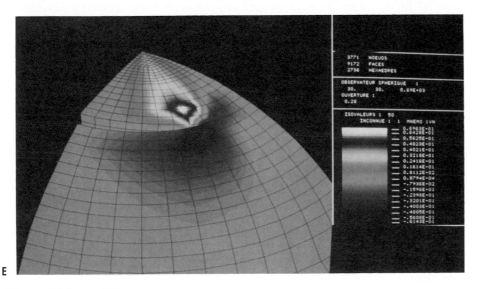

E

Figure 34-2, cont'd
C, Before surgery there is more meridional stress concentrated around the limbus and peripheral cornea (yellow, green) than in the paracentral and central areas (blue). **D,** After arcuate keratotomy, the limbal stress is not disturbed (yellow, green), but there is an increased stress at the ends of the incision (red, yellow spot). **E,** Shear stress. Meridional/hoop stress is one of three types of shear stress; it demonstrates major changes in the area near the end of the incision with no change elsewhere. (See insert for color versions of these illustrations.)

The size of the elements across the thickness of the cornea and sclera was altered to simulate different depths of the incisions; the anterior element was always used to simulate the incision by duplicating the nodes of two neighboring elements in a stress-free mesh (that is, intraocular pressure = 0). The shape was then computed by varying the intraocular pressure. The posterior elements were left intact.

Graphic representation of finite element model

In the figures depicting the finite element mesh, the number of pictorial rectangles does not correspond to the number of brick elements actually present in the finite element model; rather, the pictorial rectangles represent connections of some of the nodes within the bricks themselves. In the cross section pictorial figures, some exaggeration of the displacement of the corneal surface has been made because the displacement is so small that without this exaggeration it would not be visually apparent.

The four types of stresses that we studied in these models have been described in detail in Chapter 29, Preliminary Computer Simulation of Radial Keratotomy. The stresses are hoop (circumferential) stress, meridional (radial) stress, normal (perpendicular) stress, and three shear stresses. The advanced computer program used for arcuate keratotomy in this chapter allows us to present color-coded representations of the different distribution of these stresses (Fig. 34-2).

SIMULATION OF EFFECTS OF ARCUATE TRANSVERSE INCISIONS

We used arcuate transverse incisions rather than straight transverse incisions[13] because the arcuate incision cuts concentric to the center of the cornea across corneal tissue of nearly uniform thickness from one end to the other, whereas a straight transverse incision cuts tangential to a circular zone through cornea of varying thickness. We used either one or two symmetric arcuate incisions. We made incisions perpendicular to the vertical 90° meridian, which was simulated to have 6.00 D of astigmatism when compared with the horizontal 180° meridian parallel to the incision. We varied the length of the incisions as measured in degrees, the depth of the incisions as a percentage of corneal thickness, and the location of the incisions from the center and recorded the change in refractive power along the incised 90° meridian, along the unincised 180° meridian, and along the 135° meridian between the two.

Dioptric powers were calculated using Gullstrand's model of the eye.[9] Curvature changes were evaluated by fitting a nonaxisymmetric surface to the superficial nodes of the mesh over the central 2-mm zone.

Correlation of incision length and arc length

When an arcuate incision is made, there are two ways to express length of the incision, either in degrees of arc or as the linear length along the arc. Figure 34-3 demonstrates the relationship between angular length in degrees and arc length in millimeters. Clearly, an arcuate incision subtending an angular length of 90° is much longer when it is made along an 8-mm zone (6.28 mm) than when it is made along a 4-mm (3.14 mm) zone. Thus when the length of the incision is expressed as angular length, the location of the incision also must be given. The advantage of expressing incision length as angular length is that it is easy to measure clinically, whereas it is difficult to measure the actual arc length in millimeters.

Change in overall curvature

In the center of the clear zone, the meridian perpendicular to the incisions flattened, whereas the meridian parallel to the incisions steepened. In this central area the entire surface of the central cornea was displaced anteriorly. The

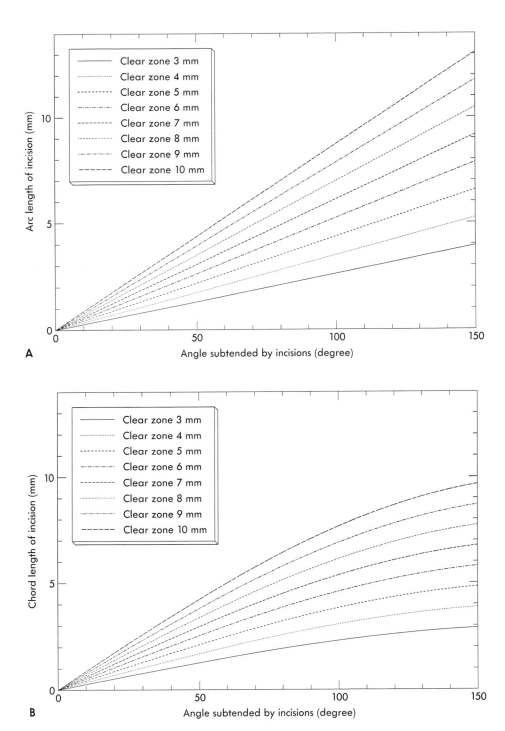

Figure 34-3
Relationship between angular length, arc length, and chord length of an incision.
A, Relationship between angle subtended by an incision and the arc length of the incision for different diameter clear zones. **B,** Relationship between angle subtended by an incision and the chord length of the incision for different diameter zones.

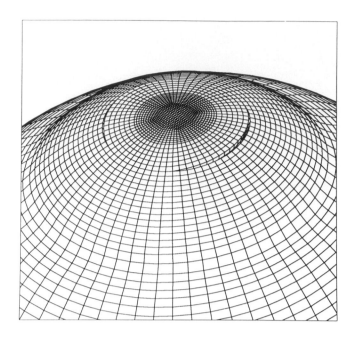

Figure 34-4
Graphic representation of effect of arcuate transverse incisions for astigmatism. A computer-generated, three-dimensional graphic model of the cornea and anterior sclera is composed of a finite element mesh, with more elements for the central 3-mm "optical" zone. Two 120° arcuate incisions at 5-mm diameter clear zone are present. The inner edge of each incision demonstrates an anterior displacement.

changes became more complex in the areas of the incisions, however. The region of the cornea on either side of the incision was displaced forward also and the curvature was steepened compared with that preoperatively. However, the configuration was different on the two sides of the incision, the central side being displaced more anteriorly and elevated greater than the outer edge of the incision (Figs. 34-4 and 34-5). The cross-sectional view of the incision showed a V configuration with the inner edge elevated more anteriorly than the outer edge. Thus, even though the general region of the incisions showed an overall steepening, the tissue adjacent to the central edge of the incision showed a localized flattening. This steepening in the region of the incisions was also present in the peripheral cornea in the incised meridian. The peripheral cornea in the meridian parallel to the incisions demonstrated a posterior displacement and a slight amount of flattening, in contrast to the central zone of the nonincised meridian.

Graphic representation of change in curvature

In the discussion that follows we represent the effect of variables (length, depth, location of incision, and so on) on the curvature of the entire cornea; that is, we represent the combined effect of the incisions on the 90° incised meridian and the 180° parallel meridian. This is comparable to a vectoral analysis of astigmatism in clinical work because it represents the total change in power in all directions on the cornea. Thus the graphs that we use combine the absolute amount of flattening in the vertical meridian and the absolute amount of steepening in the horizontal meridian to produce the total change in power in both meridians, which is plotted on the y-axis (Fig. 34-6). The graphs do not represent the change in refractive astigmatism or only the change in the incised meridian, as might be represented in graphs of results of clinical studies.

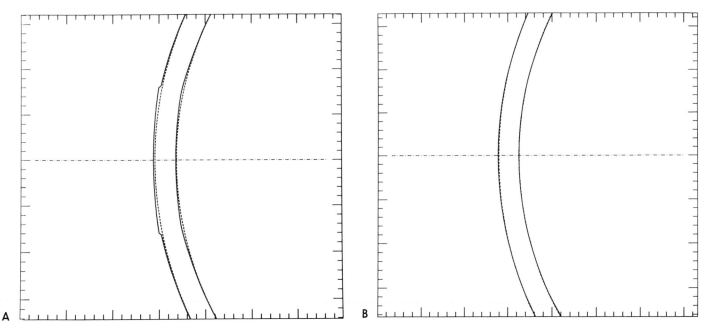

Figure 34-5
A, Cross-sectional view through the 90° incised meridian demonstrates the anterior displacement and central flattening of the cornea. The absolute amount of displacement is exaggerated for pictorial purposes (broken line, original configuration; solid line, configuration after one pair of arcuate transverse incisions). **B,** Cross-sectional view through the 180° unincised meridian demonstrates that the anterior displacement and the steepening effect on the central cornea are much less than at 90°.

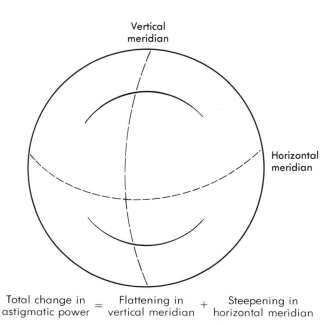

Total change in astigmatic power = Flattening in vertical meridian + Steepening in horizontal meridian

Figure 34-6
Drawing illustrates total change in power in both meridians regardless of the direction of change.

Effect of preexisting corneal curvature and astigmatism

We found no significant effect of preexisting mild and moderate corneal astigmatism on the change in refraction along any meridian for simulated standard incisions, for both mild myopic and hyperopic astigmatism (Fig. 34-7).

Effect of depth of incisions

Simulations were made using a pair of incisions of two arc lengths (60° and 120°) and three different clear zone diameters (3, 5, 7 mm).

All simulations demonstrated that deeper incisions produced a greater change in refraction. However, the amount of change at different depths depended on the diameter of the clear zone and the angular length of the incisions. In general, incisions 30% or less of corneal thickness produced small changes compared with the larger changes produced by incisions 70% depth or greater. Short incisions on the order of 60° or less demonstrated linear relationships with depth of the incision; longer incisions on the order of 120° demonstrated an exponential increase with depth (Fig. 34-8).

We demonstrated in the computer model that the effect of incision depth was a complex one, depending on the length and location of the incision; the depth of the incision had the greatest effect when the incision was long and nearer the center (see Fig. 34-8). This was in contrast to the circumstance in radial keratotomy, in which the incision depth was a simpler variable with more constant effect.[12]

In human studies[17] attempts have been made to standardize the depth of the incision by leaving 0.01 to 0.02 mm of uncut deep stromal tissue, although it was acknowledged that some variability of depth resulted from manual surgical techniques. Eye bank eye models[5,15] have achieved incision depths of 75% to 85% of corneal thickness as verified by selected histologic examination or by slit-lamp microscopy.[20,27]

Seiler and colleagues[25] used an excimer laser to make arcuate transverse excisions to study the effect of the depth of incisions in humans. This study differed from our computer simulation in numerous ways: straight transverse excisions of approximately 150 μm wide were used and viscoelastic changes and wound healing were taken into account. We simulated arcuate incisions theoretically without tissue loss and simulated instantaneous elastic changes only. Nevertheless the effect of depth in the two studies was roughly similar. Laser transverse keratotomy showed an exponential curve in which the incisions had a greatly increased effect of the depth of approximately 85% to 95%.

One advantage of computer simulation is that the depth of the theoretic incision can be determined exactly for every case and it is by definition exactly uniform from one end to the other, whereas in manual or laser cuts made in laboratory experiments or in clinical treatment, there is inherent variability in the depth of the cut along its length and from one cut to another.

Effect of length of incisions

The relative amount of refractive change increased as the length of the incisions increased. The effect was generally small for incisions subtending an arc of 30° or less. Incisions from approximately 45° to 100° long showed a greatly increased effect. Once the length reached approximately 120°, a further increase in length produced a small decrease in effect. Incisions along a larger diameter zone generally had maximum effect at a smaller angular length (approximately 100°), whereas those along a smaller diameter zone had their maximum effect at a larger angular length (approximately 120°) (Fig. 34-9). The effect of incision length on the meridian parallel to the incision was slightly different. The steepening in that meridian increased as the incision lengthened to an inflection

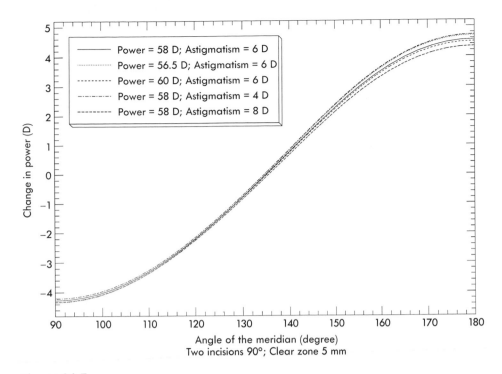

Figure 34-7

There was nearly no effect of preexisting corneal power and astigmatism on the effect of arcuate incisions. The graph represents simulation of two arcuate incisions 90% deep, subtending an arc of 90° along a clear zone diameter of 5 mm in an eye with different astigmatism and different refractive power. The y-axis indicates change in total corneal power.

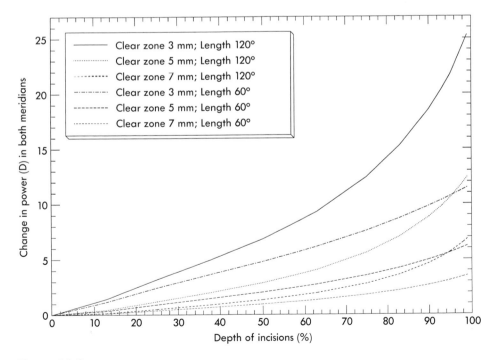

Figure 34-8

Relationship between the depth of two arcuate incisions and the change in refractive power at six different clear zone diameters and two different arc lengths of incisions, 60° and 120°. Varying the depth of the incision has a greater effect on the refraction when the incision is longer. Note that the change in power represented on the y-axis is the absolute combined values of the change in the vertical meridian plus the change in the horizontal meridian to represent the total effect of the arcuate incisions.

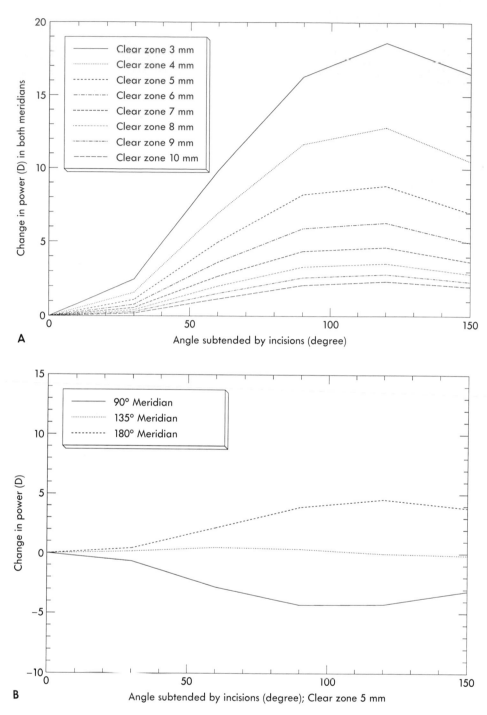

Figure 34-9

Effect of incision length. **A,** Comparison between the angular length of two arcuate incisions, 90% deep, and the change in refractive power for eight different clear zone diameters. The change in power is roughly proportionate to the length of the incision between approximately 30° and 90°. Simulation is for two arcuate incisions, 90% deep. Note that the change in power represented on the y-axis is the absolute combined values of the change in the vertical meridian plus the change in the horizontal meridian to represent the total effect of the arcuate incisions. **B,** The effect of the increase of the angular length along a single clear zone (5 mm), demonstrating the effect in the incised meridian, the unincised meridian, and the meridian in between. **C,** The steepening effect in the unincised meridian increased after the inflection point when clear zones of small diameter (for example, 3 mm) were used.

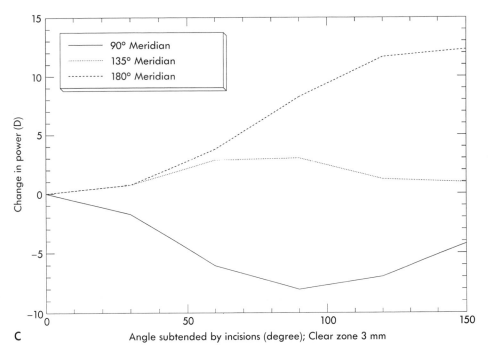

Figure 34-9, cont'd
For legend see opposite page.

point, after which a longer incision produced less steepening except in small clear zones (see Fig. 34-9, *C*).

The longer the incision, the greater the effect of its location (Fig. 34-9). An incision subtending an arc of 120° along a zone diameter of 4 mm had approximately twice the effect of an incision subtending an arc of 60° along the same 4-mm zone.

Extending the incision beyond the inflection point at small clear zones produced an overall steepening of the cornea and a general shift of the spherical equivalent refraction in a myopic direction.

We simulated the effect of incisions from 30° to 180° in length. In general, previously published[5,17,27] studies were in agreement with our simulation of the effect of incisions.

Effect of clear zone diameter

The location of the incision is commonly expressed as the diameter of the circular zone along which the arcuate incision is made. For example, the location of incisions can be designated as along the 6-mm zone, as 6 mm apart, or at a radius of 3 mm.

In general, the smaller the diameter of the clear zone, the greater the effect of the incision (Fig. 34-10). The change in refractive power in the incised meridian is roughly proportionate to the zone diameter between 3 mm and 6 mm. However, the refractive effect also depends on the length of the incision, and the optimal clear zone moves toward greater diameter when the angular length diminishes (Fig. 34-10). Longer incisions and smaller diameters produce larger changes in refraction.

All previously published studies[5,15,17,27] have found an approximate linear relationship between the diameter of the clear zone and the change in astigmatism, from diameters of approximately 5 to 8 mm, the smaller zone having a

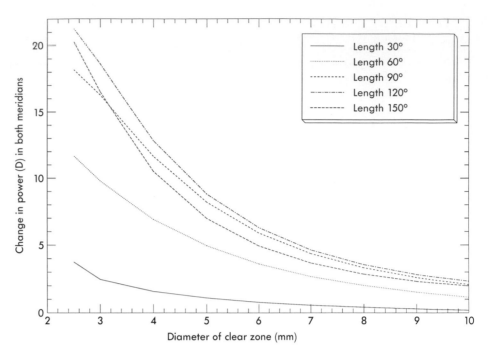

Figure 34-10
Relationship between the diameter of the clear zone and the change in refractive power for incisions of varying angular length (two arcuate incisions, 90% deep). Smaller diameter clear zones and longer incisions induce a greater change in refractive power. Effect is approximately linear between zone diameters of 3 to 7 mm— the "sweet spot." The optimal clear zone is inversely proportionate to the angular length. Note that the change in power represented on the y-axis is the absolute combined values of the change in the vertical meridian plus the change in the horizontal meridian to represent the total effect of the arcuate incisions.

greater effect. Although smaller zones are not used in human surgery because incisions would be close to the center of the cornea and more likely to produce glare, we found that the largest change was reached at a 3-mm diameter zone. It is more difficult to make an arcuate incision of a uniform depth at a small zone diameter.

Number of incisions

Most of our simulations were carried out with two arcuate incisions placed equidistantly from the center along the single circular zone perpendicular to the steep meridian at 90°. We also studied the effect of a single incision (Fig. 34-11) placed in the superior portion of the cornea perpendicular to the 90° semimeridian. This incision demonstrated an exaggerated steepening effect in the inferior semimeridian and tilting of the cornea around the visual axis with minimal change in the 180° meridian parallel to the incision. We also simulated the use of two pairs of incisions (a total of four) (Fig. 34-12) and of three pairs of incisions (a total of six), demonstrating that the additional incisions produced minor change in central corneal curvature when the first pair was of maximum optimal length (120°). The additional incisions did produce some increased steepening in the area of the incisions themselves. As more incisions were added, the peripheral incisions gaped more and there was anterior displacement of the paracentral and peripheral cornea, more on the inner side of the incisions than on the outer side.

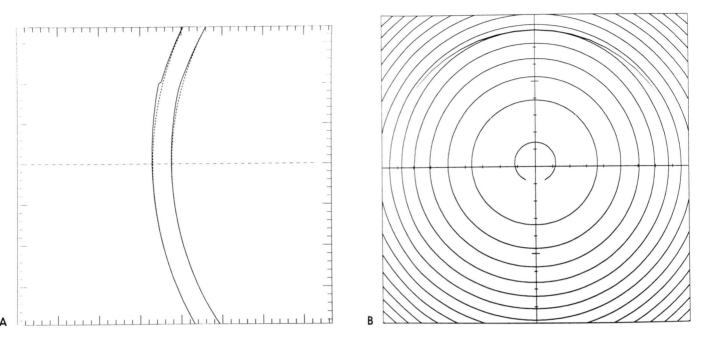

Figure 34-11
Effect of one arcuate incision on the refractive power. **A,** Drawing illustrates the effect on a cross section through the 90° incised meridian (broken line, original configuration; solid line, configuration after one arcuate transverse incision). One incision induces an asymmetric change in refractive power in the incised meridian. **B,** Computer drawing of one arcuate incision across the superior semimeridian shows displacement of the center of the cornea (the cross hairs).

Both human and eye bank eye studies report only the results of one pair of arcuate incisions. However, Lindquist and colleagues[14,21] have demonstrated that virtually all of the flattening effect in the incised meridian was achieved with the first two incisions and that the addition of more incisions parallel to the first two had a minimal additional effect on flattening, although it was possible that additional incisions may create a smoother contour of the corneal surface along that meridian. Our computer model demonstrated similar findings. Thus there seems to be little basis for using more than one pair of incisions of maximum length, depth, and location.

Effect of intraocular pressure

As the intraocular pressure increased from 7 to 25 mm Hg, there was almost a linear correlation with change in refraction (Fig. 34-13), and refractive changes were doubled in value when the intraocular pressure varied from 10 to 23 mm Hg.

This finding makes sense on the assumption that it is the intraocular pressure within the physiologic range that is the motivating force producing the change in corneal shape after incisions. However, it is at odds with clinical studies of refractive keratotomy in which the effect of intraocular pressure in the physiologic range has not been demonstrated to correlate with the refractive outcome based on regression analysis.[1,16,24] The reason for this discrepancy is unknown. Possible explanations include our inability to measure the true effect of small

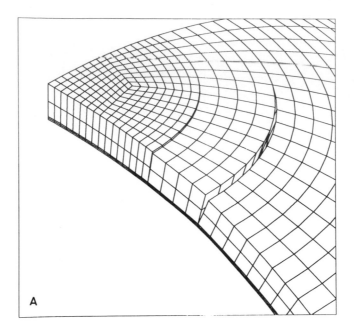

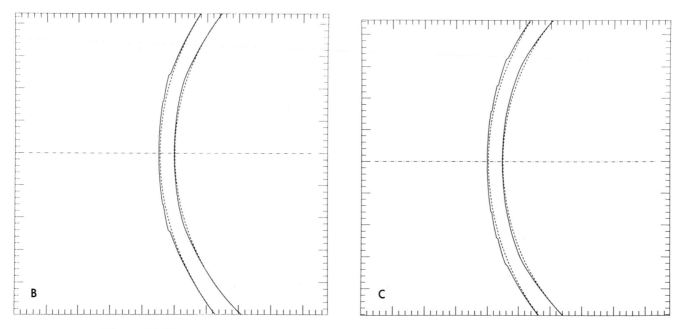

Figure 34-12

A, Mesh diagram shows two arcuate incisions along one semimeridian, 110° long, 90% deep at 4.0- and 6.0-mm diameter clear zones. There are four rectangles drawn across the thickness of the cornea. The anterior two rectangles represent one brick element that occupies 90% of the thickness of the cornea. The posterior two rectangles represent one brick element that occupies the posterior 10% of the cornea. The central portion of the tissue adjacent to the central portion of each incision is displaced slightly anteriorly compared with the tissue along the outer portion of each incision. **B,** Cross-sectional representation along the incised 90° meridian of the effect of two pairs of arcuate incisions at 4- and 6-mm clear zones. **C,** Effect of six incisions at 4-, 6-, and 8-mm clear zones. Central corneal curvature changes little with the addition of more than two incisions. Paracentral and peripheral corneal curvatures steepen a bit. Horizontal broken lines indicate geometric center of the cornea.

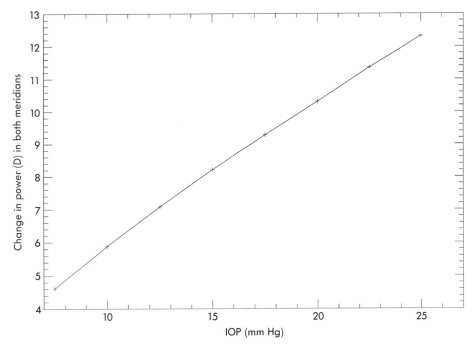

Figure 34-13
Effect of intraocular pressure on the change in refraction. The two factors have a
linear relationship. Note that the change in power represented on the y-axis is the
absolute combined values of the change in the vertical meridian plus the change in
the horizontal meridian to represent the total effect of the arcuate incisions.

changes in intraocular pressure on postoperative refraction clinically or the suggestion that the human eye in vivo does not act in accordance with the perfect
mathematic model we are describing. However, elevated intraocular pressure is
well known to enhance the effect of radial keratotomy,[4] as discussed in Chapter
13, Predictability of Refractive Keratotomy. No studies have systematically evaluated the effect of intraocular pressure on transverse incisions for astigmatism in
laboratory or human circumstances.

Refractive change in incised vs. unincised meridians—coupling effect

Arcuate incisions flattened the meridian perpendicular to the incision and
steepened the meridian parallel to the incision. This effect is known as coupling
or as the flattening to steepening ratio. With maximum incision length of 120°,
the ratio of the flattening to steepening increased as the diameter of the clear
zone increased. For example, a pair of incisions subtending an arc of approximately 120° produced a flattening to steepening ratio of 0.8:1 at a zone of 4
mm, of 0.94:1 at a zone of 5 mm, and of 1.17:1 at a zone of 8 mm (Fig. 34-14
and Table 34-1). The ratio was nearly constant for incisions along a large clear
zone (8 mm) even though the incisions subtended different degrees of arc. That
is, two incisions of different arc length along the same diameter clear zone had
the same coupling effect when the angular length varied between 30° and 150°
(Table 34-1). For incisions located in the 3- to 6.5-mm clear zones, the coupling
effect decreased rapidly as the angular length increased.

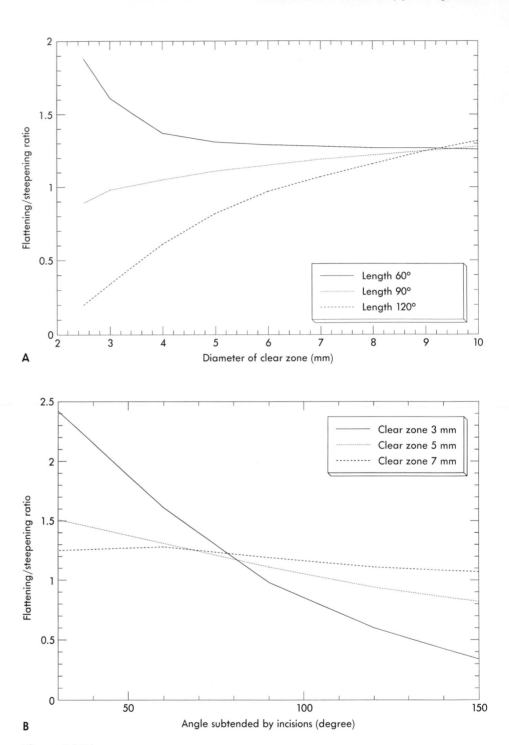

Figure 34-14
Ratio of flattening in the 90° meridian to steepening in the 180° meridian. **A** and **B,** The ratio of flattening to steepening decreases or increases depending on the clear zone diameter for a given angular length.

Table 34-1

Ratio of Flattening in Incised Vertical 90° Meridian to Steepening in Horizontal 180° Meridian

Clear zone diameter (mm)	Angle subtended by incision				
	30°	60°	90°	120°	150°
3.0	2.42	1.61	0.98	0.60	0.34
4.0	1.74	1.37	1.05	0.80	0.61
5.0	1.51	1.31	1.11	0.94	0.82
6.0	1.37	1.29	1.15	1.04	0.97
7.0	1.25	1.28	1.19	1.11	1.07
8.0	1.13	1.27	1.22	1.17	1.16
9.0	1.01	1.27	1.25	1.23	1.25
10.0	0.85	1.26	1.28	1.28	1.32

All previous studies[5,15,17,27] agree that arcuate incisions flatten the incised meridian and steepen the meridian 90° away. However, there is a difference of opinion about the flattening to steepening ratio.

For a 100° to 120° long incision at approximately a 6-mm clear zone, the reported flattening to steepening ratios were 1:1 and 1.50:1, whereas we found 1.1:1.

Effect of incision length on coupling ratio. We found that the ratio varied with the clear zone diameter and with the angular length of the incision (Fig. 34-15). For a clear zone of large diameter, the ratio was nearly constant for an angular length from 30° to 150°. The ratio for a single angular length increased with the increase of the diameter of clear zone when the angular length was 90° or more. The ratio decreased rapidly for larger zones when the incisions were short—30° to 60°.

All previously published studies indicated that the length of the incision between approximately 45° and 120° does not significantly alter the flattening to steepening ratio, and incisions longer than 120° produced a smaller flattening to steepening ratio. Our computer model predicts similar findings. Stated differently, as incisions become longer, the amount of flattening in the vertical meridian remains the same for a given diameter clear zone; however, as incisions become longer, the amount of steepening in the parallel meridian becomes greater.

Three studies in eye bank eye models have addressed the question of the coupling ratio and were in disagreement. Duffey and colleagues[5] demonstrated no effect of clear zone diameter on the coupling ratio. Lundergan et al.[15] found a variable relationship of the coupling ratio with incision length and incision number. Tripoli and colleagues[27] found a flattening to steepening ratio of approximately 1:1 for all clear zone diameters except 5 mm. Our computer simulation showed a significant effect of clear zone diameter and incision length on the coupling ratio. The practical effect of the coupling ratio is discussed in detail in Chapter 31, Keratotomy for Astigmatism, and Chapter 32, Atlas of Astigmatic Keratotomy.

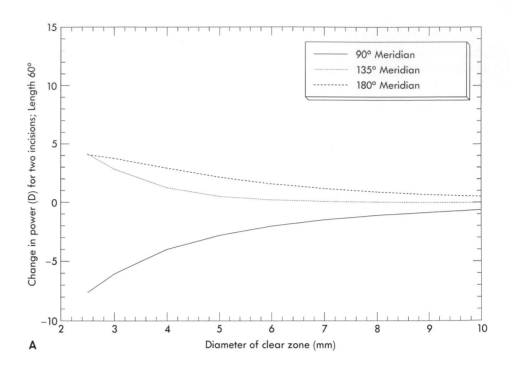

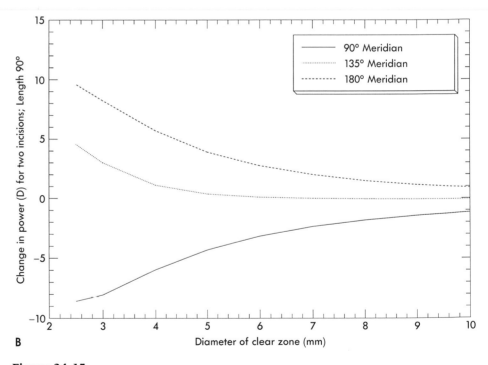

Figure 34-15
Relationship between change in refractive power in different meridians (90°, 135°, 180°) and the diameter of the clear zone for incisions of different lengths. **A,** Two incisions 60° long show minimal change as diameter of clear zone increased. **B,** Incisions 90° long show moderate effect of different zone diameter. **C,** Incisions 120° long show marked effect of zone diameter. The 90° meridian perpendicular to the incision flattens, whereas the 180° meridian parallel to the incision steepens.

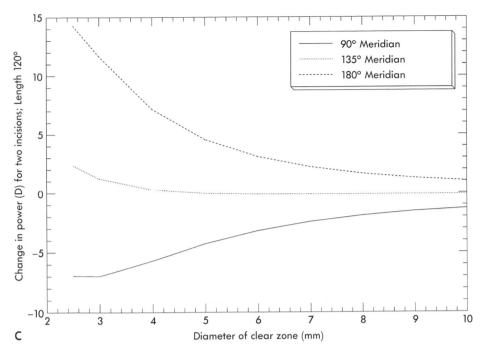

C

Figure 34-15, cont'd
For legend see opposite page.

MEANING AND APPLICATIONS OF COMPUTER SIMULATION

The similarities between the findings of our computer model and those of the human eye bank eye and human clinical case series are numerous. The similarities reinforce and encourage further development of computer simulation because they document that the mathematic simulation is close enough to clinical findings to be used as a method of testing.

The computer model has numerous strengths not available in laboratory and human models. One of the most important is its ability to create perfect and ideal surgery. In the computer model the eye is always the same in its biomechanical properties, whereas in the laboratory and clinical circumstances each eye is different in mechanical properties. Even if the eyes and surgical techniques were identical, the variable time between the operation and the postoperative measurements adds more scatter to the results. Furthermore, the precision of clinical measurements is not as great as we would like, particularly in a laboratory setting where the ocular surface is irregular. This is particularly true when measuring topographic changes with keratography.

Another major strength of the computer model is its ability to separate and analyze variables independently. We were able to simulate the effect of incisions of many lengths at many different zone diameters. This allowed us to observe an interactive effect of zone diameter on the angular length of the incision. Computer simulation allows us to manipulate each variable independently, making it easy to identify the effect of each variable on the outcome.

Our inability to accurately simulate the quantitative results achieved clinically is a reflection of our present inability to determine the exact values and elasticity coefficients of the living eye, to simulate time-dependent viscoelastic changes, and to simulate the effect of corneal wound healing. Nevertheless the similarities amply demonstrate the conceptual validity of computational mechanics as a new method of testing corneal surgery.

APPENDICES

Although most readers of this book do not "speak math," some will be interested in the concrete details of the computational methods used in our nonlinear, anisotropic computer model. Therefore we represent here in abbreviated form the mathematic approach used in our model.

Appendix A: homogenization in elasticity

Notations:

$$\Omega \subset \mathbb{R}^3 \text{ , an open bounded domain of } \mathbb{R}^3$$

$$\sigma = [\sigma_{ij}]_{1 \le i \le 3; 1 \le j \le 3} \qquad \text{the stress tensor}$$

$$e = [e_{ij}]_{1 \le i \le 3; 1 \le j \le 3} \qquad \text{the linear strain tensor}$$

$$e_{ij}(u) = \frac{1}{2}\left(\frac{\partial u_i}{\partial x_j} + \frac{\partial u_j}{\partial x_i}\right)$$

$$Y = [0,1]^3$$

$$a_{ijkh}(y) \quad Y\text{-periodic elasticity coefficients.}$$

$$\varepsilon \text{ a small parameter}$$

$$a^\varepsilon_{ijkh}(x) = a_{ijkh}\left(\frac{x}{\varepsilon}\right) \quad ; \quad x \in \Omega \; ; \; y \in Y$$

$$\tilde{f} = \frac{1}{|Y|}\int_Y f(y)\,dy \quad ; \quad \forall f \in L^1(Y) \quad \text{the mean value of f on Y}$$

$$\delta_{ij} \text{ is the Kronecker symbol: } \delta_{ij} = \begin{cases} 0 \text{ if } i \ne j \\ 1 \text{ if } i = j \end{cases}$$

We consider the problem:

$$\begin{cases} \dfrac{\partial \sigma^\varepsilon_{ij}(x)}{\partial x_j} = -f_i(x) & \text{in } \Omega \\ u^\varepsilon = 0 & \text{on } \partial_1 \Omega \\ \sigma^\varepsilon_{ij}\, n_j = F_i(x) & \text{on } \partial_2 \Omega \\ \sigma^\varepsilon_{ij}(x) = a^\varepsilon_{ijkh}(x)\, e_{kh}(u^\varepsilon) \end{cases}$$

with the usual convention of summation.
We are looking for asymptotic expansions of the following form:

$$\begin{cases} u^\varepsilon(x) = u^0(x) + \varepsilon\, u^1(x,y) + \varepsilon^2 \dots \\ e^\varepsilon_{ij} \equiv e_{ij}(u^\varepsilon) = e^0_{ij}(x,y) + \varepsilon\, e^1_{ij}(x,y) + \varepsilon^2 \dots \\ \sigma^\varepsilon_{ij} \equiv a_{ijkh}(y)\, e^\varepsilon_{kh} = \sigma^0_{ij}(x,y) + \varepsilon\, \sigma^1_{ij}(x,y) + \varepsilon^2 \dots \end{cases}$$

The classic development of homogenization leads to:

$$\widetilde{\sigma^0_{ij}} = a^h_{ijkh}\, e^\varepsilon_{khx}(u^0) = a^h_{ijkh}\, \widetilde{e^0_{kh}}$$

and the homogenized coefficients a^h_{ijkh} can be computed by the formula:

$$a^h_{ijkh} = \left\{ a_{ijlm}\left(\delta_{lk}\delta_{mk} + e_{lmy}(w^{kh})\right) \right\}^\sim$$

Where w^{kh} is the solution of the weak problem:

$$w^{kh} \in \left\{ u \; ; \; u_i \in H^1_{loc}(\mathbb{R}^3) \; , \; Y \text{ periodic} \right\} = \mathbf{V_Y} \qquad \text{such that}$$

$$\int_Y a_{ijlm} \, e_{lm}(w^{kh}) \, e_{ijy}(v) \, dy = \int_Y \frac{\partial a_{ijkh}}{\partial y_i} v_j \, dy \qquad ; \; \forall \, v \in \mathbf{V_Y}$$

When Y is partitioned into different domains, a_{ijkh} being constant on each of them, w^{kh} is the solution of the following weak problem:

$$w^{kh} \in \mathbf{V_Y} \quad ; \int_Y a_{ijlm} \, e_{lm}(w^{kh}) \, e_{ijy}(v) \, dy = - \int_\Gamma [a_{ijkh}] \, n_j v_i \, dy \qquad ; \; \forall \, v \in \mathbf{V_Y}$$

Γ is the interface between the different domains of Y, and $[a_{ijkh}]$ is the jump of a_{ijkh} on Γ.

The computation of the homogenized coefficients involves nine displacement fields (w^{kh}) $k = 1,3$; $h = 1,3$ obtained by solving an elliptic problem for each of them. This is performed numerically by the finite element method. Due to considerations of symmetry, only six problems are actually solved.

Appendix B: transverse isotropy

Notations:

$$\sigma = \left[\sigma_{ij}\right]_{1 \le i \le 3; 1 \le j \le 3} \qquad \text{the stress tensor}$$

$$\varepsilon = \left[\varepsilon_{ij}\right]_{1 \le i \le 3; 1 \le j \le 3} \qquad \text{the nonlinear strain tensor}$$

$$\varepsilon(u) = \frac{\nabla u^T . \nabla u - 1}{2}$$

For a general orthotropic material, the stress-strain relation has the following form:

$$\sigma = \begin{pmatrix} \sigma_{11} \\ \sigma_{22} \\ \sigma_{33} \\ \sigma_{23} \\ \sigma_{13} \\ \sigma_{12} \end{pmatrix} = \begin{pmatrix} a_{1111} & a_{1122} & a_{1133} & 0 & 0 & 0 \\ & a_{2222} & a_{2233} & 0 & 0 & 0 \\ & & a_{3333} & 0 & 0 & 0 \\ & & & 2a_{2323} & 0 & 0 \\ & \text{sym.} & & & 2a_{3131} & 0 \\ & & & & & 2a_{1212} \end{pmatrix} \begin{pmatrix} \varepsilon_{11} \\ \varepsilon_{22} \\ \varepsilon_{33} \\ \varepsilon_{23} \\ \varepsilon_{13} \\ \varepsilon_{12} \end{pmatrix}$$

involving nine independent constants.

For a material transversely isotropic, that is, isotropic in the direction perpendicular to the third vector X_3, we have four relations between the constants of elasticity a_{ijkh}:

$$a_{2222} = a_{1111}$$

$$a_{2233} = a_{3322} = a_{1133} = a_{3311}$$

$$a_{2323} = a_{3232} = a_{1313} = a_{3131}$$

$$2a_{1212} = 2a_{2121} = a_{1111} - a_{1122}$$

and the stress-strain relation becomes:

$$\sigma = \begin{pmatrix} \sigma_{11} \\ \sigma_{22} \\ \sigma_{33} \\ \sigma_{23} \\ \sigma_{13} \\ \sigma_{12} \end{pmatrix} = \begin{pmatrix} a_{1111} & a_{1122} & a_{1133} & 0 & 0 & 0 \\ & a_{1111} & a_{1133} & 0 & 0 & 0 \\ & & a_{3333} & 0 & 0 & 0 \\ & & & 2a_{1313} & 0 & 0 \\ & \text{sym.} & & & 2a_{1313} & 0 \\ & & & & & a_{1111}\text{-}a_{1122} \end{pmatrix} \begin{pmatrix} \varepsilon_{11} \\ \varepsilon_{22} \\ \varepsilon_{33} \\ \varepsilon_{23} \\ \varepsilon_{13} \\ \varepsilon_{12} \end{pmatrix}$$

We can write the five independent constants involved as a function of five other constants usually found in the engineering literature:

$$\begin{cases} E_1 & = \text{longitudinal modulus} \\ E_2 & = \text{transverse modulus} \\ \nu_{12}, \nu_{23} & = \text{Poisson's ratios} \\ G_{12} & = \text{shear modulus} \end{cases}$$

The expressions are:

$$\begin{cases} a_{1111} = \dfrac{E_1 (1\text{-}\nu_{12})}{(1+\nu_{12})(1\text{-}2\nu_{12})} \\[2ex] a_{1122} = \dfrac{E_1 \nu_{12}}{(1+\nu_{12})(1\text{-}2\nu_{12})} \\[2ex] a_{3333} = \dfrac{E_2 (1\text{-}\nu_{23})}{(1+\nu_{23})(1\text{-}2\nu_{23})} \\[2ex] a_{1133} = \dfrac{E_2 \nu_{23}}{(1+\nu_{23})(1\text{-}2\nu_{23})} \\[2ex] a_{1313} = G_{12} \end{cases}$$

The material becomes isotropic when:

$$\begin{cases} E_1 = E_2 = E & (\text{Young's Modulus}) \\ \nu_{12} = \nu_{23} = \nu & (\text{Poisson's ratio}) \\ G_{12} = \dfrac{E}{1+\nu} \end{cases}$$

Appendix C: homogenization of a stratified material with periodic structure

The notations are the same as in Appendices B and C.

$$\text{if} \quad A = \begin{bmatrix} \sigma_{11} & \sigma_{12} & \sigma_{22} & e_{13} & e_{23} & e_{33} \end{bmatrix}$$

$$\text{and} \quad B = \begin{bmatrix} \sigma_{13} & \sigma_{23} & \sigma_{33} & e_{11} & e_{12} & e_{22} \end{bmatrix}$$

The comportment law can be written: A = K(y). B
where K is a (6,6) matrix.

The comportment law of the homogenized material, stratified in the y direction, is then:

$$\langle A \rangle = \langle K(y) \rangle \cdot \langle B \rangle$$

where $\langle . \rangle$ is the "mean" operator.

In our case, each lamella is transversely isotropic. The plane of isotropy is perpendicular to the plane of the mean fiber of the stroma. We note θ the direction of the lamella, and we obtain:

$$\langle K(y) \rangle = \frac{1}{\pi} \int_0^{\pi} K(\theta)\, d\theta$$

We consider that each lamella is a general orthotropic material (see Appendix B), the axis of orthotropy being x,y,z. If we rotate the system of axis around Oz of an angle θ, we find the new stress-strain relation:

$$\sigma = \begin{pmatrix} \sigma_{11} \\ \sigma_{22} \\ \sigma_{33} \\ \sigma_{23} \\ \sigma_{13} \\ \sigma_{12} \end{pmatrix} = \begin{pmatrix} a^\theta_{1111} & a^\theta_{1122} & a^\theta_{1133} & 0 & 0 & a^\theta_{1112} \\ & a^\theta_{2222} & a^\theta_{2233} & 0 & 0 & a^\theta_{2212} \\ & & a^\theta_{3333} & 0 & 0 & a^\theta_{3312} \\ & & & 2a^\theta_{2323} & 2a^\theta_{2331} & 0 \\ & \text{sym.} & & & 2a^\theta_{3131} & 0 \\ & & & & & 2a^\theta_{1212} \end{pmatrix} \begin{pmatrix} \varepsilon_{11} \\ \varepsilon_{22} \\ \varepsilon_{33} \\ \varepsilon_{23} \\ \varepsilon_{13} \\ \varepsilon_{12} \end{pmatrix}$$

with

$$
\begin{cases}
a^\theta_{1111} = a_{1111}\cos^4\theta + 2\,(a_{1122} + a_{1212})\cos^2\theta\,\sin^2\theta + a_{2222}\sin^4\theta \\[4pt]
a^\theta_{2222} = a_{1111}\sin^4\theta + 2\,(a_{1122} + a_{1212})\cos^2\theta\,\sin^2\theta + a_{2222}\cos^4\theta \\[4pt]
a^\theta_{3333} = a_{3333} \\[4pt]
a^\theta_{2233} = a_{2233}\cos^2\theta + a_{3311}\sin^2\theta \\[4pt]
a^\theta_{3311} = a_{2233}\sin^2\theta + a_{3311}\cos^2\theta \\[4pt]
a^\theta_{1122} = a_{1122}\cos^4\theta + (a_{1111} + a_{2222} - 2\,a_{1212})\cos^2\theta\,\sin^2\theta + a_{1122}\sin^4\theta \\[4pt]
a^\theta_{2323} = a_{2323}\cos^2\theta + a_{3131}\sin^2\theta \\[4pt]
a^\theta_{3131} = a_{2323}\sin^2\theta + a_{3131}\cos^2\theta \\[4pt]
a^\theta_{1212} = a_{1212}\cos^4\theta + 2\,(a_{1111} + a_{2222} - a_{1212} - 2\,a_{1122})\cos^2\theta\,\sin^2\theta + a_{1212}\sin^4\theta \\[4pt]
a^\theta_{2331} = (a_{2323} - a_{3131})\sin\theta\,\cos\theta \\[4pt]
a^\theta_{3312} = (a_{2233} - a_{3311})\sin\theta\,\cos\theta \\[4pt]
a^\theta_{2212} = \sin\theta\,\cos\theta\left[(a_{1122} + a_{1212})(\sin^2\theta - \cos^2\theta) + a_{2222}\cos^2\theta - a_{1111}\sin^2\theta\right] \\[4pt]
a^\theta_{1112} = \sin\theta\,\cos\theta\left[(a_{1122} + a_{1212})(\cos^2\theta - \sin^2\theta) + a_{2222}\sin^2\theta - a_{1111}\cos^2\theta\right]
\end{cases}
$$

The expression for K (θ) is then:

$$K(\theta) = \begin{pmatrix} 0 & 0 & K_{13} & K_{14} & K_{15} & K_{16} \\ 0 & 0 & K_{23} & K_{24} & K_{25} & K_{26} \\ 0 & 0 & K_{33} & K_{34} & K_{35} & K_{36} \\ K_{41} & K_{42} & 0 & 0 & 0 & 0 \\ K_{51} & K_{52} & 0 & 0 & 0 & 0 \\ 0 & 0 & K_{63} & K_{64} & K_{65} & K_{66} \end{pmatrix}$$

with

$$K_{13} = -K_{64} = \frac{a^{\theta}_{1133}}{a_{3333}}$$

$$K_{23} = -K_{65} = \frac{a^{\theta}_{3312}}{a_{3333}}$$

$$K_{33} = -K_{66} = \frac{a^{\theta}_{3322}}{a_{3333}}$$

$$K_{63} = \frac{1}{a_{3333}}$$

$$K_{14} = a^{\theta}_{1111} - \frac{a^{\theta}_{3311} \, a^{\theta}_{3311}}{a_{3333}}$$

$$K_{25} = a^{\theta}_{1212} - \frac{a^{\theta}_{3312} \, a^{\theta}_{3312}}{a_{3333}}$$

$$K_{36} = a^{\theta}_{2222} - \frac{a^{\theta}_{3322} \, a^{\theta}_{3322}}{a_{3333}}$$

$$K_{15} = K_{24} = a^{\theta}_{1112} - \frac{a^{\theta}_{3312} \, a^{\theta}_{3311}}{a_{3333}}$$

$$K_{16} = K_{34} = a^{\theta}_{1122} - \frac{a^{\theta}_{3322} \, a^{\theta}_{3311}}{a_{3333}}$$

$$K_{26} = K_{35} = a^{\theta}_{2212} - \frac{a^{\theta}_{3312} \, a^{\theta}_{3322}}{a_{3333}}$$

$$K_{41} = \frac{a^{\theta}_{2323}}{a^{\theta}_{2323} \, a^{\theta}_{3131} - {a^{\theta}_{2331}}^2}$$

$$K_{52} = \frac{a^{\theta}_{3131}}{a^{\theta}_{2323} \, a^{\theta}_{3131} - {a^{\theta}_{2331}}^2}$$

$$K_{42} = K_{51} = \frac{-a^{\theta}_{2331}}{a^{\theta}_{2323} \, a^{\theta}_{3131} - {a^{\theta}_{2331}}^2}$$

Then, after the computation of the mean value of each of K's component, we find the homogenized coefficients. Their expressions are:

$$a^h_{1111} = a^h_{2222} = \frac{3}{8}\left(a_{1111} + a_{2222}\right) - \frac{1}{8}\left(\frac{a_{2233}^2 + a_{3311}^2}{a_{3333}}\right) + \frac{1}{4}\left(a_{1122} + a_{1212} + \frac{a_{2233}\,a_{3311}}{a_{3333}}\right)$$

$$a^h_{3333} = a_{3333}$$

$$a^h_{2233} = a^h_{3311} = \frac{1}{2}\left(a_{2233} + a_{3311}\right)$$

$$a^h_{1122} = \frac{1}{2}\left(a_{1111} + a_{2222}\right) + \frac{1}{8}\left(\frac{a_{2233}^2 + a_{3311}^2}{a_{3333}}\right) - \frac{1}{4}\left(a_{1212} + \frac{a_{2233}\,a_{3311}}{a_{3333}}\right) + \frac{3}{4}\,a_{1122}$$

$$a^h_{2323} = a^h_{3131} = \frac{2\,a_{2323}\,a_{3131}}{a_{2323} - a_{3131}}$$

$$a^h_{1212} = \frac{1}{2}\left(a_{1212} - a_{1122}\right) + \frac{1}{4}\left(a_{1111} + a_{2222}\right) - \frac{1}{8}\frac{\left(a_{2233} - a_{3311}\right)^2}{a_{3333}}$$

REFERENCES

1. Arrowsmith PN and Marks RG: Evaluating the predictability of radial keratotomy, Ophthalmology 1985;92:1237-1243.
2. Battaglioli JL and Kamm RD: Measurements of the compressive properties of the scleral tissue, Invest Ophthalmol Vis Sci 1984;25:59-65.
3. Bensoussan A, Lions JL, and Papanicolaou G: Asymptomatic analysis for periodic structures, Amsterdam, 1978, North Holland.
4. Busin M, Yau C, Avni I, et al: The effect of changes in intraocular pressure on corneal curvature after radial keratotomy in the rabbit eye, Ophthalmology 1986;93:331-334.
5. Duffey RJ, Vivant NJ, HJungwon T, Hofmann RF, and Lindstrom RL: Paired arcuate keratotomy: a surgical approach to mixed and myopic astigmatism, Arch Ophthalmol 1988;106:1130-1135.
6. Dumontet H: Homogenization d'un materiau a structure periodique stratifiee, de comportement elastique lineaire et non-lineaire et viscoelastique, Compte rendu de l'Academie des Sciences, 1982, 2eme semestre, T295, pp 633-636.
7. Fung YC: Biomechanics, New York, 1981, Springer-Verlag.
8. Greene PR: Mechanical considerations in myopia, Am J Optom Physiol Opt 1980;57:902-914.
9. Gullstrand A: Helmholtz's treatise on physiological optics, New York, 1924, Optical Society of America.
10. Hanna KD, Jouve FE, Bercovier MH, and Waring GO: Computer simulation of lamellar keratotomy and myopic keratomileusis, J Refract Surg 1988;4:222-231.
11. Hanna KD, Jouve FE, Ciarlet PG, and Waring GO: Computer simulation of arcuate and radial incisions involving the corneoscleral limbus, Eye 1989;3:227-239.
12. Hanna KD and Jouve FE: Preliminary computer simulation of the effects of radial keratotomy, Arch Ophthalmol 1989;107:911-918.
13. Hofmann R: The surgical correction of idiopathic astigmatism. In Sanders DR, Hofmann RF, and Salz JJ, editors: Refractive corneal surgery, Thorofare, NJ, 1986, Slack, Inc, pp 243-289.
14. Lindquist TD, Rubenstein JB, Rice SW, Williams PA, and Lindstrom RL: Trapezoidal astigmatic keratotomy: quantification in human cadaver eyes, Arch Ophthalmol 1986;104:1534-1539.
15. Lundergan MK and Rowsey JJ: Relaxing incisions and corneal topography, Ophthalmology 1985;92:1226-1236.
16. Lynn MJ, Waring GO, Sperduto RD, and the PERK Study Group: Factors affecting outcome and predictability of radial keratotomy in the PERK study, Arch Ophthalmol 1987;106:42-51.
17. Merlin U: Curved keratotomy procedure for congenital astigmatism, J Refract Surg 1987;3:92-97.
18. Nimni ME: Collagen: biochemistry, vol 1, Boca Raton, Fla, 1988, CRC Press, Inc, p 46.
19. Nyquist GW: Rheology of the cornea: experimental techniques and results, Exp Eye Res 1968;7:183-188.
20. Pouliquen Y: Fine structure of the corneal stroma, Cornea 1984;3:168-177.
21. Rubenstein JB, Lindquist TD, and Lindstrom RL: A graded technique of trapezoidal astigmatic keratotomy, Invest Ophthalmol Vis Sci 1987;28(suppl):224.
22. Sanchez PE: Non-homogeneous media and vibration theory, New York, 1980, Springer-Verlag.
23. Sanchez-Palencia E and Zaoui A, editors: Homogenization techniques for composite media: lectures delivered at the CISM International Center for Mechanical Sciences, Udine, Italy, July 1-5, New York, 1987, 1985, Springer-Verlag.
24. Sanders D, Deitz M, and Gallagher D: Factors affecting predictability of radial keratotomy, Ophthalmology 1985;92:1237-1243.
25. Seiler T, Bende T, Wollensak J, and Trokel S: Excimer laser keratectomy for correction of astigmatism, Am J Ophthalmol 1988;105:117-224.
26. Southhall JPC: Introduction to physiological optics, New York, 1961, Dover Publishing, Inc.
27. Tripoli NK, Cohen KL, and Holman RE: Corneal topographic response to circumferential keratotomies, J Refract Surg 1987;3:129-136.

Appendices

Prospective Evaluation of Radial Keratotomy (PERK) Study: Design and Surgical Technique

The results of the PERK study are scattered throughout this book, but the design of the study and the surgical technique are not described. We present this information here in summary form. Details are available in the published papers. The background and development of the PERK study are presented in Chapter 8, Development of Refractive Keratotomy in the United States, 1978-1990.

ELIGIBILITY CRITERIA

To enter the study a patient must have fulfilled the following eligibility requirements:

1. The patient had been offered spectacles and contact lenses and preferred to have radial keratotomy. The patient read and understood the booklet, "Radial Keratotomy—an Explanation for Study Patients," and understood that an optical correction could be necessary after surgery, that there were potential complications, that a presbyopic correction could be needed earlier than without surgery, and that a successful outcome would not necessarily ensure improved social or professional achievement. The patient had signed an informed consent form.

2. The patient was 21 years of age or older. This is equal to or over the age of majority in the United States. After this age, progression of physiologic myopia is extremely rare, although early keratoconus may go undetected.

3. There was no residual, recurrent, or active ocular disease or abnormality in either eye.

4. The patient had bilateral physiologic myopia without ophthalmoscopic signs of progressive myopia.

5. The visual acuity in each eye was correctable to at least 20/20 with spectacles or contact lenses.

6. The spherical equivalent of the current cycloplegic refraction was between −2.00 and −8.00 D inclusive, with 1.50 D or less of refractive astigmatism in each eye. We selected these arbitrary limits because under 2.00 D the chance of overcorrection becomes much greater and the visual disability is only moderately severe, and because over 8.00 D there is less chance of obtaining emmetropia after radial keratotomy. Since the study was designed to evaluate the effect of radial keratotomy on spherical myopia and since there is no provision for surgical techniques to correct astigmatism, no more than 1.50 D of astigmatism could be present.

7. There could be no more than 4.00 D difference in the spherical equivalent of the refractive error between the two eyes. This helped eliminate individuals with unilateral progressive or pathologic myopia.

8. The spherical portion of the refraction in each eye had not changed more than ±0.50 D during the previous year, or more than ±1.00 D during the previous 3 years, as documented by previous clinical records. This criterion helped eliminate individuals with progressive myopia.

9. If the patient wore contact lenses regularly, the contact lenses were removed and central keratometry readings had to be stable within ±0.50 D with regularly shaped mires on three separate measurements at least 1 week apart. Myopic individuals who wore hard or soft contact lenses and had corneal warpage could not enter the study, since only a stable regular corneal surface can provide an adequate baseline for judging the effects of radial keratotomy.

10. Individuals with systemic diseases that are likely to influence corneal healing or affect reliable follow-up in the study were excluded. These exclusions included mental retardation, systemic connective tissue diseases, severe atopic disease, and drugs such as systemic glucocorticoids.

11. The patient had to live in the greater metropolitan area of the PERK clinical center where the surgery was done. Preferably, the patient lived in stable socioeconomic conditions, increasing the likelihood that he or she would remain in the study for the full 5 years.

OPERATIVE PROCEDURE

Surgeons at all nine clinical centers used a single standardized operative technique. The investigators selected the instruments and surgical techniques that reflected the state of the art at the commencement of the study.

At eight centers one investigator performed all surgery, and at one center three investigators divided the cases. Most of the surgeons had formal training in anterior segment surgery beyond their residency. At the outset the individual surgeon's experience with radial keratotomy varied from no cases to over 600. This varied background—a situation simulating that in the ophthalmic community—helped define the role of surgical experience in the effectiveness of the procedure.

The PERK surgeons derived the technique from five sources: (1) Svyatoslav N. Fyodorov, M.D., with whom the Project Chairperson studied for 1 week; (2)

instruction given at two PERK practical laboratory surgical training sessions under the guidance of American surgeons with experience in radial keratotomy (Leo D. Bores, M.D., Santa Fe, NM; William D. Myers, M.D., Royal Oaks, MI; John W. Cowden, M.D., Detroit, MI); (3) information gained from a detailed questionnaire on surgical technique sent to 17 surgeons actively performing radial keratotomy; (4) techniques described in scientific meetings and seminars; and (5) personal experience of surgeons in the PERK study.

All surgeons observed radial keratotomy cases before performing their own first case. Surgeons who had performed fewer than 10 cases were assisted in at least their first three cases by a surgeon who had performed more than 25 cases. Each surgeon then performed 10 or more initial cases, and each had to achieve an incision depth of at least 75% of corneal thickness in two of three successive cases as documented by the independent examiner's drawings on the postoperative data forms before commencement of the final 50 cases.

As a reference for each surgeon, the surgical technique was detailed in the Manual of Procedures and was also recorded on a videotape distributed to each center. An ophthalmologist from the Clinic Monitoring Group observed each surgeon and verified that each adhered to the technique described in the protocol.

Instruments are described in Chapter 15, Surgical Instruments Used in Refractive Keratotomy, and the surgical techniques are illustrated in Chapter 17, Surgical Techniques of Radial Keratotomy. Surgery was performed in an outpatient or inpatient operating room using an operating microscope.

No mydriatic drops were used, since a small pupil helps prevent accidental misplacement of the visual axis and reduces photophobia during surgery. Topical 0.5% proparacaine provided anesthesia, using as little medication as possible on the cornea. The cornea was kept slightly moist with balanced salt solution throughout the procedure.

To mark the visual axis, an imaginary line that connects the patient's foveola with the visual object, the surgeon asked the patient to fixate the coiled filament of the coaxial microscope light. Closing one eye, the surgeon placed a mark in the corneal epithelium with a hypodermic needle at the opposite end of the light reflection (to compensate for the disparity of the convergence angle). The mark is made at one width of the light reflection inferior to the reflection itself (to compensate for the 7° prismatic displacement of the light by the microscope). (See Sternberg EB, Waring GO: Comparison of Two Methods of Marking the Visual

Axis on the Cornea During Radial Keratotomy, Am J Ophthalmol 1983;96:605-608.)

The surgeon selected the diameter of the central clear zone on the basis of the spherical equivalent of the preoperative cycloplegic refraction: -2.00 to -3.12 D = 4 mm; -3.25 to -4.37 D = 3.5 mm, and -4.50 to -8.00 D = 3 mm. A dull marking trephine, (Katena marking trephines with cross hairs, Katena Products, Inc., E. Hanover, NJ), placed on the cornea so that the intersection of the cross hairs within the trephine coincided with the visual axis mark, made a circular indentation in the epithelium.

The surgeon then measured the corneal thickness with the ultrasonic pachometer (Kremer Accutome Corneometer, Instruments for Medicine, Santa Barbara, CA), placing the sterile probe tip perpendicular to the cornea centrally and at the 3, 6, 9, and 12 o'clock meridians just outside the circular trephine mark. Readings were taken until two out of three were identical. This intraoperative pachometry had two advantages: it included changes in corneal thickness that might occur during the procedure, such as thinning from evaporation, and it measured corneal thickness in the area where the incisions were made— paracentrally.

After gaining experience with a variety of metal-bladed and diamond-bladed knives, some of the PERK surgeons designed a knife for use in this study (KOI diamond knife with micrometer, KOI Associates, Frazer, PA). The gem-quality diamond blade had a 45° cutting angle. The blade extended between two parallel footplates, each forming a smooth flat surface 1.27 mm wide, so that the knife slid like a ski over the cornea during the incision. The cutting edge of the blade extended in front of the footplates so that the blade engaged the tissue directly without the footplate compressing or displacing it.

The diamond blade length was advanced by a screw-type micrometer calibrated in 10-μm units and was set equal to the thinnest of the four paracentral pachometry readings. The surgeon verified the length with a blade gauge (KOI [coin] gauge, KOI Associates, Frazer, PA). The handle of the knife had slots designed to fit precisely between posts on the gauge platform. In this location, the diamond blade extended over the rim of a coin-shaped disc, the outside edge of which abutted on the footplate. The thickness of the rim was calibrated in 10-μm units, and the surgeon turned the disc until the area of the rim that was calibrated to the desired blade length underlay the blade. Using the highest microscopic power, the surgeon aligned the tip of the blade with the edge of the rim and, if necessary, adjusted the micrometer of the knife handle to achieve the exact desired blade length.

The micrometer knife handle–coin gauge combination had advantages. Presetting the blade length with the micrometer shortened the surgical procedure. The calibrated metal rim that verified the blade length was more accurate than the groove used in many gauge blocks, since the tip of the blade could be aligned precisely with the edge of the metal rim, rather than aimed approximately over the center of a relatively wide groove.

The surgeon made eight radial incisions spaced equidistant around the cornea. We selected eight incisions on the basis of theoretical, laboratory, and clinical considerations that demonstrate that eight incisions achieve 80% or more of the effect of 16 incisions. With eight incisions the cornea remained more rigid during the procedure, there were fewer scars and potentially less glare, there would be fewer overcorrections, and there was the option of performing additional incisions between the previous ones should an undercorrection occur. The surgeon followed a standard sequence for the incisions, which minimizes variation in technique among surgeons and helps analysis of incision depth and corneal perforations. The sequence of incisions in terms of clock hours around the cornea from the frontal view were (1) 9:00, (2) 12:00, (3) 6:00, (4) 3:00, (5) 4:30, (6) 1:30, (7) 7:30, and (8) 10:30. Incisions extended from the edge of the trephine mark to the vascular arcade of the corneal limbus.

The surgeon fixated the globe at the limbus with a double-pronged forceps to decrease torsion (Bores fixation forceps, Katena Products, Inc., E. Hanover, NJ). Each incision was made 180° away from the fixation point. The surgeon aligned the posterior dull edge of the knife blade with the circular epithelial mark, held the knife handle perpendicular to the cornea, and plunged the blade into the stroma with enough force to produce slight indentation of the cornea. After holding the blade in place for 2 or 3 seconds to ensure maximum penetration, the surgeon pulled the knife toward the limbus in a single, smooth, uniform, moderately slow movement, exerting mild pressure on the cornea and maintaining the handle perpendicular to the surface.

If perforation of the cornea occurred, the surgeon used his discretion to choose from three alternatives: (1) proceed with the operation if the perforation was small and the anterior chamber remained formed, (2) stop the operation if the eye became soft but the anterior chamber remained formed, or (3) close the perforation with interrupted 10-0 nylon sutures if the anterior chamber shallowed and stop the operation. Patients with incomplete procedures were followed according to protocol, and approximately 8 weeks after surgery the operation was completed if desired.

The surgeon gently irrigated each wound with balanced salt solution to remove any blood or epithelial cells that entered the wound. He used a thin metal "dipstick" gauge to verify the uniformity of the incisions, recutting those that were too short or had an irregular depth, but made no attempt to measure the depth of the incisions intraoperatively, since corneal swelling and tissue displacement interfered with the accuracy of that measurement. Topical 0.3% gentamicin and a mydriatic-cycloplegic were instilled, followed by application of a mild pressure patch. Systemic analgesics were used when needed for postoperative pain.

The surgeon then recorded all details of the procedure on the PERK form. This was sent to the Coordinating Center.

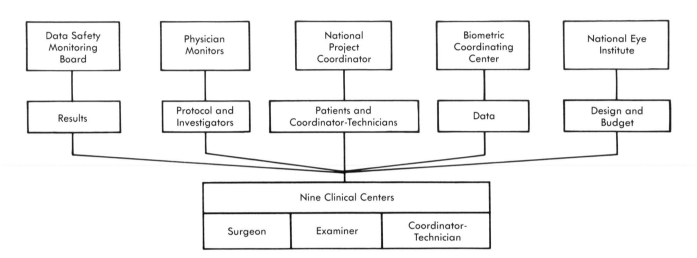

Figure A1-1

Monitors in the PERK study. In each clinical center surgeons performed radial keratotomy, and an examiner-investigator and a coordinator-technician gathered the preoperative and postoperative data. The five monitoring groups displayed across the top of the figure supervised the areas indicated beneath them. (From Waring GO, Moffitt SD, Gelender H, et al: Rationale for and design of the National Eye Institute Prospective Evaluation of Radial Keratotomy (PERK) study, Ophthalmology 1983;90:40.)

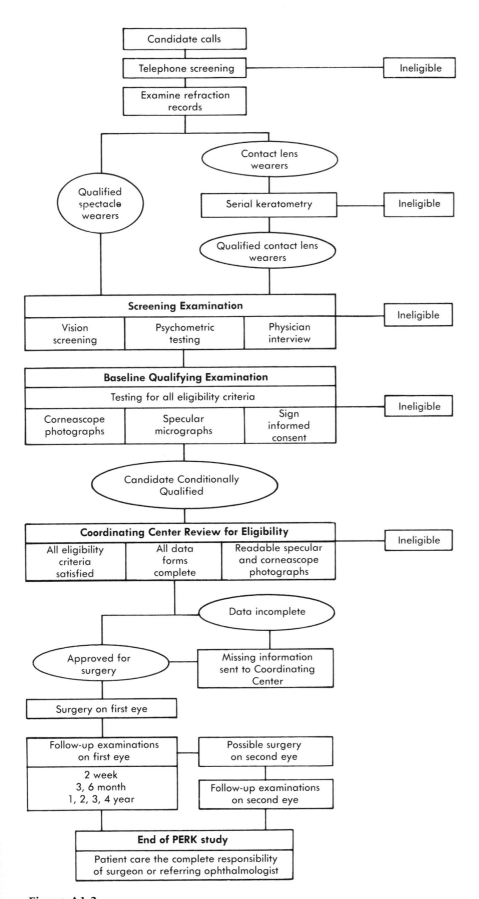

Figure A1-2

Flow of patients and data in the PERK study. (From Waring GO, Moffitt SD, Gelender H, et al: Rationale for and design of the National Eye Institute Prospective Evaluation of Radial Keratotomy (PERK) study, Ophthalmology 1983;90:40.)

Statements on Radial Keratotomy

In 1988 three medical societies issued statements on radial keratotomy for myopia: the International Society of Refractive Keratoplasty (Board of Directors of the International Society of Refractive Keratoplasty: Statement on Radial Keratotomy in 1988, J Refract Surg 1988;4:80-90); the American Medical Association (American Medical Association: Questions and Answers: Radial Keratotomy for Simple Myopia—Diagnostic and Therapeutic Technology Assessment [DATTA], JAMA 1988;260:264-267); and the American Academy of Ophthalmology (American Academy of Ophthalmology: Radial Keratotomy for Myopia, Ophthalmology 1989;96:671-687). Although all three statements covered essentially the same data base and published information, the orientation and opinions expressed in each one are different. (See Chapter 8, Development of Refractive Keratotomy in the United States, 1978-1990.) We reproduce here the International Society of Refractive Keratoplasty statement as published. Although this statement was written in 1988, its fundamental outline, premises, and conclusions are valid in the early 1990s. Omitted is detailed information on radial keratotomy with four incisions using a titrated technique of repeated operations. The statement is useful for patients requiring factual, detailed information, for physicians seeking a brief summary of radial keratotomy, and for insurance companies evaluating the procedure. In addition to its thorough background and description of the surgery and outcome, the statement concludes that radial keratotomy is not cosmetic surgery and that it is not investigational or experimental. Table 1 compares three studies, which are presented in more detail in Chapter 21, Results of Refractive Keratotomy.

Statement on Radial Keratotomy in 1988

By the Board of Directors of the International Society of Refractive Keratoplasty*

Since radial keratotomy for myopia was first done in the United States in 1978, the operation has been the subject of interest and lively debate among ophthalmologists and myopic individuals alike, spawning thousands of articles in the news media and hundreds of scientific articles. Ophthalmic surgeons around the world have performed hundreds of thousands of radial keratotomies over the past decade.

The International Society of Refractive Keratoplasty, formally incorporated in 1979, is an organization of ophthalmic surgeons with a special interest in refractive eye surgery—operations designed to correct or improve myopia (nearsightedness), hyperopia (farsightedness), and astigmatism. Radial keratotomy is the most commonly performed of these procedures.

To assess the strengths and weaknesses of radial keratotomy surgery in the management of myopia in 1988, the Board of Directors of the International Society of Refractive Keratoplasty has approved the following statement, which also contains tables that compare three major studies of radial keratotomy and a bibliography. The statement is intended to provide a general summary and survey of radial keratotomy for the interested ophthalmologist and lay person. It is not intended to resolve all controversies about the procedure, to provide standards of care for the community, or to serve as an informed consent document in patient care. More exhaustive reviews of the surgery and its results are available.[1-4]

This evaluation is based on the ethical premise spelled out in the American Academy of Ophthalmology code of ethics: "It is the duty of an ophthalmologist to place the patient's welfare and rights above all other considerations."[5]

HISTORY OF RADIAL KERATOTOMY

Approximately one fourth of the world's population is myopic.[6] Radial keratotomy for myopia has developed slowly over the past century.[7] The use of surgical incisions to alter corneal curvature began in the late 19th century, when Snellen,[8] Bates,[9] and Lans[10,11] described methods to reduce astigmatism, but their observations remained unappreciated by the profession.

Sato, in Japan in the late 1930s, observed that spontaneous breaks in Descemet's membrane in keratoconus flattened the cornea and reduced myopia.[12,13] IIc suggested making surgical incisions in the posterior cornea to treat astigmatism and myopia, a suggestion that led to extensive laboratory and clinical experimentation. This resulted in the description by Sato and

*Daniele Aron-Rosa, MD, Perry S. Binder, MD, Michael R. Deitz, MD, Daniel S. Durrie, MD, Richard Elander, MD, Miles H. Friedlander, MD, Richard L. Lindstrom, MD, Ezra Maguen, MD, Albert C. Neumann, MD, Larry F. Rich, MD, James J. Salz, MD, David J. Schanzlin, MD, Theo Seiler, MD, PhD, George W. Tate, Jr., MD, Spencer P. Thornton, MD, Richard A. Villaseñor, MD, George O. Waring III, MD, and Theodore P. Werblin, MD, PhD.

Akiyama of an operation that consisted of approximately 35 posterior and 40 anterior, equally spaced, radial incisions to reduce myopia.[14,15] In 177 eyes there was an average decrease of 3.10 diopters (range +0.37 to −9 D) within the first year after surgery. Sato's technique had two drawbacks: it was technically difficult and it damaged the corneal endothelium. This endothelial damage produced corneal edema in many eyes, which appeared an average of 20 years after the operation.[16-18]

In the early 1970s ophthalmologists in the Soviet Union, including Beliaev,[19] Yenaliev,[20] and Fyodorov and Durnev,[21-24] modified Sato's technique, making radial incisions only in the anterior peripheral cornea and sclera. Fyodorov and Durnev attempted to improve the predictability in individual patients by devising a multifactorial formula that used patient and surgical variables.[25] The most important factor was to vary the diameter of the central clear zone, making it as small as 3 mm.

In 1978, Bores, Myers, and Cowden began performing radial keratotomy in the United States,[26,27] using Fyodorov's techniques. Since then, the procedure has been modified extensively as a result of laboratory and clinical experimentation and technological innovation, including ultrasonic pachymeters and crystal-bladed micrometer knives.[1-4]

To assess the efficacy, safety, predictability, and stability of radial keratotomy, the National Eye Institute funded the Prospective Evaluation of Radial Keratotomy (PERK) Study in 1980, a collaborative effort among university-based and private ophthalmologists in nine clinical centers. The design of the study,[28] results at 1[29] and 3[30] years, and the outcome of substudies[30-43] have been presented.

Another collaborative effort among private ophthalmologists and university-based statisticians emerged in 1981 as the Analysis of Radial Keratotomy (ARK) Study Group. Although the group disbanded, the investigators have continued to publish their surgical techniques and findings with 1- to 5-year follow-up.[44-56]

Other clinicians and researchers also have published their findings.[24,25,57-68]

In recent years, controversy has surrounded attempts to categorize the level of development of radial keratotomy: is the operation investigational, experimental, in development, or an accepted procedure? This question is not easy to answer because, in contrast to drugs and devices, which are regulated by the Food and Drug Administration, there is no federal regulation of surgical procedures and no national standards for classifying their acceptance by physicians. This is particularly true for procedures in which techniques are rapidly changing, such as radial keratot-

omy. In the late 1970s and early 1980s there were many discussions on whether to designate radial keratotomy experimental or investigational. *Webster's Ninth New Collegiate Dictionary* (1987 edition) defines "investigational" as the process of observing or studying by close examination and systematic inquiry, and defines "experimental" as an operation carried out under controlled conditions in order to discover an unknown effect or law. The terms "experimental" and "investigational" have often been confused.* Clinical trials are currently defined as forms of human experimentation.[69,70]

In the early 1980s, there was disagreement about the status of radial keratotomy. The International Society of Refractive Keratoplasty considered radial keratotomy to be investigational. Since then, extensive laboratory and clinical information has been published in the peer-reviewed ophthalmic literature, clearly characterizing the risks and benefits of radial keratotomy, as indicated in the bibliography and Tables 1 and 2. Therefore, the International Society of Radial Keratotomy no longer considers radial keratotomy to be either experimental or investigational. In the absence of well-defined standards in the ophthalmic profession for accepted surgical procedures, opinions among ophthalmologists still differ about the role of radial keratotomy in clinical practice.

ALTERNATIVES FOR MANAGEMENT OF MYOPIA
Spectacles and contact lenses

There are many methods of managing myopia, and a discussion of them is beyond the scope of this document. Time has shown spectacles to be a safe, effective, and economic method of correction. They are safer now that impact-resistant lenses are required, but they have functional and cosmetic drawbacks for many patients. Contact lenses are useful devices for vision correction. Contact lens technology continues to improve, and patients who were unable to be fit only a few years ago can now often be fit effectively. However, contact lenses may cause complications such as warpage and vascularization of the cornea, endothelial cell loss, and microbial keratitis, which may require discontinuation of the lenses and may lead to visual loss.[71,72] Orthokeratology, a procedure designed to flatten the cornea by contact lens wear, has been studied in a prospective trial, but is not a predictably effective method of managing myopia.[73]

Refractive surgery

In contrast to spectacles and contact lenses, refractive surgery (including radial keratotomy) attempts to

---

*FDA-sponsored studies on IOL implantation have been labeled investigational.

correct myopia permanently, but with an important limitation: while both spectacles and contact lenses can be changed easily to meet the changing visual needs of an individual, refractive surgery is neither readily reversed nor easily modified.

Other refractive corneal procedures, including keratomileusis[74,75] and epikeratoplasty,[76,77] have been used to correct higher amounts of myopia. The complexity of keratomileusis limits its widespread application. Epikeratoplasty for myopia is currently being further evaluated. Implantation of intracorneal hydrogel and polysulfone plastic lenticules is undergoing refinement in the laboratory[78-85] and in patients,[86,87] as is laser corneal surgery.[88-92] None of these refractive corneal procedures is entirely predictable and free from complications.

Keratotomy for astigmatism

Keratotomy to treat astigmatism is sometimes performed in conjunction with radial keratotomy to treat myopia.[3,93] However, the surgical management of astigmatism is complex and beyond the scope of this document.

PATIENT MOTIVATION

Approximately 75% of the patients in two studies,[36,50] who were interviewed about their reasons for seeking radial keratotomy, stated that they wished to see well without physical dependence on spectacles or contact lenses. This was interpreted as reflecting their desire for normal bodily function independent of external prosthetic appliances. Patients also seek radial keratotomy to improve their performance in a profession or sport, to improve cosmetic appearance, or for simple convenience.

The number of patients who seek radial keratotomy is strongly influenced by external forces, including the news media, the experience of friends, and the attitudes of eye care professionals. The more positive and enthusiastic each of these three forces is, the more likely an individual patient is to seek radial keratotomy. For example, a recent survey of 4,219 ophthalmologists by a health research organization found that the prevalence of cataract surgery was evenly distributed in four geographic regions of the United States. However, 83% of radial keratotomy operations were done in the southern and western regions, with only 17% being done in the northern and central regions, indicating the marked variation in practice patterns among ophthalmologists.[94]

Radial keratotomy changes the major function of the eye—the formation of a clear image on the retina. It is designed to improve unaided visual acuity and visual function, but is not designed to improve visual acuity beyond the level achievable with glasses or contact lenses. However, published studies indicate that radial keratotomy may occasionally result in improved spectacle acuity. Therefore, radial keratotomy is functional surgery, not cosmetic surgery, because it changes the major function of the eye and not its appearance. The majority of patients indicate that their motivation for having radial keratotomy surgery is functional—to see well without glasses or contact lenses—although some patients elect to have the surgery to improve their appearance without spectacles—a cosmetic motivation.[36,50]

CRITERIA FOR PATIENT SELECTION AND INFORMED CONSENT

Published studies indicate that radial keratotomy achieves the best uncorrected visual acuity in patients who have myopia up to approximately 6 D. In patients with 6 to 12 D of myopia, the response to surgery is more variable.[3,4,29,45,46,48,49,60-63] However, radial keratotomy has corrected the refractive error in carefully selected cases of myopia from −6 to −12 D.[26,46,61,62] The effect of the surgery is influenced by patient's age.[32,51,53]

Candidates for radial keratotomy should have stable, non-progressive myopia,[28] as indicated by examination of previous refractions, by temporarily stopping the wear of contact lenses to detect corneal warpage, and by ophthalmoscopic examination to detect changes of degenerative myopia. Concurrent astigmatism should be considered. The cornea should be essentially normal, as determined by slit-lamp microscopy. Individuals with systemic diseases likely to influence corneal healing, such as connective tissue diseases or diseases that require systemic corticosteroids, may be poor candidates. Radial keratotomy may be contraindicated in eyes with severe or uncontrolled external disease. Eyes with uveitis, glaucoma, and lens or retinal disorders require special consideration.

Patients with low to moderate myopia typically have an intact, functioning visual system and an anatomically normal globe. The only abnormality is optical, the refractive error of myopia. Because radial keratotomy is an elective operation that attempts to correct this abnormal optical function and because the refractive error can be managed by alternative methods with minimal risk, it is essential for the surgeon to honestly inform the patient of known risks, benefits, and possible outcomes of the surgery, and to be sure the patient has a balanced, realistic understanding of this information. The surgeon assumes responsibility for obtaining the proper informed consent and is advised to do this well in advance of the time of surgery.[95]

Patients must understand that the outcome of surgery cannot be precisely predicted for an individual eye, that spectacles or contact lenses may still be required for best vision after the surgery, and that contact lens wear may be more difficult because of changes in the shape of the cornea.[96] All patients should be made aware that the surgery does not alter the normal aging process of the eye, which usually requires the use of reading glasses after the age of 40 or 45. Patients over 40 must realize that they may exchange dependence on distance spectacles for dependence on spectacles for near vision.

Patients who seek radial keratotomy to help them achieve specific occupational goals should insure that the surgical correction of myopia will satisfy the employer. They should know the probability of achieving the desired level of visual acuity for their occupation and they must know whether or not the employer will hire a person who has had radial keratotomy. For example, an individual seeking to be a pilot in the United States Air Force must have 20/20 or better uncorrected visual acuity in each eye with no myopic refractive error. Even if these stringent criteria were met after radial keratotomy, the Air Force currently has a policy of not hiring individuals who have had this surgery.

RADIAL KERATOTOMY SURGERY
Training of surgeons in radial keratotomy

Learning to do radial keratotomy imposes a special responsibility on the surgeon because the procedure is elective and requires meticulous accuracy. Most surgeons will follow a series of steps: (1) assimilation of oral presentations at ophthalmic meetings and study of the scientific literature; (2) completion of one or more courses that involve laboratory practice; (3) observation of cases being done by an experienced surgeon; (4) obtaining assistance from an experienced surgeon in the first few cases; (5) continual monitoring and follow-up of results obtained and consultation with colleagues to improve outcome in future cases.

Surgical techniques and factors that affect outcome

Radial keratotomy is a surgical art in which evolving techniques vary among surgeons. The radial incisions weaken the paracentral and peripheral cornea and produce a flattening (increased radius of curvature) of the central cornea, thereby reducing myopia. The variation in surgical instruments and techniques as well as the biological variability among patients create an inherent unpredictability in the outcome of radial keratotomy for individual eyes. Some of the instruments and techniques that may differ among surgeons include the style of diamond knife blade and configuration of the knife footplates, the accuracy of ultrasonic pachymeters, the control of intraocular

pressure during surgery by fixation instruments,[90] the direction of the incisions (centrifugal vs centripetal), and the manual technique of making each incision.[3] There is no available method to control corneal wound healing after the surgery.

There are three principal surgical variables that the surgeon can control in an attempt to achieve a more accurate result.[1,16,26,32,51-53,61,98-100] The first is the diameter of the central clear zone, with smaller diameter clear zones (no less than 2.75 mm) producing greater flattening of the cornea than larger ones (no greater than 5.0 mm). The second variable is the number of incisions, which usually varies from four to 16. Most of the flattening of the central cornea is achieved with the first few incisions; succeeding incisions have progressively less effect. The third is the depth of the incisions, with deeper incisions generally producing a greater central flattening.

There are two principal patient variables that clearly affect outcome: the amount of myopia and the age of the patient. This is because (1) the correction of a greater amount of myopia requires a smaller central clear zone, deeper incisions, and a greater number of incisions; and (2) the greater the patient's age, the greater the effect tends to be with the same surgical technique. It is more difficult to assess the effect of other patient characteristics on the results of surgery. These characteristics include: corneal curvature, preoperative intraocular pressure, patient's sex, corneal thickness, ocular rigidity, corneal diameter, and axial length of the globe.[32,51,53]

How the surgeon should use these surgical and patient factors to achieve the optimal result for an individual patient is an area of continued study in which the answers differ among surgeons. Alternatives range from simple surgical plans that use a fixed number of incisions cut to a fixed percentage of the corneal thickness and vary the diameter of the clear zone according to the amount of myopia,[28] to complex nomograms and formulas that incorporate many preoperative factors to change all three surgical variables. At least six nomograms and formulas have been programmed as computer software and are being sold in software-hardware packages.[2,101,102] Since each of these algorithms was derived by study of one surgeon's technique, and since recommendations for surgery on a specific patient can differ substantially, the ophthalmologist must realize that these are approximate guides, each best used with the technique on which it was based.

The outcome of surgery on the first eye may influence the surgical technique to be used on the second, especially if the first eye is markedly overcorrected or undercorrected.

Reoperations

If an eye has residual myopia after one operation, some surgeons will perform a second radial keratotomy.[41,103-105] The techniques of reoperations are less standardized than those for an initial radial keratotomy. The effectiveness and predictability are less than that of the initial operations. Although reoperations can be effective in reducing residual myopia and/or astigmatism, they have the potential to produce or increase corneal astigmatism—both regular and irregular—and in some cases may have no effect or may increase the amount of myopia. Proposed techniques include making additional incisions between the initial ones, making second incisions in the area of the initial corneal scars, opening the initial wounds and incising them again, and recutting only the paracentral part of the initial incisions.

Overcorrections may be managed by opening the wounds and suturing them shut, a laboratory technique that requires clinical study.[106]

RESULTS

The ideal result of radial keratotomy is not precisely defined, but some surgeons think that leaving the patient slightly myopic is an advantage because it will decrease the onset of symptomatic presbyopia and because patients with residual myopia after radial keratotomy see better uncorrected than patients with a similar refractive error who have not had keratotomy surgery.[22]

Published studies

Different types of information have been published about radial keratotomy since 1979, including anecdotal reports, experiences with early techniques,[24,26,57,64] clinical series,[25,58-61,65,66,100] cooperative studies,[44-51,54-56,63,107,108] a multicenter clinical trial,[28-39] and detailed descriptions of complications.[40,95,109-111]

Comparing the published results of these reports is difficult. In most series the surgeon varied the surgical plan from case to case in an attempt to improve outcome, making it difficult to determine exactly how the results were achieved and difficult to test whether they can be replicated. The PERK Study, in contrast, tested a single, defined technique of radial keratotomy, but did not make adjustments for any variables other than the patient's refraction and corneal thickness. These differences in technique and surgical protocol explain in part why reported results have varied widely. For example, the percent of eyes that achieved a refraction between −1 and +1 D at 6 to 12 months postoperatively covers a broad range: 39%,[63] 43%,[59] 58%,[49] 60%,[45] 61%,[48] and 100%.[25]

An accurate representation of the results of radial keratotomy can be gleaned from three published studies (Tables 1 and 2)[30,54,56] that have common elements: involvement of investigators in private practice and university centers, prospective data gathering, and analysis by independent biostatisticians. Even though the surgical techniques and the methods of reporting the results in each of these studies varied markedly, a reasonable comparison can be made (Tables 1 and 2). To facilitate this comparison, the data in the PERK study were recomputed so that the baseline refraction groups were similar in all three studies.

Predictability of results

All surgeons would like to be able to predict the residual refractive error and the uncorrected visual acuity in their patients after radial keratotomy. Unfortunately, current techniques of surgery do not allow accurate prediction of outcome in individual eyes. Three studies of predictability[32,51,53] have concluded that 90% of the eyes will have a residual refractive error in the range of approximately ±2 D around the predicted result (Tables 1 and 2). The patient must weigh the advantage of this less accurate but permanent surgical improvement against the more accurate but temporary improvement of contact lenses and spectacles.

COMPLICATIONS OR SIDE EFFECTS

The potential complications can be divided into three groups: (1) signs and symptoms that occur temporarily as part of the procedure; (2) signs and symptoms that persist but do not decrease best corrected visual acuity; and (3) complications that potentially or actually disrupt visual function.

Temporary sequelae

Pain, including foreign body sensation, aching, or throbbing, lasts 24 to 48 hours in many patients, often requiring analgesics. Bothersome glare occurs commonly for a few months after surgery,[27,31,45] occasionally persisting for a year or more.[35,109] Both diurnal fluctuation in vision and variation in vision from one day to the next occur with decreasing severity during the first year, but may persist for many years.[35,109,112-113]

Complications or side effects that do not reduce corrected visual acuity

Unplanned undercorrection and overcorrection are the most frequent complications of radial keratotomy (Tables 1 and 2). Those patients made hyperopic under age 40 may be asymptomatic, but will experience symptomatic presbyopia (reduced ability to focus on near objects, as in reading) earlier than they would have without surgery. Once they become presbyopic, some will require a correction for both distance and

Table 1

Comparison of Protocols for Three Studies of Radial Keratotomy

	PERK Study[28,30]	Arrowsmith and Marks[49,54]	Deitz and Sanders[55]
Design of study			
Replicable surgical protocol	Yes	No	No
Sample size determination	Yes	No	No
Study monitors	Yes	No	No
Data gathered by independent physician monitors	Yes	No	No
Selection criteria	Yes	Yes	Yes
Consecutive eyes	Yes	Yes	Yes
Independent statistical analysis	Yes	Yes	Yes
Examination conditions	Standardized	Office practice	Office practice
Reoperations included in data (% of eyes)	No—6-month values used	Yes (11%)	None (Deitz, personal communication)
Population and follow-up			
Dates of surgery	March 1982-Oct 1983	Dec 1980-Aug 1981	Jan 1982-May 1985
Follow-up time	3 years	5 years	1 year
Range	33-42 months	4.7-6.0 years	14 ± 4 months
Number of patients operated	435	101	458
Number of eyes operated	435	122	972
Percent of eyes reported	96%	78%	68%
Surgery			
Number of surgeons	10	1	1
Preoperative variables	Refraction	Refraction, keratometry, ocular rigidity, corneal diameter, surgeon's coefficient (informal relationship)	Refraction, age, keratometry, applanation, IOP, corneal diameter, sex (Deitz, personal communication)
Clear zone diameter (mm) and baseline refraction (D)	Circular—100% −2.00 to −3.12 = 4.0, 30% −3.25 to −4.37 = 3.5, 34% −4.50 to −8.00 = 3.0, 36%	Circular: 3.0 to 5.0—82% Elliptical—12% Elliptical + radial or transverse—6%	Circular: 2.7 to 6—100% 2.7-3—17% 3.0-3.49—22% 3.5-3.99—20% 4.0-6.0—41%
Instruments			
Knife blade	Diamond (single-edge)	Steel	Diamond (double-edge)
Knife handle	Micrometer	Micrometer	Micrometer
Surgical technique			
Eight incisions	100%	8 incis.—56% 16 incis.—44%	89%
Direction of incision	Clear zone to limbus	Limbus to clear zone	Clear zone to limbus
Ultrasonic pachymetry	Intraoperative, 1640 m/sec, paracentral	Preoperative, 1610 m/sec, paracentral	Preoperative, 1640 m/sec, paracentral and central (Deitz, personal communication)
Length of blade	100% of thinnest paracentral	85% to 95% of estimated average paracentral reading	106% of paracentral 108% of central (Deitz, personal communication)
Single pass incisions	100%	42%	65% <6D—essentially all
Deepening incisions	No	Single deepening—47% Double deepening—11% Freehand dissection—1%	Recutting without further blade extension, eyes >6D, 79% (Deitz, personal communication)
Transverse incisions for astigmatism	No	Yes	16% (Deitz, personal communication)
Postoperative corticosteroids	No	Yes	Yes (Deitz, personal communication)

Table 2

Comparison of Results of Three Studies of Radial Keratotomy

	PERK Study[28,30]	Arrowsmith and Marks[49,54]	Deitz and Sanders[55]
Refraction			
Method	Cycloplegic	NR	Cycloplegic (Deitz, personal communication)
Percent of total eyes ±1.00 D	66%	54%	76%
Percent of eyes ±1.00 D in three baseline refraction groups			
Lower (1.50-3.00 D)*	76%	75%	90%
Middle (3.12-6.00 D)†	55%	50%	76%
Higher (6.12-10.00 D)‡	21%	38%	53%
Percent of total overcorrected >1.00 D	16%	33%	13%
Percent of total undercorrected >1.00 D	26%	13%	12%
Visual acuity			
Percent of total eyes ≥20/40	76%	76%	88%
Percent of eyes ≥20/40 in three baseline refraction groups			
Lower (1.50-3.00 D)*	91%	NR	96%
Middle (3.12-6.00 D)†	81%	NR	89%
Higher (6.12-10.00 D)‡	60%	NR	77%
Predictability[32,52,53]			
Patient population for predictability studies	435	156	170
Dates of surgery	March 1982-Oct 1983	Dec 1980-Aug 1981	Dec 1982-Aug 1983
Number of eyes reported	411	97	124
Percent of original population reported	95%	62%	73%
Follow-up time	1 year	4 years	3 months
Percent of eyes in range of refraction around predicted outcome			
±1.00 D	69%	48%	84%
±1.50 D	86%	NR	94%
±2.00 D	95%	78%	NR
Width of 90% prediction interval	4.00 D	NR	NR
Complications			
Percent of corneal perforations	2%	35%	7%-11% (Deitz, personal communication)
Loss of best corrected visual acuity			
Loss of two or more Snellen lines	1.4%	NR	0.3%
Loss to less than 20/20	2%	6%	5%
Moderate to severe subjective glare	No increase over baseline	0	NR
Moderate to severe subjective fluctuating vision	11% increase over baseline	1%	NR
Vision-threatening complications			
Corneal erosion	1	0	0
Delayed bacterial keratitis	2	0	1 (Deitz, personal communication)
Stability			
Population—number of eyes	341 (90% follow-up)[131]	122 (78% follow-up)	165 (74% follow-up)[107]
Time interval	6 mos. to 4 years	1 to 5 years	1 to 3-4 years
Percent of eyes with refractive change ≥1 D	28%	NR	35%
Percent of eyes with continued effect of surgery	24%	NR	31%

NR, Not reported
*PERK, 1.00-3.12 D; Arrowsmith, 1.5-2.9 D; Deitz, 0.6-3.00
†PERK, 3.12-6.00 D; Arrowsmith, 3.0-5.9 D; Deitz, 3.1-6.0 D
‡PERK, 6.12-8.00 D; Arrowsmith, 6.0-9.9 D; Deitz, 6.1-11.9 D

near. Powers and colleagues found that 26% of patients still wore corrective lenses full time, and 14% part time, approximately 2 years after surgery.[50]

An increase in astigmatism of 1 to 3 D occurs in 2% to 11% of eyes.[29,46,48,109]

Rigid gas permeable contact lenses can be fit in the majority of patients after radial keratotomy, but with more difficulty than on normal corneas because the paracentral steepening of the cornea tends to decenter the lens. Soft contact lenses, especially extended wear, often induce vascularization of the keratotomy scars.

Epithelial inclusion cysts and other debris can be seen with the slit lamp in the scars in some cases, but do not seem to alter the visual results. The scars themselves become less dense over 2 to 3 years after surgery in most patients, as the corneal stroma adjacent to the incision remodels and becomes more transparent.[34] A visually insignificant, horizontal, yellow-brown epithelial iron line appears in many cases at the junction of the middle and inferior thirds of the cornea, with fingers extending between the ends of the incisions, probably as a result of mild irregular astigmatism created by the scars.[39] Map-shaped epithelial basement membrane changes can occur after radial keratotomy, but are infrequently associated with clinical symptoms or epithelial erosions.[37]

Laboratory studies have demonstrated mild damage to the corneal endothelium beneath the keratotomy incisions.[114,115] Central endothelial cell counts in humans show a decrease of less than 10%, but greater if corneal perforation occurred at surgery.[116] Specular micrographs of endothelial cells in the area of the incisions in humans 1 year after surgery have not shown a progressive decrease in cell count or progressive abnormality in cell morphology.[117] Longer follow-up in individual eyes is necessary to determine whether there is progressive endothelial cell loss over many years.

Complications that potentially reduce visual function

Decrease of best corrected spectacle visual acuity by two lines or more may occur in about 1% of patients after radial keratotomy. Most of the loss occurs at more refined levels of visual acuity, such as loss from 20/10 preoperatively to 20/20 postoperatively. A few patients are not correctable back to at least 20/20.[29,30,47,55] But as noted previously, best-corrected spectacle visual acuity is improved in some patients.

Irregular astigmatism can cause persistent ghost images or monocular diplopia contributing to decreased visual function.

Mild to moderate glare occasionally persists beyond the usual 3 to 6 months.[27,29,31,45] The majority of patients see radiating lines around lights at night, but these do not usually disrupt visual function. Disability glare, defined as glare that disrupts daily activities, occurs rarely,[29] but a few patients find it necessary to curtail night driving, to use sunglasses, or to change their occupation.[109]

Binocular vision may be disrupted following radial keratotomy. Problems of anisometropia due to asymmetrical correction, induced astigmatism, or surgery on only one eye can lead to double vision, spatial disorientation, or loss of fine depth perception.[100] Attempts to relieve these problems include additional surgery or contact lenses.

Potentially blinding complications may occur after radial keratotomy. Perforation of the cornea during surgery can lead to endophthalmitis,[118] epithelial ingrowth,[119] and traumatic cataract.[120-122] A retrobulbar anesthetic can damage the optic nerve, producing optic atrophy, or perforate the often elongated myopic globe[109]; as a result, most surgeons use either topical or peribulbar anesthetic. Bacterial keratitis may occur, both immediately after surgery—as might be expected from any corneal incision—and delayed 1 to 3 years after surgery—presumably because the epithelium in the incision scars heals slowly and is constantly turning over,[40,111] creating a site for bacterial adherence.

The incisions permanently weaken the cornea,[123-125] and traumatic rupture of the cornea at the keratotomy scars has occurred[126] (Binder PS, Waring GO, Arrowsmith PA, et al, personal communication), although there are reports of severe ocular trauma without disruption of the wounds.[127]

Ocular surgery after radial keratotomy

Patients may require further ocular surgery sometime during their life after radial keratotomy, and the presence of the weakened keratotomy scars may make the subsequent surgical procedure and postoperative course more difficult. For example, penetrating keratoplasty done within a few years after radial keratotomy often produces opening of the scars during trephination.[128] Little is published on the course of other ocular surgery after radial keratotomy.

STABILITY OF REFRACTION AFTER RADIAL KERATOTOMY

The unsutured wounds in the avascular cornea heal slowly, requiring at least 4 to 5 years to completely eject the epithelial plug[107,123,124,129,130] and to remodel the stroma adjacent to the incision scar.[34] Persistent diurnal fluctuation of vision occurs up to 3 years after surgery, and some patients notice it as long as 5 years after surgery. However, it is seldom enough to require a separate optical correction during the day.

Some instability of the refractive correction may persist for 4 to 5 years after surgery in some eyes. The change in refraction between 1 and 4 years after surgery has been reported from 1 to 3 D in 10% to 30% of eyes.[30,31,35,107,112,113] The majority of eyes showing a change in refraction have demonstrated a continued flattening of the central cornea, resulting in either a decrease in myopia or an increase in hyperopia. The determination of whether there is a clinically meaningful, systematic progression of the effect of radial keratotomy in individual eyes over many years requires further study.

PATIENT SATISFACTION

Patient satisfaction with radial keratotomy depends primarily on the postoperative visual acuity and stability of vision.[35,50] Two psychological studies of patient satisfaction found 71%[50] and 48%[35] "very satisfied" and 10% and 13% "dissatisfied."

SUMMARY

We summarize here the foregoing review of radial keratotomy. This summary is not intended to replace the entire document and should not be taken out of context of the whole review.

The operation of radial keratotomy for myopia is the most commonly performed refractive surgical procedure. Most patients who elect to have radial keratotomy do so to avoid being dependent on the artificial devices of glasses or contact lenses. Others seek the surgery for occupational, athletic, or cosmetic reasons. The operation is undergoing continued development, and several variations in technique have gained acceptance by radial keratotomy surgeons, but the exact surgical technique varies among surgeons.

Published data indicate that radial keratotomy achieves satisfactory uncorrected visual acuity in the majority of patients who have non-progressive, low to moderate amounts of myopia. The exact amount of correction cannot be predicted for an individual patient, resulting in overcorrections and undercorrections, and patients may still require the use of glasses or contact lenses after surgery. This variability of the refractive outcome stems from several factors, including: (1) the biological difference from one individual to another; (2) the variation in surgical techniques among surgeons; and (3) the difficulty of one surgeon making all incisions uniformly. As advances in the surgery occur, some ophthalmologists are reporting series of cases with improved uniformity and predictability of outcome.

The potential of this procedure to render good uncorrected visual acuity must be weighed against its known risks. Refractive side effects include anisometropia (imbalanced vision), increased astigmatism, and early symptomatic presbyopia (loss of near focus in middle age) in overcorrected patients. Other side effects include prolonged unstable vision and mild glare. Complications that produce loss of vision are extremely rare. These include ocular infections and increased risk of rupture of the cornea following severe trauma.

Radial keratotomy alters the optical function, not the appearance of the eye; therefore, the surgery itself is not cosmetic. It is elective surgery, because other alternatives are available for the management of myopia, including glasses, contact lenses, and other refractive keratoplasty procedures. A well-informed myopic patient can prudently select the best alternative treatment—either surgical or optical—on the basis of his or her personal needs, with the help of an ophthalmologist who explains both the risks and benefits of the available modes of correction.

Ten years ago, radial keratotomy was considered an experimental-investigational procedure. It has now been proven effective in reducing myopia in both clinical and laboratory studies, and its potential complications have been well delineated; therefore, the International Society of Refractive Keratoplasty no longer considers it either experimental or investigational.

REFERENCES

1. Waring GO: The changing status of radial keratotomy for myopia. Part 1 and 2. Journal of Refractive Surgery 1985;1:81-86, 1:119-137.

2. Sanders DR, Hofmann RF, Salz JR (eds): Refractive Corneal Surgery. Thorofare, New Jersey, Slack, Incorporated, 1986.

3. Sanders DR (ed): Radial Keratotomy Surgical Techniques. Thorofare, New Jersey, Slack, Incorporated, 1986.

4. Waring GO: Keratotomy for Myopia and Astigmatism. St. Louis, C.V. Mosby Company, to be published.

5. American Academy of Ophthalmology: By-laws, Code of Ethics and Standing Rules. AAO, 1988, principle 7, p 13.

6. Curtin BJ: The Myopias: Basic Science and Clinical Management. Philadelphia, Harper and Row, 1985.

7. Waring GO: Development and evaluation of refractive surgical procedures. Part 1: Five stages in the continuum of development. Part 2: Practical implementation of formal clinical trials. Journal of Refractive Surgery 1987; 3:140-157, 3:173-184.

8. Snellen H: Die richtung der Hauptmeridiane des astigmatischen Auges. Archiv fur Ophthalmologie 1869; 15: 199-207.

9. Bates WH: A suggestion of an operation to correct astigmatism. Arch Ophthalmol 1894;23:9-13.

10. Lans LJ: Experimentelle Untersuchungen uber Entstehung von Astigmatismus durch nicht-perforirende Corneawunden. Albrecht Von Graefes Arch Ophthalmol 1898;45:117-152.

11. Waring GO: The Lans distinguished refractive surgery lecture (editorial). Journal of Refractive Surgery 1987; 3:115-116.

12. Sato T: Treatment of conical cornea (incision of Descemet's membrane). Acta Soc Ophthalmol Jpn 1939; 43:544-555.

13. Akiyama K: Study of surgical treatment for myopia. (Second Report) Animal experiment. Acta Soc Ophthalmol Jpn 1955;59:294-312.

14. Sato T, Akiyama K, Shibata H: A new surgical approach to myopia. Am J Ophthalmol 1953;36:823-829.

15. Akiyama K: The surgical treatment for myopia. (Third Report) Anterior and posterior incisions. Acta Soc Ophthalmol Jpn 1955;59:797-835.

16. Yamaguchi T, Kanai A, Tanaka M, et al: Bullous keratopathy after anterior-posterior radial keratotomy for myopia and myopic astigmatism. Am J Ophthalmol 1982;93:600-606.

17. Kanai A, Yamaguchi T, Yajima Y, et al: The fine structure of bullous keratopathy after anteroposterior incision of the cornea for myopia. Folia Ophthalmol Jpn 1979;30:841-849.

18. Beatty RF, Smith RE: 30-year follow-up of posterior radial keratotomy. Am J Ophthalmol 1987;103(Pt 1):330-331.

19. Beliaev VS, Ilyina TS: Scleroplasty in the treatment of progressive myopia. Vestn Oftalmol 1972;3:60-63.

20. Yenaliev FS: Experience in surgical treatment of myopia. Vestn Oftalmol 1978;3:52.

21. Fyodorov SN, Durnev VV: Anterior keratotomy method application with the purpose of surgical correction of myopia, in Pressing Problems of Ophthalmosurgery. Moscow, 1977, pp 47-48.

22. Durnev VV: Decrease of corneal refraction by anterior keratotomy method with the purpose of surgical correction of myopia of mild moderate degree, in Proceedings of the First Congress of Ophthalmologists of Transcaucasia. Tbilisi, 1976, pp 129-132.

23. Durnev VV, Ermoshin AS: Determination of dependence between length of anterior radial nonperforating incision of cornea and their effectiveness, in Transactions of the Fifth All-Union Conference of Inventors and Rationalizers in Ophthalmology Field. Moscow, 1976, pp 106-108.

24. Fyodorov SN, Durnev VV: Operation of dosaged dissection of corneal circular ligament in cases of myopia of a mild degree. Ann Ophthalmol 1979; 11:1885-1890.

25. Hecht SD, Jamara RJ: Prospective evaluation of radial keratotomy using the Fyodorov formula: Preliminary report. Ann Ophthalmol 1982;14:319-330.

26. Bores LD, Myers W, Cowden J: Radial keratotomy: An analysis of the American experience. Ann Ophthalmol 1981;13:941-948.

27. Bores LD: Historical review and clinical results of radial keratotomy, in Binder PS (ed): Refractive corneal surgery: The correction of aphakia, hyperopia and myopia. Int Ophthalmol Clin 1983;23:93-118.

28. Waring GO, Moffitt SD, Gelender H, et al: Rationale for and design of the National Eye Institute Prospective Evaluation of Radial Keratotomy (PERK) study. Ophthalmology 1983;90:40-58.

29. Waring GO, Lynn MJ, Gelender H, et al: Results of the Prospective Evaluation of Radial Keratotomy (PERK) study 1 year after radial keratotomy. Ophthalmology 1985;92:177-198.

30. Waring GO, Lynn MJ, Culbertson W, et al: Three year results of the Prospective Evaluation of Radial Keratotomy (PERK) study. Ophthalmology 1987; 94:1339-1354.

31. Waring GO, Laibson P, Lindstrom R, et al: Changes in refraction, keratometry, and visual acuity during the first year after radial keratotomy in the PERK study. Invest Ophthalmol Vis Sci 1985;26(suppl):202.

32. Lynn MJ, Waring GO, Sperduto RD, et al: Factors affecting outcome and predictability of radial keratotomy in the PERK study. Arch Ophthalmol 1987;105:42-51.

33. Santos VR, Waring GO, Lynn MJ, et al: Relationship between refractive error and visual acuity in the Prospective Evaluation of Radial Keratotomy (PERK) study. Arch Ophthalmol 1987; 105:86-92.

34. Steinberg EB, Waring GO, Wilson LA: Slit-lamp microscopic study of corneal wound healing after radial keratotomy in the PERK study. Am J Ophthalmol 1985;100:218-224.

35. Bourque LB, Cosand BB, Drews C, et al: Reported patient satisfaction, fluctuation of vision, and glare among patients 1 year after surgery in the PERK study. Arch Ophthalmol 1986;104: 356-363.

36. Bourque LB, Rubenstein R, Cosand B, et al: Psychosocial characteristics of candidates for the Prospective Evaluation of Radial Keratotomy (PERK) study. Arch Ophthalmol 1984;102: 1187-1192.

37. Nelson JD, Williams P, Lindstrom RL, et al: Map-fingerprint-dot changes in the corneal epithelial basement membrane following radial keratotomy. Ophthalmology 1985;92:199-205.

38. Schanzlin DJ, Santos VR, Waring GO, et al: Diurnal change in refraction, corneal curvature, visual acuity, and intraocular pressure after radial keratotomy in the PERK study. Ophthalmology 1986;93:167-175.

39. Steinberg EB, Wilson LA, Waring GO, et al: Stellate iron line in the corneal epithelium after radial keratotomy. Am J Ophthalmol 98:416-421.

40. Mandelbaum S, Waring GO, Forster RK, et al: Late development of ulcerative keratitis in radial keratotomy scars. Arch Ophthalmol 1986;104: 1156-1160.

41. Cowden JW, Lynn MJ, Waring GO, et al: Repeated radial keratotomy in the Prospective Evaluation of Radial Keratotomy study. Am J Ophthalmol 1987;103:423-431.

42. Lynn MJ, Waring GO, the PERK Study Group: Stability of refraction after radial keratotomy compared with unoperated eyes in the PERK study. Invest Ophthalmol Vis Sci 1987;28 (suppl):223.

43. Ginsburg AP, Waring GO, Steinberg EB, et al: Contrast sensitivity under photopic conditions in the PERK study. Am J Ophthalmol, to be published.

44. Sanders DR, Arrowsmith PN, Deitz MR, et al: Radial Keratotomy. Thorofare, New Jersey, Slack, Incorporated, 1984, pp 1-121.

45. Deitz MR, Sanders DR, Marks RG: Radial keratotomy: An overview of the Kansas City study. Ophthalmology 1984;91:467-477.

46. Arrowsmith PN, Marks RG: Visual, refractive, and keratometric results of radial keratotomy; one-year follow-up. Arch Ophthalmol 1984;102:1612-1617.

47. Arrowsmith PN, Marks RG: Visual, refractive, and keratometric results of radial keratotomy. A two-year follow-up. Arch Ophthalmol 1987;105:76-80.

48. Sawelson H, Marks RG: Two year results of radial keratotomy. Arch Ophthalmol 1985;103:505-510.

49. Arrowsmith PN, Sanders DR, Marks RG: Visual, refractive, and keratometric results of radial keratotomy. Arch Ophthalmol 1983;101:873-881.

50. Powers MK, Meyerowitz BE, Arrowsmith PN, et al: Psychosocial findings in radial keratotomy patients 2 years after surgery. Ophthalmology 1984; 91:1193-1198.

51. Arrowsmith PN, Marks RG: Evaluating the predictability of radial keratotomy. Ophthalmology 1985;92:331-338.

52. Arrowsmith PN, Marks RG: Four-year update on predictability of radial keratotomy. Journal of Refractive Surgery 1988;4:37-45.

53. Sanders DR, Deitz MR, Gallagher D: Factors affecting the predictability of radial keratotomy. Ophthalmology 1985;92:1237-1243.

54. Arrowsmith PN, Marks RG: Five-year effectiveness and safety of radial keratotomy surgery. Ophthalmology 1987; 94(suppl):97.

55. Deitz MR, Sanders DR, Raanan MG: A consecutive series (1982-1985) of radial keratotomies performed with the diamond blade. Am J Ophthalmol 1987;103:417-422.

56. Sawelson H, Marks RG: Three-year results of radial keratotomy. Arch Ophthalmol 1987;105:81-85.

57. Reddy PS, Reddy PR: Anterior keratotomy. Ophthalmic Surg 1980;11:765-767.

58. Hoffer KJ, Darrin JJ, Petit TH, et al: Three years experience with radial keratotomy: The UCLA study. Ophthalmology 1983;90:627-636.

59. Nirankari VS, Katzen LE, Karesh JW, et al: Ongoing prospective clinical study of radial keratotomy. Ophthalmology 1983;90:637-641.

60. Rowsey JJ, Balyeat HD, Rabinovitch B, et al: Predicting the results of radial keratotomy. Ophthalmology 1983;90: 642-654.

61. Neumann AC, Osher RH, Fenzl RE: Radial keratotomy: A comprehensive evaluation. Doc Ophthalmol 1984;56: 275-301.

62. Salz JJ, Salz MS: Results of four- and eight-incision radial keratotomy for 6 to 11 diopters of myopia. Journal of Refractive Surgery 1988;4:46-50.

63. Kremer FB, Marks RG: Radial keratotomy: Prospective evaluation of safety and efficacy. Ophthalmic Surg 1983; 14:925-930.

64. Cowden JW: Radial keratotomy. A retrospective study of cases observed at the Kresge Eye Institute for 6 months. Arch Ophthalmol 1982;100: 578-580.

65. Shepard DD: Radial keratotomy: Analysis of efficacy and predictability in 1,058 consecutive cases. Part I: Efficacy. Journal of Cataract and Refractive Surgery 1986;12:632-643.

66. Shepard DD: Radial keratotomy: Analysis of efficacy and predictability in 1,058 consecutive cases. Part II: Predictability. Journal of Cataract and Refractive Surgery 1987;13:32-34.

67. Lavery FL: Comparative results of 200 consecutive radial keratotomy cases using three different nomograms. Journal of Refractive Surgery 1987; 3:88-91.

68. Minezo JL, Cisneros A, Harto M: Cirugia de la Miopia. Barcelona, Spain, Salvat Editores, 1986.

69. Silverman WA: Human Experimentation: A Guided Step Into the Unknown. New York, Oxford University Press, 1985.

70. Meinert C: Clinical Trials: Design, Conduct, and Analysis. New York, Oxford University Press, 1986.

71. Galentine PG, Cohen EG, Laibson PR, et al: Corneal ulcers associated with contact lens wear. Arch Ophthalmol 1984;102:891-894.

72. Ormerod LD, Smith RE: Contact lens-associated microbial keratitis. Arch Ophthalmol 1986;104:79-83.

73. Polse KA, Brand RJ, Vastine DW, et al: Corneal change accompanying orthokeratology. Plastic or elastic? Results of a randomized controlled clinical trial. Arch Ophthalmol 1983; 101:1873-1878.

74. Swinger CA, Barker BA: Prospective evaluation of myopic keratomileusis. Ophthalmology 1984;91:785-792.

75. Krumeich JH, Swinger CA: Nonfreeze epikeratophakia for the correction of myopia. Am J Ophthalmol 1987;103: 397-403.

76. Werblin TP, Klyce SK: Epikeratophakia surgical correction of myopia. Curr Eye Res 1981;1:591-597.

77. McDonald MB, Kaufman HE, Aquavella JV, et al: The nationwide study of epikeratophakia for myopia. Am J Ophthalmol 1987;103:375-383.

78. Werblin TP, Peiffer RL, Fryczkowski AW: Myopic hydrogel keratophakia: Preliminary report. Cornea 1985;3: 197-204.

79. Werblin TP, Peiffer RL, Patel AS: Myopic hydrogel keratophakia: Improvements in lens design. Cornea 1987; 6(3):197-201.

80. Binder PS, Zavala EY, Deg JK, et al: Alloplastic implants for the correction of refractive errors. Ophthalmology 1984;91:806-814.

81. Binder PS, Zavala EY, Deg JK: Hydrogel refractive keratoplasty. Lens removal and exchanges. Cornea 1983; 2:119-125.

82. Beekhuis WH, McCarey BE, Waring GO, et al: Hydrogel keratophakia: A microkeratome dissection in the monkey model. Br J Ophthalmol 1986; 70:192-198.

83. Beekhuis WH, McCarey BE, van Rij G, et al: Complications of hydrogel intracorneal lenses in monkeys. Arch Ophthalmol 1987;105:116-122.

84. Koenig SB, Hamano T, Yamaguchi T, et al: Refractive keratoplasty with hydrogel implants in primates. Ophthalmic Surg 1984;15:225-229.

85. Lane SL, Cameron JD, Lindstrom RL, et al: Polysulfone corneal lenses. Journal of Cataract and Refractive Surgery 1986;12:50-60.

86. Choyce P: The correction of refractive errors with polysulfone corneal inlays. Trans Ophthalmol Soc UK 1985;104: 332-342.

87. Kirkness CM, Steele ADM, Garner A: Polysulfone corneal inlays. Adverse reactions: A preliminary report. Trans Ophthalmol Soc UK 1985;104:343-350.

88. Marshall J, Trokel S, Rothery S, et al: Photoablative reprofiling of the cornea using an excimer laser: Photorefractive keratectomy. Lasers in Ophthalmology 1986;1:21-48.

89. Hanna KD, Chastang JC, Pouliquen Y, et al: Excimer laser keratectomy for myopia with a rotating slit delivery system. Arch Ophthalmol 1988;106: 245-250.

90. Waring GO, Fantes F: Challenges in laser corneal surgery. Unpublished.

91. Puliafito CA, Stern D, Kruger R, et al: High speed photography of excimer laser ablation of the cornea. Arch Ophthalmol 1987;105:1255-1259.

92. Seiler T, Bende T, Wollensak J, et al: Excimer laser for correction of astigmatism. Am J Ophthalmol 1988;105: 117-124.

93. Thornton SP, Sanders DR: Graded non-intersecting transverse incisions for correction of idiopathic astigmatism. Journal of Cataract and Refractive Surgery 1987;13:27-31.

94. Health Products Research Report I67, August 12, 1987.

95. Bettman JW: Radial keratotomy: Factors in medicolegal claims. Surv Ophthalmol 1986;30:2676-2679.

96. Shivitz IA, Russell BM, Arrowsmith PN, et al: Optical correction of postoperative radial keratotomy patients with contact lenses. CLAO J 1987;12:59-62.

97. Mendelsohn AD, Parel J-M, Dennis JJ, et al: Intraocular pressure during radial keratotomy. Journal of Refractive Surgery 1987;3:79-103.

98. Salz JJ, Rowsey JJ, Caroline P, et al: A study of optical zone size and incision redeepening in experimental radial keratotomy. Arch Ophthalmol 1985; 103:590-594.

99. O'Donnell FE: Short incision radial keratotomy: A comparative study in rabbits. Journal of Refractive Surgery 1987;3:22-27.

100. Spigelman AV, Williams PA, Nichols BD, et al: Four incision radial keratotomy. Journal of Cataract and Refractive Surgery 1988;14:125-128.

101. Sanders DR: Computerized radial keratotomy predictability programs, in Sanders DR, Hofmann RF, Salz JJ (eds): Refractive Corneal Surgery. Thorofare, New Jersey, Slack, Incorporated, 1986, pp 93-107.

102. Thornton SP: Thornton guide for radial keratotomy incisions and optical zone size. Journal of Refractive Surgery 1985;1:29-33.

103. Cowden JW, Weber B: Repeat radial keratotomy in monkeys. Ophthalmology 1983;90:251-256.

104. Villaseñor RA, Cox KC: Radial keratotomy: Reoperations. Journal of Refractive Surgery 1985;1:35-37.

105. Hofmann RF: Reoperations after radial and astigmatic keratotomy. Journal of Refractive Surgery 1987;3:119-128.

106. Lindquist TD, Rubenstein JB, Lindstrom RL: Correction of hyperopia following radial keratotomy: Quantification in human cadaver eyes. Ophthalmic Surg 1987;18:432-437.

107. Deitz MR, Sanders DR: Progressive hyperopia with long-term follow-up of radial keratotomy. Arch Ophthalmol 1985;103:782-784.

108. Salz JJ, Villaseñor RA, Elander R, et al: Four incision radial keratotomy for low to moderate myopia. Ophthalmology 1985;92(suppl 2):73.

109. O'Day DM, Feman SS, Elliott JH: Visual impairment following radial keratotomy: A cluster of cases. Ophthalmology 1986;93:319-326.

110. Cross WD, Head WJH: Complications of radial keratotomy, in Sanders DR, Hofmann RF, Salz JJ (eds): Refractive Corneal Surgery. Thorofare, New Jersey, Slack, Incorporated, 1986, pp 347-400.

111. Shivitz IA, Arrowsmith PN: Delayed keratitis after radial keratotomy. Arch Ophthalmol 1986;104:1153-1155.

112. Richmond RD: Special report: Radial keratotomy as seen through operated eyes. Journal of Refractive Surgery 1987;3:22-27.

113. Wyzinski P: Diurnal cycle of refraction after radial keratotomy. Ophthalmology 1987;94:120-124.

114. Binder PS, Stainer GA, Zavala EY, et al: Acute morphologic features of radial keratotomy. Arch Ophthalmol 1983;101:1113-1116.

115. Yamaguchi T, Kaufman H, Fukushima A, et al: Histologic and electron microscopic assessment of endothelial damage produced by anterior radial keratotomy in the monkey cornea. Am J Ophthalmol 1981;92:313-327.

116. Chiba K, Oak SS, Tsubota K, et al: Morphometric analysis of corneal endothelium following radial keratotomy. Journal of Cataract and Refractive Surgery 1987;13:263-267.

117. McRae SM, Matsuda M, Rich LF: The effect of radial keratotomy on the corneal endothelium. Am J Ophthalmol 1985;100:538-542.

118. Gelender H, Flynn HW, Mandelbaum SH: Bacterial endophthalmitis resulting from radial keratotomy. Am J Ophthalmol 1982;93:323-326.

119. Binder PS: Presumed epithelial ingrowth following radial keratotomy. CLAO J 1986;12:247-250.

120. Baldone JA, Franklin RM: Cataract following radial keratotomy. Ann Ophthalmol 1983;15:416-418.

121. Gelender H, Gelber EC: Cataract following radial keratotomy. Arch Ophthalmol 1983;101:1229-1231.

122. Stark WJ, Martin NF, Maumenee AE: Radial keratotomy. II. A risky procedure of unproven long-term success. Surv Ophthalmol 1983/84;28(101):106-111.

123. Ingraham HJ, Guber D, Green WR: Radial keratotomy: Clinical pathologic case report. Arch Ophthalmol 1985;103:683-688.

124. Yamaguchi T, Tamaki K, Kaufman HE, et al: Histologic study of a pair of human corneas after anterior radial keratotomy. Am J Ophthalmol 1985;100:281-292.

125. McKnight SJ, Fitz J, Giangiacomo J: Corneal rupture following radial keratotomy in cats subjected to BB gun injury. Ophthalmic Surg 1988;19:165-167.

126. Simons KB, Linsalata RP: Ruptured globe following blunt trauma after radial keratotomy: A case report. Ophthalmology 1987;94(suppl):148.

127. Spivack L: Case report: Radial keratotomy incisions remain intact despite facial trauma from plane crash. Journal of Refractive Surgery 1987;3:59-60.

128. Beatty RF, Robin JB, Schanzlin DJ: Penetrating keratoplasty after radial keratotomy. Journal of Refractive Surgery 1986;2:207-214.

129. Binder PS, Nayak SK, Deg JK, et al: An ultrastructural and histochemical study of long-term wound healing after radial keratotomy. Am J Ophthalmol 1987;103(Pt 2):432-440.

130. Deg JK, Zavala EY, Binder PS: Delayed corneal wound healing following radial keratotomy. Ophthalmology 1985;92:743-750.

131. Lynn MJ, Waring GO, Arentsen J, et al: Prospective Evaluation of Radial Keratotomy (PERK) Study: Results after 4 years of surgery (Abstract). Invest Ophthalmol Vis Sci 1988;29:310.

Index

A

Ablation, laser; *see* Laser ablation
Abrasion, epithelial, 633, Plate 17-26
Absorption spectrum in cornea, 677, 678
AC/A; *see* Accommodative convergence/accommodation ratio
Accommodation amplitude, 997
Accommodative convergence/accommodation ratio, 9, 329
Accutome pachometer, 426
Accutome probe, 416
A.C.E. keratometer, 72
Acetaminophen, 639, Plate 17-27
Acid mucopolysaccharides, 28
Acta Ophthalmologica, 232-233
Actin, 22
Adenosine triphosphatase-bicarbonate pump, 30
Advertising of health care, 283-286
Advisory opinion of code of ethics, 286
Age
  clear zone diameter and, 395
  predictability and, 355-357
    computerized, 394
  in prediction interval, 374-376
  refraction and, 356
    spherical equivalent, 362-363
    stability of, 319-321
  results and, 996
Agranovsky AA, 840-844
Ak-Taine; *see* Proparacaine
Akcon; *see* Naphthazoline
Akiyama K, 143, 204
Albalon; *see* Naphthazoline
Alcaine; *see* Proparacaine
Alcon 55 Villasenor pachometer, 428, 429
Alcon Biophysique pachometer, 428
Allergan-Humphrey pachometer, 428, 429
AMark formula, 384-385, 389-391
American Academy of Ophthalmology's ad hoc Ophthalmic Procedures Assessment Committee, 274
American Medical Association's Diagnostic and Therapeutic Technology Assessment program, 274
Ametropia, 38-39
  laboratory evaluation and, 156
Amoils keratometer, 72
Analgesics, postoperative, 639, Plate 17-27
Analysis of Radial Keratotomy Study, 246
Anatomic landmarks, 1214-1215
Anatomy of cornea, 17-35; *see also* Corneal anatomy and physiology

Ancillary treatments, unnecessary, 637, Plate 17-27
Anesthesia, 510, 525-530, Plate 17-1, Plate 17-5
  complications of, 867-869
  general, 528-529, Plate 17-5
  in history of keratotomy, 251
  moistening ocular surface and, 562, Plate 17-13
  peribulbar, 869
  results and, 993
  retrobulbar, 868-869
  topical, 868
    surgical instruments and supplies and, 408
Angled flat-tipped razor blade, 250
Angled knife handle, 461
Angled probe handle, 415
Animals, laboratory, 155-157
Aniseikonia, 849-851
Anisometropia, 849-851, 882-883
  after bilateral radial keratotomy, 857-860
Anisophoria, 850
Anisotropy, 1251
Anterior Eye Analysis System, 73
Anterior keratomileusis, 163
Anterior keratotomy in Soviet Union; *see* Soviet Union
Anterior-posterior keratotomy, 179-187
  clinical course after, 208
  development of, 179-187
  histopathology in, 215, 216, 217
  incision for, 199-208
    anteroposterior corneal, 199, 200
    comb-type posterior corneal, 200-201
    corneal interlayer separation and posterior tangential, 201-202
    radial, 202-208, 204-208
    tangential posterior half-corneal, 199
  in keratoconus, 208
  long-term follow-up of, 212-215
  in monkeys, 217
  in rabbits, 187-197
  Sato on corneal incisions in, 209-211
  surgical plan of, 197-198
Anterior radial keratotomy of Fyodorov, 222-232; *see also* Fyodorov anterior radial keratotomy
Antibiotics
  concluding operation and, 636, Plate 17-27
  in corneal perforations, 871
  preoperative, 520, Plate 17-3
  prophylactic, 639, Plate 17-27
Antitrust conspiracy, 262-267